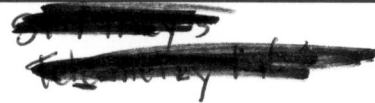
...sher,
...extbooks
...ose, RN, BSN, MEd

...tor
...eau

...tor
...bard

...ions Editor
...Kardish Fischer, RN, BSN

...ciate Acquisitions Editors
...uise Quinn, Betsy K. Snyder

...enior Clinical Editor
...arlene Ciranowicz, RN, MSN, CDE

Clinical Editor
Maryann Foley, RN, BSN

Drug Information Editor
Kenneth Wieland, RPh, PharmD

Copy Editors
Diane M. Armento, Traci Ginnona, Janet Hodgson, Karyn Newell

Designers
Stephanie Peters (senior associate art director), Matie Patterson (assistant art director)

Typography
Diane Paluba (manager), Elizabeth Bergman, Joyce Rossi Biletz, Phyllis Marron, Valerie Rosenberger

Manufacturing
Deborah Meiris (director), T.A. Landis

The clinical procedures described and recommended in this publication are based on research and consultation with nursing, medical, and legal authorities. To the best of our knowledge, these procedures reflect currently accepted practice; nevertheless, they can't be considered absolute and universal recommendations. For individual application, all recommendations must be considered in light of the patient's clinical condition and, before administration of new or infrequently used drugs, in light of the latest package-insert information. The authors and the publisher disclaim responsibility for any adverse effects resulting directly or indirectly from the suggested procedures, from any undetected errors, or from the reader's misunderstanding of the text.

...photocopy items for in-house use, or the internal or specific clients, is granted ... corporation for users ... Copyright Clearance ...ctional Reporting ... the base fee of ...75 per page, is paid directly to CCC, 27 Congress St., Salem, Mass. 01970. For those organizations that have been granted a photocopy license by CCC, a separate system of payment has been arranged. The fee code for users of the Transactional Reporting Service is 087434817X/96 $00.00 + $.75.

Ⓡ A member of the Reed Elsevier plc group

NDH-011095
ISSN 0273-320X
ISBN 0-87434-817-X

metoclopramide HCl	midazolam HCl	morphine sulfate	nalbuphine HCl	pentazocine lactate	pentobarbital Na	perphenazine	phenobarbital Na	prochlorperazine edisylate	promazine HCl	promethazine HCl	ranitidine HCl	scopolamine HBr	secobarbital Na	sodium bicarbonate	thiethylperazine maleate	thiopental Na	
P	Y	P	Y	P	P	Y			P	P	P	Y	P				atropine sulfate
	Y	Y		Y	N		N				Y	N				N	benzquinamide HCl
	Y	Y		Y	N	Y		Y		Y					Y		butorphanol tartrate
P	Y	P		P	N	Y		Y	P	P	Y	P				N	chlorpromazine HCl
Y	Y	Y	Y	Y	N	Y		Y	Y	Y		Y	N				cimetidine HCl
																	codeine phosphate
P	N	P		P	N	Y		N	N	N	Y	P				N	dimenhydrinate
Y	Y	P		P	N	Y		P	P	P	Y	P				N	diphenhydramine HCl
P	Y	P	Y	P	N	Y		P	P	P		P					droperidol
P	Y	P		P	N	Y		P	P	P	Y	P					fentanyl citrate
	Y	Y		N	N			Y	Y	Y	Y	Y	N	N		N	glycopyrrolate
P₍₅₎		N*		N			P₍₅₎		N								heparin Na
	Y			Y	Y			N*		Y	Y	Y			Y		hydromorphone HCl
P	Y	Y	Y	Y	N			P	P	P	N	Y					hydroxyzine HCl
P	Y	N		P	N	P		P	P	Y	Y	P				N	meperidine HCl
■	Y	P		P		P		P	P	P	Y	P			N		metoclopramide HCl
Y	■	Y	Y			N	N		N	Y	N	Y	N			Y	midazolam HCl
P	Y	■		P	N*	Y		P*	P	P*	Y	P				N	morphine sulfate
Y			■	N		Y			Y	Y	Y				Y		nalbuphine HCl
P		P		■	N	Y		P	Y	Y	Y	P					pentazocine lactate
N	N	N*	N	N	■	N		N	N	N		Y		Y		Y	pentobarbital Na
P	N	Y		Y	N	■		Y				Y					perphenazine
							■	N			N						phenobarbital Na
P	N	P*	Y	P	N	Y		■	P	P	Y	P				N	prochlorperazine edisylate
P	Y	Y		Y	N			P	■	P	P						promazine HCl
P	Y	P*	Y	Y	N			P	P	■	Y	P				N	promethazine HCl
Y	N	Y	Y	Y		Y	N	Y	P	Y	■	Y			Y		ranitidine HCl
P	Y	P	Y	P	Y			P		P	Y	■				Y	scopolamine HBr
													■				secobarbital Na
N			Y											■		N	sodium bicarbonate
Y	Y		Y								Y				■		thiethylperazine maleate
N			Y				N	N			Y		N			■	thiopental Na

Nursing

DRUG

HANDBOOK®

STAFF

Senior Publi...
Trade and ...
Minnie B. R...

Senior Ed...
Dave/Mor...

Art ...
John ...

Acc...
Pat...

As...
Lo...

S...
M...

NU...
SPRINGHO...
SPRINGHOUSE...

CONTENTS

Autonomic Nervous System Drugs

Respiratory Tract Drugs

Gastrointestinal Tract Drugs

Hormonal Agents

CONSULTANTS, REVIEWERS, AND ADVISORS

At the time of publication, the clinical consultants, pharmacy reviewers, and advisors held the following positions.

Clinical Consultants

Marlene Ciranowicz, RN, MSN, CDE, Independent Consultant, Dresher, Pa.

Michael R. Cohen, RPh, MS, FASHP, President, Institute for Safe Medication Practices, Warminster, Pa.

Robert A. Cohen, RPh, Pharmacist, Norristown, Pa.

Patricia A. Diehl, RN, BSN, MA, Associate Professor of Nursing, Robert C. Byrd Health Sciences Center, West Virginia University, Morgantown

Maryann Foley, RN, BSN, Independent Consultant, Flourtown, Pa.

Nancy L. Subolish, RPh, Assistant Director, Pharmacy Department, Doylestown (Pa.) Hospital

Barbara McVan, RN, Publisher, Springhouse Corporation

Kenneth Wieland, RPh, PharmD, Director of Pharmacy, Chestnut Hill (Pa.) Hospital

Pharmacy Reviewers

Douglas R. Allington, RPh, PharmD, Clinical Assistant Professor, School of Pharmacy and Allied Health, University of Montana, Missoula

Alan Caspi, PharmD, MBA, Director of Pharmacy, Lenox Hill Hospital, New York

Sandra L. Chase, PharmD, Drug Information Specialist, Department of Pharmacy, Thomas Jefferson University Hospital, Philadelphia

Douglas D. DeCarolis, RPh, PharmD, Inpatient Clinical Coordinator, Minneapolis Veterans' Administration, Medical Center

Mark J. Ellison, PharmD, FCP, BCPS, Assistant Director, Glaxo Research Institute, Research Triangle Park, N.C.

Rebecca S. Finley, PharmD, MS, Associate Professor, University of Maryland Cancer Center, Baltimore

Mary Beth Gross, PharmD, FASCP, Manager, Pharmacy, Mercy Hospital Medical Center; Associate Professor of Pharmacy, Drake University, Des Moines, Iowa

Cary E. Johnson, PharmD, Associate Professor of Pharmacy, Clinical Pharmacist-Pediatrics, College of Pharmacy, University of Michigan, Ann Arbor

Marie C. Kelly, RPh, Staff Pharmacist, Magee Women's Hospital, Pittsburgh

Joseph A. Koestner, PharmD, Clinical Pharmacist-Trauma, Pharmacy Department, Vanderbilt University Hospital, Nashville, Tenn.

Denise H. Rhoney, PharmD, Clinical Research Fellow, University of North Carolina at Chapel Hill

Donna J. Schroeder, PharmD, Director, Drug Information Anaylsis Services, Division of Clinical Pharmacy, University of California at San Francisco

Joel Shuster, PharmD, Clinical Associate Professor, School of Pharmacy, Temple University; Clinical Pharmacist Medical College of Pennsylvania, Philadelphia

Joseph F. Steiner, RPh, PharmD, Professor of Clinical Pharmacy, School of Human Medicine and Pharmacy, University of Wyoming, Casper

Candy Tsourounis, PharmD, Resident in Drug Information, University of California at San Francisco

Special thanks to the following, who have made major contributions or have contributed to the previous edition: Mary Ann Cali-Ascani, RNC, MSN, OCN; Alan D. Barreuther, RPh, PharmD; Terri L. Craig, RPh, PharmD; Nancy G. Evans, RN, BSN, CGRN; Walter Carl Faubion, RN, MHSA; Terry Matthew Foster, RN, BSN, CCRN, CEN; Joel Glucroft, PhD; Shirley A. Grieshaber, RN; Sandra Hardee Hak, PharmD; Roseann Hendrickson, RN: James R. Hildebrand, RPh, PharmD; Laurel M. Janney, PharmD; Karen Landis, RN, MS, CCRN; Mark S. Luer, PharmD; Rosemarie Marinaro, RN,C, MSN; Chris Platt Moldovanyi, RN, MSN; David R. Pipher, RPh, PharmD; Mark S. Roth, RPh, MS; Nancy V. Runta, RN, BSN, CCRN; Debra L. Ryan, RN, MN, CCRN; J. Michael Spivey, RPh, PharmD, BCPS; Daya R. Varma, MD, PhD; Christy W. Whitley, MA, PharmD; Allison P. Winecoff, PharmD.

ACKNOWLEDGMENTS

We would like to thank the following companies for granting us permission to include their drugs in the full-color photoguide.

Abbott Laboratories
Biaxin®
Depakote®
Depakote® Sprinkle
E.E.S.®
Ery-Tab®
Erythromycin Base
  Filmtab®
Hytrin®
PCE® Disperstab®

Astra Merck
Prilosec®

Boots Pharmaceuticals, Inc.
E-Mycin®
Synthroid®

Bristol-Myers Squibb Company
BuSpar®
Capoten®
Cefzil®
Duricef®
Estrace®
Pravachol®
Sumycin®
Veetids®

Burroughs Wellcome Co.
Lanoxin®
Zovirax®

Ciba-Geigy Pharmaceuticals
Lopressor®
Lotensin®
Ritalin®
Tegretol®
Voltaren®

Daniels Pharmaceuticals, Inc.
Levoxyl®

Dupont/Merck
Coumadin®
Percocet®
Sinemet®
Sinemet® CR

Eli Lilly and Company
Axid®
Ceclor®
Darvocet-N® 100
Lorabid®
Prozac®

Ethex Corporation
potassium chloride

Forest Pharmaceutical, Inc.
Armour® Thyroid
Lorcet® 10/650

Glaxo Inc.
Ceftin®
Zantac®
Zantac® EFFERdose

Goldline Laboratories, Inc.
verapamil hydrochloride

Hoechst-Roussel Pharmaceuticals Inc.
Altace®
DiaBeta®
Lasix®
Trental®

Hoffman-La Roche, Inc.
Bumex®
Klonopin®
Naprosyn®
Toradol®
Valium®

Janssen Pharmaceutical, Inc.
Hismanal®
Propulsid®

Knoll Pharmaceutical Company
Vicodin®
Vicodin ES®

Lederle Laboratories, Division of American Cyanamid Company
atenolol
Maxzide®
Maxzide®-25 mg
Suprax®
Verelan®

Lemmon Company
acetaminophen with codeine
  (300 mg/30 mg)
Cotrim® D.S.

Marion Merrill Dow, Inc.
Carafate®
Cardizem®
Cardizem® CD
Cardizem® SR
Seldane®
Seldane-D®

MD Pharmaceutical, Inc.
methylphenidate
  hydrochloride

Merck & Co., Inc.
Mevacor®
Pepcid®
Prinivil®
Vasotec®
Zocor®

Miles, Inc.
Adalat®
Cipro®

Mylan Pharmaceuticals Inc.
amitriptyline hydrochloride
cyclobenzaprine
  hydrochloride
doxepin hydrochloride
propoxyphene napsylate
  with acetaminophen

Novopharm USA Inc., Division of Novopharm Limited
amoxicillin trihydrate

Ortho/McNeil Pharmaceutical
Floxin®
Tylenol® with Codeine
  No. 3

Proctor and Gamble Pharmaceuticals
Macrobid®
Macrodantin®

Purepac Pharmaceutical Co.
acetaminophen with codeine
  (300 mg/60 mg)

Rhône-Poulenc Rorer Pharmaceuticals Inc.
Dilacor XR®
Lozol®
Slo-bid® Gyrocaps®

A.H. Robins Company
Micro-K Extencaps®

Roxane Laboratories, Inc.
Roxicet™

Rugby Laboratories, Inc.
dicyclomine hydrochloride

**Sandoz Pharmaceuticals
Corporation**
DynaCirc®
Fiorinal® with Codeine
Pamelor®

**Schein Pharmaceutical,
Inc.**
nortriptyline hydrochloride

**Schering-Plough
Corporation**
Claritin®
K-Dur®
Theo-Dur®

G.D. Searle & Company
Ambien®
Calan®

**SmithKline Beecham
Pharmaceuticals**
Amoxil®
Augmentin®
Compazine®
Compazine® Spansule®
Dyazide®
Paxil®
Relafen®
Tagamet®
Tagamet® Tiltab®

**Solvay Pharmaceuticals,
Inc.**
Orasone®

The Upjohn Company
Ansaid®
Deltasone®
Glynase®
Halcion®
Micronase®
Motrin®
Ogen®
Provera®
Xanax®

**U.S. Pharmaceuticals
Group
Pfizer Inc.**
Cardura®
Glucotrol®
Glucotrol XL™
Norvasc®
Procardia XL®
Zithromax®
Zoloft®

**Warner-Lambert
Company**
Accupril®
Dilantin®
Dilantin® Kapseals®
gemfibrozil
Lopid®
Nitrostat®

Watson Laboratories, Inc.
hydrocodone bitartrate and
   acetaminophen

**Whitby Pharmaceuticals,
Inc.**
Lortab®

Winsor Corporation
ibuprofen

Wyeth-Ayerst Laboratories
Ativan®
Inderal®
Lodine®
Premarin®

Zeneca Pharmaceuticals
Nolvadex®
Tenormin®
Zestril®

How to use *Nursing96 Drug Handbook*

Nursing96 Drug Handbook is meant to fill a very special need. It represents a joint effort by pharmacists and nurses to provide the nursing profession with drug information that focuses on what nurses need to know. With this in mind, it emphasizes clinical aspects and does not attempt to replace detailed pharmacology texts. Also, the information is arranged in a format designed to make it readily accessible.

Photoguide to tablets and capsules
To make drug identification easier for nurses and to enhance patient safety, *Nursing96 Drug Handbook* offers a brand-new photoguide to the most commonly prescribed tablets and capsules. Shown in actual-size, full-color photographs, the drugs are arranged alphabetically for quick reference, along with their most common dosage strengths. Page references to the drugs appear in boldface type in the Index.

Introductory information
Chapter 2 explains, in a general way, how drugs work. It also tells about adverse reactions and gives general guidelines about drug use in pregnancy and the presence of drugs in breast milk. Chapters 3 and 4 discuss the unique problems of administering drugs to children and elderly patients and offer guidelines to minimize problems in these areas. Chapter 5 discusses drug therapy as it relates to the nursing process.

Drug information
In chapters 6 to 100, all drugs are classified according to their approved therapeutic uses. Drugs that have multiple therapeutic uses are classified according to their most common

use; they are also listed (with a cross-reference to the major drug entry) in drug groups that share their secondary applications. For example, nadolol, a beta-adrenergic blocker, is described in the chapter that covers antianginals because its major therapeutic application is the management of angina pectoris; because it is less commonly used to treat hypertension, it is listed among the generic drugs grouped as antihypertensives with a cross-reference to Chapter 22, Antianginals.

Such classification by therapeutic use offers several advantages. It helps the reader identify an unknown drug by its clinical application alone. At the same time, it automatically identifies all other drugs that share the same use and provides easy comparison of their dosages and effects. Thereby, it quickly identifies potential pharmaco-therapeutic alternatives for patients who cannot tolerate or fail to respond to a particular drug.

Each chapter, representing a major therapeutic use, begins with an alphabetically arranged list of the generic names of drugs described in that chapter. This is followed by a list of selected combination products in which these drugs are found. Specific information on each drug is arranged under the following headings: *How Supplied; Action; Onset, Peak, Duration; Indications & Dosage; Adverse Reactions; Interactions; Contraindications;* and *Nursing Considerations.*

In each drug entry, the drug's generic name is immediately followed by an alphabetized list of its brand names. A trade name followed by an open diamond indicates a drug that is available in preparations that do not require a prescription (◊). Brands available *only* in Canada are designated with a dagger (†); those available *only* in Australia, with a double dagger (‡). A brand name with no symbol after it is available in the United States, Canada, and possibly Australia. The mention of a brand name in no way implies endorsement of that product or guarantees its legality. If a drug is a controlled substance, that is indicated (example: Controlled Substance Schedule II). Drugs regulated under the jurisdiction of the Controlled Substances Act of 1970 are divided into the following groups, or schedules.

• Schedule I (C-I): High abuse potential and no accepted medical use — for example, heroin, marijuana, and LSD.

• Schedule II (C-II): High abuse potential with severe dependence liability — for example, narcotics, amphetamines, dronabinol, and some barbiturates.

• Schedule III (C-III): Less abuse potential than schedule II drugs and moderate dependence liability — for example, nonbarbiturate sedatives, nonamphetamine stimulants, and limited amounts of certain narcotics.

• Schedule IV (C-IV): Less abuse potential than schedule III drugs and limited dependence liability — for example, some sedatives, antianxiety agents, nonnarcotic analgesics.

• Schedule V (C-V): Limited abuse potential. Primarily small amounts of narcotics, such as codeine, used as antitussives or antidiarrheals. Under federal law, limited quantities of certain C-V drugs may be purchased without a prescription directly from a pharmacist if allowed under specific state statutes. The purchaser must be at least age 18 and must furnish suitable identification. All such transactions must be recorded by the dispensing pharmacist.

Each systemically absorbed drug has been assigned a pregnancy risk category based upon available clinical and preclinical information. The Pregnancy Risk Category parallels the five Pregnancy Categories (A, B, C, D, and X) assigned by the Food and Drug Administration to reflect a drug's potential to cause birth defects. Although drugs are best avoided during pregnancy, this rating system permits rapid assessment of the risk-benefit ratio should drug administration to a pregnant woman become necessary. Drugs in category A are generally considered safe to use in pregnancy; drugs in category X are generally contraindicated.

• A: Adequate studies in pregnant women have failed to show a risk to the fetus.

• B: Animal studies have not shown a risk to the fetus, but controlled studies have not been conducted in pregnant women; or animal studies have shown an adverse effect on the fetus, but adequate studies in pregnant women have not shown a risk to the fetus.

• C: Animal studies have shown an adverse effect on the fetus, but adequate studies have not been conducted in humans. The benefits from use in pregnant women may be acceptable despite potential risks.

• D: The drug may cause risk to the human fetus, but the potential benefits of use in pregnant women may be acceptable despite the risks.

• X: Studies in animals or humans show fetal abnormalities, or adverse reaction reports indicate evidence of fetal risk. The risks involved clearly outweigh potential benefits.

• NR: Not rated.

The section titled *How Supplied* lists the preparations available for each drug (for example, tablets, capsules, solutions for injection), specifying available dosage forms and strengths. Dosage strengths available *only* in Canada are designated with a dagger (†); those available *only* in

Australia, with a double dagger (‡). Preparations that do not require a prescription are marked with an open diamond (◊).

The section titled *Action* succinctly describes the mechanism of action — that is, how the drug provides its therapeutic effect. For example, although all antihypertensives lower blood pressure, they don't all do so by the same pharmacologic process.

The section titled *Onset, Peak, Duration* describes the onset, peak (described in terms of effect or peak blood level), and duration of drug action for each route of administration, if data are available or applicable. Values listed for onset, peak, and duration are for patients with normal renal function, unless specified otherwise.

The section titled *Indications & Dosage* lists general dosage information for adults (including recommended geriatric dosages, when available) and children, as applicable. Children's dosages are usually indicated in terms of mg/kg daily. Dosage instructions reflect current clinical trends in therapeutics and can't be considered as absolute and universal recommendations. For individual application, dosage instructions must be considered in light of the patient's clinical condition.

The section titled *Adverse Reactions* lists each drug's commonly observed adverse reactions (and selected rare ones if life-threatening). The most common adverse reactions are in *italic* type; life-threatening reactions are in ***bold italic*** type. An exception to this rule is an adverse reaction that, although normally considered hazardous, has been reported to be mild and reversible with the drug in question. For example, thrombocytopenia is considered a life-threatening adverse reaction to plicamycin but a mild and reversible reaction to methyldopa. Hence, thrombocytopenia listed as an

adverse reaction to plicamyc... bold italics, whereas the same re... tion under methyldopa is not. Advers reactions are grouped according to the body system in which they appear.

The next section, *Interactions,* lists each drug's confirmed, *clinically significant* interactions with other drugs (additive effects, potentiated effects, and antagonistic effects) or foods, with specific suggestions for avoiding dangerous drug or food interactions (for example, by reducing doses or monitoring food intake). Drug interactions are listed under the drug that is adversely affected. For example, magnesium trisilicate, an ingredient in antacids, interacts with tetracycline to cause decreased absorption of tetracycline. Therefore, this interaction is listed under tetracycline. To check on the possible effects of using two or more drugs simultaneously, refer to the interaction entry for *each* of the drugs in question.

The section titled *Contraindications* lists any conditions, especially diseases, in which the use of the drug is undesirable.

The final section, *Nursing Considerations,* lists recommendations for cautious use, followed by other useful information, such as monitoring techniques and suggestions for prevention and treatment of adverse reactions. Also included are suggestions for patient comfort, for patient teaching, and for preparing, administering, and storing each drug. Recommendations for I.V. use are highlighted by **boldface** type.

Alcohol and tartrazine content

Many liquid drug preparations for oral use contain alcohol. Although the slight sedative effect that alcohol produces is not harmful in most patients — and can sometimes be beneficial — alcohol ingestion can be undesirable and even dangerous in some circumstances. Alcohol-containing

...e given very cautiously... patients who are:
...taking potent CNS ...ch as barbiturates ...that may produce a disulfiram type reaction (such as chlorpropamide, metronidazole, and furazolidone)

• taking disulfiram as part of a treatment program for their alcoholism. Such patients, upon ingestion of alcohol, will exhibit severe symptoms that may include blurred vision, confusion, dyspnea, flushing, sweating, and tachycardia.

To help prevent inadvertent exposure to alcohol, this volume signals alcohol content with a single asterisk (*) after each brand of a liquid preparation that may contain it. In many of the preparations so marked, the alcohol content is small. Nevertheless, these drugs should be avoided in patients who are susceptible to adverse effects upon exposure to alcohol.

Tartrazine dye, also known as FD&C Yellow No. 5, is a common coloring agent in some foods and drugs. Usually harmless, it can provoke a severe allergic reaction in susceptible persons. For this reason, most drug manufacturers have begun to eliminate tartrazine from their products, but many drugs still contain it.

The incidence of tartrazine sensitivity is estimated at approximately 1 in 10,000 in the general population but somewhat higher in persons with asthma and/or sensitivity to aspirin. Why this is so is unknown. The most common symptoms of tartrazine sensitivity are urticaria, rhinorrhea, asthma, and angioedema. Acutely sensitive persons may develop allergic vascular purpura, tachycardia, dyspnea, and chest pain. These allergic symptoms typically subside spontaneously upon discontinuation of the tartrazine-containing drug but may require treatment with antihistamines or epinephrine.

Avoiding exposure to tartrazine is not simply a matter of avoiding yellow-colored drugs because this substance may be present in many other color blends, such as turquoise, green, and maroon. This volume signals tartrazine content with a double asterisk (**) after each brand that may contain it. If you suspect tartrazine sensitivity in a patient receiving such a drug, inform the doctor and contact the manufacturer to determine which dosage forms contain tartrazine.

A guide to abbreviations

ACE	angiotensin-converting enzyme
ADH	antidiuretic hormone
AIDS	acquired immunodeficiency syndrome
ALT	alanine aminotransferase
AST	aspartate aminotransferase
AV	atrioventricular
b.i.d.	twice daily
BUN	blood urea nitrogen
cAMP	cyclic 3', 5' adenosine monophosphate
CBC	complete blood count
CHF	congestive heart failure
CK	creatine kinase
CMV	cytomegalovirus
CNS	central nervous system
COPD	chronic obstructive pulmonary disease
CSF	cerebrospinal fluid
CV	cardiovascular
CVA	cerebrovascular accident
D₅W	dextrose 5% in water
DNA	deoxyribonucleic acid
ECG	electrocardiogram
EEG	electroencephalogram
EENT	eyes, ears, nose, throat
FDA	Food and Drug Administration
g	gram
G	gauge
GFR	glomerular filtration rate

GI	gastrointestinal	**SIADH**	syndrome of inappropriate antidiuretic hormone
GU	genitourinary		
G6PD	glucose-6-phosphate dehydrogenase	**S.L.**	sublingual
		T_3	triiodothyronine
H_1	histamine$_1$	T_4	thyroxine
H_2	histamine$_2$	**t.i.d.**	three times daily
HIV	human immunodeficiency virus	**UCE**	urea cycle enzymopathy
		USP	United States Pharmacopeia
h.s.	at bedtime	**WBC**	white blood cell
I.D.	intradermal		
I.M.	intramuscular		
IND	investigational new drug		
IPPB	intermittent positive-pressure breathing		
IU	international unit		
I.V.	intravenous		
kg	kilogram		
M	molar		
m²	square meter		
MAO	monoamine oxidase		
mcg	microgram		
mEq	milliequivalent		
mg	milligram		
MI	myocardial infarction		
ml	milliliter		
mm³	cubic millimeter		
Na	sodium		
NaCl	sodium chloride		
NSAID	nonsteroidal anti-inflammatory drug		
OTC	over the counter		
PABA	para-aminobenzoic acid		
P.O.	by mouth		
P.R.	by rectum		
p.r.n.	as needed		
PT	prothrombin time		
PTT	partial thromboplastin time		
PVCs	premature ventricular contractions		
q	every		
q.d.	every day		
q.i.d.	four times daily		
q.o.d.	every other day		
RBC	red blood cell		
RDA	recommended daily allowance		
REM	rapid eye movement		
RNA	ribonucleic acid		
RSV	respiratory syncytial virus		
SA	sinoatrial		
S.C.	subcutaneous		

2

Drug actions, reactions, and interactions explained

Administration of any drug provokes a series of physicochemical events within the body. The first event, when a drug combines with cellular drug receptors, is known as the drug action. What follows as a result of this action of the drug is known as the drug effect. Depending on the number of different cellular drug receptors affected by a given drug, a drug effect can be local, systemic, or both. Obviously, a local effect follows application to the skin; however, transdermal absorption can produce systemic effects. Moreover, local effects can follow systemic absorption. For example, the antipeptic ulcer drug cimetidine acts solely by blocking histamine receptor cells in the parietal cells of the stomach. This is known as a local drug effect because the drug action is sharply limited to one area and does not spread to other parts of the body. On the other hand, diphenhydramine produces a systemic effect in that it blocks histamine receptors in widespread areas of the body. In other words, local drug effects are specific to a limited number of organ systems, whereas systemic drug effects are generalized and affect different and diverse organ systems.

Four important drug properties
1. Absorption
Before a drug can act within the body, it must be absorbed into the bloodstream—usually after oral administration, the most frequently used route. Before a drug contained in a tablet or capsule can be absorbed, the dosage form must disintegrate—that is, break into smaller particles. Then, these smaller particles can dissolve in gastric juices. Only after so dissolving can a drug be absorbed. Most absorption of orally administered drugs occurs in the small intestine, where the mucosal villi provide extensive surface area. Once absorbed and circulated in the bloodstream, it is bioavailable, or ready to produce a drug effect. Whether such absorption is complete or partial depends on several factors: the drug's physicochemical effects, its dosage form, its route of administration, its interactions with other substances in the GI tract, and various patient characteristics. These same factors also determine the speed of absorption. Thus, oral solutions and elixirs, which bypass the need for disintegration and dissolution, are usually absorbed more rapidly. Some tablets have enteric coatings that prevent disintegration in the acidic environment of the stomach; others may have coatings of varying thickness that delay release of the drug.

Drugs administered intramuscularly must first be absorbed through the muscle into the bloodstream. Rectal suppositories must dissolve to be absorbed through the rectal mucosa. Drugs administered intravenously, which are injected directly into the bloodstream, are completely and immediately bioavailable.
2. Distribution
After absorption, a drug moves from the bloodstream into various fluids and tissues within the body; this is distribution. Individual patient variations can greatly alter the amount of drug that is distributed throughout the body. For example, in an edematous patient, a given dose must be distributed to a larger volume than in a nonedematous patient; the amount of

drug must sometimes be increased to account for this. Remember, the dose should be decreased when the edema is corrected. Conversely, in an extremely dehydrated patient, the drug will be distributed to a much smaller volume, so the dose must then be decreased. The total area to which a drug is distributed is known as volume of distribution. Patients who are particularly obese may present another problem when considering drug distribution. Some drugs — such as digoxin, gentamicin, and tobramycin — are not well distributed to fatty tissue. Therefore, dosing based on actual body weight may lead to overdose and serious toxicity. In some cases, dosing must be based on lean body weight, which may be estimated from actuarial tables that give average weight range for height.

3. Metabolism
Most drugs are metabolized in the liver. Hepatic diseases may affect one or more of the metabolic functions of the liver. Therefore, in patients with hepatic disease, the metabolism of a drug may be increased, decreased, or unchanged. Clearly, all patients with hepatic disease must be monitored closely for drug effect and toxicity.

The rate at which a drug is metabolized varies with the individual. In some patients, drugs are metabolized so quickly that their blood and tissue levels prove therapeutically inadequate. In others, the rate of metabolism is so slow that ordinary doses can produce toxic results.

4. Excretion
The body eliminates drugs by metabolism (usually hepatic) and excretion (usually renal). Drug excretion refers to the movement of a drug or its metabolites from the tissues back into circulation and from the circulation into the organs of excretion. Although most drugs are excreted by the kidneys, some drugs can be eliminated via the lungs, exocrine glands (sweat, salivary, or mammary), kidneys, liver, skin, and intestinal tract. Drugs may also be removed artificially by direct interventions, such as peritoneal dialysis or hemodialysis.

Other modifying factors
An important factor that influences a drug's action and effect is its *binding to plasma proteins,* especially albumin, and other tissue components. Because only a free, unbound drug can act in the body, such binding greatly influences effectiveness and duration of effect.

The *patient's age* is another important factor. Elderly patients usually have decreased hepatic function, less muscle mass, and diminished renal function. Consequently, they need lower doses and sometimes longer dosage intervals to avoid toxicity. With similar consequences, neonates have underdeveloped metabolic enzyme systems and inadequate renal function. They need highly individualized dosages and careful monitoring.

Underlying disease can also markedly affect drug action and effect. For example, acidosis may cause insulin resistance. Genetic diseases, such as G6PD deficiency and hepatic porphyria, may turn drugs into toxins with serious consequences. Patients with G6PD deficiency may develop hemolytic anemia when given sulfonamides or a number of other drugs. A genetically susceptible patient can develop an acute porphyria attack if given a barbiturate. Also, patients who have highly active hepatic enzyme systems (for example, rapid acetylators), when treated with isoniazid, can develop hepatitis from the rapid intrahepatic buildup of a toxic metabolite.

Things to consider about administration

• *Dosage forms do matter.* Some tablets and capsules are too large to be easily swallowed by very ill patients. You may then request an oral solution or elixir of the same drug, but bear in mind that because a liquid is more easily and completely absorbed, it produces higher blood levels than a tablet. When a potentially toxic drug (such as digoxin) is given, the increased amount absorbed could cause toxicity. Sometimes a change in dosage form requires a change in dosage.

• *Routes of administration are not therapeutically interchangeable.* For example, phenytoin is readily absorbed orally but is slowly and erratically absorbed intramuscularly. On the other hand, gentamicin must be given parenterally because oral administration yields inadequate blood levels to treat systemic infections.

• *Improper storage can alter a drug's potency.* Most drugs should be stored in tight containers protected from direct sunlight and extremes in temperature and humidity that can cause them to deteriorate. Some may require special storage conditions, such as refrigeration.

• *The timing of drug administration can be important.* Sometimes, giving an oral drug during or shortly after mealtime decreases the amount of drug absorbed. This is not clinically significant with most drugs and may in fact be desirable with irritating drugs, such as aspirin. But penicillins and tetracyclines should not be scheduled for administration at mealtimes because certain foods can inactivate them. If in doubt about the effect of food on a certain drug, check with the pharmacist.

• *Consider the patient's age, height, and weight.* The doctor will need this information when calculating the dosage for many drugs. It should be accurately recorded on the patient's chart.

This chart should also include current laboratory data, especially renal and liver function studies, so the doctor can adjust the dosage as needed.

• *Watch for metabolic changes.* Monitor for any physiologic change (depressed respiratory function, acidosis or alkalosis) that might alter drug effect.

• *Know the patient's history.* Whenever possible, obtain a comprehensive family history from the patient or his family. Ask about past reactions to drugs, possible genetic traits that might alter drug response, and the current use of other drugs. Multiple drug therapy can cause drug interactions that can dramatically change the effects of many drugs.

Drug interactions

When one drug administered in combination with or shortly after another drug alters the effect of one or both drugs, this is known as a drug interaction. Usually, the effect of one drug is increased or decreased. For instance, one drug may inhibit or stimulate the metabolism or excretion of the other; or it may release another from plasma protein-binding sites, freeing it for further action.

Combination therapy is based on drug interaction. One drug, for example, may be given to potentiate another. Probenecid, which blocks the excretion of penicillin, is sometimes given with penicillin to maintain adequate blood levels of penicillin for a longer period. Often, two drugs with similar actions are given together precisely because of the additive effect that results. For instance, aspirin and codeine, both analgesics, are often given in combination because together they provide greater pain relief than either alone.

Drug interactions are sometimes used to prevent or antagonize certain adverse reactions. Hydrochlorothiazide and spironolactone, both diuretics, are often administered in combination because the former is potassium-depleting, whereas the latter is potassium-sparing.

But not all drug interactions are beneficial. Multiple drugs can interact to produce effects that are often undesirable and sometimes hazardous. Harmful drug interactions decrease efficacy or increase toxicity. A hypertensive patient well controlled with guanethidine may see his blood pressure rise to its former high level if he takes the antidepressant amitriptyline at the same time. Such a drug effect is known as antagonism. Drug combinations that produce these effects should be avoided if possible. Another kind of inhibiting effect occurs when a tetracycline drug is administered with calcium- or magnesium-containing drugs or foods (such as antacids or milk). These combine with tetracycline in the GI tract and cause inadequate absorption of tetracycline.

Adverse reactions

Any drug effect other than what is therapeutically intended can be called an adverse reaction. It may be expected and benign, or unexpected and potentially harmful. Mild, but *predictable,* adverse reactions are sometimes called side effects. Drowsiness caused by antihistamines is an example of this. During hay fever season, a patient may have to contend with this drowsiness to get relief from hay fever symptoms. In such a case, the dosage may be adjusted up or down to balance therapeutic effects with side effects.

An adverse reaction may be tolerated for a necessary therapeutic effect, or it may be hazardous and unacceptable and require discontinuation of the drug. Some adverse reactions subside with continued use. As an example, the drowsiness associated with methyldopa and the orthostatic hypotension associated with prazosin usu-

ally subside after several days, as the patient develops a tolerance to these effects. But many adverse reactions are dosage-related and lessen or disappear only if the dosage is reduced. Although most adverse reactions are not therapeutically desirable, an occasional one can be put to clinical use. An outstanding example of this is the drowsiness associated with diphenhydramine, which makes it clinically useful as a mild hypnotic.

Hypersensitivity, a term sometimes used interchangeably with drug allergy, is the result of an antigen-antibody immune reaction that occurs in the body when a drug is given to a susceptible patient. One of the most dangerous of all drug hypersensitivities is penicillin allergy. In its severest form, penicillin anaphylaxis can rapidly become fatal.

Rarely, idiosyncratic reactions occur. These are highly unpredictable, individual, and unusual. Probably the best known idiosyncratic drug reaction is the aplastic anemia caused by the antibiotic chloramphenicol. This reaction appears in only 1 out of 40,000 patients, but when it does, it can be fatal. A more common idiosyncratic reaction is extreme sensitivity to very low doses of a drug, or insensitivity to higher-than-normal doses.

To deal with adverse reactions correctly, you need to be alert to even minor changes in the patient's clinical status. Such minor changes may be an early warning of pending toxicity. Listen to the patient's complaints about his reactions to a drug, and consider each complaint objectively. You may be able to reduce adverse reactions in several ways. Obviously, dosage reduction often helps. But often so does a simple rescheduling of the same dose. For example, pseudoephedrine may produce stimulation that will be no problem if it's given early in the day; similarly, the drowsiness that occurs with antihistamines or tranquilizers can be totally harmless if the dose is given at bedtime. Most important, your patient needs to be told what adverse reactions to expect so he won't become worried or even stop taking the drug on his own. Of course, the patient should report any unusual or unexpected adverse reactions to the doctor.

Recognizing drug allergies or serious idiosyncratic reactions can sometimes be lifesaving. Ask each patient about drugs he is taking or has taken in the past and what, if any, unusual reactions he experienced from taking them. If a patient claims to be allergic to a drug, ask him to tell you exactly what happens when he takes it. He may be calling a harmless side effect such as upset stomach an allergic reaction, or he may have a true tendency toward anaphylaxis. In either case, you and the doctor need to know this. Of course, you must record and report any clinical changes throughout the patient's hospital stay. If you suspect a severe adverse reaction, withhold the drug until you can check with the pharmacist and the doctor.

Toxic reactions
Chronic drug toxicities are generally caused by the cumulative effect and resulting buildup of the drug in the body. These effects may be extensions of the desired therapeutic effect. For example, guanethidine-induced norepinephrine depletion produces a desired antihypertensive effect, but in larger doses, this action often produces orthostatic hypotension.

Drug toxicities typically occur when drug blood levels rise due to impaired metabolism or excretion. For example, blood levels of theophylline rise when hepatic dysfunction impairs metabolism of the drug. Similarly, digoxin toxicity can follow impaired renal function because digoxin is eliminated from the body almost ex-

clusively by the kidneys (via glomerular filtration). Of course, toxic blood levels also follow excessive dosage. Aspirin tinnitus is usually a sign that the safe dose has been exceeded.

Most drug toxicities are predictable and dosage-related; fortunately, most are also readily reversible upon dosage adjustment. So be sure to monitor patients carefully for physiologic changes that might alter drug effect. Watch especially for impaired hepatic and renal function. Warn the patient about signs of pending toxicity, and tell him what to do if a toxic reaction occurs. Also, be sure to emphasize the importance of taking a drug exactly as prescribed. Warn the patient about serious problems that could arise if he changes the dose or the schedule for taking it.

Drugs and pregnancy
Ever since the thalidomide tragedy of the late 1950s—when thousands of malformed infants were born after their mothers used this mild sedative-hypnotic during pregnancy—use of drugs during pregnancy has been a source of serious medical concern and controversy. To identify drugs that may cause such teratogenic effects, preclinical drug studies always include tests on pregnant laboratory animals. These tests point out gross teratogenicity but do not clearly establish safety. Because different species react to drugs in different ways, animal studies do not rule out possible teratogenic effects in humans. For example, the preliminary studies on thalidomide gave no warning of teratogenic effects, and it was subsequently released for general use in Europe.

What about the placental barrier? Once thought to protect the fetus from drug effects, the placenta isn't actually much of a barrier at all. Except for drugs with exceptionally large molecular structure, almost every drug administered to a pregnant woman crosses the placenta and enters the fetal circulation. An example of a drug with a large molecular size is heparin, the injectable anticoagulant. Theoretically, then, heparin could be used in a pregnant woman without fear of harming the fetus — but even heparin carries a warning for cautious use in pregnancy. Conversely, just because a drug crosses the placenta doesn't necessarily mean it's harmful to the fetus.

Actually, only one factor — stage of fetal development — seems clearly related to exaggerated risk during pregnancy. During two stages of pregnancy — the first and the third trimesters — the fetus is especially vulnerable to damage from maternal use of drugs. During these times, *all* drugs should be given with extreme caution.

The most sensitive period for drug-induced fetal malformation is the first trimester, when fetal organs are differentiating (organogenesis). During this time, *all* drugs should be withheld unless doing so would jeopardize the mother's health. Theoretically, during this sensitive time, even aspirin could harm the fetus. So, strongly advise your patient to avoid *all* self-prescribed drugs during early pregnancy. The other time of special fetal sensitivity to drugs is the last trimester. The reason? At birth, when separated from his mother, the neonate must rely on his own metabolism to eliminate any remaining drug. Because his detoxifying systems are not fully developed, any residual drug may take a long time to be metabolized — and thus may induce prolonged toxic reactions. Consequently, drugs should be used only when absolutely necessary during the last 3 months of pregnancy.

Of course, in many circumstances, pregnant women must continue to take certain drugs. For example, a woman with a seizure disorder that is well controlled with an anticonvulsant should continue to take the drug even during pregnancy. Similarly, a pregnant woman with a bacterial infection must receive antibiotics. In such cases, the potential risk to the fetus is outweighed by the mother's need. The relative risk to the fetus is expressed by the drug's pregnancy risk category (see Chapter 1).

Following these general guidelines can prevent indiscriminate and potentially harmful use of drugs in pregnancy:

● Before a drug is prescribed for a woman of childbearing age, she should be asked the date of her last menstrual period and whether she may be pregnant. If a drug is a known teratogen (for example, isotretinoin), some manufacturers may recommend special precautions to ensure that the drug not be given to a female of childbearing age until pregnancy is ruled out.
● Especially during the first and the third trimesters, a pregnant patient should avoid *all* drugs except those *essential* to maintain the pregnancy or maternal health.
● Topical drugs are not exempt from the warning against indiscriminate use during pregnancy. Many topically applied drugs can be absorbed in large enough amounts to be harmful to the fetus.
● When a pregnant patient needs *any* drug, the doctor should prescribe the *safest* possible drug in the *lowest* possible dose to minimize any harmful effect to the fetus.
● Every pregnant patient should check with her doctor before taking *any* drug.

Drugs and lactation
Most drugs a mother takes appear in breast milk. Drug levels in breast milk tend to be high when blood levels are high — generally, shortly after taking each dose. Therefore, the mother should be advised to breast-feed *before* taking medication, not *after*.

Nevertheless, with very few exceptions, a mother who wishes to breast-feed may continue to do so with her doctor's permission. However, breast-feeding should be temporarily interrupted and replaced with bottle-feeding when the mother must take tetracyclines, chloramphenicol, sulfonamides (during first 2 weeks postpartum), oral anticoagulants, iodine-containing drugs, or antineoplastics.

To protect her infant, a breast-feeding mother should avoid taking drugs indiscriminately. If she needs to take a drug, she should first check with her doctor to be sure of taking the safest drug at the lowest dose.

What to teach patients about proper use of drugs
The following general guidelines will help to ensure that the patient gets maximal therapeutic benefits and avoids adverse reactions, accidental overdose, or potentially harmful changes in effectiveness:

• Store drugs in their original containers, at room temperature (unless directed otherwise), in places that are not accessible to children or exposed to sunlight. Avoid storage in the bathroom medicine cabinet or the glove compartment or trunk of an automobile, where extremes of temperature and humidity will cause them to deteriorate.

• Learn the trade name and generic name of any drug you are taking. Be sure to tell doctors, dentists, or other health care professionals you see regularly that you are taking it. Before taking any drug, be sure you have informed your doctor, nurse, or pharmacist about any unusual reactions you've had to drugs in the past and about your allergies to foods and other substances, any special medical problems, and any drugs you've taken over the last few weeks, including any OTC drugs.

• Always read the label before taking any drug, and take the drug exactly as prescribed at the recommended dosage and for the duration of treatment. Never share prescription drugs.

• When using a drug prescribed for occasional or prolonged use, check the container for an expiration date.

• To avoid potentially harmful changes in effectiveness, do not change brands of a drug without medical approval. Certain generic preparations are not precisely equivalent in effect to brand-name preparations of the same drug.

• Never mix different drugs in a single container, and don't remove any drug from its original container or remove the label. Relying on your memory to identify a drug and specific directions for its use is hazardous.

• Discard any drugs that are outdated or no longer needed.

• Before you have any surgery (including dental surgery), tell the doctor about all the drugs that you have been taking.

• Be sure to tell the doctor, nurse, or pharmacist about any adverse reactions you've experienced while taking a drug.

• If you or someone else has taken an overdose, call your doctor, poison control center, or pharmacist immediately. Keep syrup of ipecac in your home to induce vomiting, but induce vomiting only if one of these professionals advises you to do so.

• Try to have all your prescriptions filled at the same pharmacy so that the pharmacist can identify and warn against potentially harmful drug interactions. Inform the pharmacist of any OTC drugs you're taking.

3

Drug therapy in children

A child's absorption, distribution, metabolism, and excretion processes undergo profound changes that affect drug dosage. To ensure optimal drug effect and minimal toxicity, consider these factors when administering drugs to a child.

Absorption

Drug absorption in children depends on the form of the drug; its physical properties; other drugs or substances, such as food, taken simultaneously; physiologic changes; and concurrent disease.

• The pH of neonatal gastric fluid is neutral or slightly acidic and becomes more acidic as the infant matures. This affects drug absorption. For example, nafcillin and penicillin G are better absorbed in an infant than in an adult because of low gastric acidity.

• Various infant formulas or milk products may increase gastric pH and impede absorption of acidic drugs. So, if possible, give a child oral medications on an empty stomach.

• Gastric emptying time and transit time through the small intestine — which is longer in children than in adults — can affect absorption. Also, intestinal hypermotility (as in diarrhea) can diminish the drug's absorption.

• A child's comparatively thin epidermis allows increased absorption of topical drugs.

Distribution

As with absorption, changes in body weight and physiology during childhood can significantly influence a drug's distribution and effects. In a premature infant, body fluid makes up about 85% of total body weight; in a full-term infant, 55% to 70%; and in an adult, 50% to 55%. Extracellular fluid (mostly blood) constitutes 40% of a neonate's body weight, compared with 20% in an adult. Intracellular fluid remains fairly constant throughout life and has little effect on drug dosage.

Extracellular fluid volume influences a water-soluble drug's concentration and effect because most drugs travel through extracellular fluid to reach their receptors. Children have a larger proportion of fluid to solid body weight, so their distribution area is proportionately greater.

Because the proportion of fat to lean body mass increases with age, the distribution of fat-soluble drugs is more limited in children than adults. As a result, a drug's lipid or water solubility affects the dosage for a child.

Binding to plasma proteins
As the result of a decrease in albumin concentration or intermolecular attraction between drug and plasma protein, many drugs are less bound to plasma proteins in infants than in adults.

Furthermore, preparations that bind plasma proteins may displace endogenous compounds, such as bilirubin or free fatty acids. Conversely, an endogenous compound may displace a weakly bound drug. For example, displacement of bound bilirubin can cause a rise in unbound bilirubin, which can lead to increased risk of kernicterus at normal bilirubin levels.

Since only an unbound, or free, drug has a pharmacologic effect, any alteration in ratio of a protein-bound to an unbound active drug can greatly influence its effect.

Several diseases and disorders, such as nephrotic syndrome and malnutrition, can also decrease plasma protein and increase the concentration of an unbound drug, intensifying the drug's effect or producing toxicity.

Metabolism

A neonate's ability to metabolize a drug depends on the integrity of the hepatic enzyme system, the intrauterine exposure to the drug, and the nature of the drug itself.

Certain metabolic mechanisms are underdeveloped in neonates. Glucuronidation is a metabolic process that renders most drugs more water soluble, thereby facilitating renal excretion. This process is insufficiently developed to permit full pediatric doses until the infant is 1 month old. Because of this, the use of chloramphenicol in a neonate may cause gray syndrome, illustrating the infant's inability to metabolize the drug. Use of chloramphenicol in neonates, therefore, requires decreased dosage (25 mg/kg/day) and monitoring of blood levels.

Conversely, intrauterine exposure to drugs may induce precocious development of hepatic enzyme mechanisms, increasing the infant's capacity to metabolize potentially harmful substances.

Older children can metabolize some drugs (theophylline, for example) more rapidly than adults. This ability may come from their increased hepatic metabolic activity. Larger doses than those recommended for adults may be required.

Also, preparations given concurrently to a child may alter hepatic metabolism and induce production of hepatic enzymes. Phenobarbital, for example, can induce hepatic enzyme production and accelerate metabolism of drugs given concurrently.

Excretion

Renal excretion of a drug is the net effect of glomerular filtration, active tubular secretion, and passive tubular reabsorption. Because so many drugs are excreted in the urine, the degree of renal development or presence of renal disease can profoundly affect a child's dosage requirements.

If a child is unable to excrete a drug renally, drug accumulation and possible toxicity may result unless the dosage is reduced.

Physiologically, an infant's kidneys differ from an adult's in that they have:
● high resistance to blood flow and receive a smaller proportion of cardiac output
● incomplete glomerular and tubular development and short, incomplete loops of Henle (A child's glomerular filtration reaches adult values by ages 2½ to 5 months; his tubular secretion may reach adult values by ages 7 to 12 months.)
● low glomerular filtration rate (Penicillins are eliminated by this route.)
● decreased ability to concentrate urine or reabsorb various filtered compounds
● reduced ability of the proximal tubules to secrete organic acids.

Both children and adults have diurnal variations in urine pH that correlate with sleep-awake patterns.

Calculating and monitoring pediatric dosages

When calculating pediatric dosages, don't use formulas that modify adult dosages: a child is not a scaled-down version of an adult. Pediatric dosages should be calculated on the basis of either body weight (mg/kg) or body surface area (mg/m²).
● Reevaluate dosages at regular intervals to ensure necessary adjustments as the child develops.
● Although body surface area provides a useful standard for adults and older children, don't use it in premature or full-term infants. Use the body weight method instead.

• Don't exceed the maximum adult dosage when calculating amounts per kilogram of body weight (except with certain drugs, such as theophylline, if indicated).

• Obtain an accurate maternal drug history – prescription and nonprescription drugs, vitamins, and herbs or other health foods taken during pregnancy.

• Drugs passed through breast milk can also have adverse effects on the breast-feeding infant. Before a drug is prescribed for a breast-feeding mother, the potential effects on the infant should be investigated. For example, sulfonamides given to a breast-feeding mother for a urinary tract infection appear in breast milk and may cause kernicterus at lower-than-normal levels of unconjugated bilirubin. Also, high concentrations of isoniazid appear in breast milk. Since this drug is metabolized by the liver, an infant's immature hepatic enzyme mechanisms cannot metabolize the drug, and the infant may suffer CNS toxicity.

Oral medications

• *When giving oral medication to an infant,* administer it in liquid form if possible. For accuracy, measure and give the preparation by syringe; never use a vial or cup.

• Lift the patient's head to prevent aspiration of the medication, and press down on his chin to prevent choking.

• You may also place the drug in a nipple and allow the infant to suck the contents.

• *If the patient is a toddler,* explain how you're going to give him the medication. If possible, have the parents enlist the child's cooperation.

• Don't mix medication with food or call it "candy" even if it has a pleasant taste.

• Let the child drink liquid medication from a calibrated medication cup rather than from a spoon: it's easier and more accurate. If the preparation is available only in tablet form, crush it and mix it with a compatible syrup. (Check with the pharmacist to verify that the tablet can be crushed without compromising its effectiveness.)

• *If the patient is an older child* who can swallow a tablet or capsule by himself, have him place the medication on the back of his tongue and swallow it with water or fruit juice. Remember, milk or milk products may interfere with drug absorption.

I.V. infusions

When administering I.V. infusions to children, note the following special considerations.

Protecting the insertion site

In infants, use a peripheral vein or a scalp vein in the temporal region for I.V. infusions. The scalp vein is safest in that the needle is not likely to be dislodged; however, the head must be shaved around the site. Temporary disfigurement may also result from the needle and infiltrated fluids. For these reasons, the scalp veins are not used as frequently today as they were in the past.

The extremities are the most accessible insertion sites; however, since patients tend to move about, take these precautions:

• Protect the insertion site to prevent catheter or needle dislodgment.

• Use a padded arm board to minimize dislodgment. Remove the arm board during range-of-motion exercises.

• Place the clamp out of the child's reach; if extension tubing is used to allow the child greater mobility, securely tape the connection.

• Restrain the child only when necessary.

• To allay anxiety, give a simple explanation to the child who must be restrained while asleep.

Maintaining flow rate and fluid balance

While administering an I.V. infusion to a child, monitor flow rate and check the patient's condition and insertion site at least hourly — more frequently if indicated.

Adjust the flow rate only while the patient is composed; crying and emotional upset can constrict blood vessels. Flow rate may vary if a pump isn't used. Flow should be adequate because some drugs (calcium, for example) can be very irritating at low flow rates. Infants, small children, and children with compromised cardiopulmonary status are particularly vulnerable to fluid overload with I.V. medication administration. To prevent this problem and help ensure that a limited amount of fluid is infused in a controlled manner, use a volume-control set (a volume-control device in the I.V. tubing) and an infusion pump or a syringe. Do not place more than 2 hours worth of I.V. fluid at a time in the volume-control set.

I.M. injections

I.M. injections are preferred when the drug cannot be given by other parenteral routes and rapid absorption is necessary.

• In children under age 2, the vastus lateralis muscle is the preferred injection site; in older children, either the ventrogluteal area or the gluteus medius muscle can be used.

• To determine correct needle size, consider the patient's age, muscle mass, and nutritional status and the drug's viscosity; record and rotate injection sites.

• Explain to the patient that the injection will hurt, but that the medication will help him. Restrain him during the injection, if needed, and comfort him afterward.

Topical medications and inhalants

• Use ear drops warmed to room temperature; cold drops can cause considerable pain and possibly vertigo.

• To administer drops, turn the patient on his side, with the affected ear up. If he is under age 3, pull the pinna down and back; if he is over age 3, pull the pinna up and back.

• Avoid using inhalants in very young children: obtaining their cooperation is difficult.

• Before attempting to administer medication through a metered-dose nebulizer to an older child, explain the inhaler to him. Then have him hold the nebulizer upside down and close his lips around the mouthpiece. Have him exhale; pinch his nostrils shut; and when he starts to inhale, release one dose of medication into his mouth. Tell the patient to continue inhaling until his lungs feel full.

• Most inhaled agents are not useful if taken orally; therefore, if you doubt the patient's ability to use the inhalant correctly, don't use it.

• Use topical corticosteroids with caution because chronic steroid use in children has been associated with delayed growth. When topical corticosteroids are used on the diaper area of infants, avoid covering this area with plastic or rubber pants, which will act as an occlusive dressing and enhance systemic absorption.

Parenteral nutrition

I.V. nutrition is given to patients who can't or won't take adequate food orally and patients with hypermetabolic conditions who need supplementation. The latter group includes premature infants and children who have burns or other major trauma, intractable diarrhea, malabsorption syndromes, GI abnormalities, emotional disorders (such as anorexia nervosa), and congenital abnormalities.

Before fat emulsions are administered to infants and children, however, potential benefits must be weighed against possible risks.

Fats — supplied as 10% or 20% emulsions — are administered both peripherally and centrally. Their use is limited by the child's ability to metabolize them. An infant or a child with a diseased liver cannot efficiently metabolize fats, for example.

Some fats, however, must be supplied both to prevent essential fatty acid deficiency and to permit normal growth and development. A minimum of calories (2% to 4%) must be supplied as linoleic acid — an essential fatty acid found in lipids. In infants, fats are essential for normal neurologic development.

Nevertheless, fat solutions may decrease oxygen perfusion and may adversely affect children with pulmonary disease. This risk can be minimized by supplying only the minimum fat needed for essential fatty acid requirements and not the usual intake of 40% to 50% of the child's total calories.

Fatty acids can also displace bilirubin bound to serum albumin, causing a rise in free, unconjugated bilirubin and an increased risk of kernicterus. However, fat solutions may interfere with some bilirubin assays and cause falsely elevated levels. To avoid this complication, a blood sample should be drawn 4 hours after infusion of the lipid emulsion; or if the emulsion is introduced over 24 hours, the blood sample should be centrifuged before the assay is performed.

Drug therapy in elderly patients

If you're providing drug therapy for elderly patients, you'll want to understand physiologic and pharmacokinetic changes that may alter appropriate drug dosage or cause common adverse reactions or compliance problems in elderly patients.

Physiologic changes affecting drug action

As a person ages, gradual physiologic changes occur. Some of these age-related changes may alter the therapeutic and toxic effects of medications.

Body composition
Proportions of fat, lean tissue, and water in the body change with age. Total body mass and lean body mass tend to decrease; the proportion of body fat tends to increase.

Varying from person to person, these changes in body composition affect the relationship between a drug's concentration and distribution in the body.

For example, a water-soluble drug, such as gentamicin, is not distributed to fat. Since there's relatively less lean tissue in an elderly person, more drug remains in the blood.

GI function
In elderly patients, decreases in gastric acid secretion and GI motility slow the emptying of stomach contents and the movement of intestinal contents through the entire tract. Furthermore, research suggests that elderly patients may have more difficulty absorbing medications. This is a particularly significant problem with drugs having a narrow therapeutic range, such as digoxin, in which any change in absorption can be crucial.

Hepatic function
The liver's ability to metabolize certain drugs decreases with age. This is caused by diminished blood flow to the liver, which results from the age-related decrease in cardiac output and from the diminished activity of certain liver enzymes. When an elderly patient takes certain sleep medications, such as secobarbital, the liver's reduced ability to metabolize the drug may produce a hangover effect the next morning.

Decreased hepatic function may cause:
• more intense drug effects due to higher blood levels
• longer-lasting drug effects due to prolonged blood concentrations
• greater incidence of drug toxicity.

Renal function
Although an elderly person's renal function is usually sufficient to eliminate excess body fluid and waste, the ability to eliminate some medications may be reduced by 50% or more.

Many medications commonly used by elderly patients, such as digoxin, are excreted primarily through the kidneys. If the kidneys' ability to excrete the drug is decreased, high blood concentrations may result. Digoxin toxicity, therefore, is relatively common in elderly patients who are not receiving a reduced digoxin dosage that accommodates decreased renal function.

Drug dosages can be modified to compensate for age-related decreases in renal function. Aided by laboratory tests, such as blood urea nitrogen and serum creatinine, doctors may adjust medication dosages so the patient receives the expected therapeutic benefits without the risk of toxicity. Observe your patient for signs of toxicity. A patient taking digoxin, for example, may experience anorexia, nausea, vomiting, or confusion.

Adverse drug reactions
As compared with younger people, elderly patients experience twice as many adverse drug reactions relating to greater drug consumption, poor compliance, and physiologic changes.

Signs and symptoms of adverse drug reactions — confusion, weakness, and lethargy — are often mistakenly attributed to senility or disease. If the adverse reaction isn't identified, the patient may continue to receive the drug. Furthermore, he may receive unnecessary additional medication to treat complications caused by the original medication. This can sometimes result in a pattern of inappropriate and excessive medication use.

Although any medication can cause adverse reactions, most of the serious reactions in the elderly are caused by relatively few medications. Be particularly alert for toxicities resulting from diuretics, antihypertensives, digoxin, corticosteroids, sleeping aids, and nonprescription drugs.

Diuretic toxicity
Because total body water content decreases with age, normal dosages of potassium-wasting diuretics, such as hydrochlorothiazide and furosemide, may result in fluid loss and even dehydration in an elderly patient.

These diuretics may deplete serum potassium, causing weakness in the patient; and they may raise blood uric acid and glucose levels, complicating preexisting gout and diabetes mellitus.

Antihypertensive toxicity
Many elderly people experience lightheadedness or fainting when using antihypertensive medications, partly in response to atherosclerosis and decreased elasticity of the blood vessels. Antihypertensive drugs lower blood pressure too rapidly, resulting in insufficient blood flow to the brain. This may cause dizziness, fainting, or even stroke.

Consequently, dosages of antihypertensive drugs must be carefully individualized. In elderly patients, too aggressive treatment of high blood pressure may do more harm than good, so treatment goals should be reasonable. Although bringing blood pressure down to 120/85 mm Hg may be appropriate in a young hypertensive patient, a more reasonable goal for an elderly hypertensive patient might be 150/95 mm Hg.

Digoxin toxicity
As the body's renal function and rate of excretion decline, digoxin concentrations in the blood may build to toxic levels, causing nausea, vomiting, diarrhea, and — most serious — cardiac arrhythmias. Try to prevent severe toxicity by observing your patient for early signs, such as appetite loss, confusion, or depression.

Corticosteroid toxicity
Elderly patients on corticosteroids may experience short-term effects, including fluid retention and psychological manifestations ranging from mild euphoria to acute psychotic reactions. Long-term toxic effects, such as osteoporosis, can be especially severe in elderly patients who have been taking prednisone or related steroidal compounds for months or even years. To prevent serious toxicity, carefully monitor patients on long-term regimens. Observe them for subtle changes in appearance, mood, and mobility, as well as for signs of impaired healing and fluid and electrolyte disturbances.

Sleeping aid toxicity
Sedatives or sleeping aids, such as

flurazepam, may cause excessive sedation or residual drowsiness. Keep in mind that ingestion of alcohol may exaggerate such depressant effects, even if the sleeping aid was taken the previous evening.

Nonprescription drug toxicity
When aspirin and aspirin-containing analgesics are used in moderation, toxicity is minimal, but prolonged ingestion may cause GI irritation and gradual blood loss resulting in severe anemia. Although anemia from chronic aspirin consumption can affect all age-groups, elderly patients may be less able to compensate because of their already reduced iron stores.

Laxatives may cause diarrhea in elderly patients who are extremely sensitive to such drugs as bisacodyl. Chronic oral use of mineral oil as a lubricating laxative may result in lipid pneumonia from aspiration of small residual oil droplets in the patient's mouth.

Patient noncompliance
Poor compliance can be a problem with patients of any age. However, in elderly patients, specific factors linked to aging — such as diminished visual acuity, hearing loss, forgetfulness, the common need for multiple drug therapy, and various socioeconomic factors — can combine to make compliance a special problem. Approximately one-third of elderly patients fail to comply with their prescribed drug therapy. They may fail to take prescribed doses or to follow the correct schedule; they may take medications prescribed for previous disorders, discontinue medications prematurely, or use p.r.n. medications indiscriminately.

Review your patient's medication regimen with him. Be sure he understands the medication amount and the time and frequency of doses. Also,

explain how he should take each medication — that is, with food or water or by itself.

Give your patient whatever help you can to avoid drug therapy problems, and refer him to the doctor or pharmacist if he needs further information.

Drug therapy and the nursing process

The nursing process guides nursing decisions about drug administration to ensure the patient's safety and meet medical and legal standards. This five-step process provides thorough assessment, appropriate nursing diagnosis, effective planning, correct interventions, and constant evaluation.

First step: Assessment
During assessment, the nurse focuses on direct data collection by:
• obtaining a drug history from the patient, parent, spouse, or significant other
• reviewing the patient's medical history
• performing a physical examination
• obtaining and interpreting relevant laboratory or diagnostic test results.

Drug history
Data collection begins at admission to the hospital or in an outpatient setting with specific questions about the patient's background, including allergies, medical history, habits, socioeconomic status, lifestyle and beliefs, and sensory deficits. These aspects of the patient's background can significantly influence drug therapy.

Allergies
The patient's allergy profile includes reactions to both drugs and food. Information about allergic reactions must specify the drug; a description of the reaction; its situation, time, and setting; and any contributing factors. Examples of contributing factors include concurrent use of stimulants, tobacco, alcohol, or illegal drugs, or a significant change in nutritional patterns. Asking the patient to describe his allergic reaction is especially important to help determine whether the patient reacts adversely or simply dislikes taking the drug.

Allergies to foods can also affect drug therapy. For example, allergies to shellfish can contraindicate use of drugs that contain iodine or are by-products of shellfish. Allergies to eggs are significant in patients who are to receive vaccines, which are commonly derived from chick embryos.

Prescription drugs
The patient's drug history should explore the following:
• the reason for using the drug
• the patient's knowledge of the appropriate dosage
• the patient's knowledge about determining effectiveness of the drug (if appropriate), potential adverse effects, what to do about adverse effects, and when to contact the doctor
• route of administration
• the pattern of administration at home
• use of OTC drugs
• cognitive status.

Note any special monitoring the patient must perform, such as blood glucose monitoring before insulin administration or checking radial pulse rate before taking digoxin. Make sure the patient is performing such procedures correctly and that the results are within acceptable limits.

Discuss the effects of drug therapy with the patient and determine if new symptoms or unpredicted adverse reactions have developed. Noting the patient's pattern of administration may provide insight into why a particular drug regimen succeeds or fails.

OTC drugs
A comprehensive drug history should

also list any OTC drugs the patient is taking. Many OTC drugs can inhibit or potentiate the effects of a pre-scribed drug. For example, aspirin potentiates the anticoagulant effects of warfarin.

OTC drugs include a wide range of products from common aspirin and nutritional supplements to various sprays and cleansing agents. The patient may not think of these as drugs, so the nurse may have to name types of products to get an accurate re-sponse.

Dosage and frequency of use are just as important as the type of OTC product. One aspirin tablet taken once a day may have no effect on concomi-tant drug therapy; however, a higher dosage (such as that used for arthritis) could profoundly influence therapy.

Medical history
In gathering the medical history, note any chronic diseases or disorders the patient may have and record the fol-lowing information for each:
• date of diagnosis
• initial prescribed treatment
• current treatment
• the doctor in charge.

Careful attention to this part of the medical history can uncover one of the most important problems with drug therapy — conflicting and incom-patible drug regimens. The patient who does not have a family doctor to oversee and coordinate all care may seek the care of several specialists who may prescribe drug treatment without knowing what other drugs the patient is taking. A carefully detailed medical history can uncover such problems. The nurse who identifies such conflicting or overlapping drug therapy must call them to the appro-priate doctor's attention and then teach the patient about the impor-tance of informing caregivers about all drugs he is taking.

Habits
Carefully consider dietary habits and the nontherapeutic use of drugs.

Certain foods can directly affect the effectiveness of many drugs. For example, a person who is taking the anticoagulant warfarin should not in-crease his intake of green leafy vege-tables because they contain levels of vitamin K that can antagonize the drug's anticoagulant effect.

Nontherapeutic use of drugs can profoundly affect a patient's health and impair the effectiveness of drug therapy. Consider the possible use of alcohol, tobacco, caffeine, and illegal drugs, such as marijuana, cocaine, and heroin. For example, if the patient uses alcohol, note the frequency of use, the amount, and the type of alco-hol consumed. Carefully document the intake of stimulants, such as caf-feine, because they significantly af-fect a patient's cardiovascular status and nervous system. Record the type of stimulant, the frequency of intake, and the amount consumed.

For the patient who uses tobacco, document the following information:
• the number of years the patient has used tobacco
• the kind of tobacco the patient smokes (cigarettes, cigar, or pipe) or chews
• how many cigarettes or cigars the patient smokes per day, or how much and how long he chews tobacco daily
• the brand of tobacco the patient smokes or chews.

Defining the patient's use of illegal drugs may be difficult. However, the nurse who suspects such use should encourage the patient to discuss it honestly, emphasizing that these drugs have profound effects that may cause serious drug interactions. If the patient admits using illegal drugs, document the drug, the amount and frequency of use, and the route of ad-ministration.

Socioeconomic status
Note the patient's age, educational level, occupation, and insurance coverage. These factors may be significant to compliance and to an effective plan of care. The patient's age, for example, can determine whom to include in the care (parents or other family members) and the level of information that is appropriate for teaching the patient.

Knowing the patient's educational background and occupation helps you select interventions at an appropriate level, plan a drug regimen that fits the patient's daily routine, and encourage compliance. Knowing the patient's insurance status may help you anticipate the need for financial assistance and counseling. Remember that noncompliance commonly results from inability to afford medications.

Lifestyle and beliefs
Support systems, marital status, childbearing status, attitudes toward health and health care, use of the health care system, and daily patterns of activities all affect the plan of care and patient compliance. For example, an 18-year-old single parent who is a high-school dropout on medical assistance and has no family support will probably require more teaching and support to gain a commitment and compliance than a 40-year-old affluent professional who has family support, can understand why she needs the drug, and can readily pay for it.

Sensory deficits
Any sensory deficit can significantly shape an appropriate plan of care. For example, impaired vision, paralysis of one or more extremities, loss of a limb, or loss of sensation in an extremity can impair the patient's ability to administer a subcutaneous injection, break a scored tablet, or open a medication container. Color blindness may cause difficulty in distinguishing between two medications. Hearing impairment can complicate effective patient instruction. Any sensory deficit requires careful consideration in any plan of prescribed drug therapy.

Clinical status
Two other factors can profoundly influence drug therapy: the patient's cognitive status and the systemic effects of the prescribed drugs. A patient's intact cognitive abilities ensure that he can understand and implement the actions necessary for compliance. During the interview, note if the patient is alert and oriented, if he is able to interact appropriately with people, and if his conversation is appropriate. Consider whether the patient can think clearly and express his thoughts coherently. Finally, check both short-term and long-term memory because the patient needs both to follow a specified drug regimen. If such evaluation identifies a cognitive deficit, determine the probable cause, which can range from a transient drug-related effect to permanent neurologic impairment, and then determine whether or not the patient can carry out the prescribed drug regimen. If not, the nurse must find another way to ensure that the patient receives the prescribed therapy.

After completing the drug history, perform a physical examination to assess those body systems that may be affected by a particular drug the patient is taking or that may be prescribed. Every drug has a desired effect on a body system, but it may have an undesired effect on another. For example, chemotherapeutic agents destroy cancerous cells, but they also affect normal cells and typically cause the patient to experience hair loss, diarrhea, or nausea. Therefore, examine the patient for expected drug effects; also closely monitor the patient for potentially harmful adverse effects.

Second step: Formulating a nursing diagnosis

Using information gathered during assessment, define any potential or actual drug-related problems by formulating each in a relevant nursing diagnosis. The most common problem statements related to drug therapy are *Knowledge deficit, Noncompliance,* and *Altered Health Maintenance.*

Third step: Planning

Nursing diagnoses provide the framework for planning interventions and outcome criteria (patient goals).

Outcome criteria
Outcome criteria state the desired patient behaviors or responses that should result from nursing care. Such criteria should be measurable and objective, concise, realistic for the patient, and attainable by nursing management; they should express patient behavior in terms of expectations and specify a time frame. A typical outcome statement is "Before discharge, the patient verbalizes major adverse effects related to his chemotherapy."

Fourth step: Intervention

After developing the outcome criteria, the nurse determines the interventions needed to help the patient reach the desired behavior or goals. Drug-related interventions may focus on patient teaching for a drug's action, adverse effects, scheduling, steps to avoid or treat a drug reaction, or drug administration techniques.

Appropriate interventions related to drug therapy will also include administration procedures and techniques, legal and ethical concerns, patient teaching, and any concerns related to special groups of patients (geriatric, pediatric, pregnant, or breast-feeding patients). Such interventions may be independent nursing actions, such as turning a bedridden patient every 2 hours, or may be nursing actions that require a doctor's order.

Fifth step: Evaluation

The final component of the nursing process, evaluation, is a formal and systematic process for determining the effectiveness of nursing care. This process enables the nurse to determine whether outcome criteria were met and thereby make informed decisions about subsequent interventions. For example, if the patient experienced relief of headache within 1 hour after the nurse administered a p.r.n. analgesic, the outcome criterion was met. If the headache was the same or worse, the outcome criterion was not met and requires a new assessment, which may result in a new plan of care or may yield new data that invalidate the nursing diagnosis or suggest new nursing interventions that are more specific or more acceptable to the patient. This assessment could lead to a higher dosage, a different analgesic, or a reevaluation of the cause.

Evaluation enables the nurse to design and implement a revised plan of care, to continuously reevaluate outcome criteria, and to plan again until each nursing diagnosis is successfully completed.

6

Amebicides and antiprotozoals

atovaquone
chloroquine hydrochloride
  (See Chapter 9, ANTIMALARIALS.)
chloroquine phosphate
  (See Chapter 9, ANTIMALARIALS.)
eflornithine hydrochloride
iodoquinol
metronidazole
metronidazole hydrochloride
paromomycin sulfate
pentamidine isethionate

COMBINATION PRODUCTS
None.

---

atovaquone
Mepron
Pregnancy Risk Category: C

HOW SUPPLIED
Tablets: 250 mg

ACTION
Unknown. Appears to interfere with electron transport in protozoal mitochondria, inhibiting enzymes needed for the synthesis of nucleic acids and adenosine triphosphate.

ONSET, PEAK, DURATION
Onset and duration unknown. Two peak plasma levels occur after an oral dose, suggesting enterohepatic recycling. The first occurs after 1 to 8 hours; the second occurs after 1 to 4 days.

INDICATIONS & DOSAGE
Mild to moderate Pneumocystis carinii *pneumonia in patients who cannot tolerate co-trimoxazole –*
Adults: 750 mg P.O. t.i.d. for 21 days.

ADVERSE REACTIONS
CNS: *headache, insomnia,* asthenia, dizziness.
EENT: *cough.*
GI: *nausea, diarrhea, vomiting,* constipation, abdominal pain.
Skin: *rash,* pruritus.
Other: *fever,* oral monilia.

INTERACTIONS
None significant.

CONTRAINDICATIONS
Contraindicated in patients with hypersensitivity to the drug.

NURSING CONSIDERATIONS
● Use cautiously in breast-feeding patients. In animal studies, substantial amounts of drug were excreted in breast milk.
● Because drug is highly bound to plasma protein (greater than 99.9%), also use cautiously with other highly protein-bound drugs.
● Because of the risk of other concurrent pulmonary infections, monitor patients closely during therapy.
● Instruct patient to take drug with meals because food enhances absorption significantly.

---

eflornithine hydrochloride (DFMO)
Ornidyl
Pregnancy Risk Category: C

HOW SUPPLIED
Injection (concentrate): 200 mg/ml

ACTION
Specifically and irreversibly inhibits the enzyme ornithine decarboxylase and limits the availability of substrate

---

for certain amines necessary for cell differentiation and division.

ONSET, PEAK, DURATION
Onset immediate with I.V. infusion. Serum levels peak immediately after an I.V. infusion. Duration unknown.

INDICATIONS & DOSAGE
Meningoencephalitic stage of Trypanosoma brucei gambiense *(sleeping sickness)* –
Adults: 100 mg/kg by I.V. infusion q 6 hours for 14 days.

ADVERSE REACTIONS
CNS: *seizures, hearing impairment, dizziness, headache, asthenia.*
GI: diarrhea, vomiting, abdominal pain, anorexia.
Hematologic: *anemia, leukopenia, thrombocytopenia, myelosuppression,* eosinophilia.
Other: facial edema, alopecia.

INTERACTIONS
None significant.

CONTRAINDICATIONS
Contraindicated in patients with hypersensitivity to the drug.

NURSING CONSIDERATIONS
● Use cautiously in patients with impaired renal function because most (about 80%) of the drug is excreted unchanged in the urine.
● Keep in mind that myelosuppression is a common and serious adverse reaction that is reversible when therapy is discontinued. Close patient monitoring is essential. Perform CBC and platelet counts before initiation of therapy, twice weekly during therapy, and weekly after the drug is discontinued until hematologic parameters return to pretreatment levels.
● Impose seizure precautions because seizures occurred in about 8% of patients receiving the drug during clinical trials.

● Obtain serial audiograms when feasible. Some patients have experienced hearing impairment.
● Monitor the patient for at least 24 months after treatment.
● **I.V. use:** Know that the infusion concentrate is hypertonic and must be diluted before administration. Dilute with sterile water for injection and follow strict aseptic technique. To prepare infusion, dilute one part drug to four parts sterile water for injection by adding 25 ml (5,000 mg or 5 g) of the concentrate to each of four bags containing 100 ml of sterile water. After dilution, the final concentration of each bag will be 5,000 mg/125 ml or 40 mg/ml. Use within 24 hours.
● Administer infusion over 45 minutes. Do not administer other drugs with the infusion.
● To minimize the risk of microbial growth, store diluted drug in refrigerator (39° F [4° C]).
● Be aware that the undiluted concentrate may be stored at room temperature (below 86° F [30° C]), but protect from light and freezing.

---

iodoquinol
(diiodohydroxyquin)
Diodoquin†, Diquinol, Yodoquinol, Yodoxin
Pregnancy Risk Category: C

HOW SUPPLIED
Tablets: 210 mg, 650 mg
Powder: 25 g

ACTION
Unknown. It is an iodine derivative with amebicidal activity in the intestinal lumen.

ONSET, PEAK, DURATION
Unknown.

INDICATIONS & DOSAGE
Intestinal amebiasis –
Adults: 630 to 650 mg P.O. t.i.d. af-

---

*Liquid form contains alcohol.
**May contain tartrazine.
Common reactions are in italics; ***life-threatening,*** in bold italics.

ter meals for 20 days. Total daily dosage should not exceed 2 g.

Children: usual dosage is 30 to 40 mg/kg of body weight daily in two to three divided doses for 20 days.

Additional doses should not be repeated before a resting interval of 2 to 3 weeks.

ADVERSE REACTIONS

CNS: neurotoxicity (dose-related), dysesthesia, weakness, vertigo, malaise, headache, agitation, retrograde amnesia, ataxia, *peripheral neuropathy.*

EENT: *optic neuritis,* optic atrophy, loss of vision.

GI: anorexia, nausea, vomiting, abdominal cramps, diarrhea, increased motility, constipation, epigastric burning and pain, gastritis, anal irritation and itching.

Hematologic: *agranulocytosis.*

Skin: pruritus, hives, papular and pustular eruptions, urticaria, discoloration of hair and nails.

Other: thyroid enlargement, fever, chills, generalized furunculosis, alopecia.

INTERACTIONS

None significant.

CONTRAINDICATIONS

Contraindicated in patients with hypersensitivity to 8-hydroxyquinoline derivatives or iodine-containing preparations. Iodoquinol causes liver damage in such patients. Also contraindicated in patients with hepatic or renal disease or preexisting optic neuropathy.

NURSING CONSIDERATIONS

• Use cautiously in patients with thyroid diseases.

• If the patient has difficulty swallowing, crush tablets and mix with applesauce or chocolate syrup.

• Record fluid intake and output, and color and amount of stool. Send warm specimens to laboratory for analysis.

• Watch for diarrhea during the first 2 or 3 days; notify the doctor if diarrhea continues.

• Be aware that iodoquinol may interfere with thyroid function tests for up to 6 months after drug discontinuation.

• Recommend that patient have periodic ophthalmic examinations during treatment.

• Advise the patient not to discontinue the drug prematurely. Tell him to notify the doctor if skin rash occurs.

• To help prevent reinfestation, teach the patient about the need for personal hygiene, especially good hand-washing technique. Encourage the patient not to prepare food for others until stools are negative.

metronidazole

Apo-Metronidazole†, Flagyl, Metric-21, Metrogyl‡, Metrozine‡, Neo-Metric†, Novonidazol†, PMS Metronidazole†, Protostat, Trikacide†

metronidazole hydrochloride

Flagyl I.V. RTU, Metro I.V., Novonidazol†

Pregnancy Risk Category: B

HOW SUPPLIED

Tablets: 200 mg‡, 250 mg, 400 mg‡, 500 mg

Oral suspension (benzoyl metronidazole): 200 mg/5 ml‡

Injection: 500 mg/100 ml ready to use

Powder for injection: 500-mg single-dose vials

ACTION

A direct-acting trichomonacide and amebicide that works at both intestinal and extraintestinal sites.

ONSET, PEAK, DURATION
Onset occurs immediately after I.V infusion, unknown after oral administration. Peak plasma levels occur immediately after I.V. infusion and within 1 to 2 hours of oral administration. Duration unknown.

INDICATIONS & DOSAGE
Amebic hepatic abscess –
Adults: 500 to 750 mg P.O. t.i.d. for 5 to 10 days.
Children: 35 to 50 mg/kg daily (in three doses) for 10 days.
Intestinal amebiasis –
Adults: 750 mg P.O. t.i.d. for 5 to 10 days.
Children: 35 to 50 mg/kg daily (in three doses) for 10 days. Therapy followed with oral iodoquinol.
Trichomoniasis –
Adults: 250 mg P.O. t.i.d. for 7 days or 2 g P.O. in single dose (may give the 2-g dose in two 1-g doses, each on the same day); 4 to 6 weeks should elapse between courses of therapy.
Children: 5 mg/kg dose P.O. t.i.d. for 7 days.
Refractory trichomoniasis –
Adults: 250 mg P.O. b.i.d. for 10 days.
Bacterial infections caused by anaerobic microorganisms –
Adults: loading dose is 15 mg/kg I.V. infused over 1 hour (approximately 1 g for a 70-kg adult). Maintenance dose is 7.5 mg/kg I.V. or P.O. q 6 hours (approximately 500 mg for a 70-kg adult). The first maintenance dose should be administered 6 hours after the loading dose. Maximum dosage not to exceed 4 g daily.
Giardiasis –
Adults: 250 mg P.O. t.i.d. for 5 to 7 days or 2 g P.O. once daily for 3 days.
Children: 5 mg/kg P.O. t.i.d. for 5 to 7 days.
Prevention of postoperative infection in contaminated or potentially contaminated colorectal surgery –
Adults: 15 mg/kg I.V. infused over 30 to 60 minutes and completed approximately 1 hour before surgery. Then, 7.5 mg/kg I.V. infused over 30 to 60 minutes at 6 and 12 hours after the initial dose.

ADVERSE REACTIONS
CNS: vertigo, headache, ataxia, incoordination, confusion, irritability, depression, restlessness, weakness, fatigue, drowsiness, insomnia, sensory neuropathy, paresthesia of extremities, psychic stimulation, *seizures,* neuropathy.
CV: ECG change (flattened T wave), edema (with I.V. RTU preparation).
GI: abdominal cramping, stomatitis, *nausea, vomiting, anorexia,* diarrhea, constipation, proctitis, dry mouth.
GU: darkened urine, polyuria, dysuria, pyuria, incontinence, cystitis, decreased libido, dyspareunia, dryness of vagina and vulva, sense of pelvic pressure.
Hematologic: transient leukopenia, neutropenia.
Skin: pruritus, flushing, rash.
Other: overgrowth of nonsusceptible organisms, especially *Candida* (glossitis, furry tongue), metallic taste, fever, gynecomastia, thrombophlebitis after I.V. infusion.

INTERACTIONS
Cimetidine: increased risk of metronidazole toxicity because of inhibited hepatic metabolism. Monitor closely.
Disulfiram: acute psychoses and confusional states. Don't use together.
Ethanol: disulfiram-like reaction (nausea, vomiting, headache, cramps, flushing). Don't use together.
Lithium: increased lithium levels resulting in possible toxicity. Monitor serum lithium levels closely.
Oral anticoagulants: increased anticoagulant effects. Monitor closely.
Phenytoin, phenobarbital: decreased metronidazole effectiveness because of increased hepatic clearance. Monitor closely.

---

*Liquid form contains alcohol.   *Common* reactions are in italics; *life-threatening,* in bold italics.
**May contain tartrazine.

CONTRAINDICATIONS
Contraindicated in patients with hypersensitivity to the drug or other nitroimidazole derivatives.

NURSING CONSIDERATIONS
• Use cautiously in patients with a history of blood dyscrasia or CNS disorder and in patients with retinal or visual field changes. Also use cautiously in patients with hepatic disease or alcoholism and in conjunction with known hepatotoxic drugs.
• If indicated during pregnancy for trichomoniasis, be aware that the 7-day regimen is preferred over the 2-g single-dose regimen.
• Give oral form with meals to minimize GI distress.
• **I.V. use:** Keep in mind that no preparation is necessary for RTU (ready to use). To prepare lyophilized vials of metronidazole, add 4.4 ml of sterile water for injection, bacteriostatic water for injection, sterile 0.9% sodium chloride injection, or bacteriostatic 0.9% sodium chloride injection. The reconstituted drug contains 100 mg/ml. Add the contents of the vial to 100 ml of D_5W, lactated Ringer's injection, or 0.9% sodium chloride for a final concentration of 5 mg/ml. The resulting highly acidic solution must be neutralized before administering. Carefully add 5 mEq sodium bicarbonate for each 500 mg metronidazole; carbon dioxide gas will form that may need to be vented.
• Infuse drug over at least 1 hour. Don't give I.V. push.
• Don't refrigerate the neutralized diluted solution. Precipitation may occur. If Flagyl I.V. RTU is refrigerated, crystals may form. These will disappear after the solution is gently warmed to room temperature.
• Observe carefully for edema, especially in patients also receiving corticosteroids, because Flagyl I.V. RTU may cause sodium retention.
• Record number and character of

stools when used in the treatment of amebiasis. Metronidazole should be used only after *Trichomonas vaginalis* has been confirmed by wet smear or culture or *Entamoeba histolytica* has been identified. Asymptomatic sexual partners of patients being treated for *T. vaginalis* infection should be treated simultaneously to avoid reinfection. Instruct the patient in proper hygiene.
• Tell the patient to avoid alcohol or alcohol-containing medications during therapy and for at least 48 hours after therapy is completed.
• Tell the patient metallic taste and dark or red-brown urine may occur.

paromomycin sulfate
Humatin

Pregnancy Risk Category: NR

HOW SUPPLIED
Capsules: 250 mg

ACTION
Unknown but it acts as an intestinal amebicide. It appears to inhibit protein synthesis in susceptible bacteria at the 30S segment of the ribosome.

ONSET, PEAK, DURATION
Unknown.

INDICATIONS & DOSAGE
Intestinal amebiasis, acute and chronic –
Adults and children: 25 to 35 mg/kg daily P.O. in three doses with meals for 5 to 10 days.
Tapeworms (fish, beef, pork, dog) –
Adults: 1 g P.O. q 15 minutes for four doses.
Children: 11 mg/kg P.O. q 15 minutes for four doses.

ADVERSE REACTIONS
CNS: headache, vertigo.
EENT: ototoxicity.
GI: anorexia, *nausea, vomiting, epi-*

gastric pain and burning, abdominal cramps, diarrhea, constipation, increased motility, steatorrhea, pruritus ani, malabsorption syndrome.
GU: hematuria, nephrotoxicity.
Hematologic: eosinophilia.
Skin: rash, exanthema, pruritus.
Other: overgrowth of nonsusceptible organisms.

INTERACTIONS
None significant.

CONTRAINDICATIONS
Contraindicated in patients with hypersensitivity to the drug and in those with impaired renal function or intestinal obstruction.

NURSING CONSIDERATIONS
• Use cautiously in patients with ulcerative lesions of the bowel to avoid inadvertent absorption and resulting renal toxicity. Poorly absorbed orally, but will accumulate in patients with renal impairment or ulcerative lesions.
• Ask about history of sensitivity to drug before giving first dose.
• Administer with meals.
• Be aware that criterion of cure is absence of amebae in stools examined weekly for 6 weeks after treatment and thereafter at monthly intervals for 2 years. Examine feces of family members or suspected contacts.
• Be aware that patient should avoid high doses or prolonged therapy.
• Watch for signs of superinfection (continued fever and other signs of new infections, especially monilial infections).
• Notify doctor if ringing in ears, hearing impairment, or dizziness occurs.
• To help prevent reinfestation, teach patient about the need for personal hygiene, especially good hand-washing technique. Instruct patient to refrain from preparing food for others until stools are negative.

pentamidine isethionate
NebuPent, Pentacarinat, Pentam 300, Pneumopent
Pregnancy Risk Category: C

HOW SUPPLIED
Injection: 300-mg vial
Aerosol: 300-mg vial

ACTION
Interferes with biosynthesis of DNA, RNA, phospholipids, and proteins in susceptible organisms.

ONSET, PEAK, DURATION
Unknown except peak serum levels occur ½ to 1 hour after I.M. injection, immediately after I.V. infusion.

INDICATIONS & DOSAGE
Pneumocystis carinii *pneumonia* –
Adults and children: 4 mg/kg I.V. or I.M. once daily for 14 days.
Prevention of P. carinii *pneumonia in high-risk individuals* –
Adults: 300 mg by inhalation (using a Respirgard II nebulizer) once every 4 weeks.

ADVERSE REACTIONS
CNS: confusion, hallucinations.
CV: *hypotension,* tachycardia.
GI: nausea, anorexia, metallic taste.
GU: *elevated serum creatinine,* renal toxicity.
Hematologic: *leukopenia,* thrombocytopenia, anemia.
Hepatic: elevated liver enzymes.
Respiratory: cough, **bronchospasm.**
Skin: rash, facial flushing, pruritus.
Other: fever, ***hypoglycemia,*** hyperglycemia, hypocalcemia, *sterile abscess, pain or induration at injection site.*

INTERACTIONS
Aminoglycosides, amphotericin B, capreomycin, cisplatin, colistin, methoxyflurane, polymyxin B, vancomycin: increased risk of nephrotoxicity.

---

*Liquid form contains alcohol.   *Common* reactions are in italics; ***life-threatening,*** in bold italics.
**May contain tartrazine.

CONTRAINDICATIONS
Contraindicated in patients with a history of an anaphylactic reaction to the drug.

NURSING CONSIDERATIONS
● Use cautiously in patients with hypertension, hypotension, hypoglycemia, hypocalcemia, leukopenia, thrombocytopenia, anemia, or hepatic or renal dysfunction.
● Administer the aerosol form only by the Respirgard II nebulizer manufactured by Marquest. Dosage recommendations are based on the particle size and delivery rate of this device. To administer aerosol, mix the contents of one vial in 6 ml of sterile water for injection. *Do not* use 0.9% sodium chloride solution because it will cause precipitation. Do not mix with other drugs.
● Do not use low-pressure (< 20 psi) compressors. The flow rate should be 5 to 7 liters/minute from a 40- to 50-psi air or oxygen source.
● **I.V. use:** Reconstitute drug with 3 ml of sterile water for injection. Then dilute in 50 to 250 ml of D_5W. Inject over at least 60 minutes.
● To minimize risk of hypotension, infuse drug slowly with the patient lying down. Closely monitor blood pressure.
● For I.M. injection, reconstitute drug with 3 ml of sterile water for a solution containing 100 mg/ml; administer deeply. Expect pain and induration to occur.
● Monitor blood glucose, serum calcium, serum creatinine, and BUN levels daily. After parenteral administration, blood glucose level may decrease initially; hypoglycemia may be severe in 5% to 10% of patients. This may be followed by hyperglycemia and insulin-dependent diabetes mellitus, which may be permanent.
● In patients with AIDS, be aware that pentamidine may produce less severe adverse reactions than co-tri-moxazole, the alternative treatment, and may be the treatment of choice.
● Instruct the patient to use the aerosol device until the chamber is empty, which may take up to 45 minutes.

7

Anthelmintics

mebendazole
niclosamide
oxamniquine
piperazine adipate
praziquantel
pyrantel embonate
pyrantel pamoate
thiabendazole

COMBINATION PRODUCTS
None.

---

mebendazole
Vermox

Pregnancy Risk Category: C

HOW SUPPLIED
Tablets (chewable): 100 mg
Oral suspension: 100 mg/5 ml‡

ACTION
Selectively and irreversibly inhibits
uptake of glucose and other nutrients
in susceptible helminths.

ONSET, PEAK, DURATION
Onset unknown. Plasma levels peak
in 2 to 5 hours. Duration varies with
GI transit time.

INDICATIONS & DOSAGE
Pinworm –
Adults and children over 2 years:
100 mg P.O. as a single dose. If infection persists 3 weeks later, treatment
is repeated.
Roundworm, whipworm, hookworm –
Adults and children over 2 years:
100 mg P.O. b.i.d. for 3 days. If infection persists 3 weeks later, treatment is repeated.

ADVERSE REACTIONS
GI: occasional, transient abdominal
pain and diarrhea in massive infection
and expulsion of worms.

INTERACTIONS
Cimetidine: increased plasma concentrations of mebendazole. Monitor
closely.

CONTRAINDICATIONS
Contraindicated in patients with hypersensitivity to the drug.

NURSING CONSIDERATIONS
• Be aware that tablets may be
chewed, swallowed whole, or crushed
and mixed with food.
• Administer the drug to all family
members, as prescribed, to decrease
the risk of spreading the infection.
• Know that no dietary restrictions,
laxatives, or enemas are necessary.
• Teach the patient about personal hygiene, especially good hand-washing
technique. To avoid reinfection, teach
the patient to wash perianal area
daily, to change undergarments and
bedclothes daily, and to wash hands
and clean fingernails before meals
and after bowel movements. Advise
the patient to refrain from preparing
food for others during infestation.

---

niclosamide
Niclocide, Yomesan‡

Pregnancy Risk Category: B

HOW SUPPLIED
Tablets (chewable): 500 mg

ACTION
Inhibits oxidative phosphorylation in
tapeworms.

---

*Liquid form contains alcohol.   *Common* reactions are in italics; *life-threatening*, in bold italics.
**May contain tartrazine.

ONSET, PEAK, DURATION
Unknown.

INDICATIONS & DOSAGE
Tapeworms (fish, beef, and pork) –
Adults: 4 tablets (2 g) chewed thoroughly as a single dose.
Children over 2 years and more than 34 kg: 3 tablets (1.5 g) chewed thoroughly as a single dose.
Children over 2 years and 11 to 34 kg: 2 tablets (1 g) chewed thoroughly as a single dose.
Dwarf tapeworm –
Adults: 4 tablets chewed thoroughly, daily for 7 days.
Children over 2 years and more than 34 kg: 3 tablets (1.5 g) chewed thoroughly on the first day, then 2 tablets (1 g) daily for the next 6 days.
Children over 2 years and 11 to 34 kg: 2 tablets (1 g) chewed thoroughly on the first day, then 1 (0.5 g) tablet daily for the next 6 days.

ADVERSE REACTIONS
CNS: drowsiness, dizziness, headache.
EENT: oral irritation, bad taste in mouth.
GI: *nausea, vomiting, anorexia,* diarrhea.
Skin: rash, pruritus ani.

INTERACTIONS
None significant.

CONTRAINDICATIONS
Contraindicated in patients with hypersensitivity to the drug.

NURSING CONSIDERATIONS
• Expect to administer an antiemetic before treatment as ordered. Many clinicians also give a laxative 2 hours after a dose to expel the killed worms and prevent migration of ova into the stomach.
• When treating dwarf tapeworms, urge the patient to drink fruit juices. This helps to eliminate the accumulated intestinal mucus under which the tapeworms lodge.
• Be aware that the patient is not considered cured until the stool has been negative for tapeworms for at least 3 months.
• Instruct patients to take tablets as a single dose after breakfast.
• Instruct the patient to chew tablets thoroughly and to wash down with water; for children, crush and mix the tablets with water or applesauce.
• Teach the patient about personal hygiene, especially good hand-washing technique. Advise the patient to refrain from preparing food for others during infestation.

---

oxamniquine
Vansil

Pregnancy Risk Category: C

HOW SUPPLIED
Capsules: 250 mg

ACTION
Unknown although it reduces the egg load of *Schistosoma mansoni.*

ONSET, PEAK, DURATION
Onset and duration unknown. Plasma levels peak within 1 to 1½ hours.

INDICATIONS & DOSAGE
Schistosomiasis caused by S. mansoni, *Western Hemisphere strains* –
Adults and children over 30 kg: 15 mg/kg given as a single oral dose.
Children under 30 kg: 10 mg/kg P.O., followed by 10 mg/kg P.O. 2 to 8 hours later.
Schistosomiasis caused by S. mansoni, *East and Central African strains* –
Adults and children: 30 mg/kg given as a single oral dose or in two equally divided doses over 1 to 2 days.
Schistosomiasis caused by S. mansoni, *in Sudan, Uganda, and Zaire* –
Adults and children: 40 mg/kg given

---

as a single oral dose or in two equally divided doses over 1 to 2 days.
Schistosomiasis caused by S. mansoni, *in Egypt, South Africa, and Zimbabwe* –

Adults and children: 60 mg/kg given as 15 mg/kg b.i.d. for 2 days or 20 mg/kg b.i.d. for 3 days.

ADVERSE REACTIONS
CNS: seizures, *dizziness, drowsiness, headache.*
GI: nausea, vomiting, abdominal pain, anorexia.
Skin: urticaria.

INTERACTIONS
None significant.

CONTRAINDICATIONS
Contraindicated in patients with hypersensitivity to the drug.

NURSING CONSIDERATIONS
● Use cautiously in patients with a history of epilepsy because, in rare cases, seizures have been observed within the first few hours after ingestion.
● Administer drug after meals to improve GI tolerance.
● Keep in mind that although *S. mansoni* infection is rare in the United States and Canada, travelers or immigrants from such areas as Puerto Rico, Latin America, and Africa may have contracted the infection from contaminated water.
● Warn patient that oxamniquine may cause a reddish discoloration of the urine.
● Instruct the patient to avoid driving and other hazardous activities during treatment.

piperazine adipate
Entacyl†

Pregnancy Risk Category: NR

HOW SUPPLIED
Oral suspension: 600 mg/5 ml†
Granules: 2 g/packet

ACTION
Blocks neuromuscular action, paralyzing the worm and causing its expulsion by normal peristalsis.

ONSET, PEAK, DURATION
Onset and duration is highly variable. Time to peak concentration is 2 to 4 hours.

INDICATIONS & DOSAGE
Enterobiasis (pinworm) –
Adults and children: 65 mg/kg P.O. daily for 7 to 8 days. Maximum daily dosage is 2.5 g. Alternatively, adults 2 g P.O. daily for 7 days, and children 1 g/m² P.O. daily for 7 days. Some clinicians order according to body weight:
Children under 7 kg: 250 mg P.O. daily for 7 days.
Children 7 to 14 kg: 500 mg P.O. daily for 7 days.
Children 14 to 27 kg: 1 g P.O. daily for 7 days.
Children over 27 kg and adults: 2 g P.O. daily for 7 days.
Ascariasis (roundworm) –
Adults: 3.5 g P.O. in single doses for 2 consecutive days.
Children: 75 mg/kg or 2 g/m² P.O. daily for 2 consecutive days. Maximum daily dosage is 3.5 g.
Alternatively, dosage given according to body weight:
Children under 14 kg: 1 g P.O. daily for 2 days.
Children 14 to 23 kg: 2 g P.O. daily for 2 days.
Children 23 to 45 kg: 3 g P.O. daily for 2 days.
Children over 45 kg and adults: 3.5 g P.O. daily for 2 days.
Some clinicians continue treatment for 4 days in patients with massive infestation. Treatment may be repeated in 1 week if necessary.

---

*Liquid form contains alcohol.   Common *reactions are in italics; ***life-threatening***, in bold italics.
**May contain tartrazine.

ADVERSE REACTIONS
CNS: ataxia, tremor, choreiform movements, muscular weakness, myoclonus, hyporeflexia, paresthesia, seizures, sense of detachment, EEG abnormalities, memory defect, *headache, vertigo.*
EENT: nystagmus, blurred vision, paralytic strabismus, cataracts with visual impairment, lacrimation, difficulty in focusing, rhinorrhea.
GI: *nausea, vomiting,* diarrhea, abdominal cramps.
Skin: urticaria, photodermatitis, *erythema multiforme,* purpura, eczematous skin reactions.
Other: arthralgia, fever, bronchospasm, *hemolytic anemia.*

INTERACTIONS
Pyrantel pamoate: possible antagonism. Don't administer together.

CONTRAINDICATIONS
Contraindicated in patients with hypersensitivity to the drug and in those with hepatic or renal impairment or seizure disorders.

NURSING CONSIDERATIONS
• Use cautiously in patients with severe malnutrition or anemia.
• Monitor the patient for CNS or GI reactions; be prepared to discontinue the drug if any occur.
• Be aware that no dietary restrictions, laxatives, or enemas are necessary.
• Be aware that drug should be administered to all family members, as prescribed, to decrease risk of spreading infection.
• Be aware that because of potential neurotoxicity, prolonged or repeated treatment (especially in children) is avoided.
• Tell patients that piperazine may be taken with food; but, for best absorption, tell the patient to take on empty stomach.
• Teach the patient about personal hy-

giene, especially good hand-washing technique. To avoid reinfection, teach the patient to wash perianal area, to change undergarments and bedclothes daily, and to wash hands and clean fingernails before meals and after bowel movements. Advise the patient to refrain from preparing food for others during infestation.

praziquantel
Biltricide

Pregnancy Risk Category: B

HOW SUPPLIED
Tablets: 600 mg

ACTION
Causes a contraction of schistosomes by a specific effect on the permeability of the cell membrane.

ONSET, PEAK, DURATION
Onset and duration unknown. Time to peak serum concentration is 1 to 3 hours.

INDICATIONS & DOSAGE
Schistosomiasis caused by Schistosoma mekongi, S. japonicum, S. mansoni, *and* S. haematobium—
Adults and children 4 years and older: 20 mg/kg P.O. t.i.d. as a 1-day treatment. The interval between doses should be 4 to 6 hours.
Clonorchiasis caused by Clonorchis sinensis, *opisthorchiasis caused by* Opisthorchis viverrini—
Adults and children 4 years and older: 25 mg/kg t.i.d. as a 1-day treatment.

ADVERSE REACTIONS
CNS: *drowsiness, malaise,* headache, dizziness.
GI: abdominal discomfort, nausea.
Hepatic: minimal increase in liver enzymes.
Skin: urticaria.
Other: fever.

INTERACTIONS
None significant.

CONTRAINDICATIONS
Contraindicated in patients with hypersensitivity to the drug and in those with ocular cysticercosis because destruction of the eye parasite may cause permanent eye damage.

NURSING CONSIDERATIONS
• Keep in mind that praziquantel is effective for several different species of *Schistosoma*.
• Know that praziquantel may also be effective against liver flukes.
• Be aware that adverse reactions may be more frequent or serious in patients with a heavy worm burden.
• For overdose, a fast-acting laxative is given.
• Advise the patient to take the tablet during meals and to wash down the unchewed tablet.
• Warn the patient that the tablets taste bitter. Keeping them in the mouth may cause gagging or vomiting.
• Tell the patient to avoid hazardous activities on the day of treatment and the day after because praziquantel may produce drowsiness.

---

pyrantel embonate
Anthel‡, Combantrin‡, Early Bird‡

pyrantel pamoate
Antiminth, Combantrin†, Reese's Pinworm Medicine

Pregnancy Risk Category: NR

HOW SUPPLIED
pyrantel embonate
Tablets: 125 mg‡, 250 mg‡
Oral suspension: 50 mg/ml‡
Granules: 100 mg/g‡
Squares (chocolate-flavored): 100 mg‡
pyrantel pamoate
Tablets: 125 mg†
Oral suspension: 50 mg/ml

ACTION
Blocks neuromuscular action, paralyzing the worm and causing its expulsion by normal peristalsis.

ONSET, PEAK, DURATION
Onset is highly variable. Plasma levels peak within 1 to 3 hours. Duration varies with GI transit time and extent of infestation.

INDICATIONS & DOSAGE
Roundworm and pinworm –
Adults and children over 2 years:
11 mg/kg P.O. given as a single dose. Maximum dosage is 1 g. For pinworm, dosage should be repeated in 2 weeks.

ADVERSE REACTIONS
CNS: headache, dizziness, drowsiness, insomnia.
GI: anorexia, nausea, vomiting, gastralgia, cramps, diarrhea, tenesmus.
Hepatic: transient elevation of AST.
Skin: rash.
Other: fever, weakness.

INTERACTIONS
Piperazine salts: possible antagonism; don't give together.

CONTRAINDICATIONS
Contraindicated in patients with hypersensitivity to the drug.

NURSING CONSIDERATIONS
• Use cautiously in patients with severe malnutrition or anemia or in patients with hepatic dysfunction.
• Be aware that no dietary restrictions, laxatives, or enemas are needed.
• Be aware that drug should be administered to all family members, as prescribed, to prevent risk of spreading infection.
• Advise the patient that pyrantel may be taken with food, milk, or fruit juices. Shake suspension well.
• Teach the patient about personal hy-

---

*Liquid form contains alcohol.   *Common reactions are in italics; **life-threatening**, in bold italics.*
**May contain tartrazine.

giene, especially good hand-washing technique. To avoid reinfection, teach the patient to wash perianal area daily, to change undergarments and bedclothes daily, and to wash hands and clean fingernails before meals and after bowel movements. Advise the patient to refrain from preparing food for others during infestation.

thiabendazole
Mintezol

Pregnancy Risk Category: C

HOW SUPPLIED
Tablets (chewable): 500 mg
Oral suspension: 500 mg/5 ml

ACTION
Unknown, but the drug appears to inhibit the helminth-specific enzyme fumarate reductase.

ONSET, PEAK, DURATION
Onset and duration unknown. Plasma levels peak in 1 to 2 hours.

INDICATIONS & DOSAGE
Cutaneous infestations with larva migrans (creeping eruption) –
Adults and children: 25 mg/kg P.O. b.i.d. for 2 to 5 days. Maximum dosage is 3 g daily. If lesions persist after 2 days, course is repeated.
Pinworm –
Adults and children: 25 mg/kg P.O. in 2 doses daily for 1 day; repeated in 7 days.
Roundworm, threadworm, whipworm –
Adults and children: 25 mg/kg P.O. in 2 doses daily for 2 successive days.
Trichinosis –
Adults and children: 25 mg/kg P.O. in 2 doses daily for 2 to 4 successive days.

ADVERSE REACTIONS
CNS: impaired mental alertness, impaired coordination, *drowsiness, fatigue,* giddiness, *headache,* dizziness.
CV: *hypotension.*
GI: *anorexia, nausea, vomiting,* diarrhea, epigastric distress.
Skin: *rash, pruritus, erythema multiforme.*
Other: lymphadenopathy, fever, flushing, chills.

INTERACTIONS
Theophylline: may impair hepatic metabolism of theophylline, increasing risk of toxicity. Monitor patient closely.

CONTRAINDICATIONS
Contraindicated in patients with hypersensitivity to the drug.

NURSING CONSIDERATIONS
• Use cautiously in patients with hepatic or renal dysfunction, severe malnutrition, and anemia and in patients who are vomiting.
• Be aware that drug should be administered to all family members, as prescribed, to prevent risk of spreading infection.
• Be aware that no dietary restrictions, laxatives, or enemas are necessary. However, know that supportive therapy is indicated for anemic, dehydrated, or malnourished patients.
• Teach patient to take drug after meals. For oral suspension, shake before measuring dose. For tablets, advise patient to chew before swallowing.
• Advise the patient to avoid hazardous activities, such as driving, because drug may cause drowsiness.
• Teach patient about personal hygiene, especially good hand-washing technique. To avoid reinfection, teach patient to wash perianal area daily, change undergarments and bedclothes daily, and wash hands and clean fingernails before meals and after bowel movements. Tell patient not to prepare food for others during infestation.

8
Antifungals

amphotericin B
fluconazole
flucytosine
griseofulvin microsize
griseofulvin ultramicrosize
itraconazole
ketoconazole
miconazole
nystatin

COMBINATION PRODUCTS
None.

---

amphotericin B
Fungilin Oral‡, Fungizone
Intravenous

Pregnancy Risk Category: B

HOW SUPPLIED
Tablets: 100 mg‡
Oral suspension: 100 mg/ml‡
Lozenges: 10 mg‡
Injection: 50-mg lyophilized cake

ACTION
Unknown. Probably acts by binding to sterol in the fungal cell membrane, altering cell permeability and allowing leakage of intracellular components.

ONSET, PEAK, DURATION
Onset is immediate and serum levels peak immediately after I.V. infusion. Onset, peak, and duration are unknown after oral administration.

INDICATIONS & DOSAGE
Systemic fungal infections (histoplasmosis, coccidioidomycosis, blastomycosis, cryptococcosis, disseminated moniliasis, aspergillosis, phycomycosis), meningitis —
Adults: initially, 1 mg in 250 ml of D₅W infused over 2 to 4 hours; or 0.25 mg/kg daily by slow infusion

over 6 hours. Daily dosage is gradually increased, as patient tolerance develops, to maximum 1 mg/kg daily. Therapy must not exceed 1.5 mg/kg daily. If drug is discontinued for 1 week or more, drug is resumed with initial dose and increased gradually.
Infections of the GI tract caused by Candida albicans —
Adults: 100 mg P.O. q.i.d. for 2 weeks.
Oral and perioral candidal infections —
Adults: 1 lozenge q.i.d. for 7 to 14 days. Lozenge should be allowed to dissolve slowly.

ADVERSE REACTIONS
CNS: headache, peripheral neuropathy; with intrathecal administration — peripheral nerve pain, paresthesia.
CV: hypotension, ***cardiac arrhythmias, asystole.***
GI: *anorexia, weight loss, nausea,* vomiting, dyspepsia, diarrhea, epigastric cramps.
GU: abnormal renal function with hypokalemia, azotemia, hyposthenuria, hypomagnesemia, renal tubular acidosis, nephrocalcinosis; with large doses — permanent renal impairment, anuria, oliguria.
Hematologic: normochromic, normocytic anemia.
Other: arthralgia, burning, stinging, irritation, tissue damage with extravasation, phlebitis, thrombophlebitis, pain at injection site, myalgia, muscle weakness secondary to hypokalemia, *fever, chills,* malaise, generalized pain.

INTERACTIONS
Corticosteroids: enhanced potassium depletion. Monitor serum potassium levels.

Digitalis glycosides: increased risk of digitalis toxicity in potassium-depleted patients. Monitor closely.
Flucytosine: synergistic effect; may cause increased toxicity of flucytosine. Monitor closely.
Other nephrotoxic drugs, such as antibiotics or antineoplastic agents: may cause additive renal toxicity. Administer cautiously.

CONTRAINDICATIONS
Contraindicated in patients with hypersensitivity to the drug.

NURSING CONSIDERATIONS
• Use cautiously in patients with impaired renal function.
• To reduce severe adverse reactions, be aware that the patient may receive premedication with antipyretics, antihistamines, antiemetics, or small doses of corticosteroids; addition of phosphate buffer and heparin to the solution; and alternate-day schedule. For severe reactions, discontinue the drug and notify the doctor.
• Give parenterally only in hospitalized patients, under close supervision, when diagnosis of potentially fatal fungal infection has been confirmed.
• Monitor fluid intake and output; report change in urine appearance or volume. Monitor BUN and serum creatinine (or creatinine clearance) at least weekly. Kidney damage typically reversible if drug is stopped at first sign of dysfunction.
• Obtain liver and renal function studies weekly, if ordered. If BUN exceeds 40 mg/100 ml, or if serum creatinine exceeds 3 mg/100 ml, doctor may reduce or stop drug until renal function improves. Monitor CBC weekly. Drug may be stopped if alkaline phosphatase or bilirubin levels increase.
• Monitor potassium levels closely, and report signs of hypokalemia. Check calcium and magnesium levels twice weekly, as ordered.

• **I.V. use:** Be prepared to administer an initial test dose as prescribed. 1 mg is added to 50 to 250 ml of D_5W and infused over 20 to 30 minutes; monitor the patient's pulse, respiratory rate, temperature, and blood pressure for at least 4 hours. Keep in mind that some clinicians give this test dose more slowly, over a 4-hour period.
• Use an infusion pump and in-line filter with mean pore diameter larger than 1 micron. Infuse over 6 hours; rapid infusion may cause cardiovascular collapse. Warn patient of possible discomfort at the site and of other potential adverse reactions that may occur during the several months of probable therapy.
• Use I.V. sites in distal veins. If veins become thrombosed, alternate administration sites.
• Monitor vital signs every 30 minutes; fever, shaking chills, and hypotension may appear 1 to 2 hours after start of I.V. infusion and should subside within 4 hours of discontinuation.
• Be aware that reconstituted solution is stable for 1 week under refrigeration or 24 hours at room temperature. It has 8-hour stability in room light.
• Give antibiotics separately; don't mix or piggyback with amphotericin B.
• Know that amphotericin B appears to be compatible with limited amounts of heparin sodium, hydrocortisone sodium succinate, and methylprednisolone sodium succinate.
• Store the dry form at 2° to 8° C (35.6° to 46.4° F). Protect from light. Reconstitute with 10 ml of sterile water only. To avoid precipitation, do not mix with solutions containing sodium chloride, other electrolytes, or bacteriostatic agents such as benzyl alcohol. Do not use if solution contains precipitate or foreign matter.

---

†Available in Canada only. ‡Available in Australia only. ◊Available OTC.

fluconazole
Diflucan

Pregnancy Risk Category: C

HOW SUPPLIED
Tablets: 50 mg, 100 mg, 150 mg, 200 mg
Powder for oral suspension: 10 mg/ml
Injection: 200 mg/100 ml, 400 mg/200 ml

ACTION
Inhibits fungal cytochrome P-450, an enzyme responsible for fungal sterol synthesis, and weakens fungal cell walls.

ONSET, PEAK, DURATION
Onset immediate with I.V. administration; unknown with oral administration. Peak serum levels occur immediately after I.V. infusion, 1 to 2 hours after oral administration. Duration unknown.

INDICATIONS & DOSAGE
Oropharyngeal candidiasis –
Adults: 200 mg P.O. or I.V. on the first day, followed by 100 mg once daily. Therapy should continue for at least 2 weeks.
Esophageal candidiasis –
Adults: 200 mg P.O. or I.V. on the first day, followed by 100 mg once daily. Higher doses (up to 400 mg daily) have been used, depending on the patient's condition and tolerance of treatment. Patients should receive the drug for at least 3 weeks and for 2 weeks after symptoms resolve.
Systemic candidiasis –
Adults: 400 mg P.O. or I.V. on the first day, followed by 200 mg once daily. Treatment should continue for at least 4 weeks or for 2 weeks after symptoms resolve.
Cryptococcal meningitis –
Adults: 400 mg P.O. or I.V. on the first day, followed by 200 mg once daily. Higher doses (up to 400 mg

daily) may be used. Treatment should continue for 10 to 12 weeks after CSF cultures are negative.
Prevention of candidiasis in bone marrow transplant –
Adults: 400 mg. P.O. or I.V. once daily. Start prophylaxis several days before anticipated granulocytopenia. Continue therapy for 7 days after the neutrophil count rises above 1,000 cells/mm^3.
Suppression of relapse of cryptococcal meningitis in patients with AIDS –
Adults: 200 mg P.O. or I.V. daily.
   In patients with renal failure: If creatinine clearance is 21 to 50 ml/minute, dosage is reduced by 50%. If creatinine clearance is 11 to 20 ml/minute, dosage is reduced by 75%. Patients receiving regular hemodialysis treatment should receive the usual dose after each dialysis session.

ADVERSE REACTIONS
CNS: headache, dizziness.
GI: *nausea,* vomiting, abdominal pain, diarrhea.
Hepatic: hepatotoxicity (rare), elevated enzymes.
Skin: rash, **Stevens-Johnson syndrome (rare)**.

INTERACTIONS
Cyclosporine, phenytoin: may increase plasma concentrations of these drugs. Monitor serum cyclosporine or phenytoin levels.
Isoniazid, phenytoin, rifampin, valproic acid, oral sulfonylureas: increased incidence of abnormally elevated hepatic transaminases. Monitor closely.
Oral antidiabetic agents (tolbutamide, glyburide, glipizide): may increase plasma concentrations of these drugs. Monitor for enhanced hypoglycemic effect.
Rifampin: enhanced metabolism of fluconazole. Monitor for lack of response.

---

*Liquid form contains alcohol.
**May contain tartrazine.

Common reactions are in italics; *life-threatening,* in bold italics.

Warfarin: increased risk of bleeding. Monitor PT.

CONTRAINDICATIONS
Contraindicated in patients with hypersensitivity to the drug.

NURSING CONSIDERATIONS
• As a safeguard, use cautiously in patients with hypersensitivity to other antifungal azole compounds, although no information exists regarding cross-sensitivity.
• Do not remove protective overwrap from I.V. bags of fluconazole until just before use, to ensure product sterility. The plastic container may show some opacity from moisture absorbed during sterilization. This is normal, will not affect the drug, and will diminish over time.
• **I.V. use:** Administer by continuous infusion at a rate not to exceed 200 mg/hour. Use an infusion pump. To prevent air embolism, do not connect in series with other infusions. Do not add any other drugs to the solution.
• Periodically monitor liver function during prolonged therapy, as ordered. Although adverse hepatic effects are rare, they can be serious.
• If the patient develops mild rash, monitor closely. Discontinue drug if lesions progress and notify doctor.
• Keep in mind that the incidence of adverse reactions appears to be greater in HIV-infected patients.
• Keep in mind that safety and effectiveness in children have not been established, but a few children ages 3 to 13 have received 3 to 6 mg/kg/day.

---

flucytosine
(5-fluorocytosine, 5-FC)
Ancobon, Ancotil†

Pregnancy Risk Category: C

HOW SUPPLIED
Capsules: 250 mg, 500 mg

ACTION
Unknown. Appears to penetrate fungal cells — where it is converted to fluorouracil, a known metabolic antagonist — and cause defective protein synthesis.

ONSET, PEAK, DURATION
Onset and duration unknown. Serum levels peak within 1 to 2 hours after oral dose.

INDICATIONS & DOSAGE
Severe fungal infections caused by susceptible strains of Candida *(including septicemia, endocarditis, urinary tract and pulmonary infections) and* Cryptococcus *(meningitis, pulmonary infection, and possible urinary tract infections)—*
Adults and children over 50 kg: 50 to 150 mg/kg daily P.O. q 6 hours.
Adults and children under 50 kg: 1.5 to 4.5 g/m²/day P.O. in four divided doses.
   Severe infections, such as meningitis, may require doses up to 250 mg/kg.

ADVERSE REACTIONS
CNS: dizziness, drowsiness, confusion, headache, vertigo.
GI: *nausea, vomiting, diarrhea,* abdominal bloating.
Hematologic: anemia, *leukopenia, bone marrow suppression, thrombocytopenia.*
Hepatic: elevated liver enzymes (ALT, AST); elevated serum alkaline phosphatase, BUN, or creatinine.
Skin: occasional rash.

INTERACTIONS
Amphotericin B: synergistic effects and possibly enhanced toxicity when used together. Monitor patient closely.

CONTRAINDICATIONS
Contraindicated in patients with hypersensitivity to the drug.

---

†Available in Canada only.   ‡Available in Australia only.   ◇ Available OTC.

NURSING CONSIDERATIONS

• Use with extreme caution in patients with impaired hepatic or renal function or bone marrow suppression.
• Before therapy, obtain hematologic tests and renal and liver function studies, as ordered. Also, ensure that susceptibility tests establishing that organism is flucytosine-sensitive are on the chart.
• Administer capsules over a 15-minute period to reduce adverse GI reactions.
• Monitor blood, liver, and renal function studies frequently during therapy; obtain susceptibility tests weekly, as ordered, to monitor drug resistance.
• Monitor fluid intake and output; report any marked change.
• If possible, regularly perform blood level assays of drug, as ordered, to maintain flucytosine at therapeutic level (25 to 120 mcg/ml). Higher blood levels may be toxic.
• Inform the patient that adequate therapeutic response may take weeks or months.

---

griseofulvin microsize
Fulcin‡, Fulvicin-U/F, Grifulvin V, Grisactin, Grisovin‡, Grisovin 500‡, Grisovin-FP

griseofulvin ultramicrosize
Fulvicin P/G, Grisactin Ultra, Griseostatin‡, Gris-PEG

Pregnancy Risk Category: NR

HOW SUPPLIED
griseofulvin microsize
Tablets: 250 mg, 500 mg
Capsules: 125 mg, 250 mg
Oral suspension: 125 mg/5ml
griseofulvin ultramicrosize
Tablets: 125 mg, 165 mg, 250 mg, 330 mg

ACTION
An antifungal antibiotic derived from *Penicillium* that arrests fungal cell activity by disrupting its mitotic spindle structure.

ONSET, PEAK, DURATION
Onest and duration unknown. Serum levels peak within 4 to 8 hours after oral dose.

INDICATIONS & DOSAGE
Ringworm infections of skin, hair, nails (tinea corporis, tinea capitis) when caused by Trichophyton, Microsporum, *or* Epidermophyton —
Adults: 500 mg (microsize) P.O. daily in single or divided doses. Severe infections may require up to 1 g daily. Alternatively, 330 to 375 mg ultramicrosize daily in single or divided doses.
Tinea pedis and tinea unguium —
Adults: 0.75 to 1 g (microsize) P.O. daily. Alternatively, 660 to 750 mg ultramicrosize P.O. daily in divided doses.
Children: 11 mg/kg/day (microsize) P.O. Alternatively, 7.3 mg/kg/day of the ultramicrosize.

ADVERSE REACTIONS
CNS: headache (in early stages of treatment), transient decrease in hearing, fatigue with large doses, occasional mental confusion, impaired performance of routine activities, psychotic symptoms, dizziness, insomnia.
GI: nausea, vomiting, excessive thirst, flatulence, diarrhea.
Hematologic: leukopenia, *granulocytopenia* (requires discontinuation of drug), porphyria.
Skin: rash, urticaria, photosensitivity, *toxic epidermal necrolysis* (rare).
Other: estrogen-like effects in children, oral thrush, hypersensitivity reactions (rash, *angioedema, serum sickness-like reactions*), lupuslike

---

*Liquid form contains alcohol.
**May contain tartrazine.

Common reactions are in italics; *life-threatening,* in bold italics.

syndrome or exacerbation of existing lupus erythematosus.

INTERACTIONS
Coumarin anticoagulants: decreased effectiveness. Monitor PT when used concurrently.
Ethanol: may cause tachycardia, diaphoresis, and flushing. Avoid ethanol.
Oral contraceptives: decreased effectiveness. Suggest alternative methods of contraception.
Phenobarbital: decreased griseofulvin blood levels due to decreased absorption or increased metabolism. Avoid using together or administer griseofulvin t.i.d.

CONTRAINDICATIONS
• Contraindicated in patients with hypersensitivity to the drug and in those with porphyria or hepatocellular failure.
• Also contraindicated in pregnant patients or women who intend to become pregnant during therapy.

NURSING CONSIDERATIONS
• Use cautiously in penicillin-sensitive patients because griseofulvin is a penicillin derivative.
• Because of potential toxicity, know that drug is used only when topical treatment fails to arrest mycotic disease.
• Obtain laboratory tests as ordered to confirm diagnosis of infecting organism. Continue drug until clinical and laboratory examinations confirm complete eradication.
• Be aware that because griseofulvin ultramicrosize is dispersed in polyethylene glycol, it is absorbed more rapidly and completely than microsize preparations and is effective at one-half to two-thirds the usual griseofulvin dose.
• Administer after a high-fat meal to enhance absorption and minimize GI distress.
• Assess hematologic, renal, and hepatic function periodically during prolonged therapy, as ordered.
• Keep in mind that effective treatment of tinea pedis may require concomitant use of a topical agent.
• Advise the patient that prolonged treatment may be needed to control infection and prevent relapse, even if symptoms abate in first few days of therapy. Tell the patient to keep skin clean and dry and to maintain good hygiene.
• Caution the patient to avoid intense sunlight.

---

itraconazole
Sporanox

Pregnancy Risk Category: C

HOW SUPPLIED
Capsules: 100 mg

ACTION
Interferes with fungal cell-wall synthesis by inhibiting the formation of ergosterol, a vital component, and increasing cell-wall permeability that makes the fungus susceptible to osmotic instability.

ONSET, PEAK, DURATION
Unknown.

INDICATIONS & DOSAGE
Pulmonary and extrapulmonary blastomycosis; histoplasmosis –
Adults: 200 mg P.O. daily. Dosage increased as needed and tolerated in 100-mg increments to a maximum of 400 mg daily. Dosages that exceed 200 mg daily should be given in two divided doses. Treatment should continue for a minimum of 3 months. In life-threatening illness, a loading dose of 200 mg t.i.d. is administered for 3 days.
Aspergillosis –
Adults: 200 to 400 mg P.O. daily.

ADVERSE REACTIONS
GI: nausea, vomiting, diarrhea, abdominal pain, anorexia.
Skin: rash, pruritus.
Other: edema, fatigue, fever, malaise.

INTERACTIONS
Cyclosporine, digoxin: possible increased plasma levels of these drugs. Monitor plasma levels closely.
H$_2$-receptor antagonists, antacids, rifampin, phenytoin: possible lowered itraconazole plasma levels. Avoid concomitant use.
Isoniazid: may decrease plasma levels of itraconazole. Monitor closely.
Oral anticoagulants: possible enhanced anticoagulant effects. Monitor PT closely.
Oral antidiabetic agents: similar antifungals have caused hypoglycemia. Monitor blood glucose levels closely.
Terfenadine, astemizole: inhibited metabolism of these antihistamines, resulting in elevated blood levels and risk of serious cardiac toxicity. Never administer together.

CONTRAINDICATIONS
Contraindicated in patients with hypersensitivity to the drug, in patients receiving terfenadine or astemizole, and in breast-feeding patients because drug is excreted in breast milk.

NURSING CONSIDERATIONS
• Use cautiously in patients with hypochlorhydria because they may not absorb the drug as readily as patients with normal gastric acidity. Because hypochlorhydria can accompany HIV infection, also use cautiously in HIV-infected patients.
• Use cautiously in patients receiving other highly bound medications because itraconazole and its metabolite are more than 99% bound to plasma proteins.
• Perform baseline liver function

tests, as ordered, and monitor periodically.
• Teach patients to recognize and report the signs and symptoms of liver disease (anorexia, dark urine, pale stools, unusual fatigue, or jaundice).
• Tell the patient to take drug with food to ensure maximal absorption.

---

ketoconazole
Nizoral

Pregnancy Risk Category: C

HOW SUPPLIED
Tablets: 200 mg
Oral suspension: 100 mg/5 ml†

ACTION
Inhibits purine transport and DNA, RNA, and protein synthesis; increases cell-wall permeability, making the fungus more susceptible to osmotic pressure.

ONSET, PEAK, DURATION
Onset and duration unknown. Serum levels peak within 1 to 2 hours after oral dose.

INDICATIONS & DOSAGE
Systemic candidiasis, chronic mucocandidiasis, oral thrush, candiduria, coccidioidomycosis, histoplasmosis, chromomycosis, and paracoccidioidomycosis; severe cutaneous dermatophyte infections resistant to therapy with topical or oral griseofulvin –
Adults and children over 40 kg: initially, 200 mg P.O. daily in a single dose. Dosage may be increased to 400 mg once daily in patients who don't respond to lower dosage.
Children 2 years and over: 3.3 to 6.6 mg/kg P.O. daily as a single dose.

ADVERSE REACTIONS
CNS: headache, nervousness, dizziness.
GI: *nausea, vomiting,* abdominal pain, diarrhea, constipation.

---

*Liquid form contains alcohol.   *Common* reactions are in italics; *life-threatening*, in bold italics.
**May contain tartrazine.

Hepatic: elevated liver enzymes, or *fatal hepatotoxicity*.
Skin: itching.
Other: gynecomastia with tenderness.

INTERACTIONS
Antacids, anticholinergics, H_2 blockers: decreased absorption of ketoconazole. Wait at least 2 hours after ketoconazole dose before administering these drugs.
Astemizole, terfenadine: may increase plasma levels of these drugs, precipitating CV events. Monitor closely.
Cisapride: may cause ventricular arrhythmias. Avoid concomitant use.
Rifampin, isoniazid: increased ketoconazole metabolism. Monitor for decreased antifungal effect.

CONTRAINDICATIONS
Contraindicated in patients with hypersensitivity to the drug and in those taking terfenadine or astemizole.

NURSING CONSIDERATIONS
• Use cautiously in patients with hepatic disease and in those who are taking other hepatotoxic drugs.
• Because of the potential for serious hepatotoxicity, be aware that ketoconazole should not be used for less serious conditions, such as fungus infections of the skin or nails.
• Monitor for elevated liver enzymes and nausea that does not subside, as well as for unusual fatigue, jaundice, dark urine, or pale stools — all signs of possible hepatotoxicity.
• Keep in mind that much larger doses (up to 800 mg/day) can be used to treat fungal meningitis and intracerebral fungal lesions.
• Instruct the patient to dissolve each tablet in 4 ml aqueous solution of 0.2 N hydrochloric acid, sip the mixture through a glass or plastic straw (to avoid contact with teeth), and end the procedure with a glass of water because ketoconazole requires gastric acidity for dissolution and absorption. Decreased bioavailability has been reported in patients with conditions associated with hypochlorhydria, such as AIDS.
• Make sure the patient understands that treatment should be continued until all clinical and laboratory tests indicate that active fungal infection has subsided. If drug is discontinued too soon, infection will recur. Minimum treatment for candidiasis is 7 to 14 days; for other systemic fungal infections, 6 months; for resistant dermatophyte infections, at least 4 weeks.
• Reassure the patient that, although nausea is common early in therapy, it will subside. To minimize nausea, divide the daily dosage into two doses. Taking with meals also helps to decrease nausea.

miconazole
Monistat I.V.
Pregnancy Risk Category: C

HOW SUPPLIED
Injection: 10 mg/ml

ACTION
Inhibits purine transport and DNA, RNA, and protein synthesis; increases cell-wall permeability, making the fungus more susceptible to osmotic pressure.

ONSET, PEAK, DURATION
Onset immediate. Plasma levels peak immediately after I.V. infusion. Duration unknown.

INDICATIONS & DOSAGE
Systemic fungal infections (coccidioidomycosis, candidiasis, cryptococcosis, paracoccidioidomycosis), chronic mucocutaneous candidiasis —
Adults: 200 to 3,600 mg/day I.V. Dosages may vary with diagnosis and with infective agent. Daily dosage

may be divided over 3 infusions, 200 to 1,200 mg per infusion. Dilute in at least 200 ml of 0.9% sodium chloride. Repeated courses may be needed because of relapse or reinfection.
Children 1 year and over: 20 to 40 mg/kg/day I.V. Do not exceed 15 mg/kg per infusion.
Fungal meningitis –
Adults: 20 mg intrathecally as an adjunct to I.V. administration, q 3 to 7 days.

ADVERSE REACTIONS
CNS: dizziness, drowsiness.
GI: *nausea, vomiting,* diarrhea.
Hematologic: transient decreases in hematocrit, thrombocytopenia.
Skin: *pruritic rash.*
Other: *anaphylactoid reactions,* fever, chills, transient decrease in serum sodium, phlebitis at injection site.

INTERACTIONS
Oral anticoagulants: enhanced anticoagulant effect. Monitor closely.

CONTRAINDICATIONS
Contraindicated in patients with hypersensitivity to the drug.

NURSING CONSIDERATIONS
• Use cautiously because the drug is dissolved in a vehicle containing polyoxyl 35 castor oil, a substance known to cause anaphylactoid reactions. Give the first dose under continuous medical supervision with emergency resuscitative equipment immediately available. Subsequent doses may be administered on an outpatient basis in selected patients.
• To lessen adverse GI reactions, do not administer at mealtimes.
• Know that premedication with an antiemetic may lessen nausea and vomiting.
• **I.V. use:** Be aware that I.V. miconazole has been replaced largely by newer drugs that are better tolerated.

• Dilute infusion with at least 200 ml of 0.9% sodium chloride solution and infuse over 30 to 60 minutes. Rapid I.V. injection of undiluted miconazole may produce arrhythmias.
• For intrathecal use, administer drug undiluted using a subcutaneous intrathecal (Ommaya) reservoir. Alternatively, be aware that the drug may be given by lumbar or cisternal puncture.
• Monitor levels of hemoglobin, hematocrit, electrolytes, and lipids regularly. Transient elevations in serum cholesterol and triglycerides may be caused by castor oil vehicle.
• In treatment of fungal meningitis and urinary bladder infections, assist with supplemental intrathecal administration and bladder irrigation, respectively.
• Inform patient that pruritic rash may persist for weeks after drug is discontinued. Keep in mind that pruritus may be controlled with diphenhydramine.
• Inform the patient that adequate therapeutic response may take weeks or months.

nystatin
Mycostatin*, Nadostine†, Nilstat, Nystex*

Pregnancy Risk Category: NR

HOW SUPPLIED
Tablets: 500,000 units
Oral suspension: 100,000 units/ml
Vaginal suppositories: 100,000 units

ACTION
Unknown. Probably acts by binding to sterols in the fungal cell membrane, altering cell permeability and allowing leakage of intracellular components.

ONSET, PEAK, DURATION
Not applicable because drug is not absorbed.

---

*Liquid form contains alcohol.   *Common* reactions are in italics; *life-threatening,* in bold italics.
**May contain tartrazine.

INDICATIONS & DOSAGE

GI infections –
Adults: 500,000 to 1 million units as oral tablets t.i.d.
Oral, vaginal, and intestinal infections caused by Candida albicans (Monilia) *and other* Candida *species –*
Adults: 400,000 to 600,000 units oral suspension q.i.d. for oral candidiasis.
Children and infants over 3 months: 250,000 to 500,000 units oral suspension q.i.d.
Neonates and premature infants: 100,000 units oral suspension q.i.d.
Vaginal infections –
Adults: 100,000 units, as vaginal tablets, inserted high into vagina, daily or b.i.d. for 14 days.

ADVERSE REACTIONS

GI: transient nausea, vomiting, diarrhea (usually with large oral dosage).

INTERACTIONS

None significant.

CONTRAINDICATIONS

Contraindicated in patients with hypersensitivity to the drug.

NURSING CONSIDERATIONS

● Keep in mind that nystatin is not effective against systemic infections.
● Know that vaginal tablets can be used by pregnant patients up to 6 weeks before term to treat maternal infection that may cause thrush in neonates.
● For treatment of oral candidiasis (thrush): After the mouth is clean of food debris, have the patient hold suspension in mouth for several minutes before swallowing. When treating infants, swab medication on oral mucosa. Instruct the patient in good oral hygiene techniques. Tell the patient overuse of mouthwash or having poorly fitting dentures, especially in older patients, may alter flora and promote infection.

● For treatment of oral candidiasis, be aware that immunosuppressed patients are sometimes instructed by the doctor to suck on vaginal tablets (100,000 units) because this provides prolonged contact with oral mucosa.
● Advise the patient to continue medication for at least 2 days after symptoms disappear to ensure against reinfection. Consult the doctor for exact length of therapy.
● Instruct patient to continue therapy during menstruation.
● Explain that predisposing factors of vaginal infection include use of antibiotics, oral contraceptives, and corticosteroids; diabetes; reinfection by sexual partner; and tight-fitting panty hose. Encourage the patient to use cotton (not synthetic) underpants.
● Instruct the patient in careful hygiene for affected areas, including cleansing perineal area from front to back after defecation.
● Nystatin is virtually nontoxic and nonsensitizing when used orally, vaginally, or topically, but advise the patient to report redness, swelling, or irritation.

9

Antimalarials

chloroquine hydrochloride
chloroquine phosphate
chloroquine sulphate
doxycycline
(See Chapter 14, TETRACYCLINES.)
hydroxychloroquine sulfate
mefloquine hydrochloride
primaquine phosphate
pyrimethamine
pyrimethamine with sulfadoxine

COMBINATION PRODUCTS
ARALEN PHOSPHATE WITH PRIMA-
QUINE PHOSPHATE: chloroquine
phosphate 500 mg (300 mg base) and
primaquine phosphate 79 mg (45 mg
base).

---

chloroquine hydrochloride
Aralen HCl, Chlorquin‡

chloroquine phosphate
Aralen Phosphate, Chlorquin‡

chloroquine sulphate
Nivaquine‡

Pregnancy Risk Category: NR

HOW SUPPLIED
chloroquine hydrochloride
Injection: 50 mg/ml (40-mg/ml base)
chloroquine phosphate
Tablets: 250 mg (150-mg base), 500
mg (300-mg base)
chloroquine sulphate
Tablets: 200 mg (150-mg base)
Syrup: 68 mg (50-mg base)/5 ml

ACTION
Unknown. As an antimalarial, chloroquine may bind to and alter the properties of DNA in susceptible parasites.

ONSET, PEAK, DURATION
Onset and duration unknown. Peak
levels occur 30 minutes after parenteral administration and within 1 to 3
hours after oral administration.

INDICATIONS & DOSAGE
Acute malarial attacks caused by
Plasmodium vivax, P. malariae, P.
ovale, *and susceptible strains of* P.
falciparum—
Adults: initially, 600 mg (base) P.O.,
then 300 mg at 6, 24, and 48 hours.
Or 160 to 200 mg (base) I.M. initially; repeated in 6 hours p.r.n. Patient should be switched to oral therapy as soon as possible.
Children: initially, 10 mg (base)/kg
P.O., then 5 mg (base)/kg at 6, 24,
and 48 hours (do not exceed adult
dose). Or 5 mg (base)/kg I.M. initially; repeated in 6 hours p.r.n. Do
not exceed 10 mg (base)/kg/24 hours.
Patient should be switched to oral
therapy as soon as possible.
Malaria prophylaxis—
Adults and children: 5 mg (base)/kg
P.O. (not to exceed 300 mg) weekly
on the same day (begun 2 weeks before probable exposure and continued
for 4 to 6 weeks afterward). If treatment begins after exposure, the initial
dose is doubled (600 mg for adults,
10 mg/kg for children) in 2 divided
doses P.O. 6 hours apart.
Extraintestinal amebiasis—
Adults: 1 g (600-mg base) chloroquine phosphate P.O. daily for 2 days;
then 500 mg (300-mg base) daily for
at least 2 to 3 weeks. Treatment is
usually combined with an intestinal
amebicide.
Children: 16 mg/kg chloroquine
phosphate (10 mg/kg base) P.O. once
daily for 2 to 3 weeks. Maximum dos-

---

age is 500 mg chloroquine phosphate (300-mg base) daily.

ADVERSE REACTIONS
CNS: mild and transient headache, neuromyopathy, psychic stimulation, fatigue, irritability, nightmares, seizures, dizziness.
CV: hypotension, ECG changes.
EENT: *visual disturbances* (blurred vision; difficulty in focusing; reversible corneal changes; typically irreversible, sometimes progressive or delayed retinal changes, such as narrowing of arterioles; macular lesions; pallor of optic disk; optic atrophy; patchy retinal pigmentation, typically leading to blindness); ototoxicity (nerve deafness, vertigo, tinnitus).
GI: anorexia, abdominal cramps, diarrhea, nausea, vomiting, stomatitis.
Hematologic: *agranulocytosis, aplastic anemia,* hemolytic anemia, thrombocytopenia.
Skin: pruritus, lichen planus eruptions, skin and mucosal pigmentary changes, pleomorphic skin eruptions.

INTERACTIONS
Cimetidine: decreased hepatic metabolism of chloroquine. Monitor for toxicity.
Magnesium and aluminum salts, kaolin: decreased GI absorption. Separate administration times.

CONTRAINDICATIONS
Contraindicated in patients with hypersensitivity to the drug and in those with retinal or visual field changes or porphyria.

NURSING CONSIDERATIONS
• Use with extreme caution in patients with severe GI, neurologic, or blood disorders.
• Use cautiously in patients with hepatic disease or alcoholism because drug concentrates in liver, and in those with G6PD deficiency or psoriasis because drug may exacerbate these conditions.
• Ensure baseline and periodic ophthalmic examinations are performed. Check periodically for ocular muscle weakness after long-term use.
• Assist patient with obtaining audiometric examinations before, during, and after therapy, especially if long-term.
• Monitor CBCs and liver function studies periodically during long-term therapy as ordered; if a severe blood disorder not attributable to the disease develops, drug may need to be discontinued.
• Assess the patient for possible overdose, which can quickly lead to toxic symptoms: headache, drowsiness, visual disturbances, cardiovascular collapse, and seizures, followed by cardiopulmonary arrest. Children are extremely susceptible to toxicity; avoid long-term treatment.
• To enhance compliance for prophylaxis, advise the patient to take drug immediately before or after meals on same day each week.
• Instruct the patient to avoid excessive sun exposure to prevent exacerbation of drug-induced dermatoses.
• Tell the patient to report blurred vision, increased sensitivity to light, or muscle weakness.

hydroxychloroquine sulfate
Plaquenil

Pregnancy Risk Category: NR

HOW SUPPLIED
Tablets: 200 mg (155-mg base)

ACTION
Unknown. May bind to and alter the properties of DNA in susceptible organisms.

ONSET, PEAK, DURATION
Onset and duration unknown. Plasma levels peak within 2 to 4½ hours.

INDICATIONS & DOSAGE

Suppressive prophylaxis of malaria attacks caused by Plasmodium vivax, P. malariae, P. ovale, *and susceptible strains of* P. falciparum—

Adults and children: for suppression—5 mg (base)/kg P.O. (not to exceed 310 mg) weekly on same day of the week (begin 2 weeks before entering and continue for 8 weeks after leaving endemic area). If not started before exposure, initial dose is doubled (620 mg for adults, 10 mg/kg for children) in 2 divided doses P.O. 6 hours apart.

Acute malarial attacks—

Adults: initially, 800 mg (sulfate) P.O., then 400 mg after 6 to 8 hours, then 400 mg daily for 2 days (total 2 g sulfate salt).

Children: 13 mg/kg (sulfate) P.O., then 6.5 mg/kg 6 hours later, then 6.5 mg/kg daily for 2 days.

Lupus erythematosus (chronic discoid and systemic)—

Adults: 400 mg (sulfate) P.O. daily or b.i.d., continued for several weeks or months, depending on response. Prolonged maintenance dosage—200 to 400 mg (sulfate) daily.

Rheumatoid arthritis—

Adults: initially, 400 to 600 mg (sulfate) P.O. daily. When good response occurs (usually in 4 to 12 weeks), dosage is cut in half.

ADVERSE REACTIONS

CNS: irritability, nightmares, ataxia, seizures, psychic stimulation, toxic psychosis, vertigo, nystagmus, lassitude, fatigue, dizziness, hypoactive deep tendon reflexes, skeletal muscle weakness.

EENT: visual disturbances (blurred vision; difficulty in focusing; reversible corneal changes; typically irreversible, sometimes progressive or delayed retinal changes, such as narrowing of arterioles; macular lesions; pallor of optic disk; optic atrophy; visual field defects; patchy retinal pigmenta-tion, commonly leading to blindness), ototoxicity (irreversible nerve deafness, tinnitus, labyrinthitis).

GI: anorexia, abdominal cramps, diarrhea, nausea, vomiting.

Hematologic: *agranulocytosis, leukopenia,* thrombocytopenia, *hemolysis in patients with G6PD deficiency, aplastic anemia.*

Skin: pruritus, lichen planus eruptions, skin and mucosal pigmentary changes, pleomorphic skin eruptions.

Other: weight loss, alopecia, bleaching of hair.

INTERACTIONS

Cimetidine: decreased hepatic metabolism of hydroxychloroquine. Monitor for toxicity.

Magnesium and aluminum salts, kaolin: decreased GI absorption. Separate administration times.

CONTRAINDICATIONS

Contraindicated in patients with hypersensitivity to the drug, in long-term therapy for children, and in patients with retinal or visual field changes or porphyria.

NURSING CONSIDERATIONS

• Use with extreme caution in patients with severe GI, neurologic, or blood disorders.

• Use cautiously in patients with hepatic disease or alcoholism because drug concentrates in liver, and in those with G6PD deficiency or psoriasis because drug may exacerbate these conditions.

• Ensure baseline and periodic ophthalmic examinations are performed. Check periodically for ocular muscle weakness after long-term use.

• Assist patient with obtaining audiometric examinations before, during, and after therapy, especially if long-term.

• Monitor CBCs and liver function studies periodically during long-term therapy, as ordered; if severe blood

---

Liquid form contains alcohol.   Common reactions are in italics; *life-threatening,* in bold italics.
**May contain tartrazine.

disorder not attributable to disease develops, drug may need to be discontinued.

• Assess the patient for possible overdose, which can quickly lead to toxic symptoms: headache, drowsiness, visual disturbances, cardiovascular collapse, and seizures, followed by cardiopulmonary arrest. Children are extremely susceptible to toxicity; long-term treatment should be avoided.

• To enhance compliance for prophylaxis, advise the patient to take hydroxychloroquine immediately before or after meals on same day each week.

mefloquine hydrochloride
Lariam, Mephaquin

Pregnancy Risk Category: C

HOW SUPPLIED
Tablets: 250 mg

ACTION
Unknown. Antimalarial activity may be related to its ability to form complexes with hemin.

ONSET, PEAK, DURATION
Onset and duration unknown. Time to peak concentrations is 7 to 24 hours.

INDICATIONS & DOSAGE
Acute malaria infections caused by mefloquine-sensitive strains of Plasmodium falciparum *or* P. vivax —
Adults: 1,250 mg P.O. as a single dose. Patients with *P. vivax* infections should receive subsequent therapy with primaquine or other 8-aminoquinolines to avoid relapse after treatment of the initial infection.
Malaria prophylaxis —
Adults: 250 mg P.O. once weekly. Prophylaxis should be initiated 1 week before entering endemic area, and continued for 4 weeks after return from such areas. After the patient returns to an area without malaria after

a prolonged stay in an endemic area, prophylaxis ends after three doses.

ADVERSE REACTIONS
CNS: dizziness, syncope, headache, transient emotional disturbances (rare).
CV: extrasystoles.
EENT: tinnitus.
GI: loss of appetite, vomiting, *nausea,* loose stools, diarrhea, GI discomfort.
Skin: rash.
Other: fatigue, fever, chills.

INTERACTIONS
Quinine, chloroquine: increased risk of seizures.
Quinine, quinidine, beta-adrenergic blocking agents: ECG abnormalities and cardiac arrest may occur. Avoid concomitant use.
Valproic acid: decreased valproic acid blood levels and loss of seizure control at start of mefloquine therapy. Monitor anticonvulsant blood levels.

CONTRAINDICATIONS
Contraindicated in patients with hypersensitivity to mefloquine or related compounds.

NURSING CONSIDERATIONS
• Use cautiously in patients with cardiac disease or seizure disorders.
• Because the health risks from concomitant administration of quinine and mefloquine are great, be aware that mefloquine therapy should not begin sooner than 12 hours after the last dose of quinine or quinidine.
• Keep in mind that patients with infections caused by *P. vivax* are at high risk for relapse because the drug does not eliminate the hepatic phase (exoerythrocytic parasites). Follow-up therapy with primaquine is advisable.
• Monitor liver function tests periodically as ordered.
• In cases of suspected overdose, induce vomiting or perform gastric la-

vage as appropriate because of potential for cardiotoxicity. Animal studies reveal that mefloquine has cardiac actions similar to quinidine and quinine.
• Advise the patient to take the drug on the same day of the week when using it for prophylaxis.
• Tell the patient not to take the drug on an empty stomach and always to take it with a full glass (at least 8 oz [240 ml]) of water.
• Advise patients to use caution when performing hazardous activities that require alertness and coordination because dizziness, disturbed sense of balance, and neuropsychiatric reactions may occur.
• Instruct patients taking mefloquine prophylaxis to discontinue the drug if they notice signs or symptoms of impending toxicity, such as unexplained anxiety, depression, confusion, or restlessness, and notify their doctor.
• Recommend to the patient undergoing long-term therapy to have periodic ophthalmic examinations because ocular lesions have been noted in laboratory animals.

---

primaquine phosphate
Pregnancy Risk Category: NR

HOW SUPPLIED
Tablets: 7.5 mg (base)‡, 15 mg (base)

ACTION
Unknown. It may be effective because of the drug's ability to bind to and alter the properties of DNA.

ONSET, PEAK, DURATION
Onset and duration unknown. Plasma levels peak in 2 to 3 hours.

INDICATIONS & DOSAGE
Radical cure of relapsing Plasmodium vivax *malaria, eliminating symptoms and infection completely; prevention of relapse –*
Adults: 15 mg (base) P.O. daily for

14 days. (26.3-mg tablet = 15 mg of base.)

ADVERSE REACTIONS
CNS: headache.
EENT: disturbances of visual accommodation.
GI: nausea, vomiting, epigastric distress, abdominal cramps.
Hematologic: leukopenia, *hemolytic anemia in G6PD deficiency,* methemoglobinemia in NADH methemoglobin reductase deficiency, leukocytosis, mild anemia, *granulocytopenia, agranulocytosis.*
Skin: urticaria.

INTERACTIONS
Magnesium and aluminum salts: decreased GI absorption. Separate administration times.
Quinacrine: enhanced toxicity of primaquine. Don't use together.

CONTRAINDICATIONS
Contraindicated in patients with systemic diseases in which granulocytopenia may develop (such as lupus erythematosus or rheumatoid arthritis) and in those taking bone marrow suppressants and potentially hemolytic drugs.

NURSING CONSIDERATIONS
• Use cautiously in patients with previous idiosyncratic reaction (manifested by hemolytic anemia, methemoglobinemia, or leukopenia); in those with a family or personal history of favism; and in those with erythrocytic G6PD deficiency or NADH methemoglobin reductase deficiency.
• Administer drug with meals.
• Keep in mind that when administering the drug, a fast-acting antimalarial (such as chloroquine) is used to reduce possibility of drug-resistant strains.
• Obtain frequent blood studies and urine examinations as ordered in

---

*Liquid form contains alcohol.   *Common* reactions are in italics; *life-threatening,* in bold italics.
**May contain tartrazine.

light-skinned patients taking more than 30 mg (base) daily, dark-skinned patients taking more than 15 mg (base) daily, and patients with severe anemia or suspected sensitivity.
• Monitor patient for sudden fall in hemoglobin concentration, erythrocyte or leukocyte count, or marked darkening of the urine, which suggests impending hemolytic reactions. Discontinue drug immediately and notify the doctor.

---

pyrimethamine
Daraprim

pyrimethamine with sulfadoxine
Fansidar

Pregnancy Risk Category: C

HOW SUPPLIED
pyrimethamine
Tablets: 25 mg
pyrimethamine with sulfadoxine
Tablets: pyrimethamine 25 mg, sulfadoxine 500 mg

ACTION
Inhibits the enzyme dihydrofolate reductase, thereby impeding reduction of dihydrofolic acid to tetrahydrofolic acid. Sulfadoxine competitively inhibits use of PABA.

ONSET, PEAK, DURATION
Onset and duration unknown. When administered alone, pyrimethamine serum levels peak 2 to 6 hours after oral dose. When given as the combination product, serum pyrimethamine levels peak 1½ to 8 hours and sulfadoxine levels peak 2½ to 6 hours after oral dose.

INDICATIONS & DOSAGE
Malaria prophylaxis and transmission control (pyrimethamine) –
Adults and children over 10 years: 25 mg P.O. weekly.

Children 4 to 10 years: 12.5 mg P.O. weekly.
Children under 4 years: 6.25 mg P.O. weekly.
Needs to be continued in all agegroups at least 10 weeks after leaving endemic areas.
Acute attacks of malaria (Fansidar) –
Adults: 2 to 3 tablets as a single dose, either alone or in sequence with quinine or primaquine.
Children 9 to 14 years: 2 tablets.
Children 4 to 8 years: 1 tablet.
Children under 4 years: ½ tablet.
Malaria prophylaxis (Fansidar) –
Adults: 1 tablet weekly, or 2 tablets q 2 weeks.
Children 9 to 14 years: ¾ tablet weekly, or 1½ tablets q 2 weeks.
Children 4 to 8 years: ½ tablet weekly, or 1 tablet q 2 weeks.
Children under 4 years: ¼ tablet weekly, or ½ tablet q 2 weeks.
Acute attacks of malaria (pyrimethamine) –
Adults and children over 15 years: 25 mg P.O. daily for 2 days.
Children under 15 years: 12.5 mg P.O. daily for 2 days.
Not recommended alone in nonimmune patients; should be used with faster-acting antimalarials, such as chloroquine, for 2 days to initiate transmission control and suppressive cure.
Toxoplasmosis (pyrimethamine) –
Adults: initially, 100 mg P.O., then 25 mg P.O. daily for 4 to 5 weeks; at the same time, 1 g sulfadiazine is given P.O. q 6 hours.
Children: initially, 1 mg/kg P.O. (not to exceed 100 mg) in two equally divided doses for 2 to 4 days, then 0.5 mg/kg daily for 4 weeks, along with 100 mg sulfadiazine/kg P.O. daily, divided q 6 hours.

ADVERSE REACTIONS
CNS: stimulation and seizures (acute toxicity).

---

†Available in Canada only.   ‡Available in Australia only.   ◇Available OTC.

GI: anorexia, vomiting, diarrhea, atrophic glossitis.
Hematologic: *agranulocytosis, aplastic anemia,* megaloblastic anemia, bone marrow suppression, leukopenia, thrombocytopenia, pancytopenia.
Skin: rash, *erythema multiforme (Stevens-Johnson syndrome), toxic epidermal necrolysis.*

INTERACTIONS

Folic acid and PABA: decreased antitoxoplasmic effects. May require dosage adjustment.
Sulfonamides, co-trimoxazole, methotrexate: increased risk of bone marrow suppression. Don't use together.

CONTRAINDICATIONS

• Pyrimethamine is contraindicated in patients with hypersensitivity to the drug and in patients with megaloblastic anemia caused by folic acid deficiency. Fansidar is contraindicated in patients with porphyria because it contains sulfadoxine, a sulfonamide.
• Repeated use of Fansidar is contraindicated in patients with severe renal insufficiency, marked liver parenchymal damage or blood dyscrasias, known hypersensitivity to pyrimethamine or sulfonamides, documented megaloblastic anemia due to folate deficiency; infants under 2 months; in pregnancy at term; and during breastfeeding.

NURSING CONSIDERATIONS

• Use cautiously in patients with impaired hepatic or renal function, severe allergy or bronchial asthma, or G6PD deficiency.
• Use cautiously in patients with seizure disorders; smaller doses may be needed. Also use cautiously after treatment with chloroquine.
• Give with meals to minimize GI distress.
• Obtain twice-weekly blood counts, including platelets, as ordered, for the patient with toxoplasmosis because dosages used approach toxic levels. If signs of folic acid or folinic acid deficiency develop, dosage should be reduced or discontinued while the patient receives parenteral folinic acid (leucovorin) until blood counts become normal.
• Keep in mind that, when used to treat toxoplasmosis in patients with AIDS, therapy may need to be continued for several months. Chronic suppressive therapy for the lifetime of the patient may also be necessary.
• Because of the possibility of severe skin reactions, keep in mind that Fansidar should be used only in regions where chloroquine-resistant malaria is prevalent and only when the traveler plans to stay in the region longer than 3 weeks.
• Warn patients taking Fansidar to stop drug and notify doctor at first sign of skin rash.
• Instruct the patient to take the first prophylactic dose of Fansidar 1 to 2 days before traveling to an endemic area.

Liquid form contains alcohol.   Common reactions are in italics; *life-threatening,* in bold italics.
**May contain tartrazine.

10

Antituberculars and antileprotics

aminosalicylate sodium
capreomycin sulfate
clofazimine
cycloserine
dapsone
ethambutol hydrochloride
ethionamide
isoniazid
pyrazinamide
rifampin
streptomycin sulfate
(See Chapter 11, AMINOGLYCOSIDES.)

COMBINATION PRODUCTS
RIFAMATE: isoniazid 150 mg and rifampin 300 mg.
RIFATER: isoniazid 50 mg, rifampin 120 mg, and pyrazinamide 300 mg.
RIMACTANE/INH DUAL PACK: thirty 300-mg isoniazid tablets and sixty 300-mg rifampin capsules.

---

aminosalicylate sodium (para-amino salicylate, PAS)
Nemasol Sodium†, Sodium P.A.S., Tubasal

Pregnancy Risk Category: NR

HOW SUPPLIED
Tablets: 500 mg

ACTION
Unknown. Believed to suppress growth and reproduction of *Mycobacterium tuberculosis* by competitively inhibiting the formation of folic acid.

ONSET, PEAK, DURATION
Onset and duration unknown. Serum levels peak within 1 to 2 hours.

INDICATIONS & DOSAGE
Adjunctive treatment of tuberculosis –
Adults: 3.3 to 4 g P.O. q 8 hours, or 5 to 6 g every 12 hours. Maximum daily dosage is 20 g. Must be taken with other antitubercular agents.
Children: 50 to 75 mg/kg P.O. q 6 hours or 66.7 to 100 mg/kg q 8 hours. Maximum daily dosage is 12 g. Must be taken with other antitubercular agents.

ADVERSE REACTIONS
GI: abdominal pain, nausea, vomiting, diarrhea, anorexia.
GU: crystalluria.
Hematologic: *hemolytic anemia.*
Hepatic: *hepatitis.*
Skin: rash.
Other: hypersensitivity reactions (eosinophilia, joint pain, fever), mononucleosis-like syndrome, goiter or myxedema (with long-term therapy).

INTERACTIONS
Aminobenzoate derivatives: decreased absorption of aminosalicylate sodium from the GI tract. Avoid concomitant use.
Cyanocobalamin (vitamin B_{12}): decreased absorption of vitamin B_{12} from the GI tract. Provide parenteral supplement as ordered.
Digoxin: may cause decreased absorption of digoxin. Monitor closely.
Probenecid, sulfinpyrazone: decreased excretion of aminosalicylate sodium, resulting in toxicity. Monitor closely.
Rifampin: may impair the absorption of rifampin. Separate administration times by at least 6 hours.
Warfarin, other anticoagulants: enhanced anticoagulant effect. Monitor for bleeding.

---

†Available in Canada only.   ‡Available in Australia only.   ◊ Available OTC.

CONTRAINDICATIONS
Contraindicated in patients with hypersensitivity to the drug, other salicylates, or sulfonamides.

NURSING CONSIDERATIONS
• Use cautiously in patients with peptic ulcer or other GI disease, and in patients with CHF. Also use cautiously in patients who may become pregnant because the drug may be teratogenic.
• Be aware that urine glucose determinations may be false-positive with copper sulfate tests (Benedict's solution, Clinitest); glucose enzymatic tests (Clinistix, Tes-Tape) are not affected.
• Advise the patient to take the drug with meals or antacids to minimize GI adverse effects. Children may tolerate this drug better than adults.
• Tell the patient to report back pain; pain during urination; unusual bruising or bleeding; fever or sore throat; yellow eyes, sclera, or skin; or severe joint pain.
• Encourage the patient to comply with therapy, which may last several months.
• Instruct the patient to store drug away from heat, humidity, or direct sunlight. Tell the patient not to take tablets that are discolored.

---

capreomycin sulfate
Capastat Sulfate

Pregnancy Risk Category: C

HOW SUPPLIED
Injection: 1 g/vial

ACTION
Unknown.

ONSET, PEAK, DURATION
Onset and duration unknown. Plasma levels peak 1 to 2 hours after I.M. injection.

INDICATIONS & DOSAGE
Adjunctive treatment of tuberculosis –
Adults: 15 mg/kg/day up to 1 g I.M. daily injected deeply into large muscle mass for 60 to 120 days; then 1 g two to three times weekly for 18 to 24 months. Maximum dosage should not exceed 20 mg/kg/day. Must be given in conjunction with another antitubercular drug.

ADVERSE REACTIONS
CNS: headache, *neuromuscular blockade.*
EENT: *ototoxicity* (tinnitus, vertigo, hearing loss).
GU: *nephrotoxicity* (elevated BUN and nonprotein nitrogen levels, casts, RBC counts, leukocytes; tubular necrosis; proteinuria; decreased creatinine clearance).
Hematologic: eosinophilia, leukocytosis, leukopenia.
Other: hypokalemia; alkalosis; hepatotoxicity; pain, induration, excessive bleeding, and sterile abscesses at injection site.

INTERACTIONS
Nephrotoxic or ototoxic drugs such as aminoglycosides, colistin, polymyxin B, or vancomycin: increased risk of additive toxicity. Avoid concomitant use.

CONTRAINDICATIONS
Contraindicated in patients with hypersensitivity to the drug.

NURSING CONSIDERATIONS
• Use with extreme caution in patients receiving other ototoxic or nephrotoxic drugs.
• Use cautiously in patients with impaired renal function, history of allergies, or hearing impairment.
• Assess patient's renal function and hearing before beginning therapy.
• Be aware that capreomycin is considered a "second-line" drug in the treatment of tuberculosis and should

---

*Liquid form contains alcohol.
**May contain tartrazine.   *Common* reactions are in italics; *life-threatening*, in bold italics.

always be administered with other antitubercular agents to prevent the development of resistant organisms.

• Give deep I.M. to minimize local reactions. Apply ice to injection site p.r.n. for pain. Know that drug is never given I.V. because this route may cause neuromuscular blockade.

• Evaluate patient's hearing every 1 to 2 weeks after beginning therapy. Notify the doctor if the patient complains of tinnitus, vertigo, or hearing impairment.

• Monitor renal function during therapy; notify the doctor if function decreases. In renal impairment, dosage must be reduced.

• Be aware that straw- or dark-colored solution after reconstitution does not indicate a loss in potency. Do not administer solutions that contain a precipitate.

---

clofazimine
Lamprene

Pregnancy Risk Category: C

HOW SUPPLIED
Capsules: 50 mg, 100 mg

ACTION
Unknown. Thought to inhibit mycobacterial growth by binding preferentially to mycobacterial DNA. Also has anti-inflammatory effects that suppress skin reactions of erythema nodosum leprosum.

ONSET, PEAK, DURATION
Onset and duration unknown. With chronic therapy, time to peak concentration is 1 to 6 hours.

INDICATIONS & DOSAGE
Dapsone-resistant leprosy (Hansen's disease) –
Adults: 100 mg P.O. daily in combination with other antileprotics for 3 years. Then, clofazimine *alone,* 100 mg daily.

Erythema nodosum leprosum –
Adults: 100 to 200 mg P.O. daily for up to 3 months. Dosage is tapered to 100 mg daily as soon as possible. Dosages above 200 mg daily are not recommended.

ADVERSE REACTIONS
EENT: conjunctival and corneal pigmentation.
GI: *epigastric pain, diarrhea, nausea, vomiting, GI intolerance, bowel obstruction, GI bleeding.*
Skin: *pink to brownish black pigmentation, ichthyosis and dryness,* rash, itching.
Other: *splenic infarction,* discolored body fluids and excrement.

INTERACTIONS
Dapsone: impaired anti-inflammatory effects of clofazimine; no intervention appears necessary.
Isoniazid: may decrease skin levels and increase serum and urine levels of clofazimine. Monitor for decreased effectiveness.
Rifampin: decreased rifampin bioavailability. Monitor for decreased effectiveness.

CONTRAINDICATIONS
None known.

NURSING CONSIDERATIONS
• Use cautiously in patients with GI dysfunction, such as abdominal pain and diarrhea.
• Be aware that doses that exceed 100 mg daily should be given for as short a period as possible and only under close medical supervision.
• If the patient complains of colic, burning abdominal pain, or any other GI symptom, report this to the doctor, who may reduce the dose or increase the interval between doses.
• Advise the patient to take the drug with meals or milk.
• Warn the patient that clofazimine may discolor skin, body fluids, and

---

excrement. The color ranges from red to brownish black. Reassure the patient that the unsightly skin discoloration is reversible but may not disappear until several months or years after drug treatment ends.
• Recommend application of skin oil or cream to help reverse skin dryness or ichthyosis.

cycloserine
Seromycin

Pregnancy Risk Category: C

HOW SUPPLIED
Capsules: 250 mg

ACTION
Inhibits cell-wall biosynthesis by interfering with the bacterial use of amino acids (bacteriostatic).

ONSET, PEAK, DURATION
Onset and duration unknown. Serum levels peak 3 to 4 hours after oral dose.

INDICATIONS & DOSAGE
Adjunctive treatment in pulmonary or extrapulmonary tuberculosis –
Adults: initially, 250 mg P.O. q 12 hours for 2 weeks; then, if blood levels are below 25 to 30 mcg/ml and no toxicity has developed, dose is increased to 250 mg q 8 hours for 2 weeks. If optimum blood levels are still not achieved, and no toxicity has developed, then dose is increased to 250 mg q 6 hours. Maximum dosage is 1 g/day. If CNS toxicity occurs, drug is discontinued for 1 week, then resumed at 250 mg daily for 2 weeks. If no serious toxic effects occur, dosage is increased by 250-mg increments q 10 days until blood level of 25 to 30 mcg/ml is obtained.

ADVERSE REACTIONS
CNS: *seizures,* drowsiness, headache, tremor, dysarthria, vertigo, confu-

sion, loss of memory, ***possible suicidal tendencies*** and other psychotic symptoms, *nervousness, hallucinations, depression,* hyperirritability, paresthesia, paresis, hyperreflexia.
Other: hypersensitivity reactions (allergic dermatitis).

INTERACTIONS
Ethanol or ethionamide: increased risk of CNS toxicity (seizures).
Isoniazid: monitor for CNS toxicity (dizziness or drowsiness).

CONTRAINDICATIONS
Contraindicated in patients with hypersensitivity to the drug and in those with seizure disorders, depression or severe anxiety, psychosis, severe renal insufficiency, or excessive concurrent use of alcohol.

NURSING CONSIDERATIONS
• Use cautiously in patients with impaired renal function; reduced dosage is required.
• Obtain specimen for culture and sensitivity tests before therapy begins and periodically thereafter to detect possible resistance.
• Know that cycloserine is considered a "second-line" drug in the treatment of tuberculosis and should always be administered with other antitubercular agents to prevent the development of resistant organisms.
• Monitor serum cycloserine levels periodically as ordered, especially in patients receiving high doses (more than 500 mg daily) because toxic reactions may occur with blood levels above 30 mcg/ml.
• Monitor results of hematologic tests and renal and liver function studies.
• Observe for psychotic symptoms, hallucinations, and possible suicidal tendencies.
• Administer pyridoxine, anticonvulsants, tranquilizers, or sedatives, as ordered, to relieve adverse reactions.
• Warn the patient to avoid alcohol,

---

*Liquid form contains alcohol.
May contain tartrazine.   *Common* reactions are in italics; ***life-threatening,* in bold italics.

which may cause serious neurologic reactions.

---

dapsone
Avlosulfon†, Dapsone 100‡

Pregnancy Risk Category: C

HOW SUPPLIED
Tablets: 25 mg, 100 mg

ACTION
Unknown. May inhibit folic acid biosynthesis in susceptible organisms (bacteriostatic).

ONSET, PEAK, DURATION
Onset and duration unknown. Plasma levels peak 4 to 8 hours after oral dose.

INDICATIONS & DOSAGE
All forms of leprosy (Hansen's disease) –
Adults: 100 mg P.O. daily, indefinitely; give with rifampin 600 mg daily for 6 months.
Children: 1.4 mg/kg P.O. daily.
Dermatitis herpetiformis –
Adults: 50 mg P.O. daily; increased to 300 mg daily as needed.

ADVERSE REACTIONS
CNS: insomnia, psychosis, headache, dizziness, lethargy, severe malaise, paresthesia, peripheral neuropathy (with loss of motor function).
EENT: tinnitus, allergic rhinitis.
GI: anorexia, abdominal pain, nausea, vomiting.
Hematologic: *aplastic anemia, agranulocytosis, hemolytic anemia,* methemoglobinemia, possible leukopenia.
Hepatic: hepatitis, cholestatic jaundice.
Skin: allergic dermatitis (generalized or fixed maculopapular rash).

INTERACTIONS
Folic acid antagonists, such as methotrexate: increased risk of adverse hematologic reactions. Avoid concomitant use.
Rifampin: increased hepatic metabolism of dapsone. Monitor for lack of efficacy.

CONTRAINDICATIONS
Contraindicated in patients with hypersensitivity to the drug.

NURSING CONSIDERATIONS
• Use cautiously in patients with chronic renal, hepatic, or CV disease; refractory types of anemia; and G6PD deficiency.
• Obtain CBC before therapy to establish a baseline value, as ordered.
• Monitor CBC weekly for the first month, monthly for 6 months, and semiannually thereafter.
• Be prepared to reduce or temporarily discontinue if hemoglobin falls below 9 g/dl; if WBC count falls below 5,000/mm³; or if RBC count falls below 2.5 million/mm³ or remains low.
• If generalized, diffuse dermatitis occurs, notify doctor and prepare to interrupt therapy regimen.
• Administer antihistamines as ordered to combat dapsone-induced allergic dermatitis.
• Monitor for signs and symptoms of erythema nodosum reaction, which may occur during therapy as a result of *Mycobacterium leprae* bacilli (malaise, fever, painful inflammatory induration in the skin and mucosa, iritis, and neuritis). In severe cases, therapy should be stopped and glucocorticoids given cautiously.
• Instruct breast-feeding patients to report cyanosis in infants, which indicates high sulfone level.

---

†Available in Canada only.   ‡Available in Australia only.   ◊Available OTC.

ethambutol hydrochloride
Etibi†, Myambutol

Pregnancy Risk Category: NR

HOW SUPPLIED
Tablets: 100 mg, 400 mg

ACTION
Unknown. Appears to interfere with the synthesis of one or more metabolites of susceptible bacteria, altering cellular metabolism during cell division (bacteriostatic).

ONSET, PEAK, DURATION
Onset and duration unknown. Plasma levels peak within 2 to 4 hours of oral dose.

INDICATIONS & DOSAGE
Adjunctive treatment in pulmonary tuberculosis –
Adults and children over 13 years: for patients who have not received previous antitubercular therapy, 15 mg/kg P.O. daily in a single dose.
Re-treatment: 25 mg/kg P.O. daily as a single dose for 60 days with at least one other antitubercular drug; then decreased to 15 mg/kg/day as a single dose.

ADVERSE REACTIONS
CNS: headache, dizziness, mental confusion, possible hallucinations, peripheral neuritis (numbness and tingling of extremities).
EENT: optic neuritis (vision loss and loss of color discrimination, especially red and green).
GI: anorexia, nausea, vomiting, abdominal pain.
Other: *anaphylactoid reactions,* fever, malaise, bloody sputum, *elevated uric acid level.*

INTERACTIONS
Aluminum salts: may delay and reduce absorption of ethambutol. Separate administration times by several hours.

CONTRAINDICATIONS
Contraindicated in patients with hypersensitivity to the drug, in those with optic neuritis, and in children under 13 years.

NURSING CONSIDERATIONS
• Use cautiously in patients with impaired renal function, cataracts, recurrent eye inflammations, gout, and diabetic retinopathy.
• Perform visual acuity and color discrimination tests and obtain AST and ALT levels, as ordered, before therapy.
• Anticipate dosage reduction in patients with impaired renal function.
• Know that ethambutol should always be administered with other antitubercular agents to prevent the development of resistant organisms.
• Monitor AST and ALT levels every 2 to 4 weeks, as ordered, and perform visual acuity and color discrimination tests during treatment.
• Monitor serum uric acid level as ordered; observe the patient for symptoms of gout.
• Reassure the patient that visual disturbances will disappear several weeks to months after drug is stopped.

ethionamide
Trecator-SC

Pregnancy Risk Category: NR

HOW SUPPLIED
Tablets: 250 mg

ACTION
Unknown. Probably inhibits peptide synthesis.

ONSET, PEAK, DURATION
Onset and duration unknown. Plasma levels peak in approximately 1.8 hours.

INDICATIONS & DOSAGE
Adjunctive treatment in pulmonary or extrapulmonary tuberculosis (when primary therapy with streptomycin or isoniazid cannot be used or has failed) –
Adults: 500 mg to 1 g P.O. daily in divided doses. Concomitant administration of other antitubercular drugs and pyridoxine recommended.
Children: 15 to 20 mg/kg P.O. daily in three to four doses. Maximum dosage is 1 g daily.

ADVERSE REACTIONS
CNS: asthenia, drowsiness, *peripheral neuritis,* psychic disturbances (especially mental depression).
CV: postural hypotension.
GI: *anorexia,* metallic taste, nausea, vomiting, sialorrhea, *epigastric distress,* diarrhea, stomatitis, weight loss.
Hematologic: thrombocytopenia.
Hepatic: jaundice, hepatitis, elevated AST and ALT.
Skin: rash, *exfoliative dermatitis.*

INTERACTIONS
None significant.

CONTRAINDICATIONS
Contraindicated in patients with hypersensitivity to the drug or severe liver damage.

NURSING CONSIDERATIONS
• Use cautiously in patients with diabetes mellitus.
• Obtain culture and sensitivity tests, as ordered, before starting therapy.
• Remember that ethionamide should always be administered with other antitubercular agents to prevent the development of resistant organisms.
• Give with meals or antacids to min-

imize GI effects. The patient may require an antiemetic.
• Monitor hepatic function every 2 to 4 weeks.
• If skin rash occurs, withhold drug and notify doctor; condition may progress to exfoliative dermatitis.
• Be aware that pyridoxine may be ordered to prevent neuropathy.
• Instruct the patient to take this drug exactly as prescribed; warn against discontinuing drug without the doctor's consent.
• Warn against excess alcohol ingestion, which may make the patient more vulnerable to liver damage.

isoniazid (isonicotinic acid hydride, INH)
Isotamine†, Laniazid, Nydrazid**, PMS-Isoniazid†, Tubizid
Pregnancy Risk Category: NR

HOW SUPPLIED
Tablets: 50 mg, 100 mg, 300 mg
Oral solution: 50 mg/5 ml
Injection: 100 mg/ml

ACTION
Unknown. Appears to inhibit cell-wall biosynthesis by interfering with lipid and DNA synthesis (bactericidal).

ONSET, PEAK, DURATION
Onset and duration unknown. Plasma levels peak within 1 to 2 hours of oral or I.M. administration.

INDICATIONS & DOSAGE
Actively growing tubercle bacilli –
Adults: 5 mg/kg P.O. or I.M. daily in a single dose, up to 300 mg/day, continued for 6 months to 2 years.
Infants and children: 10 to 20 mg/kg P.O. or I.M. daily in a single dose, up to 300 to 500 mg/day, continued long enough to prevent relapse. Concomitant administration of at least one other antitubercular drug is recommended.

Prevention of tubercle bacilli in those closely exposed to tuberculosis or those with positive skin test whose chest X-rays and bacteriologic studies are consistent with nonprogressive tuberculosis –

Adults: 300 mg P.O. daily in a single dose, continued for 6 months to 1 year.

Infants and children: 10 mg/kg P.O. daily in a single dose, up to 300 mg/day, continued for 1 year.

ADVERSE REACTIONS

CNS: *peripheral neuropathy* (especially in patients who are malnourished, alcoholic, diabetic, or slow acetylators), usually preceded by paresthesia of hands and feet; psychosis.

GI: nausea, vomiting, epigastric distress, constipation, mouth dryness.

Hematologic: *agranulocytosis, hemolytic anemia, aplastic anemia,* eosinophilia, leukopenia, neutropenia, thrombocytopenia, methemoglobinemia, pyridoxine-responsive hypochromic anemia.

Hepatic: hepatitis, occasionally severe and sometimes fatal, especially in elderly patients.

Other: rheumatic syndrome and lupuslike syndrome, hypersensitivity reactions (fever, rash, lymphadenopathy, vasculitis), hyperglycemia, metabolic acidosis, irritation at I.M. injection site.

INTERACTIONS

Aluminum-containing antacids and laxatives: may decrease the rate and amount of isoniazid absorbed. Give isoniazid at least 1 hour before antacid or laxative.

Carbamazepine: increased risk of isoniazid hepatotoxicity. Use together cautiously.

Corticosteroids: may decrease therapeutic effectiveness of isoniazid. Monitor need for larger isoniazid dose.

Disulfiram: may cause neurologic symptoms, including changes in behavior and coordination. Avoid concomitant use.

Ethanol: may be associated with increased incidence of isoniazid-related hepatitis. Avoid concomitant use.

Phenytoin, carbamazepine: increased plasma levels of these anticonvulsants. Monitor closely.

CONTRAINDICATIONS

Contraindicated in patients with acute hepatic disease or isoniazid-associated liver damage.

NURSING CONSIDERATIONS

• Use cautiously in patients with chronic non-isoniazid-associated liver disease, seizure disorders (especially in those taking phenytoin), severe renal impairment, and chronic alcoholism and in elderly patients.

• Be aware that isoniazid should always be administered with other antitubercular agents to prevent the development of resistant organisms.

• Keep in mind that isoniazid pharmacokinetics may vary among patients because its metabolism occurs in the liver by genetically controlled acetylation. Fast acetylators metabolize the drug up to five times as fast as slow acetylators. About 50% of blacks and whites are slow acetylators; over 80% of Chinese, Japanese, and Eskimos are fast acetylators.

• Monitor hepatic function closely for changes.

• Administer pyridoxine, as ordered, to prevent peripheral neuropathy, especially in malnourished patients.

• Instruct the patient to take this drug exactly as prescribed; warn against discontinuing drug without the doctor's consent.

• Advise the patient to take with food if GI irritation occurs.

• Tell the patient to notify the doctor immediately if symptoms of liver impairment occur (loss of appetite, fatigue, malaise, jaundice, dark urine).

---

*Liquid form contains alcohol.
**May contain tartrazine.

Common reactions are in italics; *life-threatening,* in bold italics.

• Advise the patient to avoid alcoholic beverages while taking this drug.

• Encourage the patient to fully comply with treatment, which may take months or years.

pyrazinamide
PMS Pyrazinamide†, Tebrazid†, Zinamide‡

Pregnancy Risk Category: C

HOW SUPPLIED
Tablets: 500 mg

ACTION
Unknown.

ONSET, PEAK, DURATION
Onset and duration unknown. Serum levels peak in 1 to 2 hours.

INDICATIONS & DOSAGE
Adjunctive treatment of tuberculosis (when primary and secondary antitubercular drugs cannot be used or have failed)—
Adults: 15 to 30 mg/kg P.O. once daily. Maximum dosage is 2 g daily.

ADVERSE REACTIONS
GI: anorexia, nausea, vomiting, diarrhea.
GU: dysuria.
Hematologic: sideroblastic anemia, possible bleeding tendency due to thrombocytopenia.
Other: malaise, fever, arthralgia, hepatitis, interference with control in diabetes mellitus, *hyperuricemia.*

INTERACTIONS
None significant.

CONTRAINDICATIONS
Contraindicated in patients with hypersensitivity to the drug or severe hepatic disease.

NURSING CONSIDERATIONS
• Use cautiously in patients with diabetes mellitus, renal failure, or gout.

• Be aware that pyrazinamide should always be administered with other antitubercular agents to prevent the development of resistant organisms.

• Keep in mind that a reduced dosage is needed in patients with renal impairment because nearly 100% of the drug is excreted in urine.

• Question doses that exceed 35 mg/kg because they may cause liver damage.

• Monitor hematopoietic studies and serum uric acid levels, as ordered.

• Monitor liver function studies; examine for jaundice and liver tenderness or enlargement before and frequently during therapy.

• Watch closely for signs of gout and of liver impairment (loss of appetite, fatigue, malaise, jaundice, dark urine, and liver tenderness). Notify the doctor at once.

• When used with surgical management of tuberculosis, pyrazinamide is started 1 to 2 weeks before surgery and continued for 4 to 6 weeks postoperatively.

• Be aware that patients with concomitant HIV infections may require longer courses of therapy.

rifampin (rifampicin)
Rifadin, Rifadin IV, Rimactane, Rimycin‡, Rofact†

Pregnancy Risk Category: C

HOW SUPPLIED
Capsules: 150 mg, 300 mg
Injection: 600 mg

ACTION
Inhibits DNA-dependent RNA polymerase, thus impairing RNA synthesis (bactericidal).

ONSET, PEAK, DURATION
Onset and duration unknown. Serum levels peak 2 to 4 hours after oral dose.

INDICATIONS & DOSAGE
Pulmonary tuberculosis –
Adults: 600 mg P.O. or I.V. daily in single dose 1 hour before or 2 hours after meals.
Children over 5 years: 10 to 20 mg/ kg P.O. or I.V. daily in single dose 1 hour before or 2 hours after meals. Maximum dosage is 600 mg daily. Concomitant administration with other antitubercular agents is recommended.
Meningococcal carriers –
Adults: 600 mg P.O. or I.V. b.i.d. for 2 days, or 600 mg P.O. or I.V. once daily for 4 days.
Children 1 month to 12 years: 10 mg/kg P.O. or I.V. b.i.d. for 2 days, not to exceed 600 mg/day, or 10 to 20 mg/kg once daily for 4 days.
Neonates: 5 mg/kg P.O. or I.V. b.i.d. for 2 days.
Prophylaxis of Haemophilus influenzae type b –
Adults and children: 20 mg/kg P.O. daily for 4 days, not to exceed 600 mg/day.

ADVERSE REACTIONS
CNS: headache, fatigue, *drowsiness,* ataxia, dizziness, mental confusion, generalized numbness.
GI: epigastric distress, anorexia, nausea, vomiting, abdominal pain, diarrhea, flatulence, sore mouth and tongue.
Hematologic: eosinophilia, thrombocytopenia, transient leukopenia, *hemolytic anemia.*
Hepatic: *serious hepatotoxicity* as well as *transient abnormalities in liver function tests.*
Skin: pruritus, urticaria, rash.
Other: flulike syndrome, discoloration of body fluids, hyperuricemia.

INTERACTIONS
Anticoagulants, corticosteroids, cyclosporine, digitalis glycosides, quinidine, oral contraceptives, sulfonylureas, dapsone, narcotics, analgesics, methadone, barbiturates, diazepam, verapamil, beta-adrenergic blockers, clofibrate, progestins, disopyramide, mexiletine, theophylline, chloramphenicol, and anticonvulsants: reduced effectiveness of these drugs. Monitor closely.
Ethanol: may increase risk of hepatotoxicity. Avoid use.
Ketoconazole, para-aminosalicylate sodium: may interfere with absorption of rifampin. Give these drugs 8 to 12 hours apart.
Probenecid: may increase rifampin levels. Use cautiously.

CONTRAINDICATIONS
Contraindicated in patients with hypersensitivity to the drug.

NURSING CONSIDERATIONS
• Use cautiously in patients with liver disease.
• Be aware that concomitant treatment with at least one other antitubercular agent is recommended.
• Give 1 hour before or 2 hours after meals for optimal absorption; however, if GI irritation occurs, the patient may take rifampin with meals.
• **I.V. use:** Reconstitute vial with 10 ml of sterile water for injection to make a solution containing 60 mg/ml. Add to 100 ml of D_5W and infuse over 30 minutes, or add to 500 ml of D_5W and infuse over 3 hours. When dextrose is contraindicated, drug may be diluted with 0.9% sodium chloride injection. Do not use other I.V. solutions.
• Monitor hepatic function, hematopoietic studies, and serum uric acid levels, as ordered.
• Watch closely for signs of hepatic impairment. Notify the doctor if present.

---

*Liquid form contains alcohol.   *Common* reactions are in italics; *life-threatening,* in bold italics.
**May contain tartrazine.

- May cause hemorrhage in neonates of rifampin-treated mothers.
- Warn the patient about drowsiness and possible red-orange discoloration of urine, feces, saliva, sweat, sputum, and tears. Soft contact lenses may be permanently stained.
- Advise the patient to avoid alcoholic beverages while taking this drug.

11

Aminoglycosides

amikacin sulfate
gentamicin sulfate
kanamycin sulfate
neomycin sulfate
netilmicin sulfate
streptomycin sulfate
tobramycin sulfate

COMBINATION PRODUCTS
NEOSPORIN G.U. IRRIGANT: 40 mg
neomycin sulfate and 200,000 units
polymyxin B sulfate/ml.

---

amikacin sulfate
Amikin

Pregnancy Risk Category: D

HOW SUPPLIED
Injection: 50 mg/ml, 250 mg/ml

ACTION
Inhibits protein synthesis by binding
directly to the 30S ribosomal subunit.
Generally bactericidal.

ONSET, PEAK, DURATION
Onset immediate after I.V. infusion;
unknown after I.M. injection. Peak
serum levels occur immediately after
I.V. infusion, 1 hour after I.M. injection. Measurable serum levels persist
for 8 to 12 hours.

INDICATIONS & DOSAGE
*Serious infections caused by sensitive
strains of* Pseudomonas aeruginosa,
Escherichia coli, Proteus, Klebsiella,
Serratia, Enterobacter, Acinetobacter, Providencia, Citrobacter, Staphylococcus; *meningitis* –
Adults and children: 15 mg/kg/day
divided q 8 to 12 hours I.M. or I.V.
infusion (in 100 to 200 ml of D_5W or
0.9% NaCl run in over 30 to 60 minutes).

Neonates: initially, loading dose of
10 mg/kg I.V., followed by 7.5 mg/kg
q 12 hours.
*Uncomplicated urinary tract infec-
tions* –
Adults: 250 mg I.M. or I.V. b.i.d.
In impaired renal function –
Adults: initially, 7.5 mg/kg. Subsequent doses and frequency determined by blood amikacin levels and
renal function studies.

ADVERSE REACTIONS
CNS: headache, lethargy, ***neuromuscular blockade.***
EENT: *ototoxicity (tinnitus, vertigo,
hearing loss).*
GU: *nephrotoxicity (cells or casts in
urine, oliguria, proteinuria, decreased creatinine clearance, increased BUN and serum creatinine
levels).*
Other: hypersensitivity reactions
(anaphylaxis), hepatic necrosis.

INTERACTIONS
Cephalothin: increased nephrotoxicity. Use together cautiously.
Dimenhydrinate: may mask symptoms of ototoxicity. Use with caution.
*General anesthetics, neuromuscular
blocking agents:* may potentiate neuromuscular blockade.
Indomethacin: may increase serum
trough and peak levels of amikacin.
Monitor serum amikacin levels
closely.
*I.V. loop diuretics (such as furose-
mide):* increased ototoxicity. Use cautiously.
*Other aminoglycosides, acyclovir,
amphotericin B, cisplatin, methoxyflurane, vancomycin:* increased nephrotoxicity. Use together cautiously.
Parenteral penicillins (such as ticar-

---

*Liquid form contains alcohol.
**May contain tartrazine.

Common reactions are in italics; **life-threatening,** in bold italics.

cillin): amikacin inactivation in vitro. Don't mix together.

CONTRAINDICATIONS
Contraindicated in patients with hypersensitivity to the drug or other aminoglycosides.

NURSING CONSIDERATIONS
• Use cautiously in patients with impaired renal function or neuromuscular disorders, in neonates and infants, and in elderly patients.
• Obtain specimen for culture and sensitivity tests before first dose. Therapy may begin pending results.
• Evaluate patient's hearing before beginning therapy.
• Weigh the patient and review baseline renal function studies before therapy begins.
• **I.V. use:** After I.V. infusion, flush line with 0.9% sodium chloride solution or D₅W.
• Obtain blood for peak amikacin level 1 hour after I.M. injection and 30 minutes to 1 hour after infusion ends; for trough levels, draw blood just before next dose. Don't collect blood in a heparinized tube because heparin is incompatible with aminoglycosides.
• Be aware that peak blood levels that are above 35 mcg/ml and trough levels that are above 10 mcg/ml may be associated with a higher incidence of toxicity.
• Monitor renal function (output, specific gravity, urinalysis, BUN and creatinine levels, and creatinine clearance). Notify the doctor of signs of decreasing renal function.
• Evaluate the patient's hearing during therapy. Notify the doctor if the patient complains of tinnitus, vertigo, or hearing loss.
• Encourage adequate fluid intake; patient should be well hydrated while taking drug to minimize chemical irritation of the renal tubules.
• Watch for superinfection (continued

fever and other signs of new infections, especially of upper respiratory tract).
• Keep in mind that therapy is usually continued for 7 to 10 days.
• Know that if no response occurs after 3 to 5 days, therapy may be stopped and new specimens obtained for culture and sensitivity testing.
• Be aware that potency of drug is not affected if solution turns light yellow.

---

gentamicin sulfate
Cidomycin†‡, Garamycin, Gentamicin Sulfate ADD-Vantage, Jenamicin

Pregnancy Risk Category: NR

HOW SUPPLIED
Injection: 40 mg/ml (adult), 10 mg/ml (pediatric), 2 mg/ml (intrathecal)
I.V. infusion (premixed): 40 mg, 60 mg, 70 mg, 80 mg, 90 mg, 100 mg, available in 0.9% sodium chloride solution

ACTION
Inhibits protein synthesis by binding directly to the 30S ribosomal subunit. Usually bactericidal.

ONSET, PEAK, DURATION
Onset immediate after I.V. administration, unknown after I.M. administration. Peak serum levels occur in 30 to 90 minutes. Duration unknown.

INDICATIONS & DOSAGE
Serious infections caused by sensitive strains of Pseudomonas aeruginosa, Escherichia coli, Proteus, Klebsiella, Serratia, Enterobacter, Citrobacter, Staphylococcus —
Adults: 3 mg/kg daily in divided doses I.M. or I.V. infusion q 8 hours (in 50 to 200 ml of 0.9% sodium chloride solution or D₅W infused over 30 minutes to 2 hours). For life-threatening infections, the patient may receive

up to 5 mg/kg daily in three to four divided doses.
Children: 2 to 2.5 mg/kg q 8 hours I.M. or by I.V. infusion.
Neonates over 1 week or infants: 7.5 mg/kg daily in divided doses q 8 hours.
Neonates under 1 week and preterm infants: 2.5 mg/kg I.V. q 12 hours.
Meningitis –
Adults: systemic therapy as above; 4 to 8 mg intrathecally daily also may be used.
Children and infants over 3 months: systemic therapy as above; 1 to 2 mg intrathecally daily may also be used.
Endocarditis prophylaxis for GI or GU procedure or surgery –
Adults: 1.5 mg/kg I.M. or I.V. 30 minutes before procedure or surgery. Maximum dosage is 80 mg. Given with ampicillin (vancomycin in penicillin-allergic patients). Repeated in 8 hours.
Children: 2 mg/kg I.M. or I.V. 30 minutes before procedure or surgery. Maximum dosage is 80 mg. Given with ampicillin (vancomycin in penicillin-allergic patients). After 8 hours, half the initial dose is given.
Posthemodialysis to maintain therapeutic blood levels –
Adults: 1 to 1.7 mg/kg I.M. or by I.V. infusion after each dialysis.
Children: 2 to 2.5 mg/kg I.M. or by I.V. infusion after each dialysis.

ADVERSE REACTIONS
CNS: headache, lethargy, ***neuromuscular blockade***.
EENT: *ototoxicity (tinnitus, vertigo, hearing loss).*
GU: *nephrotoxicity (cells or casts in the urine; oliguria; proteinuria; decreased creatinine clearance; increased BUN, nonprotein nitrogen, and serum creatinine levels).*
Other: hypersensitivity reactions.

INTERACTIONS
Cephalothin: increased nephrotoxicity. Use together cautiously.
Dimenhydrinate: may mask symptoms of ototoxicity. Use with caution.
General anesthetics, neuromuscular blockers: may potentiate neuromuscular blockade.
Indomethacin: may increase serum peak and trough levels of gentamicin. Monitor serum gentamicin levels closely.
I.V. loop diuretics (such as furosemide): increased ototoxicity. Use cautiously.
Other aminoglycosides, amphotericin B, acyclovir, cisplatin, methoxyflurane, vancomycin: increased ototoxicity and nephrotoxicity. Use together cautiously.
Parenteral penicillins (such as ampicillin and ticarcillin): gentamicin inactivation in vitro. Don't mix together.

CONTRAINDICATIONS
Contraindicated in patients with hypersensitivity to the drug or other aminoglycosides.

NURSING CONSIDERATIONS
• Use cautiously in neonates, infants, elderly patients, and patients with impaired renal function or neuromuscular disorders.
• Obtain specimen for culture and sensitivity tests before giving first dose.
• Evaluate patient's hearing before beginning therapy.
• Weigh the patient and review baseline renal function studies before therapy begins.
• **I.V. use:** When giving by intermittent I.V. infusion, dilute with 50 to 200 ml of D_5W or 0.9% sodium chloride injection and infuse over 30 minutes to 2 hours. After completing I.V. infusion, flush the line with 0.9% sodium chloride solution or D_5W.
• Use preservative-free formulations

---

*Liquid form contains alcohol.
May contain tartrazine.   *Common* reactions are in italics; ***life-threatening*, in bold italics.

of gentamicin when intrathecal route is ordered.

• Obtain blood for peak gentamicin level 1 hour after I.M. injection and 30 minutes to 1 hour after I.V. infusion; for trough levels, draw blood just before next dose. Don't collect blood in a heparinized tube because heparin is incompatible with aminoglycosides.

• Be aware that peak blood levels above 12 mcg/ml and trough levels above 2 mcg/ml may be associated with higher incidence of toxicity.

• Monitor renal function (output, specific gravity, urinalysis, BUN and creatinine levels, and creatinine clearance). Notify the doctor of signs of decreasing renal function.

• Evaluate the patient's hearing during therapy. Notify the doctor if the patient complains of tinnitus, vertigo, or hearing loss.

• Know that hemodialysis (8 hours) removes up to 50% of drug from blood.

• Watch for superinfection (continued fever and other signs of new infections, especially of upper respiratory tract).

• Know that therapy usually continues for 7 to 10 days. If no response occurs in 3 to 5 days, therapy may be stopped and new specimens obtained for culture and sensitivity testing.

• Encourage adequate fluid intake; patient should be well hydrated while taking drug to minimize chemical irritation of the renal tubules.

---

kanamycin sulfate
Kanasig‡, Kantrex
Pregnancy Risk Category: D

HOW SUPPLIED
Capsules: 500 mg
Injection: 37.5 mg/ml (pediatric), 250 mg/ml, 333 mg/ml

ACTION
Inhibits protein synthesis by binding directly to the 30S ribosomal subunit. Generally bactericidal.

ONSET, PEAK, DURATION
Onset immediate after I.V. infusion, unknown after I.M. or oral administration. Peak serum levels occur immediately after I.V. infusion, 1 hour after I.M. injection. Measurable serum levels persist for 8 to 12 hours.

INDICATIONS & DOSAGE
Serious infections caused by sensitive strains of Escherichia coli, Proteus, Enterobacter aerogenes, Klebsiella pneumoniae, Serratia marcescens, Acinetobacter—
Adults and children with normal renal function: 15 mg/kg/day divided q 8 to 12 hours I.M. or I.V. Maximum daily dosage is 1.5 g.
Neonates: 15 mg/kg/day divided q 12 hours I.M. or I.V..
Adjunctive treatment in hepatic coma—
Adults: 8 to 12 g P.O. daily in divided doses.
Preoperative bowel sterilization—
Adults: 1 g P.O. q 1 hour for four doses, then q 4 hours for four doses; or 1 g P.O. q 1 hour for four doses, then q 6 hours for 36 to 72 hours.
Intraperitoneal irrigation—
500 mg in 20 ml sterile distilled water instilled via catheter into wound after patient has recovered from anesthesia and neuromuscular blocker effects.
Wound irrigation—
Up to 2.5 mg/ml in 0.9% sodium chloride solution.
Inhalation—
250 mg diluted with 3 ml of 0.9% sodium chloride solution and nebulized two to four times per day.

ADVERSE REACTIONS
CNS: headache, lethargy, *neuromuscular blockade.*

EENT: *ototoxicity (tinnitus, vertigo, hearing loss).*
GU: *nephrotoxicity (cells or casts in the urine, oliguria, proteinuria, decreased creatinine clearance, increased BUN and serum creatinine levels).*
Other: hypersensitivity reactions *(anaphylaxis).*

INTERACTIONS
Cephalothin: increased nephrotoxicity. Use together cautiously.
Dimenhydrinate: may mask symptoms of ototoxicity. Use with caution.
General anesthetics, neuromuscular blocking agents: may potentiate neuromuscular blockade.
I.V. loop diuretics (such as furosemide): increased ototoxicity. Use cautiously.
Other aminoglycosides, acyclovir, amphotericin B, cisplatin, methoxyflurane, vancomycin: increased nephrotoxicity. Don't use together.
Parenteral penicillins (such as ticarcillin): kanamycin inactivation in vitro. Don't mix together.

CONTRAINDICATIONS
Contraindicated for oral use in patients with intestinal obstruction and in treatment of systemic infection. Also contraindicated in patients with hypersensitivity to the drug or other aminoglycosides.

NURSING CONSIDERATIONS
• Use cautiously in patients with impaired renal function or neuromuscular disorders and in elderly patients.
• Obtain specimen for culture and sensitivity tests before first dose. Therapy may begin pending results.
• Evaluate patient's hearing before beginning therapy.
• Weigh the patient and review baseline renal function studies before therapy.
• **I.V. use:** Dilute 500 mg of the drug per 200 ml of 0.9% sodium chloride

solution or D₅W and infuse over 30 to 60 minutes.
• For I.M. administration, inject deeply into upper outer quadrant of buttocks. Rotate injection sites.
• Obtain peak and trough levels as ordered. Be aware that peak blood levels over 30 mcg/ml and trough levels over 10 mcg/ml may be associated with increased incidence of toxicity.
• Monitor renal function (output, specific gravity, urinalysis, BUN and creatinine levels, and creatinine clearance). Notify the doctor of signs of decreasing renal function.
• Evaluate the patient's hearing during therapy. Notify the doctor if the patient complains of tinnitus, vertigo, or hearing loss.
• Encourage adequate fluid intake; patient should be well hydrated while taking drug to minimize chemical irritation of the renal tubules.
• Watch for superinfection (continued fever and other signs of new infection, especially of upper respiratory tract).
• Know that if no response occurs in 3 to 5 days, therapy may be stopped and new specimens obtained for culture and sensitivity testing.

---

neomycin sulfate
Mycifradin, Neo-fradin, Neosulf‡, Neo-Tabs

Pregnancy Risk Category: NR

HOW SUPPLIED
Tablets: 500 mg
Oral solution: 125 mg/5 ml

ACTION
Inhibits protein synthesis by binding directly to the 30S ribosomal subunit. Generally bactericidal.

ONSET, PEAK, DURATION
Onset unknown. Peak plasma levels occur in 1 to 4 hours. The drug is usually detectable in plasma for about 8 hours.

INDICATIONS & DOSAGE

Infectious diarrhea caused by enteropathogenic Escherichia coli —
Adults: 50 mg/kg daily P.O. in four divided doses for 2 to 3 days.
Children: 50 to 100 mg/kg daily P.O. divided q 4 to 6 hours for 2 to 3 days.
Suppression of intestinal bacteria preoperatively —
Adults: 1 g P.O. q 1 hour for four doses, then 1 g q 4 hours for the balance of the 24 hours. A saline cathartic should precede therapy.
Children: 40 to 100 mg/kg daily P.O. divided q 4 to 6 hours. First dose should follow saline cathartic.
Adjunctive treatment in hepatic coma —
Adults: 1 to 3 g P.O. q.i.d. for 5 to 6 days; or 200 ml of 1% solution or 100 ml of 2% solution as enema retained for 20 to 60 minutes q 6 hours.

ADVERSE REACTIONS

CNS: headache, lethargy.
EENT: *ototoxicity (tinnitus, vertigo, hearing loss).*
GI: nausea, vomiting.
GU: *nephrotoxicity (cells or casts in the urine, oliguria, proteinuria, decreased creatinine clearance, increased BUN and serum creatinine levels).*
Skin: rash, urticaria.
Other: hypersensitivity reactions *(anaphylaxis).*

INTERACTIONS

Cephalothin: increased nephrotoxicity. Use together cautiously.
Digoxin: decreased digoxin absorption. Monitor closely.
Dimenhydrinate: may mask symptoms of ototoxicity. Use with caution.
I.V. loop diuretics (such as furosemide): increased ototoxicity. Use cautiously.
Oral anticoagulants: inhibited vitamin K-producing bacteria; may potentiate anticoagulant effect.
Other aminoglycosides, acyclovir, *amphotericin B, cisplatin, methoxyflurane, vancomycin:* increased nephrotoxicity. Use together cautiously.

CONTRAINDICATIONS

Contraindicated in patients with hypersensitivity to other aminoglycosides and in those with intestinal obstruction.

NURSING CONSIDERATIONS

• Use cautiously in patients with impaired renal function, neuromuscular disorders, or ulcerative bowel lesions and in elderly patients. Never administer parenterally.
• Evaluate patient's hearing before beginning therapy.
• Monitor renal function (output, specific gravity, urinalysis, BUN and creatinine levels, and creatinine clearance). Notify the doctor of signs of decreasing renal function.
• Evaluate patient's hearing during prolonged therapy. Notify the doctor if the patient complains of tinnitus, vertigo, or hearing loss. Onset of deafness may occur several weeks after drug is stopped.
• Watch for superinfection (fever or other signs of new infection).
• In adjunctive treatment of hepatic coma, decrease the patient's dietary protein and assess neurologic status frequently during therapy.
• Encourage adequate fluid intake; patient should be well hydrated while taking drug to minimize chemical irritation of the renal tubules.
• For preoperative disinfection, provide a low-residue diet and a cathartic immediately before oral administration of neomycin, as ordered.
• Keep in mind that the ototoxic and nephrotoxic properties of neomycin limit its usefulness.
• Know that neomycin is nonabsorbable at recommended dosage. However, more than 4 g/day may be systemically absorbed and lead to nephrotoxicity.

• Be aware that drug is available in combination with polymyxin B as a urinary bladder irrigant.

netilmicin sulfate
Netromycin

Pregnancy Risk Category: D

HOW SUPPLIED
Injection: 25 mg/ml†, 50 mg/ml†, 100 mg/ml

ACTION
Inhibits protein synthesis by binding directly to the 30S ribosomal subunit. Generally bactericidal.

ONSET, PEAK, DURATION
Onset immediate after I.V. infusion, unknown after I.M. injection. Peak serum levels occur immediately after I.V. infusion, 30 minutes to 1 hour after I.M. injection. Measurable serum levels persist for 8 to 12 hours.

INDICATIONS & DOSAGE
Serious infections caused by sensitive strains of Pseudomonas aeruginosa, Escherichia coli, Proteus, Klebsiella, Serratia, Enterobacter, Citrobacter, Staphylococcus —
Adults and children over age 12: 3 to 6.5 mg/kg/day by I.M. injection or I.V. infusion. May be given q 12 hours to treat serious urinary tract infections and q 8 to 12 hours to treat serious systemic infections.
Infants and children age 6 weeks to 12: 5.5 to 8 mg/kg/day by I.M. injection or I.V. infusion given either as 1.8 to 2.7 mg/kg q 8 hours or as 2.7 to 4 mg/kg q 12 hours.
Neonates under age 6 weeks: 4 to 6.5 mg/kg/day by I.M. injection or I.V. infusion given as 2 to 3.25 mg/kg q 12 hours.
Complicated UTIs —
Adults (normal renal function): 3 to 4 mg/kg/day by I.M. injection or I.V.

infusion divided into two equal doses given q 12 hours.

ADVERSE REACTIONS
CNS: headache, lethargy, *neuromuscular blockade*.
EENT: *ototoxicity (tinnitus, vertigo, hearing loss)*.
GU: *nephrotoxicity (cells or casts in the urine; oliguria; proteinuria; decreased creatinine clearance; increased BUN, nonprotein nitrogen, and serum creatinine levels)*.
Other: hypersensitivity reactions **(anaphylaxis)**.

INTERACTIONS
Cephalothin: increased nephrotoxicity. Use together cautiously.
Dimenhydrinate: may mask symptoms of ototoxicity. Use cautiously.
General anesthetics, neuromuscular blocking agents: may potentiate neuromuscular blockade.
I.V. loop diuretics (such as furosemide): increased ototoxicity. Use cautiously.
Other aminoglycosides, acyclovir, amphotericin B, cisplatin, methoxyflurane, vancomycin: increased nephrotoxicity. Use together cautiously.
Parenteral penicillins (such as ticarcillin): netilmicin inactivation. Don't mix together.

CONTRAINDICATIONS
Contraindicated in patients with hypersensitivity to the drug or other aminoglycosides.

NURSING CONSIDERATIONS
• Use cautiously in patients with impaired renal function or neuromuscular disorders and in neonates, infants, and elderly patients. Commercially available form contains sulfites, which may cause an allergic reaction in certain individuals.
• Obtain specimen for culture and sensitivity tests before first dose. Therapy may begin pending results.

• Weigh the patient and review baseline renal function studies before therapy begins.

• Evaluate the patient's hearing before beginning therapy.

• **I.V. use:** After completing I.V. infusion, flush the line with 0.9% sodium chloride solution or D_5W.

• Obtain blood for peak netilmicin level 1 hour after I.M. injection and 30 minutes to 1 hour after infusion ends; for trough levels, draw blood just before next dose. Don't draw blood in a heparinized tube because heparin is incompatible with aminoglycosides.

• Be aware that blood levels above 16 mcg/ml and trough levels above 4 mcg/ml may be associated with higher incidence of toxicity.

• Monitor renal function (output, specific gravity, urinalysis, BUN and creatinine levels, and creatinine clearance) as ordered. Notify the doctor of signs of decreasing renal function.

• Evaluate the patient's hearing during therapy. Notify the doctor if the patient complains of tinnitus, vertigo, or hearing loss. However, some studies show that this drug is less ototoxic than other aminoglycosides.

• Watch for superinfection (continued fever and other signs of new infections, especially of upper respiratory tract).

• Encourage adequate fluid intake, patient should be well hydrated while taking drug to minimize chemical irritation of the renal tubules.

• Know that therapy usually continues for 7 to 10 days. If no response occurs in 3 to 5 days, therapy may be stopped and new specimens obtained for culture and sensitivity testing.

---

streptomycin sulfate

Pregnancy Risk Category: D

HOW SUPPLIED
Injection: 400 mg/ml, 500 mg/ml, 1-g vial, 5-g vial

ACTION
Inhibits protein synthesis by binding directly to the 30S ribosomal subunit. Generally bactericidal.

ONSET, PEAK, DURATION
Onset and duration unknown. Serum levels peak 1 to 2 hours after I.M. injection.

INDICATIONS & DOSAGE
Streptococcal endocarditis –
Adults: 1 g q 12 hours I.M. for 1 week, then 500 mg q 12 hours for 1 week, given with penicillin. Patients over 60 years should receive 500 mg I.M. q 12 hours for entire 2 weeks.
Primary and adjunctive treatment in tuberculosis –
Adults: 1 g or 15 mg/kg I.M. daily for 2 to 3 months, then 1 g two or three times a week.
Children: 20 to 40 mg/kg I.M. daily in divided doses injected deeply into large muscle mass. Given concurrently with other antitubercular agents, but *not* with capreomycin. Continued until sputum specimen becomes negative.
Enterococcal endocarditis –
Adults: 1 g I.M. q 12 hours for 2 weeks, then 500 mg I.M. q 12 hours for 4 weeks, given with penicillin.
Tularemia –
Adults: 1 to 2 g I.M. daily in divided doses injected deep into upper outer quadrant of buttocks. Continued until patient is afebrile for 5 to 7 days.

ADVERSE REACTIONS
CNS: headache, *neuromuscular blockade*.
EENT: *ototoxicity (tinnitus, vertigo, hearing loss)*.
GU: some nephrotoxicity (not nearly as frequent as with other aminoglycosides).

Skin: *exfoliative dermatitis.*
Other: pain, irritation, and sterile abscesses at injection site; hypersensitivity reactions (rash, fever, urticaria, and angioedema); *transient agranulocytosis.*

INTERACTIONS
Cephalothin: increased nephrotoxicity. Use together cautiously.
Dimenhydrinate: may mask symptoms of streptomycin-induced ototoxicity. Use together cautiously.
General anesthetics, neuromuscular blockers: may potentiate neuromuscular blockade.
I.V. loop diuretics (such as furosemide): increased ototoxicity. Use together cautiously.
Other aminoglycosides, acyclovir, amphotericin B, cisplatin, methoxyflurane, vancomycin: increased nephrotoxicity. Use together cautiously.

CONTRAINDICATIONS
Contraindicated in patients with hypersensitivity to the drug or other aminoglycosides and in patients with labyrinthine disease. Never administer intravenously.

NURSING CONSIDERATIONS
• Use cautiously in patients with impaired renal function or neuromuscular disorders and in elderly patients.
• Obtain specimen for culture and sensitivity tests before first dose except when treating tuberculosis. Therapy may begin pending results.
• Evaluate patient's hearing before beginning therapy.
• Protect hands when preparing because drug is irritating.
• For I.M. administration, inject deeply into upper outer quadrant of buttocks. Rotate injection sites.
• Obtain blood for peak streptomycin level 1 to 2 hours after I.M. injection; for trough levels, draw blood just before next dose. Don't use a heparin-

ized tube because heparin is incompatible with aminoglycosides.
• Evaluate the patient's hearing during and 6 months after therapy. Notify the doctor if the patient complains of hearing loss, roaring noises, or fullness in ears.
• Watch for signs of superinfection (continued fever and other signs of new infections).
• Encourage adequate fluid intake; patient should be well hydrated while taking drug to minimize chemical irritation of the renal tubules.
• Be aware that in primary treatment of tuberculosis, streptomycin is discontinued when sputum becomes negative.

---

tobramycin sulfate
Nebcin

Pregnancy Risk Category: D

HOW SUPPLIED
Injection: 40 mg/ml, 10 mg/ml (pediatric)
Powder for injection: 30 mg/ml after reconstitution
Premixed parenteral injection for I.V. infusion: 60 mg or 80 mg in 0.9% sodium chloride

ACTION
Inhibits protein synthesis by binding directly to the 30S ribosomal subunit. Generally bactericidal.

ONSET, PEAK, DURATION
Onset immediate after I.V. infusion, unknown after I.M. injection. Peak serum levels occur immediately after I.V. infusion, 30 to 90 minutes after I.M. injection. Measurable serum levels persist for about 8 hours after I.M. or I.V. administration.

INDICATIONS & DOSAGE
Serious infections caused by sensitive strains of Escherichia coli, Proteus, Klebsiella, Enterobacter, Serratia,

---

*Liquid form contains alcohol.   *Common* reactions are in italics; *life-threatening*, in bold italics.
**May contain tartrazine.

Staphylococcus aureus, Pseudomonas, Citrobacter, Providencia —
Adults: 3 mg/kg I.M. or I.V. daily divided q 8 hours. Up to 5 mg/kg daily divided q 6 to 8 hours for life-threatening infections.
Children: 6 to 7.5 mg/kg I.M. or I.V. daily in three or four equally divided doses.
Neonates under 1 week or premature infants: Up to 4 mg/kg/day I.V. or I.M. in two equal doses q 12 hours.

ADVERSE REACTIONS
CNS: headache, lethargy, *neuromuscular blockade.*
EENT: *ototoxicity (tinnitus, vertigo, hearing loss).*
GU: *nephrotoxicity (cells or casts in the urine, oliguria, proteinuria, decreased creatinine clearance, increased BUN and serum creatinine levels).*
Other: hypersensitivity reactions *(anaphylaxis).*

INTERACTIONS
Cephalothin: increased nephrotoxicity. Use together cautiously.
Dimenhydrinate: may mask symptoms of ototoxicity. Use with caution.
General anesthetics, neuromuscular blocking agents: may potentiate neuromuscular blockade.
I.V. loop diuretics (such as furosemide): increased ototoxicity. Use together cautiously.
Other aminoglycosides, acyclovir, amphotericin B, cisplatin, methoxyflurane, vancomycin: increased nephrotoxicity. Use together cautiously.
Parenteral penicillins (such as ticarcillin): tobramycin inactivation in vitro. Don't mix together.

CONTRAINDICATIONS
Contraindicated in patients with hypersensitivity to the drug or other aminoglycosides.

NURSING CONSIDERATIONS
● Use cautiously in patients with impaired renal function or neuromuscular disorders and in elderly patients.
● Obtain specimen for culture and sensitivity tests before first dose. Therapy may begin pending results.
● Weigh the patient and review baseline renal function studies before starting therapy.
● Evaluate patient's hearing before beginning therapy.
● **I.V. use:** Dilute in 50 to 100 ml of 0.9% sodium chloride solution or D_5W for adults and in less volume for children. Infuse over 20 to 60 minutes. After I.V. infusion, flush line with 0.9% sodium chloride solution or D_5W.
● Obtain blood for peak tobramycin level 1 hour after I.M. injection and 30 minutes to 1 hour after infusion ends; draw blood for trough level just before next dose. Don't collect blood in a heparinized tube because heparin is incompatible with aminoglycosides.
● Be aware that blood levels over 12 mcg/ml and trough levels above 2 mcg/ml may be associated with increased incidence of toxicity.
● Monitor renal function (output, specific gravity, urinalysis, BUN and creatinine levels, and creatinine clearance). Notify the doctor of signs of decreasing renal function.
● Evaluate the patient's hearing during therapy. Notify the doctor if the patient complains of tinnitus, vertigo, or hearing loss.
● Watch for signs of superinfection (continued fever and other signs of new infections).
● Encourage adequate fluid intake; patient should be well hydrated while taking drug to minimize chemical irritation of the renal tubules.
● Be aware that if no response occurs in 3 to 5 days, therapy may be stopped and new specimens obtained for culture and sensitivity testing.

---

amoxicillin/clavulanate
  potassium
amoxicillin trihydrate
ampicillin
ampicillin sodium
ampicillin trihydrate
ampicillin sodium/sulbactam
  sodium
bacampicillin hydrochloride
carbenicillin indanyl sodium
cloxacillin sodium
dicloxacillin sodium
methicillin sodium
mezlocillin sodium
nafcillin sodium
oxacillin sodium
penicillin G benzathine
penicillin G potassium
penicillin G procaine
penicillin G sodium
penicillin V
penicillin V potassium
piperacillin sodium
piperacillin sodium and
  tazobactam sodium
ticarcillin disodium
ticarcillin disodium/clavulanate
  potassium

COMBINATION PRODUCTS

AUGMENTIN, CLAVULIN†: amoxicillin 250 mg and clavulanate potassium 125 mg per tablet; amoxicillin 500 mg and clavulanate potassium 125 mg per tablet; amoxicillin 125 mg and clavulanate potassium 31.5 mg per chewable tablet; amoxicillin 250 mg and clavulanate potassium 62.5 mg per chewable tablet; amoxicillin 125 mg and clavulanate potassium 31.5 mg per 5 ml oral suspension; amoxicillin 250 mg and clavulanate potassium 62.5 mg per 5 ml oral suspension.
POLYCILLIN-PRB: ampicillin trihydrate 3.5 g and probenecid 1 g per bottle.

PRINCIPEN WITH PROBENECID: ampicillin trihydrate 3.5 g and probenecid 1 g per bottle.

---

amoxicillin/clavulanate potassium (amoxycillin/ clavulanate potassium)
Augmentin, Clavulin†

Pregnancy Risk Category: B

HOW SUPPLIED
Tablets (chewable): 125 mg amoxicillin trihydrate, 31.25 mg clavulanic acid; 250 mg amoxicillin trihydrate, 62.5 mg clavulanic acid
Tablets (film-coated): 250 mg amoxicillin trihydrate, 125 mg clavulanic acid; 500 mg amoxicillin trihydrate, 125 mg clavulanic acid
Oral suspension: 125 mg amoxicillin trihydrate and 31.25 mg clavulanic acid/5 ml (after reconstitution); 250 mg amoxicillin trihydrate and 62.5 mg clavulanic acid/5 ml (after reconstitution)

ACTION
An aminopenicillin that prevents bacterial cell-wall synthesis during replication. Clavulanic acid increases amoxicillin effectiveness by inactivating beta lactamases, which destroy amoxicillin.

ONSET, PEAK, DURATION
Onset unknown. Serum levels peak in 1 to 2½ hours. Serum concentrations are usually low or undetectable 6 to 8 hours after oral administration.

INDICATIONS & DOSAGE
Lower respiratory infections, otitis media, sinusitis, skin and skin structure infections, and urinary tract infections caused by susceptible strains

---

*Liquid form contains alcohol.
**May contain tartrazine.

Common reactions are in italics; *life-threatening,* in bold italics.

of gram-positive and gram-negative organisms —

Adults: 250 mg (based on the amoxicillin component) P.O. q 8 hours. For more severe infections, 500 mg q 8 hours.

Children: 20 to 40 mg/kg (based on the amoxicillin component) P.O. daily in divided doses q 8 hours.

ADVERSE REACTIONS

GI: *nausea,* vomiting, *diarrhea.*
Hematologic: anemia, thrombocytopenia, thrombocytopenic purpura, eosinophilia, leukopenia.
Other: hypersensitivity reactions (erythematous maculopapular rash, urticaria, **anaphylaxis**), overgrowth of nonsusceptible organisms.

INTERACTIONS

Allopurinol: increased incidence of skin rash.
Probenecid: increased blood levels of amoxicillin and other penicillins. Probenecid may be used for this purpose.

CONTRAINDICATIONS

Contraindicated in patients with hypersensitivity to the drug or other penicillins and in those with a previous history of amoxicillin-associated cholestatic jaundice or hepatic dysfunction.

NURSING CONSIDERATIONS

● Use cautiously in patients with other drug allergies, especially to cephalosporins (possible cross-sensitivity), and in those with mononucleosis (high incidence of maculopapular rash).
● Before giving, ask the patient about any allergic reactions to penicillin. However, a negative history of penicillin allergy is no guarantee against an allergic reaction.
● Obtain specimen for culture and sensitivity tests before first dose. Therapy may begin pending results.
● Give with food to prevent GI dis-

tress. Incidence of adverse GI effects, especially diarrhea, is greater than with amoxicillin alone.
● Give drug at least 1 hour before bacteriostatic antibiotics.
● Observe closely. With large doses and prolonged therapy, bacterial or fungal superinfection may occur, especially in elderly, debilitated, or immunosuppressed patients.
● Know that both the "250" and "500" tablets contain the same amount of clavulanic acid (125 mg). Therefore, two "250" tablets are not equivalent to one "500" tablet.
● Be aware that this drug combination is particularly useful in clinical settings with high prevalence of amoxicillin-resistant organisms.
● After reconstitution, refrigerate the oral suspension and discard after 10 days.
● Know that urine glucose determinations may be false-positive with copper sulfate tests (Benedict's solution, Clinitest); glucose enzymatic tests (Clinistix, Tes-Tape) are not affected.
● Tell the patient to take entire quantity of drug exactly as prescribed, even after he feels better.

---

amoxicillin trihydrate (amoxycillin trihydrate)

Alphamox‡, Amoxil, Apo-Amoxi†, Cilamox‡, Ibiamox‡, Larotid, Moxacin‡, Novamoxin†, Nu-Amoxi†, Polymox, Trimox, Wymox

Pregnancy Risk Category: NR

HOW SUPPLIED

Tablets (chewable): 125 mg, 250 mg
Capsules: 250 mg, 500 mg
Oral suspension: 50 mg/ml (pediatric drops), 125 mg/5 ml, 250 mg/5 ml (after reconstitution)

ACTION

An aminopenicillin that inhibits cell-wall synthesis during bacterial multiplication; bacteria resist amoxicillin

---

†Available in Canada only.   ‡Available in Australia only.   ◇Available OTC.

by producing penicillinases—enzymes that hydrolyze amoxicillin.

ONSET, PEAK, DURATION
Onset unknown. Serum levels peak within 1 to 2 hours. Serum concentrations are usually low or undetectable 6 to 8 hours after oral administration.

INDICATIONS & DOSAGE
Systemic infections, acute and chronic urinary tract infections caused by susceptible strains of gram-positive and gram-negative organisms—
Adults and children 20 kg or over: 250 to 500 mg P.O. q 8 hours.
Children under 20 kg: 20 mg/kg P.O. daily in divided doses q 8 hours; in severe infection, 40 mg/kg P.O. daily in divided doses q 8 hours or 500 mg to 1 g/m^2 P.O. in divided doses q 8 hours.
Uncomplicated gonorrhea—
Adults and children over 45 kg: 3 g P.O. with 1 g probenecid given as a single dose.
Endocarditis prophylaxis for dental procedures—
Adults: initially, 3 g P.O. 1 hour before procedure; then 1.5 g 6 hours later.
Children: initially, 50 mg/kg P.O. 1 hour before procedure; then half the initial dose 6 hours later.

ADVERSE REACTIONS
GI: *nausea,* vomiting, *diarrhea.*
Hematologic: anemia, thrombocytopenia, thrombocytopenic purpura, eosinophilia, leukopenia.
Other: hypersensitivity reactions (erythematous maculopapular rash, urticaria, ***anaphylaxis),*** overgrowth of nonsusceptible organisms.

INTERACTIONS
Allopurinol: increased incidence of skin rash.
Probenecid: increased blood levels of amoxicillin and other penicillins. Probenecid may be used for this purpose.

CONTRAINDICATIONS
Contraindicated in patients with hypersensitivity to the drug or other penicillins.

NURSING CONSIDERATIONS
• Use cautiously in patients with other drug allergies, especially to cephalosporins (possible cross-sensitivity), and in those with mononucleosis (high incidence of maculopapular rash).
• Before giving, ask the patient about any allergic reactions to penicillin. However, a negative history of penicillin allergy is no guarantee against an allergic reaction.
• Obtain specimen for culture and sensitivity tests before first dose. Therapy may begin pending results.
• Give with food to prevent GI distress.
• Give amoxicillin at least 1 hour before bacteriostatic antibiotics.
• Observe closely. With large doses and prolonged therapy, bacterial or fungal superinfection may occur, especially in elderly, debilitated, or immunosuppressed patients.
• Store Trimox oral suspension at room temperature for up to 2 weeks. Be sure to check individual product labels for storage information.
• Be aware that urine glucose determinations may be false-positive with copper sulfate tests (Benedict's solution, Clinitest); glucose enzymatic tests (Clinistix, Tes-Tape) are not affected.
• Keep in mind that amoxicillin generally causes diarrhea less often than ampicillin.
• Tell the patient to take entire quantity of medication exactly as prescribed, even after he feels better.
• Warn the patient never to use leftover amoxicillin for a new illness or to share it with family and friends.
• Tell the patient to call the doctor if rash, fever, or chills develop. A rash is the most common allergic reaction,

---

*Liquid form contains alcohol.
**May contain tartrazine.*

*Common reactions are in italics; **life-threatening,** in bold italics.*

especially when the patient is also taking allopurinol.

---

ampicillin
Apo-Ampi†, Novo Ampicillin†, Nu-Ampi†, Omnipen, Principen

ampicillin sodium
Ampicin†, Ampicyn Injection‡, Omnipen-N, Penbritin†, Polycillin-N, Totacillin-N

ampicillin trihydrate
Ampicyn Oral‡, D-Amp, Omnipen, Penbritin‡, Polycillin, Principen-250, Principen-500, Totacillin

Pregnancy Risk Category: B

HOW SUPPLIED
Capsules: 250 mg, 500 mg
Oral suspension: 100 mg/ml (pediatric drops), 125 mg/5 ml, 250 mg/5 ml, 500 mg/5 ml (after reconstitution)
Injection: 125 mg, 250 mg, 500 mg, 1 g, 2 g
Infusion: 500 mg, 1 g, 2 g
Pharmacy bulk package: 10-g vial

ACTION
An aminopenicillin that inhibits cell-wall synthesis during microorganism multiplication; bacteria resist ampicillin by producing penicillinases — enzymes that hydrolyze ampicillin.

ONSET, PEAK, DURATION
Onset immediate after I.V. administration, unknown after I.M. injection. Peak plasma levels occur immediately after I.V. administration, within 1 hour of I.M. administration, and within 2 hours of oral administration. Serum levels are usually low or undetectable 6 to 8 hours after oral administration.

INDICATIONS & DOSAGE
Systemic infections and acute and chronic urinary tract infections caused by susceptible strains of gram-positive and gram-negative organisms—
Adults and children 20 kg or over: 250 to 500 mg P.O. q 6 hours; or 2 to 12 g I.M. or I.V. daily, in divided doses q 4 to 6 hours.
Children 20 kg or less: 50 to 100 mg/kg P.O. daily, in divided doses q 6 hours; or 100 to 200 mg/kg I.M. or I.V. daily, in divided doses q 6 hours.
Meningitis —
Adults: 8 to 14 g I.V. daily in divided doses q 3 to 4 hours.
Children: up to 300 mg/kg I.V. daily in divided doses q 3 to 4 hours.
Uncomplicated gonorrhea —
Adults and children over 45 kg: 3.5 g P.O. with 1 g probenecid given as a single dose.
Endocarditis prophylaxis for dental procedures —
Adults: 1 to 2 g I.M. or I.V. with gentamicin 30 minutes before procedure, then repeated 6 hours afer initial dose.
Children 50 mg/kg I.M. or I.V. with gentamicin 2 mg/kg 30 minutes before procedure; half the initial dose is given 6 hours later.

ADVERSE REACTIONS
GI: *nausea,* vomiting, *diarrhea,* glossitis, stomatitis.
Hematologic: anemia, thrombocytopenia, thrombocytopenic purpura, eosinophilia, leukopenia.
Other: hypersensitivity reactions (erythematous maculopapular rash, urticaria, *anaphylaxis*), overgrowth of nonsusceptible organisms, pain at injection site, vein irritation, thrombophlebitis.

INTERACTIONS
Allopurinol: increased incidence of skin rash.
Probenecid: increased blood levels of ampicillin and other penicillins. Probenecid may be used for this purpose.

CONTRAINDICATIONS
Contraindicated in patients with hypersensitivity to the drug or other penicillins.

NURSING CONSIDERATIONS
• Use cautiously in patients with other drug allergies, especially to cephalosporins (possible cross-sensitivity), or in those with mononucleosis (high incidence of maculopapular rash).
• Before giving, ask the patient about any allergic reactions to penicillin. However, a negative history of penicillin allergy is no guarantee against a future allergic reaction.
• Obtain specimen for culture and sensitivity tests before first dose. Therapy may begin pending results.
• **I.V. use:** For I.V. injection, reconstitute using bacteriostatic water for injection. Use 5 ml for the 125-mg, 250-mg, or 500-mg vials; 7.4 ml for the 1-g vials; or 14.8 ml for the 2-g vials. Give direct I.V. injections over 3 to 5 minutes for doses of 500 mg or less; over 10 to 15 minutes for larger doses. Don't exceed a rate of 100 mg/minute. Alternatively, dilute in 50 or 100 ml of 0.9% sodium chloride injection and give by intermittent infusion over 15 to 30 minutes. Don't mix with solutions containing dextrose or fructose because these solutions promote rapid breakdown of ampicillin.
• Use initial dilution within 1 hour. Follow manufacturer's directions for stability data when ampicillin is further diluted for I.V. infusion.
• Give I.V. intermittently to prevent vein irritation. Change site every 48 hours.
• Don't give I.M. or I.V. unless prescribed and infection is severe or patient can't take oral dose.
• Give 1 to 2 hours before or 2 to 3 hours after meals. When given orally, drug may cause GI disturbances. Food may interfere with absorption.

• Give ampicillin at least 1 hour before bacteriostatic antibiotics.
• Observe closely. With large doses or prolonged therapy, bacterial or fungal superinfection may occur, especially in elderly, debilitated, or immunosuppressed patients.
• Know that dosage should be altered in patients with impaired renal function.
• Be aware that in pediatric meningitis, ampicillin may be given concurrently with parenteral chloramphenicol for 24 hours pending cultures.
• Keep in mind that urine glucose determinations may be false-positive with copper sulfate tests (Benedict's solution, Clinitest); glucose enzymatic tests (Clinistix, Tes-Tape) are not affected.
• Tell the patient to take entire quantity of medication exactly as prescribed, even after he feels better.
• Tell the patient to call the doctor if rash, fever, or chills develop. A rash is the most common allergic reaction, especially if the patient is also taking allopurinol.
• Warn the patient never to use leftover ampicillin for a new illness or to share it with family and friends.

ampicillin sodium/ sulbactam sodium
Unasyn

Pregnancy Risk Category: B

HOW SUPPLIED
Injection: vials and piggyback vials containing 1.5 g (1 g ampicillin sodium with 0.5 g sulbactam sodium) and 3 g (2 g ampicillin sodium with 1 g sulbactam sodium)

ACTION
Ampicillin (an aminopenicillin) inhibits cell-wall synthesis during microorganism multiplication; sulbactam inactivates bacterial beta-lactamase, the enzyme that inactivates am-

---

*Liquid form contains alcohol.   *Common* reactions are in italics; *life-threatening*, in bold italics.
**May contain tartrazine.

picillin and provides bacterial resistance to it.

ONSET, PEAK, DURATION
Onset immediate after I.V. administration, unknown after I.M. injection. Peak serum levels occur immediately after I.V. adminstration, unknown after I.M. injection. Duration unknown.

INDICATIONS & DOSAGE
Intra-abdominal, gynecologic, and skin structure infections caused by susceptible strains –
Adults: dosage expressed as total drug (each 1.5-g vial contains 1 g ampicillin sodium and 0.5 g sulbactam sodium) – 1.5 to 3 g I.M. or I.V. q 6 hours. Maximum daily dosage is 4 g sulbactam (12 g of the combined drugs).

ADVERSE REACTIONS
GI: *nausea,* vomiting, *diarrhea,* glossitis, stomatitis.
Hematologic: anemia, thrombocytopenia, thrombocytopenic purpura, eosinophilia, leukopenia.
Other: hypersensitivity reactions (erythematous maculopapular rash, urticaria, ***anaphylaxis***), overgrowth of nonsusceptible organisms, pain at injection site, vein irritation, thrombophlebitis.

INTERACTIONS
Allopurinol: increased incidence of skin rash.
Probenecid: increased levels of ampicillin. Probenecid may be used for this purpose.

CONTRAINDICATIONS
Contraindicated in patients with hypersensitivity to the drug or other penicillins.

NURSING CONSIDERATIONS
• Use cautiously in patients with other drug allergies, especially to cephalosporins (possible cross-sensitivity), or in those with mononucleosis (high incidence of maculopapular rash).
• Before giving, ask the patient about any allergic reactions to penicillin. However, a negative history of penicillin allergy is no guarantee against a future allergic reaction.
• Obtain specimen for culture and sensitivity tests before first dose. Therapy may begin pending results.
• **I.V. use:** When preparing I.V. injection, reconstitute powder with any of the following diluents: 0.9% sodium chloride solution, D_5W, lactated Ringer's injection, ⅙ M sodium lactate, dextrose 5% and 0.45% sodium chloride injection, and 10% invert sugar. Stability varies with diluent, temperature, and concentration of solution.
• After reconstitution, allow vials to stand for a few minutes for foam to dissipate. This will permit visual inspection of contents for particles.
• Give I.V. dose by slow injection (over 10 to 15 minutes), or dilute in 50 to 100 ml of a compatible diluent and infuse over 15 to 30 minutes. If permitted, give intermittently to prevent vein irritation. Change site every 48 hours.
• When giving I.V., don't add or mix with other drugs because they might prove physically or chemically incompatible.
• For I.M. injection, reconstitute with sterile water for injection or 0.5% or 2% lidocaine hydrochloride injection. Add 3.2 ml to a 1.5-g vial (or 6.4 ml to a 3-g vial) to yield a concentration of 375 mg/ml. Administer deeply.
• Give drug at least 1 hour before bacteriostatic antibiotics.
• Observe closely. With large doses and prolonged therapy, bacterial or fungal superinfection may occur, especially in elderly, debilitated, or immunosuppressed patients.
• Know that dosage should be altered

in patients with impaired renal function.

• Keep in mind that urine glucose determinations may be false-positive with copper sulfate tests (Benedict's solution, Clinitest); glucose enzymatic tests (Clinistix, Tes-Tape) are not affected.

• Tell the patient to call the doctor if rash, fever, or chills develop. A rash is the most common allergic reaction.

bacampicillin hydrochloride
Penglobe†, Spectrobid

Pregnancy Risk Category: B

HOW SUPPLIED
Tablets: 400 mg
Oral suspension: 125 mg/5 ml (after reconstitution)

ACTION
An aminopenicillin that inhibits cell-wall synthesis during microorganism multiplication; bacteria resist bacampicillin by producing penicillinases — enzymes that hydrolyze its active form (ampicillin).

ONSET, PEAK, DURATION
Onset unknown. Plasma levels peak within 30 to 90 minutes. Serum concentrations are usually low or undetectable 6 to 8 hours later.

INDICATIONS & DOSAGE
Upper respiratory tract infections and otitis media caused by streptococci, pneumococci, staphylococci, and Haemophilus influenzae; *urinary tract infections caused by* Escherichia coli, Proteus mirabilis, *and* Enterococcus faecalis; *skin infections caused by streptococci and susceptible staphylococci —*
Adults and children over 25 kg: 400 mg P.O. q 12 hours.
Children 25 kg or less: 25 mg/kg/day P.O. in divided doses q 12 hours.

Lower respiratory tract infections; other severe infections —
Adults and children over 25 kg: 800 mg P.O. q 12 hours.
Children 25 kg or less: 50 mg/kg/day P.O. in divided doses q 12 hours.
Gonorrhea —
Adults: 1.6 g P.O. plus 1 g probenecid given as a single dose.

ADVERSE REACTIONS
GI: *nausea,* vomiting, *diarrhea,* glossitis, stomatitis.
Hematologic: anemia, thrombocytopenia, thrombocytopenic purpura, eosinophilia, leukopenia.
Other: hypersensitivity reactions (erythematous maculopapular rash, urticaria, ***anaphylaxis***), overgrowth of nonsusceptible organisms.

INTERACTIONS
Allopurinol: increased incidence of skin rash.
Disulfiram: possible disulfiram-alcohol reaction. Do not give together.
Probenecid: increased blood levels of bacampicillin or other penicillins. Probenecid may be used for this purpose.

CONTRAINDICATIONS
Contraindicated in patients with hypersensitivity to the drug or other penicillins.

NURSING CONSIDERATIONS
• Use cautiously in patients with other drug allergies, especially to cephalosporins (possible cross-sensitivity), or in those with mononucleosis (high incidence of maculopapular rash).
• Before giving, ask the patient about any allergic reactions to penicillin. However, a negative history of penicillin allergy is no guarantee against an allergic reaction.
• Obtain specimen for culture and sensitivity tests before first dose. Therapy may begin pending results.

---

*Liquid form contains alcohol.   Common reactions are in italics; **life-threatening**, in bold italics.
**May contain tartrazine.

• Unlike ampicillin, administer bacampicillin with meals without fear of diminished drug absorption.
• Give bacampicillin at least 1 hour before bacteriostatic antibiotics.
• Observe closely. With large doses and prolonged therapy, bacterial or fungal superinfection may occur, especially in elderly, debilitated, or immunosuppressed patients.
• Know that diarrhea may occur less frequently with bacampicillin than with ampicillin.
• Be aware that bacampicillin is specially formulated to produce high blood levels of antibiotic when administered twice daily.
• Keep in mind that urine glucose determinations may be false-positive with copper sulfate tests (Benedict's solution, Clinitest); glucose enzymatic tests (Clinistix, Tes-Tape) are not affected.
• Tell the patient to take entire quantity of medication as prescribed, even after he feels better.
• Warn the patient never to use leftover bacampicillin for a new illness or to share it with family and friends.
• Tell the patient to call the doctor if rash, fever, or chills develop. A rash is the most common allergic reaction.

---

carbenicillin indanyl sodium
Geocillin, Geopen Oral†

Pregnancy Risk Category: B

HOW SUPPLIED
Tablets: 382 mg

ACTION
An extended-spectrum penicillin that inhibits cell-wall synthesis during microorganism multiplication; bacteria resist carbenicillin by producing penicillinases—enzymes that hydrolyze its active form.

ONSET, PEAK, DURATION
Onset unknown. Serum levels peak within 30 minutes. Serum carbenicillin concentrations are generally low or undetectable 6 hours after a dose.

INDICATIONS & DOSAGE
Urinary tract infection and prostatitis caused by susceptible strains of gram-negative organisms –
Adults: 382 to 764 mg P.O. q.i.d.
Not recommended for children.

ADVERSE REACTIONS
GI: *nausea,* vomiting, *diarrhea, flatulence, abdominal cramps, unpleasant taste.*
Hematologic: leukopenia, neutropenia, eosinophilia, ***hemolytic anemia,*** thrombocytopenia.
Other: hypersensitivity reactions (rash, chills, fever, urticaria, pruritus, ***anaphylaxis***), overgrowth of nonsusceptible organisms.

INTERACTIONS
None significant.

CONTRAINDICATIONS
Contraindicated in patients with hypersensitivity to the drug or other penicillins.

NURSING CONSIDERATIONS
• Use cautiously in patients with other drug allergies, especially to cephalosporins (possible cross-sensitivity).
• Before giving, ask the patient about any allergic reactions to penicillin. However, a negative history of penicillin allergy is no guarantee against a future allergic reaction.
• Obtain specimen for culture and sensitivity tests before first dose. Therapy may begin pending results.
• Know that drug is used only in patients whose creatinine clearance values are 10 ml/minute or more.
• Give 1 to 2 hours before or 2 to 3

---

hours after meals because food may interfere with absorption.

• Observe closely. With large doses or prolonged therapy, bacterial or fungal superinfection may occur, especially in elderly, debilitated, or immunosuppressed patients.

• Keep in mind that urine glucose determinations may be false-positive with copper sulfate tests (Benedict's solution, Clinitest); glucose enzymatic tests (Clinistix, Tes-Tape) are not affected.

• Be aware that carbenicillin may also interfere with the direct results of Coombs' test and certain tests for serum uric acid.

• Tell the patient to take all of the medication exactly as prescribed, even after he feels better.

• Tell the patient to call the doctor if rash, fever, or chills develop. A rash is the most common allergic reaction.

• Warn the patient never to use leftover carbenicillin for a new illness or to share it with family and friends.

---

cloxacillin sodium

Alclox‡, Apo-Cloxi†, Austrastaph‡, Cloxapen, Novocloxin†, Nu-Cloxi†, Orbenin†, Orbenin Injection‡, Tegopen

Pregnancy Risk Category: B

HOW SUPPLIED
Capsules: 250 mg, 500 mg
Oral solution: 125 mg/5 ml (after reconstitution)

ACTION
A penicillinase-resistant penicillin that inhibits cell-wall synthesis during microorganism multiplication; bacteria resist penicillins by producing penicillinases—enzymes that convert penicillins to inactive penicilloic acid. Cloxacillin resists these enzymes.

ONSET, PEAK, DURATION
Onset unknown. Plasma levels peak within ½ to 2 hours. Drug concentrations are generally low 6 hours after a dose.

INDICATIONS & DOSAGE
Systemic infections caused by penicillinase-producing staphylococci—
Adults and children over 20 kg: 250 to 500 mg P.O. q 6 hours.
Children 20 kg or less: 50 to 100 mg/kg P.O. daily, in divided doses q 6 hours.

ADVERSE REACTIONS
GI: *nausea,* vomiting, *epigastric distress, diarrhea.*
Hematologic: eosinophilia.
Other: hypersensitivity reactions (rash, urticaria, chills, fever, sneezing, wheezing, ***anaphylaxis***), intrahepatic cholestasis, overgrowth of nonsusceptible organisms.

INTERACTIONS
Probenecid: increased blood levels of cloxacillin and other penicillins. Probenecid may be used for this purpose.

CONTRAINDICATIONS
Contraindicated in patients with hypersensitivity to the drug or other penicillins.

NURSING CONSIDERATIONS
• Use cautiously in patients with other drug allergies, especially to cephalosporins (possible cross-sensitivity), or in those with mononucleosis (high incidence of maculopapular rash).

• Before giving, ask the patient about any allergic reactions to penicillin. However, a negative history of penicillin allergy is no guarantee against a future allergic reaction.

• Obtain specimen for culture and sensitivity tests before first dose. Therapy may begin pending results.

• Give 1 to 2 hours before or 2 to 3

---

hours after meals. Drug may cause GI disturbances. Food may interfere with its absorption.
• Give cloxacillin at least 1 hour before bacteriostatic antibiotics.
• As ordered, periodically assess renal, hepatic, and hematopoietic function in patients receiving long-term therapy.
• Observe closely. With large doses and prolonged therapy, bacterial or fungal superinfection may occur, especially in elderly, debilitated, or immunosuppressed patients.
• Keep in mind that cloxacillin may falsely elevate or cause false-positive results with certain tests for urine or serum proteins.
• Tell the patient to take entire quantity of medication exactly as prescribed, even after he feels better.
• Tell the patient to call the doctor if rash, fever, or chills develop. A rash is the most common allergic reaction.
• Instruct patient to take each dose with a full glass of water, not with fruit juice or carbonated beverage, because their acid will inactivate the drug.
• Warn the patient never to use left-over cloxacillin for a new illness or to share it with family and friends.

dicloxacillin sodium
Dycill, Dynapen, Pathocil
Pregnancy Risk Category: NR

HOW SUPPLIED
Capsules: 125 mg, 250 mg, 500 mg
Oral suspension: 62.5 mg/5 ml (after reconstitution)

ACTION
A penicillinase-resistant penicillin that inhibits cell-wall synthesis during microorganism multiplication; bacteria resist penicillins by producing penicillinases — enzymes that convert penicillins to inactive penicilloic

acid. Dicloxacillin resists these enzymes.

ONSET, PEAK, DURATION
Onset unknown. Plasma levels peak within ½ to 2 hours. Drug concentrations are generally low 6 hours after a dose.

INDICATIONS & DOSAGE
Systemic infections caused by penicillinase-producing staphylococci –
Adults and children over 40 kg: 125 to 250 mg P.O. q 6 hours.
Children 40 kg or less: 25 to 50 mg/kg P.O. daily, in divided doses q 6 hours.

ADVERSE REACTIONS
CNS: neuromuscular irritability, seizures.
GI: *nausea,* vomiting, *epigastric distress,* flatulence, *diarrhea.*
Hematologic: eosinophilia.
Other: hypersensitivity reactions (pruritus, urticaria, rash, ***anaphylaxis***), overgrowth of nonsusceptible organisms.

INTERACTIONS
Probenecid: increased blood levels of dicloxacillin and other penicillins. Probenecid may be used for this purpose.

CONTRAINDICATIONS
Contraindicated in patients with hypersensitivity to the drug or other penicillins.

NURSING CONSIDERATIONS
• Use cautiously in patients with other drug allergies, especially to cephalosporins (possible cross-sensitivity), or in those with mononucleosis (high incidence of maculopapular rash).
• Before giving, ask the patient about any allergic reactions to penicillin. However, a negative history of peni-

---

cillin allergy is no guarantee against a
future allergic reaction.
• Obtain specimen for culture and
sensitivity tests before first dose.
Therapy may begin pending results.
• Give 1 to 2 hours before or 2 to 3
hours after meals. Drug may cause GI
disturbances. Food may interfere with
absorption.
• Give dicloxacillin at least 1 hour before bacteriostatic antibiotics.
• As ordered, periodically assess
renal, hepatic, and hematopoietic
function in patients receiving long-
term therapy.
• Observe closely. With large doses
and prolonged therapy, bacterial or
fungal superinfection may occur, especially in elderly, debilitated, or immunosuppressed patients.
• Tell the patient to take entire quantity of medication exactly as prescribed, even after he feels better.
• Tell the patient to call the doctor if
rash, fever, or chills develop. A rash
is the most common allergic reaction.
• Warn the patient never to use leftover dicloxacillin for a new illness or
to share it with family and friends.

---

methicillin sodium
Metin‡, Staphcillin

Pregnancy Risk Category: B

HOW SUPPLIED
Injection: 1 g, 4 g, 6 g
I.V. infusion piggyback: 1 g
Pharmacy bulk package: 10 g

ACTION
A penicillinase-resistant penicillin
that inhibits cell-wall synthesis during
microorganism multiplication; bacteria resist penicillins by producing
penicillinases—enzymes that convert
penicillins to inactive penicilloic
acid. Methicillin resists these enzymes.

ONSET, PEAK, DURATION
Onset immediate after I.V. administration, unknown after I.M. administration. Peak serum levels occur immediately after I.V. infusion, within
30 to 60 minutes of I.M. injection.
Drug concentrations undetectable 6
hours after an I.M. dose.

INDICATIONS & DOSAGE
*Systemic infections caused by penicil-
linase-producing staphylococci—*
Adults and children over 40 kg: 4 to
12 g I.M. or I.V. daily, in divided
doses q 4 to 6 hours.
Children 40 kg and less: 100 to 300
mg/kg I.M. or I.V. daily, in divided
doses q 4 to 6 hours.

ADVERSE REACTIONS
CNS: neuropathy, *seizures with high
doses.*
GI: glossitis, stomatitis.
Hematologic: *agranulocytosis, eosinophilia,* hemolytic anemia, transient neutropenia.
GU: interstitial nephritis.
Other: hypersensitivity reactions
(chills, fever, edema, rash, urticaria,
anaphylaxis), overgrowth of nonsusceptible organisms, vein irritation,
thrombophlebitis.

INTERACTIONS
Probenecid: increased blood levels of
methicillin and other penicillins. Probenecid may be used for this purpose.

CONTRAINDICATIONS
Contraindicated in patients with hypersensitivity to the drug or other
penicillins.

NURSING CONSIDERATIONS
• Use cautiously in patients with
other drug allergies, especially to
cephalosporins (possible cross-sensitivity), and in infants.
• Before giving, ask the patient about
any allergic reactions to penicillin.
However, a negative history of peni-

---

*Liquid form contains alcohol.
**May contain tartrazine.   *Common* reactions are in italics; *life-threatening,* in bold italics.

cillin allergy is no guarantee against a future allergic reaction.

• Obtain specimen for culture and sensitivity tests before first dose. Therapy may begin pending results.

• **I.V. use:** Reconstitute vials using sterile water for injection or 0.9% sodium chloride injection. For 1-g vials, use 1.5 ml of diluent; for 4-g vials, 5.7 ml of diluent; and for 6-g vials, 8.6 ml of diluent. For direct injection, further dilute each 500 mg drug with 35 ml of 0.9% sodium chloride injection and inject at a rate of 10 ml/minute into the tubing of a free-flowing compatible I.V. solution. For intermittent infusion, dilute to a maximum concentration of 2 to 20 mg/ml and infuse over 20 to 30 minutes.

• Give I.V. intermittently to prevent vein irritation. Change site every 48 hours.

• For I.M. administration, inject reconstituted drug deeply into the gluteus maximus to avoid sciatic nerve injury.

• Give methicillin at least 1 hour before bacteriostatic antibiotics.

• As ordered, periodically assess hepatic, renal, and hematopoietic function in patients receiving long-term therapy.

• Closely monitor renal function. Urinalysis should be done frequently to detect interstitial nephritis.

• Institute seizure precautions. Patients with high blood levels of this drug may develop seizures.

• Observe closely. With large doses and prolonged therapy, bacterial or fungal superinfection may occur, especially in elderly, debilitated, or immunosuppressed patients.

---

mezlocillin sodium
Mezlin

Pregnancy Risk Category: B

HOW SUPPLIED
Injection: 1 g, 2 g, 3 g, 4 g
Pharmacy bulk package: 20 g

ACTION
An extended-spectrum penicillin that inhibits cell-wall synthesis during microorganism multiplication; bacteria resist mezlocillin by producing penicillinases — enzymes that hydrolyze mezlocillin.

ONSET, PEAK, DURATION
Onset immediate after I.V. administration, unknown after I.M. injection. Peak serum levels occur immediately after I.V. administration, within 45 to 90 minutes of I.M. injection. Duration unknown.

INDICATIONS & DOSAGE
Systemic infections caused by susceptible strains of gram-positive and especially gram-negative organisms (including Proteus *and* Pseudomonas aeruginosa) —
Adults: 200 to 300 mg/kg daily I.V. or I.M. in four to six divided doses. Usual dose is 3 g q 4 hours or 4 g q 6 hours. For very serious infections, up to 24 g daily may be administered.
Children up to 12 years: 50 mg/kg q 4 hours by I.V. infusion or direct I.V. injection.

ADVERSE REACTIONS
CNS: neuromuscular irritability.
GI: nausea, diarrhea.
Hematologic: *bleeding with high doses,* neutropenia, thrombocytopenia, eosinophilia, leukopenia, *hemolytic anemia.*
Other: hypersensitivity reactions (*anaphylaxis,* edema, fever, chills, rash, pruritus, urticaria), overgrowth of nonsusceptible organisms, *hypokalemia,* pain at injection site, vein irritation, phlebitis.

INTERACTIONS
Aminoglycoside antibiotics (such as gentamicin and tobramycin): chemically incompatible. Don't mix together in I.V. solution. Give 1 hour apart, especially in patients with renal insufficiency.
Probenecid: increased blood levels of mezlocillin. Probenecid may be used for this purpose.

CONTRAINDICATIONS
Contraindicated in patients with hypersensitivity to the drug or other penicillins.

NURSING CONSIDERATIONS
• Use cautiously in patients with other drug allergies, especially to cephalosporins (possible cross-sensitivity), or in those with bleeding tendencies, uremia, or hypokalemia.
• Before giving, ask the patient about any allergic reactions to penicillin. A negative history of penicillin allergy, however, is no guarantee against future allergic reaction.
• Obtain specimen for culture and sensitivity tests before first dose. Therapy may begin pending results.
• **I.V. use:** Reconstitute vials with at least 10 ml/g of drug using sterile water for injection, D5W, or 0.9% sodium chloride injection. Solutions with a concentration not exceeding 10% may be given by direct injection over 3 to 5 minutes. Alternatively, dilute in about 50 to 100 ml of suitable I.V. solution and give by intermittent infusion over 30 minutes.
• Give I.V. intermittently to prevent vein irritation. Change site every 48 hours.
• When giving I.M., don't give more than 2 g per injection. Inject deeply and slowly (12 to 15 seconds) into the body of a large muscle.
• Give mezlocillin at least 1 hour before bacteriostatic antibiotics.
• Check CBC and platelet counts frequently, as ordered. Drug may cause thrombocytopenia.
• Monitor serum potassium level.
• Institute seizure precautions. Patients with high serum levels of this drug may have seizures.
• Observe closely. With large doses and prolonged therapy, bacterial or fungal superinfection may occur, especially in elderly, debilitated, or immunosuppressed patients.
• Be aware that dosage should be altered in patients with impaired renal function.
• Be aware that drug is almost always used with another antibiotic, such as gentamicin.
• Be aware that mezlocillin may interfere with positive direct antiglobulin (Coomb's) test results. Drug may also interfere with certain tests for serum and urine proteins; tests that use bromphenol blue (Albustix, Albutest) are not affected.

---

nafcillin sodium
Nafcil, Nallpen, Unipen
Pregnancy Risk Category: B

HOW SUPPLIED
Tablets: 500 mg
Capsules: 250 mg
Oral solution: 250 mg/5 ml (after reconstitution)
Injection: 500 mg, 1 g, 2 g
I.V. infusion piggyback: 1 g, 2 g
Pharmacy bulk package: 10 g

ACTION
A penicillinase-resistant penicillin that inhibits cell-wall synthesis during microorganism multiplication; bacteria resist penicillins by producing penicillinases — enzymes that hydrolyze penicillins. Nafcillin resists these enzymes.

ONSET, PEAK, DURATION
Onset immediate after I.V. administration, unknown after I.M. injection.

Peak serum levels occur immediately after I.V. administration, within 30 to 60 minutes of I.M. injection, ½ to 2 hours after oral administration. Duration unknown.

INDICATIONS & DOSAGE

Systemic infections caused by penicillinase-producing staphylococci –
Adults: 250 to 500 mg P.O. q 4 to 6 hours (more severe infections may be treated with 1 g P.O. q 4 to 6 hours); or 2 to 12 g I.M. or I.V. daily in divided doses q 4 to 6 hours.
Children older than 1 month: 50 to 100 mg/kg P.O. daily, in divided doses q 6 hours; or 100 to 200 mg/kg I.M. or I.V. daily in divided doses q 4 to 6 hours.

ADVERSE REACTIONS

GI: *nausea,* vomiting, diarrhea.
Hematologic: transient leukopenia, neutropenia, granulocytopenia, ***thrombocytopenia*** with high doses.
Other: hypersensitivity reactions (chills, fever, rash, pruritus, urticaria, ***anaphylaxis***), vein irritation, thrombophlebitis.

INTERACTIONS

Aminoglycosides: synergistic effect; monitor closely. Chemical and physical incompatibility; do not mix together in same I.V. solution.
Probenecid: increased blood levels of nafcillin. Probenecid may be used for this purpose.
Rifampin: dose-dependent antagonism. Monitor closely.
Warfarin: increased risk of bleeding when used with I.V. nafcillin. Monitor closely.

CONTRAINDICATIONS

Contraindicated in patients with hypersensitivity to the drug or other penicillins.

NURSING CONSIDERATIONS

● Use cautiously in patients with other drug allergies, especially to cephalosporins (possible cross-sensitivity), or in those with GI distress.
● Before giving, ask the patient about any allergic reactions to penicillin. However, a negative history of penicillin allergy is no guarantee against a future allergic reaction.
● Obtain specimen for culture and sensitivity tests before first dose. Therapy may begin pending results.
● Give 1 to 2 hours before or 2 to 3 hours after meals. When given orally, drug may cause GI disturbances. Food may interfere with absorption.
● **I.V. use:** Reconstitute piggyback containers according to manufacturer's instructions. Reconstitute 500-mg, 1-g, or 2-g vials using sterile water for injection, D_5W, or 0.9% sodium chloride injection. Add 1.7 ml for each 500 mg of drug. Reconstituted drug may be given I.M. Alternatively, dilute with 15 to 30 ml of sterile water for injection or 0.45% or 0.9% sodium chloride injection, and give by direct injection into a vein or into the tubing of a free-flowing I.V. solution over 5 to 10 minutes. Or dilute drug to a concentration of 2 to 40 mg/ml and give by intermittent I.V. infusion over 30 to 60 minutes.
● Avoid continuous I.V. infusions to prevent vein irritation. Change site every 48 hours.
● Give nafcillin at least 1 hour before bacteriostatic antibiotics.
● Observe closely. With large doses and prolonged therapy, bacterial or fungal superinfection may occur, especially in elderly, debilitated, or immunosuppressed patients.
● Keep in mind that nafcillin may falsely elevate or cause false-positive results with certain tests for urine or serum proteins.
● Tell the patient to take entire quantity of medication exactly as prescribed, even after he feels better.

---

†Available in Canada only.   ‡Available in Australia only.   ◊Available OTC.

• Tell the patient to call the doctor if rash, fever, or chills develop. A rash is the most common allergic reaction.

oxacillin sodium
Bactocill, Prostaphlin

Pregnancy Risk Category: B

HOW SUPPLIED
Capsules: 250 mg, 500 mg
Oral solution: 250 mg/5 ml (after reconstitution)
Injection: 250 mg, 500 mg, 1 g, 2 g, 4 g
I.V. infusion: 1 g, 2 g, 4 g
Pharmacy bulk package: 4 g, 10 g

ACTION
A penicillinase-resistant penicillin that inhibits cell-wall synthesis during microrganism multiplication; bacteria resist penicillins by producing penicillinases — enzymes that convert penicillins to inactive penicilloic acid. Oxacillin resists these enzymes.

ONSET, PEAK, DURATION
Onset immediate after I.V. administration, unknown after I.M. injection. Peak serum levels occur immediately after I.V. administration, within ½ to 2 hours of oral dose, within 30 minutes of an I.M. dose. Duration unknown.

INDICATIONS & DOSAGE
Systemic infections caused by penicillinase-producing staphylococci —
Adults and children over 40 kg: 500 mg P.O. q 4 to 6 hours; or 2 to 12 g I.M. or I.V. daily, in divided doses q 4 to 6 hours.
Children 40 kg or less: 50 to 100 mg/ kg P.O. daily, in divided doses q 6 hours; or 100 to 200 mg/kg I.M. or I.V. daily, in divided doses q 4 to 6 hours.

ADVERSE REACTIONS
CNS: neuropathy, neuromuscular irritability, *seizures.*
GI: oral lesions.
GU: interstitial nephritis, transient hematuria, proteinuria.
Hematologic: granulocytopenia, thrombocytopenia, eosinophilia, *hemolytic anemia,* transient neutropenia.
Other: hypersensitivity reactions (fever, chills, rash, urticaria, *anaphylaxis*), overgrowth of nonsusceptible organisms, hepatitis, elevated liver enzymes, *thrombophlebitis.*

INTERACTIONS
Aminoglycosides: possible synergistic effect; monitor closely. Chemical and physical incompatibility; do not mix together in the same I.V. solution.
Probenecid: increased blood levels of oxacillin and other penicillins. Probenecid may be used for this purpose.
Rifampin: possible antagonism. Monitor closely.

CONTRAINDICATIONS
Contraindicated in patients with hypersensitivity to the drug or other penicillins.

NURSING CONSIDERATIONS
• Use cautiously in patients with other drug allergies, especially to cephalosporins (possible cross-sensitivity); in premature neonates; and in infants.
• Before giving, ask the patient about any allergic reactions to penicillin. However, a negative history of penicillin allergy is no guarantee against a future allergic reaction.
• Obtain specimen for culture and sensitivity tests before first dose. Therapy may begin pending results.
• **I.V. use:** For direct I.V. injection, reconstitute vials with sterile water for injection or 0.9% sodium chloride injection. Use 5 ml of diluent for a 250- or 500-mg vial, 10 ml of diluent

---

*Liquid form contains alcohol.
**May contain tartrazine.

Common reactions are in italics; *life-threatening,* in bold italics.

for a 1-g vial, 20 ml of diluent for a 2-g vial, or 40 ml of diluent for a 4-g vial. When the solution is clear, withdraw the ordered dose and inject over 10 minutes. When giving by piggyback injection, reconstitute the 1-g piggyback vial with 20 to 100 ml of diluent; reconstitute the 2-g vial with 19 to 99 ml of diluent. For intermittent infusion, further dilute the drug to a concentration of 5 to 40 mg/ml.

• To prevent vein irritation, avoid continuous infusions. Change site every 48 hours.

• Don't give I.M. or I.V. unless ordered and infection is severe or the patient can't take oral dose.

• Give 1 to 2 hours before or 2 to 3 hours after meals. When given orally, drug may cause GI disturbances. Food may interfere with absorption.

• Give oxacillin at least 1 hour before bacteriostatic antibiotics.

• Monitor periodic liver function studies; watch for elevated AST and ALT levels.

• Observe closely. With large doses and prolonged therapy, bacterial or fungal superinfection may occur, especially in elderly, debilitated, or immunosuppressed patients.

• Keep in mind that oxacillin may falsely elevate or cause false-positive results with certain tests for urine or serum proteins.

• Tell the patient to take entire quantity of medication exactly as prescribed, even after he feels better.

• Tell the patient to call the doctor if rash, fever, or chills develop. A rash is the most common allergic reaction.

penicillin G benzathine (benzylpenicillin benzathine)

Bicillin L-A, Permapen

Pregnancy Risk Category: B

HOW SUPPLIED
Injection: 300,000 units/ml, 600,000 units/ml

ACTION
A natural penicillin that inhibits cell-wall synthesis during microorganism multiplication; bacteria resist penicillins by producing penicillinases — enzymes that convert penicillins to inactive penicilloic acid.

ONSET, PEAK, DURATION
Onset unknown. Serum levels peak 13 to 24 hours after I.M. injection. Detectable in serum 1 to 4 weeks after I.M. injection.

INDICATIONS & DOSAGE
Congenital syphilis —
Children under 2 years: 50,000 units/kg I.M. as a single dose.
Group A streptococcal upper respiratory infections —
Adults: 1.2 million units I.M. as a single injection.
Children over 27 kg: 900,000 units I.M. as a single injection.
Children under 27 kg: 300,000 to 600,000 units I.M. as a single injection.
Prophylaxis of poststreptococcal rheumatic fever —
Adults and children: 1.2 million units I.M. once monthly or 600,000 units twice monthly.
Syphilis of less than 1 year's duration —
Adults: 2.4 million units I.M. as a single dose.
Syphilis of more than 1 year's duration —
Adults: 2.4 million units I.M. weekly for 3 successive weeks.

ADVERSE REACTIONS
CNS: neuropathy, *seizures* with high doses.
Hematologic: eosinophilia, hemolytic anemia, thrombocytopenia, leukopenia.

Other: hypersensitivity reactions (maculopapular and *exfoliative dermatitis*, chills, fever, edema, *anaphylaxis*), pain and sterile abscess at injection site.

INTERACTIONS
Aminoglycosides: physical and/or chemical incompatibility. Administer separately.
Colestipol: decreased serum concentrations of penicillin G benzathine. Administer penicillin G benzathine 1 hour before or 4 hours after colestipol.
Probenecid: increased blood levels of penicillin. Probenecid may be used for this purpose.

CONTRAINDICATIONS
Contraindicated in patients with hypersensitivity to the drug or other penicillins.

NURSING CONSIDERATIONS
• Use cautiously in patients with other drug allergies, especially to cephalosporins (possible cross-sensitivity).
• Before giving, ask the patient about any allergic reactions to penicillin. However, a negative history of penicillin allergy is no guarantee against a future allergic reaction.
• Obtain specimen for culture and sensitivity tests before first dose. Therapy may begin pending results.
• Shake medication well before injection.
• Never give I.V. — inadvertent I.V. administration has caused cardiac arrest and death.
• Inject deeply into upper outer quadrant of buttocks in adults; in midlateral thigh in infants and small children. Avoid injection into or near major nerves or blood vessels to prevent permanent neurovascular damage.
• Give penicillin G benzathine at least 1 hour before bacteriostatic antibiotics.

• Know that drug's extremely slow absorption time makes allergic reactions difficult to treat.
• Observe closely. With large doses and prolonged therapy, bacterial or fungal superinfection may occur, especially in elderly, debilitated, or immunosuppressed patients.
• Tell the patient to call the doctor if rash, fever, or chills develop. Fever and eosinophilia are the most common allergic reactions.

penicillin G potassium (benzylpenicillin potassium)
Megacillin†, Pfizerpen

Pregnancy Risk Category: B

HOW SUPPLIED
Tablets: 500,000 units†
Oral suspension: 250,000 units†, 500,000 units†
Injection: 1 million units, 5 million units, 10 million units, 20 million units

ACTION
A natural penicillin that inhibits cell-wall synthesis during microorganism multiplication; bacteria resist penicillins by producing penicillinases — enzymes that convert penicillins to inactive penicilloic acid.

ONSET, PEAK, DURATION
Onset immediate after I.V. infusion, unknown after I.M. injection. Peak serum levels occur immediately after I.V. infusion, within 15 to 30 minutes of I.M. injection, within ½ to 1 hour of oral dose. Duration unknown.

INDICATIONS & DOSAGE
Moderate to severe systemic infections —
Adults: highly individualized; 1.6 to 3.2 million units P.O. daily in divided doses q 6 hours; 1.2 to 24 million

---

*Liquid form contains alcohol.   *Common* reactions are in italics; *life-threatening*, in bold italics.
**May contain tartrazine.

units I.M. or I.V. daily in divided doses q 4 hours.

Children: 25,000 to 100,000 units/kg P.O. daily in divided doses q 6 hours; or 25,000 to 300,000 units/kg I.M. or I.V. daily in divided doses q 4 hours.

ADVERSE REACTIONS
CNS: neuropathy, *seizures* with high doses.
Hematologic: *hemolytic anemia,* leukopenia, thrombocytopenia.
Other: hypersensitivity reactions (rash, urticaria, maculopapular eruptions, *exfoliative dermatitis,* chills, fever, edema, *anaphylaxis*), overgrowth of nonsusceptible organisms, possible severe potassium poisoning with high doses (hyperreflexia, *seizures, coma*), thrombophlebitis, pain at injection site.

INTERACTIONS
Aminoglycosides: physical and/or chemical incompatibility. Administer separately.
Colestipol: decreased serum concentrations of penicillin G potassium. Administer penicillin G potassium 1 hour before or 4 hours after colestipol.
Potassium-sparing diuretics: possible increased risk of hyperkalemia. Do not use together.
Probenecid: increased blood levels of penicillin. Probenecid may be used for this purpose.

CONTRAINDICATIONS
Contraindicated in patients with hypersensitivity to the drug or other penicillins.

NURSING CONSIDERATIONS
• Use cautiously in patients with other drug allergies, especially to cephalosporins (possible cross-sensitivity).
• Before giving, ask the patient about any allergic reactions to penicillin. However, a negative history of penicillin allergy is no guarantee against a future allergic reaction.
• Obtain specimen for culture and sensitivity tests before first dose. Therapy may begin pending results.
• **I.V. use:** Reconstitute vials with sterile water for injection, D₅W, or 0.9% sodium chloride injection. Volume of diluent varies with manufacturer.
• Use a continuous I.V. infusion when large doses are required (10 million units or more). Otherwise, give via intermittent I.V. infusion over 1 to 2 hours.
• For I.M. injection, administer deeply into large muscle; may be extremely painful.
• Give 1 to 2 hours before or 2 to 3 hours after meals. When given orally, drug may cause GI disturbances. Food may interfere with absorption.
• Give penicillin G potassium at least 1 hour before bacteriostatic antibiotics.
• Monitor renal function closely. Patients with poor renal function are predisposed to high blood levels.
• Observe closely. With large doses and prolonged therapy, bacterial or fungal superinfection may occur, especially in elderly, debilitated, or immunosuppressed patients.
• Institute seizure precautions. Patients with high blood levels of this drug may develop seizures.
• Tell the patient to take entire amount of medication exactly as prescribed, even after he feels better.
• Warn the patient never to use leftover penicillin for a new illness or to share penicillin with family and friends.
• Tell the patient to call the doctor if rash, fever, or chills develop. A rash is the most common allergic reaction.

penicillin G procaine
(benzylpenicillin procaine)
Ayercillin†, Crysticillin-300 A.S.,
Pfizerpen-AS, Wycillin

Pregnancy Risk Category: B

HOW SUPPLIED
Injection: 300,000 units/ml, 500,000
units/ml, 600,000 units/ml

ACTION
A natural penicillin that inhibits cell-
wall synthesis during microorganism
multiplication; bacteria resist penicillins by producing penicillinases — enzymes that convert penicillins to inactive penicilloic acid.

ONSET, PEAK, DURATION
Onset unknown. Serum levels peak 1
to 4 hours after I.M. dose. Drug persists in serum for 1 to 2 days; after
high doses, for 5 days.

INDICATIONS & DOSAGE
*Moderate to severe systemic infec-
tions —*
Adults: 600,000 to 1.2 million units
I.M. daily in a single dose.
Children over 1 month: 25,000 to
50,000 units/kg I.M. daily in a single
dose.
Uncomplicated gonorrhea —
Adults and children over age 12: 1 g
probenecid; after 30 minutes, 4.8 mil-
lion units of penicillin G procaine
I.M., divided between two injection
sites.
Pneumococcal pneumonia —
Adults and children over age 12:
600,000 units to 1.2 million units
I.M. daily for 7 to 10 days.

ADVERSE REACTIONS
CNS: *seizures.*
Hematologic: thrombocytopenia, *hemolytic anemia,* leukopenia.
Other: arthralgia, hypersensitivity
reactions (rash, urticaria, chills, fever, edema, prostration, *anaphy-*

laxis), overgrowth of nonsusceptible
organisms.

INTERACTIONS
Aminoglycosides: physical and/or
chemical incompatibility. Administer
separately.
Colestipol: decreased serum concentrations of penicillin G procaine. Administer penicillin G procaine 1 hour
before or 4 hours after colestipol.
Probenecid: increased blood levels of
penicillin. Probenecid may be used
for this purpose.

CONTRAINDICATIONS
Contraindicated in patients with hypersensitivity to the drug or other
penicillins.

NURSING CONSIDERATIONS
• Use cautiously in patients with
other drug allergies, especially to
cephalosporins (possible cross-sensitivity). Some formulations contain
sulfites, which may cause allergic reactions in sensitive persons.
• Before giving, ask the patient about
any allergic reactions to penicillin.
However, a negative history of penicillin allergy is no guarantee against a
future allergic reaction.
• Obtain specimen for culture and
sensitivity tests before first dose.
Therapy may begin pending results.
• Give deep I.M. in upper outer
quadrant of buttocks in adults; in midlateral thigh in small children. Do not
give subcutaneously. Don't massage
injection site. Avoid injection near
major nerves or blood vessels to prevent permanent neurovascular damage.
• Never give I.V. — inadvertent I.V.
administration has caused death from
CNS toxicity caused by procaine.
• Give penicillin G procaine at least
1 hour before bacteriostatic antibiotics.
• Know that because of drug's slow

---

*Liquid form contains alcohol.   *Common* reactions are in italics; *life-threatening,* in bold italics.
**May contain tartrazine.

absorption rate, allergic reactions are hard to treat.
- Monitor renal and hematopoietic function periodically, as ordered.
- Observe closely. With large doses and prolonged therapy, bacterial or fungal superinfection may occur, especially in elderly, debilitated, or immunosuppressed patients.
- Tell the patient to call the doctor if rash, fever, or chills develop. A rash is the most common allergic reaction.

penicillin G sodium (benzylpenicillin sodium)
Crystapen†

Pregnancy Risk Category: B

HOW SUPPLIED
Injection: 5 million-units vial

ACTION
A natural penicillin that inhibits cell-wall synthesis during active multiplication; bacteria resist penicillins by producing penicillinases — enzymes that convert penicillins to inactive penicilloic acid.

ONSET, PEAK, DURATION
Onset immediate after I.V. administration, unknown after I.M. injection. Peak serum levels occur 15 to 30 minutes after I.M. injection, immediately after I.V. administration. Duration unknown.

INDICATIONS & DOSAGE
Moderate to severe systemic infections –
Adults: 1.2 to 24 million units daily I.M. or I.V. in divided doses q 4 to 6 hours.
Children: 25,000 to 300,000 units/kg daily I.M. or I.V. in divided doses q 4 to 6 hours.
Endocarditis prophylaxis for dental surgery –
Adults and children over 27 kg: 2 million units I.V. or I.M. 30 to 60 minutes before procedure; then 1 million units 6 hours later.

ADVERSE REACTIONS
CNS: neuropathy, *seizures.*
CV: *CHF* with high doses.
Hematologic: hemolytic anemia, leukopenia, thrombocytopenia.
Other: arthralgia, hypersensitivity reactions (*exfoliative dermatitis,* urticaria, *anaphylaxis*), overgrowth of nonsusceptible organisms, vein irritation, pain at injection site, thrombophlebitis.

INTERACTIONS
Aminoglycosides: physical and/or chemical incompatibility. Administer separately.
Colestipol: decreased serum concentrations of penicillin G sodium. Administer penicillin G sodium 1 hour before or 4 hours after colestipol.
Probenecid: increased blood levels of penicillin. Probenecid may be used for this purpose.

CONTRAINDICATIONS
- Contraindicated in patients with hypersensitivity to the drug or other penicillins and in patients on sodium-restricted diets.
- Use cautiously in patients with other drug allergies, especially to cephalosporins (possible cross-allergenicity).

NURSING CONSIDERATIONS
- Use cautiously in patients with other drug allergies, especially to cephalosporins (possible cross-allergenicity).
- Before giving, ask the patient about any allergic reactions to penicillin. However, a negative history of penicillin allergy is no guarantee against a future allergic reaction.
- Obtain specimen for culture and sensitivity tests before first dose. Therapy may begin pending results.
- **I.V. use:** Reconstitute vials with

sterile water for injection, 0.9% sodium chloride injection, or D₅W. Check manufacturer's instructions for volume of diluent necessary to produce desired drug concentration.
• For patients receiving 10 million units of drug or more daily, dilute in 1 to 2 liters of compatible solution and administer over 24 hours. Otherwise, give by intermittent I.V. infusion: Dilute drug in 50 to 100 ml and give over 1 to 2 hours q 4 to 6 hours.
• In neonates and children, give divided doses usually over 15 to 30 minutes.
• Give penicillin G sodium at least 1 hour before bacteriostatic antibiotics.
• Observe closely. With large doses and prolonged therapy, bacterial or fungal superinfection may occur, especially in elderly, debilitated, or immunosuppressed patients.
• Institute seizure precautions. Patients with high blood levels of this drug may develop seizures.

---

penicillin V
(phenoxymethyl penicillin)

penicillin V potassium
(phenoxymethylpenicillin potassium)
Abbocillin VK‡, Apo-Pen-VK†, Beepen-VK, Betapen-VK, Cilicane VK‡, Ledercillin VK, Nadopen-V-200†, Nadopen-V-400†, Nadopen-VK†, NovoPen-VK†, Nu-Pen VK†, Pen Vee, Pen Vee K, PVF K†, PVK‡, Robicillin VK, V-Cillin K, VC-K, Veetids**

Pregnancy Risk Category: B

HOW SUPPLIED
penicillin V
Tablets: 250 mg, 500 mg
Oral suspension: 125 mg/5 ml, 250 mg/5 ml (after reconstitution)
penicillin V potassium
Tablets: 125 mg, 250 mg, 500 mg
Tablets (film-coated): 250 mg, 500 mg

Capsules: 250 mg‡
Oral suspension: 125 mg/5 ml, 250 mg/5 ml (after reconstitution)

ACTION
A natural penicillin that inhibits cell-wall synthesis during microorganism multiplication; bacteria resist penicillins by producing penicillinases—enzymes that convert penicillins to inactive penicilloic acid.

ONSET, PEAK, DURATION
Onset and duration unknown. Serum levels peak within 30 to 60 minutes.

INDICATIONS & DOSAGE
Mild to moderate systemic infections—
Adults: 250 to 500 mg (400,000 to 800,000 units) P.O. q 6 hours.
Children: 15 to 50 mg/kg (25,000 to 90,000 units/kg) P.O. daily, in divided doses q 6 to 8 hours.
Endocarditis prophylaxis for dental surgery—
Adults: 2 g P.O. 30 to 60 minutes before procedure; then 1 g 6 hours afterward.
Children under 30 kg: half of the adult dose.

ADVERSE REACTIONS
CNS: neuropathy.
GI: *epigastric distress,* vomiting, diarrhea, *nausea.*
Hematologic: eosinophilia, hemolytic anemia, leukopenia, thrombocytopenia.
Other: hypersensitivity reactions (rash, urticaria, chills, fever, edema, **anaphylaxis**), overgrowth of nonsusceptible organisms.

INTERACTIONS
Oral contraceptives containing estrogen: decreased effectiveness of oral contraceptive. Monitor for breakthrough bleeding.
Probenecid: increased blood levels of penicillin. Probenecid may be used for this purpose.

---

*Liquid form contains alcohol.
**May contain tartrazine.
Common reactions are in italics; *life-threatening,* in bold italics.

CONTRAINDICATIONS

Contraindicated in patients with hypersensitivity to the drug or other penicillins.

NURSING CONSIDERATIONS

• Use cautiously in patients with other drug allergies, especially to cephalosporins (possible cross-sensitivity), or in those with GI disturbances.
• Before giving, ask the patient about any allergic reactions to penicillins. However, a negative history of penicillin allergy is no guarantee against a future allergic reaction.
• Obtain specimen for culture and sensitivity tests before first dose. Therapy may begin pending results.
• Give 1 to 2 hours before or 2 to 3 hours after meals. May cause GI disturbances. Food may interfere with absorption.
• Give penicillin V at least 1 hour before bacteriostatic antibiotics.
• As ordered, periodically assess renal and hematopoietic function in patients receiving long-term therapy.
• Observe closely. With large doses and prolonged therapy, bacterial or fungal superinfection may occur, especially in elderly, debilitated, or immunosuppressed patients.
• Be aware that The American Heart Association considers amoxicillin the preferred agent for endocarditis prophylaxis because GI absorption is better and serum levels are sustained longer. Penicillin V is considered an alternative agent.
• Tell the patient to take entire quantity of medication exactly as prescribed, even after he feels better.
• Tell the patient to take each dose with a full glass of water only because the acid in fruit juice or a carbonated beverage will inactivate the drug.
• Warn the patient never to use leftover penicillin for a new illness or to share penicillin with family and friends.

• Tell the patient to call the doctor if rash, fever, or chills develop. A rash is the most common allergic reaction.

---

piperacillin sodium
Pipracil, Pipril‡

Pregnancy Risk Category: B

HOW SUPPLIED
Injection: 2 g, 3 g, 4 g
Pharmacy bulk package: 40 g

ACTION
Extended-spectrum penicillin that inhibits cell-wall synthesis during microorganism multiplication; bacteria resist penicillins by producing penicillinases — enzymes that convert penicillins to inactive penicilloic acid.

ONSET, PEAK, DURATION
Onset immediate after I.V. administration, unknown after I.M. injection. Peak serum levels occur immediately after I.V. adminstration, within 30 to 50 minutes of I.M. dose. Duration unknown.

INDICATIONS & DOSAGE
Systemic infections caused by susceptible strains of gram-positive and especially gram-negative organisms (including Proteus *and* Pseudomonas aeruginosa)—
Adults and children over 12 years: 100 to 300 mg/kg daily in divided doses q 4 to 6 hours I.V. or I.M. Doses for children under 12 years not established.
Prophylaxis of surgical infections—
Adults: 2 g I.V., given 30 to 60 minutes before surgery. Dose may be repeated during surgery and once or twice more after surgery.

ADVERSE REACTIONS
CNS: neuromuscular irritability, *seizures,* headache, dizziness.
GI: nausea, diarrhea.
Hematologic: *bleeding with high*

---

doses, neutropenia, eosinophilia, leukopenia, *thrombocytopenia.*
Other: *hypokalemia,* hypersensitivity reactions (edema, fever, chills, rash, pruritus, urticaria, ***anaphylaxis***), overgrowth of nonsusceptible organisms, pain at injection site, vein irritation, phlebitis.

INTERACTIONS
Aminoglycoside antibiotics (such as gentamicin and tobramycin): chemically incompatible. Don't mix in the same I.V. container.
Probenecid: increased blood levels of piperacillin. Probenecid may be used for this purpose.

CONTRAINDICATIONS
Contraindicated in patients with hypersensitivity to the drug or other penicillins.

NURSING CONSIDERATIONS
• Use cautiously in patients with other drug allergies, especially to cephalosporins (possible cross-sensitivity), or in those with bleeding tendencies, uremia, and hypokalemia.
• Before giving, ask the patient about any allergic reactions to penicillin. However, a negative history of penicillin allergy is no guarantee against a future allergic reaction.
• Obtain specimen for culture and sensitivity tests before first dose. Therapy may begin pending results.
• **I.V. use:** Reconstitute each gram of drug with 5 ml of diluent, such as sterile or bacteriostatic water for injection, 0.9% sodium chloride injection (with or without preservative), D_5W, or dextrose 5% in 0.9% sodium chloride injection. Shake until dissolved. Inject reconstituted solution directly into a vein or into the tubing of a free-flowing I.V. solution over 3 to 5 minutes. Alternatively, dilute with at least 50 ml of a compatible I.V. solution and give by intermittent infusion over 30 minutes.

• Avoid continuous infusions to prevent vein irritation. Change site every 48 hours.
• For I.M. injection, reconstituted with sterile or bacteriostatic water for injection, 0.9% sodium chloride injection (with or without preservative), or 0.5% to 1% lidocaine hydrochloride. Add 2 ml of diluent for each gram of drug. Final solution will contain 1 g/2.5 ml.
• Give piperacillin at least 1 hour before bacteriostatic antibiotics.
• Check CBC and platelet counts frequently, as ordered. Drug may cause thrombocytopenia.
• Monitor serum potassium level.
• Institute seizure precautions. Patients with high serum levels of this drug may have seizures.
• Observe closely. With large doses and prolonged therapy, bacterial or fungal superinfection may occur, especially in elderly, debilitated, or immunosuppressed patients.
• Know that dosage should be altered in patients with impaired renal function.
• Be aware that cystic fibrosis patients tend to be most susceptible to fever or rash.
• Be aware that drug may be better suited for patients on sodium-free diets than ticarcillin (contains 1.85 mEq sodium/g of piperacillin).
• Keep in mind that piperacillin is typically used with another antibiotic, such as gentamicin.

---

piperacillin sodium and tazobactam sodium
Zosyn

Pregnancy Risk Category: B

HOW SUPPLIED
Powder for injection: 2 g piperacillin and 0.25 g tazobactam per vial, 3 g piperacillin and 0.375 g tazobactam per vial, 4 g piperacillin and 0.5 g tazobactam per vial

---

Pharmacy bulk package: 40.5 g

ACTION
Piperacillin is an extended-spectrum penicillin that inhibits cell-wall synthesis during microorganism multiplication; tazobactam increases piperacillin effectiveness by inactivating beta lactamases, which destroy penicillins.

ONSET, PEAK, DURATION
Onset immediate after I.V. infusion. Plasma levels peak immediately after I.V. infusion. Duration unknown.

INDICATIONS & DOSAGE
Appendicitis (complicated by rupture or abscess) and peritonitis caused by Escherichia coli, Bacteroides fragilis, B. ovatus, B. thetaiotaomicron, *or* B. vulgatus; *skin and skin structure infections caused by* Staphylococcus aureus; *postpartum endometritis or pelvic inflammatory disease caused by* E. coli; *moderately severe community-acquired pneumonia caused by* Haemophilus influenzae –
Adults: 3 g piperacillin and 0.375 g tazobactam I.V. q 6 hours.
In patients with renal impairment –
Adults: if creatinine clearance is 20 to 40 ml/minute, 2 g piperacillin and 0.25 g tazobactam I.V. q 6 hours. If creatinine clearance is below 20 ml/minute, 2 g piperacillin and 0.25 g tazobactam I.V. q 8 hours.

ADVERSE REACTIONS
CNS: *headache, insomnia,* agitation, dizziness, anxiety.
CV: hypertension, tachycardia, chest pain, edema.
EENT: rhinitis.
GI: *diarrhea, nausea, constipation,* vomiting, dyspepsia, stool changes, abdominal pain.
Respiratory: dyspnea.
Skin: rash (including maculopapular, bullous, urticarial, and eczematoid), pruritus.

Other: fever; pain; moniliasis; inflammation, phlebitis at I.V. site.

INTERACTIONS
Aminoglycoside antibiotics (such as gentamicin and tobramycin): chemically incompatible. Don't mix in the same I.V. container.
Probenecid: increased blood levels of piperacillin. Probenecid may be used for this purpose.
Vercuronium: prolongation of neuromuscular blockage. Monitor closely.

CONTRAINDICATIONS
Contraindicated in patients with hypersensitivity to the drug or other penicillins.

NURSING CONSIDERATIONS
● Use cautiously in patients with other drug allergies, especially to cephalosporins (possible cross-sensitivity), or in those with bleeding tendencies, uremia, and hypokalemia.
● Obtain specimen for culture and sensitivity tests before first dose. Therapy may begin pending results.
● **I.V. use:** Reconstitute each gram of piperacillin with 5 ml of diluent, such as sterile or bacteriostatic water for injection, 0.9% sodium chloride injection, bacteriostatic 0.9% sodium chloride injection, D_5W, dextrose 5% in 0.9% sodium chloride injection, or dextran 6% in 0.9% sodium chloride injection. Don't use lactated Ringer's injection. Shake until dissolved. Further dilute to a final volume of 50 ml before infusion.
● Infuse over at least 30 minutes. Discontinue any primary infusion during administration if possible. Don't mix with other drugs.
● Use drug immediately after reconstitution. Discard unused drug after 24 hours if held at room temperature; 48 hours if refrigerated. Once diluted, drug is stable in I.V. bags for 24 hours at room temperature or 1 week if refrigerated.

• Change I.V. site every 48 hours.
• Because hemodialysis removes 6% of the piperacillin dose and 21% of the tazobactam dose, be aware that supplemental doses may be needed after hemodialysis.
• With large doses and prolonged therapy, bacterial and fungal superinfection may occur, especially in elderly, debilitated, or immunosuppressed patients.

ticarcillin disodium
Ticar, Ticillin‡

Pregnancy Risk Category: NR

HOW SUPPLIED
Injection: 1 g, 3 g, 6 g
I.V. infusion: 3 g
Pharmacy bulk package: 20 g, 30 g

ACTION
An extended-spectrum penicillin that inhibits cell-wall synthesis during microorganism multiplication; bacteria resist penicillins by producing penicillinases — enzymes that convert penicillins to inactive penicilloic acid.

ONSET, PEAK, DURATION
Onset immediate after I.V. administration, unknown after I.M. injection. Peak serum levels occur immediately after I.V. administration, within 30 to 75 minutes of I.M. injection. Duration unknown.

INDICATIONS & DOSAGE
Severe systemic infections caused by susceptible strains of gram-positive and especially gram-negative organisms (including Pseudomonas *and* Proteus) —
Adults: 18 g I.V. or I.M. daily, in divided doses q 4 to 6 hours.
Children: 50 to 300 mg/kg I.V. or I.M. daily, in divided doses q 4 to 6 hours.

ADVERSE REACTIONS
CNS: *seizures,* neuromuscular excitability.
GI: nausea, diarrhea.
Hematologic: leukopenia, neutropenia, eosinophilia, *thrombocytopenia,* hemolytic anemia.
Other: hypersensitivity reactions (rash, pruritus, urticaria, chills, fever, edema, ***anaphylaxis***), overgrowth of nonsusceptible organisms, hypokalemia, pain at injection site, vein irritation, phlebitis.

INTERACTIONS
Aminoglycoside antibiotics (such as gentamicin and tobramycin): chemically incompatible. Don't mix in the same I.V. container.
Lithium: altered renal elimination of lithium. Monitor serum lithium levels closely.
Probenecid: increased blood levels of ticarcillin and other penicillins. Probenecid may be used for this purpose.

CONTRAINDICATIONS
Contraindicated in patients with hypersensitivity to the drug or other penicillins.

NURSING CONSIDERATIONS
• Use cautiously in patients with other drug allergies, especially to cephalosporins (possible cross-sensitivity), or in those with impaired renal function, hemorrhagic conditions, hypokalemia, or sodium restrictions (contains 5.2 to 6.5 mEq sodium/g).
• Before giving, ask the patient about any allergic reactions to penicillin. However, a negative history of penicillin allergy is no guarantee against a future allergic reaction.
• Obtain specimen for culture and sensitivity tests before first dose. Therapy may begin pending results.
• **I.V. use:** Reconstitute vials using D_5W, 0.9% sodium chloride injection, sterile water for injection, or other compatible solution. Add 4 ml of dilu-

---

*Liquid form contains alcohol.
**May contain tartrazine.

Common reactions are in italics; ***life-threatening,*** in bold italics.

ent for each gram of drug. Further dilute to a maximum concentration of 50 mg/ml and inject slowly directly into a vein or into the tubing of a free-flowing I.V. solution. Alternatively, dilute to a concentration of 10 to 100 mg/ml and give by intermittent infusion over 30 to 120 minutes in adults or 10 to 20 minutes in neonates.

• Avoid continuous infusion to prevent vein irritation. Change site every 48 hours.

• For I.M. injection, reconstitute vials using sterile water for injection, 0.9% sodium chloride injection, or lidocaine 1% (without epinephrine). Use 2 ml diluent for each gram of drug. Administer deep I.M. into large muscle. Don't exceed 2 g per injection.

• Give ticarcillin at least 1 hour before bacteriostatic antibiotics.

• Monitor serum potassium.

• Check CBC and platelet counts frequently, as ordered. Drug may cause thrombocytopenia.

• Institute seizure precautions. Patients with high blood levels of ticarcillin may develop seizures.

• Be aware that ticarcillin is typically used with another antibiotic, such as gentamicin.

• Observe closely. With large doses and prolonged therapy, bacterial or fungal superinfection may occur, especially in elderly, debilitated, or immunosuppressed patients.

• Know that dosage should be decreased in patients with impaired renal function.

ticarcillin disodium/ clavulanate potassium

Timentin

Pregnancy Risk Category: B

HOW SUPPLIED
Injection: 3 g ticarcillin and 100 mg clavulanic acid
Pharmacy bulk package: 31 g

ACTION
Ticarcillin is an extended-spectrum penicillin that inhibits cell-wall synthesis during microorganism replication; clavulanic acid increases ticarcillin's effectiveness by inactivating beta lactamases, which destroy ticarcillin.

ONSET, PEAK, DURATION
Onset immediate after I.V. infusion. Peak serum levels occur immediately after I.V. infusion. Duration unknown.

INDICATIONS & DOSAGE
Lower respiratory tract, urinary tract, bone and joint, and skin and skin structure infections and septicemia when caused by beta-lacta-mase-producing strains of bacteria or by ticarcillin-susceptible organisms—
Adults: 3.1 g (3 g ticarcillin and 100 mg clavulanate acid) administered by I.V. infusion q 4 to 6 hours.

ADVERSE REACTIONS
CNS: *seizures,* neuromuscular excitability.
GI: nausea, diarrhea.
Hematologic: leukopenia, neutropenia, eosinophilia, *thrombocytopenia,* hemolytic anemia.
Other: hypersensitivity reactions (rash, pruritus, urticaria, chills, fever, edema, ***anaphylaxis***), overgrowth of nonsusceptible organisms, hypokalemia, pain at injection site, vein irritation, phlebitis.

INTERACTIONS
Aminoglycoside antibiotics (such as gentamicin and tobramycin): chemically incompatible. Don't mix in the same I.V. container.
Probenecid: increased blood levels of ticarcillin. Probenecid may be used for this purpose.

CONTRAINDICATIONS

Contraindicated in patients with hypersensitivity to the drug or other penicillins.

NURSING CONSIDERATIONS

• Use cautiously in patients with other drug allergies, especially to cephalosporins (possible cross-sensitivity), and in those with impaired renal function, hemorrhagic condition, hypokalemia, or sodium restrictions (contains 4.5 mEq sodium/g).

• Before giving, ask the patient about any allergic reactions to penicillin. However, a negative history of penicillin allergy is no guarantee against a future allergic reaction.

• Obtain specimen for culture and sensitivity tests before first dose. Therapy may begin pending results.

• **I.V. use:** Reconstitute drug with 13 ml of sterile water for injection or 0.9% sodium chloride injection. Further dilute to a maximum of 10 to 100 mg/ml (based on ticarcillin component) and administer by I.V. infusion over 30 minutes. In fluid-restricted patients, dilute to a maximum of $48 - g$/ml if using D_5W, 43 mg/ml if using 0.9% sodium chloride injection, or 86 mg/ml if using sterile water for injection.

• Give drug at least 1 hour before bacteriostatic antibiotics.

• Check CBC and platelet counts frequently, as ordered. Drug may cause thrombocytopenia.

• Observe closely. With large doses and prolonged therapy, bacterial or fungal superinfection may occur, especially in elderly, debilitated, or immunosuppressed patients.

• Know that dosage should be decreased in patients with impaired renal function.

---

*Liquid form contains alcohol.   *Common* reactions are in italics; ***life-threatening***, in bold italics.
**May contain tartrazine.

Cephalosporins

cefaclor
cefadroxil monohydrate
cefamandole nafate
cefazolin sodium
cefixime
cefmetazole sodium
cefonicid sodium
cefoperazone sodium
cefotaxime sodium
cefotetan disodium
cefoxitin sodium
cefpodoxime proxetil
cefprozil
ceftazidime
ceftizoxime sodium
ceftriaxone sodium
cefuroxime axetil
cefuroxime sodium
cephalexin hydrochloride
cephalexin monohydrate
cephalothin sodium
cephapirin sodium
cephradine
loracarbef

COMBINATION PRODUCTS
None.

cefaclor
Ceclor

Pregnancy Risk Category: B

HOW SUPPLIED
Capsules: 250 mg, 500 mg
Oral suspension: 125 mg/5 ml, 250 mg/5 ml, 187 mg/5 ml, 375 mg/5 ml

ACTION
A second-generation cephalosporin that inhibits cell-wall synthesis, promoting osmotic instability; usually bactericidal.

ONSET, PEAK, DURATION
Onset and duration unknown. Peak levels occur within 30 to 60 minutes.

INDICATIONS & DOSAGE
Respiratory or urinary tract, skin, and soft-tissue infections and otitis media caused by Haemophilus influenzae, Streptococcus pneumoniae, S. pyogenes, Escherichia coli, Proteus mirabilis, Klebsiella *species, and staphylococci*—
Adults: 250 to 500 mg P.O. q 8 hours. For pharyngitis or otitis media, daily dosage may be given in two equally divided doses q 12 hours.
Children: 20 mg/kg daily P.O. in divided doses q 8 hours. For pharyngitis or otitis media, daily dosage may be given in two equally divided doses q 12 hours. In more serious infections, 40 mg/kg daily are recommended, not to exceed 1 g daily.

ADVERSE REACTIONS
CNS: dizziness, headache, somnolence, malaise.
GI: *nausea,* vomiting, *diarrhea,* anorexia, dyspepsia, abdominal cramps, pseudomembranous colitis, oral candidiasis.
GU: red and white cells in urine, vaginal moniliasis, vaginitis.
Hematologic: transient leukopenia, lymphocytosis, anemia, eosinophilia.
Skin: *maculopapular rash,* dermatitis.
Other: hypersensitivity reactions (serum sickness, *anaphylaxis*), fever, transient increases in liver enzymes.

INTERACTIONS
Chloramphenicol: antagonistic effect. Do not use together.
Probenecid: may inhibit excretion and increase blood levels of cefaclor.

CONTRAINDICATIONS
Contraindicated in patients with hypersensitivity to other cephalosporins.

NURSING CONSIDERATIONS
• Use cautiously in patients with impaired renal function or a history of sensitivity to penicillin.
• Obtain specimen for culture and sensitivity tests before first dose. Therapy may begin pending test results.
• With large doses or prolonged therapy, monitor for superinfection, especially in high-risk patients.
• Store reconstituted suspension in refrigerator. Stable for 14 days if refrigerated. Shake well before using.
• Keep in mind that from 40% to 75% of patients receiving cephalosporins show a false-positive direct Coombs' test.
• Be aware that urine glucose determinations may be false-positive with copper sulfate tests (Clinitest); glucose enzymatic tests (Clinistix, Tes-Tape) are not affected.
• Tell patient that drug may be taken with meals.
• Tell the patient to take entire amount of medication exactly as prescribed, even after he feels better.
• Tell patient to call the doctor if skin rash develops.

---

cefadroxil monohydrate
Duricef, Ultracef

Pregnancy Risk Category: B

HOW SUPPLIED
Tablets: 1 g
Capsules: 500 mg
Oral suspension: 125 mg/5 ml, 250 mg/5 ml, 500 mg/5 ml

ACTION
A first-generation cephalosporin that inhibits cell-wall synthesis, promoting osmotic instability; usually bactericidal.

ONSET, PEAK, DURATION
Onset and duration unknown. Serum levels peak within 1 to 2 hours after an oral dose.

INDICATIONS & DOSAGE
Urinary tract infections caused by Escherichia coli, Proteus mirabilis, *and* Klebsiella *species; skin and soft-tissue infections; and streptococcal pharyngitis* —
Adults: 500 mg to 2 g P.O. daily, depending on infection being treated. Usually given once daily or b.i.d.
Children: 30 mg/kg P.O. daily in two divided doses.

ADVERSE REACTIONS
CNS: dizziness, headache, malaise, paresthesia.
GI: pseudomembranous colitis, *nausea,* anorexia, vomiting, *diarrhea,* glossitis, *dyspepsia,* abdominal cramps, anal pruritus, tenesmus, oral candidiasis.
GU: genital pruritus, moniliasis.
Hematologic: transient neutropenia, eosinophilia, leukopenia, anemia.
Skin: *maculopapular and erythematous rashes.*
Other: hypersensitivity reactions (serum sickness, ***anaphylaxis***), transient increases in liver enzymes, dyspnea.

INTERACTIONS
Probenecid: may inhibit excretion and increase blood levels of cefadroxil.

CONTRAINDICATIONS
Contraindicated in patients with hypersensitivity to the drug or other cephalosporins.

NURSING CONSIDERATIONS
• Use cautiously in patients with a history of sensitivity to penicillin. Also use cautiously in patients with impaired renal function; dosage adjustments may be necessary.
• Obtain specimen for culture and

---

*Liquid form contains alcohol.   *Common* reactions are in italics; ***life-threatening,*** in bold italics.
**May contain tartrazine.

sensitivity tests before first dose. Therapy may begin pending test results.

• With large doses or prolonged therapy, monitor for superinfection, especially in high-risk patients.

• Know that the drug's longer half-life permits once- or twice-daily dosing.

• Keep in mind from 40% to 75% of patients receiving cephalosporins show a false-positive direct Coombs' test.

• Be aware that urine glucose determinations may be false-positive with copper sulfate tests (Clinitest); glucose enzymatic tests (Clinistix, Tes-Tape) are not affected.

• Be aware that if creatinine clearance is below 50 ml/minute, dosage interval should be lengthened so drug doesn't accumulate.

• Because absorption is not delayed by presence of food, tell the patient to take with food or milk to lessen GI discomfort.

• Tell the patient to take entire amount of medication exactly as prescribed, even after he feels better.

• Advise the patient to call the doctor if skin rash develops.

---

cefamandole nafate
Mandol

Pregnancy Risk Category: B

HOW SUPPLIED
Injection: 1 g, 2 g
Pharmacy bulk package: 10 g

ACTION
A second-generation cephalosporin that inhibits cell-wall synthesis, promoting osmotic instability; usually bactericidal.

ONSET, PEAK, DURATION
Onset immediate after I.V. adminstration, unknown after I.M. injection. Peak serum levels occur 30 minutes to 2 hours after I.M. injection, immediately after I.V. administration. Duration unknown.

INDICATIONS & DOSAGE
Perioperative prophylaxis in contaminated surgery —
Adults: 1 to 2 g I.M. or I.V. 30 to 60 minutes before surgery; then 1 to 2 g I.M. or I.V. q 6 hours for 24 hours.
Children 3 months and older: 12.5 to 25 mg/kg I.M. or I.V. 30 to 60 minutes before surgery; then 12.5 to 25 mg/kg I.M. or I.V. q 6 hours for 24 hours.
Note: In cases where infection could be devastating, prophylaxis may be continued for 3 days.
Serious infections of respiratory and GU tracts; skin, soft-tissue, bone, and joint infections; septicemia; and peritonitis caused by Escherichia coli *and other coliform bacteria,* Staphylococcus aureus *(penicillinase- and non-penicillinase-producing),* S. epidermidis, *group A beta-hemolytic streptococci,* Klebsiella, Haemophilus influenzae, Proteus mirabilis, *and* Enterobacter —
Adults: 500 mg to 1 g q 4 to 8 hours. In life-threatening infections, up to 2 g q 4 hours may be needed.
Infants and children: 50 to 100 mg/kg daily in equally divided doses q 4 to 8 hours. May be increased to total daily dosage of 150 mg/kg, not to exceed maximum adult dosage.

ADVERSE REACTIONS
CNS: headache, malaise, paresthesia, dizziness.
GI: pseudomembranous colitis, nausea, anorexia, vomiting, *diarrhea,* glossitis, dyspepsia, abdominal cramps, tenesmus, anal pruritus, oral candidiasis.
GU: genital pruritus and moniliasis.
Hematologic: transient neutropenia, eosinophilia, hemolytic anemia, *hypoprothrombinemia,* bleeding.

---

† Available in Canada only.   ‡ Available in Australia only.   ◇ Available OTC.

Skin: *maculopapular and erythematous rashes, urticaria.*
Other: hypersensitivity reactions (serum sickness, ***anaphylaxis***); transient increases in liver enzymes; dyspnea; at injection site — *pain, induration, sterile abscesses,* temperature elevation, tissue sloughing; with I.V. injection — *phlebitis, thrombophlebitis.*

INTERACTIONS
Aminoglycosides: incompatible when mixed together. Administer at a different site.
Aspirin, oral anticoagulants: increased risk of bleeding. Monitor for bleeding.
Ethanol: possible disulfiram-like reaction. Warn patient not to drink alcohol for several days after discontinuing cefamandole.
Probenecid: may inhibit excretion and increase serum levels of cefamandole. Sometimes used for this effect.

CONTRAINDICATIONS
Contraindicated in patients with hypersensitivity to the drug or other cephalosporins.

NURSING CONSIDERATIONS
• Use cautiously in patients with a history of sensitivity to penicillin. Also use cautiously and with dosage adjustments in patients with renal failure.
• Obtain specimen for culture and sensitivity tests before first dose. Therapy may begin pending test results.
• **I.V. use:** Reconstitute 1 g with 10 ml of sterile water for injection, D_5W, or 0.9% sodium chloride for injection. To give by direct injection, inject into a large vein or into the tubing of a free-flowing I.V. solution over 3 to 5 minutes. If using sterile water, dilute to 20 ml to avoid giving a hypertonic solution.
• After reconstitution, remember that drug is stable for 24 hours at room temperature; for 96 hours under refrigeration.
• For intermittent injection, dilute to 100 ml using a compatible solution.
• Don't mix with I.V. infusions containing calcium ions (chemically incompatible).
• For I.M. administration, inject deeply into a large muscle mass, such as the gluteus maximus or the lateral aspect of the thigh. I.M. cefamandole is not as painful as I.M. cefoxitin and doesn't require addition of lidocaine.
• With large doses or prolonged therapy, monitor for superinfection, especially in high-risk patients.
• Monitor for signs of bleeding. The chemical structure of this drug includes the methylthiotetrazole side chain that has been associated with bleeding disorders. Vitamin K can promptly reverse bleeding if it occurs.
• Be aware that drug is not as effective as cefoxitin in treating anaerobic infections. Cefamandole offers little advantage over previously available drugs.
• Know that from 40% to 75% of patients receiving cephalosporins show a false-positive direct Coombs' test.
• Keep in mind that urine glucose determinations may be false-positive with copper sulfate tests (Clinitest); glucose enzymatic tests (Clinistix, Tes-Tape) are not affected.

cefazolin sodium
Ancef, Kefzol, Zolicef
Pregnancy Risk Category: B

HOW SUPPLIED
Injection (parenteral): 500 mg, 1 g
Infusion: 500 mg/50 ml vial, 500 mg/ 100 ml vial
Pharmacy bulk package: 5 g, 10 g, 20 g

ACTION
A first-generation cephalosporin that inhibits cell-wall synthesis, promot-

---

*Liquid form contains alcohol.   *Common* reactions are in italics; **life-threatening**, in bold italics.
**May contain tartrazine.

ing osmotic instability; usually bactericidal.

ONSET, PEAK, DURATION
Onset immediate after I.V. administration, unknown after I.M. injection. Plasma levels peak within 1 to 2 hours after I.M. injection, immediately after I.V. adminstration. Duration unknown.

INDICATIONS & DOSAGE
Perioperative prophylaxis in contaminated surgery –
Adults: 1 g I.M. or I.V. 30 to 60 minutes before surgery; then 0.5 to 1 g I.M. or I.V. q 6 to 8 hours for 24 hours. In long operations (> 2 hours), another 0.5 to 1 g dose may be administered intraoperatively.
Note: In cases where infection would be devastating, prophylaxis may be continued for 3 to 5 days.
Serious infections of respiratory, biliary, and GU tracts; skin, soft-tissue, bone, and joint infections; septicemia; and endocarditis caused by Escherichia coli, *Enterobacteriaceae, gonococci,* Haemophilus influenzae, Klebsiella, Proteus mirabilis, Staphylococcus aureus, Streptococcus pneumoniae, *and group A beta-hemolytic streptococci* –
Adults: 250 mg I.M. or I.V. q 8 hours to 1.5 g q 6 hours. Maximum 12 g/ day in life-threatening situations.
Children over 1 month: 25 to 50 mg/ kg or 1.25 g/m^2 daily I.M. or I.V. in three or four divided doses. In severe infections, dosage may be increased to 100 mg/kg/day.

ADVERSE REACTIONS
CNS: dizziness, headache, malaise, paresthesia.
GI: pseudomembranous colitis, nausea, anorexia, vomiting, *diarrhea,* glossitis, dyspepsia, abdominal cramps, anal pruritus, tenesmus, oral candidiasis.
GU: genital pruritus and moniliasis, vaginitis.
Hematologic: transient neutropenia, leukopenia, eosinophilia, anemia.
Skin: *maculopapular and erythematous rashes, urticaria.*
Other: hypersensitivity reactions (serum sickness, **anaphylaxis**); transient increases in liver enzymes; dyspnea; at injection site —*pain, induration, sterile abscesses, tissue sloughing;* with I.V. injection —*phlebitis, thrombophlebitis.*

INTERACTIONS
Probenecid: may inhibit excretion and increase blood levels of cefazolin.

CONTRAINDICATIONS
Contraindicated in patients with hypersensitivity to other cephalosporins.

NURSING CONSIDERATIONS
● Use cautiously in patients with a history of sensitivity to penicillin. Also use cautiously and with dosage adjustments in patients with renal failure.
● Obtain specimen for culture and sensitivity tests before first dose. Therapy may begin pending test results.
● **I.V. use:** Reconstitute with sterile water, bacteriostatic water, or 0.9% sodium chloride solution as follows: 2 ml to 500-mg vial; 2.5 ml to 1-g vial. Shake well until dissolved. Resultant concentration: 225 mg/ml or 330 mg/ml, respectively.
● Know that reconstituted cefazolin is stable for 24 hours at room temperature or 96 hours under refrigeration.
● For direct injection, further dilute Ancef with 5 ml or Kefzol with 10 ml, of sterile water for injection. Inject into a large vein or into the tubing of a free-flowing I.V. solution over 3 to 5 minutes. For intermittent infusion, add reconstituted drug to 50 to 100 ml of compatible solution or use premixed solution. Commercially avail-

---

†Available in Canada only. ‡Available in Australia only. ◇Available OTC.

able frozen solutions of cefazolin in
D_5W should be given only by intermittent or continuous I.V. infusion.
• Alternate injection sites if I.V. therapy lasts longer than 3 days. Use of
small I.V. needles in the larger available veins may be preferable.
• After reconstitution, inject I.M.
drug without further dilution. Not as
painful as other cephalosporins. Injection should be given deeply into a
large muscle mass, such as the gluteus
maximus or the lateral aspect of the
thigh.
• With large doses or prolonged therapy, monitor for superinfection, especially in high-risk patients.
• Be aware that dose and dosing interval will be adjusted if creatinine
clearance is below 55 ml/minute.
• Know that because of long duration
of effect, most infections can be
treated with a dose q 8 hours.
• Keep in mind that from 40% to 75%
of patients receiving cephalosporins
show a false-positive direct Coombs'
test.
• Be aware that urine glucose determinations may be false-positive with
copper sulfate tests (Clinitest); glucose enzymatic tests (Clinistix, Tes-
Tape) are not affected.

cefixime
Suprax

Pregnancy Risk Category: B

HOW SUPPLIED
Tablets: 200 mg, 400 mg
Oral suspension: 100 mg/5 ml (after
reconstitution)

ACTION
A third-generation cephalosporin that
inhibits cell-wall synthesis, promoting osmotic instability; usually bactericidal.

ONSET, PEAK, DURATION
Onset and duration unknown. Serum
levels peak within 3.1 to 4.4 hours after an oral dose. Peak serum concentrations are approximately 15% to
50% higher when administered as oral
suspension rather than tablets.

INDICATIONS & DOSAGE
*Uncomplicated urinary tract infec-
tions caused by* Escherichia coli *and*
Proteus mirabilis; *otitis media caused
by* Haemophilus influenzae *(beta-lactamase positive and negative strains),*
Moraxella (Branhamella) catarrhalis,
and Streptococcus pyogenes; *pharyngitis and tonsillitis caused by* S. pyogenes; *acute bronchitis and acute exacerbations of chronic bronchitis
caused by* S. pneumoniae *and* H. influenzae *(beta-lactamase positive and
negative strains)* –
**Adults and children over 12 years or
weighing over 50 kg:** 400 mg/day
P.O. as a single 400-mg tablet or 200
mg q 12 hours.
**Children 12 years and younger or
weighing 50 kg or less:** 8 mg/kg/day
suspension P.O. as a single daily dose
or 4 mg/kg q 12 hours.
Uncomplicated gonorrhea caused by
Neisseria gonorrhoeae –
Adults: 400 mg P.O. as a single dose.

ADVERSE REACTIONS
CNS: headaches, dizziness, nervousness, malaise, fatigue, somnolence,
insomnia.
GI: *diarrhea,* loose stools, abdominal
pain, nausea, vomiting, dyspepsia,
flatulence, pseudomembranous colitis.
GU: genital pruritus, vaginitis, genital candidiasis, transient increases in
BUN and serum creatinine levels.
Hematologic: thrombocytopenia,
leukopenia, eosinophilia.
Skin: pruritus, rash, urticaria.
Other: drug fever, transient increases
in liver enzymes, hypersensitivity re-

---

*Liquid form contains alcohol.   *Common* reactions are in italics; ***life-threatening***, in bold italics.
**May contain tartrazine.

actions (serum sickness, *anaphylaxis*).

INTERACTIONS
Probenecid: may inhibit excretion and increase blood levels of cefixime.
Salicylates: may displace cefixime from plasma protein-binding sites. Clinical significance is unknown.

CONTRAINDICATIONS
Contraindicated in patients with hypersensitivity to the drug or other cephalosporins.

NURSING CONSIDERATIONS
• Use cautiously and with reduced dosage in patients with renal dysfunction; reduced dosage is necessary in patients with creatinine clearance below 60 ml/minute. Also use cautiously in patients with a history of sensitivity to penicillin.
• Obtain specimen for culture and sensitivity tests before first dose. Therapy may begin pending test results.
• To prepare oral suspension: add required amount of water to powder in two portions. Shake well after each addition. After mixing, suspension is stable for 14 days. No need to refrigerate, but keep tightly closed. Shake well before using.
• With large doses or prolonged therapy, monitor for superinfection, especially in high-risk patients.
• Know that from 40% to 75% of patients receiving cephalosporins show a false-positive direct Coombs' test.
• Keep in mind that urine glucose determinations may be false-positive with copper sulfate tests (Clinitest); glucose enzymatic tests (Clinistix, Tes-Tape) are not affected.
• Tell the patient to take all of the medication prescribed, even after he feels better.
• Tell the patient to call the doctor if skin rash develops.

cefmetazole sodium (cefmetazone)
Zefazone

Pregnancy Risk Category: B

HOW SUPPLIED
Injection: 1 g, 2 g

ACTION
A semisynthetic cephamycin antibiotic pharmacologically similar to second-generation cephalosporins that inhibits cell-wall synthesis, promoting osmotic instability; usually bactericidal.

ONSET, PEAK, DURATION
Onset and duration unknown. Plasma levels peak immediately after I.V. administration.

INDICATIONS & DOSAGE
Lower respiratory tract infections caused by Streptococcus pneumoniae, Staphylococcus aureus *(penicillinase- and non-penicillinase-producing strains),* Escherichia coli, *and* Haemophilus influenzae *(non-penicillinase-producing strains); intra-abdominal infections caused by* E. coli *or* Bacteroides fragilis; *skin and skin-structure infections caused by* S. aureus *(penicillinase- and non-penicillinase-producing strains),* Staph. epidermidis, Streptococcus pyogenes, Strep. agalactiae, E. coli, Proteus mirabilis, Klebsiella pneumoniae, *and* B. fragilis —
Adults: 2 g I.V. q 6 to 12 hours for 5 to 14 days.
Urinary tract infections caused by E. coli —
Adults: 2 g I.V. q 12 hours.
Prophylaxis in patients undergoing vaginal hysterectomy —
Adults: 2 g I.V. 30 to 90 minutes before surgery as a single dose; or 1 g I.V. 30 to 90 minutes before surgery, repeated in 8 and 16 hours.

---

†Available in Canada only.   ‡Available in Australia only.   ◊Available OTC.

Prophylaxis in patients undergoing abdominal hysterectomy—
Adults: 1 g I.V. 30 to 90 minutes before surgery, repeated in 8 and 16 hours.
Prophylaxis in patients undergoing cesarean section—
Adults: 2 g I.V. as a single dose after clamping cord; or 1 g I.V. after clamping cord, repeated in 8 and 16 hours.
Prophylaxis in patients undergoing colorectal surgery—
Adults: 2 g I.V. as a single dose 30 to 90 minutes before surgery. Some clinicians follow with additional 2-g doses in 8 and 16 hours.
Prophylaxis in patients undergoing cholecystectomy (high risk)—
Adults: 1 g I.V. 30 to 90 minutes before surgery, repeated in 8 and 16 hours.

ADVERSE REACTIONS
CNS: headache.
CV: *shock,* hypotension.
EENT: epistaxis.
GI: nausea, vomiting, *diarrhea,* epigastric pain, pseudomembranous colitis.
GU: vaginitis.
Respiratory: pleural effusion, dyspnea, respiratory distress.
Skin: rash, pruritus, generalized erythema.
Other: fever, bacterial or fungal superinfection, hypersensitivity reactions (serum sickness, ***anaphylaxis***), altered color perception, pain at injection site, phlebitis.

INTERACTIONS
Aminoglycosides: potential increased risk of nephrotoxicity. Monitor closely.
Ethanol: possible disulfiram-like reaction. Should be avoided for 24 hours before and after administration of cefmetazole.
Probenecid: may inhibit excretion and

increase blood levels of cefmetazole. Sometimes used for this effect.

CONTRAINDICATIONS
Contraindicated in patients with hypersensitivity to the drug or other cephalosporins.

NURSING CONSIDERATIONS
• Use cautiously in patients with a history of sensitivity to penicillin.
• Obtain specimen for culture and sensitivity tests before first dose. Therapy may begin pending test results.
• **I.V. use:** Reconstitute with bacteriostatic water for injection, sterile water for injection, or 0.9% sodium chloride injection. After reconstitution, drug may be further diluted to concentrations ranging from 1 to 20 mg/ml by adding it to 0.9% sodium chloride injection, D_5W, or lactated Ringer's injection. Reconstituted or dilute solutions are stable for 24 hours at room temperature (77° F [25° C]) or 1 week if refrigerated at 46° F (8° C).
• Monitor patient for bacterial and fungal superinfections. Prolonged use may result in overgrowth of nonsusceptible organisms.
• Monitor PT and administer vitamin K as ordered. The chemical structure of this drug includes the methylthiotetrazole side chain that has been associated with bleeding disorders. However, such bleeding has not been reported with this drug.
• Know that from 40% to 75% of patients receiving cephalosporins show a false-positive direct Coombs' test.
• Keep in mind that urine glucose determinations may be false-positive with copper sulfate tests (Clinitest); glucose enzymatic tests (Clinistix, Tes-Tape) are not affected.

---

*Liquid form contains alcohol.   *Common* reactions are in italics; *life-threatening,* in bold italics.
**May contain tartrazine.

cefonicid sodium
Monocid

Pregnancy Risk Category: B

HOW SUPPLIED
Injection: 500 mg, 1 g
Infusion: 1 g/100 ml
Pharmacy bulk package: 10 g

ACTION
A second-generation cephalosporin that inhibits cell-wall synthesis, promoting osmotic instability; usually bactericidal.

ONSET, PEAK, DURATION
Onset immediate after I.V. administration, unknown after I.M. injection. Plasma levels peak within 1 to 2 hours after I.M. injection, immediately after I.V. administration. Duration unknown.

INDICATIONS & DOSAGE
Perioperative prophylaxis in contaminated surgery –
Adults: 1 g I.M. or I.V. 30 to 60 minutes before surgery; then 1 g I.M. or I.V. daily for 2 days after surgery.
Serious infections of the lower respiratory and urinary tracts, skin and skin-structure infections, septicemia, bone and joint infections, and perioperative prophylaxis. Susceptible microorganisms include Streptococcus pneumoniae, Klebsiella pneumoniae, Escherichia coli, Haemophilus influenzae, Proteus mirabilis, Staphylococcus aureus, Staph. epidermidis, *and* Strep. pyogenes –
Adults: usual dosage is 1 g I.V. or I.M. q 24 hours. In life-threatening infections, 2 g q 24 hours.

ADVERSE REACTIONS
CNS: dizziness, headache, malaise, paresthesia.
GI: pseudomembranous colitis, nausea, anorexia, vomiting, diarrhea, glossitis, dyspepsia, abdominal cramps, anal pruritus, tenesmus, oral candidiasis.
GU: genital pruritus and moniliasis, vaginitis.
Hematologic: transient neutropenia, leukopenia, eosinophilia, anemia.
Skin: *maculopapular and erythematous rashes, urticaria.*
Other: dyspnea; hypersensitivity reactions (serum sickness, **anaphylaxis**); at injection site – *pain, induration, sterile abscesses, tissue sloughing;* with I.V. injection – *phlebitis, thrombophlebitis.*

INTERACTIONS
Aminoglycosides: potential increased risk of nephrotoxicity. Monitor closely.
Probenecid: may inhibit excretion and increase blood levels of cefonicid.

CONTRAINDICATIONS
Contraindicated in patients with hypersensitivity to the drug or other cephalosporins.

NURSING CONSIDERATIONS
• Use cautiously in patients with a history of sensitivity to penicillin. Also use cautiously and with dosage adjustments in patients with renal failure.
• Obtain specimen for culture and sensitivity tests before first dose. Therapy may begin pending test results.
• **I.V. use:** Reconstitute 500-mg vial with 2 ml of sterile water for injection (yields a concentration of 220 mg/ml) and 1-g vial with 2.5 ml of sterile water for injection (yields a concentration of 325 mg/ml). Shake well. Reconstitute piggyback vials with 50 to 100 ml of sterile water for injection, bacteriostatic water for injection, or 0.9% sodium chloride.
• For I.M. use, when administering 2-g I.M. doses once daily, divide the dose equally and inject deeply into large muscle masses, such as the glu-

teus maximus or the lateral aspect of the thigh.
• With large doses or prolonged therapy, monitor for superinfection, especially in high-risk patients.
• Be aware that the chemical structure of this drug includes the methylthiotetrazole side chain that has been associated with bleeding disorders. However, such bleeding has not been reported with this drug.
• Know that from 40% to 75% of patients receiving cephalosporins show a false-positive direct Coombs' test.
• Keep in mind that urine glucose determinations may be false-positive with copper sulfate tests (Clinitest); glucose enzymatic tests (Clinistix, Tes-Tape) are not affected.
• Be aware that dosing interval will be adjusted for patients with renal impairment.

---

cefoperazone sodium
Cefobid

Pregnancy Risk Category: B

HOW SUPPLIED
Infusion: 1 g, 2 g piggyback
Parenteral: 1 g, 2 g
Pharmacy bulk package: 10-g vial

ACTION
A third-generation cephalosporin that inhibits cell-wall synthesis, promoting osmotic instability; usually bactericidal.

ONSET, PEAK, DURATION
Onset immediate after I.V. administration, unknown after I.M. injection. Serum levels peak 1 to 2 hours after I.M. injection, immediately after I.V. administration. Duration unknown.

INDICATIONS & DOSAGE
Serious infections of the respiratory tract; intra-abdominal, gynecologic, and skin infections; bacteremia; and septicemia. Susceptible microorgan-

isms include Streptococcus pneumoniae *and* S. pyogenes; Staphylococcus aureus *(penicillinase- and non-penicillinase-producing) and* S. epidermidis; *enterococci;* Escherichia coli; Klebsiella; Haemophilus influenzae; Enterobacter; Citrobacter; Proteus; *some* Pseudomonas, *including* P. aeruginosa; *and* Bacteroides fragilis —
Adults: usual dosage is 1 to 2 g q 12 hours I.M. or I.V. In severe infections or in infections caused by less sensitive organisms, the total daily dosage or frequency may be increased up to 16 g/day in certain situations.

ADVERSE REACTIONS
CNS: headache, malaise, paresthesia, dizziness.
GI: pseudomembranous colitis, nausea, anorexia, vomiting, *diarrhea,* glossitis, dyspepsia, abdominal cramps, tenesmus, anal pruritus, oral candidiasis.
GU: genital pruritus and moniliasis.
Hematologic: transient neutropenia, eosinophilia, hemolytic anemia, hypoprothrombinemia, bleeding.
Skin: *maculopapular and erythematous rashes,* urticaria.
Other: dyspnea; mildly elevated liver enzymes; hypersensitivity reactions (serum sickness, ***anaphylaxis***); at injection site — *pain, induration, sterile abscesses, temperature elevation, tissue sloughing;* with I.V. injection — *phlebitis, thrombophlebitis.*

INTERACTIONS
Ethanol: possible disulfiram-like reaction. Warn patients not to drink alcohol for several days after discontinuing cefoperazone.
Probenecid: may inhibit excretion and increase blood levels of cefoperazone.

CONTRAINDICATIONS
Contraindicated in patients with hypersensitivity to the drug or other cephalosporins.

---

*Liquid form contains alcohol.
**May contain tartrazine.

*Common reactions are in italics; **life-threatening,** in bold italics.

NURSING CONSIDERATIONS
• Use cautiously in patients with impaired renal function or with a history of sensitivity to penicillin.
• Doses of 4 g/day should be given cautiously to patients with hepatic disease or biliary obstruction. Higher dosages require monitoring of serum levels.
• Obtain specimen for culture and sensitivity tests before first dose. Therapy may begin pending test results.
• **I.V. use:** Reconstitute 1- or 2-g vial with a minimum of 2.8 ml of compatible I.V. solution; the manufacturer recommends using 5 ml/g. Give by direct injection into a large vein or into the tubing of a free-flowing I.V. solution over 3 to 5 minutes. When giving by intermittent infusion, add reconstituted drug to 20 to 40 ml of a compatible I.V. solution and infuse over 15 to 30 minutes.
• To prepare drug for I.M. injection: using the 1-g vial, dissolve drug with 2 ml of sterile water for injection; then add 0.6 ml of 2% lidocaine hydrochloride for a final concentration of 333 mg/ml. Alternatively, dissolve drug with 2.8 ml of sterile water for injection; then add 1 ml of 2% lidocaine hydrochloride for a final concentration of 250 mg/ml. When using the 2-g vial, dissolve drug with 3.8 ml of sterile water for injection; then add 1.2 ml of 2% lidocaine hydrochloride for a final concentration of 333 mg/ml. Alternatively, dissolve drug with 5.4 ml of sterile water for injection; then add 1.8 ml of 2% lidocaine hydrochloride for a final concentration of 250 mg/ml.
• For I.M. administration, inject deeply into a large muscle mass, such as the gluteus maximus or the lateral aspect of the thigh.
• With large doses or prolonged therapy, monitor for superinfection, especially in high-risk patients.
• Monitor PT regularly. The chemical structure of this drug includes the methylthiotetrazole side chain that has been associated with bleeding disorders. Vitamin K promptly reverses bleeding if it occurs.
• Be aware that because of high degree of biliary excretion, cefoperazone may increase the risk of diarrhea over other cephalosporins.
• Know that from 40% to 75% of patients receiving cephalosporins show a false-positive direct Coombs' test.
• Keep in mind urine glucose determinations may be false-positive with copper sulfate tests (Clinitest); glucose enzymatic tests (Clinistix, Tes-Tape) are not affected.

---

cefotaxime sodium
Claforan

Pregnancy Risk Category: B

HOW SUPPLIED
Injection: 500 mg, 1 g, 2 g
Infusion: 1 g, 2 g
Pharmacy bulk package: 10-g vial

ACTION
A third-generation cephalosporin that inhibits cell-wall synthesis, promoting osmotic instability; usually bactericidal.

ONSET, PEAK, DURATION
Onset immediate after I.V. administration, unknown after I.M. injection. Serum levels peak 30 minutes after I.M. injection, immediately after I.V. administration. Duration unknown.

INDICATIONS & DOSAGE
Perioperative prophylaxis in contaminated surgery –
Adults: 1 g I.M. or I.V. 30 to 60 minutes before surgery. Patients undergoing bowel surgery should receive preoperative mechanical cleansing and a nonabsorbable anti-infective agent such as neomycin. Patients undergoing cesarean section should receive 1

g I.M. or I.V. as soon as the umbilical cord is clamped, followed by 1 g I.M. or I.V. 6 and 12 hours later.

Serious infections of the lower respiratory and urinary tracts, CNS, skin, bone, and joints; gynecologic and intra-abdominal infections; bacteremia; and septicemia. Susceptible microorganisms include streptococci, including Streptococcus pneumoniae *and* S. pyogenes; Staphylococcus aureus *(penicillinase- and non-penicillinase-producing) and* S. epidermidis; Escherichia coli; Klebsiella; Haemophilus influenzae; Enterobacter; Proteus; *and* Peptostreptococcus—

Adults: usual dose is 1 g I.V. or I.M. q 6 to 8 hours. Up to 12 g daily can be administered in life-threatening infections.

Children weighing 50 kg or more: the usual adult dose but dosage should not exceed 12 g daily.

Children 1 month to 12 years weighing less than 50 kg: 50 to 180 mg/kg/day I.M. or I.V. in four to six divided doses.

Neonates to 1 week: 50 mg/kg I.V. q 12 hours.

Neonates 1 to 4 weeks: 50 mg/kg I.V. q 6 to 8 hours.

ADVERSE REACTIONS
CNS: headache, malaise, paresthesia, dizziness.
GI: pseudomembranous colitis, nausea, anorexia, vomiting, *diarrhea,* glossitis, dyspepsia, abdominal cramps, tenesmus, anal pruritus, oral candidiasis.
GU: genital pruritus and moniliasis.
Hematologic: transient neutropenia, eosinophilia, hemolytic anemia.
Skin: *maculopapular and erythematous rashes, urticaria.*
Other: hypersensitivity reactions (serum sickness, ***anaphylaxis***); transient increases in liver enzymes; dyspnea; elevated temperature; at injection site—*pain, induration, sterile abscesses, temperature elevation, tissue sloughing;* with I.V. injection—*phlebitis, thrombophlebitis.*

INTERACTIONS
Aminoglycosides: may increase risk of nephrotoxicity. Monitor closely.
Probenecid: may inhibit excretion and increase blood levels of cefotaxime. Use together cautiously.

CONTRAINDICATIONS
Contraindicated in patients with hypersensitivity to the drug or other cephalosporins.

NURSING CONSIDERATIONS
• Use cautiously in patients with a history of sensitivity to penicillin. Also use cautiously and with dosage adjustments in patients with renal failure.
• Obtain specimen for culture and sensitivity tests before first dose. Therapy may begin pending test results.
• **I.V. use:** For direct injection, reconstitute 500-mg, 1-g, or 2-g vials with 10 ml of sterile water for injection. Solutions containing 1 g/14 ml are isotonic. Inject drug into a large vein or into the tubing of a free-flowing I.V. solution over 3 to 5 minutes.
• For I.V. infusion, reconstitute infusion vials with 50 to 100 ml of D_5W or 0.9% sodium chloride solution. Infuse drug over 20 to 30 minutes. Interrupt flow of primary I.V. solution during infusion.
• For I.M. administration, inject deeply into a large muscle mass, such as the gluteus maximus or the lateral aspect of the thigh.
• With large doses or prolonged therapy, monitor for superinfection, especially in high-risk patients.
• Know that from 40% to 75% of patients receiving cephalosporins show a false-positive direct Coomb's test.
• Keep in mind that urine glucose determinations may be false-positive with copper sulfate tests (Clinitest);

---

*Liquid form contains alcohol.
**May contain tartrazine.

Common reactions are in italics; ***life-threatening,*** in bold italics.

glucose enzymatic tests (Clinistix, Tes-Tape) are not affected.

cefotetan disodium
Cefotan

Pregnancy Risk Category: B

HOW SUPPLIED
Injection: 1 g, 2 g
Infusion: 1 g, 2 g piggyback
Pharmacy bulk package: 10-g vial

ACTION
A semisynthetic cephamycin antibiotic that is pharmacologically similar to the second-generation cephalosporins. Inhibits cell-wall synthesis, promoting osmotic instability; usually bactericidal.

ONSET, PEAK, DURATION
Onset immediate after I.V. administration, unknown after I.M. injection. Peak serum levels occur 1½ to 3 hours after I.M. injection, immediately after I.V. administration. Duration unknown.

INDICATIONS & DOSAGE
Serious urinary tract and lower respiratory tract infections and gynecologic, skin and skin-structure, intra-abdominal, and bone and joint infections caused by susceptible streptococci, Staphylococcus aureus *(penicillinase- and non-penicillinase-producing) and* S. epidermidis, Escherichia coli, Klebsiella, Enterobacter, Proteus, Haemophilus influenzae, Neisseria gonorrhoeae, *and* Bacteroides, *including* B. fragilis; *and perioperative prophylaxis—*
Adults: 1 to 2 g I.V. or I.M. q 12 hours for 5 to 10 days. Up to 6 g daily in life-threatening infections.

ADVERSE REACTIONS
CNS: headache, malaise, paresthesia, dizziness.
GI: pseudomembranous colitis, nausea, anorexia, vomiting, *diarrhea,* glossitis, dyspepsia, abdominal cramps, tenesmus, anal pruritus.
GU: genital pruritus and moniliasis.
Hematologic: transient neutropenia, eosinophilia, hemolytic anemia, hypoprothrombinemia, bleeding.
Skin: *maculopapular and erythematous rashes, urticaria.*
Other: hypersensitivity reactions (serum sickness, *anaphylaxis*); transient increases in liver enzymes; dyspnea; elevated temperature; at injection site—*pain, induration, sterile abscesses, tissue sloughing;* with I.V. injection—*phlebitis, thrombophlebitis.*

INTERACTIONS
Aminoglycosides: possible synergistic effect and possible increased risk of nephrotoxicity. Use with caution.
Ethanol: possible disulfiram-like reaction. Warn patients not to drink alcohol for several days after discontinuing cefotetan.
Probenecid: may inhibit excretion and increase blood levels of cefotetan. Sometimes used for this effect.

CONTRAINDICATIONS
Contraindicated in patients with hypersensitivity to the drug or other cephalosporins.

NURSING CONSIDERATIONS
● Use cautiously in patients with a history of sensitivity to penicillin. Also use cautiously and with dosage adjustments in patients with renal failure.
● Obtain specimen for culture and sensitivity tests before first dose. Therapy may begin pending test results.
● **I.V. use:** Reconstitute with sterile water for injection. Then may be mixed with 50 to 100 ml of D₅W or 0.9% sodium chloride solution. Interrupt flow of primary I.V. solution during cefotetan infusion.
● Reconstitute I.M. injection with

sterile water or bacteriostatic water for injection, 0.9% sodium chloride for injection, or 0.5% or 1% lidocaine hydrochloride. Shake to dissolve and let stand until clear.

• Know that reconstituted solution remains stable for 24 hours at room temperature or 96 hours if refrigerated.

• With large doses or prolonged therapy, monitor for superinfection, especially in high-risk patients.

• Know that the chemical structure of this drug includes the methylthio-tetrazole side chain that has been associated with bleeding disorders. However, such bleeding has not been reported with this drug.

• Be aware that from 40% to 75% of patients receiving cephalosporins show a false-positive direct Coombs' test.

• Keep in mind that urine glucose determinations may be false-positive with copper sulfate tests (Clinitest); glucose enzymatic tests (Clinistix, Tes-Tape) are not affected.

---

cefoxitin sodium
Mefoxin

Pregnancy Risk Category: B

HOW SUPPLIED
Injection: 1 g, 2 g
Infusion: 1 g, 2 g in 50-ml or 100-ml container
Pharmacy bulk package: 10 g

ACTION
A semisynthetic cephamycin antibiotic that is pharmacologically similar to the second-generation cephalosporins. Inhibits cell-wall synthesis, promoting osmotic instability; usually bactericidal.

ONSET, PEAK, DURATION
Onset immediate after I.V. administration, unknown after I.M. injection. Serum levels peak within 20 to 30 minutes after I.M. injection, immediately after I.V. administration. Duration unknown.

INDICATIONS & DOSAGE
Serious infections of respiratory and GU tracts, skin, soft-tissue, bone, and joint infections, and bloodstream and intra-abdominal infections caused by susceptible Escherichia coli *and other coliform bacteria,* Staphylococcus aureus *(penicillinase- and non-penicillinase-producing) and* S. epidermidis, *streptococci,* Klebsiella, Haemophilus influenzae, *and* Bacteroides, *including* B. fragilis; *and perioperative prophylaxis—*
Adults: 1 to 2 g q 6 to 8 hours for uncomplicated forms of infection. Up to 12 g daily in life-threatening infections.
Children over 3 months: 80 to 160 mg/kg daily given in four to six equally divided doses. Maximum daily dose is 12 g.
Prophylactic use in surgery—
Adults: 2 g I.M. or I.V. 30 to 60 minutes before surgery, then 2 g I.M. or I.V. q 6 hours for 24 hours (72 hours after prosthetic arthroplasty).
Children 3 months or older: 30 to 40 mg/kg I.M. or I.V. 30 to 60 minutes before surgery then 30 to 40 mg/kg q 6 hours for 24 hours (72 hours after prosthetic arthroplasty).

ADVERSE REACTIONS
CNS: headache, malaise, paresthesia, dizziness.
GI: pseudomembranous colitis, nausea, anorexia, vomiting, *diarrhea,* glossitis, dyspepsia, abdominal cramps, tenesmus, anal pruritus, oral candidiasis.
GU: genital pruritus and moniliasis.
Hematologic: transient neutropenia, eosinophilia, *hemolytic anemia.*
Skin: *maculopapular and erythematous rashes, urticaria.*
Other: hypersensitivity reactions (serum sickness, ***anaphylaxis***); tran-

---

*Liquid form contains alcohol.
**May contain tartrazine.

Common reactions are in italics; *life-threatening,* in bold italics.

sient increases in liver enzymes; dyspnea; elevated temperature; at injection site —*pain, induration, sterile abscesses, tissue sloughing;* with I.V. injection —*phlebitis, thrombophlebitis.*

INTERACTIONS
Nephrotoxic agents: possible increased risk of nephrotoxicity. Monitor closely.
Probenecid: may inhibit excretion and increase blood levels of cefoxitin. Sometimes used for this effect.

CONTRAINDICATIONS
Contraindicated in patients with hypersensitivity to the drug or other cephalosporins.

NURSING CONSIDERATIONS
● Use cautiously in patients with a history of sensitivity to penicillin. Also use cautiously and with dosage adjustments in patients with renal failure.
● Obtain specimen for culture and sensitivity tests before first dose. Therapy may begin pending test results.
● **I.V. use:** Reconstitute 1 g with at least 10 ml of sterile water for injection and 2 g with 10 to 20 ml of sterile water for injection. Solutions of dextrose 5% and 0.9% sodium chloride for injection can also be used. For direct injection, inject drug into a large vein or into the tubing of a free-flowing I.V. solution over 3 to 5 minutes. For intermittent infusion, add reconstituted drug to 50 or 100 ml of dextrose 5% or 10% in water or 0.9% sodium chloride injection. Interrupt flow of primary I.V. solution during infusion.
● Reconstitute I.M. injection with 0.5% or 1% lidocaine hydrochloride (without epinephrine) to minimize pain. Inject deeply into a large muscle mass, such as the gluteus maximus or the lateral aspect of the thigh.
● After reconstitution, store for 24

hours at room temperature or 1 week under refrigeration.
● Assess I.V. site frequently. Associated with development of thrombophlebitis.
● With large doses or prolonged therapy, monitor for superinfection, especially in high-risk patients.
● Be aware that from 40% to 75% of patients receiving cephalosporins show a false-positive direct Coombs' test.
● Keep in mind that urine glucose determinations may be false-positive with copper sulfate tests (Clinitest); glucose enzymatic tests (Clinistix, Tes-Tape) are not affected.

cefpodoxime proxetil
Vantin

Pregnancy Risk Category: B

HOW SUPPLIED
Tablets (film-coated): 100 mg, 200 mg
Oral suspension: 50 mg/5 ml, 100 mg/5 ml in 100-ml bottles

ACTION
A second-generation cephalosporin that inhibits cell-wall synthesis, promoting osmotic instability; usually bactericidal.

ONSET, PEAK, DURATION
Onset and duration unknown. Serum levels peak 2 to 3 hours after an oral dose.

INDICATIONS & DOSAGE
Acute, community-acquired pneumonia caused by non-beta-lactamase-producing strains of Haemophilus influenzae *or* Streptococcus pneumoniae —
Adults and children 13 years and older: 200 mg P.O. q 12 hours for 14 days.
Acute bacterial exacerbation of chronic bronchitis caused by S. pneumoniae, H. influenzae *(non-beta-lac-*

tamase-producing strains only), or Moraxella (Branhamella) catarrhalis—
Adults and children 13 years and older: 200 mg P.O. q 12 hours for 10 days.
Uncomplicated gonorrhea in men and women; rectal gonococcal infections in women—
Adults and children 13 years and older: 200 mg P.O. as a single dose. Follow with doxycycline 100 mg P.O. b.i.d. for 7 days.
Uncomplicated skin and skin-structure infections caused by Staphylococcus aureus *or* Strep. pyogenes—
Adults and children 13 years and older: 400 mg P.O. q 12 hours for 7 to 14 days.
Acute otitis media caused by S. pneumoniae, H. influenzae, *or* M. catarrhalis—
Children 6 months and over: 5 mg/kg (not to exceed 200 mg) P.O. q 12 hours for 10 days.
Pharyngitis or tonsillitis caused by S. pyogenes—
Adults: 100 mg P.O. q 12 hours for 10 days.
Children 6 months and over: 5 mg/kg (not to exceed 100 mg) P.O. q 12 hours for 10 days.
Uncomplicated urinary tract infections caused by Escherichia coli, Klebsiella pneumoniae, Proteus mirabilis, *or* Staph. saprophyticus—
Adults: 100 mg P.O. q 12 hours for 7 days.
   In patients with renal failure: Know that when creatinine clearance is below 30 ml/minute/1.73 m², dosage interval should be increased to q 24 hours. Patients receiving dialysis should get the drug three times weekly, after dialysis.

ADVERSE REACTIONS
CNS: headache.
GI: *diarrhea,* nausea, vomiting, abdominal pain.
GU: vaginal fungal infections.

Skin: rash.
Other: hypersensitivity reactions *(anaphylaxis).*

INTERACTIONS
Antacids, H₂ antagonists: decreased absorption of cefpodoxime. Avoid concomitant use.
Probenecid: decreased excretion of cefpodoxime. Monitor for toxicity.

CONTRAINDICATIONS
Contraindicated in patients with hypersensitivity to the drug or other cephalosporins. Safety and efficacy in children under age 6 months have not been established.

NURSING CONSIDERATIONS
• Use cautiously in patients with a history of penicillin hypersensitivity because of the risk of cross-sensitivity and in patients receiving nephrotoxic drugs because other cephalosporins have been shown to have nephrotoxic potential. Because drug is excreted in human breast milk, also use cautiously in breast-feeding women.
• Obtain specimen for culture and sensitivity tests before first dose. Therapy may begin pending test results.
• Administer drug with food to enhance absorption. Shake well before using.
• Store suspension in the refrigerator (36° to 46° F [2° to 8° C]). Discard unused portion after 14 days.
• Monitor for signs and symptoms of superinfection. May cause overgrowth of nonsusceptible bacteria or fungi.
• Know that from 40% to 75% of patients receiving cephalosporins show a false-positive direct Coombs' test.
• Keep in mind that urine glucose determinations may be false-positive with copper sulfate tests (Clinitest); glucose enzymatic tests (Clinistix, Tes-Tape) are not affected.

*Liquid form contains alcohol.   *Common* reactions are in italics; *life-threatening,* in bold italics.
**May contain tartrazine.

cefprozil
Cefzil

Pregnancy Risk Category: B

HOW SUPPLIED
Tablets: 250 mg, 500 mg
Oral suspension: 125 mg/5 ml, 250 mg/5 ml

ACTION
A second-generation cephalosporin that interferes with cell-wall synthesis during microorganism replication, leading to osmotic instability and cell lysis (bactericidal).

ONSET, PEAK, DURATION
Onset and duration unknown. Serum levels peak within 1½ hours after an oral dose.

INDICATIONS & DOSAGE
Pharyngitis or tonsillitis caused by Streptococcus pyogenes —
Adults and children 13 years and older: 500 mg P.O. daily for at least 10 days.
Otitis media caused by S. pneumoniae, Haemophilus influenzae, *and* Moraxella (Branhamella) catarrhalis —
Infants and children 6 months to 12 years: 15 mg/kg P.O. q 12 hours for 10 days.
Secondary bacterial infections of acute bronchitis and acute bacterial exacerbation of chronic bronchitis caused by S. pneumoniae, H. influenzae, *and* M. catarrhalis —
Adults and children 13 years and older: 500 mg P.O. q 12 hours for 10 days.
Uncomplicated skin and skin-structure infections caused by Staphylococcus aureus *and* S. pyogenes —
Adults and children 13 years and older: 250 mg P.O. b.i.d., or 500 mg daily to b.i.d.

ADVERSE REACTIONS
CNS: dizziness, hyperactivity, headache, nervousness, insomnia.
GI: *diarrhea, nausea,* vomiting, abdominal pain.
GU: elevated BUN level, elevated serum creatinine level, genital pruritus, vaginitis.
Hematologic: decreased leukocyte count, eosinophilia.
Hepatic: elevated liver enzymes, cholestatic jaundice (rare).
Skin: rash, urticaria, diaper rash.
Other: superinfection, hypersensitivity reactions (serum sickness, *anaphylaxis*).

INTERACTIONS
Aminoglycosides: potential increased risk of nephrotoxicity. Monitor closely.
Probenecid: may inhibit excretion and increase blood levels of cefprozil.

CONTRAINDICATIONS
Contraindicated in patients with hypersensitivity to the drug or other cephalosporins.

NURSING CONSIDERATIONS
• Use cautiously in patients with a history of sensitivity to penicillin. Also use cautiously in patients with impaired hepatic or renal function. Know that patients with creatinine clearance less than 30 ml/minute should receive 50% of usual dose.
• Obtain specimen for culture and sensitivity tests before first dose. Therapy may begin pending test results.
• Administer after hemodialysis treatment is completed; drug is removed by hemodialysis.
• Know that from 40% to 75% of patients receiving cephalosporins show a false-positive direct Coombs' test.
• Keep in mind that urine glucose determinations may be false-positive with copper sulfate tests (Clinitest);

---

†Available in Canada only.   ‡Available in Australia only.   ◊Available OTC.

glucose enzymatic tests (Clinistix, Tes-Tape) are not affected.
- Monitor for signs and symptoms of superinfection. May cause overgrowth of nonsusceptible bacteria or fungi.
- Tell the patient to shake suspension well before measuring dose.
- Tell patient that oral suspensions contain the drug in a bubble-gum flavored vehicle to improve palatability and compliance in children. Reconstituted suspension should be stored in the refrigerator, and unused drug should be discarded after 14 days.
- Tell the patient to take all of the medication as prescribed, even after he feels better.

ceftazidime
Ceptaz, Fortaz, Magnacef†, Pentacef, Tazicef, Tazidime

Pregnancy Risk Category: B

HOW SUPPLIED
Injection (with sodium carbonate): 500 mg, 1 g, 2 g; 6 g (pharmacy bulk package)
Injection (with arginine): 1 g, 2 g; 6 g, 10 g (pharmacy bulk package)
Infusion: 1 g, 2 g in 50-ml and 100-ml vials (premixed)

ACTION
A third-generation cephalosporin that inhibits cell-wall synthesis, promoting osmotic instability; usually bactericidal.

ONSET, PEAK, DURATION
Onset immediate after I.V. administration, unknown after I.M. injection. Peak serum levels occur within 1 hour after I.M. injection, immediately after I.V. administration. In women, peak serum concentrations may be lower after I.M. injection into the gluteus maximus than into the vastus lateralis. Duration unknown.

INDICATIONS & DOSAGE
Serious infections of the lower respiratory and urinary tracts; gynecologic, intra-abdominal, CNS, and skin infections; bacteremia; and septicemia. Among susceptible microorganisms are streptococci, including Streptococcus pneumoniae *and* S. pyogenes; Staphylococcus aureus *(penicillinase- and non-penicillinase-producing);* Escherichia coli; Klebsiella; Proteus; Enterobacter; Haemophilus influenzae; Pseudomonas; *and some strains of* Bacteroides—
Adults and children 12 years and older: 1 g I.V. or I.M. q 8 to 12 hours; up to 6 g daily in life-threatening infections.
Children 1 month to 12 years: 30 to 50 mg/kg I.V. q 8 hours.
Neonates 0 to 4 weeks: 30 mg/kg I.V. q 12 hours.

ADVERSE REACTIONS
CNS: headache, dizziness.
GI: pseudomembranous colitis, nausea, vomiting, diarrhea, dysgeusia, abdominal cramps.
GU: genital pruritus and moniliasis.
Hematologic: eosinophilia; thrombocytosis, leukopenia.
Skin: *maculopapular and erythematous rashes, urticaria.*
Other: hypersensitivity reactions (serum sickness, **anaphylaxis**); transient elevation in liver enzymes; dyspnea; elevated temperature; at injection site—*pain, induration, sterile abscesses, tissue sloughing;* with I.V. injection—*phlebitis, thrombophlebitis.*

INTERACTIONS
Chloramphenicol: antagonistic effect. Avoid concomitant use.

CONTRAINDICATIONS
Contraindicated in patients with hypersensitivity to the drug or other cephalosporins.

NURSING CONSIDERATIONS

• Use cautiously in patients with a history of sensitivity to penicillin. Also use cautiously and with dosage adjustments in patients with renal failure.

• Obtain specimen for culture and sensitivity tests before first dose. Therapy may begin pending test results.

• **I.V. use:** Reconstitute sodium carbonate-containing solutions with sterile water for injection. Add 5 ml to a 500-mg vial; 10 ml to a 1-g or 2-g vial. Shake well to dissolve drug. Carbon dioxide is released during dissolution, and a positive pressure will develop in the vial. Reconstitute arginine-containing solutions with 10 ml of sterile water for injection. This formulation won't release gas bubbles. Each brand of ceftazidime includes specific instructions for reconstitution. Read and follow these instructions carefully.

• For I.M. administration, inject deeply into a large muscle mass, such as the gluteus maximus or the lateral aspect of the thigh.

• With large doses or prolonged therapy, monitor for superinfection, especially in high-risk patients.

• Keep in mind that commercially available preparations contain either sodium carbonate (Fortaz, Magnicef, Tazicef, Tazidime) or arginine (Ceptaz, Pentacef) to facilitate dissolution of drug. Safety and efficacy of arginine-containing solutions in children 12 years and under have not been established.

• Be aware that from 40% to 75% of patients receiving cephalosporins show a false-positive direct Coombs' test.

• Keep in mind that urine glucose determinations may be false-positive with copper sulfate tests (Clinitest); glucose enzymatic tests (Clinistix, Tes-Tape) are not affected.

• Know that ceftazidime is removed by hemodialysis; a supplemental dose of the drug is indicated after each dialysis period, as ordered.

---

ceftizoxime sodium
Cefizox

Pregnancy Risk Category: B

HOW SUPPLIED
Injection: 500 mg, 1 g, 2 g
Infusion: 1 g, 2 g in 100-mg vials or in 50 ml of D_5W
Pharmacy bulk package: 10 g

ACTION
A third-generation cephalosporin that inhibits cell-wall synthesis, promoting osmotic instability; usually bactericidal.

ONSET, PEAK, DURATION
Onset immediate after I.V. administration, unknown after I.M. injection. Serum levels peak ½ to 1½ hours after I.M. injection, immediately after I.V. administration. Duration unknown.

INDICATIONS & DOSAGE
Serious infections of the lower respiratory and urinary tracts, gynecologic infections, bacteremia, septicemia, meningitis, intra-abdominal infections, bone and joint infections, and skin infections. Among susceptible microorganisms are streptococci, including Streptococcus pneumoniae *and* S. pyogenes; Staphylococcus aureus *(penicillinase- and non-penicillinase-producing) and* S. epidermidis; Escherichia coli; Klebsiella; Haemophilus influenzae; Enterobacter; Proteus; *some* Pseudomonas; *and* Peptostreptococcus—
Adults: usual dosage is 1 to 2 g I.V. or I.M. q 8 to 12 hours. In life-threatening infections, up to 2 g q 4 hours.
Children over 6 months: 33 to 50 mg/kg I.V. q 6 to 8 hours. For serious infections, up to 200 mg/kg/day in di-

vided doses may be used. Don't exceed 12 g/day.

ADVERSE REACTIONS
CNS: headache, malaise, paresthesia, dizziness.
GI: pseudomembranous colitis, nausea, anorexia, vomiting, *diarrhea,* glossitis, dyspepsia, abdominal cramps, tenesmus, anal pruritus.
GU: genital pruritus and moniliasis.
Hematologic: transient neutropenia, eosinophilia, hemolytic anemia.
Skin: *maculopapular and erythematous rashes, urticaria.*
Other: hypersensitivity reactions (serum sickness, *anaphylaxis*); dyspnea; elevated temperature; at injection site—*pain, induration, sterile abscesses, tissue sloughing;* with I.V. injection—*phlebitis, thrombophlebitis.*

INTERACTIONS
Probenecid: may inhibit excretion and increase blood levels of ceftizoxime. Sometimes used for this effect.

CONTRAINDICATIONS
Contraindicated in patients with hypersensitivity to ceftizoxime or other cephalosporins.

NURSING CONSIDERATIONS
• Use cautiously in patients with a history of sensitivity to penicillin. Also use cautiously and with dosage adjustments in patients with renal failure.
• Obtain specimen for culture and sensitivity tests before first dose. Therapy may begin pending test results.
• **I.V. use:** To reconstitute powder, add 5 ml of sterile water to a 500-mg vial, 10 ml to a 1-g vial, or 20 ml to a 2-g vial. Reconstitute piggyback vials with 50 to 100 ml of 0.9% sodium chloride solution or D_5W. Shake vial well.
• For I.M. administration, inject deeply into a large muscle mass, such

as the gluteus maximus or the lateral aspect of the thigh. Larger doses (2 g) should be divided and administered at two separate sites.
• With large doses or prolonged therapy, monitor for superinfection, especially in high-risk patients.
• Know that from 40% to 75% of patients receiving cephalosporins show a false-positive direct Coombs' test.
• Keep in mind that urine glucose determinations may be false-positive with copper sulfate tests (Clinitest); glucose enzymatic tests (Clinistix, Tes-Tape) are not affected.

ceftriaxone sodium
Rocephin

Pregnancy Risk Category: B

HOW SUPPLIED
Injection: 250 mg, 500 mg, 1 g, 2 g
Infusion: 1 g, 2 g
Pharmacy bulk package: 10 g

ACTION
A third-generation cephalosporin that inhibits cell-wall synthesis, promoting osmotic instability; usually bactericidal.

ONSET, PEAK, DURATION
Onset immediate after I.V. administration, unknown after I.M. injection. Peak serum levels occur 1½ to 4 hours after I.M. injection, immediately after I.V. adminstration. Duration unknown.

INDICATIONS & DOSAGE
Uncomplicated gonococcal vulvovaginitis, urethritis, or proctitis—
Adults: 250 mg I.M. as a single dose, followed with 100 mg of doxycycline P.O. q 12 hours for 7 days.
Children: 125 mg I.M. as a single dose.
Serious infections of the lower respiratory and urinary tracts; gynecologic, bone and joint, intra-abdominal, and

---

skin infections; bacteremia; septicemia; and Lyme disease caused by
such susceptible microorganisms as
streptococci, including Streptococcus
pneumoniae and S. pyogenes; Staphylococcus aureus (penicillinase- and
non-penicillinase-producing) and S.
epidermidis; Escherichia coli; Klebsiella; Haemophilus influenzae; Neisseria meningitidis; N. gonorrhoeae;
Enterobacter; Proteus; Pseudomonas;
Peptostreptococcus, and Serratia
marcescens—

Adults and children over 12 years: 1
to 2 g I.M. or I.V. daily or in equally
divided doses b.i.d. Total daily dosage should not exceed 4 g.
Children 12 years and under: 50 to
75 mg/kg, not to exceed 2 g/day,
given in divided doses q 12 hours.
Meningitis—
Adults and children: 100 mg/kg
given in divided doses q 12 hours.
May give loading dose of 75 mg/kg,
not to exceed 4 g.
Preoperative prophylaxis—
Adults: 1 g I.V. as a single dose ½ to
2 hours before surgery.

ADVERSE REACTIONS
CNS: headache, dizziness.
GI: pseudomembranous colitis, nau-
sea, vomiting, diarrhea, dysgeusia.
GU: genital pruritus and moniliasis.
Hematologic: eosinophilia, thrombo-
cytosis, leukopenia.
Skin: pain, induration, or tenderness
at injection site; phlebitis; *rash.*
Other: hypersensitivity reactions
(serum sickness, *anaphylaxis*), ele-
vated temperature.

INTERACTIONS
Probenecid: high doses (1 or 2 g/day)
may enhance hepatic clearance of ceftriaxone and shorten half-life. Avoid
concomitant use.

CONTRAINDICATIONS
Contraindicated in patients with hypersensitivity to ceftriaxone or other
cephalosporins.

NURSING CONSIDERATIONS
• Use cautiously in patients with a
history of sensitivity to penicillin.
• Obtain specimen for culture and
sensitivity tests before first dose.
Therapy may begin pending test results.
• **I.V. use:** Reconstitute with sterile
water for injection, 0.9% sodium
chloride injection, dextrose 5% or
10% injection, or a combination of sodium chloride and dextrose injection
and other compatible solutions. Reconstitute by adding 2.4 ml of diluent
to the 250-mg vial, 4.8 ml to the
500-mg vial, 9.6 ml to the 1-g vial,
and 19.2 ml to the 2-g vial. All reconstituted solutions yield a concentration that averages 100 mg/ml. After
reconstitution, dilute further for intermittent infusion to desired concentration. I.V. dilutions are stable for 24
hours at room temperature.
• For I.M. administration, inject
deeply into a large muscle mass, such
as the gluteus maximus or the lateral
aspect of the thigh.
• With large doses or prolonged therapy, monitor for superinfection, especially in high-risk patients.
• Know that dosage adjustment usually is not needed in patients with
renal insufficiency.
• Know that from 40% to 75% of patients receiving cephalosporins show
a false-positive direct Coombs' test.
• Keep in mind that urine glucose determinations may be false-positive
with copper sulfate tests (Clinitest);
glucose enzymatic tests (Clinistix,
Tes-Tape) are not affected.
• Be aware that drug commonly is
used in home antibiotic programs for
outpatient treatment of serious infections, such as osteomyelitis.

cefuroxime axetil
Ceftin

cefuroxime sodium
Kefurox, Zinacef

Pregnancy Risk Category: B

HOW SUPPLIED
cefuroxime axetil
Tablets: 125 mg, 250 mg, 500 mg
Suspension: 125 mg/5 mL
cefuroxime sodium
Injection: 750 mg, 1.5 g
Infusion: 750 mg, 1.5 g premixed, frozen solution
Pharmacy bulk package: 7.5 g

ACTION
A second-generation cephalosporin that inhibits cell-wall synthesis, promoting osmotic instability; usually bactericidal.

ONSET, PEAK, DURATION
Onset is immediate after I.V. administration, unknown after oral and I.M. administration. Peak serum levels occur within 2 hours after oral administration, 15 to 60 minutes after I.M. injection, immediately after I.V. administration. Duration unknown.

INDICATIONS & DOSAGE
Injectable form is for serious infections of the lower respiratory and urinary tracts; skin and skin-structure infections; bone and joint infections; septicemia; meningitis; and gonorrhea; and for perioperative prophylaxis; oral form is used to treat otitis media, pharyngitis, tonsillitis, infections of the urinary and lower respiratory tracts, and skin and skin-structure infections. Among susceptible organisms are Streptococcus pneumoniae *and* S. pyogenes, Haemophilus influenzae, Klebsiella, Staphylococcus aureus, Escherichia coli, Enterobacter, *and* Neisseria gonorrhoeae —
Adults and children 12 years and older: usual dosage of cefuroxime sodium is 750 mg to 1.5 g I.M. or I.V. q 8 hours for 5 to 10 days. For life-threatening infections and infections caused by less susceptible organisms, 1.5 g I.M. or I.V. q 6 hours; for bacterial meningitis, up to 3 g I.V. q 8 hours.

Alternatively, administer 250 mg of cefuroxime axetil P.O. q 12 hours. For severe infections, dosage may be increased to 500 mg q 12 hours.
Children and infants over 3 months: 50 to 100 mg/kg/day cefuroxime sodium I.M. or I.V. in equally divided doses q 6 to 8 hours. Higher doses are administered when treating meningitis. Alternatively, 125 mg of cefuroxime axetil P.O. q 12 hours; for bacterial meningitis, 200 to 240 mg/kg I.V. in divided doses q 6 to 8 hours.
Uncomplicated urinary tract infections —
Adults: 125 to 250 mg P.O. q 12 hours.
Otitis media —
Children under 2 years: 125 mg P.O. q 12 hours.
Children 2 years and over: 250 mg P.O. q 12 hours.
Perioperative prophylaxis —
Adults: 1.5 g I.V. 30 to 60 minutes before surgery; in lengthy operations, 750 mg I.V. or I.M. q 8 hours. For open-heart surgery, 1.5 g I.V. at induction of anesthesia and then q 12 hours for a total dosage of 6 g.

ADVERSE REACTIONS
CNS: headache, malaise, paresthesia, dizziness.
GI: pseudomembranous colitis, nausea, anorexia, vomiting, *diarrhea,* glossitis, dyspepsia, abdominal cramps, tenesmus, anal pruritus.
GU: genital pruritus and moniliasis.
Hematologic: transient neutropenia, eosinophilia, ***hemolytic anemia,*** decrease in hemoglobin and hematocrit.
Skin: *maculopapular and erythematous rashes, urticaria.*

Liquid form contains alcohol.   *Common reactions are in italics; **life-threatening,** in bold italics.*
**May contain tartrazine.

Other: transient increases in liver enzymes; hypersensitivity reactions (serum sickness, *anaphylaxis*); dyspnea; at injection site — *pain, induration, sterile abscesses, temperature elevation, tissue sloughing;* with I.V. injection — *phlebitis, thrombophlebitis.*

INTERACTIONS
Diuretics: increased risk of adverse renal reactions. Monitor closely.
Probenecid: may inhibit excretion and increase blood levels of cefuroxime. Sometimes used for this effect.

CONTRAINDICATIONS
Contraindicated in patients with hypersensitivity to cefuroxime or other cephalosporins.

NURSING CONSIDERATIONS
• Use cautiously in patients with history of sensitivity to penicillin. Also use cautiously and with reduced dosage in patients with impaired renal function.
• Obtain specimen for culture and sensitivity tests before first dose. Therapy may begin pending test results.
• **I.V. use:** For each 750-mg vial of Kefurox, reconstitute with 9 ml of sterile water for injection. Withdraw 8 ml from the vial for the proper dose. For each 1.5-g vial of Kefurox, reconstitute with 16 ml of sterile water for injection; withdraw entire contents of vial for a dose. For each 750-mg vial of Zinacef, reconstitute with 8 ml of sterile water for injection; for each 1.5-g vial, reconstitute with 16 ml. In each case, withdraw entire contents of vial for a dose.
• To give by direct injection, inject into a large vein or into the tubing of a free-flowing I.V. solution over 3 to 5 minutes.
• For intermittent infusion, add reconstituted drug to 100 ml D₅W, 0.9% sodium chloride injection, or other compatible I.V. solution. Infuse over 15 to 60 minutes.
• For I.M. administration, inject deeply into a large muscle mass, such as the gluteus maximus or the lateral aspect of the thigh.
• Know that absorption of cefuroxime axetil is enhanced by food.
• Keep in mind that cefuroxime axetil is available only in tablet form, which may be crushed for patients who cannot swallow tablets. Tablets may be allowed to dissolve in small amounts of apple, orange, or grape juice or chocolate milk. However, the drug has a bitter taste that is difficult to mask, even with food.
• With large doses or prolonged therapy, monitor for superinfection, especially in high-risk patients.
• Know that from 40% to 75% of patients receiving cephalosporins show a false-positive direct Coombs' test.
• Keep in mind that urine glucose determinations may be false-positive with copper sulfate tests (Clinitest); glucose enzymatic tests (Clinistix, Tes-Tape) are not affected.

cephalexin hydrochloride
Keftab

cephalexin monohydrate
Apo-Cephalex†, Cefanex, Ceporex†‡, C-Lexin, Keflet, Keflex, Novolexin†, Nu-Cephalex‡
Pregnancy Risk Category: B

HOW SUPPLIED
cephalexin hydrochloride
Tablets: 250 mg, 500 mg
cephalexin monohydrate
Tablets: 250 mg, 500 mg, 1 g
Capsules: 250 mg, 500 mg
Oral suspension: 100 mg/5 ml, 125 mg/5 ml, 250 mg/5 ml

ACTION
A first-generation cephalosporin that inhibits cell-wall synthesis, promot-

---

ing osmotic instability; usually bactericidal.

ONSET, PEAK, DURATION
Onset unknown. Serum levels peak within 1 hour. Duration unknown.

INDICATIONS & DOSAGE
Respiratory tract, GI tract, skin, soft-tissue, bone, and joint infections and otitis media caused by Escherichia coli *and other coliform bacteria, group A beta-hemolytic streptococci,* Haemophilus influenzae, Klebsiella, Moraxella (Branhamella) catarrhalis, Proteus mirabilis, Streptococcus pneumoniae, *and staphylococci* –
Adults: 250 mg to 1 g P.O. q 6 hours.
Children: 6 to 12 mg/kg P.O. q 6 hours (monohydrate only). Maximum 25 mg/kg q 6 hours.

ADVERSE REACTIONS
CNS: dizziness, headache, malaise, paresthesia.
GI: pseudomembranous colitis, *nausea, anorexia,* vomiting, *diarrhea,* glossitis, dyspepsia, abdominal cramps, anal pruritus, tenesmus, oral candidiasis.
GU: genital pruritus and moniliasis, vaginitis.
Hematologic: transient neutropenia, eosinophilia, anemia.
Skin: *maculopapular and erythematous rashes, urticaria.*
Other: transient increases in liver enzymes, hypersensitivity reactions (serum sickness, ***anaphylaxis***), dyspnea.

INTERACTIONS
Probenecid: may increase blood levels of cephalosporins. Sometimes used for this effect.

CONTRAINDICATIONS
Contraindicated in patients with hypersensitivity to cephalosporins.

NURSING CONSIDERATIONS
• Use cautiously in patients with impaired renal function or with a history of sensitivity to penicillin. Ask the patient if he has had any reaction to previous cephalosporin or penicillin therapy before administering first dose.
• Obtain specimen for culture and sensitivity tests before first dose. Therapy may begin pending test results.
• To prepare oral suspension: Add required amount of water to powder in two portions. Shake well after each addition. After mixing, store in refrigerator. The mixture will remain stable for 14 days without significant loss of potency. Keep tightly closed and shake well before using.
• With large doses or prolonged therapy, monitor for superinfection, especially in high-risk patients.
• Know that from 40% to 75% of patients receiving cephalosporins show a false-positive direct Coombs' test, but only a few of these indicate hemolytic anemia.
• Keep in mind that urine glucose determinations may be false-positive with copper sulfate tests (Clinitest); glucose enzymatic tests (Clinistix, Tes-Tape) are not affected.
• Know that group A beta-hemolytic streptococcal infections should be treated for a minimum of 10 days.
• Tell the patient to take all of the medication exactly as prescribed, even after he feels better.
• Tell the patient to take drug with food or milk to lessen GI discomfort.
• Instruct the patient to call the doctor if skin rash develops.

---

cephalothin sodium
Ceporacin†‡, Keflin
Pregnancy Risk Category: B

HOW SUPPLIED
Injection: 1 g, 2 g, 4 g
Infusion: 1 g/50 ml, 2 g/50 ml, 1 g/dl, 2 g/dl
Pharmacy bulk package: 20 g

ACTION
A first-generation cephalosporin that inhibits cell-wall synthesis, promoting osmotic instability; usually bactericidal.

ONSET, PEAK, DURATION
Onset immediate after I.V. administration, unknown after I.M. injection. Serum levels peak within 30 minutes of I.M. injection, immediately after I.V. administration. Duration unknown.

INDICATIONS & DOSAGE
Serious infections of respiratory, GU, or GI tract; skin and soft-tissue infections (including peritonitis); bone and joint infections; septicemia; and endocarditis caused by such susceptible organisms as Escherichia coli *and other coliform bacteria,* Enterobacteriaceae, enterococci, gonococci, group A beta-hemolytic streptococci, *Haemophilus influenzae,* Klebsiella, *Proteus mirabilis,* Salmonella, Staphylococcus aureus, Shigella, Streptococcus pneumoniae *and* S. viridans, *and staphylococci; and perioperative prophylaxis* –
Adults: 500 mg to 1 g I.M. or I.V. (or intraperitoneally) q 4 to 6 hours; in life-threatening infections, up to 2 g q 4 hours.
Children: 80 to 160 mg/kg/day I.V. in divided doses q 4 or 6 hours. Dose should be proportionately less in accordance with age, weight, and severity of infection.
Perioperative prophylaxis in contaminated or potentially contaminated surgery –
Adults: 1 to 2 g I.V. 30 to 60 minutes before surgery and 1 to 2 g q 6 h postoperatively for 24 hours.

Children: 20 to 30 mg/kg I.V. 30 to 60 minutes before surgery and q 6 hours postoperatively for 24 hours

ADVERSE REACTIONS
CNS: headache, malaise, paresthesia, dizziness.
GI: pseudomembranous colitis, nausea, anorexia, vomiting, *diarrhea*, glossitis, dyspepsia, abdominal cramps, tenesmus, anal pruritus, oral candidiasis.
GU: nephrotoxicity, genital pruritus and moniliasis.
Hematologic: transient neutropenia, eosinophilia, *hemolytic anemia.*
Skin: *maculopapular and erythematous rashes, urticaria.*
Other: transient increases in liver enzymes; hypersensitivity reactions (serum sickness, *anaphylaxis*); dyspnea; fever; at injection site – *pain, induration, sterile abscesses, tissue sloughing;* with I.V. injection – *phlebitis, thrombophlebitis.*

INTERACTIONS
Probenecid: may increase blood levels of cephalosporins. Use together cautiously.

CONTRAINDICATIONS
Contraindicated in patients with hypersensitivity to cephalothin or other cephalosporins.

NURSING CONSIDERATIONS
• *Use cautiously* in patients with impaired renal function and in those with a history of sensitivity to penicillin.
• Obtain specimen for culture and sensitivity tests before first dose. Therapy may begin pending test results.
• **I.V. use:** When giving this drug I.V., check frequently for vein irritation and phlebitis. Alternate injection sites if I.V. therapy lasts longer than 3 days. Use of small I.V. needles in the larger available veins may be prefera-

---

†Available in Canada only.   ‡Available in Australia only.   ◊ Available OTC.

ble. Addition of a small concentration of heparin (100 units) or hydrocortisone (10 to 25 mg) may reduce incidence of phlebitis.

• For I.V. administration, dilute contents of 2-g vial with at least 20 ml of sterile water for injection, dextrose 5% injection, or 0.9% sodium chloride injection and add to one of following I.V. solutions: dextrose 5% injection, dextrose 5% in lactated Ringer's injection, Ionosol B in D_5W, lactated Ringer's injection, Normosol-N in D_5W, Plasma-Lyte injection, Plasma-Lyte-N injection in dextrose 5%, Ringer's injection, or Plasma-Lyte-N in 0.9% sodium chloride injection. Choose solution and fluid volume according to patient's fluid and electrolyte status.

• Know that I.V. route is preferable in severe or life-threatening infections.

• For I.M. administration, reconstitute each gram of cephalothin sodium with 4 ml of sterile water for injection, providing 500 mg in each 2.2 ml. If vial contents don't dissolve completely, add an additional 0.2 to 0.4 ml of diluent, and warm contents slightly. Inject deeply into a large muscle mass, such as the gluteus maximus or the lateral aspect of the thigh.

• Avoid I.M. route if possible; drug causes severe pain when administered I.M.

• With large doses or prolonged therapy, monitor for superinfection, especially in high-risk patients.

• Know that from 40% to 75% of patients receiving cephalosporins show a false-positive direct Coombs' test; only a few of these indicate hemolytic anemia.

• Keep in mind that urine glucose determinations may be false-positive with copper sulfate tests (Clinitest); glucose enzymatic tests (Clinistix, Tes-Tape) are not affected.

cephapirin sodium
Cefadyl

Pregnancy Risk Category: B

HOW SUPPLIED
Injection: 500-mg, 1-g, 2-g vials; 1-g, 2-g, 4-g piggyback vials
Pharmacy bulk package: 20 g

ACTION
Synthetic first-generation cephalosporin that inhibits cell-wall synthesis, promoting osmotic instability; usually bactericidal.

ONSET, PEAK, DURATION
Onset immediate after I.V. administration, unknown after I.M. injection. Serum levels peak within 30 minutes of I.M. injection, immediately after I.V. administration. Duration unknown.

INDICATIONS & DOSAGE
Perioperative prophylaxis in contaminated or potentially contaminated surgery—
Adults: 1 to 2 g I.M. or I.V. 30 to 60 minutes before surgery; then 1 to 2 g I.M. or I.V. q 6 hours for 24 hours. In procedures longer than 2 hours, additional doses may be given during surgery. In cases where infection would be devastating, prophylaxis may be continued for 3 to 5 days.
Serious infections of respiratory, GU, or GI tract; skin and soft-tissue infections; bone and joint infections (including osteomyelitis); septicemia; and endocarditis caused by Streptococcus pneumoniae, Escherichia coli, *group A beta-hemolytic streptococci,* Haemophilus influenzae, Klebsiella, Proteus mirabilis, Staphylococcus aureus, *and* Strep. viridans—
Adults: 500 mg to 1 g I.M. or I.V. q 4 to 6 hours. In life-threatening infections, up to 12 g/day may be used.
Children over 3 months: 10 to 20 mg/kg I.V. or I.M. q 6 hours; dose de-

---

Liquid form contains alcohol.   *Common* reactions are in italics; ***life-threatening,*** in bold italics.
**May contain tartrazine.

pends on age, weight, and severity of infection.

Patients with reduced renal function: may be treated adequately with a lower dose (7.5 to 15 mg/kg q 12 hours), depending on causative organism and severity of function. Patients with severely reduced renal function who are scheduled for dialysis should receive same dose just before dialysis and q 12 hours thereafter.

ADVERSE REACTIONS
CNS: dizziness, headache, malaise, paresthesia.
GI: pseudomembranous colitis, nausea, anorexia, vomiting, *diarrhea,* glossitis, dyspepsia, abdominal cramps, tenesmus, anal pruritus, oral candidiasis.
GU: genital pruritus and moniliasis, vaginitis.
Hematologic: transient neutropenia, eosinophilia, anemia.
Skin: *maculopapular and erythematous rashes, urticaria.*
Other: transient increases in liver enzymes; hypersensitivity reactions (serum sickness, **anaphylaxis**); dyspnea; at injection site—*pain, induration, sterile abscesses, tissue sloughing;* with I.V. injection—*phlebitis, thrombophlebitis.*

INTERACTIONS
Probenecid: may increase blood levels of cephalosporins. Sometimes used for this effect.

CONTRAINDICATIONS
Contraindicated in patients with hypersensitivity to cephapirin or other cephalosporins.

NURSING CONSIDERATIONS
• Use cautiously in patients with a history of sensitivity to penicillin.
• Obtain specimen for culture and sensitivity tests before first dose. Therapy may begin pending test results.

• **I.V. use:** Prepare I.V. infusion using dextrose injection, sodium chloride injection, or bacteriostatic water for injection as diluent: 20 ml yields 1 g/ 10 ml; 50 ml yields 1 g/25 ml; 100 ml yields 1 g/50 ml.
• When using I.V. infusion with Y-tubing, dilute 4-g vial with 40 ml of diluent. During infusion of cephapirin solution, stop other solution. Check volume of cephapirin solution carefully so that calculated dose is infused.
• When giving this drug I.V., check frequently for vein irritation and phlebitis. Alternate injection sites if I.V. therapy lasts longer than 3 days. Use of small I.V. needles in the larger available veins may be preferable.
• For I.M. use, reconstitute 1-g vial with 2 ml of sterile water for injection or bacteriostatic water for injection so that 1.2 ml contains 500 mg of cephapirin. Prepare patient for painful I.M. injection. Inject deeply into a large muscle mass, such as the gluteus maximus or the lateral aspect of the thigh.
• Store reconstituted cephapirin for 10 days under refrigeration and for 24 hours at room temperature.
• With large doses or prolonged therapy, monitor for superinfection, especially in high-risk patients.
• Know that from 40% to 75% of patients receiving cephalosporins show a false-positive direct Coombs' test, but only a few indicate hemolytic anemia.
• Keep in mind that urine glucose determinations may be false-positive with copper sulfate tests (Clinitest); glucose enzymatic tests (Clinistix, Tes-Tape) are not affected.

cephradine
Anspor, Velosef**

Pregnancy Risk Category: B

HOW SUPPLIED
Capsules: 250 mg, 500 mg
Oral suspension: 125 mg/5 ml, 250 mg/5 ml

ACTION
First-generation cephalosporin that inhibits cell-wall synthesis, promoting osmotic instability; usually bactericidal.

ONSET, PEAK, DURATION
Onset and duration unknown. Serum levels peak within 1 hour after oral dose.

INDICATIONS & DOSAGE
Serious infections of respiratory, GU, or GI tract; skin and soft-tissue infections; bone and joint infections; septicemia; endocarditis; and otitis media caused by such susceptible organisms as Escherichia coli *and other coliform bacteria, group A beta-hemolytic streptococci,* Haemophilus influenzae, Klebsiella, Proteus mirabilis, Staphylococcus aureus, Streptococcus pneumoniae, Strep. viridans, *and staphylococci; and perioperative prophylaxis* –
Adults: 250 to 500 mg P.O. q 6 hours.
Children over 9 months: 25 to 50 mg/kg P.O. daily in divided doses.
Otitis media –
75 to 100 mg/kg P.O. daily. Don't exceed 4 g daily.
All patients, regardless of age and weight: larger doses (up to 1 g q.i.d.) may be given for severe or chronic infections.

ADVERSE REACTIONS
CNS: dizziness, headache, malaise, paresthesia.
GI: pseudomembranous colitis, *nausea, anorexia,* vomiting, heartburn, glossitis, dyspepsia, abdominal cramping, *diarrhea,* tenesmus, anal pruritus, oral candidiasis.
GU: genital pruritus and moniliasis, vaginitis.

Hematologic: transient neutropenia, eosinophilia.
Skin: *maculopapular and erythematous rashes, urticaria.*
Other: transient increases in liver enzymes, hypersensitivity reactions (serum sickness, ***anaphylaxis***), dyspnea.

INTERACTIONS
Probenecid: may increase blood levels of cephalosporins. Sometimes used for this effect.

CONTRAINDICATIONS
Contraindicated in patients with hypersensitivity to cephradine and to other cephalosporins.

NURSING CONSIDERATIONS
• Use cautiously in patients with impaired renal function or with a history of sensitivity to penicillin.
• Obtain specimen for culture and sensitivity tests before first dose. Therapy may begin pending test results.
• Know that group A beta-hemolytic streptococcal infections should be treated for a minimum of 10 days.
• Be aware that from 40% to 75% of patients receiving cephalosporins show a false-positive direct Coombs' test, but only a few indicate hemolytic anemia.
• Keep in mind that urine glucose determinations may be false-positive with copper sulfate tests (Clinitest); glucose enzymatic tests (Clinistix, Tes-Tape) are not affected.
• With large doses or prolonged therapy, monitor for superinfection, especially in high-risk patients.
• Tell the patient to take drug with food or milk to lessen GI discomfort.
• Tell the patient to take all of the medication exactly as prescribed, even after he feels better.

loracarbef
Lorabid

Pregnancy Risk Category: B

HOW SUPPLIED
Pulvules: 200 mg, 400 mg
Powder for oral suspension: 100 mg/5 ml, 200 mg/5 ml in 50-ml and 100-ml bottles

ACTION
A synthetic beta-lactam antibiotic of the carbacephem class with actions similar to the second-generation cephalosporins. Inhibits cell-wall synthesis, promoting osmotic instability; usually bactericidal.

ONSET, PEAK, DURATION
Onset and duration unknown. Serum levels peak 30 minutes to 1 hour after an oral dose.

INDICATIONS & DOSAGE
Secondary bacterial infections of acute bronchitis –
Adults: 200 to 400 mg P.O. q 12 hours for 7 days.
Acute bacterial exacerbations of chronic bronchitis –
Adults: 400 mg P.O. q 12 hours for 7 days.
Pneumonia –
Adults: 400 mg P.O. q 12 hours for 14 days.
Pharyngitis, sinusitis, or tonsillitis –
Adults: 200 to 400 mg P.O. q 12 hours for 10 days.
Children: 15 mg/kg P.O. daily in divided doses q 12 hours for 10 days.
Acute otitis media –
Children: 30 mg/kg (oral suspension) P.O. daily in divided doses q 12 hours for 10 days.
Uncomplicated skin and skin-structure infections –
Adults: 200 mg P.O. q 12 hours for 7 days.
Impetigo –

Children: 15 mg/kg P.O. daily in divided doses q 12 hours for 7 days.
Uncomplicated cystitis –
Adults: 200 mg P.O. daily for 7 days.
Uncomplicated pyelonephritis –
Adults: 400 mg P.O. q 12 hours for 14 days.

Patients with a creatinine clearance greater than or equal to 50 ml/minute/1.73 m^2 don't require dose and interval changes. Patients with a creatinine clearance of 10 to 49 ml/minute/1.73 m^2 should receive half of the usual dose at the same interval; with a creatinine clearance below 10 ml/minute/1.73 m^2, the usual dose q 3 to 5 days. Hemodialysis patients require another dose after dialysis.

ADVERSE REACTIONS
CNS: headache, somnolence, nervousness, insomnia, dizziness.
CV: vasodilation.
GI: diarrhea, nausea, vomiting, abdominal pain, anorexia, pseudomembranous colitis.
GU: vaginal candidiasis or moniliasis, transient increases in BUN and creatinine levels.
Hematologic: transient thrombocytopenia, leukopenia, eosinophilia.
Skin: rash, urticaria, pruritus, *erythema multiforme.*
Other: hypersensitivity reactions, including *anaphylaxis;* transient elevations in AST, ALT, and alkaline phosphatase levels.

INTERACTIONS
Probenecid: decreased excretion of loracarbef, causing increased plasma levels. Monitor for toxicity.

CONTRAINDICATIONS
Contraindicated in patients with hypersensitivity to the drug or other cephalosporins and in patients with diarrhea caused by pseudomembranous colitis.

NURSING CONSIDERATIONS

• Use cautiously in pregnant or breast-feeding women. Safety and efficacy have not been established in infants under 6 months.

• Obtain specimen for culture and sensitivity tests before first dose. Therapy may begin pending test results.

• To reconstitute powder for oral suspension, add 30 ml of water in two portions to the 50-ml bottle or 60 ml of water in two portions to the 100-ml bottle; shake after each addition.

• After reconstitution, store oral suspension for 14 days at room temperature (59° to 86° F [15° to 30° C]).

• Monitor for signs and symptoms of superinfection. May cause overgrowth of nonsusceptible bacteria or fungi.

• Monitor the patient for seizures. Beta-lactam antibiotics may trigger seizures in susceptible patients, especially when given without dosage modification to those with renal impairment. If seizures occur, discontinue drug and notify the doctor. Administer anticonvulsants as ordered.

• For otitis media, be alert that the more rapidly absorbed oral suspension produces higher peak plasma levels than do the capsules.

• Know that from 40% to 75% of patients receiving cephalosporins show a false-positive direct Coombs' test; only a few of these indicate hemolytic anemia.

• Tell the patient to take drug on an empty stomach, at least 1 hour before or 2 hours after meals.

• Tell the patient to take all of the medication prescribed, even after he feels better.

• Instruct the patient to discard unused portion after 14 days.

---

*Liquid form contains alcohol.
**May contain tartrazine.

Common reactions are in italics; *life-threatening,* in bold italics.

demeclocycline hydrochloride
doxycycline
doxycycline hyclate
doxycycline hydrochloride
minocycline hydrochloride
oxytetracycline hydrochloride
tetracycline hydrochloride

COMBINATION PRODUCTS
UROBIOTIC-250: oxytetracycline hydrochloride 250 mg, sulfamethizole 250 mg, and phenazopyridine hydrochloride 50 mg.

demeclocycline hydrochloride
Declomycin, Ledermycin‡

Pregnancy Risk Category: NR

HOW SUPPLIED
Tablets: 150 mg, 300 mg
Capsules: 150 mg

ACTION
Unknown. Thought to exert bacteriostatic effect by binding to the 30S ribosomal subunit of microorganisms, thus inhibiting protein synthesis.

ONSET, PEAK, DURATION
Onset and duration unknown. Serum levels peak within 3 to 4 hours after oral dose.

INDICATIONS & DOSAGE
Infections caused by susceptible gram-negative and gram-positive organisms, including Haemophilus ducreyi, Rickettsiae, Mycoplasma pneumoniae, Yersinia pestis, Campylobacter fetus. *Also indicated for the organism causing psittacosis, lymphogranuloma venereum, granuloma inguinale, relapsing fever, and trachoma* –

Adults: 150 mg P.O. q 6 hours or 300 mg P.O. q 12 hours.
Children over age 8: 6 to 12 mg/kg P.O. daily, in divided doses q 6 to 12 hours.
Gonorrhea –
Adults: initially, 600 mg P.O.; then 300 mg P.O. q 12 hours for 4 days (total 3 g).

ADVERSE REACTIONS
CNS: *intracranial hypertension* (pseudotumor cerebri).
CV: pericarditis.
EENT: dysphagia, glossitis.
GI: anorexia, *nausea, vomiting, diarrhea,* enterocolitis, anogenital inflammation.
Hematologic: neutropenia, eosinophilia, thrombocytopenia, *hemolytic anemia.*
Skin: *maculopapular and erythematous rashes, photosensitivity, increased pigmentation, urticaria.*
Other: hypersensitivity reactions *(anaphylaxis),* elevated liver enzymes, *increased BUN level,* diabetes insipidus syndrome (polyuria, polydipsia, weakness), permanent tooth discoloration or bone growth retardation if used in children under age 8.

INTERACTIONS
Antacids (including sodium bicarbonate) and laxatives containing aluminum, magnesium, or calcium; antidiarrheals; food, milk, or other dairy products: decreased antibiotic absorption. Give antibiotic 1 hour before or 2 hours after any of the above.
Ferrous sulfate and other iron products, zinc: decreased antibiotic absorption. Give antibiotic 3 hours after or 2 hours before iron administration.
Methoxyflurane: may cause nephro-

toxicity with tetracyclines. Monitor carefully.
Oral anticoagulants: increased anticoagulant effect. Monitor PT and adjust dosage as ordered.
Oral contraceptives: decreased contraceptive effectiveness and increased risk of breakthrough bleeding. Use a nonhormonal birth control method.
Penicillins: may interfere with bactericidal action of penicillins. Avoid using together.

CONTRAINDICATIONS
Contraindicated in patients with hypersensitivity to the drug or other tetracyclines.

NURSING CONSIDERATIONS
Use cautiously in patients with impaired renal or hepatic function. Use of these drugs during last half of pregnancy and in children under age 8 may cause permanent discoloration of teeth, enamel defects, and bone growth retardation.
• Obtain specimen for culture and sensitivity tests before first dose. Therapy may begin pending test results.
• Check expiration date. Outdated or deteriorated tetracyclines have been associated with reversible nephrotoxicity (Fanconi's syndrome).
• Don't expose these drugs to light or heat; store in tight container.
• With large doses or prolonged therapy, monitor for superinfection, especially in high-risk patients.
• Check the patient's tongue for signs of monilia infection. Stress good oral hygiene.
• Be aware that demeclocycline may cause false-negative reading of glucose enzymatic tests (Clinistix, Tes-Tape).
• Warn the patient to avoid direct sunlight and ultraviolet light. A sunscreen may help prevent photosensitivity reactions. Photosensitivity persists for some time after discontinuation of drug.
• Explain to the patient that drug's effectiveness is reduced when taken with milk or other dairy products, food, antacids, or iron products. Tell him to take each dose with a full glass of water on an empty stomach, at least 1 hour before or 2 hours after meals, and to remain standing for 90 seconds after ingestion. Give at least 1 hour before bedtime to prevent esophagitis.
• Instruct the patient to take entire amount of medication, exactly as prescribed, even after he feels better.

doxycycline
Doxylin‡, Vibramycin

doxycycline hyclate
Apo-Doxy†, Doryx, Doxy-Caps, Doxycin†, Doxy-Tabs, Monodox, Novodoxylin†, Vibramycin, Vibra-Tabs

doxycycline hydrochloride
Cyclidox‡, Doryx‡, Vibramycin‡, Vibramycin IV, Vibra-Tabs 50‡

Pregnancy Risk Category: D

HOW SUPPLIED
doxycycline
Tablets: 50 mg‡, 100 mg‡
Oral suspension: 25 mg/5 ml
Syrup: 50 mg/5 ml
doxycycline hyclate
Tablets: 50 mg, 100 mg
Capsules: 50 mg, 100 mg
Capsules (coated pellets): 100 mg
Injection: 100 mg, 200 mg
doxycycline hydrochloride
Tablets: 50 mg‡, 100 mg‡
Capsules: 50 mg‡, 100 mg‡, 250 mg‡
Injection: 100 mg‡
Powder for injection: 200 mg

ACTION
Unknown. Thought to exert bacteriostatic effect by binding to the 30S ri-

bosomal subunit of microorganisms, thus inhibiting protein synthesis.

ONSET, PEAK, DURATION

Onset immediate after I.V. administration, unknown after oral administration. Serum levels peak within 1½ to 4 hours after oral dose; not clearly defined for I.V. use. Duration unknown.

INDICATIONS & DOSAGE

Infections caused by sensitive gram-negative and gram-positive organisms, including Rickettsiae, Chlamydia, *and* Mycoplasma, *and the organisms that cause trachoma and Lyme disease* –

Adults: 100 mg P.O. q 12 hours on first day, then 100 mg P.O. daily; or 200 mg I.V. on first day in one or two infusions, then 100 to 200 mg I.V. daily.

Children over age 8 and under 45 kg: 4.4 mg/kg P.O. or I.V. daily, in divided doses q 12 hours on first day; then 2.2 to 4.4 mg/kg daily. For children over 45 kg, dosage is same as for adults.

Give I.V. infusion slowly (minimum 1 hour). Infusion must be completed within 12 hours (within 6 hours in lactated Ringer's solution or dextrose 5% in lactated Ringer's solution).

Gonorrhea in patients allergic to penicillin –

Adults: 200 mg P.O. initially, followed by 100 mg P.O. h.s. and 100 mg P.O. b.i.d. for 3 days; or 300 mg P.O. initially and repeat dose in 1 hour.

Primary or secondary syphilis in patients allergic to penicillin –

Adults: 300 mg P.O. daily in divided doses for at least 10 days.

Uncomplicated urethral, endocervical, or rectal infections caused by Chlamydia trachomatis *or* Ureaplasma urealyticum –

Adults: 100 mg P.O. b.i.d. for at least 7 days.

Prophylaxis of malaria –

Adults: 100 mg P.O. daily.

Children over 8 years: 2 mg/kg P.O. once daily. Dosage should not exceed adult dose.

Note: Prophylaxis should begin 1 to 2 days before travel to malarious area and be continued throughout travel and for 4 weeks after.

ADVERSE REACTIONS

CNS: *intracranial hypertension* (pseudotumor cerebri).

CV: pericarditis.

EENT: sore throat, glossitis, dysphagia.

GI: anorexia, *epigastric distress, nausea,* vomiting, *diarrhea,* oral candidiasis, enterocolitis, anogenital inflammation.

Hematologic: neutropenia, eosinophilia.

Skin: *maculopapular and erythematous rashes, photosensitivity, increased pigmentation, urticaria.*

Other: hypersensitivity reactions *(anaphylaxis)*; elevated liver enzymes; permanent discoloration of teeth, enamel defects, bone growth retardation if used in children under age 8; superinfection; thrombophlebitis.

INTERACTIONS

Antacids (including sodium bicarbonate) and laxatives containing aluminum, magnesium, or calcium; antidiarrheals: decreased antibiotic absorption. Give antibiotic 1 hour before or 2 hours after any of the above.

Ferrous sulfate and other iron products, zinc: decreased antibiotic absorption. Give drug 3 hours after or 2 hours before iron administration.

Methoxyflurane: may cause nephrotoxicity with tetracyclines. Monitor carefully.

Oral anticoagulants: increased anti-

coagulant effect. Monitor PT and adjust dosage as ordered.
Oral contraceptives: decreased contraceptive effectiveness and increased risk of breakthrough bleeding. Use a nonhormonal form of birth control.
Penicillins: may interfere with bactericidal action of penicillins. Avoid using together.
Phenobarbital, carbamazepine, alcohol: decreased antibiotic effect. Avoid if possible.

CONTRAINDICATIONS
Contraindicated in patients with hypersensitivity to the drug or other tetracyclines.

NURSING CONSIDERATIONS
• Use cautiously in patients with impaired renal or hepatic function. Use of these drugs during last half of pregnancy and in children under age 8 may cause permanent discoloration of teeth, enamel defects, and bone growth retardation.
• Obtain specimen for culture and sensitivity tests before first dose. Therapy may begin pending test results.
• Check expiration date. Outdated or deteriorated tetracyclines have been associated with reversible nephrotoxicity (Fanconi's syndrome).
• Administer with milk or food if adverse GI reactions develop.
• **I.V. use:** Reconstitute powder for injection with sterile water for injection. Use 10 ml in 100-mg vial and 20 ml in 200-mg vial. Dilute solution to 100 to 1,000 ml for I.V. infusion. Avoid extravasation. Don't infuse solutions that are more concentrated than 1 mg/ml. Monitor I.V. infusion site for signs of thrombophlebitis, which may occur with I.V. administration.
• Don't expose drug to light or heat. Protect it from sunlight during infusion.
• Know that reconstituted injectable

solution is stable for 72 hours if refrigerated.
• Be alert that parenteral form may cause false-positive reading of copper sulfate tests (Clinitest). All forms may cause false-negative reading of glucose enzymatic tests (Clinistix, Tes-Tape).
• With large doses or prolonged therapy, monitor for superinfection, especially in high-risk patients.
• Check the patient's tongue for signs of fungal infection. Stress good oral hygiene.
• Know that doxycycline may be used cautiously in patients with renal impairment; doesn't accumulate or cause a significant rise in BUN levels.
• Tell the patient to take entire amount of medication exactly as prescribed, even after he feels better.
• Tell patient not to take oral tablets or capsules within 1 hour of bedtime because of possible dysphagia.
• Tell the patient to use a sunscreen and avoid strong sunlight during therapy to prevent photosensitivity reactions.

---

minocycline hydrochloride
Dynacin, Minocin*, Minomycin‡, Minomycin IV‡

Pregnancy Risk Category: D

HOW SUPPLIED
Tablets (film-coated): 50 mg, 100 mg
Capsules: 50 mg, 100 mg
Oral suspension: 50 mg/5 ml
Injection: 100 mg

ACTION
Unknown. Thought to exert bacteriostatic effect by binding to the 30S ribosomal subunit of microorganisms, thus inhibiting protein synthesis.

ONSET, PEAK, DURATION
Onset immediate after I.V. administration, unknown after oral administration. Serum levels peak immedi-

---

ately after I.V. administration, within 1 to 4 hours after oral dose. Duration unknown.

INDICATIONS & DOSAGE

Infections caused by sensitive gram-negative and gram-positive organisms, trachoma, amebiasis—
Adults: 200 mg I.V.; then 100 mg I.V. q 12 hours. Not to exceed 400 mg/day. Or 200 mg P.O. initially; then 100 mg P.O. q 12 hours. Some clinicians use 100 or 200 mg P.O. initially, followed by 50 mg q.i.d.
Children over 8 years: initially, 4 mg/kg P.O. or I.V., followed by 2 mg/kg q 12 hours.
Given I.V. in 500- to 1,000-ml solution without calcium, and administered over 6 hours.
Gonorrhea in patients sensitive to penicillin—
Adults: initially, 200 mg P.O.; then 100 mg q 12 hours for at least 4 days.
Syphilis in patients sensitive to penicillin—
Adults: initially, 200 mg P.O.; then 100 mg q 12 hours for 10 to 15 days.
Meningococcal carrier state—
100 mg P.O. q 12 hours for 5 days.
Uncomplicated urethral, endocervical, or rectal infection caused by Chlamydia trachomatis *or* Ureaplasma urealyticum—
Adults: 100 mg P.O. b.i.d. for at least 7 days.
Uncomplicated gonococcal urethritis in men—
Adults: 100 mg P.O. b.i.d. for 5 days.

ADVERSE REACTIONS

CNS: *light-headedness, dizziness from vestibular toxicity;* **intracranial hypertension** (pseudotumor cerebri).
CV: pericarditis.
EENT: dysphagia, glossitis.
GI: *anorexia,* epigastric distress, oral candidiasis, *nausea,* vomiting, *diarrhea,* enterocolitis, inflammatory lesions in anogenital region.

Hematologic: neutropenia, eosinophilia.
Skin: *maculopapular and erythematous rashes, photosensitivity, increased pigmentation, urticaria.*
Other: hypersensitivity reactions *(anaphylaxis);* elevated liver enzymes; increased BUN level; permanent discoloration of teeth, enamel defects, and bone growth retardation if used in children under age 8; superinfection; *thrombophlebitis.*

INTERACTIONS

Antacids (including sodium bicarbonate) and laxatives containing aluminum, magnesium, or calcium; antidiarrheals: decreased antibiotic absorption. Give antibiotic 1 hour before or 2 hours after any of the above.
Ferrous sulfate and other iron products, zinc: decreased antibiotic absorption. Give drug 3 hours after or 2 hours before iron administration.
Methoxyflurane: may cause nephrotoxicity with tetracyclines. Monitor carefully.
Oral anticoagulants: increased anticoagulant effect. Monitor PT and adjust dosage as ordered.
Oral contraceptives: decreased contraceptive effectiveness and increased risk of breakthrough bleeding. Use a nonhormonal form of birth control.
Penicillins: may interfere with bactericidal action of penicillins. Avoid using together.

CONTRAINDICATIONS

Contraindicated in patients with hypersensitivity to the drug or other tetracyclines.

NURSING CONSIDERATIONS

• Use cautiously in patients with impaired renal or hepatic function. Use of these drugs during last half of pregnancy and in children under age 8 may cause permanent discoloration of teeth, enamel defects, and bone growth retardation.

• Obtain specimen for culture and sensitivity tests before first dose. Therapy may begin pending test results.

• Check expiration date. Outdated or deteriorated tetracyclines have been associated with reversible nephrotoxicity (Fanconi's syndrome).

• Don't expose these drugs to light or heat. Keep cap tightly closed.

• **I.V. use:** Reconstitute 100-mg of powder with 5-ml of sterile water for injection, with further dilution of 500 to 1,000 ml for I.V. infusion. Stable for 24 hours at room temperature.

• Be aware that patient may develop thrombophlebitis with I.V. administration of this drug. Avoid extravasation. Switch to oral therapy as soon as possible.

• With large doses or prolonged therapy, monitor for superinfection, especially in high-risk patients.

• Check the patient's tongue for signs of monilia infection. Stress good oral hygiene.

• Be aware that the drug may cause tooth discoloration in young adults. Observe for brown pigmentation, and inform the doctor if it occurs.

• Know that parenteral form may cause false-positive reading of copper sulfate tests (Clinitest). All forms may cause false-negative reading of glucose enzymatic tests (Clinistix, Tes-Tape).

• Tell the patient that the drug may be taken with food. Tell the patient to take entire amount of medication exactly as prescribed, even after he feels better.

• Tell the patient to take oral form of drug with a full glass of water. Don't take within 1 hour of bedtime to avoid esophagitis.

• Warn the patient to avoid driving or other hazardous tasks until the adverse CNS effects of the drug are known.

• Warn the patient to avoid direct sunlight and ultraviolet light. A sunscreen may help prevent photosensitivity reactions.

---

oxytetracycline hydrochloride
Terramycin, Tija

Pregnancy Risk Category: NR

HOW SUPPLIED
Capsules: 250 mg
Injection: 50 mg/ml, 125 mg/ml (with lidocaine 2%)

ACTION
Unknown. Thought to exert bacteriostatic effect by binding to the 30S ribosomal subunit of microorganisms, thus inhibiting protein synthesis.

ONSET, PEAK, DURATION
Onset and duration unknown. Serum levels peak within 2 to 4 hours after oral dose, unknown after I.M. injection.

INDICATIONS & DOSAGE
Infections caused by sensitive gram-negative and gram-positive organisms, trachoma, rickettsiae –
Adults: 1 to 2 g P.O. in four divided doses, 100 mg I.M. q 8 to 12 hours, or 250 mg I.M. as a single dose.
Children over 8 years: 25 to 50 mg/kg P.O. daily, in divided doses q 6 hours; 15 to 25 mg/kg I.M. daily, in divided doses q 8 to 12 hours.
Brucellosis –
Adults: 500 mg P.O. q.i.d. for 3 weeks combined with 1 g of streptomycin I.M. q 12 hours first week, once daily second week.
Syphilis in patients sensitive to penicillin –
Adults: 30 to 40 g total dosage P.O., divided equally over 10 to 15 days.
Gonorrhea in patients sensitive to penicillin –
Adults: initially, 1.5 g P.O., followed by 0.5 g q.i.d., for a total of 9 g.

ADVERSE REACTIONS

CNS: *intracranial hypertension* (pseudotumor cerebri).
CV: pericarditis.
EENT: dysphagia, glossitis.
GI: *anorexia, nausea,* vomiting, *diarrhea,* oral candidiasis, enterocolitis, anogenital inflammation.
Hematologic: neutropenia, eosinophilia.
Skin: *maculopapular and erythematous rashes, urticaria, photosensitivity, increased pigmentation.*
Other: hypersensitivity reactions *(anaphylaxis);* elevated liver enzymes; permanent discoloration of teeth, enamel defects, and bone growth retardation if used in children under age 8; superinfection; increased BUN levels; *irritation after I.M. injection; thrombophlebitis.*

INTERACTIONS

Antacids (including sodium bicarbonate) and laxatives containing aluminum, magnesium, or calcium; antidiarrheals; food, milk, or other dairy products: decreased antibiotic absorption. Give antibiotic 1 hour before or 2 hours after any of the above.
Ferrous sulfate and other iron products, zinc: decreased antibiotic absorption. Give antibiotic 3 hours after or 2 hours before iron administration.
Methoxyflurane: may cause nephrotoxicity with tetracyclines. Monitor carefully.
Oral anticoagulants: increased anticoagulant effect. Monitor PT and adjust dosage as ordered.
Oral contraceptives: decreased contraceptive effectiveness and increased risk of breakthrough bleeding. Use a nonhormonal form of birth control.
Penicillins: may interfere with bactericidal action of penicillins. Avoid using together.

CONTRAINDICATIONS

Contraindicated in patients with hypersensitivity to the drug or other tetracyclines.

NURSING CONSIDERATIONS

• Use cautiously in patients with impaired renal or hepatic function. Use of these drugs during last half of pregnancy and in children under age 8 may cause permanent discoloration of teeth, enamel defects, and bone growth retardation.
• Obtain specimen for culture and sensitivity tests before first dose. Therapy may begin pending test results.
• Check expiration date. Outdated or deteriorated oxytetracyclines have been associated with reversible nephrotoxicity (Fanconi's syndrome).
• Don't expose these drugs to light or heat.
• For I.M. administration, inject deeply into a large muscle mass. Warn the patient that it may be painful. Rotate sites. I.M. preparations contain a local anesthetic; ask the patient about hypersensitivity reactions to local anesthetics.
• With large doses or prolonged therapy, monitor for superinfection, especially in high-risk patients.
• Check the patient's tongue for signs of fungal infection. Stress good oral hygiene.
• Know that parenteral form may cause false-positive reading of copper sulfate tests (Clinitest). All forms may cause false-negative reading of glucose enzymatic tests (Clinistix, Tes-Tape).
• Explain to the patient that drug's effectiveness is reduced when taken with milk or other dairy products, food, antacids, or iron products. Tell him to take each dose with a full glass of water on an empty stomach, at least 1 hour before or 2 hours after meals. Give at least 1 hour before bedtime to prevent esophagitis.

• Tell the patient to take entire amount of medication exactly as prescribed, even after he feels better.
• Warn the patient to avoid direct sunlight and ultraviolet light. A sunscreen may help prevent photosensitivity reactions. Photosensitivity persists for considerable time after discontinuation of drug.

tetracycline hydrochloride
Achromycin V, Apo-Tetra†, Austramycin V‡, Hostacycline P‡, Nor-Tet, Novotetra†, Panmycin**, Panmycin P‡, Robitet, Sumycin, Tetracap, Tetralan, Tetralean†

Pregnancy Risk Category: NR

HOW SUPPLIED
Tablets: 250 mg, 500 mg
Capsules: 100 mg, 250 mg, 500 mg
Oral suspension: 125 mg/5 ml

ACTION
Unknown. Thought to exert bacteriostatic effect by binding to the 30S ribosomal subunit of microorganisms, thus inhibiting protein synthesis.

ONSET, PEAK, DURATION
Onset and duration unknown. Serum levels peak within 2 to 4 hours.

INDICATIONS & DOSAGE
Infections caused by sensitive gram-negative and gram-positive organisms, including Rickettsiae, Chlamydia, Mycoplasma, and organisms that cause trachoma–
Adults: 250 to 500 mg P.O. q 6 hours.
Children over 8 years: 25 to 50 mg/kg P.O. daily, in divided doses q 6 hours.
Uncomplicated urethral, endocervical, or rectal infection caused by Chlamydia trachomatis–
Adults: 500 mg P.O. q.i.d. for at least 7 days.
Brucellosis–
Adults: 500 mg P.O. q 6 hours for 3

weeks combined with 1 g of streptomycin I.M. q 12 hours first week; daily, the second week.
Gonorrhea in patients sensitive to penicillin–
Adults: initially, 1.5 g P.O.; then 500 mg q 6 hours for a total dose of 9 g.
Syphilis in patients sensitive to penicillin–
Adults: total of 30 to 40 g P.O. in equally divided doses over 10 to 15 days.
Acne–
Adults and adolescents: initially, 250 mg P.O. q 6 hours; then 125 to 500 mg daily or every other day.

ADVERSE REACTIONS
CNS: dizziness, headache, ***intracranial hypertension*** (pseudotumor cerebri).
CV: pericarditis.
EENT: sore throat, glossitis, dysphagia.
GI: anorexia, *epigastric distress, nausea,* vomiting, *diarrhea,* esophagitis, oral candidiasis, stomatitis, enterocolitis, inflammatory lesions in anogenital region.
Hematologic: neutropenia, eosinophilia.
Skin: *candidal superinfection, maculopapular and erythematous rashes, urticaria, photosensitivity, increased pigmentation.*
Other: hypersensitivity reactions, elevated liver enzymes, *increased BUN levels, permanent discoloration of teeth, enamel defects, and retardation of bone growth if used in children under age 8.*

INTERACTIONS
Antacids (including sodium bicarbonate) and laxatives containing aluminum, magnesium, or calcium; antidiarrheals containing kaolin, pectin, or bismuth subsalicylate; food, milk, or other dairy products: decreased antibiotic absorption. Give antibiotic 1

hour before or 2 hours after any of the above.

Ferrous sulfate and other iron products, zinc: decreased antibiotic absorption. Give tetracyclines 3 hours after or 2 hours before iron administration.

Lithium carbonate: may alter serum lithium levels.

Methoxyflurane: may cause severe nephrotoxicity with tetracyclines. Monitor carefully.

Oral anticoagulants: potentiated anticoagulant effects. Monitor PT and adjust anticoagulant dosage as ordered.

Oral contraceptives: decreased contraceptive effectiveness and increased risk of breakthrough bleeding. Use a nonhormonal form of birth control.

Penicillins: may interfere with bactericidal action of penicillins. Avoid using together.

CONTRAINDICATIONS
Contraindicated in patients with hypersensitivity to tetracyclines.

NURSING CONSIDERATIONS
• Use with extreme caution in patients with impaired renal or hepatic function. Also use with extreme caution (if at all) during last half of pregnancy and in children under age 8 because drug may cause permanent discoloration of teeth, enamel defects, and bone growth retardation.
• Obtain specimen for culture and sensitivity tests before giving first dose. Therapy may begin pending test results.
• Check expiration date. Outdated or deteriorated tetracyclines have been associated with reversible nephrotoxicity (Fanconi's syndrome).
• Don't expose drug to light or heat.
• With large doses or prolonged therapy, monitor for superinfection, especially in high-risk patients.
• Check the patient's tongue for signs of monilia infection. Stress good oral hygiene.

• Know that drug may cause false-negative reading with glucose enzymatic tests (Clinistix, Tes-Tape).
• Explain to the patient that effectiveness is reduced when taken with milk or other dairy products, food, antacids, or iron products. Tell him to take each dose with a full glass of water on an empty stomach, at least 1 hour before or 2 hours after meals. Give at least 1 hour before bedtime to prevent esophagitis.
• Tell the patient to take drug exactly as prescribed, even after he feels better, and to take entire amount prescribed.
• Warn the patient to avoid direct sunlight and ultraviolet light. A sunscreen may help prevent photosensitivity reactions. Photosensitivity persists after discontinuation of drug.

15

Sulfonamides

co-trimoxazole
sulfadiazine
sulfamethoxazole
sulfisoxazole

COMBINATION PRODUCTS

AZO GANTANOL, AZO SULFAMETH-
OXAZOLE†, URO GANTANOL†:
sulfamethoxazole 500 mg and phenazopyridine hydrochloride 100 mg.
AZO GANTRISIN, AZO SULFISOXA-
ZOLE: sulfisoxazole 500 mg and phenazopyridine hydrochloride 50 mg.
PEDIAZOLE: sulfisoxazole 600 mg
and erythromycin ethylsuccinate 200
mg per 5 ml.
TRIPLE SULFA: sulfadiazine 167 mg,
sulfamerazine 167 mg, and sulfa-
methazine 167 mg.

---

co-trimoxazole
(sulfamethoxazole-
trimethoprim)

Apo-Sulfatrim†, Apo-Sulfatrim DS†,
Bactrim*, Bactrim DS, Bactrim I.V.
Infusion, Cotrim, Cotrim D.S.,
Novotrimel†, Novotrimel DS†,
Protrin†, Protrin DF†, Resprim‡,
Roubac†, Roubac DS†, Septra*,
Septra DS, Septra I.V. Infusion,
Septrin‡, SMZ-TMP,
Sulfamethoprim, Sulfamethoprim
DS, Sulmeprim, Trib‡, Uroplus DS,
Uroplus SS

*Pregnancy Risk Category: C
(contraindicated at term)*

HOW SUPPLIED

Tablets: trimethoprim 80 mg and
sulfamethoxazole 400 mg; trimethoprim 160 mg and sulfamethoxazole
800 mg
Oral suspension: trimethoprim 40 mg
and sulfamethoxazole 200 mg/5 ml
Injection: trimethoprim 16 mg and

sulfamethoxazole 80 mg/ml (5 ml/am-
pule)

ACTION

Sulfamethoxazole component inhibits
the formation of dihydrofolic acid
from PABA; the trimethoprim component inhibits dihydrofolate reductase.
Both decrease bacterial folic acid synthesis.

ONSET, PEAK, DURATION

Onset immediate after I.V. administration, unknown after oral administration. Serum levels peak 1 to 4
hours after an oral dose or immediately after an I.V. infusion. Duration
unknown.

INDICATIONS & DOSAGE

*Urinary tract infections and shigel-
losis –*

Adults: 160 mg trimethoprim/800 mg
sulfamethoxazole (double strength
tablet) P.O. q 12 hours for 10 to 14
days in urinary tract infections and for
5 days in shigellosis. For simple cystitis or acute urethral syndrome, one to
three double-strength tablets may be
given as a single dose. If indicated,
I.V. infusion is given: 8 to 10 mg/kg/
day (based on trimethoprim component) in two to four divided doses q 6,
8, or 12 hours for up to 14 days. Maximum daily dose is 960 mg trimethoprim.
Children 2 months and over: 8 mg/
kg trimethoprim/40 mg/kg sulfamethoxazole P.O. per 24 hours, in two divided doses q 12 hours (10 days for
urinary tract infections; 5 days, for
shigellosis). If indicated, I.V. infusion
is given: 8 to 10 mg/kg/day (based on
trimethoprim component) in two to
four divided doses q 6, 8, or 12 hours.
Adult dose should not be exceeded.

---

*Liquid form contains alcohol.
**May contain tartrazine.

*Common reactions are in italics; **life-threatening,** in bold italics.*

Otitis media in patients with penicillin allergy or penicillin-resistant infections —
Children 2 months and over: 8 mg/kg trimethoprim/40 mg/kg sulfamethoxazole P.O. per 24 hours, in two divided doses q 12 hours for 10 days.
Pneumocystis carinii *pneumonia —*
Adults and children 2 months and over: 20 mg/kg trimethoprim/100 mg/kg sulfamethoxazole P.O. per 24 hours, in equally divided doses q 6 hours for 14 days. If indicated, I.V. infusion may be given 15 to 20 mg/kg/day (based on trimethoprim component) in three or four divided doses q 6 to 8 hours for up to 14 days.
Chronic bronchitis —
Adults: 160 mg trimethoprim/800 mg sulfamethoxazole P.O. q 12 hours for 10 to 14 days. Not recommended for infants under 2 months old.
Traveler's diarrhea —
Adults: 160 mg trimethoprim/800 mg sulfamethoxazole P.O. b.i.d. for 3 to 5 days. Some patients may require 2 days of therapy or less.
Urinary tract infections in males with prostatitis —
Adults: 160 mg trimethoprim/800 mg sulfamethoxazole P.O. b.i.d. for 3 to 6 months.
Chronic urinary tract infections —
Adults: 40 mg trimethoprim/200 mg sulfamethoxazole (½ tablet) or 80 mg trimethoprim/400 mg sulfamethoxazole P.O. daily or three times a week for 3 to 6 months.

ADVERSE REACTIONS
CNS: headache, mental depression, seizures, hallucinations, ataxia, nervousness, fatigue, muscle weakness, vertigo, insomnia.
GI: *nausea, vomiting, diarrhea,* abdominal pain, anorexia, stomatitis.
GU: *toxic nephrosis with oliguria and anuria,* crystalluria, hematuria.
Hematologic: *agranulocytosis, aplastic anemia,* megaloblastic anemia, thrombocytopenia, leukopenia, *hemolytic anemia.*
Hepatic: jaundice.
Skin: *erythema multiforme (Stevens-Johnson syndrome), generalized skin eruption, epidermal necrolysis, exfoliative dermatitis,* photosensitivity, urticaria, pruritus.
Other: hypersensitivity reactions (*serum sickness, drug fever, anaphylaxis*), thrombophlebitis.

INTERACTIONS
Oral anticoagulants: increased anticoagulant effect. Monitor for bleeding.
Oral antidiabetic agents: increased hypoglycemic effect. Monitor blood glucose levels.
Oral contraceptives: decreased contraceptive effectiveness and increased risk of breakthrough bleeding. Suggest a nonhormonal form of contraception.
Phenytoin: may inhibit hepatic metabolism of phenytoin. Monitor closely.

CONTRAINDICATIONS
Contraindicated in patients with hypersensitivity to trimethoprim or sulfonamides, severe renal impairment (creatinine clearance less than 15 ml/minute), or porphyria; in megaloblastic anemia caused by folate deficiency; and in pregnant women at term.

NURSING CONSIDERATIONS
• Use cautiously and in reduced dosages in patients with impaired hepatic or renal function (creatinine clearance of 15 to 30 ml/minute), severe allergy or bronchial asthma, G6PD deficiency, and blood dyscrasia.
• Obtain specimen for culture and sensitivity tests before first dose. Therapy may begin pending results.
• Note that the "DS" or" DF" product means "double strength."
• **I.V. use:** Dilute I.V. infusion in D_5W before administration. Don't mix with other drugs or solutions. In-

fuse slowly over 60 to 90 minutes. Don't give by rapid infusion or bolus injection. Don't refrigerate.
• Never administer I.M.
• Promptly report complaints of skin rash, sore throat, fever, or mouth sores—early signs of blood dyscrasia.
• Watch for superinfection (fever or other signs of new infection).
• Be aware that adverse reactions, especially hypersensitivity reactions, rash, and fever, occur much more frequently in AIDS patients.
• Tell the patient to take entire amount of medication exactly as prescribed, even if he feels better.

sulfadiazine
Microsulfon

Pregnancy Risk Category: C (contraindicated at term)

HOW SUPPLIED
Tablets: 500 mg

ACTION
Inhibits formation of dihydrofolic acid from PABA, decreasing bacterial folic acid synthesis.

ONSET, PEAK, DURATION
Onset and duration unknown. Serum levels peak within 6 hours of an oral dose.

INDICATIONS & DOSAGE
Urinary tract infection–
Adults: initially, 2 to 4 g P.O., then 2 to 4 g daily in three to six doses q 24 hours.
Children 2 months and over: initially, 75 mg/kg or 2 g/m² P.O., then 150 mg/kg or 4 g/m² P.O. in four to six divided doses daily. Maximum daily dosage is 6 g.
Rheumatic fever prophylaxis, as an alternative to penicillin–
Children over 30 kg: 1 g P.O. daily.
Children under 30 kg: 500 mg P.O. daily.

Adjunctive treatment in toxoplasmosis–
Adults: 2 to 8 g P.O. daily. Usually give with pyrimethamine.
Children: 100 to 200 mg/kg P.O. daily. Usually given with pyrimethamine.

ADVERSE REACTIONS
CNS: headache, mental depression, convulsions, hallucinations.
GI: *nausea, vomiting, diarrhea,* abdominal pain, anorexia, stomatitis.
GU: *toxic nephrosis* with oliguria and anuria, crystalluria, hematuria.
Hematologic: *agranulocytosis, aplastic anemia,* megaloblastic anemia, thrombocytopenia, leukopenia, *hemolytic anemia.*
Skin: *erythema multiforme (Stevens-Johnson syndrome), generalized skin eruption, epidermal necrolysis, exfoliative dermatitis,* photosensitivity, urticaria, pruritus.
Other: hypersensitivity reactions (*serum sickness, drug fever, anaphylaxis*), jaundice, local irritation, extravasation.

INTERACTIONS
Oral anticoagulants: increased anticoagulant effect. Monitor for bleeding.
Oral antidiabetic agents: increased hypoglycemic effect. Monitor blood glucose levels.
Oral contraceptives: decreased contraceptive effectiveness and increased risk of breakthrough bleeding. Suggest a nonhormonal form of contraception.
PABA-containing drugs: inhibited antibacterial action. Don't use together.

CONTRAINDICATIONS
Contraindicated in patients with hypersensitivity to sulfonamides, in those with porphyria, in infants under age 2 months (except in congenital

---

*Liquid form contains alcohol.
**May contain tartrazine.

Common reactions are in italics; *life-threatening*, in bold italics.

toxoplasmosis), in pregnant women at term, and during breast-feeding.

NURSING CONSIDERATIONS

• Use cautiously and in reduced doses in patients with impaired hepatic or renal function, bronchial asthma, history of multiple allergies, G6PD deficiency, and blood dyscrasia.
• Obtain specimen for culture and sensitivity tests before first dose. Therapy may begin pending results.
• Give drug on schedule to maintain constant blood level.
• Monitor for signs of blood dyscrasia (purpura, ecchymosis, sore throat, fever, and pallor). Report them immediately.
• Monitor urine cultures, CBCs, and urinalyses before and during therapy, as ordered.
• Watch for superinfection (fever or other signs of new infection).
• Be aware that folic or folinic acid may be used during rest periods in toxoplasmosis therapy to reverse hematopoietic depression or anemia associated with pyrimethamine and sulfadiazine.
• Tell the patient to drink a full glass of water with each dose and to drink plenty of water throughout the day to prevent crystalluria. Monitor fluid intake and output. Intake should be sufficient to produce output of 1,500 ml daily (between 3,000 and 4,000 ml daily for adults). To prevent crystalluria, sodium bicarbonate may be administered to alkalinize urine. Monitor urine pH daily.
• Tell the patient to take entire amount of medication exactly as prescribed, even if he feels better.
• Warn the patient to avoid direct sunlight and ultraviolet light to prevent photosensitivity reaction.

sulfamethoxazole (sulphamethoxazole)

Apo-Sulfamethoxazole†, Gantanol, Gantanol DS

Pregnancy Risk Category: C (contraindicated at term)

HOW SUPPLIED
Tablets: 500 mg
Oral suspension: 500 mg/5 ml

ACTION
Inhibits formation of dihydrofolic acid from PABA, decreasing bacterial folic acid synthesis.

ONSET, PEAK, DURATION
Onset and duration unknown. Serum levels peak within 2 hours of an oral dose.

INDICATIONS & DOSAGE
Urinary tract and systemic infections –
Adults: initially, 2 g P.O., then 1 g P.O. b.i.d. up to t.i.d. for severe infections.
Children and infants over 2 months: initially, 50 to 60 mg/kg P.O., then 25 to 30 mg/kg b.i.d. Maximum dosage should not exceed 75 mg/kg daily.

ADVERSE REACTIONS
CNS: headache, mental depression, seizures, hallucinations.
GI: *nausea, vomiting, diarrhea,* abdominal pain, anorexia, stomatitis.
GU: *toxic nephrosis with oliguria and anuria,* crystalluria, hematuria.
Hematologic: *agranulocytosis, aplastic anemia,* megaloblastic anemia, thrombocytopenia, leukopenia, *hemolytic anemia.*
Skin: *erythema multiforme (Stevens-Johnson syndrome), generalized skin eruption, epidermal necrolysis, exfoliative dermatitis,* photosensitivity, urticaria, pruritus.
Other: hypersensitivity reactions

---

*(serum sickness, drug fever, **anaphylaxis**), jaundice.*

INTERACTIONS
Oral anticoagulants: increased anticoagulant effect. Monitor for bleeding.
Oral antidiabetic agents: increased hypoglycemic effect. Monitor blood glucose levels.
Oral contraceptives: decreased contraceptive effectiveness and increased risk of breakthrough bleeding. Suggest a nonhormonal form of contraception.
PABA-containing drugs: inhibited antibacterial action. Don't use together.
Phenytoin: may increase phenytoin effect. Monitor closely.

CONTRAINDICATIONS
Contraindicated in patients with hypersensitivity to sulfonamides; in those with porphyria, in infants under age 2 months (except in congenital toxoplasmosis), in pregnant women at term, and during breast-feeding.

NURSING CONSIDERATIONS
• Use cautiously and in reduced dosages in patients with impaired hepatic or renal function, severe allergy or bronchial asthma, G6PD deficiency, and blood dyscrasia.
• Obtain specimen for culture and sensitivity tests before first dose. Therapy may begin pending results.
• Monitor urine cultures, CBCs, and urinalyses before and during therapy, as ordered.
• Watch for superinfection (fever or other signs of new infection).
• Intake should be sufficient to produce output of 1,500 ml daily (between 3,000 and 4,000 ml daily for adults). To help prevent crystalluria, sodium bicarbonate may be administered to alkalinize urine. Monitor urine pH daily.
• Tell the patient to drink a full glass

of water with each dose and to drink plenty of water during the day to prevent crystalluria. Monitor fluid intake and output.
• Tell the patient to take entire amount of medication exactly as prescribed, even if he feels better.
• Instruct the patient to report early signs of blood dyscrasia (sore throat, fever, and pallor) to the doctor immediately.
• Warn the patient to avoid direct sunlight and ultraviolet light to prevent photosensitivity reaction.

---

sulfisoxazole (sulfafurazole, sulphafurazole)
Azo-Sulfisoxazole†‡, Gantrisin, Novosoxazole†

Pregnancy Risk Category: C (contraindicated at term)

HOW SUPPLIED
Tablets: 500 mg
Liquid: 500 mg/5 ml

ACTION
Inhibits formation of dihydrofolic acid from PABA, decreasing bacterial folic acid synthesis.

ONSET, PEAK, DURATION
Onset and duration unknown. Serum levels peak in 2 to 4 hours.

INDICATIONS & DOSAGE
Urinary tract and systemic infections –
Adults: initially, 2 to 4 g P.O., then 4 to 8 g in 24 hours divided in four to six doses.
Children over 2 months: initially, 75 mg/kg P.O. daily or 2 g/m² P.O. daily in divided doses q 6 hours, then 150 mg/kg or 4 g/m² P.O. daily in divided doses q 6 hours.

ADVERSE REACTIONS
CNS: headache, mental depression, *seizures,* hallucinations.
GI: *nausea, vomiting, diarrhea,* abdominal pain, anorexia, stomatitis.
GU: *toxic nephrosis with oliguria and anuria,* crystalluria, hematuria.
Hematologic: *agranulocytosis, aplastic anemia,* megaloblastic anemia, thrombocytopenia, leukopenia, *hemolytic anemia.*
Skin: *erythema multiforme, generalized skin eruption, epidermal necrolysis, exfoliative dermatitis,* photosensitivity, urticaria, pruritus.
Other: hypersensitivity reactions (*serum sickness, drug fever, anaphylaxis*), jaundice.

INTERACTIONS
Oral anticoagulants: increased anticoagulant effect. Monitor for bleeding.
Oral antidiabetic agents: increased hypoglycemic effect. Monitor blood glucose levels.
Oral contraceptives: decreased contraceptive effectiveness, increased risk of breakthrough bleeding. Suggest a nonhormonal form of contraception.
PABA-containing drugs: inhibited antibacterial action. Don't use together.

CONTRAINDICATIONS
Contraindicated in patients with hypersensitivity to sulfonamines, in infants under age 2 months (except in congenital toxoplasmosis), in pregnant women at term, and during breast-feeding.

NURSING CONSIDERATIONS
• Use cautiously in patients with impaired hepatic or renal function, severe allergy or bronchial asthma, and G6PD deficiency.
• Obtain specimen for culture and sensitivity tests before first dose. Therapy may begin pending results.
• Monitor urine cultures, CBCs, PT, and urinalyses before and during therapy, as ordered.
• When drug is given preoperatively, be aware that the patient should receive a low-residue diet and a minimal number of enemas and cathartics.
• Watch for superinfection (fever or other signs of new infection).
• Monitor fluid intake and output. Maintain intake between 3,000 and 4,000 ml daily for adults to produce output of 1,500 ml daily. Sodium bicarbonate may be administered to alkalinize urine. Monitor urine pH daily.
• Tell the patient to drink a full glass of water with each dose and to drink plenty of water each day to prevent crystalluria.
• Tell the patient to take entire amount of medication exactly as prescribed, even if he feels better.
• Warn the patient to avoid sunlight to prevent photosensitivity reaction.
• Tell the patient to report early signs of blood dyscrasia (sore throat, fever, and pallor) immediately to the doctor.

16

Fluoroquinolones

cinoxacin
ciprofloxacin
enoxacin
lomefloxacin hydrochloride
nalidixic acid
norfloxacin
ofloxacin

COMBINATION PRODUCTS
None.

cinoxacin
Cinobac

Pregnancy Risk Category: B

HOW SUPPLIED
Capsules: 250 mg, 500 mg

ACTION
Inhibits microbial DNA synthesis.

ONSET, PEAK, DURATION
Onset unknown. Plasma levels peak within 2 hours of an oral dose; urine levels peak in 2 to 4 hours. Urine levels of the drug remain sufficient for antimicrobial effect for at least 12 hours after a dose.

INDICATIONS & DOSAGE
Initial and recurrent urinary tract infections caused by susceptible strains of Escherichia coli, Klebsiella, Enterobacter, Proteus mirabilis, P. vulgaris, P. Serratia, *and* Citrobacter—
Adults and children over 12 years:
1 g P.O. daily, in two to four divided doses for 7 to 14 days.
   Not recommended for children under 18 years.

ADVERSE REACTIONS
CNS: *dizziness, headache,* drowsiness, insomnia, *seizures*.
EENT: tinnitus.

GI: *nausea, vomiting, abdominal pain,* diarrhea, distorted taste.
Skin: rash, urticaria, pruritus, photosensitivity.
Other: elevated liver enzymes.

INTERACTIONS
Oral anticoagulants: increased anticoagulant effect. Monitor for bleeding.
Probenecid: may decrease urine levels of cinoxacin by inhibiting renal tubular secretion. Monitor for increased toxicity and reduced antibacterial effectiveness.
Theophylline, caffeine: increased effects of these drugs. Monitor closely.

CONTRAINDICATIONS
Contraindicated in patients with hypersensitivity to the drug or other fluoroquinolones.

NURSING CONSIDERATIONS
• Use cautiously in patients with impaired renal and hepatic function.
• Obtain clean-catch urine specimen for culture and sensitivity tests before starting therapy and repeat p.r.n. Therapy may begin pending results.
• Give cinoxacin with meals to help decrease adverse GI reactions.
• Report adverse CNS reactions to the doctor immediately. They indicate serious toxicity and usually mean that administration of drug should be stopped.
• Know that high urine levels permit twice-daily dosing.
• Remind the patient to take entire amount of this drug as prescribed, even when he feels better.
• Warn the patient about photosensitizing effects of the drug, and advise him to avoid bright sunlight and to wear sunblock.

*Liquid form contains alcohol.
**May contain tartrazine.
Common reactions are in italics; *life-threatening*, in bold italics.

ciprofloxacin
Cipro, Cipro I.V., Ciproxin‡

Pregnancy Risk Category: C

HOW SUPPLIED
Tablets: 250 mg, 500 mg, 750 mg
Infusion (premixed): 200 mg in 100 ml D$_5$W, 400 mg in 200 ml D$_5$W
Injection: 200 mg, 400 mg

ACTION
Unknown. Bactericidal effects may result from drug's inhibiting bacterial DNA gyrase and preventing replication in susceptible bacteria.

ONSET, PEAK, DURATION
Onset immediate after I.V. administration, unknown after oral administration. Serum levels peak 0.5 to 2.3 hours after oral administration immediately after I.V. administration. Duration unknown.

INDICATIONS & DOSAGE
Mild to moderate urinary tract infections –
Adults: 250 mg P.O. or 200 mg I.V. q 12 hours.
Severe or complicated urinary tract infections; mild to moderate bone and joint infections; mild to moderate respiratory tract infections; mild to moderate skin and skin-structure infections; infectious diarrhea –
Adults: 500 mg P.O. or 400 mg I.V. q 12 hours.
Severe or complicated bone or joint infections; severe respiratory tract infections; severe skin and skin-structure infections –
Adults: 750 mg P.O. q 12 hours.
Uncomplicated cervical or urethral gonorrhea due to Neisseria gonorrhoeae –
Adults: 250 mg P.O. as single dose.

ADVERSE REACTIONS
CNS: headache, restlessness, tremor, light-headedness, confusion, hallucinations, *seizures,* paresthesia.
GI: *nausea, diarrhea,* vomiting, abdominal pain or discomfort, oral candidiasis.
GU: crystalluria, increased serum creatinine and BUN levels, interstitial nephritis.
Musculoskeletal: arthralgia, joint or back pain, joint inflammation, joint stiffness, achiness, neck or chest pain.
Other: *rash;* eosinophilia; photosensitivity; elevated liver enzymes; with I.V. administration – thrombophlebitis, burning, pruritus, erythema, swelling.

INTERACTIONS
Antacids containing magnesium hydroxide or aluminum hydroxide, sucralfate, iron supplements: decreased ciprofloxacin absorption. Separate administration by at least 2 hours.
Caffeine: increased effect of caffeine. Monitor closely.
Probenecid: may elevate serum level of ciprofloxacin. Monitor for toxicity.
Theophylline: increased plasma theophylline concentrations and prolonged theophylline half-life. Monitor blood levels of theophylline and observe for adverse effects.

CONTRAINDICATIONS
Contraindicated in patients sensitive to fluoroquinolone antibiotics.

NURSING CONSIDERATIONS
• Use cautiously in patients with CNS disorders, such as severe cerebral arteriosclerosis or seizure disorders, and in those at an increased risk for seizures. May cause CNS stimulation.
• Obtain specimen for culture and sensitivity tests before first dose. Therapy may begin pending results.
• Administer oral form 2 hours after a meal or 2 hours before or after taking antacids, sucralfate, or products that

---

contain iron (such as vitamins with mineral supplements). Food does not affect absorption but may delay peak serum levels.

• **I.V. use:** Dilute drug using D_5W or 0.9% sodium chloride injection to a final concentration of 1 to 2 mg/ml before use. Infuse slowly (over 1 hour) into a large vein.

• Be aware that dosage adjustments are necessary in patients with renal dysfunction.

• Know that long-term therapy may result in overgrowth of organisms resistant to ciprofloxacin.

• Advise the patient to drink plenty of fluids to reduce the risk of crystalluria.

• Warn the patient to avoid hazardous tasks that require alertness, such as driving, until CNS effects of the drug are known.

• Advise the patient to avoid caffeine while taking the drug because of potential for cumulative caffeine effects.

• Advise the patient that hypersensitivity reactions may occur even after first dose. If he notices a skin rash or any allergic reaction, he should stop taking the drug immediately and notify the doctor.

• Instruct the patient to discontinue breast-feeding during treatment or be treated with another drug. Drug is excreted in breast milk.

---

enoxacin
Penetrex

Pregnancy Risk Category: C

HOW SUPPLIED
Tablets: 200 mg, 400 mg

ACTION
Inhibits bacterial DNA synthesis, mainly by blocking DNA gyrase. Bactericidal.

ONSET, PEAK, DURATION
Onset and duration unknown. Serum levels peak in 1 to 3 hours.

INDICATIONS & DOSAGE
Uncomplicated urinary tract infections –
Adults: 200 mg P.O. q 12 hours for 7 days.
Severe or complicated urinary tract infections –
Adults: 400 mg P.O. q 12 hours for 14 days.
Uncomplicated urethral or endocervical gonorrhea –
Adults: 400 mg P.O. as a single dose. Doxycycline therapy may follow to treat possible coexisting chlamydial infection.
In patients with renal failure –
If creatinine clearance is 30 ml/minute or less, therapy started with usual initial dose. Subsequent doses are decreased by 50%.

ADVERSE REACTIONS
CNS: headache, restlessness, tremor, light-headedness, confusion, hallucinations, *seizures.*
GI: *nausea, diarrhea,* vomiting, abdominal pain or discomfort, oral candidiasis.
GU: crystalluria.
Other: *rash,* photosensitivity, eosinophilia, dyspnea, cough, elevated liver enzymes.

INTERACTIONS
Aminophylline, cyclosporine, caffeine, theophylline: increased levels of these drugs because of decreased metabolism. Use together cautiously.
Antacids containing magnesium hydroxide or aluminum hydroxide, oral iron supplements, sucralfate: decreased enoxacin absorption. Separate administration times by at least 2 hours.
Oral anticoagulants: increased anticoagulant effect. Use together cautiously.

---

*Liquid form contains alcohol.   *Common* reactions are in italics; *life-threatening,* in bold italics.
**May contain tartrazine.

CONTRAINDICATIONS
Contraindicated in patients with hypersensitivity to the drug or other fluoroquinolone antibiotics.

NURSING CONSIDERATIONS
• Use cautiously in patients with CNS disorders, such as severe cerebral arteriosclerosis or seizure disorders, and in those at increased risk for seizures. May cause CNS stimulation.
• Use cautiously and with dosage adjustments in patients with impaired renal or hepatic function.
• Obtain specimen for culture and sensitivity tests before first dose. Therapy may begin pending results.
• Have patients being treated for gonorrhea obtain an initial serologic test for syphilis before therapy starts. Drug has not been shown to be effective in treating syphilis and may mask signs and symptoms of infection. Have the patient repeat the serologic test in 1 to 3 months.
• Administer 2 hours after a meal or 2 hours before or after antacids containing magnesium hydroxide or aluminum hydroxide, sucralfate, or products that contain iron (such as vitamins with mineral supplements).
• Monitor closely for superinfection.
• Be aware that similar drugs have been known to cause severe phototoxicity reactions. Advise the patient to avoid overexposure to direct sunlight while taking drug and to use a sunblock and wear protective clothing while outdoors.
• Warn the patient not to drink beverages containing caffeine while taking enoxacin. Drug inhibits the metabolism of caffeine and can result in toxicity.
• Advise the patient to liberally increase fluid intake while taking drug because similar drugs have caused urine microcrystal formation.
• Warn the patient to avoid driving and hazardous activities until adverse CNS effects of the drug are known because drug can cause light-headedness or dizziness.

---

lomefloxacin hydrochloride
Maxaquin

Pregnancy Risk Category: C

HOW SUPPLIED
Tablets (film-coated): 400 mg

ACTION
Inhibits bacterial DNA gyrase, an enzyme necessary for bacterial replication (bactericidal).

ONSET, PEAK, DURATION
Onset and duration unknown. Plasma levels peak 1½ hours after an oral dose.

INDICATIONS & DOSAGE
Acute bacterial exacerbations of chronic bronchitis caused by Haemophilus influenzae *or* Moraxella (Branhamella) catarrhalis—
Adults: 400 mg P.O. daily for 10 days.
Uncomplicated urinary tract infections (cystitis) caused by Escherichia coli, Klebsiella pneumoniae, Proteus mirabilis, *or* Staphylococcus saprophyticus—
Adults: 400 mg P.O. daily for 10 days.
Complicated urinary tract infections caused by E. coli, K. pneumoniae, P. mirabilis, *or* Pseudomonas aeruginosa; *possibly effective against infections caused by* Citrobacter diversus *or* Enterobacter cloacae—
Adults: 400 mg P.O. daily for 14 days.
Prophylaxis of infections after transurethral surgical procedures—
Adults: 400 mg P.O. as a single dose 2 to 6 hours before surgery.
  Patients with a creatinine clearance of 10 to 40 ml/minute should receive a loading dose of 400 mg P.O. on the first day, followed by 200 mg daily for

the duration of therapy. Hemodialysis removes negligible amounts of the drug.

ADVERSE REACTIONS

CNS: *dizziness, headache,* abnormal dreams, fatigue, malaise, asthenia, agitation, anorexia, anxiety, confusion, depersonalization, depression, increased appetite, insomnia, nervousness, somnolence, *seizures, coma,* hyperkinesia, tremor, vertigo, paresthesia, arthralgia, myalgia, asthenia.

CV: flushing, hypotension, hypertension, edema, syncope, arrhythmia, tachycardia, bradycardia, extrasystoles, cyanosis, angina pectoris, *MI, cardiac failure, pulmonary embolisms,* cerebrovascular disorder, cardiomyopathy, phlebitis.

EENT: epistaxis, abnormal vision, conjunctivitis, eye pain, earache, tinnitus, tongue discoloration.

GI: *diarrhea, nausea,* dry mouth, intermenstrual bleeding, leukorrhea, vaginitis, abdominal pain, dyspepsia, vomiting, flatulence, constipation, inflammation, dysphagia, bleeding.

GU: dysuria, hematuria, anuria, epididymitis, orchitis, vaginal moniliasis, perineal pain.

Hematologic: thrombocythemia, thrombocytopenia, lymphadenopathy, increased fibrinolysis.

Respiratory: cough, dyspnea, chest pain, *bronchospasm,* respiratory disorder, respiratory infection, increased sputum, stridor.

Skin: pruritus, skin disorder, skin exfoliation, eczema, rash, urticaria, *photosensitivity.*

Other: *anaphylaxis,* increased sweating, taste perversion, leg cramps, myalgia, thirst, fatigue, chest or back pain, malaise, chills, allergic reaction, facial edema, influenza-like symptoms, decreased heat tolerance, hypoglycemia, elevated liver enyzmes, gout.

INTERACTIONS

Antacids, sucralfate: impaired absorption after binding with lomefloxacin in the GI tract. Administer no less than 4 hours before or 2 hours after a dose.

Cimetidine: increased half-life of other fluoroquinolones when administered to patients taking cimetidine; lomefloxacin has not been tested. Monitor for toxicity.

Probenecid: decreased excretion of lomefloxacin. Monitor for toxicity.

Warfarin, cyclosporine: increased effects or serum levels when combined with other fluoroquinolones; lomefloxacin has not been tested. Monitor for toxicity.

CONTRAINDICATIONS

Contraindicated in patients with hypersensitivity to lomefloxacin or other fluoroquinolones.

NURSING CONSIDERATIONS

• Use cautiously in patients with known or suspected CNS disorders, such as seizure disorder or cerebral arteriosclerosis, that may predispose the patient to seizures.

• Obtain culture and sensitivity tests before first dose. Therapy may begin pending results.

• Administer on an empty stomach.

• Be aware that although most fluoroquinolones exhibit photosensitizing effects, early studies suggest that photosensitization and phototoxicity are more common with lomefloxacin. Some animal studies suggest that prolonged use of the drug may predispose subjects to skin cancers.

• Keep in mind that prolonged use may result in overgrowth of organisms resistant to lomefloxacin.

• Advise the patient that hypersensitivity reactions may occur even after first dose. If skin rash or other allergic reaction occurs, the patient should stop taking the drug and notify the doctor.

---

*Liquid form contains alcohol.   *Common* reactions are in italics; *life-threatening,* in bold italics.
**May contain tartrazine.

• Warn patient to avoid driving and hazardous tasks until CNS effects of drug are known. Drug may cause dizziness or light-headedness.
• Advise the patient to wear protective clothing, use a sunblock, and avoid prolonged exposure to sunlight during treatment and for a few days after therapy ends. If sunburn occurs, the patient should call the doctor as soon as possible.

---

nalidixic acid
NegGram

Pregnancy Risk Category: B (safe use in first trimester not known)

HOW SUPPLIED
Tablets: 250 mg, 500 mg, 1 g
Oral suspension: 250 mg/5 ml

ACTION
Inhibits microbial DNA synthesis by bacterial DNA gyrase.

ONSET, PEAK, DURATION
Onset and duration unknown. Serum levels peak 1 to 2 hours after an oral dose. Urine levels peak 3 to 4 hours after a dose.

INDICATIONS & DOSAGE
Acute and chronic urinary tract infections caused by susceptible gram-negative organisms (Proteus, Klebsiella, Enterobacter, *and* Escherichia coli)—
Adults: 1 g P.O. q.i.d. for 7 to 14 days; 2 g daily for long-term use.
Children over 3 months: 55 mg/kg P.O. daily divided q.i.d. for 7 to 14 days; 33 mg/kg daily for long-term use.

ADVERSE REACTIONS
CNS: drowsiness, weakness, headache, dizziness, vertigo, *seizures,* malaise, confusion, hallucinations.
EENT: sensitivity to light, change in color perception, diplopia, blurred vision.

GI: *abdominal pain, nausea, vomiting,* diarrhea.
Hematologic: eosinophilia, *leukopenia, thrombocytopenia.*
Skin: pruritus, photosensitivity, urticaria, rash.
Other: angioedema, fever, chills, *increased intracranial pressure and bulging fontanelles in infants and children.*

INTERACTIONS
Oral anticoagulants: Increased anticoagulant effect. Monitor for bleeding.

CONTRAINDICATIONS
Contraindicated in patients with hypersensitivity to the drug, in those with seizure disorders, and in infants under age 3 months.

NURSING CONSIDERATIONS
• Use with extreme caution in prepubertal children; erosion of cartilage of immature animals has been reported.
• Use cautiously in patients with impaired hepatic or renal function or with severe cerebral arteriosclerosis.
• Use cautiously in patients with pulmonary disease because nalidixic acid may increase respiratory depression in those with respiratory impairment.
• Obtain specimen for culture and sensitivity tests before starting therapy and repeat p.r.n. Therapy may begin pending results.
• Monitor CBC, renal, and liver function studies during long-term therapy, as ordered.
• Be aware that resistant bacteria may emerge within the first 48 hours of therapy.
• Know that drug may cause a false-positive Clinitest reaction. Use Clinistix or Tes-Tape to monitor urine glucose. Also gives false elevations in urine vanillylmandelic acid and 17-ketosteroids. Tests should be repeated after therapy is completed.

• Tell the patient to avoid undue exposure to sunlight because of photosensitivity. The patient may continue to be photosensitive for as long as 3 months after therapy ends.

• Tell the patient to report visual disturbances; these usually disappear with reduced dose.

norfloxacin
Noroxin

Pregnancy Risk Category: C

HOW SUPPLIED
Tablets: 400 mg

ACTION
Inhibits bacterial DNA synthesis, mainly by blocking DNA gyrase. Bactericidal.

ONSET, PEAK, DURATION
Onset and duration unknown. Plasma levels peak within 1 to 2 hours of an oral dose.

INDICATIONS & DOSAGE
Complicated or uncomplicated urinary tract infections caused by susceptible strains of Escherichia coli, Klebsiella, Enterobacter, Proteus, Pseudomonas aeruginosa, Citrobacter, Staphylococcus aureus *(and* epidermidis*), and group D streptococci –*
Adults: for uncomplicated infections, 400 mg P.O. b.i.d. for 7 to 10 days. For complicated infections, 400 mg b.i.d. for 10 to 21 days.
Cystitis caused by E. coli, Klebsiella pneumoniae, *or* Proteus mirabilis –
Adults: 400 mg P.O. b.i.d. for 3 days.
Acute, uncomplicated gonorrhea –
Adults: 800 mg P.O. as a single dose, followed by doxycycline therapy to treat any coexisting chlamydial infection. Adults with creatinine clearance ≤ 30 ml/minute should receive 400 mg once daily.

ADVERSE REACTIONS
CNS: fatigue, somnolence, headache, dizziness, *seizures.*
GI: nausea, constipation, flatulence, heartburn, dry mouth.
GU: increased serum creatinine and BUN levels, crystalluria.
Hematologic: eosinophilia.
Skin: rash, photosensitivity.
Musculoskeletal: arthralgia, arthritis, myalgia, joint swelling.
Other: *hypersensitivity reactions* (rash, anaphylactoid reactions), transient elevations of AST and ALT, fever.

INTERACTIONS
Antacids, iron products, sucralfate: may hinder absorption. Separate administration times by 2 hours.
Cyclosporine: increased serum concentrations of cyclosporine. Monitor serum levels.
Nitrofurantoin: decreased norfloxacin effectiveness. Don't use together.
Oral anticoagulants: increased anticoagulant effect. monitor closely.
Probenecid: may increase serum levels of norfloxacin by decreasing its excretion. Monitor for toxicity.
Theophylline: possibly impaired theophylline metabolism, resulting in increased plasma levels and risk of toxicity. Monitor closely.

CONTRAINDICATIONS
Contraindicated in patients with hypersensitivity to fluoroquinolones.

NURSING CONSIDERATIONS
• Use cautiously in patients with conditions that may predispose them to seizure disorders, such as cerebral arteriosclerosis. Also use cautiously in those with renal impairment.
• Advise the patient to take the drug 1 hour before or 2 hours after meals because food, antacids, iron products, and sucralfate may hinder absorption.
• Warn the patient not to exceed the recommended dosages and to drink

---

*Liquid form contains alcohol.
**May contain tartrazine.
Common reactions are in italics; *life-threatening,* in bold italics.

several glasses of water throughout the day to maintain hydration and adequate urine output.

• Because norfloxacin may cause dizziness, warn the patient to avoid hazardous activities that require alertness and good coordination until the CNS effects of the drug are known.

ofloxacin
Floxin

Pregnancy Risk Category: C

HOW SUPPLIED
Tablets: 200 mg, 300 mg, 400 mg
Injection: 20 mg/ml, 40 mg/ml; 4 mg/ml premixed in D_5W

ACTION
Unknown. Thought to inhibit bacterial DNA gyrase and prevent DNA replication in susceptible bacteria.

ONSET, PEAK, DURATION
Onset immediate after I.V. infusion, unknown after oral administration. Plasma levels peak immediately after an I.V. infusion, within 1 to 2 hours after an oral dose.

INDICATIONS & DOSAGE
Lower respiratory tract infections caused by susceptible strains of Haemophilus influenzae *or* Streptococcus pneumoniae —
Adults: 400 mg I.V. or P.O. q 12 hours for 10 days.
Cervicitis or urethritis caused by Chlamydia trachomatis *or* Neisseria gonorrhoeae —
Adults: 300 mg I.V. or P.O. q 12 hours for 7 days.
Acute, uncomplicated gonorrhea —
Adults: 400 mg I.V. or P.O. as a single dose.
Mild-to-moderate skin and skin structure infections caused by susceptible strains of Staphylococcus aureus, Staph. epidermidis, Streptococcus pyogenes, *or* Proteus mirabilis —

Adults: 400 mg I.V. or P.O. q 12 hours for 10 days.
Cystitis caused by Escherichia coli *or* Klebsiella pneumoniae —
Adults: 200 mg I.V. or P.O. q 12 hours for 3 days.
Urinary tract infections caused by susceptible strains of Citrobacter diversus, Enterobacter aerogenes, E. coli, P. mirabilis, *or* Pseudomonas aeruginosa —
Adults: 200 mg I.V. or P.O. q 12 hours for 7 days. Complicated infections may require therapy for 10 days.
Prostatitis caused by E. coli —
Adults: 300 mg I.V. or P.O. q 12 hours for 6 weeks.

If creatinine clearance is 10 to 50 ml/minute, dosage interval is decreased to once q 24 hours. If creatinine clearance is < 10 ml/minute, half the recommended dose is given q 24 hours.

ADVERSE REACTIONS
CNS: headache, dizziness, fatigue, lethargy, malaise, drowsiness, sleep disorders, nervousness, light-headedness, insomnia, *seizures*.
CV: chest pain.
GI: nausea, anorexia, abdominal pain or discomfort, diarrhea, vomiting, dry mouth, flatulence, dysgeusia.
GU: vaginitis, vaginal discharge, genital pruritus.
Hematologic: eosinophilia.
Musculoskeletal: trunk pain, transient arthralgia, myalgia.
Skin: rash, pruritus, photosensitivity.
Other: hypersensitivity reactions *(anaphylactoid reaction)*, elevated liver enzymes, visual disturbances, fever.

INTERACTIONS
Antacids containing aluminum or magnesium hydroxide, iron salts, sucralfate, products containing zinc: may interfere with the GI absorption of ofloxacin. Separate administration by at least 2 hours.

---

†Available in Canada only. ‡Available in Australia only. ◇Available OTC.

Oral anticoagulants: increased effect. Monitor for bleeding and altered PT.
Antineoplastic agents: may lower serum levels of fluoroquinolones. Monitor for lack of effect.
Theophylline: decreased clearance of theophylline with some fluoroquinolones. Monitor theophylline levels.

CONTRAINDICATIONS

Contraindicated in patients with hypersensitivity to the drug or other fluoroquinolones.

NURSING CONSIDERATIONS

● Use cautiously during pregnancy only when benefits outweigh risks to the fetus.
● Use cautiously in patients with a history of seizure disorders or other CNS diseases, such as cerebral arteriosclerosis. If patient experiences excessive CNS stimulation (restlessness, tremor, confusion, hallucinations), discontinue medication and notify doctor. Institute seizure precautions.
● Use cautiously and with dosage adjustments in patients with renal failure, as prescribed, because the drug is mainly eliminated by renal excretion.
● **I.V. use:** Dilute concentrate for injection before use. Single-use vials containing 20 or 40 mg/ml must be diluted to a maximum concentration of 4 mg/ml using a compatible I.V. solution, such as D_5W, 0.9% sodium chloride injection, D_5W in 0.9% sodium chloride injection, or sterile water for injection. Infuse over not less than 60 minutes.
● Because compatibility with other drugs is not known, don't mix ofloxacin with other drugs. If giving infusion at a Y-site, discontinue other solution during infusion.
● Monitor regular blood studies and hepatic and renal function tests during prolonged therapy as ordered.
● Know that patients treated for gonorrhea should have a serologic test for syphilis. Drug is not effective against syphilis, and treatment of gonorrhea may mask or delay symptoms of syphilis.
● Advise the patient to take the drug with plenty of fluids, but not with meals, and to avoid antacids, sucralfate, and products containing iron or zinc for at least 2 hours before or after each dose.
● Because the drug may cause lightheadedness, warn patient to avoid hazardous tasks such as driving until the adverse CNS effects are known.
● Advise the patient to use sunblock and protective clothing to avoid photosensitivity reactions.
● Tell the patient to stop drug and notify the doctor if a rash or other signs of hypersensitivity reactions develop.

---

*Liquid form contains alcohol.
**May contain tartrazine.

Common reactions are in italics; ***life-threatening,*** in bold italics.

17
Antivirals

acyclovir sodium
amantadine hydrochloride
didanosine
famciclovir
foscarnet sodium
ganciclovir
ribavirin
rimantadine
stavudine
vidarabine monohydrate
zalcitabine
zidovudine

COMBINATION PRODUCTS
None.

---

acyclovir sodium
Zovirax

Pregnancy Risk Category: C

HOW SUPPLIED
Capsules: 200 mg
Tablets: 400 mg, 800 mg
Suspension: 200 mg/5 ml
Injection: 500 mg/vial, 1 g/vial

ACTION
Becomes incorporated into viral DNA
and inhibits viral multiplication.

ONSET, PEAK, DURATION
Onset immediate after I.V. infusion,
unknown after oral administration.
Serum levels peak immediately after
I.V. infusion, within 1.7 hours of oral
dose. Duration unknown.

INDICATIONS & DOSAGE
*Initial and recurrent episodes of mu-
cocutaneous herpes simplex virus
(HSV-1 and HSV-2) infections in immunocompromised patients; severe
initial episodes of herpes genitalis in
patients who are not immunocompromised –*

Adults and children over age 11: 5
mg/kg, given at a constant rate over a
period of 1 hour by I.V. q 8 hours for 7
days (5 days for herpes genitalis).
Children under age 12: 250 mg/m²,
given at a constant rate over a period
of 1 hour by I.V. q 8 hours for 7 days
(5 days for herpes genitalis).
Initial genital herpes –
Adults: 200 mg P.O. q 4 hours while
awake (a total of 5 capsules daily).
Treatment should continue for 10
days.
*Intermittent therapy for recurrent gen-
ital herpes –*
Adults: 200 mg P.O. q 4 hours while
awake (a total of 5 capsules daily).
Treatment should continue for 5 days.
Initiate therapy at the first sign of recurrence.
*Chronic suppressive therapy for recur-
rent genital herpes –*
Adults: 200 mg P.O. t.i.d. or 400 mg
b.i.d. for 6 to 12 months.
Chicken pox –
Adults and children: 20 mg/kg P.O.
q.i.d. for 5 days. Therapy should be
started as soon as symptoms appear.

ADVERSE REACTIONS
CNS: (associated with I.V. dosage):
*headache, encephalopathic changes
(lethargy, obtundation, tremor, confusion, hallucinations, agitation, seizures, coma).*
CV: hypotension.
GI: *nausea, vomiting,* diarrhea.
GU: *transient elevations of serum creatinine levels,* hematuria.
Skin: rash, itching.
Other: *inflammation, vesicular eruptions, and phlebitis at injection site.*

INTERACTIONS
Probenecid: increased acyclovir blood
levels. Monitor for possible toxicity.

---

†Available in Canada only. ‡Available in Australia only. ◇ Available OTC.

Zidovudine: may cause drowsiness or lethargy. Use together cautiously.

CONTRAINDICATIONS
Contraindicated in patients with hypersensitivity to the drug.

NURSING CONSIDERATIONS
• Use cautiously in patients with underlying neurologic problems, renal disease, or dehydration and in those receiving other nephrotoxic drugs.
• **I.V. use:** Administer I.V. infusion over at least 1 hour to prevent renal tubular damage. Bolus injection, dehydration (decreased urine output), preexisting renal disease, and the concomitant use of other nephrotoxic drugs increase the risk of renal toxicity.
• Don't give by bolus injection or administer I.M. or S.C.
• Be alert that concentrated solutions (10 mg/ml or more) may be associated with a higher incidence of phlebitis.
• Encourage fluid intake because the patient must be adequately hydrated during acyclovir infusion.
• Notify the doctor if serum creatinine level does not return to normal within a few days. He may increase hydration, adjust dose, or discontinue acyclovir. It is recommended that acyclovir be administered in a reduced dosage to patients with impaired renal function.
• Know that encephalopathic changes are more likely in patients with neurologic disorders or in those who have had neurologic reactions to cytotoxic drugs.
• Keep in mind that Burroughs-Wellcome, the manufacturer, maintains an ongoing registry of women exposed to the drug during pregnancy. Follow-up studies to date have not shown an increased risk for birth defects for infants born to patients exposed to the drug during pregnancy. Health care providers are encouraged to report

such exposures to the registrar at (800) 722-9292.
• Instruct the patient that drug is effective in managing herpes infection but does not eliminate or cure it. Warn the patient that acyclovir will not prevent spread of infection to others.
• Urge the patient to recognize early symptoms of herpes infection (such as tingling, itching, or pain) so he can take acyclovir before the infection fully develops.

---

amantadine hydrochloride
Antadine‡, Symadine, Symmetrel

Pregnancy Risk Category: C

HOW SUPPLIED
Capsules: 100 mg
Syrup: 50 mg/5 ml

ACTION
Unknown. Appears to interfere with influenza A virus penetration into susceptible cells. In parkinsonism, its action is unknown.

ONSET, PEAK, DURATION
Onset for antidyskinetic symptoms usually within 48 hours, unknown for antiviral activity. Peak plasma levels occur 2 to 4 hours after an oral dose. Duration unknown.

INDICATIONS & DOSAGE
Prophylaxis or symptomatic treatment of influenza type A virus, respiratory tract illnesses –
Adults up to 64 years and children 10 years and over: 200 mg P.O. daily in a single dose or divided b.i.d.
Children 1 to 9 years: 4.4 to 8.8 mg/kg P.O. daily, as a single dose or divided b.i.d. Maximum dose is 150 mg daily.
Adults over 64 years: 100 mg P.O. once daily.
    Treatment should continue for 24 to 48 hours after symptoms disappear.

---

*Liquid form contains alcohol.   *Common* reactions are in italics; *life-threatening,* in **bold italics.**
**May contain tartrazine.

Prophylaxis should start as soon as possible after initial exposure and continue for at least 10 days after exposure. May continue prophylactic treatment up to 90 days for repeated or suspected exposures if influenza vaccine unavailable. If used with influenza vaccine, dose is continued for 2 to 3 weeks until protection from vaccine develops.

Drug-induced extrapyramidal reactions–

Adults: 100 mg P.O. b.i.d., up to 300 mg daily in divided doses. Patient may benefit from as much as 400 mg daily, but dosages over 200 mg must be closely supervised.

Idiopathic parkinsonism, parkinsonian syndrome–

Adults: 100 mg P.O. b.i.d.; in patients who are seriously ill or receiving other antiparkinsonian drugs, 100 mg daily for at least 1 week, then 100 mg b.i.d., p.r.n.

ADVERSE REACTIONS
CNS: depression, fatigue, confusion, dizziness, psychosis, hallucinations, anxiety, *irritability,* ataxia, *insomnia,* weakness, headache, light-headedness, difficulty concentrating.
CV: peripheral edema, orthostatic hypotension, *CHF.*
GI: anorexia, nausea, constipation, vomiting, dry mouth.
GU: urine retention.
Skin: *livedo reticularis* (with prolonged use).

INTERACTIONS
Anticholinergics: increased adverse anticholinergic effects. Use together cautiously.
CNS stimulants: additive CNS stimulation. Use together cautiously.
Hydrochlorothiazide, triamterene: increased levels of amantadine. Use together cautiously.

CONTRAINDICATIONS
Contraindicated in patients with hypersensitivity to the drug.

NURSING CONSIDERATIONS
• Use cautiously in those with seizure disorders, CHF, peripheral edema, hepatic disease, mental illness, eczematoid rash, renal impairment, orthostatic hypotension, and CV disease and in elderly patients. Dosage may need to be adjusted in patients with renal failure.
• Be aware that elderly patients are more susceptible to neurologic adverse effects. Taking the drug in two daily doses rather than as a single dose may reduce their incidence.
• If insomnia occurs, tell the patient to take the drug several hours before bedtime.
• If orthostatic hypotension occurs, instruct the patient not to stand or change positions too quickly.
• Instruct the patient to report adverse reactions to the doctor, especially dizziness, depression, anxiety, nausea, and urine retention.
• In the patient with parkinsonism, warn against discontinuing drug abruptly to prevent precipitating a parkinsonian crisis.

didanosine (ddI)
Videx

Pregnancy Risk Category: B

HOW SUPPLIED
Tablets (chewable): 25 mg, 50 mg, 100 mg, 150 mg
Powder for oral solution (buffered): 100 mg/packet, 167 mg/packet, 250 mg/packet, 375 mg/packet
Powder for oral solution (pediatric): 10 mg/ml in 2- and 4-g bottles

ACTION
Unknown. Appears to inhibit replication of HIV by preventing DNA replication. In addition, dideoxyadenosine

triphosphate (ddATP) inhibits the enzyme HIV-RNA dependent DNA polymerase (reverse transcriptase).

ONSET, PEAK, DURATION
Onset and duration unknown. Peak levels occur in ½ to 1 hour.

INDICATIONS & DOSAGE
Advanced HIV infection in patients who cannot tolerate or who no longer respond to zidovudine therapy –
Adults 75 kg and over: 300 mg (two 150-mg tablets) P.O. q 12 hours; or 375 mg buffered powder q 12 hours.
Adults 50 to 74 kg: 200 mg (two 100-mg tablets) P.O. q 12 hours; or 250 mg buffered powder q 12 hours.
Adults 35 to 49 kg: 125 mg (one 100-mg and one 25-mg tablet) P.O. q 12 hours; or 167 mg buffered powder q 12 hours.
Children: 200 mg/m^2 P.O. daily in divided doses q 12 hours.

ADVERSE REACTIONS
CNS: *headache,* insomnia, dizziness, **seizures,** confusion, anxiety, nervousness, hypertonia, abnormal thinking.
CV: hypertension, edema, hyperlipemia.
GI: *diarrhea, nausea, vomiting, abdominal pain,* **pancreatitis,** dry mouth, dyspepsia, flatulence.
Hepatic: liver abnormalities.
Other: *peripheral neuropathy,* rash, pruritus, asthenia, pain, myalgia, arthritis, pneumonia, infection, cough, myopathy, alopecia, increased serum uric acid levels.

INTERACTIONS
Antacids containing magnesium or aluminum hydroxides: enhanced adverse effects of the antacid component (including diarrhea or constipation) when administered with didanosine tablets or pediatric suspension. Avoid concomitant use.
Dapsone, ketoconazole, drugs that require gastric acid for adequate absorption: decreased absorption from buffering action. Administer these drugs 2 hours before didanosine.
Fluoroquinolones, tetracyclines: decreased absorption from buffering agents in didanosine tablets or antacids in pediatric suspension.
Itraconazole: decreased serum concentrations of itraconazole. Avoid concomitant use.

CONTRAINDICATIONS
Contraindicated in patients with a history of hypersensitivity to any component of the formulation.

NURSING CONSIDERATIONS
• Use cautiously in patients with a history of pancreatitis. In early studies, the drug caused pancreatitis in about 9% of all patients; fatalities have occurred. Also use cautiously in patients with peripheral neuropathy, renal or hepatic impairment, or hyperuricemia.
• Administer didanosine on an empty stomach, regardless of the dosage form used; administering the drug with meals can decrease absorption by 50%.
• Know that most patients should receive two tablets per dose.
• To administer single-dose packets containing buffered powder for oral solution, pour contents into 4 oz of water. Do not use fruit juice or other beverages that may be acidic. Stir for 2 or 3 minutes until the powder dissolves completely. Administer immediately.
• Use care when preparing the powder or crushing tablets to avoid excessive dispersal of the powder into the air.
• Keep in mind that in early clinical trials, the powder for oral solution was associated with a high incidence of diarrhea. The manufacturer suggests switching to the tablet formulation if diarrhea is a problem, although no evidence suggests that other for-

---

*Liquid form contains alcohol.   *Common* reactions are in italics; *life-threatening,* in bold italics.
**May contain tartrazine.

mulations may be associated with a lower incidence of diarrhea.

• Know that the pediatric powder for oral solution must be prepared by a pharmacist before dispensing. It must be constituted with Purified Water, USP, then diluted with an antacid (either Mylanta Double Strength Liquid or Maalox TC Suspension) to a final concentration of 10 mg/ml. The admixture is stable for 30 days if refrigerated (at 36° to 46° F [2° to 8° C]). Shake the solution well before measuring the dose.

• Because the tablets contain buffers that raise stomach pH to levels that prevent degradation of the active drug, instruct the patient to chew tablets thoroughly before swallowing and drink at least 1 oz of water with each dose. If the tablets are manually crushed, stir them thoroughly in 1 oz of water to disperse the particles uniformly, then have the patient drink the mixture immediately.

• Inform patients receiving a sodium-restricted diet that each two-tablet dose of didanosine contains 529 mg of sodium; each single packet of buffered powder for oral solution contains 1.38 g of sodium.

---

famciclovir
Famvir

Pregnancy Risk Category: B

HOW SUPPLIED
Tablets: 500 mg

ACTION
A guanosine nucleoside that is converted to penciclovir, which enters viral cells and inhibits DNA polymerase and viral DNA synthesis.

ONSET, PEAK, DURATION
Onset and duration unknown. Serum levels peak within 1 hour.

INDICATIONS & DOSAGE
Acute herpes zoster –
Adults: 500 mg P.O. q 8 hours.

In patients with reduced renal function: If creatinine clearance is greater than or equal to 60 ml/minute, 500 mg P.O. q 8 hours; if 40 to 59 ml/minute, 500 mg P.O. q 12 hours; if 20 to 39 ml/minute, 500 mg P.O. q 24 hours.

ADVERSE REACTIONS
CNS: *headache,* fatigue.
GI: diarrhea, *nausea,* vomiting.

INTERACTIONS
Probenecid: may increase plasma concentrations of famciclovir. Monitor patient for increased adverse effects.

CONTRAINDICATIONS
Contraindicated in patients with hypersensitivity to the drug.

NURSING CONSIDERATIONS
• Use cautiously in patients with renal or hepatic impairment. Know that dosage adjustment may be needed.
• Famciclovir may be taken without regard to meals.
• Teach patients how to prevent spread of infection to others.
• Urge patients to recognize the early symptoms of herpes infection, such as tingling, itching, or pain, and to report them. Treatment is more effective if therapy is started within 48 hours of rash onset.

---

foscarnet sodium (phosphonoformic acid)
Foscavir

Pregnancy Risk Category: C

HOW SUPPLIED
Injection: 24 mg/ml in 250- and 500-ml bottles

ACTION
Inhibits all known herpesviruses in vitro by blocking the pyrophosphate binding site on DNA polymerases and reverse transcriptases.

ONSET, PEAK, DURATION
Onset immediate. Peak levels occur immediately after I.V. infusion. Duration unknown.

INDICATIONS & DOSAGE
CMV retinitis in patients with AIDS — **Adults:** initially, 60 mg/kg I.V. as an induction treatment in patients with normal renal function. Administer I.V. over 1 hour q 8 hours for 2 to 3 weeks, depending on clinical response. Followed with a maintenance infusion of 90 mg/kg daily administered over 2 hours; this dose may be increased as needed and tolerated to 120 mg/kg daily if the disease shows signs of progression.

ADVERSE REACTIONS
CNS: *headache, seizures, fatigue, rigors, malaise, asthenia, paresthesia, dizziness, hypoesthesia, neuropathy,* tremor, ataxia, generalized spasms, dementia, stupor, sensory disturbances, meningitis, aphasia, abnormal coordination, EEG abnormalities, vertigo, *coma,* encephalopathy, abnormal gait, hypertonia, visual field defects, dyskinesia, extrapyramidal reactions, speech disorders, paralysis, peripheral neuropathy, nystagmus, *cerebral edema.*
CV: *hypertension, palpitations, ECG abnormalities, sinus tachycardia, first-degree AV block, hypotension, flushing.*
EENT: visual disturbances.
GI: *nausea, diarrhea, vomiting, abdominal pain, anorexia,* constipation, dysphagia, rectal hemorrhage, dry mouth, melena, flatulence, ulcerative stomatitis, *pancreatitis.*
GU: *abnormal renal function, decreased creatinine clearance and in-* creased serum creatinine levels, albuminuria, dysuria, polyuria, urethral disorder, urine retention, urinary tract infections, **acute renal failure.**
Hematologic: anemia, granulocytopenia, leukopenia, **bone marrow suppression,** thrombocytopenia, platelet abnormalities, thrombocytosis, WBC count abnormalities, lymphadenopathy.
Respiratory: *cough, dyspnea,* pneumonitis, sinusitis, pharyngitis, rhinitis, respiratory insufficiency, pulmonary infiltration, stridor, pneumothorax, **bronchospasm,** hemoptysis.
Skin: *rash, increased sweating,* pruritus, skin ulceration, erythematous rash, seborrhea, skin discoloration.
Other: fever; pain; infection; sepsis; hypokalemia; hypomagnesemia; hypophosphatemia or hyperphosphatemia; hypocalcemia; leg cramps; inflammation, pain at infusion site.

INTERACTIONS
Nephrotoxic drugs such as amphotericin B, aminoglycosides: increased risk of nephrotoxicity. Avoid concomitant use.
Pentamidine: increased risk of nephrotoxicity; severe hypocalcemia has also been reported. Don't use together.
Zidovudine: possible increased incidence or severity of anemia. Monitor blood counts.

CONTRAINDICATIONS
Contraindicated in patients with hypersensitivity to the drug.

NURSING CONSIDERATIONS
• Use cautiously and with reduced dosage in patients with abnormal renal function as ordered because it will result in accumulation of the drug and enhanced toxicity. Because foscarnet is nephrotoxic, it has the potential to worsen renal impairment. Some degree of nephrotoxicity occurs in most patients treated with the drug.

---

*Liquid form contains alcohol.   *Common* reactions are in italics; **life-threatening,** in bold italics.
**May contain tartrazine.

• Obtain serum electrolyte levels and creatinine clearance before beginning therapy, as ordered.
• **I.V. use:** Use an infusion pump to administer foscarnet. To minimize renal toxicity, make sure the patient is adequately hydrated before and during the infusion.
• Do not exceed the recommended dosage, infusion rate, or frequency of administration. All doses must be individualized according to the patient's renal function.
• Monitor creatinine clearance frequently during therapy because of the drug's adverse effects on renal function. A baseline 24-hour creatinine clearance is recommended, followed by regular determinations two to three times weekly during induction and at least once every 1 to 2 weeks during maintenance. If creatinine clearance falls below 0.4 ml/minute/kg, drug should be discontinued.
• Because the drug can adversely affect important serum electrolytes such as potassium, calcium, magnesium, and phosphorus, monitor serum electrolyte levels using a schedule similar to that established for creatinine clearance. Assess the patient for tetany and seizures associated with abnormal electrolyte levels.
• Monitor the patient's hemoglobin and hematocrit levels. Anemia is common (in up to 33% of patients treated with the drug). It may be severe enough to require transfusions.
• Keep in mind that administration of the drug is associated with a dose-related transient decrease in ionized serum calcium, which may not always be reflected in the patient's laboratory values.
• Because the drug is highly toxic and toxicity is probably dose-related, keep in mind that the lowest effective maintenance dose should be used throughout therapy.
• Advise the patient to report perioral

tingling, numbness in the extremities, and paresthesia.

ganciclovir
Cytovene

Pregnancy Risk Category: C

HOW SUPPLIED
Capsules: 250 mg
Injection: 500 mg/vial

ACTION
Unknown. Thought to inhibit viral DNA synthesis of CMV.

ONSET, PEAK, DURATION
Onset immediate with I.V. infusion. Peak serum levels occur immediately after I.V. infusion. Duration unknown.

INDICATIONS & DOSAGE
CMV retinitis in immunocompromised individuals, including patients with AIDS—
Adults: induction treatment— 5 mg/kg I.V. q 12 hours for 14 to 21 days (normal renal function); maintenance treatment—5 mg/kg I.V. daily for 7 days each week, or 6 mg/kg daily for 5 days each week. Alternatively, 1,000 mg P.O. t.i.d. with food.
  Dosage is adjusted for patients with impaired renal function and is based on creatinine clearance levels.

ADVERSE REACTIONS
CNS: altered dreams, confusion, ataxia, dizziness, headache, *seizures,* behavioral changes.
CV: arrhythmias, hypotension, hypertension.
GI: nausea, vomiting, diarrhea, anorexia.
GU: hematuria, increased serum creatinine levels.
Hematologic: *granulocytopenia, thrombocytopenia.*
Other: retinal detachment in CMV retinitis patients; abnormal liver func-

---

†Available in Canada only.   ‡Available in Australia only.   ◇ Available OTC.

tion tests results; at injection site — inflammation, pain, phlebitis.

INTERACTIONS
Cytotoxic agents: increased toxic effects, especially hematologic effects and stomatitis. Monitor closely.
Imipenem/cilastatin: heightened seizure activity with concomitant use. Monitor closely.
Immunosuppressants such as azathioprine, cyclosporine, corticosteroids: Enhanced immune and bone marrow suppression. Use together cautiously.
Probenecid: increased ganciclovir blood levels. Monitor closely.
Zidovudine: increased incidence of granulocytopenia with concurrent use. Monitor closely.

CONTRAINDICATIONS
Contraindicated in patients with hypersensitivity to the drug and with an absolute neutrophil count below 500/mm³ or a platelet count below 25,000/mm³.

NURSING CONSIDERATIONS
• Use cautiously and in reduced dosage in patients with renal dysfunction.
• **I.V. use:** Administer infusion over at least 1 hour. Infusions faster than 60 minutes will result in increased toxicity. Use an infusion pump. Do not administer as an I.V. bolus.
• Do not administer S.C. or I.M.
• Use caution when preparing ganciclovir solution, which is alkaline.
• Because of the frequency of granulocytopenia and thrombocytopenia, obtain neutrophil and platelet counts every 2 days during twice-daily ganciclovir dosing and at least weekly thereafter.
• Encourage fluid intake; ganciclovir infusion therapy should be accompanied by adequate hydration.

ribavirin
Virazole
Pregnancy Risk Category: X

HOW SUPPLIED
Powder to be reconstituted for inhalation: 6 g in 100-ml glass vial

ACTION
Inhibits viral activity by an unknown mechanism, possibly by inhibiting RNA and DNA synthesis by depleting intracellular nucleotide pools.

ONSET, PEAK, DURATION
Onset immediate upon exposure to the drug. Peak levels occur immediately after an aerosol treatment. Duration unknown.

INDICATIONS & DOSAGE
Hospitalized infants and young children infected by RSV—
Infants and young children: solution in concentration of 20 mg/ml delivered via the Viratek Small Particle Aerosol Generator (SPAG-2) and mechanical ventilator or oxygen hood, face mask, or oxygen tent at a rate of about 12.5 liters of mist per minute. Treatment is carried out for 12 to 18 hours/day for at least 3, and no more than 7 days.

ADVERSE REACTIONS
CV: *cardiac arrest,* hypotension, bradycardia.
EENT: conjunctivitis.
Hematologic: anemia, reticulocytosis.
Respiratory: worsening of respiratory state, bronchospasm.
Other: rash or erythema of eyelids, transient increases in liver enzymes.

INTERACTIONS
None significant.

---

*Liquid form contains alcohol.   *Common* reactions are in italics; *life-threatening,* in bold italics.
**May contain tartrazine.

CONTRAINDICATIONS
Contraindicated in patients with hypersensitivity to the drug and in those who are or may become pregnant during treatment.

NURSING CONSIDERATIONS
• Administer ribavirin aerosol by the Viratek Small Particle Aerosol Generator (SPAG-2) only. Don't use any other aerosol-generating device.
• Use sterile USP water for injection, *not* bacteriostatic water. Water used to reconstitute this drug must not contain any antimicrobial agent.
• Discard solutions placed in the SPAG-2 unit at least every 24 hours before adding newly reconstituted solution.
• Avoid unnecessary occupational exposure to the drug. The most frequent adverse effects reported in health care personnel exposed to aerosolized ribavirin include eye irritation and headache.
• Monitor ventilator function frequently. Ribavirin may precipitate in ventilator apparatus, causing result in equipment malfunction with serious consequences.
• Monitor patients receiving ribavirin threrapy longer than 1 to 2 weeks for the development of anemia.
• Store reconstituted solutions at room temperature for 24 hours.
• Continue providing supportive respiratory and fluid management.
• Keep in mind that ribavirin aerosol is indicated only for severe lower respiratory tract infection caused by RSV. Although treatment may be started while awaiting diagnostic test results, existence of RSV infection must be eventually documented.
• Be aware that most infants and children with RSV infection don't require treatment because the disease is commonly mild and self-limiting. Infants with underlying conditions, such as prematurity or cardiopulmonary disease, get RSV in its severest form and

benefit most from treatment with ribavirin aerosol.

---

rimantadine
Flumadine

Pregnancy Risk Category: C

HOW SUPPLIED
Tablets: 100 mg
Syrup: 50 mg/5 ml
Injection: 200 mg

ACTION
Unknown. Appears to prevent viral uncoating, an early step in virus reproductive cycle.

ONSET, PEAK, DURATION
Onset and duration unknown. Peak plasma levels occur in 1 to 4 hours.

INDICATIONS & DOSAGE
Influenza A –
Adults and children age 10: 100 mg P.O. b.i.d.
Children under age 10: 5 mg/kg (not to exceed 150 mg) P.O. once a day.
Elderly patients, patients with severe hepatic or renal dysfunction: 100 mg P.O. daily.

ADVERSE REACTIONS
CNS: insomnia, headache, dizziness, nervousness, fatigue, asthenia.
EENT: eye pain, tinnitus.
GI: nausea, vomiting, anorexia, dry mouth, abdominal pain.

INTERACTIONS
None significant.

CONTRAINDICATIONS
Contraindicated in patients with hypersensitivity to the drug or amantadine.

NURSING CONSIDERATIONS
• Use cautiously in patients with renal or hepatic impairment and in patients with a history of seizures. Pregnant

---

†Available in Canada only.   ‡Available in Australia only.   ◊ Available OTC.

patients should consider the risks compared to the benefits before taking this drug.

• For influenza infections, administer therapy within 48 hours of onset of symptoms and continue for 7 days after the initial signs and symptoms occurred.

• Consider the risk to contacts of treated patients who may be subject to morbidity from influenza A. Influenza A-resistant strains can emerge during therapy. Patients taking the drug may still be able to spread the disease.

• Instruct the patient to take drug several hours before bedtime to prevent insomnia.

stavudine (2,3 didehydro-3-deoxythymidine, d4T)
Zerit

Pregnancy Risk Category: C

HOW SUPPLIED
Capsules: 15 mg, 20 mg, 30 mg, 40 mg

ACTION
A primidine nucleoside analogue that prevents replication of HIV by inhibiting the enzyme reverse transcriptase.

ONSET, PEAK, DURATION
Onset and duration unknown. Serum levels peak within 1 hour.

INDICATIONS & DOSAGE
Patients with advanced HIV infection who are intolerant or unresponsive to other antiviral therapies –
Adults weighing 60 kg or more: 40 mg P.O. q 12 hours.
Adults weighing less than 60 kg: 30 mg P.O. q 12 hours.

ADVERSE REACTIONS
CNS: *peripheral neuropathy.*
Hematologic: bone marrow suppression.

Other: myalgia, hepatotoxicity.

INTERACTIONS
Myelosuppressants: additive myelosuppression. Avoid concomitant use.

CONTRAINDICATIONS
Contraindicated in patients with hypersensitivity to the drug.

NURSING CONSIDERATIONS
• Use cautiously in patients with renal impairment or history of peripheral neuropathy. Also use cautiously in pregnant women.

• Know that peripheral neuropathy appears to be the major dose-limiting adverse effect of stavudine. It may or may not resolve after drug is discontinued.

• Periodically monitor CBC and serum levels of creatinine, AST, ALT, and alkaline phosphatase, as ordered.

• Tell the patient that the drug may be taken without regard to meals.

• Advise the patient that he cannot receive stavudine if he experienced peripheral neuropathy while receiving any other nucleoside analogue or if his treatment plan includes a cytotoxic antineoplastic agent.

• Warn the patient not to take any other drugs for HIV or AIDS (especially from the "street") unless the doctor has approved them.

• Teach the patient signs and symptoms of peripheral neuropathy – pain, burning, aching, weakness, or pins and needles in the extremities – and tell him to report these immediately.

vidarabine monohydrate (adenine arabinoside, ara-A)
Vira-A

Pregnancy Risk Category: C

HOW SUPPLIED
Concentrate for I.V. infusion: 200 mg/ml in 5-ml vial (equivalent to 187.4 mg vidarabine)

ACTION
Unknown. Appears to become incorporated into viral DNA and to inhibit viral multiplication.

ONSET, PEAK, DURATION
Onset immediate after I.V. infusion. Peak serum levels occur immediately after I.V. infusion. Duration unknown.

INDICATIONS & DOSAGE
Herpes simplex virus encephalitis –
Adults and children (including neonates): 15 mg/kg I.V. daily for 10 days. Slowly infuse the total daily dose at a constant rate over 12 to 24 hours. Avoid rapid or bolus injection.
Herpes zoster in immunosuppressed patients –
Adults: 10 mg/kg I.V. daily for 5 days.

ADVERSE REACTIONS
CNS: tremor, dizziness, hallucinations, confusion, malaise, weakness, psychosis, ataxia.
GI: *anorexia, nausea,* vomiting, diarrhea.
Hematologic: anemia, neutropenia, thrombocytopenia.
Skin: pruritus, rash.
Other: weight loss; elevated AST, bilirubin; pain and phlebitis at injection site.

INTERACTIONS
Allopurinol: reduced metabolism of vidarabine and increased risk of adverse CNS effects. Monitor closely.

CONTRAINDICATIONS
Contraindicated in patients with hypersensitivity to the drug.

NURSING CONSIDERATIONS
● Use cautiously in patients with impaired renal function. Dosage adjustment may be necessary.
● **I.V. use:** Use with a 0.45-micron (or smaller) I.V. filter. Any I.V. solution is suitable as a diluent.
● Dilute to a concentration of less than 0.5 mg/ml. Because vidarabine is not highly soluble, each milligram of drug requires 2.2 ml of I.V. solution; the maximum concentration is 450 mg/liter. Dilute just before using, and use within 48 hours.
● Don't give I.M. or S.C. because of low solubility and poor absorption. Because large volumes of solution must be administered, monitor the patient for fluid overload.
● As ordered, monitor hematologic tests, such as hemoglobin, hematocrit, WBC count, and platelet count, during therapy. Also monitor renal and liver function studies, as ordered.

---

zalcitabine
(dideoxycytidine, ddC)
HIVID

Pregnancy Risk Category: C

HOW SUPPLIED
Tablets: 0.375 mg, 0.75 mg

ACTION
Inhibits replication of HIV by blocking viral DNA synthesis.

ONSET, PEAK, DURATION
Onset and duration unknown. Peak plasma levels occur 1 to 2 hours after an oral dose.

INDICATIONS & DOSAGE
Advanced HIV infection (CD4 + T cell count below 300 cells/mm³) in patients who have demonstrated significant clinical or immunologic deterioration –
Adults and children 13 years or older who weigh at least 30 kg: 0.75

---

mg P.O. q 8 hours. Must be taken with zidovudine 200 mg P.O. q 8 hours.

ADVERSE REACTIONS
CNS: *peripheral neuropathy,* headache, fatigue, dizziness, confusion, impaired concentration, amnesia, insomnia, mental depression, tremor, hypertonia, asthenia, agitation, abnormal thinking, anxiety.
CV: cardiomyopathy, *CHF,* left ventricular hypokinesis, chest pain, hypertension, palpitation, syncope, tachycardia, atrial fibrillation.
EENT: pharyngitis, cough, ocular pain, abnormal vision, ototoxicity.
GI: nausea, vomiting, diarrhea, abdominal pain, anorexia, constipation, stomatitis, esophageal ulcer, glossitis.
Hematologic: anemia, neutropenia, leukopenia.
Skin: pruritus; night sweats; erythematous, maculopapular, or follicular rash.
Other: myalgia, arthralgia, fatigue, fever, rigors, chest pain, weight increase, *pancreatitis,* increased liver enzymes.

INTERACTIONS
Aminoglycosides, amphotericin B, foscarnet, and other drugs that may impair renal function: increased risk of nephrotoxicity. Avoid concomitant use.
Chloramphenicol, cisplatin, dapsone, disulfiram, ethionamide, glutethimide, gold salts, hydralazine, iodoquinol, isoniazid, metronidazole, nitrofurantoin, phenytoin, ribavirin, and vincristine as well as other drugs that can cause peripheral neuropathy: increased risk of peripheral neuropathy. Avoid concomitant use.
Pentamidine: increased risk of pancreatitis. Avoid concomitant use.

CONTRAINDICATIONS
Contraindicated in patients with hypersensitivity to the drug or any component of the formulation.

NURSING CONSIDERATIONS
• Use with extreme caution in patients with preexisting peripheral neuropathy.
• Use cautiously in patients with renal impairment (creatinine clearance below 55 ml/minute) because they may be at increased risk for toxicity to the drug. Dosage adjustments are necessary in patients with moderate to severe renal failure.
• Also use cautiously in patients with hepatic failure. In clinical trials, the drug regimen (zalcitabine plus zidovudine) exacerbated hepatic dysfunction in patients with preexisting liver impairment.
• Additionally, use cautiously in patients with a history of pancreatitis. Rarely, pancreatitis has been fatal in patients receiving zalcitabine. In patients receiving zalcitabine as the only treatment, pancreatitis was rare (less than 1%).
• Use cautiously in patients with baseline cardiomyopathy or history of CHF.
• Do not administer the drug with food because it decreases the rate and extent of absorption.
• Assess for signs of peripheral neuropathy, characterized by numbness and burning in the extremities, the major toxicity resulting from the drug. If drug isn't withdrawn, peripheral neuropathy can progress to sharp shooting pain or severe continuous burning pain requiring opioid analgesics. It may or may not be reversible.
• If the patient experiences symptoms that resemble peripheral neuropathy, prepare to withdraw the drug. Drug should be discontinued if symptoms are bilateral and persist beyond 72 hours. If symptoms persist or worsen beyond 1 week, drug should be permanently discontinued. However, if all findings relevant to peripheral neuropathy have resolved to minor symptoms, the drug may be reintroduced at 0.375 mg P.O. q 8 hours.

• If zalcitabine is discontinued because of toxicity, be aware that the patient should resume the recommended dose for zidovudine (100 mg q 4 hours).

• Make sure the patient understands that drug doesn't cure HIV infection and that opportunistic infections may still occur despite continued use. Review safe sex practices with the patient.

• Inform the patient that peripheral neuropathy is the major toxicity associated with this drug and that pancreatitis is the major life-threatening toxicity. Review the signs and symptoms of these adverse reactions, and instruct the patient to call the doctor promptly if any appear.

• Instruct patients of childbearing age to use an effective contraceptive while taking this drug.

zidovudine
(azidothymidine, AZT)
Apo-Zidovudine†, Novo-AZT†, Retrovir

Pregnancy Risk Category: C

HOW SUPPLIED
Capsules: 100 mg
Syrup: 50 mg/5 ml
Injection: 10 mg/ml

ACTION
Prevents replication of HIV by inhibiting the enzyme reverse transcriptase.

ONSET, PEAK, DURATION
Onset immediate after I.V. infusion, unknown after oral administration. Peak plasma levels occur in ½ to 1½ hours. Duration unknown.

INDICATIONS & DOSAGE
Symptomatic HIV infection, including AIDS –
Adults and children 12 years and
over: 100 mg P.O. q 4 hours around the clock.
Children 3 months to 12 years: 180 mg/m² P.O. q 6 hours (720 mg/m²/day), not to exceed 200 mg q 6 hours.
Selected patients with AIDS or advanced AIDS-related complex (ARC) who have a history of Pneumocystis carinii *pneumonia or a CD4 + lymphocyte count below 200 cells/mm³ –*
Adults: 1 to 2 mg/kg I.V. infused over 1 hour q 4 hours around the clock, followed by 200 mg P.O. q 4 hours around the clock when oral administration can replace parenteral administration.
Asymptomatic HIV infection –
Adults and children 12 years and over: 100 mg P.O. q 4 hours while awake (500 mg daily).
Children 3 months to 12 years: 180 mg/m² P.O. q 6 hours (720 mg/m²/day), not to exceed 200 mg q 6 hours.
To reduce risk of transmission of HIV from infected mother with a baseline CD4 + lymphocyte counts greater than 200 cells/mm³ to newborn –
Adults: 100 mg P.O. given initially between 14 and 34 weeks gestation and continued throughout pregnancy. During labor, administer loading dose of 2 mg/kg followed by continuous infusion of 1 mg/kg/hour until delivery.
Infants: 2 mg/kg P.O. (syrup) q 6 hours for 6 weeks beginning 8 to 12 hours after birth.

ADVERSE REACTIONS
CNS: *headache, seizures,* paresthesia, agitation, malaise, restlessness, insomnia, confusion, anxiety, ataxia, nystagmus.
GI: *nausea,* anorexia, abdominal pain.
Hematologic: *severe bone marrow suppression (resulting in anemia), agranulocytosis, thrombocytopenia.*
Skin: *rash,* itching.
Other: myalgia, diaphoresis, fever, taste perversion, pharyngitis, sinusi-

tis, dysuria, flu syndrome, chest pain, lactic acidosis, hepatomegaly.

INTERACTIONS
Acetaminophen, aspirin, co-trimoxazole, indomethacin: may impair hepatic metabolism of zidovudine, increasing the drug's toxicity.
Acyclovir: possible seizures, lethargy, and fatigue. Use together cautiously.
Amphotericin B, dapsone, flucytosine, pentamidine: increased risk of nephrotoxicity and bone marrow suppression. Monitor closely.
Ganciclovir: increased risk and hematologic toxicity. Monitor closely.
Other cytotoxic drugs: additive adverse effects on the bone marrow. Avoid concomitant use.
Probenecid: may decrease the renal clearance of zidovudine. Avoid concomitant use.
Ribavirin: antagonizes the antiviral activity of zidovudine against HIV. Use cautiously.

CONTRAINDICATIONS
Contraindicated in patients with hypersensitivity to the drug.

NURSING CONSIDERATIONS
• Use cautiously and with close monitoring in patients with advanced symptomatic HIV infection and in patients with severe bone marrow depression.
• Use in HIV-infected pregnant patients only when clearly needed.
• Use with caution in any patient with hepatomegaly, hepatitis, or other known risk factors for liver disease.
• **I.V. use:** Dilute before administration. Remove the calculated dose from the vial; add to D_5W to achieve a concentration that does not exceed 4 mg/ml. Infuse drug over 1 hour at a constant rate; give every 4 hours around the clock. Avoid rapid infusion or bolus injection. Adding mixture to biological or colloidal fluids (for example, blood products, protein solutions)

is not recommended. After drug is diluted, the solution is physically and chemically stable for 24 hours at room temperature and for 48 hours if refrigerated at 35.6° to 46.4° F (2° to 8° C) to minimize the risk of microbial contamination. Store undiluted vials at 59° to 77° F (15° to 25° C) and protect them from light.
• Monitor blood studies every 2 weeks, as ordered, to detect anemia or agranulocytosis. Patients may require dosage reduction or temporary discontinuation of the drug.
• Be aware that zidovudine has been shown to temporarily decrease morbidity and mortality in certain patients with AIDS or ARC.
• Know that the optimum duration of treatment as well as the dosage for optimum effectiveness and minimum toxicity is not yet known.
• Advise patients that blood transfusions may be needed during treatment. Zidovudine frequently causes a low RBC count.
• Remind patients that they *must* comply with the every-4-hour dosage schedule. Suggest ways to avoid missing doses, perhaps by using alarm clocks.
• Warn patients not to take any other drugs for AIDS (especially those available on the street) unless their doctors have approved them. Some purported AIDS cures may interfere with zidovudine's effectiveness.
• Advise pregnant, HIV-infected patients that zidovudine therapy only *reduces* the risk of HIV transmission to their newborn. Long-term risks to infants are unknown.
• Advise health care workers who consider zidovudine prophylaxis after occupational exposure (following needle-stick injury, for example) that animal and human studies have not yet proved the drug's safety or efficacy. Some clinicians do not advocate such use of zidovudine.

---

*Liquid form contains alcohol.
**May contain tartrazine.   *Common* reactions are in italics; *life-threatening,* in bold italics.

18

Macrolide anti-infectives

azithromycin
clarithromycin
erythromycin base
erythromycin estolate
erythromycin ethylsuccinate
erythromycin gluceptate
erythromycin lactobionate
erythromycin stearate

COMBINATION PRODUCTS
None.

---

azithromycin
Zithromax

Pregnancy Risk Category: B

HOW SUPPLIED
Capsules: 250 mg

ACTION
Binds to the 50S subunit of bacterial ribosomes, blocking protein synthesis; bacteriostatic or bactericidal, depending on concentration.

ONSET, PEAK, DURATION
Onset and duration unknown. Serum levels peak in young patients in 2.5 to 3.2 hours, in elderly patients in 3.8 to 4.4 hours.

INDICATIONS & DOSAGE
Acute bacterial exacerbations of COPD caused by Haemophilus influenzae, Moraxella (Branhamella) catarrhalis, *or* Streptococcus pneumoniae; *mild community-acquired pneumonia caused by* H. influenzae *or* S. pneumoniae; *uncomplicated skin and skin-structure infections caused by* Staphylococcus aureus, Strep. pyogenes, *or* Strep. agalactiae; *second-line therapy of pharyngitis or tonsillitis caused by* S. pyogenes —
Adults and adolescents age 16 and

over: 500 mg P.O. as a single dose on day 1, followed by 250 mg daily on days 2 through 5. Total dose is 1.5 g.
Nongonococcal urethritis or cervicitis caused by Chlamydia trachomatis —
Adults and adolescents age 16 and over: 1 g P.O. as a single dose.

ADVERSE REACTIONS
CNS: dizziness, vertigo, headache, fatigue, somnolence.
CV: palpitations, chest pain.
GI: *nausea, vomiting, diarrhea, abdominal pain,* dyspepsia, flatulence, melena, cholestatic jaundice.
GU: monilia, vaginitis, nephritis.
Skin: rash, photosensitivity.
Other: angioedema, pseudomembranous colitis.

INTERACTIONS
Aluminum- and magnesium-containing antacids: lowered peak plasma levels of azithromycin. Separate administration times by at least 2 hours.
Astemizole and terfenadine: potentially serious CV effects (prolongation of QT interval and ventricular tachycardia) have been associated with other macrolide anti-infectives. Monitor patient closely.
Digoxin: elevated digoxin levels. Monitor closely.
Theophylline: possibly increase plasma theophylline levels with other macrolides; effect of azithromycin is unknown. Monitor theophylline levels carefully.
Warfarin: possibly increased PT with other macrolides; effect of azithromycin is unknown. Monitor PT carefully.

CONTRAINDICATIONS
Contraindicated in patients with hypersensitivity to erythromycin or other macrolides.

---

†Available in Canada only.   ‡Available in Australia only.   ◊ Available OTC.

NURSING CONSIDERATIONS
• Use cautiously in patients with impaired hepatic function.
• Obtain specimen for culture and sensitivity tests before first dose. Therapy may begin pending results.
• Administer 1 hour before or 2 hours after meals; do not administer with antacids.
• Monitor for signs and symptoms of superinfection. May cause overgrowth of nonsusceptible bacteria or fungi.
• Tell the patient that the drug should always be taken on an empty stomach because food or antacids will decrease absorption.
• Tell the patient to take all of the medication as prescribed, even after he feels better.

---

clarithromycin
Biaxin

Pregnancy Risk Category: C

HOW SUPPLIED
Tablets: 250 mg, 500 mg
Suspension: 125 mg/5 ml, 250 mg/5 ml

ACTION
Binds to the 50S subunit of bacterial ribosomes, blocking protein synthesis; bacteriostatic or bactericidal, depending on concentration.

ONSET, PEAK, DURATION
Onset and duration unknown. Serum levels peak in 2 to 3 hours.

INDICATIONS & DOSAGE
Pharyngitis or tonsillitis caused by Streptococcus pyogenes —
Adults: 250 mg P.O. q 12 hours for 10 days.
Children: 15 mg/kg/day P.O. in divided doses q 12 hours for 10 days.
Acute maxillary sinusitis caused by S. pneumoniae —

Adults: 500 mg P.O. q 12 hours for 14 days.
Children: 15 mg/kg/day P.O. in divided doses q 12 hours for 10 days.
Acute exacerbations of chronic bronchitis caused by Moraxella (Branhamella) catarrhalis *or* S. pneumoniae; *pneumonia caused by* S. pneumoniae *or* Mycoplasma pneumoniae —
Adults: 250 mg P.O. q 12 hours for 7 to 14 days.
Acute exacerbations of chronic bronchitis caused by Haemophilus influenzae —
Adults: 500 mg P.O. q 12 hours for 7 to 14 days.
Uncomplicated skin and skin-structure infections caused by Staphylococcus aureus *or* Strep. pyogenes —
Adults: 250 mg P.O. q 12 hours for 7 to 14 days.
Children: 15 mg/kg/day P.O. in divided doses q 12 hours for 10 days.
Acute otitis media —
Children: 15 mg/kg/day P.O. in divided doses q 12 hours for 10 days.

ADVERSE REACTIONS
CNS: headache.
GI: *diarrhea, nausea, abnormal taste,* dyspepsia, abdominal pain or discomfort.

INTERACTIONS
Carbamazepine: may increase serum levels of carbamazepine. Monitor blood levels.
Terfenadine: altered metabolism of terfenadine, with prolongation of QT interval and ventricular tachycardia. Avoid concurrent use.
Theophylline: increased plasma theophylline levels possible with other macrolides; effect of clarithromycin is unknown. Monitor theophylline levels carefully.
Warfarin: increased PT possible with other macrolides; effect of clarithromycin is unknown. Monitor PT carefully.

---

*Liquid form contains alcohol. *Common* reactions are in italics; *life-threatening,* in bold italics.
**May contain tartrazine.

CONTRAINDICATIONS
Contraindicated in patients with hypersensitivity to erythromycin or other macrolides.

NURSING CONSIDERATIONS
• Use cautiously in patients with hepatic or renal impairment.
• Obtain urine specimen for culture and sensitivity tests before first dose. Therapy may begin pending results.
• Administer drug without regard to meals.
• Monitor the patient for superinfection. Drug may cause overgrowth of nonsusceptible bacteria or fungi.
• Tell the patient to take all of the medication as prescribed, even after he feels better.

---

erythromycin base
Apo-Erythro†, EMU-V‡, E-Mycin, Erybid†, ERYC, ERYC-125†, ERYC-250†, Ery-Tab, Erythromid†, Erythromycin Base Filmtab, Novorythro†, PCE Disperstab, Robimycin

erythromycin estolate
Erythrozone, Ilosone, Novorythro†

erythromycin ethylsuccinate
Apo-Erythro-ES†, EEG Dulcets‡, E.E.S., EES-400‡, EES granules‡, EryPed, Erythro, Erythrocin

erythromycin gluceptate
Ilotycin

erythromycin lactobionate
Erythrocin

erythromycin stearate
Apo-Erythro-S†, Erythrocin, Erythrocot, My-E, Novorythro†, Wintrocin, Wyamycin S

Pregnancy Risk Category: B

HOW SUPPLIED
erythromycin base
Tablets (enteric-coated): 250 mg, 333 mg, 500 mg
Tablets (filmtabs): 250 mg, 500 mg
Capsules (enteric-coated pellets): 250 mg
erythromycin estolate
Tablets: 500 mg
Capsules: 250 mg
Oral suspension: 125 mg/5 ml, 250 mg/5 ml
erythromycin ethylsuccinate
Tablets: 400 mg
Tablets (chewable): 200 mg
Oral suspension: 200 mg/5 ml, 400 mg/5 ml, 100 mg/2.5 ml
erythromycin gluceptate
Injection: 1-g vials
erythromycin lactobionate
Injection: 500-mg, 1-g vials
erythromycin stearate
Tablets (film-coated): 250 mg, 500 mg

ACTION
Inhibits bacterial protein synthesis by binding to the 50S subunit of the ribosome.

ONSET, PEAK, DURATION
Onset immediate after I.V. infusion, unknown after oral administration. Peak serum levels occur 1 to 4 hours after an oral dose or immediately after I.V. infusion. Duration unknown.

INDICATIONS & DOSAGE
Acute pelvic inflammatory disease caused by Neisseria gonorrhoeae —
Adults: 500 mg I.V. (erythromycin gluceptate, lactobionate) q 6 hours for 3 days, then 250 mg (erythromycin base, estolate, stearate) or 400 mg (erythromycin ethylsuccinate) P.O. q 6 hours for 7 days.
Endocarditis prophylaxis for dental procedures in patients allergic to penicillin —
Adults: initially, 800 mg (ethylsuccinate) or 1 g (stearate) P.O. 2 hours before procedure; then 400 mg (ethyl-

succinate) or 500 mg (stearate) P.O. 6 hours later.

Children: initially, 20 mg/kg (ethylsuccinate or stearate) P.O. 2 hours before procedure; then half the initial dose 6 hours later.

Intestinal amebiasis —

Adults: 250 mg (base, estolate, stearate) or 400 mg (ethylsuccinate) P.O. q 6 hours for 10 to 14 days.

Children: 30 to 50 mg/kg (base, estolate, ethylsuccinate, stearate) P.O. daily, in divided doses q 6 hours for 10 to 14 days.

Mild to moderately severe respiratory tract, skin, and soft-tissue infections caused by sensitive group A beta-hemolytic streptococci, Diplococcus pneumoniae, Mycoplasma pneumoniae, Corynebacterium diphtheriae, Bordetella pertussis, Listeria monocytogenes —

Adults: 250 to 500 mg (erythromycin base, estolate, stearate) P.O. q 6 hours; or 400 to 800 mg (erythromycin ethylsuccinate) P.O. q 6 hours; or 15 to 20 mg/kg I.V. daily, as continuous infusion or in divided doses q 6 hours.

Children: 30 mg/kg to 50 mg/kg (oral erythromycin salts) P.O. daily, in divided doses q 6 hours; or 15 to 20 mg/kg I.V. daily, in divided doses q 4 to 6 hours.

Syphilis —

Adults: 500 mg (erythromycin base, estolate, stearate) P.O. q.i.d. for 15 days.

Legionnaire's disease —

Adults: 500 mg to 1 g I.V. or P.O. (base, estolate, stearate) or 800 to 1,600 mg (ethylsuccinate) q 6 hours for 21 days.

Uncomplicated urethral, endocervical, or rectal infections when tetracyclines are contraindicated —

Adults: 500 mg (base, estolate, stearate) or 800 mg (ethylsuccinate) P.O. q.i.d. for at least 7 days.

Urogenital Chlamydia trachomatis *infections during pregnancy —*

Adults: 500 mg (base, estolate, stearate) P.O. q.i.d. for at least 7 days or 250 mg (base, estolate, stearate) or 400 mg (ethylsuccinate) P.O. q.i.d. for at least 14 days.

Conjunctivitis caused by C. trachomatis *in neonates —*

Neonates: 50 mg/kg P.O. daily in four divided doses for at least 2 weeks.

Pneumonia of infancy caused by C. trachomatis —

Infants: 50 mg/kg/day in four divided doses for at least 3 weeks.

ADVERSE REACTIONS
EENT: hearing loss with high I.V. doses.
GI: *abdominal pain and cramping, nausea, vomiting, diarrhea.*
Hepatic: cholestatic jaundice (with erythromycin estolate).
Skin: urticaria, rashes.
Other: overgrowth of nonsusceptible bacteria or fungi; ***anaphylaxis;*** fever; *venous irritation, thrombophlebitis after I.V. injection.*

INTERACTIONS
Astemizole, terfenadine: decreased metabolism, leading to increased levels of these antihistamines and cardiotoxicity. Avoid concomitant use.
Carbamazepine: increased carbamazepine blood levels and increased risk of toxicity. Monitor closely.
Clindamycin, lincomycin: may be antagonistic. Don't use together.
Cyclosporine: increased concentrations of cyclosporine. Monitor closely.
Midazolam and triazolam: increased effects of these drugs. Monitor closely.
Oral anticoagulants: increased anticoagulant effects. Monitor PT closely.
Theophylline: decreased erythromycin blood level and increased theophylline toxicity. Use together cautiously.

---

*Liquid form contains alcohol.
**May contain tartrazine.   *Common* reactions are in italics; *life-threatening,* in bold italics.

CONTRAINDICATIONS

Contraindicated in patients with hypersensitivity to the drug or other macrolides. Erythromycin estolate is contraindicated in patients with hepatic disease.

NURSING CONSIDERATIONS

• Use other erythromycin salts cautiously in patients with impaired hepatic function.
• Obtain urine specimen for culture and sensitivity tests before first dose. Therapy may begin pending results.
• When administering suspension, be sure to note the concentration.
• **I.V. use:** Reconstitute according to manufacturer's directions and dilute each 250 mg in at least 100 ml of 0.9% sodium chloride solution. Infuse over 1 hour.
• Do not administer erythromycin lactobionate with other drugs.
• Monitor the patient for signs and symptoms of superinfection. May cause overgrowth of nonsusceptible bacteria or fungi.
• Monitor hepatic function (increased serum levels of alkaline phosphatase, ALT, AST, and bilirubin may occur). Erythromycin estolate may cause serious hepatotoxicity in adults (reversible cholestatic jaundice).Other erythromycin salts cause hepatotoxicity to a lesser degree. The patient who develops hepatotoxicity from estolate may react similarly to treatment with any erythromycin preparation.
• Keep in mind that the drug may falsely elevate concentrations of urinary catecholamines, 17-hydroxycorticosterone, and 17-ketosteroids.
• Be aware that drug may interfere with colorimetric assays, resulting in falsely elevated AST and ALT concentrations.
• Keep in mind that coated tablets or encapsulated pellets have caused fewer instances of GI upset; they may be more tolerable in patients who cannot tolerate erythromycin.

• For best absorption, instruct the patient to take oral form of drug with full glass of water 1 hour before or 2 hours after meals. Coated tablets may be taken with meals. Tell the patient not to drink fruit juice with drug. Chewable erythromycin tablets should not be swallowed whole.
• Tell the patient to take entire amount of drug exactly as prescribed, even after he feels better.
• Instruct the patient to report adverse reactions, especially nausea, abdominal pain, and fever.

19

Miscellaneous anti-infectives

aztreonam
bacitracin
chloramphenicol
chloramphenicol palmitate
chloramphenicol sodium succinate
clindamycin hydrochloride
clindamycin palmitate hydrochloride
clindamycin phosphate
imipenem/cilastatin sodium
lincomycin hydrochloride
methenamine hippurate
methenamine mandelate
nitrofurantoin macrocrystals
nitrofurantoin microcrystals
polymyxin B sulfate
rifabutin
spectinomycin dihydrochloride
trimethoprim
trimetrexate glucuronate
vancomycin hydrochloride

COMBINATION PRODUCTS
CYSTEX: methenamine 165 mg, salicylamide 65 mg, sodium salicylate 97 mg, and benzoic acid 32 mg.
HEXALOL: methenamine 40.8 mg, phenyl salicylate 18.1 mg, atropine sulfate 0.03 mg, hyoscyamine 0.03 mg, benzoic acid 4.5 mg, and methylene blue 5.4 mg.
MACROBID: nitrofurantoin macrocrystals 25 mg and nitrofurantoin monohydrate 75 mg.
THIACIDE: methenamine mandelate 500 mg and potassium acid phosphate 250 mg.
TRAC TABS 2X: methenamine 120 mg, methylene blue 6 mg, phenyl salicylate 30 mg, atropine sulfate 0.06 mg, hyoscyamine sulfate 0.03 mg, and benzoic acid 7.5 mg.
URISEDAMINE: methenamine mandelate 500 mg and hyoscyamine 0.15 mg.
URO-PHOSPHATE: methenamine 300 mg and sodium acid phosphate 500 mg. Sugar coated.
UROQUID-ACID: methenamine mandelate 350 mg and sodium acid phosphate 200 mg.
UROQUID-ACID NO. 2: methenamine mandelate 500 mg and sodium acid phosphate 500 mg.

aztreonam
Azactam
Pregnancy Risk Category: B

HOW SUPPLIED
Injection: 500-mg, 1-g, 2-g vials

ACTION
Inhibits bacterial cell-wall synthesis, ultimately causing cell-wall destruction; bactericidal.

ONSET, PEAK, DURATION
Onset immediate after I.V. administration, unknown after I.M. injection. Serum levels peak in 0.6 to 1.3 hours after I.M. injection, immediately after I.V. infusion. Duration unknown.

INDICATIONS & DOSAGE
Urinary tract infections, lower respiratory tract infections, septicemia, skin and skin-structure infections, intra-abdominal infections, surgical infections, and gynecologic infections caused by various aerobic organisms –
Adults: 500 mg to 2 g I.V. or I.M. q 8 to 12 hours. For severe systemic or life-threatening infections, 2 g q 6 to 8 hours may be given. Maximum dosage is 8 g daily.

*Liquid form contains alcohol.
**May contain tartrazine.
Common reactions are in italics; ***life-threatening,*** in bold italics.

ADVERSE REACTIONS

CNS: *seizures,* headache, insomnia, confusion.
CV: hypotension.
GI: diarrhea, nausea, vomiting.
Hematologic: neutropenia, anemia.
Other: hypersensitivity reactions (rash, *anaphylaxis*), altered taste, halitosis, rash, transient elevation of ALT and AST, thrombophlebitis at I.V. site, discomfort and swelling at I.M. injection site.

INTERACTIONS

Aminoglycosides, beta-lactam antibiotics and other anti-infectives: synergistic effect. Monitor patient closely.
Cefoxitin, imipenem: possible antagonistic effect. Do not use together.
Furosemide, probenecid: increased serum aztreonam levels. Avoid concomitant use.

CONTRAINDICATIONS

Contraindicated in patients with hypersensitivity to the drug.

NURSING CONSIDERATIONS

• Use cautiously in elderly patients and in those with impaired renal function. Dosage adjustment may be necessary.
• Obtain urine specimen for culture and sensitivity tests before first dose. Therapy may begin pending results.
• **I.V. use:** To administer a bolus of aztreonam, inject drug slowly (over 3 to 5 minutes) directly into a vein or I.V. tubing. Give infusions over 20 minutes to 1 hour.
• Administer I.M. injections deep into a large muscle mass, such as the upper outer quadrant of the gluteus maximus or the lateral aspect of the thigh. Give doses greater than 1 g I.V.
• Observe the patient for signs of superinfection.
• Because aztreonam is ineffective against gram-positive and anaerobic organisms, anticipate using it with other antibiotics for immediate treatment of life-threatening illnesses. Aztreonam is a narrow-spectrum antibiotic, effective solely against gram-negative organisms.
• Be aware that patients who are allergic to penicillins or cephalosporins may not be allergic to aztreonam. However, close monitoring of those who have had an immediate hypersensitivity reaction to these antibiotics is recommended.

---

bacitracin

Pregnancy Risk Category: NR

HOW SUPPLIED

Injection: 10,000-unit, 50,000-unit vials

ACTION

Hinders bacterial cell-wall synthesis, damaging the bacterial plasma membrane and making the cell more vulnerable to osmotic pressure.

ONSET, PEAK, DURATION

Onset and duration unknown. Plasma levels peak within 1 hour of an I.M. injection.

INDICATIONS & DOSAGE

Pneumonia or empyema caused by susceptible staphylococci –
Infants over 2.5 kg: 1,000 units/kg I.M. daily, divided q 8 to 12 hours.
Infants under 2.5 kg: 900 units/kg I.M. daily, divided q 8 to 12 hours.

ADVERSE REACTIONS

EENT: ototoxicity.
GI: nausea, vomiting, anorexia, diarrhea, rectal itching or burning.
GU: *nephrotoxicity (albuminuria,* cylindruria, oliguria, anuria, increased BUN, *tabular and glomerular necrosis).*
Hematologic: blood dyscrasia, eosinophilia.
Skin: urticaria, rash.
Other: superinfection, fever, rash,

anaphylaxis, neuromuscular block-ade, pain at injection site.

INTERACTIONS
Nephrotoxic drugs (such as aminoglycosides): increased nephrotoxicity. Use together cautiously.
Neuromuscular blockers, inhalational anesthetics: prolonged muscle weakness. Monitor the patient for excessive muscle weakness or respiratory distress.

CONTRAINDICATIONS
Contraindicated in patients with hypersensitivity to the drug or impaired renal function.

NURSING CONSIDERATIONS
• Use cautiously in those with myasthenia gravis and neuromuscular disease.
• Obtain urine specimen for culture and sensitivity tests before first dose. Therapy may begin pending results.
• Assess baseline renal function studies before starting therapy.
• Administer by deep I.M. injection only; warn the patient that injection may be painful.
• Monitor renal function daily during therapy. Notify the doctor of any change.
• Maintain adequate fluid intake, and monitor urine output closely. If fluid intake or output decreases, notify the doctor.
• Report adverse effects to the doctor immediately.
• Provide measures to keep urine pH above 6.0 to reduce the risk of nephrotoxicity.
• Be aware that prolonged therapy may result in overgrowth of nonsusceptible organisms, especially *Candida albicans.*
• Know that concentration of bacitracin should be between 5,000 and 10,000 units/ml. Store in refrigerator. Drug is inactivated if stored at room temperature.

chloramphenicol
Chloromycetin, Novochlorocap†

chloramphenicol palmitate
Chloromycetin Palmitate

chloramphenicol sodium succinate
Chloromycetin Sodium Succinate, Pentamycetin†

Pregnancy Risk Category: NR

HOW SUPPLIED
chloramphenicol
Capsules: 250 mg, 500 mg
chloramphenicol palmitate
Oral suspension: 150 mg/5 ml
chloramphenicol sodium succinate
Injection: 1-g, 10-g vials

ACTION
Inhibits bacterial protein synthesis by binding to the 50S subunit of the ribosome; bacteriostatic.

ONSET, PEAK, DURATION
Onset immediate after I.V. administration, unknown after oral or I.M. administration. Serum levels peak immediately after I.V. administration, 1 to 3 hours after oral dose, and unknown after an I.M. injection. Duration unknown.

INDICATIONS & DOSAGE
Haemophilus influenzae *meningitis, acute* Salmonella typhi *infection, and meningitis, bacteremia, or other severe infections caused by sensitive* Salmonella *species,* Rickettsia, *lymphogranuloma, psittacosis, or various sensitive gram-negative organisms –*
Adults and children: 50 to 100 mg/kg P.O. or I.V. daily, divided q 6 hours. Maximum dosage is 100 mg/kg daily.
Premature infants, neonates 2 weeks or younger, and children and infants with immature metabolic processes: 25 mg/kg P.O. or I.V. once

---

*Liquid form contains alcohol.   *Common* reactions are in italics; *life-threatening,* in bold italics.
**May contain tartrazine.

daily. I.V. route must be used to treat meningitis.

ADVERSE REACTIONS
CNS: headache, mild depression, confusion, delirium, peripheral neuropathy with prolonged therapy.
EENT: optic neuritis (in patients with cystic fibrosis), glossitis, decreased visual acuity.
GI: nausea, vomiting, stomatitis, diarrhea, enterocolitis.
Hematologic: *aplastic anemia,* hypoplastic anemia, *granulocytopenia,* thrombocytopenia.
Other: infections from nonsusceptible organisms, hypersensitivity reactions (fever, rash, urticaria, *anaphylaxis*), jaundice, *gray syndrome in neonates, (abdominal distention, gray cyanosis, vasomotor collapse, respiratory distress, death within a few hours of onset of symptoms).*

INTERACTIONS
Chlorpropamide, dicumarol, phenobarbital, phenytoin, tolbutamide: Increased blood levels possible. Monitor for toxicity.
Iron supplements, vitamin B$_{12}$, folic acid: possible delayed response in patients with anemia. Monitor closely.

CONTRAINDICATIONS
Contraindicated in patients with hypersensitivity to the drug.

NURSING CONSIDERATIONS
• Use cautiously in patients with impaired hepatic or renal function, acute intermittent porphyria, and G6PD deficiency and with other drugs that cause bone marrow suppression or blood disorders.
• Obtain specimen for culture and sensitivity tests before first dose. Therapy may begin pending results.
• **I.V. use:** Give I.V. slowly over at least 1 minute. Check injection site daily for phlebitis and irritation.
• Reconstitute 1-g vial of powder for injection with 10 ml of sterile water for injection. Concentration will be 100 mg/ml. Stable for 30 days at room temperature, but refrigeration recommended. Do not use cloudy solutions.
• Obtain plasma concentration levels. Therapeutic plasma concentrations are 5 to 25 mcg/ml.
• Monitor CBC, platelets, serum iron, and reticulocytes before and every 2 days during therapy, as ordered. Stop drug immediately if anemia, reticulocytopenia, leukopenia, or thrombocytopenia develops and notify doctor.
• Monitor for evidence of superinfection by nonsusceptible organisms.
• Tell the patient to take medication for as long as prescribed, exactly as directed, even after he feels better.
• Instruct the patient to report adverse reactions to the doctor, especially nausea, vomiting, diarrhea, fever, confusion, sore throat, or mouth sores.

clindamycin hydrochloride
Cleocin HCl, Dalacin C†‡

clindamycin palmitate hydrochloride
Cleocin Pediatric, Dalacin C Palmitate†‡

clindamycin phosphate
Cleocin Phosphate, Dalacin C†‡, Dalacin C Phosphate

Pregnancy Risk Category: NR

HOW SUPPLIED
clindamycin hydrochloride
Capsules: 75 mg, 150 mg, 300 mg
clindamycin palmitate hydrochloride
Oral solution: 75 mg/5 ml
clindamycin phosphate
Injection: 150 mg/ml

ACTION
Inhibits bacterial protein synthesis by binding to the 50S subunit of the ribosome.

ONSET, PEAK, DURATION
Onset immediate after I.V. administration, unknown after oral and I.M. administration. Serum levels peak immediately after I.V. administration, 3 hours after an I.M. injection, or within 45 minutes to 1 hour of an oral dose. Duration unknown.

INDICATIONS & DOSAGE
Infections caused by sensitive staphylococci, streptococci, pneumococci, Bacteroides, Fusobacterium, Clostridium perfringens, *and other sensitive aerobic and anaerobic organisms –*
Adults: 150 to 450 mg P.O. q 6 hours; or 300 mg I.M. or I.V. q 6, 8, or 12 hours.
Children over 1 month: 8 to 20 mg/kg P.O. daily, in divided doses q 6 to 8 hours; or 15 to 40 mg/kg I.M. or I.V. daily, in divided doses q 6 hours.
Endocarditis prophylaxis for dental procedures in patients allergic to penicillin –
Adults: initially, 300 mg P.O. 1 hour before procedure; then 150 mg 6 hours later.
Children: initially, 10 mg/kg P.O. 1 hour before procedure; then half the initial dose 6 hours later.

ADVERSE REACTIONS
GI: *nausea,* vomiting, abdominal pain, *diarrhea,* pseudomembranous colitis, esophagitis, flatulence, anorexia, *bloody or tarry stools, dysphagia.*
Hematologic: transient leukopenia, eosinophilia, thrombocytopenia.
Skin: maculopapular rash, urticaria.
Other: unpleasant or bitter taste; **anaphylaxis;** elevated alkaline phosphatase, AST, bilirubin; *pain,* induration, *sterile abscess with I.M. injec-*tion; thrombophlebitis, erythema, and pain after I.V. administration.

INTERACTIONS
Erythromycin: may block access of clindamycin to its site of action. Don't use together.
Kaolin: decreased absorption of oral clindamycin. Separate administration times.
Neuromuscular blockers: potentiated neuromuscular blockade possible. Monitor closely.

CONTRAINDICATIONS
Contraindicated in patients with hypersensitivity to the antibiotic congener lincomycin.

NURSING CONSIDERATIONS
● Use cautiously in neonates and patients with renal or hepatic disease, asthma, history of GI disease, or significant allergies.
● Know that drug does not penetrate blood-brain barrier.
● Obtain urine specimen for culture and sensitivity tests before first dose. Therapy may begin pending results.
● **I.V. use:** When giving I.V., check site daily for phlebitis and irritation. For I.V. infusion, dilute each 300 mg in 50 ml solution, and give no faster than 30 mg/minute (over 10 to 60 minutes). Never give undiluted as a bolus.
● For I.M. administration, inject deeply. Rotate sites. Warn the patient that I.M. injection may be painful. Doses greater than 600 mg per injection are not recommended.
● Be aware that I.M. injection may raise creatine kinase in response to muscle irritation.
● Don't refrigerate reconstituted oral solution, because it will thicken. Drug is stable for 2 weeks at room temperature.
● Monitor renal, hepatic, and hematopoietic functions during prolonged therapy, as ordered.

---

*Liquid form contains alcohol.
**May contain tartrazine.

Common reactions are in italics; ***life-threatening,*** in bold italics.

• Observe the patient for signs of superinfection.
• Don't give opioid antidiarrheals to treat drug-induced diarrhea. May prolong and worsen diarrhea.
• Advise the patient taking the capsule form to take with a full glass of water to prevent dysphagia.
• Instruct the patient to report adverse reactions, especially diarrhea, to the doctor. Warn the patient not to treat such diarrhea himself.

---

imipenem/cilastatin sodium
Primaxin, Primaxin I.M.

Pregnancy Risk Category: C

HOW SUPPLIED
Injection: 250-mg, 500-mg, 750-mg vials
Powder for injection: 500 mg

ACTION
Imipenem is bactericidal and inhibits bacterial cell-wall synthesis. Cilastatin inhibits the enzymatic breakdown of imipenem in the kidneys, making it effective in the urinary tract.

ONSET, PEAK, DURATION
Onset and duration unknown. Serum levels peak immediately after I.V. infusion.

INDICATIONS & DOSAGE
Serious infections of the lower respiratory and urinary tracts, intra-abdominal and gynecologic infections, bacterial septicemia, bone and joint infections, skin and soft-tissue infections, and endocarditis. Most known microorganisms are susceptible: Staphylococcus, Streptococcus, Escherichia coli, Klebsiella, Proteus, Enterobacter, Pseudomonas aeruginosa, *and* Bacteroides, *including* B. fragilis —
Adults: 250 mg to 1 g by I.V. infusion q 6 to 8 hours. Maximum daily dosage is 50 mg/kg/day or 4 g/day, whichever is less. Alternatively, 500 to 750 mg

I.M. q 12 hours. Maximum daily dosage is 1,500 mg/day.

ADVERSE REACTIONS
CNS: *seizures,* dizziness, somnolence.
CV: hypotension.
GI: nausea, vomiting, diarrhea, *pseudomembranous colitis.*
Skin: rash, urticaria, pruritus.
Other: *hypersensitivity reactions (anaphylaxis); thrombophlebitis, pain at injection site,* fever, transient increases in liver enzymes.

INTERACTIONS
Beta-lactam antibiotics: possible in vitro antagonism. Avoid concomitant use.
Ganciclovir: may cause seizures. Avoid concomitant use.
Probenecid: increased serum concentrations of cilastatin. Avoid concomitant use.

CONTRAINDICATIONS
Contraindicated in patients with hypersensitivity to the drug.

NURSING CONSIDERATIONS
• Use cautiously in patients allergic to penicillins or cephalosporins because this drug has similar properties.
• Also use cautiously in patients who have a history of seizure disorders, especially if they also have compromised renal function. If seizures develop and persist, despite anticonvulsant therapy, notify the doctor. The drug should then be discontinued.
• Be aware that patients with impaired renal function may need a lower dose or longer intervals between doses.
• Obtain urine specimen for culture and sensitivity tests before first dose. Therapy may begin pending results.
• **I.V. use:** Don't administer by direct I.V. bolus injection. Each 250- or 500-mg dose should be given by I.V. infusion over 20 to 30 minutes. Each 1-g dose should be infused over 40 to

60 minutes. If nausea occurs, the infusion may be slowed.

• When reconstituting powder, shake until the solution is clear. Solutions may range from colorless to yellow, and variations of color within this range do not affect the drug's potency. After reconstitution, solution is stable for 10 hours at room temperature and for 48 hours when refrigerated.

• Monitor patients for bacterial or fungal superinfections and resistant infections during and after therapy.

• Keep in mind that imipenem/cilastatin has the broadest antibacterial spectrum of any available antibiotic. The drug is most valuable for empiric treatment of infections and for mixed infections that would otherwise require a combination of antibiotics, typically including an aminoglycoside.

---

lincomycin hydrochloride
Lincocin

Pregnancy Risk Category: NR

HOW SUPPLIED
Capsules: 500 mg
Pediatric capsules: 250 mg
Injection: 300 mg/ml in 2-ml and 10-ml vials and 2-ml U-Ject

ACTION
Unknown. Appears to inhibit bacterial protein synthesis by binding to the 50S subunit of the ribosome.

ONSET, PEAK, DURATION
Onset immediate after I.V. infusion, unknown after I.M. or oral administration. Peak levels occur immediately after an I.V. infusion, 30 minutes after an I.M. injection, or 2 to 4 hours after an oral dose. Duration unknown.

INDICATIONS & DOSAGE
Respiratory tract, skin and soft-tissue, and urinary tract infections; osteomyelitis, septicemia caused by sensitive

group A beta-hemolytic streptococci, pneumococci, and staphylococci—
Adults: 500 mg P.O. q 6 to 8 hours (not to exceed 8 g daily); or 600 mg I.M. daily or q 12 hours; or 600 mg to 1 g I.V. q 8 to 12 hours (not to exceed 8 g daily).
Children over 1 month: 30 to 60 mg/kg P.O. daily, in divided doses q 6 to 8 hours; or 10 mg/kg I.M. daily or in divided doses q 12 hours; or 10 to 20 mg/kg I.V. daily, in divided doses q 6 to 8 hours.

ADVERSE REACTIONS
CNS: dizziness, headache.
CV: hypotension with rapid I.V. infusion.
EENT: glossitis, tinnitus.
GI: nausea, vomiting, *pseudomembranous colitis, persistent diarrhea,* abdominal cramps, stomatitis, pruritus ani.
GU: vaginitis.
Hematologic: *neutropenia, leukopenia,* thrombocytopenia, purpura.
Skin: rashes, urticaria.
Other: hypersensitivity reactions **(anaphylaxis),** angioedema, cholestatic jaundice, pain at injection site.

INTERACTIONS
Antidiarrheals (such as kaolin, pectin, and attapulgite): reduced oral absorption of lincomycin by as much as 90%. Antidiarrheals should be avoided or given at least 2 hours before lincomycin.
Neuromuscular blockers: may potentiate neuromuscular blockade. Monitor for prolonged weakness.

CONTRAINDICATIONS
Contraindicated in patients with hypersensitivity to lincomycin or clindamycin.

NURSING CONSIDERATIONS
• Use cautiously in patients with GI disorders (especially colitis), asthma or significant allergies, hepatic or

---

*Liquid form contains alcohol.   *Common* reactions are in italics; *life-threatening,* in bold italics.
**May contain tartrazine.

renal disease, and endocrine or metabolic disorders.
• Obtain specimen for culture and sensitivity tests before first dose. Therapy may begin pending results.
• **I.V. use:** For I.V. infusion, dilute to 100 ml; infuse over 1 hour. Rapid I.V. infusion may cause hypotension and syncope. Monitor blood pressure in the patient receiving the drug parenterally.
• When giving I.V., check site daily for phlebitis and irritation and rotate infusion sites regularly.
• For I.M. administration, inject deeply. Rotate injection sites. Warn patients that I.M. injection may be painful.
• Monitor CBC and platelets. Stop drug immediately if neutropenia, leukopenia, or other blood disorders develop and notify doctor.
• Monitor hepatic function (increased levels of alkaline phosphatase, ALT, AST, or bilirubin may occur).
• Monitor for signs of bacterial and fungal superinfection, especially when therapy exceeds 10 days.
• For best absorption, instruct the patient to take drug with a full glass of water 1 hour before or 2 hours after meals.
• Advise the patient to take drug exactly as directed, even after he feels better, and to take entire amount prescribed.
• Tell the patient to report adverse reactions to the doctor, especially diarrhea. Warn him not to treat diarrhea himself because it may reflect the onset of antibiotic-associated pseudomembranous colitis.

---

methenamine hippurate
Hiprex**, Hip-Rex†, Urex

methenamine mandelate
Mandameth, Mandelamine, Sterine†

Pregnancy Risk Category: C

HOW SUPPLIED
methenamine hippurate
Tablets: 1 g
methenamine mandelate
Tablets: 500 mg, 1 g
Tablets (enteric-coated): 250 mg, 500 mg, 1 g
Tablets (film-coated): 500 mg, 1 g
Suspension: 500 mg/15 ml

ACTION
Hydrolyzed to ammonia and to formaldehyde, causing antibacterial action against gram-positive and gram-negative organisms. Mandelic and hippuric acids, with which methenamines are combined, are also antibacterial by unknown mechanisms.

ONSET, PEAK, DURATION
Onset and duration unknown. Plasma levels peak within 1 hour of administration. Urine levels of formaldehyde peak within 2 hours of administration of a film-coated tablet, or 3 to 8 hours after an enteric-coated tablet.

INDICATIONS & DOSAGE
Long-term prophylaxis or suppression of chronic urine tract infections –
Adults and children over age 12: 1 g (hippurate) P.O. q 12 hours.
Children age 6 to 12: 500 mg to 1 g (hippurate) P.O. q 12 hours.
Urinary tract infections, infected residual urine in patients with neurogenic bladder –
Adults: 1 g (mandelate) P.O. q.i.d. after meals and h.s.
Children age 6 to 12: 500 mg (mandelate) P.O. q.i.d. after meals and h.s.
Children under age 6: 50 mg/kg (mandelate) P.O. divided in four doses after meals and h.s.

ADVERSE REACTIONS
GI: nausea, vomiting, diarrhea, abdominal cramps, anorexia.
GU: with high doses, urinary tract ir-

ritation, dysuria, frequency, albuminuria, hematuria.
Skin: rashes.
Other: elevated liver enzymes.

INTERACTIONS
Acetazolamide: antagonized methenamine effect. Use together cautiously.
Sulfamethizole: forms an insoluble precipitate in acid urine. Do not administer together.
Urine alkalinizing agents: inhibited methenamine action. Don't use together.

CONTRAINDICATIONS
Contraindicated in patients with renal insufficiency, severe hepatic disease, or severe dehydration.

NURSING CONSIDERATIONS
• Administer cautiously to elderly or debilitated patients because aspiration could cause lipid pneumonia. Oral suspension contains vegetable oil.
• Obtain a clean-catch urine specimen for culture and sensitivity tests before starting therapy, and repeat as needed. Therapy may begin pending results.
• Administer after meals to minimize GI upset.
• Monitor fluid intake and output. Intake should be at least 1,500 to 2,000 ml daily.
• For best results, maintain urine pH at 5.5 or below. Use Nitrazine paper to check pH. Large doses of ascorbic acid (12 g/day) may be necessary to effectively acidify urine.
• Monitor liver function studies periodically during long-term therapy.
• If rash appears, withhold dose and contact the doctor.
• Be aware that *Proteus* and *Pseudomonas* tend to raise urine pH; urine acidifiers are usually necessary when treating these infections.
• Keep in mind that drug interferes with fluorometric procedures for determination of urine catecholamines

and vanillylmandelic acid, causing erroneously high results.
• Instruct patient to limit intake of alkaline foods, such as vegetables, milk, and peanuts. Patients may drink cranberry, plum, and prune juices. These juices or ascorbic acid may be used to acidify urine.
• Warn the patient not to take antacids, including Alka-Seltzer and sodium bicarbonate.

nitrofurantoin macrocrystals
Macrodantin

nitrofurantoin microcrystals
Apo-Nitrofurantoin†, Furadantin, Furan, Furanite, Macrodantin, Nephronex†, Nitrofan, Novofuran†

Pregnancy Risk Category: B

HOW SUPPLIED
nitrofurantoin macrocrystals
Capsules: 25 mg, 50 mg, 100 mg
nitrofurantoin microcrystals
Tablets: 50 mg, 100 mg
Capsules: 50 mg, 100 mg
Oral suspension: 25 mg/5 ml

ACTION
Unknown. Appears to interfere with bacterial enzyme systems and possibly with bacterial cell-wall formation.

ONSET, PEAK, DURATION
Unknown.

INDICATIONS & DOSAGE
Urinary tract infections caused by susceptible Escherichia coli, Staphylococcus aureus, *enterococci; certain strains of* Klebsiella, Proteus, *and* Enterobacter—
Adults and children over age 12: 50 to 100 mg P.O. q.i.d. with milk or meals.
Children 1 month to age 12: 5 to 7 mg/kg P.O. daily, divided q.i.d.

Long-term suppression therapy –
Adults: 50 to 100 mg P.O. daily h.s.
Children: 1 to 2 mg/kg P.O. daily h.s.

ADVERSE REACTIONS

CNS: peripheral neuropathy, headache, dizziness, drowsiness, *ascending polyneuropathy with high doses or renal impairment.*
GI: *anorexia, nausea, vomiting,* abdominal pain, *diarrhea.*
Hematologic: *hemolysis in patients with G6PD deficiency* (reversed after stopping drug), *agranulocytosis,* thrombocytopenia.
Skin: maculopapular, erythematous, or eczematous eruption; pruritus; urticaria; *exfoliative dermatitis; Stevens-Johnson syndrome*, hepatitis.
Other: *asthmatic attacks in patients with history of asthma;* hypersensitivity reactions *(anaphylaxis);* transient alopecia; drug fever; overgrowth of nonsusceptible organisms in the urinary tract; pulmonary sensitivity reactions (cough, chest pains, fever, chills, dyspnea).

INTERACTIONS

Magnesium-containing antacids: decreased nitrofurantoin absorption. Separate administration times by 1 hour.
Nalidixic acid, norfloxacin: possible decreased effectiveness. Avoid using together.
Probenecid, sulfinpyrazone: increased blood levels and decreased urine levels. May result in increased toxicity and lack of therapeutic effect. Don't use together.

CONTRAINDICATIONS

Contraindicated in children 1 month and under and in patients with moderate to severe renal impairment, anuria, oliguria, or creatinine clearance under 60 ml/minute.

NURSING CONSIDERATIONS

● Use cautiously in patients with renal impairment, anemia, diabetes mellitus, electrolyte abnormalities, vitamin B deficiency, debilitating disease, and G6PD deficiency.
● Obtain urine specimen for culture and sensitivity tests before starting therapy and repeat p.r.n. Therapy may begin pending results.
● Give with food or milk to minimize GI distress.
● Monitor fluid intake and output carefully. May turn urine brown or darker.
● Monitor CBC regularly.
● Monitor pulmonary status.
● Monitor the patient for signs of superinfection. Use of nitrofurantoin may result in growth of nonsusceptible organisms, especially *Pseudomonas.*
● Be aware that drug has no effect in blood or tissue outside the urinary tract.
● Know that hypersensitivity may develop when used for long-term therapy.
● Be aware that some patients may experience fewer adverse GI effects with nitrofurantoin macrocrystals.
● Keep in mind that drug may cause false-positive results with urine glucose test using copper sulfate reduction method (Clinitest) but not with glucose oxidase tests (Tes-Tape, Diastix, Clinistix).
● Know that dual-release capsules (25 mg nitrofurantoin macrocrystals combined with 75 mg nitrofurantoin monohydrate) enable patients to take drug only twice daily.
● Continue treatment for 3 days after sterile urine specimens have been obtained.
● Store drug in amber container. Keep away from metals other than stainless steel or aluminum to avoid precipitate formation. Warn patients not to use containers made of these materials.

---

†Available in Canada only.　　‡Available in Australia only.　　◊ Available OTC.

polymyxin B sulfate
Aerosporin

Pregnancy Risk Category: NR

HOW SUPPLIED
Powder for injection: 500,000-unit vials

ACTION
Hinders bacterial cell-wall synthesis, damaging the bacterial plasma membrane and making the cell more vulnerable to osmotic pressure (bactericidal).

ONSET, PEAK, DURATION
Onset immediate after I.V. infusion, unknown after I.M. injection. Peak serum levels occur immediately after I.V. infusion, within 2 hours of an I.M. injection. Duration unknown.

INDICATIONS & DOSAGE
Acute urinary tract infections or septicemia caused by sensitive Pseudomonas aeruginosa, *or when other antibiotics are ineffective or contraindicated; bacteremia caused by sensitive* Enterobacter aerogenes *and* Klebsiella pneumoniae, *or acute urinary tract infections caused by* Escherichia coli —
Adults and children over 2 years: 15,000 to 25,000 units/kg daily I.V. infusion, in divided doses q 12 hours; or 25,000 to 30,000 units/kg I.M. daily, in divided doses q 4 to 8 hours.
Meningitis caused by sensitive P. aeruginosa *or* Haemophilus influenzae *when other antibiotics ineffective or contraindicated* —
Adults and children over 2 years: 50,000 units intrathecally once daily for 3 to 4 days, then 50,000 units every other day for at least 2 weeks after CSF tests are negative and CSF sugar is normal.
Children under 2 years: 20,000 units intrathecally once daily for 3 to 4 days, then 25,000 units every other day for at least 2 weeks after cerebrospinal fluid tests are negative and cerebrospinal fluid sugar is normal.

ADVERSE REACTIONS
CNS: *neurotoxicity,* irritability, drowsiness, facial flushing, weakness, ataxia, respiratory paralysis, headache and meningeal irritation with intrathecal administration, peripheral and perioral paresthesias, **seizures, coma.**
EENT: blurred vision.
GU: *nephrotoxicity* (albuminuria, cylindruria, hematuria, proteinuria, decreased urine output, increased BUN level).
Skin: urticaria.
Other: hypersensitivity reactions (fever, **anaphylaxis**), pain at I.M. injection site.

INTERACTIONS
● *Aminoglycosides, amphotericin B, cisplatin, vancomycin, zidovudine:* increased risk of nephrotoxicity. Avoid concomitant use.
● *Neuromuscular blockers:* may potentiate neuromuscular blockade. Monitor closely.

CONTRAINDICATIONS
Contraindicated in patients with hypersensitivity to the drug.

NURSING CONSIDERATIONS
● Use cautiously in those with impaired renal function or myasthenia gravis.
● Give only to a hospitalized patient under constant supervision.
● Obtain urine specimen for culture and sensitivity tests before first dose. Therapy may begin pending results.
● **I.V. use:** When giving I.V., check site daily for phlebitis and irritation. Dilute each 500,000 units in 300 to 500 ml of D₅W; infuse over 60 to 90 minutes. Rotate I.V. sites regularly.
● Avoid administering by I.M. injection because of severe local pain. If

---

*Liquid form contains alcohol. *Common* reactions are in italics; *life-threatening*, in bold italics.
**May contain tartrazine.

I.M. route must be used, give deeply and check dosage carefully. I.M. dosage differs from I.V. dosage.
• Refrigerate parenteral solutions and use within 72 hours.
• Know that for meningitis, the drug is given intrathecally to achieve adequate CSF levels.
• Don't give solution containing local anesthetics I.V. or intrathecally.
• Monitor renal function (BUN, serum creatinine, creatinine clearance, urine output) before and during therapy, as ordered. Fluid intake should be sufficient to maintain output at 1,500 ml/day (between 3,000 and 4,000 ml/day for adults).
• Notify the doctor immediately if the patient develops fever, adverse CNS effects, rash, or symptoms of nephrotoxicity.
• If the patient is scheduled for surgery, notify anesthesiologist of preoperative treatment with this drug because it may prolong neuromuscular blockade.

---

rifabutin
Mycobutin

Pregnancy Risk Category: B

HOW SUPPLIED
Capsules: 150 mg

ACTION
Inhibits DNA-dependent RNA polymerase in susceptible bacteria, blocking bacterial protein synthesis.

ONSET, PEAK, DURATION
Onset and duration unknown. Plasma levels peak 1½ to 4 hours after an oral dose.

INDICATIONS & DOSAGE
Prevention of disseminated Mycobacterium avium *complex (MAC) in patients with advanced HIV infection* —
Adults: 300 mg P.O. daily as a single dose or divided b.i.d.

ADVERSE REACTIONS
EENT: uveitis.
GI: dyspepsia, eructation, flatulence, nausea, vomiting, abdominal pain.
GU: *discolored urine.*
Hematologic: neutropenia, leukopenia, thrombocytopenia, eosinophilia.
Skin: *rash.*
Other: fever, myalgia, myositis, taste perversion.

INTERACTIONS
Oral contraceptives: decreased effectiveness. Instruct patient to use nonhormonal forms of birth control.
Zidovudine, drugs metabolized by the liver: decreased serum levels of zidovudine. Because rifabutin, like rifampin, induces liver enzymes, it may lower serum levels of many other drugs as well. Although dosage adjustments may be necessary, further study is needed.

CONTRAINDICATIONS
Contraindicated in patients with hypersensitivity to the drug or other rifamycin derivatives (such as rifampin). Also contraindicated in patients with active tuberculosis because single-agent therapy with rifabutin increases the risk of inducing bacterial resistance to both rifabutin and rifampin.

NURSING CONSIDERATIONS
• Use cautiously in patients with preexisting neutropenia and thrombocytopenia. Perform baseline hematologic studies and repeat periodically.
• Know that high-fat meals slow the rate, but not the extent, of absorption.
• Mix with soft foods, such as applesauce, for patients who have difficulty swallowing.
• Keep in mind that no evidence exists that drug will provide effective prophylaxis against *Mycobacterium tuberculosis.* Patients requiring prophylaxis against both *M. tuberculosis*

---

and MAC may require rifampin and rifabutin.

• Tell the patient that drug or its metabolites may discolor urine, feces, sputum, saliva, tears, and skin brownish orange. Tell him to avoid wearing soft contact lenses because they may be permanently stained.

• Tell the patient to report photophobia, excessive lacrimation, or eye pain immediately. Drug may rarely cause uveitis.

---

spectinomycin dihydrochloride
Trobicin

Pregnancy Risk Category: NR

HOW SUPPLIED
Injection: 2-g vial with 3.2-ml diluent; 4-g vial with 6.2-ml diluent
Powder for injection: 2 g, 4 g

ACTION
Mechanism: Inhibits protein synthesis by binding to the 30S subunit of the ribosome.

ONSET, PEAK, DURATION
Onset and duration unknown. Serum levels peak 1 hour after a single 2-g I.M. dose, 2 hours after a single 4-g I.M. dose.

INDICATIONS & DOSAGE
Gonorrhea –
Adults: 2 to 4 g I.M. single dose injected deeply into the upper outer quadrant of the buttock.

ADVERSE REACTIONS
CNS: insomnia, dizziness, headache.
GI: nausea, vomiting.
GU: decreased urine output, decrease in creatinine clearance, increase in BUN.
Skin: urticaria, pruritus.
Other: fever, chills (may mask or delay symptoms of incubating syphilis), transient increases in liver enzymes,

decrease in hemoglobin values, pain at injection site.

INTERACTIONS
None significant.

CONTRAINDICATIONS
Contraindicated in patients with hypersensitivity to the drug.

NURSING CONSIDERATIONS
• Shake vial vigorously after reconstitution and before withdrawing dose. Store at room temperature after reconstitution and use within 24 hours.
• Use 20G needle to administer drug. Divide the 4-g dose (10 ml) into two 5-ml injections – give one in each buttock.
• Be aware that drug is not effective in the treatment of syphilis. Serologic test for syphilis should be done before treatment dose and 3 months afterward.

---

trimethoprim
Alprin‡, Proloprim, Trimpex, Triprim‡

Pregnancy Risk Category: C

HOW SUPPLIED
Tablets: 100 mg, 200 mg

ACTION
Interferes with the action of dihydrofolate reductase, inhibiting bacterial synthesis of folic acid.

ONSET, PEAK, DURATION
Onset and duration unknown. Plasma levels peak 1 to 4 hours after an oral dose.

INDICATIONS & DOSAGE
Uncomplicated urinary tract infections caused by susceptible strains of Escherichia coli, Proteus mirabilis, Klebsiella, *and* Enterobacter –
Adults: 200 mg P.O. daily as a single

---

dose or in divided doses q 12 hours for 10 days.

Not recommended for children under age 12.

ADVERSE REACTIONS
GI: *epigastric distress, nausea, vomiting,* glossitis.
Hematologic: thrombocytopenia, leukopenia, megaloblastic anemia, methemoglobinemia.
Skin: *rash, pruritus, exfoliative dermatitis.*
Other: fever.

INTERACTIONS
Phenytoin: may decrease phenytoin metabolism and increase its serum levels. Monitor for toxicity.

CONTRAINDICATIONS
Contraindicated in patients with hypersensitivity to the drug and in those with documented megaloblastic anemia caused by folate deficiency.

NURSING CONSIDERATIONS
• Use cautiously in patients with impaired hepatic function. Dosage should be decreased in patients with severely impaired renal function.
• Obtain urine specimen for culture and sensitivity tests before first dose. Therapy may begin pending results.
• Monitor CBC routinely. Clinical signs such as sore throat, fever, pallor, or purpura may be early indications of serious blood disorders. Prolonged use of trimethoprim at high doses may cause bone marrow suppression.
• Keep in mind that because resistance to trimethoprim develops rapidly when given alone, it is usually given in combination with other drugs.
• Be aware that the drug is not recommended for use in patients with creatinine clearance less than 15 ml/minute.
• Instruct the patient to take entire amount of the drug, as prescribed, even if he feels better.

---

trimetrexate glucuronate
NeuTrexin

Pregnancy Risk Category: D

HOW SUPPLIED
Injection: 25-mg vials

ACTION
Prevents reduction of folic acid to tetrahydrofolate by binding to dihydrofolate reductase.

ONSET, PEAK, DURATION
Unknown.

INDICATIONS & DOSAGE
Alternative treatment of Pneumocystis carinii *pneumonia in patients with AIDS –*
Adults: 45 mg/m^2 I.V. infusion over 60 to 90 minutes daily for 21 days, administered with 20 mg/m^2 of leucovorin I.V. or P.O. q 6 hours for 24 days.

ADVERSE REACTIONS
CNS: peripheral neuropathy.
GI: nausea, vomiting, stomatitis.
Hematologic: *neutropenia, thrombocytopenia, anemia.*
Hepatic: hepatotoxicity.
Skin: rash.

INTERACTIONS
Acetaminophen, cimetidine, clotrimazole, erythromycin, fluconazole, ketoconazole, miconazole, rifampin, rifabutin: may interfere with trimetrexate metabolism and lead to toxicity. Monitor closely.
Chloride-containing solutions, leucovorin: precipitate will form if mixed with trimetrexate. Administer separately.
Hepatotoxic, myelosuppressive, or nephrotoxic drugs: enhanced toxicity. Use together cautiously and monitor closely.

---

†Available in Canada only.   ‡Available in Australia only.   ◇Available OTC.

CONTRAINDICATIONS

Contraindicated in patients with hypersensitivity to trimetrexate, methotrexate, or leucovorin.

NURSING CONSIDERATIONS

• Use cautiously in patients with impaired hematologic, renal, or hepatic function and in women of childbearing age because the drug may cause fetal harm. Avoid using during pregnancy.

• Follow institutional policy when administering parenteral form of this drug because parenteral form is associated with carcinogenic, mutagenic, and teratogenic risks for personnel.

• **I.V. use:** Reconstitute 25-mg vial with 2 ml of D_5W or sterile water for injection to yield a solution of 12.5 mg/ml. Complete dissolution usually occurs within 30 seconds. Further dilute reconstituted solution with D_5W to yield a final concentration of 0.25 to 2 mg/ml. Infuse over 60 minutes. After reconstitution, the drug is stable at room temperature or refrigerated for 24 hours.

• Use only D_5W for I.V. infusion. Drug is incompatible with chloride-containing solutions (including 0.9% sodium chloride solution) and leucovorin.

• Flush the I.V. line with at least 10 ml of D_5W immediately before and after the trimetrexate infusion.

• Administer leucovorin either before or after trimetrexate. When giving I.V., be sure to flush the I.V. line with D_5W because the two drugs are incompatible. Leucovorin calcium may be infused over 5 to 10 minutes.

• Know that leucovorin therapy must accompany trimetrexate treatments to avoid potentially life-threatening toxicity. Leucovorin therapy must extend for 3 days beyond trimetrexate treatment.

• When calculating the oral dose of leucovorin, round dosage up to the next increment of 25 mg.

• Monitor patients closely. Many adverse effects may be decreased by adjusting the dosage of leucovorin.

• Avoid I.M. injections in patients with thrombocytopenia.

• Warn patients to watch for signs of infection (fever, sore throat, fatigue) and bleeding (easy bruising, nosebleeds, bleeding gums, melena). Take temperature daily.

• Advise women of childbearing age to avoid becoming pregnant during therapy. Also recommend consulting doctor before becoming pregnant.

---

vancomycin hydrochloride
Vancocin, Vancoled

Pregnancy Risk Category: C

HOW SUPPLIED
Capsules: 125 mg, 250 mg
Powder for oral solution: 1-g, 10-g bottles
Powder for injection: 500-mg, 1-g vials
Pharmacy bulk package: 5 g, 10 g

ACTION
Hinders bacterial cell-wall synthesis, damaging the bacterial plasma membrane and making the cell more vulnerable to osmotic pressure.

ONSET, PEAK, DURATION
Onset immediate after I.V. infusion, unknown after oral administration. Serum levels peak immediately after I.V. infusion, unknown after oral administration. Duration unknown.

INDICATIONS & DOSAGE
Severe staphylococcal infections when other antibiotics are ineffective or contraindicated—
Adults: 500 mg I.V. q 6 hours, or 1 g q 12 hours.
Children: 40 mg/kg I.V. daily, in divided doses q 6 hours.
Neonates: 10 mg/kg I.V. daily, in divided doses q 6 to 12 hours.

---

*Liquid form contains alcohol.   *Common* reactions are in italics; *life-threatening,* in bold italics.
**May contain tartrazine.

Antibiotic-associated pseudomembranous and staphylococcal enterocolitis –

Adults: 125 to 500 mg P.O. q 6 hours for 7 to 10 days.

Children: 40 mg/kg P.O. daily, in divided doses q 6 hours. Maximum daily dosage is 2 g.

Endocarditis prophylaxis for dental procedures –

Adults: 1 g I.V. slowly over 1 hour, starting 1 hour before procedure.

Children: 20 mg/kg I.V. over 1 hour, starting 1 hour before procedure.

ADVERSE REACTIONS

EENT: tinnitus, ototoxicity.

GI: nausea.

GU: nephrotoxicity.

Hematologic: transient eosinophilia, leukopenia.

Skin: "red-neck" syndrome with rapid I.V. infusion (maculopapular rash on face, neck, trunk, and extremities).

Other: chills, fever, *anaphylaxis,* superinfection, pain or thrombophlebitis with I.V. administration, necrosis.

INTERACTIONS

Aminoglycosides, amphotericin B, cisplatin, pentamidine: increased risk of nephrotoxicity and ototoxicity. Monitor closely.

CONTRAINDICATIONS

Contraindicated in patients with hypersensitivity to the drug.

NURSING CONSIDERATIONS

• Use cautiously in patients receiving other neurotoxic, nephrotoxic, or ototoxic drugs; in patients over age 60, and in those with impaired hepatic or renal function, preexisting hearing loss, or allergies to other antibiotics. Patients with renal dysfunction require dosage adjustment.

• Obtain urine specimen for culture and sensitivity tests before first dose. Therapy may begin pending results.

• Obtain hearing evaluation and renal function studies before therapy.

• **I.V. use:** For I.V. infusion, dilute in 200 ml sodium chloride injection or 5% glucose solution and infuse over 60 minutes. Check site daily for phlebitis and irritation. Report pain at infusion site. Avoid extravasation. Severe irritation and necrosis can result.

• Monitor the patient carefully for red-neck syndrome, which can occur if drug is infused too rapidly. If this reaction occurs, stop infusion and report to the doctor.

• Refrigerate I.V. solution after reconstitution and use within 96 hours.

• Do not give drug intramuscularly.

• Know that the oral preparation is stable for 2 weeks if refrigerated.

• Monitor renal function (BUN, serum creatinine, urinalysis, creatinine clearance, and urine output) during therapy. Also monitor for signs of superinfection.

• Have the patient's hearing evaluated during prolonged therapy.

• Be aware that when using the drug to treat staphylococcal endocarditis, it will be given for at least 4 weeks.

• Tell the patient to take entire amount of medication exactly as directed, even after he feels better.

• Tell the patient to stop drug immediately and report adverse reactions, especially fullness or ringing in ears.

20

Inotropics

amrinone lactate
digitoxin
digoxin
milrinone lactate

COMBINATION PRODUCTS
None.

---

amrinone lactate
Inocor

Pregnancy Risk Category: C

HOW SUPPLIED
Injection: 5 mg/ml

ACTION
Unknown. Thought to produce inotropic action by increasing cellular levels of cAMP. Produces vasodilation through a direct relaxant effect on vascular smooth muscle.

ONSET, PEAK, DURATION
Onset begins within 2 to 5 minutes. Serum levels peak in 10 minutes. Effects persist ½ to 2 hours after dose.

INDICATIONS & DOSAGE
Short-term management of CHF –
Adults: initially, 0.75 mg/kg I.V. bolus over 2 to 3 minutes. Then begin maintenance infusion of 5 to 10 mcg/kg/minute. Additional bolus of 0.75 mg/kg may be given 30 minutes after start of therapy. Total daily dosage should not exceed 10 mg/kg.

ADVERSE REACTIONS
CV: *arrhythmias,* hypotension.
GI: nausea, vomiting, cramps, diarrhea, anorexia.
Hematologic: *thrombocytopenia* (depends on dose and duration of therapy).

Hepatic: elevated enzymes, hepatotoxicity (rare).
Other: burning at injection site, hypersensitivity reactions (pericarditis, ascites, myositis vasculitis, pleuritis), fever, chest pain.

INTERACTIONS
Digitalis glycosides: enhanced inotropic effect. Beneficial drug interaction.

CONTRAINDICATIONS
Contraindicated in patients with hypersensitivity to amrinone or bisulfites.

NURSING CONSIDERATIONS
• Know that amrinone should not be used in patients with severe aortic or pulmonic valvular disease in place of surgical correction of the obstruction or during acute phase of MI.
• Use cautiously in patients with hypertrophic cardiomyopathy.
• Be aware that amrinone is primarily prescribed for patients who have not responded to therapy with digitalis glycosides, diuretics, and vasodilators.
• Expect dosage to be based on clinical response, including assessment of pulmonary artery wedge pressure and cardiac output.
• Anticipate that amrinone may be added to digitalis glycoside therapy in patients with atrial fibrillation and flutter because it enhances AV conduction and increases ventricular response rate.
• **I.V. use:** Administer amrinone with an infusion pump and use as supplied, or dilute in 0.45% or 0.9% sodium chloride to a concentration of 1 to 3 mg/ml. Use diluted solution within 24 hours.
• Don't dilute with solutions contain-

---

*Liquid form contains alcohol.   *Common* reactions are in italics; ***life-threatening,*** in bold italics.
**May contain tartrazine.

ing dextrose because a slow chemical reaction occurs over 24 hours. However, amrinone can be injected into free-flowing dextrose infusions through a Y-connector or directly into the tubing.
• Don't administer furosemide and amrinone through the same I.V. line because precipitation occurs.
• Monitor blood pressure and heart rate throughout the infusion. If the patient's blood pressure falls, slow or stop infusion and notify the doctor.
• Monitor platelet count. If it falls below 150,000/mm³, decrease dosage as ordered.
• Patients with end-stage cardiac disease may receive home treatment with an amrinone drip while awaiting heart transplantation.

digitoxin
Crystodigin, Digitaline†

Pregnancy Risk Category: C

HOW SUPPLIED
Tablets: 0.05 mg, 0.1 mg, 0.15 mg, 0.2 mg

ACTION
Inhibits sodium-potassium activated adenosine triphosphatase, promoting movement of calcium from extracellular to intracellular cytoplasm and thereby strengthening myocardial contraction. Also acts on CNS to enhance vagal tone, slowing conduction through the AV node and providing an antiarrhythmic effect.

ONSET, PEAK, DURATION
Onset occurs in ½ to 2 hours. Serum levels peak 4 to 12 hours after oral dose. Effects may persist for 3 to 4 weeks after last dose.

INDICATIONS & DOSAGE
CHF, paroxysmal supraventricular tachycardia, atrial fibrillation and flutter —

Adults and children 12 years and older: loading dose is 1.2 to 1.6 mg P.O. in divided doses over 24 hours; average maintenance dosage is 0.15 mg daily (range: 0.05 to 0.3 mg daily).
Premature infants, neonates, severely ill older infants: loading dose is 0.022 mg/kg or 0.3 to 0.35 mg/m² P.O. in divided doses over 24 hours; maintenance dosage is 0.0022 mg/kg daily.
Children 2 weeks to 1 year: loading dose is 0.045 mg/kg P.O. in divided doses over 24 hours; maintenance dosage is 0.0045 mg/kg daily.
Children 1 to 2 years: loading dose is 0.04 mg/kg P.O. in divided doses over 24 hours; maintenance dosage is 0.004 mg/kg daily.
Children 2 to 12 years: loading dose is 0.03 mg/kg or 0.75 mg/m² P.O. in divided doses over 24 hours; maintenance dosage is 0.003 mg/kg or 0.075 mg/m² daily.

ADVERSE REACTIONS
The following are signs of toxicity that may occur with all digitalis glycosides:
CNS: *fatigue, generalized muscle weakness, agitation, hallucinations,* headache, malaise, dizziness, vertigo, stupor, paresthesia.
CV: *arrhythmias* (most commonly conduction disturbances with or without AV block, PVCs, and supraventricular arrhythmias); arrhythmias may lead to increased severity of CHF and hypotension. *Toxic effects on heart may be life-threatening and require immediate attention.*
EENT: *yellow-green halos around visual images, blurred vision,* light flashes, photophobia, diplopia.
GI: *anorexia, nausea,* vomiting, diarrhea.

INTERACTIONS

Amiodarone, quinidine, verapamil: possible increased serum digitoxin levels. Monitor patient closely.

Amphotericin B, corticosteroids, diuretics (including loop diuretics, chlorthalidone, metolazone, and thiazides), ticarcillin: hypokalemia or hypomagnesemia, predisposing patient to digitalis toxicity. Monitor serum potassium and serum magnesium levels.

Antacids, kaolin-pectin, oral neomycin, sulfasalazine: decreased absorption of digitoxin. Schedule doses as far as possible from digitoxin administration.

Cholestyramine, colestipol, metoclopramide: decreased absorption of digitoxin. Monitor for decreased effect and low blood levels. Increase dosage if necessary and as ordered.

Parenteral calcium, thiazides: hypercalcemia and hypomagnesemia, predisposing patient to digitalis toxicity. Monitor serum calcium and serum magnesium levels.

Phenobarbital, phenylbutazone, phenytoin, rifampin: faster metabolism and shorter duration of digitoxin. Observe for underdigitalization.

CONTRAINDICATIONS

Contraindicated in patients with hypersensitivity to the drug; digitalis-induced toxicity; ventricular fibrillation; or ventricular tachycardia unless caused by CHF.

NURSING CONSIDERATIONS

• Use with extreme caution in elderly patients and in those with acute MI, incomplete AV block, sinus bradycardia, PVCs, chronic constrictive pericarditis, hypertrophic cardiomyopathy, severe pulmonary disease, and thyroid disease. Reduce dosage in patients with renal impairment.

• Be aware that hypothyroid patients are extremely sensitive to glycosides; hyperthyroid patients may need larger doses.

• Before administering loading dose, obtain baseline data (heart rate and rhythm, blood pressure, and electrolytes) and question the patient about recent use of digitalis glycosides (within the previous 2 to 3 weeks).

• Be aware that the loading dose is always divided over the first 24 hours unless the clinical situation indicates otherwise.

• Before giving, take apical-radial pulse for a full minute. Record and report to the doctor any significant changes (sudden increase or decrease in the pulse rate, pulse deficit, irregular beats, and, particularly, regularization of a previously irregular rhythm). If any of these changes occur, check blood pressure and obtain a 12-lead ECG.

• Monitor serum digitoxin levels. Therapeutic blood levels of digitoxin range from 25 to 35 ng/ml.

• Because digitoxin is a long-acting drug, watch for cumulative effects and signs of toxicity, especially in children and elderly patients. Ask the patient about nausea, vomiting, anorexia, visual disturbances, and other symptoms of toxicity.

• Excessive slowing of pulse rate (60 beats/minute or less) may be a sign of digitalis toxicity. Withhold drug and notify the doctor.

• For digitalis toxicity, administer agents that bind the drug in the intestine (for example, colestipol or cholestyramine). Treat arrhythmias with phenytoin I.V. or lidocaine I.V. and potentially life-threatening toxicity with specific antigen-binding fragments (such as digoxin immune FAB) as ordered.

• Monitor serum potassium level carefully. Take corrective action before hypokalemia occurs. Encourage the patient to eat potassium-rich foods.

• Withhold drug for 1 to 2 days before elective cardioversion, as ordered. Adjust dose after cardioversion.

---

*Liquid form contains alcohol.   *Common* reactions are in italics; ***life-threatening***, in bold italics.
**May contain tartrazine.

- Instruct the patient and a responsible family member about drug action, dosage regimen, pulse taking, reportable signs, and follow-up plans.
- Tell patient not to substitute one brand of digitoxin for another.

digoxin
Digoxin, Lanoxicaps, Lanoxin*, Novodigoxin†

Pregnancy Risk Category: C

HOW SUPPLIED
Tablets: 0.125 mg, 0.25 mg, 0.5 mg
Capsules: 0.05 mg, 0.1 mg, 0.2 mg
Elixir: 0.05 mg/ml
Injection: 0.05 mg/ml†, 0.1 mg/ml (pediatric), 0.25 mg/ml

ACTION
Inhibits sodium-potassium activated adenosine triphosphatase, thereby promoting movement of calcium from extracellular to intracellular cytoplasm and strengthening myocardial contraction. Also acts on CNS to enhance vagal tone, slowing conduction through the SA and AV nodes and providing an antiarrhythmic effect.

ONSET, PEAK, DURATION
Onset occurs in ½ to 2 hours after oral dose or 5 to 30 minutes after I.V. administration. Serum levels peak 2 to 6 hours after oral dose or 1 to 4 hours after I.V. administration. Effects persist 3 to 4 days after last dose.

INDICATIONS & DOSAGE
CHF, paroxysmal supraventricular tachycardia, atrial fibrillation and flutter–
Adults: loading dose is 0.5 to 1 mg I.V. or P.O. in divided doses over 24 hours; maintenance dosage is 0.125 to 0.5 mg I.V. or P.O. daily (average is 0.25 mg). Depending on patient response, larger doses may be needed for treatment of arrhythmias. Smaller

loading and maintenance doses are given to patients with impaired renal function.
Adults over 65 years: 0.125 mg P.O. daily as maintenance dose. Frail or underweight elderly patients may require only 0.0625 mg daily or 0.125 mg every other day.
Premature neonates: loading dose is 0.025 mg/kg I.V. in three divided doses over 24 hours; maintenance dosage is 0.01 mg/kg daily, divided q 12 hours.
Neonates: loading dose is 0.035 mg/kg P.O., divided q 8 hours over 24 hours; I.V. loading dose is 0.02 to 0.03 mg/kg; maintenance dosage is 0.01 mg/kg P.O. daily, divided q 12 hours.
Children 1 month to 2 years: loading dose is 0.035 to 0.06 mg/kg P.O. in three divided doses over 24 hours; I.V. loading dose is 0.03 to 0.05 mg/kg; maintenance dosage is 0.01 to 0.02 mg/kg P.O. daily, divided q 12 hours.
Children over 2 years: loading dose is 0.02 to 0.04 mg/kg P.O. daily, divided q 8 hours over 24 hours; I.V. loading dose is 0.015 to 0.035 mg/kg; maintenance dosage is 0.012 mg/kg P.O. daily, divided q 12 hours.

ADVERSE REACTIONS
The following are signs of toxicity that may occur with all digitalis glycosides:
CNS: *fatigue, generalized muscle weakness, agitation, hallucinations,* headache, malaise, dizziness, vertigo, stupor, paresthesia.
CV: *arrhythmias* (most commonly, conduction disturbances with or without AV block, PVCs, and supraventricular arrhythmias); arrythmias may lead to increased severity of CHF and hypotension. *Toxic effects on the heart may be life-threatening and require immediate attention.*
EENT: *yellow-green halos around vi-*

---

sual images, blurred vision, light flashes, photophobia, diplopia.
GI: *anorexia, nausea,* vomiting, diarrhea.

INTERACTIONS
Amiloride: inhibited digoxin effect and increased digoxin excretion. Monitor for altered digoxin effect.
Amiodarone, diltiazem, nifedipine, quinidine, verapamil: increased digoxin blood levels. Monitor for toxicity.
Amphotericin B, carbenicillin, corticosteroids, diuretics (including loop diuretics, chlorthalidone, metolazone, and thiazides), ticarcillin: hypokalemia, predisposing patient to digitalis toxicity. Monitor serum potassium levels.
Antacids, kaolin-pectin: decreased absorption of oral digoxin. Schedule doses as far as possible from oral digoxin administration.
Anticholinergics: may increase digoxin absorption of oral digoxin tablets. Monitor blood levels and observe for toxicity.
Cholestyramine, colestipol, metoclopramide: decreased absorption of oral digoxin. Monitor for decreased effect and low blood levels. Increase dosage if necessary and as ordered.
Parenteral calcium, thiazides: hypercalcemia and hypomagnesemia, predisposing patient to digitalis toxicity. Monitor serum calcium and serum magnesium levels.

CONTRAINDICATIONS
Contraindicated in patients with hypersensitivity to the drug; any digitalis-induced toxicity; ventricular fibrillation; or ventricular tachycardia unless caused by CHF.

NURSING CONSIDERATIONS
• Use with extreme caution in elderly patients and in those with acute MI, incomplete AV block, sinus bradycardia, PVCs, chronic constrictive pericarditis, hypertrophic cardiomyopa-

thy, renal insufficiency, severe pulmonary disease, or hypothyroidism. Reduce dosage in patients with renal impairment.
• Be aware that hypothyroid patients are extremely sensitive to digitalis glycosides; hyperthyroid patients may need larger doses.
• Before administering the loading dose, obtain baseline data (heart rate and rhythm, blood pressure, and electrolytes) and question the patient about recent use of digitalis glycosides (within the previous 2 to 3 weeks).
• Be aware that the loading dose is always divided over the first 24 hours unless the clinical situation indicates otherwise.
• Before giving, take apical-radial pulse for a full minute. Record and report to the doctor any significant changes (sudden increase or decrease in pulse rate, pulse deficit, irregular beats, and particularly regularization of a previously irregular rhythm). If any of these changes occurs, check blood pressure and obtain a 12-lead ECG.
• **I.V. use:** Infuse drug slowly over at least 5 minutes.
• Absorption of digoxin from parenteral route and from liquid-filled capsules is superior to absorption from tablets or elixir. Expect dosage reduction of 20% to 25% when changing from tablets or elixir to liquid-filled capsules or parenteral therapy.
• Monitor serum digoxin levels. Therapeutic blood levels of digoxin range from 0.5 to 2.0 ng/ml. Obtain blood for digoxin levels 8 hours after last oral dose.
• Excessive slowing of the pulse rate (60 beats/minute or less) may be a sign of digitalis toxicity. Withhold drug and notify the doctor.
• Monitor serum potassium levels carefully. Take corrective action before hypokalemia occurs. Encourage the patient to eat potassium-rich foods.

*Liquid form contains alcohol.   *Common* reactions are in italics; *life-threatening,* in bold italics.
**May contain tartrazine.

• Withhold drug for 1 to 2 days before elective cardioversion. Adjust dose after cardioversion.
• Instruct the patient and a responsible family member about drug action, dosage regimen, how to take pulse, reportable signs, and follow-up care.
• Tell the patient not to substitute one brand of digoxin for another.

---

milrinone lactate
Primacor

Pregnancy Risk Category: C

HOW SUPPLIED
Injection: 1 mg/ml

ACTION
Produces inotropic action by increasing cellular levels of cAMP. Produces vasodilation by directly relaxing vascular smooth muscle.

ONSET, PEAK, DURATION
Onset occurs within 5 to 15 minutes. Serum levels peak within 1 to 2 hours. Duration is 3 to 6 hours.

INDICATIONS & DOSAGE
Short-term treatment of CHF –
Adults: initial loading dose is 50 mcg/kg I.V., administered slowly over 10 minutes, followed by continuous I.V. infusion of 0.375 to 0.75 mcg/kg/minute. Adjust infusion dose according to clinical and hemodynamic responses, as ordered.
   In patients with renal failure: if creatinine clearance is 50 ml/minute or less, dosage is titrated to maximum clinical effect and not to exceed 1.13 mg/kg/day.

ADVERSE REACTIONS
CNS: headache.
CV: *ventricular arrhythmias, ventricular ectopic activity,* nonsustained ventricular tachycardia, *sustained ventricular tachycardia, ventricular fibrillation.*

INTERACTIONS
None reported.

CONTRAINDICATIONS
Contraindicated in patients with hypersensitivity to the drug.

NURSING CONSIDERATIONS
• Know that milrinone should not be used in patients with severe aortic or pulmonic valvular disease in place of surgical correction of the obstruction or during acute phase of MI.
• Use cautiously in patients with atrial flutter or fibrillation because drug slightly shortens AV node conduction time and may increase ventricular response rate. Administer a digitalis glycoside, if ordered, before beginning milrinone therapy.
• Be aware that milrinone is typically given with digoxin and diuretics.
• Be aware that inotropic agents may aggravate outflow tract obstruction in hypertrophic subaortic stenosis.
• **I.V. use:** Prepare I.V. infusion solution using 0.45% or 0.9% sodium chloride or D₅W. Prepare the 100-mcg/ml solution by adding 180 ml of diluent per 20-mg (20-ml) vial, the 150-mcg/ml solution by adding 113 ml of diluent per 20-mg (20-ml) vial, and the 200-mcg/ml solution by adding 80 ml of diluent per 20-mg (20-ml) vial.
• Be aware that improvement of cardiac output may result in enhanced urine output. Expect dosage reduction in patient's diuretic therapy as CHF improves. Remember that potassium loss may predispose patient to digitalis toxicity.
• Monitor fluid and electrolyte status, blood pressure, heart rate, and renal function during therapy. Excessive decrease in blood pressure requires discontinuation or slower rate of infusion.
• Monitor patients closely. Patients treated with milrinone have exhibited supraventricular and ventricular arrhythmias.

---

†Available in Canada only.   ‡Available in Australia only.   ◊ Available OTC.

adenosine
amiodarone hydrochloride
atropine sulfate
bretylium tosylate
disopyramide
disopyramide phosphate
esmolol hydrochloride
flecainide acetate
lidocaine hydrochloride
mexiletine hydrochloride
moricizine hydrochloride
phenytoin
   (See Chapter 30, ANTICONVULSANTS.)
phenytoin sodium
   (See Chapter 30, ANTICONVULSANTS.)
procainamide hydrochloride
propafenone hydrochloride
propranolol hydrochloride
   (See Chapter 22, ANTIANGINALS.)
quinidine bisulfate
quinidine gluconate
quinidine polygalacturonate
quinidine sulfate
sotalol
tocainide hydrochloride

COMBINATION PRODUCTS
None.

---

adenosine
Adenocard

Pregnancy Risk Category: C

HOW SUPPLIED
Injection: 3 mg/ml in 2-ml vials

ACTION
A naturally occurring nucleoside that acts on the AV node to slow conduction and inhibit reentry pathways. Adenosine is also useful in treating paroxysmal supraventricular tachycardia (PSVT) associated with accessory bypass tracts (Wolff-Parkinson-White syndrome).

ONSET, PEAK, DURATION
Onset is immediate. Peak serum levels occur immediately. Duration is extremely short although the exact time is unknown.

INDICATIONS & DOSAGE
Conversion of PSVT to sinus rhythm –
Adults: 6 mg I.V. by rapid bolus injection over 1 to 2 seconds. If PSVT is not eliminated in 1 to 2 minutes, 12 mg by rapid I.V. push may be given and repeated (if necessary). Single doses over 12 mg are not recommended.

ADVERSE REACTIONS
CNS: apprehension, back pain, blurred vision, burning sensation, dizziness, heaviness in arms, lightheadedness, neck pain, numbness, tingling in arms.
CV: chest pain, *facial flushing,* headache, hypotension, palpitations, diaphoresis.
GI: metallic taste, nausea.
Respiratory: *chest pressure, dyspnea, shortness of breath,* hyperventilation.
Other: *tightness in throat, groin pressure.*

INTERACTIONS
Carbamazepine: higher degrees of heart block may occur.
Dipyridamole: may potentiate adenosine's effects. Smaller doses may be necessary.
Methylxanthines: antagonism of adenosine's effects. Patients receiving theophylline or caffeine may require higher doses or may not respond to adenosine therapy.

---

*Liquid form contains alcohol.
**May contain tartrazine.

Common reactions are in italics; ***life-threatening,*** in bold italics.

CONTRAINDICATIONS
• Contraindicated in patients with hypersensitivity to the drug.
• Also contraindicated in patients with second- or third-degree heart block or sick sinus syndrome unless an artificial pacemaker is present because adenosine decreases conduction through the AV node and may produce transient first-, second-, or third-degree heart block. These effects are usually transient; however, patients who develop significant heart block after a dose of adenosine should not receive additional doses.

NURSING CONSIDERATIONS
• Use cautiously in patients with asthma because bronchoconstriction may occur.
• Crystals may form if solution is cold. If crystals are visible, gently warm solution to room temperature. Don't use solutions that aren't clear.
• Because adenosine contains no preservatives, discard any unused drug.
• I.V. use: Rapid I.V. injection is necessary for drug action. Administer directly into a vein if possible; when giving through an I.V. line, use the most proximal port and flush immediately and rapidly with 0.9% sodium chloride solution to ensure that the drug reaches the systemic circulation quickly.
• Monitor patient's ECG for arrhythmias. In clinical trials, more than half of the patients exhibited new arrhythmias, including sinus bradycardia or tachycardia, atrial premature contractions, various degrees of AV block, PVCs, and skipped beats, when adenosine was used to convert to normal sinus rhythm. Such arrhythmias are usually transient.

---

amiodarone hydrochloride
Aratac‡, Cordarone, Cordarone X‡

Pregnancy Risk Category: D

HOW SUPPLIED
Tablets: 100 mg†‡, 200 mg
Injection: 50 mg/ml‡

ACTION
Unknown. Thought to prolong the refractory period and action potential duration and decrease repolarization.

ONSET, PEAK, DURATION
Onset may occur in 2 to 3 days despite more rapid peak concentration, but more commonly takes 1 to 3 weeks, even with loading doses. Serum levels peak 3 to 7 hours after oral administration. Duration of antiarrhythmic effects may last for weeks or months but rate variable and unpredictable.

INDICATIONS & DOSAGE
Recurrent ventricular fibrillation and recurrent hemodynamically unstable ventricular tachycardia refractory to other antiarrhythmics –
Adults: give loading dose of 800 to 1,600 mg P.O. daily for 1 to 3 weeks until initial therapeutic response occurs, then 650 to 800 mg/day P.O. for 1 month, and then, for maintenance, 200 to 600 mg P.O. daily.
   Or, give loading dose of 5 to 10 mg/kg I.V. over 20 minutes to 2 hours using a central line. Alternatively (and where available), a loading dose of 5 mg/kg I.V. over 20 minutes to 2 hours using a central line. Then repeated 2 to 3 times in 24 hours to a maximum of 1.2 g.

ADVERSE REACTIONS
CNS: peripheral neuropathy, extrapyramidal symptoms, headache, muscle weakness, *malaise, fatigue.*
CV: bradycardia, hypotension, ***arrhythmias, CHF.***
EENT: *corneal microdeposits,* visual disturbances.
GI: *nausea, vomiting,* constipation.
Hepatic: *altered liver enzymes,* hepatic dysfunction.

---

†Available in Canada only.   ‡Available in Australia only.   ◇ Available OTC.

Respiratory: *severe pulmonary toxicity (pneumonitis, alveolitis).*
Skin: *photosensitivity,* blue-gray skin pigmentation.
Other: hypothyroidism, hyperthyroidism, gynecomastia.

INTERACTIONS

Antiarrhythmics: amiodarone may reduce the hepatic or renal clearance of certain antiarrhythmics (especially flecainide, procainamide, or quinidine); concomitant use of amiodarone with other antiarrhythmics (especially mexilitine, propafenone, quinidine, disopyramide, or procainamide) may induce torsades de pointes.
Antihypertensives: increased hypotensive effect. Use together cautiously.
Beta blockers, calcium channel blockers: increased cardiac depressant effects; may potentiate slowing of sinus node and AV conduction. Use together cautiously.
Digitalis glycosides: increased serum digoxin levels (average of 70% to 100%). Monitor digoxin levels closely and adjust dosage as ordered.
Phenytoin: may decrease phenytoin metabolism. Monitor serum phenytoin levels and adjust dosage as ordered.
Theophylline: increased theophylline levels with toxicity may occur. Monitor serum theophylline levels.
Warfarin: increased PT (average of 100% within 1 to 4 weeks of therapy). Decrease warfarin dosage 33% to 50% when amiodarone is initiated. Monitor patient closely.

CONTRAINDICATIONS

Contraindicated in patients with hypersensitivity to the drug and in those with severe sinus node disease resulting in preexisting bradycardia. Unless an artificial pacemaker is present, drug is also contraindicated in patients with second- or third-degree AV block and in those in whom bradycardia has caused syncope.

NURSING CONSIDERATIONS

• Use with extreme caution in patients receiving other antiarrhythmics.
• Use cautiously in patients with pulmonary or thyroid disease.
• Be aware that although amiodarone is often effective for treatment of arrhythmias resistant to other drug therapy, the high incidence of adverse reactions limits its use.
• Obtain baseline pulmonary, liver, and thyroid function tests.
• Administer loading doses in a hospital setting and with continuous ECG monitoring because of the slow onset of antiarrhythmic effect and risk of life-threatening arrhythmias.
• Divide oral loading dose into three equal doses and give with meals to decrease GI intolerance. Maintenance dosage may be given once daily, but may be divided into two doses taken with meals if GI intolerance occurs.
• **I.V. use:** Know that amiodarone may be given I.V. where facilities for close monitoring of cardiac function and resuscitation are available. Initial dosage of 5 mg/kg should be mixed in 250 ml of 5% dextrose solution. Repeat doses preferably should be administered through a central venous catheter. Patient should receive a maximum of 1.2 g in up to 500 ml of 5% dextrose solution daily.
• Continuously monitor cardiac status of patient receiving I.V. amiodarone.
• Monitor blood pressure and heart rate and rhythm frequently. Perform continuous ECG monitoring during initiation and alteration of dosage. Notify doctor of any significant change.
• Monitor carefully for pulmonary toxicity, which can be fatal. Incidence increases in patients receiving more than 400 mg/day.
• Monitor for symptoms of pneumonitis — exertional dyspnea, nonproductive cough, and pleuritic chest

---

Common reactions are in italics; ***life-threatening,*** in bold italics.

pain. Monitor pulmonary function tests and chest X-ray.
• Monitor liver and thyroid function tests and serum electrolytes, particularly potassium and magnesium levels.
• Recommend instillation of methylcellulose ophthalmic solution during amiodarone therapy to minimize corneal microdeposits. Within 1 to 4 months after beginning amiodarone therapy, most patients show corneal microdeposits upon slit-lamp ophthalmic examination. However, only 2% to 3% have actual vision disturbances.
• Advise patients to use a sunscreen to prevent photosensitivity reaction. Monitor for burning or tingling skin followed by erythema and possible skin blistering.
• Be aware that amiodarone's adverse effects are more prevalent at high doses but are generally reversible when drug therapy is stopped. Resolution of adverse reactions may take up to 4 months.

atropine sulfate
Pregnancy Risk Category: C

HOW SUPPLIED
Tablets: 0.4 mg, 0.6 mg
Injection: 0.05 mg/ml, 0.1 mg/ml, 0.3 mg/ml, 0.4 mg/ml, 0.5 mg/ml, 0.6 mg/ml, 0.8 mg/ml, 1 mg/ml, 1.2 mg/ml

ACTION
An anticholinergic that inhibits acetylcholine at the parasympathetic neuroeffector junction, blocking vagal effects on the SA node; this enhances conduction through the AV node and speeds heart rate.

ONSET, PEAK, DURATION
Onset occurs within 30 minutes to 1 hour with oral administration, 30 minutes with I.M. administration, and immediately with I.V. administra-

tion. Serum levels peak within 2 hours after oral administration, within 1 to 1.6 hours after I.M. administration, and within 2 to 4 minutes after I.V. administration. Duration is about 4 hours.

INDICATIONS & DOSAGE
Symptomatic bradycardia, bradyarrhythmia (junctional or escape rhythm) –
Adults: usually 0.5 to 1 mg I.V. push; repeated q 3 to 5 minutes to maximum of 2 mg as needed. Lower doses (less than 0.5 mg) can cause bradycardia.
Children: 0.01 mg/kg I.V. up to maximum of 0.4 mg; or 0.3 mg/m^2; may repeat q 4 to 6 hours.
Antidote for anticholinesterase insecticide poisoning –
Adults: 2 to 3 mg I.V. repeated q 5 to 10 minutes until muscarinic symptoms disappear or signs of atropine toxicity appear. Severe poisoning may require up to 6 mg every hour.
Children: 1 mg I.V. or I.M., then 0.5 to 1 mg I.V. or I.M. q 5 to 10 minutes until muscarinic signs disappear or signs of atropine toxicity appear.
Preoperatively for diminishing secretions and blocking cardiac vagal reflexes –
Adults and children weighing 20 kg or more: 0.4 to 0.6 mg I.M. or S.C. 45 to 60 minutes before anesthesia.
Children weighing less than 20 kg: 0.01 mg/kg I.M. or S.C. up to maximum dose of 0.4 mg 45 to 60 minutes before anesthesia.
Adjunctive treatment of peptic ulcer disease; treatment of functional GI disorders such as irritable bowel syndrome –
Adults: 0.4 to 0.6 mg P.O. q 4 to 6 hours.
Children: 0.01 mg/kg or 0.3 mg/m^2 (not to exceed 0.4 mg) q 4 to 6 hours.

ADVERSE REACTIONS
CNS: *headache, restlessness,* ataxia, disorientation, hallucinations, delir-

ium, *coma, insomnia, dizziness;* excitement, agitation, and confusion (especially in elderly patients).
CV: 1 to 2 mg—*tachycardia, palpitations;* greater than 2 mg—***tachycardia, angina.***
EENT: 1 mg—*slight mydriasis,* photophobia; 2 mg—*blurred vision, mydriasis.*
GI: *dry mouth (common even at low doses),* thirst, *constipation,* nausea, vomiting.
GU: urine retention.
Hematologic: leukocytosis.
Skin: hot, flushed skin.

INTERACTIONS
Antacids: decreased absorption of anticholinergics. Separate administration times by at least 1 hour.
Anticholinergics or drugs with anticholinergic effects, such as amantadine, glutethimide, meperidine, antiarrhythmics, antiparkinsonian agents, phenothiazines, and tricyclic antidepressants: additive anticholinergic effects. Use together cautiously.
Ketoconazole, levodopa: decreased absorption. Avoid concomitant use.
Methotrimeprazine: may produce extrapyramidal symptoms. Monitor patient carefully.
Potassium chloride wax-matrix tablets: increased risk of mucosal lesions. Use cautiously.

CONTRAINDICATIONS
Contraindicated in patients with hypersensitivity to drug, acute angle-closure glaucoma, obstructive uropathy, obstructive disease of GI tract, paralytic ileus, toxic megacolon, intestinal atony, unstable CV status in acute hemorrhage, asthma, and myasthenia gravis.

NURSING CONSIDERATIONS
• Use cautiously in patients with Down syndrome because they may be more sensitive to the drug.
• **I.V. use:** Administer by direct I.V.

into a large vein or I.V. tubing over at least 1 to 2 minutes.
• Be aware that many of the adverse reactions (such as dry mouth and constipation) vary with the dose and should be expected. They are an extension of the drug's pharmacologic activity.
• Monitor patients for paradoxical initial bradycardia, especially those receiving small doses (0.4 to 0.6 mg). This is caused by a drug effect in the CNS and usually disappears within 2 minutes.
• Watch for tachycardia in cardiac patients because it may precipitate ventricular fibrillation.
• Monitor fluid intake and urine output. Drug causes urine retention and urinary hesitancy.
• Monitor closely for urine retention in elderly men with benign prostatic hyperplasia.
• Antidote for atropine overdose is physostigmine salicylate.

bretylium tosylate
Bretylate†‡, Bretylol, Critifib‡
Pregnancy Risk Category: C

HOW SUPPLIED
Injection: 50 mg/ml

ACTION
Unknown but considered a class III antiarrhythmic that initially exerts transient adrenergic stimulation through release of norepinephrine. Subsequent depletion of norepinephrine causes adrenergic blocking actions to predominate, prolonging repolarization and increasing duration of action potential and effective refractory period.

ONSET, PEAK, DURATION
Onset occurs within a few minutes but suppression of ventricular tachycardia and ventricular fibrillation may not occur for 20 minutes to 6 hours.

Serum levels peak within 6 to 9 hours. Effects may persist 6 to 24 hours.

INDICATIONS & DOSAGE
Ventricular fibrillation or hemodynamically unstable ventricular tachycardia unresponsive to other antiarrhythmics—
Adults: 5 mg/kg by I.V. push over 1 minute. If necessary, dose increased to 10 mg/kg and repeated q 15 to 30 minutes until 30 to 35 mg/kg have been given. For continuous suppression, diluted solution administered at 1 to 2 mg/minute continuously or 5 to 10 mg/kg diluted over more than 8 minutes q 6 hours.

ADVERSE REACTIONS
CNS: *vertigo, dizziness, light-headedness, syncope* (usually secondary to hypotension).
CV: *severe hypotension (especially orthostatic),* bradycardia, anginal pain, transient arrhythmias, transient hypertension.
GI: severe nausea, vomiting (with rapid infusion).
Other: muscle atrophy and tissue necrosis with repeated injections.

INTERACTIONS
All antihypertensives: may potentiate hypotension. Monitor blood pressure.
Other antiarrhythmics: additive or antagonistic antiarrhythmic effects. Monitor for additive toxicity.
Sympathomimetics: bretylium may potentiate effects of drugs given to correct hypotension.

CONTRAINDICATIONS
Contraindicated in digitalized patients unless the arrhythmia is life-threatening, not caused by digitalis, and unresponsive to other antiarrhythmics.

NURSING CONSIDERATIONS
• Use with extreme caution in patients with fixed cardiac output (aortic stenosis and pulmonary hypertension) to avoid severe and sudden drop in blood pressure.
• Bretylium is used with other cardiac life-support measures, such as cardiopulmonary resuscitation, countershock, epinephrine, sodium bicarbonate, and lidocaine.
• **I.V. use:** When used in maintenance therapy, dilute using dextrose or sodium chloride injection before administration. Follow manufacturer's guidelines for specific dilution guidelines (varies according to dosage). When administering as a direct I.V. injection, use a 20G to 22G needle and inject over 1 minute into a vein or I.V. line containing a free-flowing, compatible solution.
• To prevent nausea and vomiting in the patient, follow dosage directions carefully.
• Keep the patient in the supine position until tolerance to hypotension develops. Tell the patient to avoid sudden postural changes.
• Monitor the patient closely. The initial release of norepinephrine caused by bretylium may induce transient hypertension and arrhythmias.
• Monitor blood pressure and heart rate and rhythm continuously. Notify doctor immediately of any significant change. If supine systolic blood pressure falls below 75 mm Hg, the doctor may order norepinephrine, dopamine, or volume expanders to raise blood pressure.
• Observe for increased anginal pain in susceptible patients.

disopyramide
Rythmodan†

disopyramide phosphate
Napamide, Norpace, Norpace CR, Rythmodan LA†

Pregnancy Risk Category: C

HOW SUPPLIED
disopyramide
Capsules: 100 mg†, 150 mg†
disopyramide phosphate
Tablets (sustained-release): 250 mg†
Capsules: 100 mg, 150 mg
Capsules (controlled-release): 100 mg, 150 mg
Injection: 10 mg/ml‡

ACTION
Unknown but the the drug is considered a class Ia antiarrhythmic that depresses phase O and prolongs the action potential. All class I drugs have membrane-stabilizing effects.

ONSET, PEAK, DURATION
Onset occurs within ½ to 3 ½ hours after an oral dose. Plasma levels peak within 2 to 2½ hours after an oral dose. Effects persist for 1½ to 8½ hours after last dose.

INDICATIONS & DOSAGE
Symptomatic PVCs (unifocal, multifocal, or coupled); ventricular tachycardia not severe enough to require cardioversion –
Adults weighing more than 50 kg: 150 mg q 6 hours with conventional capsules or 300 mg q 12 hours with extended-release preparations.
Adults weighing 50 kg or less: highly individualized.
Children under 1 year: 10 to 30 mg/kg P.O. daily.
Children 1 to 4 years: 10 to 20 mg/kg P.O. daily.
Children 4 to 12 years: 10 to 15 mg/kg P.O. daily.
Children 12 to 18 years: 6 to 15 mg/kg P.O. daily.
    For pediatric dosages, divide into equal amounts and give q 6 hours.
    Recommended dosages in advanced renal insufficiency: if creatinine clearance is 30 to 40 ml/minute, 100 mg q 8 hours; if creatinine clearance is 15 to 30 ml/minute, 100 mg q 12 hours; if creatinine clearance is < 15 ml/minute, 100 mg q 24 hours.
    For parenteral use in adults: initially, 2 mg/kg I.V. slowly (over not less than 15 minutes). Administer until arrhythmia is eliminated or patient has received 150 mg. Repeat dosage if conversion is successful but arrhythmia returns. Total I.V. dosage should not exceed 300 mg in the first hour. Follow with an I.V. infusion of 0.4 mg/kg/hour (usually 20 to 30 mg/hour) to a maximum of 800 mg/day.

ADVERSE REACTIONS
CNS: dizziness, agitation, depression, fatigue, muscle weakness, syncope.
CV: *hypotension,* **CHF, heart block,** edema, weight gain, **arrhythmias.**
EENT: *blurred vision, dry eyes, dry nose.*
GI: nausea, vomiting, anorexia, bloating, abdominal pain, *constipation, dry mouth.*
GU: urine retention, urinary hesitancy.
Hepatic: cholestatic jaundice.
Skin: rash.
Other: hypoglycemia, aches, pain.

INTERACTIONS
Antiarrhythmics: possible additive or antagonized antiarrhythmic effects.
Phenytoin: increased metabolism of disopyramide. Monitor for decreased antiarrhythmic effect.
Rifampin: Disopyramide levels may be decreased.

CONTRAINDICATIONS
Contraindicated in patients with hypersensitivity to the drug, cardiogenic shock, or second- or third-degree heart block in the absence of an artificial pacemaker.

NURSING CONSIDERATIONS
• Use with extreme caution and avoid, if possible, in patients with CHF. Use cautiously in patients with

---

*Liquid form contains alcohol.   *Common* reactions are in italics; **life-threatening,** in bold italics.
**May contain tartrazine.

underlying conduction abnormalities, urinary tract diseases (especially prostatic hypertrophy), hepatic or renal impairment, myasthenia gravis, or acute angle-closure glaucoma.
• Correct any underlying electrolyte abnormalities before therapy begins, as ordered.
• Check apical pulse before administering drug. Notify the doctor if pulse rate is slower than 60 beats/minute or faster than 120 beats/minute.
• Know that release preparations should not be used for rapid control of ventricular arrhythmias; when therapeutic blood levels must be rapidly attained; in patients with cardiomyopathy or possible cardiac decompensation; or in those with severe renal impairment.
• For administration to young children, pharmacist may prepare disopyramide suspension from 100 mg capsules using cherry syrup. Suspension should be dispensed in amber glass bottles and protected from light.
• **I.V. use:** Add 200 mg to 200 to 500 ml of a compatible solution, such as 0.9% sodium chloride or D₅W. Do not mix with other drugs; switch to oral therapy as soon as possible.
• Watch for recurrence of arrhythmias and check for adverse reactions; notify the doctor if any occur.
• Discontinue drug if heart block develops, if QRS complex widens by more than 25%, or if QT interval lengthens by more than 25% above baseline; also notify physician.
• Manage constipation with proper diet or bulk laxatives.
• When transferring patients from immediate-release to sustained-release capsules, advise them to take a sustained-release capsule 6 hours after the last immediate-release capsule was taken.
• Teach the patient the importance of taking drug on time and exactly as prescribed. This may require use of an alarm clock for night doses.

• Advise the patient to chew gum or hard candy to relieve dry mouth.

esmolol hydrochloride
Brevibloc

Pregnancy Risk Category: C

HOW SUPPLIED
Injection: 10 mg/ml, 250 mg/ml

ACTION
A class II antiarrhythmic, esmolol is an ultrashort-acting selective beta₁-adrenergic blocker that decreases heart rate, myocardial contractility, and blood pressure.

ONSET, PEAK, DURATION
Onset occurs almost immediately. Peak serum levels vary with infusion rate, but typically occur in 30 minutes. Effects begin to subside 1 to 2 minutes after infusion ends, with complete reversal of effects within 30 minutes.

INDICATIONS & DOSAGE
Supraventricular tachycardia; to control ventricular rate in patients with atrial fibrillation or flutter in perioperative, postoperative, or other emergent circumstances; noncompensatory sinus tachycardia when heart rate requires specific interventions –
Adults: loading dose is 500 mcg/kg/minute by I.V. infusion over 1 minute, followed by 4-minute maintenance infusion of 50 mcg/kg/minute. If adequate response does not occur within 5 minutes, loading dose is repeated and followed by maintenance infusion of 100 mcg/kg/minute for 4 minutes. Loading dose is repeated and maintenance infusion is increased in a stepwise fashion as needed. Maximum maintenance infusion for tachycardia is 200 mcg/kg/minute.
Management of perioperative and postoperative tachycardia or hypertension –

Adults: for perioperative treatment of tachycardia or hypertension, 80 mg (approximately 1 mg/kg) I.V. bolus over 30 seconds followed by 150 mcg/kg/minute I.V. infusion, if needed. Adjust the infusion rate as needed up to a maximum of 300 mcg/kg/minute; for postoperative treatment of tachycardia and hypertension, same as for supraventricular tachycardia.

ADVERSE REACTIONS
CNS: dizziness, somnolence, headache, agitation, fatigue.
CV: *hypotension* (sometimes with diaphoresis).
GI: *nausea,* vomiting.
Respiratory: *bronchospasm.*
Other: inflammation and induration at infusion site.

INTERACTIONS
Digoxin: esmolol may increase serum digoxin levels by 10% to 20%. Monitor serum digoxin levels.
Morphine: may increase esmolol blood levels. Titrate esmolol carefully.
Reserpine (and other catecholamine-depleting drugs): may cause additive bradycardia and hypotension. Titrate esmolol carefully.
Succinylcholine: esmolol may prolong neuromuscular blockade.

CONTRAINDICATIONS
Contraindicated in patients with sinus bradycardia, heart block greater than first-degree, cardiogenic shock, or overt heart failure.

NURSING CONSIDERATIONS
• Use cautiously in patients with impaired renal function, diabetes, or bronchospasm.
• Know that esmolol has advantages over other beta blockers in treating arrhythmias because it has an extremely short duration of action and can be accurately titrated.
• **I.V. use:** Don't give esmolol by I.V.

push; use an infusion control device. The 10-mg/ml single-dose vials may be used without diluting, but the injection concentrate (250 mg/ml) must be diluted to a maximum concentration of 10 mg/ml before infusion. Remove 20 ml from 500 ml of D_5W, lactated Ringer's solution, or 0.45% or 0.9% sodium chloride solution and add two ampules of esmolol (final concentration 10 mg/ml).
• Remember that esmolol solutions are incompatible with diazepam, furosemide, sodium bicarbonate, and thiopental sodium.
• Monitor ECG and blood pressure continuously during infusion. Up to 50% of all patients treated with esmolol develop hypotension. Monitor closely, especially if patient's pretreatment blood pressure was low.
• Hypotension can usually be reversed within 30 minutes by decreasing the dose or, if necessary, by stopping the infusion. Notify doctor if this becomes necessary.
• If a local reaction develops at the infusion site, change to another site. Avoid using butterfly needles.
• Be aware that esmolol is recommended only for short-term use, for no longer than 48 hours.
• When the patient's heart rate becomes stable, esmolol will be replaced by alternative (longer-acting) antiarrhythmics, such as propranolol, digoxin, or verapamil. A half hour after the first dose of the alternative agent is administered, reduce infusion rate by 50%. Monitor patient response and if heart rate is controlled for 1 hour after administration of the second dose of the alternative drug, discontinue esmolol infusion.

---

flecainide acetate
Tambocor

Pregnancy Risk Category: C

HOW SUPPLIED
Tablets: 50 mg, 100 mg, 150 mg
Injection: 10 mg/ml‡

ACTION
A class Ic antiarrhythmic that decreases excitability, conduction velocity, and automaticity as a result of slowed atrial, atrioventricular (AV) node, His-Purkinje system, and intraventricular conduction and causes a slight but significant prolongation of refractory periods in these tissues.

ONSET, PEAK, DURATION
Onset immediate with I.V. administration, unknown with oral administration. Serum levels peak immediately after I.V. infusion, 2 to 3 hours after oral administration. Duration unknown.

INDICATIONS & DOSAGE
Paroxysmal supraventricular tachycardia, paroxysmal atrial fibrillation or flutter in patients without structural heart disease; life-threatening ventricular arrhythmias, such as sustained ventricular tachycardia –
Adults: for paroxysmal supraventricular tachycardia, 50 mg P.O. q 12 hours. Increased in increments of 50 mg b.i.d. q 4 days. Maximum dosage is 300 mg. In patients with renal impairment (creatinine clearance ≤ 35 ml/minute), initial dosage is 100 mg once daily or 50 mg b.i.d. For life-threatening ventricular arrhythmias, 100 mg P.O. q 12 hours. Increase in increments of 50 mg b.i.d. q 4 days until efficacy is achieved. Maximum dosage is 400 mg daily for most patients.

Initial dosage for patients with CHF is 50 mg P.O. q 12 hours.

Where available, flecainide may be given by I.V. injection‡ –
Adults: 2 mg/kg I.V. push over not less than 10 minutes; or dilute the dose and administer as an infusion.

ADVERSE REACTIONS
CNS: *dizziness, headache,* fatigue, tremor.
CV: *new or worsened arrhythmias,* chest pain, *CHF, cardiac arrest.*
EENT: *blurred vision and other visual disturbances.*
GI: nausea, constipation, abdominal pain.
Other: *dyspnea,* edema, skin rash.

INTERACTIONS
Amiodarone, cimetidine: altered pharmacokinetics. Monitor for toxicity.
Digitalis glycosides: flecainide may increase plasma digoxin levels by 15% to 25%. Monitor serum digoxin levels.
Propranolol, other beta blockers: both flecainide and propranolol plasma levels increase by 20% to 30%. Monitor for propranolol and flecainide toxicity.
Urine acidifying and alkalinizing agents: extremes of urine pH may substantially alter excretion of flecainide. Monitor for flecainide toxicity or decreased effectiveness.

CONTRAINDICATIONS
Contraindicated in patients with hypersensitivity to the drug; in those with preexisting second- or third-degree AV block or right bundle branch block when associated with a left hemiblock (in the absence of an artificial pacemaker); and in those with cardiogenic shock.

NURSING CONSIDERATIONS
● Use cautiously in patients with preexisting CHF, cardiomyopathy, severe renal or hepatic disease, prolonged QT interval, sick sinus syndrome, or blood dyscrasia.
● Know that when used to prevent ventricular arrhythmias, flecainide should be reserved for patients with documented life-threatening arrhythmias.

---

†Available in Canada only. ‡Available in Australia only. ◇Available OTC.

• Check that pacing threshold was determined 1 week before and after initiating therapy in patients with pacemakers because flecainide can alter endocardial pacing thresholds.

• Correct hypokalemia or hyperkalemia as ordered before giving flecainide because these electrolyte disturbances may alter the effect of flecainide.

• Know that most patients can be adequately maintained on an every-12-hour dosing schedule, but some need to receive flecainide every 8 hours.

• **I.V. use:** When administering by I.V. push, give over at least 10 minutes. For I.V. infusion, mix only with D_5W.

• Be aware that dosage adjustments should be made only once every 3 to 4 days.

• Be aware that twice-daily dosing for flecainide enhances patient compliance.

• Because of flecainide's long half-life, its full therapeutic effect may take 3 to 5 days. Administer concomitant I.V. lidocaine as ordered for the first several days.

• Monitor serum flecainide levels, especially in patients with renal failure or CHF. Therapeutic serum levels of flecainide range from 0.2 to 1 mcg/ml. Incidence of adverse effects increases when trough blood levels exceed 1 mcg/ml.

---

lidocaine hydrochloride (lignocaine hydrochloride)
Lido Pen Auto-Injector, Xylocaine, Xylocard†‡

Pregnancy Risk Category: B

HOW SUPPLIED
Injection (for I.M. use): 300 mg/3 ml automatic injection device
Injection (for direct I.V. use): 1% (10 mg/ml), 2% (20 mg/ml)
Injection (for I.V. admixtures): 4% (40 mg/ml), 10% (100 mg/ml), 20% (200 mg/ml)
Infusion (premixed): 0.2% (2 mg/ml), 0.4% (4 mg/ml), 0.8% (8 mg/ml)

ACTION
Lidocaine, a class 1B antiarrhythmic, decreases the depolarization, automaticity, and excitability in the ventricles during the diastolic phase by a direct action on the tissues, especially the Purkinje network, without involvement of the autonomic nervous system.

ONSET, PEAK, DURATION
Onset is immediate (45 to 90 seconds) with I.V. bolus administration, 5 to 15 minutes with I.M. administration. Without a bolus loading dose, peak serum levels occur within 30 to 60 minutes of starting an I.V. infusion. After an I.M. injection, plasma levels peak in about 10 minutes. Effects of I.V. bolus dose last for 10 to 20 minutes; effective blood levels persist for about 60 minutes after an I.M. injection.

INDICATIONS & DOSAGE
Ventricular arrhythmias resulting from MI, cardiac manipulation, or digitalis glycosides –
Adults: 50 to 100 mg (1 to 1.5 mg/kg) by I.V. bolus at 25 to 50 mg/minute. Half this amount is given to elderly patients or patients under 50 kg and to those with CHF or hepatic disease. Bolus dose is repeated q 3 to 5 minutes until arrhythmias subside or adverse reactions develop. Don't exceed 300-mg total bolus during a 1-hour period. Simultaneously, constant infusion of 20 to 50 mcg/kg/minute (1 to 4 mg/minute) is begun. If single bolus has been given, smaller bolus dose may be repeated 15 to 20 minutes after start of infusion to maintain therapeutic serum level. After 24 hours of continuous infusion, rate is

---

decreased by half. Alternatively, 200 to 300 mg I.M.; followed by second I.M. dose 60 to 90 minutes later, if needed.

Children: 1 mg/kg by I.V. bolus, followed by infusion of 30 mcg/kg/minute.

ADVERSE REACTIONS
CNS: *confusion, tremor,* lethargy, somnolence, *stupor, restlessness,* slurred speech, euphoria, depression, *light-headedness,* paresthesia, muscle twitching, *seizures.*
CV: *hypotension,* bradycardia, *new or worsened arrhythmias.*
EENT: *tinnitus, blurred or double vision.*
Other: *anaphylaxis,* soreness at injection site, sensation of cold, diaphoresis.

INTERACTIONS
Beta blockers, cimetidine: decreased metabolism of lidocaine. Monitor for toxicity.
Phenytoin, procainamide, propranolol, quinidine: additive cardiac depressant effects. Monitor carefully.

CONTRAINDICATIONS
Contraindicated in patients with hypersensitivity to the amide-type local anesthetics; Adams-Stokes syndrome; Wolff-Parkinson-White syndrome; and severe degrees of SA, AV, or intraventricular block in absence of artifical pacemaker.

NURSING CONSIDERATIONS
• Use cautiously in patients with complete or second-degree heart block or sinus bradycardia; in elderly patients; in those with CHF or renal or hepatic disease; and in those who weigh under 50 kg. Reduced dosage in these patients is required.
• **I.V. use:** Patients receiving infusions must be on a cardiac monitor and must be attended *at all times.* Use an infusion control device for administering infusion precisely. Do not exceed an infusion rate of 4 mg/minute; faster rate greatly increases risk of toxicity.
• Give I.M. injections in the deltoid muscle only.
• Remind physician to test isoenzymes if I.M. route is prescribed in a patient with suspected MI. This is necessary because a patient who has received I.M. lidocaine will show a seven-fold increase in serum CK level. Such an increase originates in the skeletal muscle, not the heart.
• Monitor therapeutic serum levels as ordered. Therapeutic serum levels are 2 to 5 mcg/ml.
• Monitor patient for toxicity. In many severely ill patients, seizures may be the first clinical sign of toxicity. However, severe reactions usually are preceded by somnolence, confusion, and paresthesia.
• If signs of toxicity (such as dizziness) occur, stop drug at once and notify the doctor. Continued infusion could lead to seizures and coma. Give oxygen via nasal cannula, if not contraindicated. Keep oxygen and cardiopulmonary resuscitation equipment available.
• Monitor the patient's response, especially blood pressure and serum electrolytes, BUN, and creatinine levels, as ordered. Notify the doctor promptly if abnormalities develop.
• Discontinue infusion and notify the doctor if arrhythmias worsen or ECG changes, such as widening QRS complex or substantially prolonged PR interval, are evident.

---

mexiletine hydrochloride
Mexitil
Pregnancy Risk Category: C

HOW SUPPLIED
Capsules: 50 mg‡, 100 mg†, 150 mg, 200 mg, 250 mg
Injection: 250 mg/10 ml‡

ACTION
A class Ib antiarrhythmic, mexiletine blocks the fast sodium channel in cardiac tissues, especially the Purkinje network, without involvement of the autonomic nervous system. Reduces the rate of rise and amplitude of the action potential and decreases automaticity in the Purkinje fibers. Shortens the duration of the action potential and, to a lesser extent, decreases the effective refractory period in the Purkinje fibers.

ONSET, PEAK, DURATION
Onset occurs in ½ to 2 hours with oral administration, immediate with I.V. administration. Serum levels peak within 2 to 3 hours after oral administration, immediate after I.V. administration. Duration unknown.

INDICATIONS & DOSAGE
Refractory life-threatening ventricular arrhythmias, including ventricular tachycardia and PVCs –
Adults: 200 to 400 mg P.O. followed by 200 mg q 8 hours. Dose increased every 2 to 3 days to 400 mg q 8 hours if satisfactory control is not obtained. Patients who respond well to an every-12-hour schedule may be given up to 450 mg q 12 hours.

Where available, mexiletine may be given I.V.‡ –
Adults: loading dose is 100 to 250 mg I.V. at a rate of 25 mg/minute. Then prepare an infusion solution of 250 mg mexiletine in 500 ml of D_5W and administer the first 120 ml (60 mg) over 1 hour. If clinical response is inadequate, give another bolus of 200 mg over 10 to 20 minutes. Maintenance dosage is 0.5 mg/minute (1 ml/minute of prepared solution).

ADVERSE REACTIONS
CNS: *tremor, dizziness,* blurred vision, ataxia, diplopia, confusion, nystagmus, nervousness, headache.
CV: hypotension, bradycardia, wid-

ened QRS complex, **new or worsened arrhythmias,** palpitations, chest pain.
GI: nausea, vomiting.
Skin: rash.

INTERACTIONS
Antacids, atropine, narcotics: slowed mexilitine absorption. Monitor patient.
Cimetidine: increased or decreased mexiletine blood levels. Monitor carefully.
Methylxanthines, such as caffeine or theophylline: reduced clearance of methylxanthines, possibly resulting in toxicity. Monitor carefully.
Metoclopramide: mexiletine absorption may be accelerated. Monitor for toxicity.
Phenobarbital, phenytoin, rifampin, urine acidifiers: decreased mexiletine blood levels. Monitor carefully.
Urine alkalinizers: increased mexiletine blood levels. Monitor carefully.

CONTRAINDICATIONS
Contraindicated in patients with cardiogenic shock or preexisting second- or third-degree AV block in the absence of an artifical pacemaker.

NURSING CONSIDERATIONS
• Use cautiously in patients with preexisting first-degree heart block, a ventricular pacemaker, preexisting sinus node dysfunction, intraventricular conduction disturbances, hypotension, severe CHF, or seizure disorder.
• When changing from lidocaine to mexiletine, stop the lidocaine infusion when the first mexiletine dose is given. Keep the infusion line open, however, until the arrhythmia appears to be satisfactorily controlled.
• **I.V. use:** Mexiletine injection is compatible with 0.9% sodium chloride, D_5W, 5% sodium bicarbonate, 1/6 M sodium lactate, and 10% fructose (levulose).
• To lessen GI distress, administer oral dose with meals or antacids.

---

*Liquid form contains alcohol.   *Common* reactions are in italics; **life-threatening,** in bold italics.
**May contain tartrazine.

• If you feel the patient is a good candidate for every-12-hour therapy, notify the doctor. Twice-daily dosage enhances compliance.
• Monitor therapeutic levels, as ordered. Therapeutic levels range from 0.75 to 2 mcg/ml.
• Monitor patient for toxicity. An early sign of mexiletine toxicity is tremor, usually a fine tremor of the hands. This progresses to dizziness and later to ataxia and nystagmus as the drug's blood level increases. Question patients about these symptoms.
• Monitor blood pressure and heart rate and rhythm frequently. Notify the doctor of any significant change.

---

moricizine hydrochloride
Ethmozine

Pregnancy Risk Category: B

HOW SUPPLIED
Tablets: 200 mg, 250 mg, 300 mg

ACTION
A class I antiarrhythmic that reduces the fast inward current carried by sodium ions across myocardial cell membranes. Has potent local anesthetic activity and membrane-stabilizing effect.

ONSET, PEAK, DURATION
Onset occurs within 2 hours. Serum levels peak within ½ to 2 hours; effects peak within 10 to 14 hours. Effects persist 10 to 24 hours after the last dose.

INDICATIONS & DOSAGE
Life-threatening ventricular arrhythmias –
Adults: individualized dosage is based on clinical response and patient tolerance. Therapy should begin in the hospital. Most patients respond to 600 to 900 mg P.O. daily in divided doses q 8 hours. Daily dosage increased q 3 days by 150 mg until the desired clinical effect is seen.
  In patients with hepatic or renal impairment, 600 mg or less P.O. daily.

ADVERSE REACTIONS
CNS: *dizziness, headache, fatigue,* anxiety, hypoesthesia, asthenia, nervousness, paresthesia, sleep disorders.
CV: ***proarrhythmic events (ventricular tachycardia, PVCs),*** *ECG abnormalities (including conduction defects, sinus pause, junctional rhythm, or AV block),* **CHF,** *palpitations,* **sustained ventricular tachycardia,** *chest pain, sinus bradycardia,* **sinus arrest.**
EENT: blurred vision.
GI: *nausea, vomiting, abdominal pain, dyspepsia, diarrhea, dry mouth.*
GU: urine retention, urinary frequency, dysuria.
Respiratory: dyspnea.
Skin: rash.
Other: drug-induced fever, diaphoresis, musculoskeletal pain.

INTERACTIONS
Cimetidine: increased plasma levels of and decreased clearance of moricizine. Begin moricizine therapy at low dosage (not more than 600 mg daily) and monitor plasma levels and therapeutic effect closely.
Digoxin, propranolol: additive prolongation of the PR interval. Monitor closely.
Theophylline: increased clearance and reduced plasma levels of theophylline. Monitor plasma levels and therapeutic response; adjust theophylline dosage as needed.

CONTRAINDICATIONS
Contraindicated in patients with hypersensitivity to the drug; preexisting second- or third-degree AV block or right bundle branch block when associated with left hemiblock (bifascicular block) unless an artificial pace-

---

maker is present; and cardiogenic shock.

NURSING CONSIDERATIONS
• Know that because drug has been detected in breast milk, a decision should be made to discontinue breast-feeding or discontinue the drug, depending on drug's potential benefit to the mother.
• Use with extreme caution in patients with sick sinus syndrome because drug may cause sinus bradycardia or sinus arrest in these patients. Also use with extreme caution in patients with coronary artery disease and left ventricular dysfunction because these patients may be at risk for sudden death when treated with the drug.
• Administer cautiously to patients with liver impairment.
• Patients with hepatic or renal dysfunction will have decreased moricizine clearance. Administer cautiously and monitor effects closely.
• Know that when substituting moricizine for another antiarrhythmic, previous drug should be withdrawn for one to two of the drug's half-lives before moricizine is started. Patients who have shown a tendency to develop life-threatening arrhythmias after withdrawal of drug therapy should be hospitalized during withdrawal and adjustment to moricizine. Guidelines doctors use for starting moricizine therapy are as follows:
— disopyramide, 6 to 12 hours after the last dose.
— mexiletine, 8 to 12 hours after the last dose.
— procainamide, 3 to 6 hours after the last dose.
— propafenone, 8 to 12 hours after the last dose.
— quinidine, 6 to 12 hours after the last dose.
— tocainide, 8 to 12 hours after the last dose.
• Determine electrolyte status and

correct imbalances before therapy as ordered. Hypokalemia, hyperkalemia, and hypomagnesemia may alter the effects of the drug.

---

procainamide hydrochloride
Procainamide Durules‡, Procan SR, Promine, Pronestyl**, Pronestyl-SR

Pregnancy Risk Category: C

HOW SUPPLIED
Tablets: 250 mg, 375 mg, 500 mg
Tablets (sustained-release): 250 mg, 500 mg, 750 mg, 1,000 mg
Capsules: 250 mg, 375 mg, 500 mg
Injection: 100 mg/ml, 500 mg/ml

ACTION
A class Ia antiarrhythmic that decreases excitability, conduction velocity, automaticity, and membrane responsiveness with prolonged refractory period. Larger than usual doses may induce AV block.

ONSET, PEAK, DURATION
Onset occurs immediately with I.V. injection, 10 to 30 minutes after I.M. injection, and 2 hours after oral dose. Peak serum levels occur immediately after I.V. infusion, 15 to 60 minutes after I.M. injection, and 1 to 1½ hours after oral dose. Duration unknown.

INDICATIONS & DOSAGE
Life-threatening ventricular arrhythmias —
Adults: 100 mg by slow I.V. push q 5 minutes, no faster than 25 to 50 mg/minute until arrhythmias disappear, adverse reactions develop, or 1 g has been given. Usual effective dose is 500 to 600 mg. When arrhythmias disappear, give continuous infusion of 2 to 6 mg/minute. If arrhythmias recur, repeat bolus as above and increase infusion rate. Alternatively,

---

0.5 to 1 g I.M. q 4 to 8 hours until oral therapy begins.

For oral therapy, 50 mg/kg daily q 3 hours; average is 250 to 500 mg q 3 hours.

In patients with renal or hepatic dysfunction, decreased dosages or longer dosing intervals may be needed.

ADVERSE REACTIONS
CNS: hallucinations, confusion, *seizures,* depression, dizziness.
CV: *severe hypotension,* bradycardia, AV block, *ventricular fibrillation* (after parenteral use).
GI: with high doses — nausea, vomiting, anorexia, diarrhea, bitter taste.
Hematologic: thrombocytopenia, *neutropenia* (especially with sustained-release forms), *agranulocytosis, hemolytic anemia, increased antinuclear antibody (ANA) titer.*
Skin: *maculopapular rash.*
Other: *fever, lupuslike syndrome* (especially after prolonged administration), *myalgia.*

INTERACTIONS
Amiodarone: increased procainamide levels and toxicity; additive effects on QT interval and QRS complex. Avoid concomitant use.
Anticholinergics: additive anticholinergic effects.
Anticholinesterase agents: anticholinesterase dosage may need to be increased.
Cimetidine: may increase procainamide blood levels. Monitor for toxicity.
Neuromuscular blockers: increased skeletal muscle relaxant effects. Monitor the patient closely.

CONTRAINDICATIONS
Contraindicated in patients with hypersensitivity to procaine and related drugs; in those with complete, second-, or third-degree heart block in the absence of an artificial pace-

maker; and in patients with myasthenia gravis or systemic lupus erythematosus. Also contraindicated in patients with atypical ventricular tachycardia (torsades de pointes) because procainamide may aggravate this condition.

NURSING CONSIDERATIONS
• Use with extreme caution when treating patients with ventricular tachycardia during coronary occlusion.
• Use cautiously in patients with CHF or other conduction disturbances, such as bundle-branch heart block, sinus bradycardia, or digitalis glycoside intoxication, or with hepatic or renal insufficiency. Also use cautiously in those with preexisting blood dyscrasias or bone marrow suppression.
• **I.V. use:** Patients receiving infusions must be attended *at all times.* Use an infusion control device to administer the infusion precisely.
• Note that the vials for I.V. injection contain 1 g of drug: 100 mg/ml (10 ml) or 500 mg/ml (2 ml).
• Keep patients in the supine position during I.V. administration. If drug is given too rapidly, hypotension can occur. Watch closely for adverse reactions during infusion and notify the doctor if they occur.
• If procainamide solution becomes discolored, check with pharmacy and prepare to discard.
• Monitor blood pressure and ECG continuously during I.V. administration. Watch for prolonged QT intervals and QRS complexes, heart block, or increased arrhythmias. If these occur, withhold drug, obtain rhythm strip, and notify the doctor immediately.
• Monitor plasma levels of procainamide and its active metabolite NAPA. To suppress ventricular arrhythmias, therapeutic serum concentrations of procainamide are 4 to 8

mcg/ml; therapeutic levels of NAPA are 10 to 30 mcg/ml.
- Monitor QT interval closely in patients with renal failure.
- Hypokalemia predisposes patients to arrhythmias; therefore, monitor serum electrolytes, especially potassium level.
- Elderly patients may be more likely to develop hypotension. Monitor blood pressure carefully.
- Monitor CBC frequently during first 3 months of therapy, particularly in patients taking sustained-release dosage forms.
- Be aware that positive ANA titer is common in about 60% of patients who don't have symptoms of lupuslike syndrome. This response seems to be related to prolonged use, not dosage. May progress to systemic lupus erythematosus if drug is not discontinued.
- Instruct patients to report fever, rash, muscle pain, diarrhea, bleeding, bruises, or pleuritic chest pain.
- Stress to patients the importance of taking the drug exactly as prescribed. This may require use of an alarm clock for nighttime doses.
- Reassure patients who are taking the extended-release form of procainamide that a wax-matrix "ghost" from the tablet may be passed in the stool. The drug is completely absorbed before this occurs.

---

propafenone hydrochloride
Rythmol

Pregnancy Risk Category: C

HOW SUPPLIED
Tablets: 150 mg, 300 mg

ACTION
A class Ic antiarrhythmic, propafenone reduces the inward sodium current in Purkinje and myocardial cells. Decreases excitability, conduction velocity, and automaticity in AV nodal,
His-Purkinje, and intraventricular tissue; causes a slight but significant prolongation of refractory period in AV nodal tissue.

ONSET, PEAK, DURATION
Onset and duration unknown. Plasma levels peak within 3½ hours.

INDICATIONS & DOSAGE
Suppression of life-threatening ventricular arrhythmias, such as sustained ventricular tachycardia –
Adults: initially, 150 mg P.O. q 8 hours. Dosage may be increased at 3- to 4-day intervals to 225 mg q 8 hours, if necessary, increase dosage to 300 mg q 8 hours. Maximum daily dosage is 900 mg.

ADVERSE REACTIONS
CNS: anorexia, anxiety, ataxia, dizziness, drowsiness, fatigue, headache, insomnia, syncope, tremor, weakness.
CV: atrial fibrillation, bradycardia, bundle branch block, *CHF,* chest pain, edema, first-degree AV block, hypotension, increased QRS duration, intraventricular conduction delay, palpitations, *proarrhythmic events (ventricular tachycardia, PVCs).*
EENT: blurred vision.
GI: abdominal pain or cramps, constipation, diarrhea, dyspepsia, flatulence, nausea, vomiting, dry mouth, unusual taste.
Respiratory: dyspnea.
Skin: rash.
Other: diaphoresis, joint pain.

INTERACTIONS
Antiarrhythmics: increased risk of CHF.
Cimetidine: decreased metabolism of propafenone.
Digitalis glycosides, oral anticoagulants: propafenone may increase serum levels of these agents by about 35% to 85%, resulting in toxicity.
Local anesthetics: increased risk of CNS toxicity.

---

*Liquid form contains alcohol.   *Common* reactions are in italics; *life-threatening,* in bold italics.
**May contain tartrazine.

Metoprolol, propranolol: propafenone slows the metabolism of these agents. Adjust dosage as necessary and as ordered.
Quinidine: slowed metabolism of propafenone. Avoid concomitant use.
Rifampin: increased clearance of propafenone. Monitor closely.

CONTRAINDICATIONS
Contraindicated in patients with hypersensitivity to the drug and in those with severe or uncontrolled CHF; cardiogenic shock; SA, AV, or intraventricular disorders of impulse conduction in the absence of a pacemaker; bradycardia; marked hypotension; bronchospastic disorders; and electrolyte imbalance.

NURSING CONSIDERATIONS
• Use cautiously in patients with CHF because propafenone can exert a negative inotropic effect on the heart. Also use cautiously in patients taking other cardiac depressant drugs and in those with hepatic or renal failure.
• To minimize adverse GI reactions, administer drug with food.
• Continuous cardiac monitoring is recommended during initiation of therapy and during dosage adjustments. If PR interval or QRS complex increases by more than 25%, a reduction in dosage may be necessary.
• During concomitant use with digoxin, frequently monitor ECG and serum digoxin levels.

---

quinidine bisulfate
(66.4% quinidine base)
Biquin Durules†, Kinidin Durules‡

quinidine gluconate
(62% quinidine base)
Quinaglute Dura-Tabs, Quinalan, Quinate†

quinidine polygalacturonate
(60.5% quinidine base)
Cardioquin

quinidine sulfate
(83% quinidine base)
Apo-Quinidine†, Cin-Quin, Novoquindin†, Quine, Quinidex Extentabs, Quinora

Pregnancy Risk Category: C

HOW SUPPLIED
quinidine bisulfate
Tablets (extended-release): 250 mg†‡
quinidine gluconate
Tablets (extended-release): 324 mg, 325 mg†, 330 mg
Injection: 80 mg/ml
quinidine polygalacturonate
Tablets: 275 mg
quinidine sulfate
Tablets: 200 mg, 300 mg
Tablets (extended-release): 300 mg
Capsules: 200 mg, 300 mg
Injection: 200 mg/ml

ACTION
A class Ia antiarrhythmic, quinidine has both direct and indirect (anticholinergic) effects on cardiac tissue. Automaticity, conduction velocity, and membrane responsiveness are decreased. The effective refractory period is prolonged. The anticholinergic action reduces vagal tone.

ONSET, PEAK, DURATION
Onset is immediate with I.V. administration and 1 to 3 hours after oral administration. Peak plasma levels occur immediately after I.V. injection, within 1 to 2 hours after oral dose. Effects persist 6 to 8 hours after oral dose.

INDICATIONS & DOSAGE
Atrial flutter or fibrillation –
Adults: 200 mg quinidine sulfate or equivalent base P.O. q 2 to 3 hours for five to eight doses, with subsequent

---

daily increases until sinus rhythm is restored or toxic effects develop. Quinidine is administered only after digitalization to avoid increasing AV conduction. Maximum dosage is 3 to 4 g daily.

Paroxysmal supraventricular tachycardia –
Adults: 400 to 600 mg I.M. or P.O. gluconate q 2 to 3 hours until toxic adverse reactions develop or arrhythmia subsides.

Premature atrial and ventricular contractions; paroxysmal AV junctional rhythm; paroxysmal atrial tachycardia; paroxysmal ventricular tachycardia; maintenance after cardioversion of atrial fibrillation or flutter –
Adults: test dose is 200 mg P.O. or I.M. Quinidine sulfate or equivalent base 200 to 400 mg P.O. q 4 to 6 hours; or initially, quinidine gluconate 600 mg I.M., then up to 400 mg q 2 hours, p.r.n.; or quinidine gluconate 800 mg (10 ml of the commercially available solution) added to 40 ml of D_5W, infused I.V. at 16 mg (1 ml)/minute.
Children: test dose is 2 mg/kg; 3 to 6 mg/kg q 2 to 3 hours for five doses P.O. daily.

Severe Plasmodium falciparum *malaria –*
Adults: 10 mg/kg gluconate I.V. diluted in 250 ml of 0.9% sodium chloride and infused over 1 to 2 hours, followed by a continuous maintenance infusion of 0.02 mg/kg/minute for 72 hours or until parasitemia is reduced to less than 1%.

Patients with impaired hepatic function and those with CHF require a reduced dosage.

ADVERSE REACTIONS
CNS: *vertigo, headache, light-headedness,* confusion, restlessness, cold sweats, pallor, fainting, dementia.
CV: *PVCs; ventricular tachycardia; atypical ventricular tachycardia (torsades de pointes); severe hypoten-*
sion; SA and AV block; ventricular fibrillation, *tachycardia; aggravated CHF; ECG changes (particularly widening of QRS complex, notched P waves, widened QT interval, ST-segment depression).*
EENT: *tinnitus,* excessive salivation, blurred vision.
GI: *diarrhea, nausea, vomiting,* anorexia, abdominal pain.
Hematologic: *hemolytic anemia, thrombocytopenia, agranulocytosis.*
Hepatic: *hepatotoxicity.*
Respiratory: acute asthmatic attack, *respiratory arrest.*
Skin: rash, petechial hemorrhage of buccal mucosa, pruritus.
Other: angioedema, *fever, cinchonism.*

INTERACTIONS
Acetazolamide, antacids, sodium bicarbonate, thiazide diuretics: may increase quinidine blood levels because of alkaline urine. Monitor for increased effect.
Amiodarone, cimetidine: increased serum quinidine levels. Monitor for increased effect.
Barbiturates, phenytoin, rifampin: may lower blood levels of quinidine. Monitor for decreased quinidine effect.
Digoxin: increased serum digoxin levels after initiating quinidine therapy. Monitor closely.
Nifedipine: may decrease quinidine blood levels. Monitor carefully.
Other antiarrhythmics, such as lidocaine, phenytoin, procainamide, and propranolol: increased risk of toxicity. Use together cautiously.
Verapamil: may result in hypotension, bradycardia, or AV block. Monitor blood pressure and heart rate.
Warfarin: increased anticoagulant effect. Monitor closely.

CONTRAINDICATIONS
Contraindicated in patients with idiosyncrasy or hypersensitivity to quini-

---

*Liquid form contains alcohol.
**May contain tartrazine.
Common reactions are in italics; **life-threatening,** in bold italics.

dine or related cinchona derivatives, intraventricular conduction defects, digitalis toxicity when AV conduction is grossly impaired, and abnormal rhythms due to escape mechanisms.

NURSING CONSIDERATIONS
• Use cautiously in patients with asthma, muscle weakness, or infection accompanied by fever because hypersensitivity reactions to the drug may be masked.
• Also use cautiously in patients with hepatic or renal impairment because systemic accumulation of quinidine may occur.
• Check apical pulse rate and blood pressure before starting therapy. If you detect extremes in pulse rate, withhold drug and notify the doctor at once.
• Know that anticoagulant therapy is commonly advised before quinidine therapy in long-standing atrial fibrillation because restoration of normal sinus rhythm may result in thromboembolism caused by dislodgment of thrombi from atrial wall.
• When changing route of administration, be aware that dosage needs to be altered to compensate for variations in quinidine base content.
• Never use discolored (brownish) quinidine solution.
• Do not crush sustained-release tablets.
• When used to treat severe malaria, patients should be hospitalized in an intensive-care setting. Continuous monitoring is necessary. Decrease infusion rate if plasma quinidine level exceeds 6 mcg/ml, uncorrected QT interval exceeds 0.6 second, or QRS complex widening exceeds 25% of baseline.
• Monitor liver function tests during the first 4 to 8 weeks of therapy.
• Monitor serum quinidine levels as ordered. Therapeutic plasma levels for antiarrhythmic effects are 2 to 5 mcg/ml.

• Monitor patient response carefully. Adverse GI reactions, especially diarrhea, are signs of toxicity. Notify the doctor. Check quinidine blood levels, which are toxic when greater than 8 mcg/ml. GI symptoms may be decreased by giving drug with meals.
• Store drug away from heat and direct light.

---

sotalol
Betapace, Sotacor†‡
Pregnancy Risk Category: B

HOW SUPPLIED
Tablets: 80 mg, 160 mg, 240 mg

ACTION
A nonselective beta-adrenergic blocker that depresses sinus heart rate, slows AV conduction, decreases cardiac output, and lowers systolic and diastolic blood pressure.

ONSET, PEAK, DURATION
Onset and duration not clearly defined. Peak plasma levels occur within 2½ to 4 hours.

INDICATIONS & DOSAGE
Documented, life-threatening ventricular arrhythmias –
Adults: initially, 80 mg P.O. b.i.d. Dosage is increased q 2 to 3 days as needed and tolerated; most patients respond to daily dosage of 160 to 320 mg. A few patients with refractory arrhythmias have received as much as 640 mg daily.
   In patients with renal failure: If creatinine clearance is greater than 60 ml/minute, no adjustment in dosage interval is necessary. If creatinine clearance is 30 to 60 ml/minute, dosage interval is increased to q 24 hours; 10 to 30 ml/minute, q 36 to 48 hours; less than 10 ml/minute, individualized dosage.
Hypertension† –
Adults: 80 mg P.O. b.i.d. Dosage is

increased at weekly intervals in 80-mg increments b.i.d. as needed and tolerated. Most patients respond to daily dosage of 160 to 320 mg; patients taking 320 mg or less daily may take drug as a single morning dose.

Angina†–

Adults: 80 mg P.O. b.i.d. Dosage increased at weekly intervals in 80-mg increments b.i.d. as needed and tolerated. Most patients respond to doses of 160 mg b.i.d.; maximum daily dosage is 480 mg.

ADVERSE REACTIONS

CNS: *asthenia, headache, dizziness, weakness, fatigue.*

CV: *bradycardia, **arrhythmias, CHF, AV block, proarrhythmic events (ventricular tachycardia, PVCs).***

GI: *nausea.*

Respiratory: *dyspnea, **bronchospasm.***

INTERACTIONS

Antiarrhythmics: additive effects. Avoid concomitant use.

Antihypertensives, catecholamine-depleting drugs (such as reserpine and guanethidine): enhanced hypotensive effects. Monitor closely.

Calcium channel blockers: enhanced myocardial depression. Avoid concomitant use.

Clonidine: beta blockers may enhance the rebound effect seen after withdrawal of clonidine. Discontinue sotalol several days before withdrawing clonidine.

General anesthetics: may cause additional myocardial depression. Monitor closely.

CONTRAINDICATIONS

Contraindicated in patients with hypersensitivity to the drug, severe sinus node dysfunction, sinus bradycardia, second- and third-degree AV block in the absence of an artificial pacemaker, congenital or acquired long QT syndrome, cardiogenic shock, uncontrolled CHF, and bronchial asthma.

NURSING CONSIDERATIONS

• Use cautiously in patients with renal impairment.

• Also use cautiously in patients with diabetes mellitus. Beta blockers may mask signs and symptoms of hypoglycemia.

• Because proarrhythmic events may occur at start of therapy and during dosage adjustments, patient should be hospitalized. Facilities and personnel should be available for cardiac rhythm monitoring and interpretation of ECG.

• Note that although patients receiving I.V. lidocaine have started sotalol therapy without ill effect, other antiarrhythmic drugs should be withdrawn before therapy with sotalol. Sotalol therapy typically is delayed until two or three half-lives of the withdrawn drug have elapsed. After withdrawal of amiodarone, sotalol shouldn't be administered until the QT interval normalizes.

• Be aware that dosage should be adjusted slowly, allowing 2 to 3 days between dosage increments for adequate monitoring of QT intervals and for plasma levels of drug to reach a steady-state level.

• Monitor serum electrolytes regularly, especially if patient is receiving diuretics. Electrolyte imbalances, such as hypokalemia or hypomagnesemia, may enhance QT-interval prolongation and increase the risk of serious arrhythmias, such as torsades de pointes.

• Explain to patients the importance of taking this drug as prescribed, even when they are feeling well. Caution patients not to discontinue drug suddenly.

• Because food can interfere with absorption, tell patients to take this drug on an empty stomach, 1 hour before or 2 hours after meals.

---

tocainide hydrochloride
Tonocard

Pregnancy Risk Category: C

HOW SUPPLIED
Tablets: 400 mg, 600 mg

ACTION
A class Ib antiarrhythmic, tocainide blocks the fast sodium channel in cardiac tissues, especially the Purkinje network, without involvement of the autonomic nervous system. It reduces the rate of rise and amplitude of the action potential and decreases automaticity in the Purkinje fibers. It shortens the duration of action potential and, to a lesser extent, decreases the effective refractory period in the Purkinje fibers.

ONSET, PEAK, DURATION
Onset unknown. Plasma levels peak ½ to 2 hours after an oral dose. Duration is 8 hours.

INDICATIONS & DOSAGE
Suppression of symptomatic life-threatening ventricular arrhythmias, such as sustained ventricular tachycardia –
Adults: initially, 400 mg P.O. q 8 hours. Usual dosage is between 1,200 and 1,800 mg daily in three divided doses.

ADVERSE REACTIONS
CNS: *light-headedness, tremor,* restlessness, paresthesia, confusion, dizziness.
CV: hypotension, *new or worsened arrhythmias, CHF.*
EENT: blurred vision.
GI: *nausea, vomiting, epigastric pain,* constipation, diarrhea, anorexia.
Hematologic: *blood dyscrasia, including aplastic anemia.*
Hepatic: hepatitis.
Respiratory: *respiratory arrest, pulmonary fibrosis, pneumonitis, pulmonary edema.*

Skin: rash.

INTERACTIONS
Beta blockers: decreased myocardial contractility; increased CNS toxicity.

CONTRAINDICATIONS
Contraindicated in patients with hypersensitivity to lidocaine or other amide-type local anesthetics and in those with second- or third-degree AV block in the absence of an artificial pacemaker.

NURSING CONSIDERATIONS
• Use cautiously in patients with CHF or diminished cardiac reserve and in those with hepatic or renal impairment. These patients often may be treated effectively with a lower dose.
• Be aware that drug is considered by cardiologists as "oral lidocaine." May ease transition from I.V. lidocaine to oral antiarrhythmic therapy. Monitor the patient carefully during this transition period.
• Monitor the patient for tremor, which may indicate that the maximum dosage has been reached.
• Monitor therapeutic blood levels as ordered. Therapeutic blood levels range from 4 to 10 mcg/ml. Report deviations.
• Tell the patient to report immediately any unusual bruising or bleeding, or signs of infection. Agranulocytosis and bone marrow suppression have been reported in patients taking usual doses of the drug. Most cases have been reported within the first 12 weeks of therapy.
• Tell the patient to report sudden onset of any pulmonary symptoms, such as coughing, wheezing, or exertional dyspnea. Drug has been associated with serious pulmonary toxicity.
• Note that dizziness and falling are more likely to occur in elderly patients. Take safety precautions.

---

†Available in Canada only.　　　‡Available in Australia only.　　　◊Available OTC.

22

Antianginals

amlodipine besylate
amyl nitrate
bepridil hydrochloride
diltiazem hydrochloride
erythrityl tetranitrate
isosorbide dinitrate
isosorbide mononitrate
nadolol
nicardipine
nifedipine
nitroglycerin
pentaerythritol tetranitrate
propranolol hydrochloride
verapamil
verapamil hydrochloride

COMBINATION PRODUCTS

ANGIJEN NO. 1: pentaerythritol tetranitrate 20 mg and phenobarbital sodium 15 mg.
ARCOTRATE NO. 3: pentaerythritol tetranitrate 20 mg and phenobarbital sodium 8 mg.
BITRATE: pentaerythritol tetranitrate 15 mg and phenobarbital sodium 20 mg.
DIMYCOR: pentaerythritol tetranitrate 10 mg and phenobarbital sodium 15 mg.
NITROTYM-PLUS: nitroglycerin 2.5 mg and butabarbital sodium 48 mg.
PERBUZEM: pentaerythritol tetranitrate 10 mg and butabarbital sodium 15 mg.

---

amlodipine besylate
Norvasc

Pregnancy Risk Category: C

HOW SUPPLIED
Tablets: 2.5 mg, 5 mg, 10 mg

ACTION
Inhibits calcium ion influx across cardiac and smooth-muscle cells, thus decreasing myocardial contractility and oxygen demand. Also dilates coronary arteries and arterioles.

ONSET, PEAK, DURATION
Onset unknown. Serum levels peak in 6 to 9 hours. Effects persist for 24 hours.

INDICATIONS & DOSAGE
Chronic stable angina; vasospastic angina (Prinzmetal's [variant] angina) –
Adults: initially, 10 mg P.O. daily. Small, frail, or elderly patients or patients with hepatic insufficiency should begin therapy at 5 mg daily. Most patients require 10 mg daily for adequate therapy.
Hypertension –
Adults: initially, 5 mg P.O. daily. Small, frail, or elderly patients; patients currently receiving other antihypertensives; or patients with hepatic insufficiency should begin therapy at 2.5 mg daily. Dosage adjusted according to patient response and tolerance. Maximum daily dosage is 10 mg.

ADVERSE REACTIONS
CNS: *headache,* fatigue, somnolence.
CV: *edema,* dizziness, flushing, palpitation.
GI: nausea, abdominal pain.

INTERACTIONS
None known.

CONTRAINDICATIONS
Contraindicated in patients with hypersensitivity to the drug.

NURSING CONSIDERATIONS
• Use cautiously in patients receiving other peripheral vasodilators, especially those with severe aortic steno-

---

*Liquid form contains alcohol.
**May contain tartrazine.

Common reactions are in italics; **life-threatening,** in bold italics.

sis, and in those with CHF. Because drug is metabolized by the liver, also use cautiously and in reduced dosage in patients with severe hepatic disease.
• Sublingual nitroglycerin may be taken as needed when anginal symptoms are acute. If the patient continues nitrate therapy during titration of amlodipine dosage, urge continued compliance.
• Monitor the patient carefully. Some patients, especially those with severe obstructive coronary artery disease, have developed increased frequency, duration, or severity of angina or even acute MI after initiation of calcium channel blocker therapy or at time of dosage increase.
• Monitor blood pressure frequently during initiation of therapy. Because drug-induced vasodilation has a gradual onset, acute hypotension is rare.
• Notify the doctor if signs of CHF occur, such as swelling of hands and feet or shortness of breath.
• Caution patients to continue taking the drug, even when they are feeling better.

amyl nitrite
Pregnancy Risk Category: X

HOW SUPPLIED
Ampules (crushable): 0.18 ml, 0.3 ml

ACTION
Antianginal action unknown. Thought to be the result of a reduction in systemic and pulmonary arterial pressure (afterload) and decreased cardiac output becaue of peripheral vasodilation, rather than coronary artery dilation. Converts hemoglobin to methemoglobin (which binds cyanide) to treat cyanide poisoning.

ONSET, PEAK, DURATION
Onset occurs within 30 seconds. Peak unknown. Effects persist 3 to 5 minutes.

INDICATIONS & DOSAGE
Relief of angina pectoris –
Adults and children: 0.18 to 0.3 ml by inhalation (one glass ampule) p.r.n.
Antidote for cyanide poisoning –
0.3 ml by inhalation for 30 to 60 seconds q 5 minutes until conscious.

ADVERSE REACTIONS
CNS: *headache, sometimes with throbbing;* dizziness; weakness.
CV: *orthostatic hypotension, tachycardia,* flushing, palpitations, fainting.
GI: nausea, vomiting.
Hematologic: methemoglobinemia.
Skin: cutaneous vasodilation.
Other: hypersensitivity reactions.

INTERACTIONS
None significant.

CONTRAINDICATIONS
Contraindicated in patients with hypersensitivity to nitrites, severe anemia, angle-closure glaucoma, postural hypotension, increased intracranial pressure and in pregnant patients.

NURSING CONSIDERATIONS
• Use cautiously in patients with glaucoma (except angle-closure type which is a contraindication), volume depletion, or hypotension.
• Extinguish all cigarettes before use, or ampule may ignite.
• Wrap ampule in cloth and crush. Hold near the patient's nose and mouth so vapor is inhaled.
• Watch for orthostatic hypotension. Have the patient sit down and avoid rapid position changes while inhaling drug.
• Advise the patient that keeping the head low, deep breathing, and move-

ment of extremities may help relieve dizziness, syncope, or weakness from orthostatic hypotension.
• Store away from light.
• Be aware that drug is often abused. Claimed to have aphrodisiac benefits. Street name is "Amy."

bepridil hydrochloride
Bepadin‡, Vascor

Pregnancy Risk Category: C

HOW SUPPLIED
Tablets: 200 mg, 300 mg, 400 mg

ACTION
A calcium channel blocker that inhibits calcium ion influx across cardiac and smooth-muscle cells. This action dilates coronary arteries as well as peripheral arteries and arterioles; it may reduce heart rate, decrease myocardial contractility, and slow AV node conduction.

ONSET, PEAK, DURATION
Onset unknown. Plasma levels peak within 2 to 3 hours. Effects persist for 24 hours.

INDICATIONS & DOSAGE
Chronic stable angina in patients who cannot tolerate or who fail to respond to other agents –
Adults: initially, 200 mg P.O. daily. After 10 days, dosage increased based on response. Maintenance dosage in most patients is 300 mg/day. Maximum daily dosage is 400 mg.

ADVERSE REACTIONS
CNS: dizziness.
CV: edema, flushing, palpitations, tachycardia, *ventricular arrhythmias, including torsades de pointes, ventricular tachycardia, ventricular fibrillation.*
GI: nausea, diarrhea.
Hematologic: *agranulocytosis.*
Skin: rash.

Other: dyspnea.

INTERACTIONS
Fentanyl anesthesia: severe hypotension has been reported with concomitant use of a beta blocker and a calcium channel blocker. Inform anesthesiologist that the patient is taking a calcium channel blocker.

CONTRAINDICATIONS
Contraindicated in patients with hypersensitivity to the drug; uncompensated cardiac insufficiency, sick sinus syndrome or second- or third-degree AV block unless pacemaker is present; hypotension (< 90 mm Hg systolic); congenital QT interval prolongation; or history of serious ventricular arrhythmias. Also contraindicated in those receiving other drugs that prolong the QT interval.

NURSING CONSIDERATIONS
• Use cautiously in patients with left bundle branch block, sinus bradycardia (less than 50 beats/minute), impaired renal or hepatic function, or CHF.
• Monitor patient for adverse reactions. Bepridil is not considered a primary agent because it has been associated with severe ventricular arrhythmias, including torsades de pointes; also associated with agranulocytosis.
• Note that elderly patients may require more frequent monitoring to prevent adverse reactions.
• Tell patients to promptly report any unusual bruising or bleeding or signs of persistent infections, including sore throat, fever, or malaise.

diltiazem hydrochloride
Cardizem, Cardizem CD, Cardizem SR, Dilacor XR, Vasocardol SR‡

Pregnancy Risk Category: C

---

*Liquid form contains alcohol.   *Common* reactions are in italics; *life-threatening,* in bold italics.
**May contain tartrazine.

HOW SUPPLIED
Tablets: 30 mg, 60 mg, 90 mg, 120 mg
Capsules (extended-release; Cardizem CD): 120 mg, 180 mg, 240 mg, 300 mg
Capsules (sustained-release; Cardizem SR, Dilacor XR, Vasocardol SR‡): 60 mg, 90 mg, 120 mg, 180 mg, 240 mg
Injection: 5 mg/ml

ACTION
A calcium channel blocker that inhibits calcium ion influx across cardiac and smooth-muscle cells, decreasing myocardial contractility and oxygen demand. Also dilates coronary arteries and arterioles.

ONSET, PEAK, DURATION
Onset is about 3 minutes after I.V. bolus injection, 30 to 60 minutes after oral administration of regular tablets, 2 to 3 hours after extended- or sustained-release preparations. Peak plasma levels occur immediately after I.V. injection, 2 to 3 hours after regular tablet, 6 to 11 hours after sustained-release capsule, or 10 to 14 hours after extended-release capsule. Effects persist 1 to 3 hours after I.V. bolus, up to 10 hours after I.V. infusion, 6 to 8 hours after regular tablet, about 12 hours after sustained-release capsule, about 24 hours after extended-release capsule.

INDICATIONS & DOSAGE
Vasospastic angina (Prinzmetal's [variant] angina) and classic chronic stable angina pectoris –
Adults: 30 mg P.O. t.i.d. or q.i.d. before meals and h.s. Dosage increased gradually to maximum of 360 mg/day in divided doses. Alternatively, 120 or 180 mg (dual-release capsule). Titrated as needed and tolerated to a maximum of 480 mg daily.
Hypertension –
Adults: 60 to 120 mg P.O. b.i.d. (sustained-release capsule). Titrated to effect. Maximum recommended dosage is 360 mg/day. Alternatively, 180 to 240 mg daily (extended-release capsule) initially. Dosage adjusted as necessary.
Atrial fibrillation or flutter; paroxysmal supraventricular tachycardia –
Adults: 0.25 mg/kg as an I.V. bolus injection over 2 minutes. If response is inadequate, 0.35 mg/kg I.V. after 15 minutes and followed with a continuous infusion of 10 mg/hour. Some patients respond well to infusion rates of 5 mg/hour; the maximum dose is 15 mg/hour.

ADVERSE REACTIONS
CNS: *headache, fatigue, drowsiness,* dizziness, nervousness, depression, insomnia, confusion.
CV: *edema, arrhythmias,* flushing, bradycardia, hypotension, conduction abnormalities, *CHF.*
GI: *nausea, constipation,* vomiting, diarrhea.
GU: nocturia, polyuria.
Hepatic: transient elevation of liver enzymes.
Skin: *rash,* pruritus, photosensitivity.

INTERACTIONS
Cimetidine: may inhibit diltiazem metabolism. Monitor for toxicity.
Cyclosporine: diltiazem may increase serum cyclosporine levels, possibly by decreasing its metabolism, leading to increased risk of cyclosporine toxicity. Avoid concomitant use.
Digoxin: diltiazem may increase serum levels of digoxin. Monitor for toxicity.
Furosemide: forms a precipitate when mixed with diltiazem injection. Administer through separate I.V. lines.
Propranolol, other beta blockers: may precipitate CHF or prolong cardiac conduction time. Use together cautiously.

CONTRAINDICATIONS

Contraindicated in patients with sick sinus syndrome or second- or third-degree AV block in the absence of an artificial pacemaker, hypotension (systolic blood pressure below 90 mm Hg), hypersensitivity to the drug, acute MI, and pulmonary congestion (documented by X-ray).

NURSING CONSIDERATIONS

• Use cautiously in elderly patients because duration of action may be prolonged; in patients with CHF; and in those with impaired hepatic or renal function.
• **I.V. use:** Infusions lasting longer than 24 hours are not recommended.
• Monitor blood pressure during initiation of therapy and dosage adjustments.
• If systolic blood pressure is below 90 mm Hg or heart rate is below 60 beats/minute, withhold dose and notify the doctor.
• Assist patients with ambulation during initiation of diltiazem therapy because dizziness may occur.
• If nitrate therapy is prescribed during titration of diltiazem dosage, urge patient compliance. Sublingual nitroglycerin, especially, may be taken concomitantly as needed when anginal symptoms are acute.
• Tell patients to swallow Dilacor XR whole. Do not open, crush, or chew.

erythrityl tetranitrate
Cardilate

Pregnancy Risk Category: C

HOW SUPPLIED
Tablets (oral, sublingual): 10 mg

ACTION
Unknown. A nitrate that is thought to reduce cardiac oxygen demand by decreasing left ventricular end-diastolic pressure (preload) and, to a lesser extent, systemic vascular resistance (afterload). Drug also may increase blood flow through the collateral coronary vessels.

ONSET, PEAK, DURATION
Onset, occurs within 5 minutes of S.L. administration, 15 to 30 minutes after oral administration. Peak effects occur within 15 minutes of S.L. administation or 60 minutes of oral administration. Effective for up to 3 hours after S.L. administration, 6 hours after oral administration.

INDICATIONS & DOSAGE
Prophylaxis and long-term management of frequent or recurrent anginal pain, reduced exercise tolerance associated with angina pectoris –
Adults: 5 to 10 mg S.L. prior to each anticipated physical or emotional stress and h.s. for patients with history of nocturnal attacks; 10 mg P.O. before each meal, as well as at mid-morning and mid-afternoon, if needed, and at bedtime for patients with history of nocturnal attacks.

ADVERSE REACTIONS
CNS: *headache, sometimes with throbbing; dizziness;* weakness.
CV: *orthostatic hypotension, tachycardia, flushing, palpitations,* fainting.
GI: nausea, vomiting.
Skin: cutaneous vasodilation.
Other: hypersensitivity reactions, sublingual burning.

INTERACTIONS
Ethanol: may increase hypotension. Avoid concomitant use.

CONTRAINDICATIONS
Contraindicated in patients with hypersensitivity or idiosyncratic reactions to nitrates.

---

*Liquid form contains alcohol.
**May contain tartrazine.

Common reactions are in italics; *life-threatening,* in bold italics.

NURSING CONSIDERATIONS

• Use cautiously in patients with severe liver or renal disease, acute MI, or CHF.
• Know that to prevent development of tolerance, a nitrate-free interval of 8 to 12 hours per day has been recommended.
• Monitor blood pressure and intensity and duration of drug response.
• May cause headaches, especially at beginning of therapy; dosage may need to be reduced temporarily, but tolerance usually develops. Treat headache with aspirin or acetaminophen.
• Caution patients to take medication regularly, as prescribed, and to keep it accessible at all times.
• Advise patients that abrupt discontinuation of drug causes coronary vasospasm.
• Tell patients to take an S.L. tablet at the first sign of an attack. The tablet should be wet with saliva and placed under the tongue until completely absorbed, and the patient should sit down and rest. Dose may be repeated every 10 to 15 minutes for a maximum of three doses. If drug doesn't provide relief, medical help should be obtained promptly.
• Patients who complain of tingling sensation with drug placed S.L. may try holding tablets in the buccal pouch.
• Advise patients to take oral tablets on an empty stomach, either ½ hour before or 1 to 2 hours after meals, and to swallow oral tablets whole.
• To minimize orthostatic hypotension, patients should change to upright position slowly. Advise patients to go up and down stairs carefully and to lie down at the first sign of dizziness.
• Tell patient to store drug in a cool place, in a tightly closed container, away from light. To ensure freshness, replace supply every 3 months. Remove cotton from container because it absorbs drug.

---

isosorbide dinitrate
Apo-ISDN†, Cedocard-SR†, Coradur†, Coronex†, Dilatrate-SR, Iso-Bid, Isonate, Isorbid, Isordil, Isotrate, Nitro-Spray‡, Novosorbide†, Sorbitrate, Sorbitrate SA

isosorbide mononitrate
Imdur, Ismo, Monoket
Pregnancy Risk Category: C

HOW SUPPLIED
isosorbide dinitrate
Tablets: 5 mg, 10 mg, 20 mg, 30 mg, 40 mg
Tablets (chewable): 5 mg, 10 mg
Tablets (sublingual): 2.5 mg, 5 mg, 10 mg
Tablets (sustained-release): 40 mg
Capsules: 40 mg
Capsules (sustained-release): 40 mg
Topical spray: 10%‡, 12.5 mg/metered spray‡
isosorbide mononitrate
Tablets: 10 mg, 20 mg
Tablets (extended-release): 60 mg

ACTION
Not completely known. A nitrate that is thought to reduce cardiac oxygen demand by decreasing left ventricular end-diastolic pressure (preload) and, to a lesser extent, systemic vascular resistance (afterload). Drug also may increase blood flow through the collateral coronary vessels.

Most of isosorbide dinitrate's pharmacologic activity is attributed to its active metabolite, isosorbide mononitrate.

ONSET, PEAK, DURATION
Onset and peak levels occur as follows: isosorbide dinitrate — 2 to 5 minutes after administration of S.L. or chewable form, 15 to 40 minutes

after oral form, 30 minutes after extended-release form. Isosorbide mononitrate — 60 minutes. Duration is as follows: isosorbide dinitrate — effective for 1 to 2 hours after administration of S.L. form, 1 to 2 hours after chewable form, 4 to 6 hours after oral form, 12 hours after extended-release form. Isosorbide mononitrate — not determined.

INDICATIONS & DOSAGE
Acute anginal attacks (S.L. and chewable tablets of isosorbide dinitrate only), prophylaxis in situations likely to cause anginal attacks —
Adults: *S.L. form* — 2.5 to 5 mg under the tongue for prompt relief of anginal pain, repeated q 5 to 10 minutes (maximum of three doses for each 30-minute period). For prophylaxis, 2.5 to 10 mg q 2 to 3 hours.
Chewable form — 5 to 10 mg p.r.n. for acute attack or q 2 to 3 hours for prophylaxis, but only after initial test dose of 5 mg to determine risk of severe hypotension.
Oral form (isosorbide dinitrate) — 5 to 30 mg P.O. t.i.d. or q.i.d. for prophylaxis only (use smallest effective dose); 40 mg P.O. (sustained-release form) q 6 to 12 hours.
Oral form (isosorbide mononitrate) — 30 mg to 60 mg P.O. once daily upon arising; increased to 120 mg once daily after several days, if needed.
Topical form‡(where available) — initially, 2 sprays to the chest in the morning from a distance of about 8″ (20 cm). Rub solution in. Increase dosage gradually as needed to 2 to 5 sprays, daily or b.i.d. (in the morning and h.s.).

ADVERSE REACTIONS
CNS: *headache, sometimes with throbbing; dizziness;* weakness.
CV: *orthostatic hypotension, tachycardia, palpitations, ankle edema,* fainting.
GI: nausea, vomiting.

Skin: cutaneous vasodilation, *flushing.*
Other: hypersensitivity reactions, sublingual burning.

INTERACTIONS
Antihypertensives: possibly increased hypotensive effects. Monitor closely during initial therapy.
Ethanol: may increase hypotension. Avoid concomitant use.

CONTRAINDICATIONS
Contraindicated in patients with hypersensitivity or idiosyncrasy to nitrates; severe hypotension; shock; or acute MI with low left ventricular filling pressure.

NURSING CONSIDERATIONS
• Use cautiously in patients with blood volume depletion (such as that resulting from diuretic therapy) or mild hypotension.
• Know that to prevent development of tolerance, a nitrate-free interval of 8 to 12 hours per day has been recommended. The dosage regimen for isosorbide mononitrate (one tablet upon awakening with the second dose in 7 hours, or one extended-release tablet daily) is intended to minimize nitrate tolerance by providing a substantial nitrate-free interval.
• Monitor blood pressure and intensity and duration of drug response.
• Caution patients to take medication regularly, as prescribed, and to keep it accessible at all times.
• Advise patients that abrupt discontinuation of drug causes coronary vasospasms.
• Tell patients to take an S.L. tablet at the first sign of an attack. The tablet should be wet with saliva and placed under the tongue until completely absorbed, and the patient should sit down and rest until pain subsides. Dose may be repeated every 10 to 15 minutes for a maximum of three doses. If drug doesn't provide relief,

---

*Liquid form contains alcohol.   *Common* reactions are in italics; *life-threatening*, in bold italics.
**May contain tartrazine.

medical help should be obtained promptly.

• Patients who complain of tingling sensation with the drug placed S.L. may try holding a tablet in the buccal pouch.

• Warn the patient not to confuse S.L. with oral form.

• Teach the patient taking oral form of isosorbide dinitrate to take oral tablet on an empty stomach, either ½ before or 1 to 2 hours after meals; to swallow oral tablets whole; and to chew chewable tablets thoroughly before swallowing.

• Tell patients to minimize orthostatic hypotension by changing to upright position slowly. Advise patients to go up and down stairs carefully and to lie down at the first sign of dizziness.

• May cause headaches, especially at beginning of therapy. Dosage may need to be reduced temporarily, but tolerance usually develops. Treat headache with aspirin or acetaminophen.

• Tell patients to store drug in a cool place, in a tightly closed container, away from light.

nadolol
Corgard, Syn-Nadolol†

Pregnancy Risk Category: C

HOW SUPPLIED
Tablets: 20 mg, 40 mg, 80 mg, 120 mg, 160 mg

ACTION
A beta-adrenergic blocker that reduces cardiac oxygen demand by blocking catecholamine-induced increases in heart rate, blood pressure, and force of myocardial contraction. Depresses renin secretion.

ONSET, PEAK, DURATION
Onset and duration unknown. Plasma levels peak within 2 to 4 hours.

INDICATIONS & DOSAGE
Angina pectoris –
Adults: 40 mg P.O. once daily, initially. Dosage increased in 40 to 80 mg increments until optimum response occurs. Usual maintenance dosage range is 40 to 240 mg once daily.
Hypertension –
Adults: 40 mg P.O. once daily, initially. Dosage increased in 40 to 80 mg increments until optimum response occurs. Usual maintenance dosage range is 40 to 320 mg once daily. Doses of 640 mg may be necessary in rare cases.

ADVERSE REACTIONS
CNS: fatigue, lethargy.
CV: *bradycardia, hypotension, CHF,* peripheral vascular disease.
GI: nausea, vomiting, diarrhea.
Respiratory: *increased airway resistance.*
Skin: rash.
Other: fever.

INTERACTIONS
Antihypertensives: enhanced antihypertensive effect.
Digitalis glycosides: excessive bradycardia and additive effects on AV conduction. Use together cautiously.
Epinephrine: severe vasoconstriction and reflex bradycardia. Monitor blood pressure and observe the patient carefully.
Insulin, oral antidiabetic agents: can alter dosage requirements in previously stabilized diabetics patients. Observe the patient carefully.
NSAIDs: decreased antihypertensive effect. Monitor blood pressure and adjust dosage.

CONTRAINDICATIONS
Contraindicated in patients with bronchial asthma, sinus bradycardia and greater than first-degree heart block, and cardiogenic shock.

NURSING CONSIDERATIONS

• Use cautiously in patients with heart failure, chronic bronchitis, emphysema, or renal or hepatic impairment and in patients undergoing major surgery involving general anesthesia. Also use cautiously in diabetic patients because beta-adrenergic blockers may mask certain signs and symptoms of hypoglycemia.
• Always check the patient's apical pulse before giving drug. If slower than 60 beats/minute, withhold drug and call the doctor.
• Monitor blood pressure frequently. If the patient develops severe hypotension, administer a vasopressor, as prescribed.
• Know that abrupt discontinuation can exacerbate angina and MI. Dosage should be reduced gradually over 1 to 2 weeks.
• Be aware that nadolol masks common signs of shock and hyperthyroidism.
• Explain to patients the importance of taking the drug as prescribed, even when they are feeling well. Caution patients not to discontinue the drug suddenly.

nicardipine
Cardene, Cardene IV, Cardene SR
Pregnancy Risk Category: C

HOW SUPPLIED
Capsules (immediate-release): 20 mg, 30 mg
Capsules (sustained-release): 30 mg, 45 mg, 60 mg
Injection: 2.5 mg/ml

ACTION
A calcium channel blocker that inhibits calcium ion influx across cardiac and smooth-muscle cells, decreasing myocardial contractility and oxygen demand. Also dilates coronary arteries and arterioles.

ONSET, PEAK, DURATION
Onset is immediate with I.V. administration, within 20 minutes for both oral formulations. Serum levels peak within minutes after I.V. injection, within ½ to 2 hours after immediate-release capsules, 1 to 4 hours after sustained-release capsule. Effects of immediate-release product persist for 6 to 8 hours, of sustained-release preparation, up to 12 hours; rapid decline after cessation of I.V. infusion.

INDICATIONS & DOSAGE
Chronic stable angina (used alone or in combination with other antianginal agents)—
Adults: initially, 20 mg P.O. t.i.d. (immediate-release only). Dosage titrated according to patient response every 3 days. Usual dosage range is 20 to 40 mg t.i.d.
Hypertension—
Adults: initially, 20 to 40 mg P.O. t.i.d. (immediate-release) or 30 mg b.i.d. (sustained-release). Dosage increased according to patient response. Alternatively, for patients unable to take oral nicardipine, 50 ml/hour (5 mg/hour) I.V. infusion initially; then increased by 25 ml/hour (2.5 mg/hour) every 15 minutes up to a maximum of 150 ml/hour (15 mg/hour).

ADVERSE REACTIONS
CNS: *dizziness, light-headedness, headache, paresthesia, drowsiness, asthenia.*
CV: *peripheral edema, palpitations,* angina, tachycardia.
GI: nausea, abdominal discomfort, dry mouth.
Skin: rash, *flushing.*

INTERACTIONS
Antihypertensives: enhanced antihypertensive effect. Monitor patient closely.
Beta blockers: may increase cardiac depressant effects. Monitor the patient closely.

*Liquid form contains alcohol.   *Common* reactions are in italics; **life-threatening,** in bold italics.
**May contain tartrazine.

Cimetidine: may decrease metabolism of calcium channel blockers. Monitor for increased pharmacologic effect.
Cyclosporine: nicardipine may increase plasma levels of cyclosporine. Monitor for toxicity.
Theophylline: pharmacologic effects of theophylline may be enhanced. Monitor for toxicity.

CONTRAINDICATIONS
Contraindicated in patients with hypersensitivity to the drug and in those with advanced aortic stenosis.

NURSING CONSIDERATIONS
• Use cautiously in patients with cardiac conduction disturbances, hypotension, CHF, and impaired hepatic and renal function.
• **I.V. use:** When switching to oral therapy other than nicardipine, initiate therapy upon discontinuation of the infusion. If oral nicardipine is to be used, administer first dose of t.i.d. regimen 1 hour prior to discontinuation of infusion.
• Adjust infusion rate if hypotension or tachycardia occurs, as ordered.
• Measure blood pressure frequently during initial therapy. Maximum blood pressure response occurs about 1 hour after dosing with the immediate-release form and 2 to 4 hours with the sustained-release form. Check for potential orthostatic hypotension. Because large swings in blood pressure may occur based on blood level of drug, assess adequacy of antihypertensive effect 8 hours after dosing.
• Advise the patient to report chest pain immediately. Some patients may experience increased frequency, severity, or duration of chest pain at beginning of therapy or during dosage adjustments. The mechanism for this adverse reaction is not known.

nifedipine
Adalat, Adalat CC, Adalat FT†, Adalat P.A.†, Nu-Nifed†, Procardia, Procardia XL

Pregnancy Risk Category: C

HOW SUPPLIED
Tablets (extended-release): 30 mg, 60 mg, 90 mg
Capsules: 10 mg, 20 mg

ACTION
Unknown. Thought to inhibit calcium ion influx across cardiac and smooth-muscle cells, decreasing myocardial contractility and oxygen demand. Also may dilate coronary arteries and arterioles.

ONSET, PEAK, DURATION
Onset occurs in 20 minutes. Serum levels peak in about 30 to 60 minutes for capsules, 1 to 2 hours for tablets. Effects persist for 4 to 8 hours for capsules; 12 to 24 hours for extended-release formulations.

INDICATIONS & DOSAGE
Vasospastic angina (also called Prinzmetal's [variant] angina) and classic chronic stable angina pectoris –
Adults: starting dose is 10 mg P.O. t.i.d. Usual effective dose range is 10 to 20 mg t.i.d. Some patients may require up to 30 mg q.i.d. Maximum daily dosage is 180 mg.
Hypertension –
Adults: 30 or 60 mg P.O. (extended-release form only) once daily. Titrated over a 7- to 14-day period. Doses larger than 90 mg are not recommended.

ADVERSE REACTIONS
CNS: *dizziness, light-headedness, flushing, headache,* weakness, syncope.
CV: peripheral edema, hypotension, palpitations.
EENT: nasal congestion.

GI: *nausea, heartburn,* diarrhea.
Respiratory: dyspnea.
Other: muscle cramps, hypokalemia.

INTERACTIONS
Cimetidine, ranitidine: decreased nifedipine metabolism.
Propranolol, other beta blockers: may cause hypotension and heart failure. Use together cautiously.

CONTRAINDICATIONS
Contraindicated in patients with hypersensitivity to the drug.

NURSING CONSIDERATIONS
• Use cautiously in patients with CHF or hypotension; also use cautiously in elderly patients because duration of action may be prolonged. Use extended-release tablets cautiously in patients with severe GI narrowing because obstructive symptoms may occur.
• When a rapid response to the drug is desired, instruct the patient to bite and swallow the capsule. If he is unable to chew capsules, the liquid can be withdrawn by puncturing the capsule with a needle and squeezing the contents into the mouth. When using these methods, continuous blood pressure and ECG monitoring is recommended.
• Despite the widespread S.L. use of nifedipine capsules, this route of administration should be avoided. Peak serum levels are lower and it takes longer for peak levels to occur than when capsules are bitten and swallowed.
• Monitor blood pressure regularly, especially in patients who also are taking beta blockers or antihypertensives.
• Monitor serum potassium level regularly, as ordered.
• If the patient is kept on nitrate therapy while nifedipine dosage is being titrated, urge continued compliance. S.L. nitroglycerin, especially, may be taken as needed when anginal symptoms are acute.
• Patient may briefly develop anginal exacerbation when beginning drug therapy or when dosage is increased. Reassure him that this symptom is temporary.
• Instruct the patient to swallow extended-release tablets without breaking, crushing, or chewing.
• Reassure the patient who is taking the extended-release form of the drug that a wax-matrix "ghost" from the tablet may be passed in the stool. Drug is completely absorbed before this occurs.
• Warn the patient not to switch brands. Procardia XL and Adalat CC are not therapeutically equivalent because of major differences in their pharmacokinetics.
• Tell patient to protect capsules from direct light and moisture and to store at room temperature.
• Be aware that although rebound effect hasn't been observed when drug is stopped, dosage should still be reduced slowly under doctor's supervision.

nitroglycerin (glyceryl trinitrate)
Anginine‡, Deponit, GTN-Pohl‡, Minitran, Nitradisc‡, Nitro-Bid, Nitro-Bid I.V., Nitrocine, Nitrodisc, Nitro-Dur, Nitrogard, Nitroglyn, Nitroject, Nitrol, Nitrolingual, Nitrong, Nitrostat, Transderm-Nitro, Transderm-Nitro‡, Tridil

Pregnancy Risk Category: C

HOW SUPPLIED
Tablets (buccal): 1 mg, 2 mg, 3 mg
Tablets (sublingual): 0.15 mg ($1/400$ gr), 0.3 mg ($1/200$ gr), 0.4 mg ($1/150$ gr), 0.6 mg ($1/100$ gr)
Tablets (sustained-release): 2.5 mg, 2.6 mg, 6.5 mg, 9 mg, 13 mg
Capsules (sustained-release): 2.5 mg, 6.5 mg, 9 mg, 13 mg

Aerosol (translingual): 0.4 mg metered spray
Topical: 2% ointment
Transdermal: 2.5 mg, 5 mg, 7.5 mg, 10 mg, 15 mg per 24-hour system
Injection: 0.5 mg/ml, 0.8 mg/ml, 1 mg/ml, 5 mg/ml, 10 mg/ml

ACTION
A nitrate that reduces cardiac oxygen demand by decreasing left ventricular end-diastolic pressure (preload) and, to a lesser extent, systemic vascular resistance (afterload). Also increases blood flow through the collateral coronary vessels.

ONSET, PEAK, DURATION
Onset and peak immediate after I.V. form, 1 to 3 minutes after S.L. form, 2 to 4 minutes after translingual form, 3 minutes after buccal form, 20 to 45 minutes after oral form, 30 minutes after topical ointment, 30 minutes after transdermal system. With I.V. form, effects last 3 to 5 minutes; with S.L. form, 30 to 60 minutes; with translingual form, 30 to 60 minutes; with buccal form, 5 hours; with oral form, 8 to 12 hours; with topical ointment, 4 to 8 hours; with transdermal system, up to 24 hours with system in place (otherwise, effects last several minutes after removal).

INDICATIONS & DOSAGE
Prophylaxis against chronic anginal attacks –
Adults: 2.5 mg or 2.6 mg sustained-release (capsule) q 8 to 12 hours; titrated upward to an effective dose increasing by 2.5- or 2.6-mg increments 2 to 4 times daily. Or, use of 2% ointment: Dosage started with ½″ ointment, increasing by ½″ increments until headache occurs, then decreasing to previous dose. Range of dosage with ointment is ½″ to 5″. Usual dose is 1″ to 2″. Alternatively, transdermal disc or pad (Nitrodisc, Nitro-Dur, or Transderm-Nitro) 0.2 to 0.4 mg/hour once daily.
Acute angina pectoris, prophylaxis to prevent or minimize anginal attacks when taken immediately before stressful events –
Adults: 1 S.L. tablet (gr ¼₀₀, ½₀₀, ⅟₁₅₀, ⅟₁₀₀) dissolved under the tongue or in the buccal pouch as soon as angina begins. Repeat q 5 minutes, if needed, for 15 minutes. Or, using Nitrolingual spray, one or two sprays into mouth, preferably onto or under the tongue. Repeat q 3 to 5 minutes if needed, to a maximum of three doses within a 15-minute period. Or, 1 to 3 mg transmucosally q 3 to 5 hours during waking hours.
Hypertension associated with surgery; CHF associated with MI; angina pectoris in acute situations; to produce controlled hypotension during surgery (by I.V. infusion) –
Adults: initial infusion rate is 5 mcg/minute. Increased as needed, by 5 mcg/minute q 3 to 5 minutes until a response is noted. If a 20 mcg/minute rate doesn't produce a response, dosage is increased by as much as 20 mcg/minute q 3 to 5 minutes. Up to 100 mcg/minute may be needed.

ADVERSE REACTIONS
CNS: *headache, sometimes with throbbing; dizziness;* weakness.
CV: *orthostatic hypotension, tachycardia, flushing, palpitations,* fainting.
GI: nausea, vomiting.
Skin: cutaneous vasodilation, contact dermatitis (patch), rash.
Other: hypersensitivity reactions, sublingual burning.

INTERACTIONS
Antihypertensives: possibly enhanced hypotensive effect. Monitor closely.
Ethanol: possible increased hypotension. Advise the patient to avoid use of ethanol.

CONTRAINDICATIONS

• Contraindicated in patients with hypersensitivity to nitrates and in those with early MI (sublingual nitroglycerin), severe anemia, increased intracranial pressure, angle-closure glaucoma, postural hypotension, and allergy to adhesives (transdermal).

• I.V. nitroglycerin is contraindicated in patients with hypersensitivity to I.V. form, cardiac tamponade, restrictive cardiomyopathy, or constrictive pericarditis.

NURSING CONSIDERATIONS

• Use cautiously in patients with hypotension or volume depletion.

• **I.V. use:** Dilute with D_5W or 0.9% sodium chloride injection. Concentration should not exceed 400 mcg/ml. Always administer with an infusion control device and titrate to desired response. Also, always mix in glass bottles and avoid use of I.V. filters because drug binds to plastic. Regular polyvinyl chloride (PVC) tubing can bind up to 80% of the drug, making it necessary to infuse higher dosages. A special nonabsorbent (non-PVC) tubing is available from the manufacturer; patients receive more drug when these infusion sets are used. Always use the same type of infusion set when changing I.V. lines.

• When changing the concentration of nitroglycerin infusion, flush the I.V. administration set with 15 to 20 ml of the new concentration before use. This will clear the line of the old drug solution.

• Closely monitor vital signs during infusion. Be particularly aware of blood pressure, especially if the drug is being used in a patient with an MI. Excessive hypotension may worsen the MI.

• To apply ointment, measure the prescribed amount on the application paper; then place the paper on any nonhairy area. Do not rub in. Cover with plastic film to aid absorption and to protect clothing. If using Tape-Surrounded Appli-Ruler (TSAR) system, keep the TSAR on skin to protect patient's clothing and to ensure that ointment remains in place. Remove all excess ointment from previous site before applying the next dose. Avoid getting ointment on fingers.

• Know that transdermal dosage forms can be applied to any nonhairy part of the skin except distal parts of the arms or legs (absorption will not be maximal at from distal sites).

• Be sure to remove transdermal patch before defibrillation. Because of its aluminum backing, the electric current may cause the patch to explode.

• When stopping transdermal treatment of angina, gradually reduce the dose and frequency of application over 4 to 6 weeks, as ordered.

• Monitor blood pressure and intensity and duration of drug response.

• May cause headaches, especially at beginning of therapy. Dosage may need to be reduced temporarily, but tolerance usually develops. Treat headache with aspirin or acetaminophen.

• Tolerance to the drug can be minimized with a 10- to 12-hour nitrate-free interval. To achieve this, remove transdermal system in the early evening and apply a new system the next morning or omit the last daily dose of a buccal, sustained-release, or ointment form. Check with the doctor for alterations in dosage regimen if tolerance is suspected.

• Tell the patient to take an S.L. tablet at the first sign of an attack. The tablet should be wet with saliva and placed under the tongue until completely absorbed, and the patient should sit down and rest until pain subsides. Dose may be repeated every 10 to 15 minutes for a maximum of three doses. If drug doesn't provide relief, medical help should be obtained promptly.

---

*Liquid form contains alcohol.
**May contain tartrazine.

Common reactions are in italics; *life-threatening*, in bold italics.

• Patient who complains of a tingling sensation with the drug placed S.L. may try holding a tablet in the buccal pouch.

• Tell the patient to take oral tablets on an empty stomach, either 30 minutes before or 1 to 2 hours after meals; to swallow oral tablets whole; and not to chew tablets.

• Remind the patient who is using translingual aerosol form that he should *not* inhale the spray, but should release it onto or under the tongue. Also tell him to wait about 10 seconds or so before swallowing.

• Tell the patient to place the transmucosal tablet between the lip and gum above the incisors, or between the cheek and gum. Tablets should be be swallowed or chewed.

• Caution the patient to take nitroglycerin regularly, as prescribed, and to have it accessible at all times.

• Advise the patient that abrupt discontinuation of drug causes coronary vasospasms.

• An additional dose may be taken before anticipated stress or at bedtime if angina is nocturnal.

• Instruct the patient to use caution when wearing transdermal patch near microwave oven. Leaking radiation may heat patch's metallic backing and cause burns.

• Advise the patient to avoid alcoholic beverages.

• To minimize orthostatic hypotension, tell the patient to change to upright position slowly. Advise him to go up and down stairs carefully and to lie down at the first sign of dizziness.

• Tell the patient to store drug in cool, dark place in a tightly closed container. To ensure freshness, replace supply of S.L. tablets every 3 months. Remove cotton from container because it absorbs drug.

• Tell the patient to store S.L. tablets in original container or other container specifically approved for this use and to carry the container in a jacket pocket or purse, not in a pocket close to the body.

pentaerythritol tetranitrate
Dilar, Duotrate, Naptrate, Pentritol, Pentylan, Peritrate, Peritrate Forte†, Peritrate SA, PETN

Pregnancy Risk Category: C

HOW SUPPLIED
Tablets: 10 mg, 20 mg, 40 mg
Tablets (sustained-release): 80 mg
Capsules (sustained-release): 30 mg, 45 mg

ACTION
Reduces cardiac oxygen demand by decreasing left ventricular end-diastolic pressure (preload) and, to a lesser extent, systemic vascular resistance (afterload). Also increases blood flow through the collateral coronary vessels.

ONSET, PEAK, DURATION
Onset occurs 30 minutes after oral tablets, 1 hour or more after sustained-release forms. Peak levels unknown. Effects persist for 4 to 5 hours after oral tablets; 12 hours after sustained-release forms.

INDICATIONS & DOSAGE
Prophylaxis against angina pectoris –
Adults: 10 to 20 mg P.O. t.i.d. or q.i.d.; titrated upward as needed to 40 mg P.O. q.i.d. ½ before or 1 hour after meals and h.s.; or 30 to 80 mg sustained-release form P.O. b.i.d. on empty stomach.

ADVERSE REACTIONS
CNS: *headache, sometimes with throbbing; dizziness;* weakness.
CV: *orthostatic hypotension, tachycardia, flushing, palpitations,* fainting.
GI: nausea, vomiting.
Skin: cutaneous vasodilation.
Other: hypersensitivity reactions.

INTERACTIONS
Antihypertensives: possible enhanced hypotensive effect. Monitor closely.
Ethanol: may increase hypotension. Avoid concomitant use.

CONTRAINDICATIONS
Contraindicated in patients with hypersensitivity to nitrates, severe anemia, increased intracranial pressure, angle-closure glaucoma, or postural hypotension.

NURSING CONSIDERATIONS
• Use cautiously in patients with volume depletion or glaucoma (except angle-closure type).
• Monitor blood pressure and intensity and duration of drug response.
• May cause headaches, especially at beginning of therapy. Dosage may need to be reduced temporarily, but tolerance usually develops. Treat headache with aspirin or acetaminophen.
• Warn patient that drug is not to be used for relief of acute anginal attacks.
• Caution the patient to take medication regularly, as prescribed, and to have it accessible at all times.
• Tell patient additional doses may be taken before anticipated stress or at bedtime for nocturnal angina.
• Advise the patient that abrupt discontinuation of drug causes coronary vasospasm.
• To minimize orthostatic hypotension, tell the patient to change to upright position slowly. Advise him to go up and down stairs carefully and to lie down at the first sign of dizziness.
• Instruct patient to store drug in a cool place, in a tightly covered container away from light.

propranolol hydrochloride
Apo-Propranolol†, Deralin‡, Detensol†, Inderal, Inderal LA, Novopranol†, pms-Propranolol†

Pregnancy Risk Category: C

HOW SUPPLIED
Tablets: 10 mg, 20 mg, 40 mg, 60 mg, 80 mg, 90 mg
Capsules (extended-release): 60 mg, 80 mg, 120 mg, 160 mg
Oral solution: 4 mg/ml, 8 mg/ml, 80 mg/ml (concentrate)
Injection: 1 mg/ml

ACTION
A nonselective beta-adrenergic blocker that reduces cardiac oxygen demand by blocking catecholamine-induced increases in heart rate, blood pressure, and force of myocardial contraction. Depresses renin secretion and prevents vasodilation of cerebral arteries.

ONSET, PEAK, DURATION
Onset occurs within1 minute after I.V. injection, 30 minutes after oral administration. Peak plasma levels occur 60 to 90 minutes after oral administration or immediately after I.V. injection. Effects persist for about 12 hours after oral administration. Drug undetectable in the plasma 5 minutes after I.V. bolus administration.

INDICATIONS & DOSAGE
Angina pectoris –
Adults: 10 to 20 mg P.O. t.i.d. or q.i.d. Or one 80-mg extended-release capsule daily. Dosage increased at 7- to 10-day intervals. The average optimum dosage is 160 to 240 mg daily.
Mortality reduction after MI –
Adults: 180 to 240 mg P.O. daily in divided doses beginning 5 to 21 days after MI has occurred. Usually administered t.i.d. or q.i.d.
Supraventricular, ventricular, and atrial arrhythmias; tachyarrhythmias

---

caused by excessive catecholamine action during anesthesia, hyperthyroidism, or pheochromocytoma –
Adults: 0.5 to 3 mg by slow I.V. push, not to exceed 1 mg/minute. After 3 mg have been given, another dose may be given in 2 minutes; subsequent doses, no sooner than q 4 hours. May be diluted and infused slowly. Usual maintenance dosage is 10 to 30 mg P.O. t.i.d. or q.i.d.
Hypertension –
Adults: initially, 80 mg P.O. daily in two to four divided doses or the extended-release form once daily. Increased at 3- to 7-day intervals to maximum daily dosage of 640 mg. Usual maintenance dosage is 160 to 480 mg daily.
Prevention of frequent, severe, uncontrollable, or disabling migraine or vascular headache –
Adults: initially, 80 mg P.O. daily in divided doses or 1 extended-release capsule daily. Usual maintenance dosage is 160 to 240 mg daily, t.i.d. or q.i.d.
Essential tremor –
Adults: 40 mg (tablets, oral solution) P.O. b.i.d. Usual maintenance dosage is 120 to 320 mg daily in 3 divided doses.
Hypertrophic subaortic stenosis –
Adults: 20 to 40 mg P.O. t.i.d. or q.i.d., or 80 to 160 mg extended-release capsules once daily.
Adjunct therapy in pheochromocytoma –
Adults: 60 mg P.O. daily in divided doses in conjunction with an alpha-adrenergic blocker 3 days prior to surgery.

ADVERSE REACTIONS
CNS: *fatigue, lethargy,* vivid dreams, hallucinations, mental depression.
CV: *bradycardia, hypotension, CHF,* intermittent claudication.
GI: nausea, vomiting, diarrhea.
Respiratory: *increased airway resistance.*

Skin: rash.
Other: fever, arthralgia.

INTERACTIONS
Aminophylline: antagonized beta-blocking effects of propranolol. Use together cautiously.
Cimetidine: inhibits propranolol's metabolism. Monitor for increased beta-blocking effect.
Digitalis glycosides, diltiazem, verapamil: hypotension, bradycardia, and increased depressant effect on myocardium. Use together cautiously.
Epinephrine: severe vasoconstriction. Monitor blood pressure and observe the patient carefully.
Glucagon, isoproterenol: antagonized propranolol effect. May be used therapeutically and in emergencies.
Insulin, oral antidiabetic agents: can alter requirements for these drugs in previously stabilized diabetics. Monitor for hypoglycemia.

CONTRAINDICATIONS
Contraindicated in patients with bronchial asthma, sinus bradycardia and heart block greater than first-degree, cardiogenic shock, and CHF (unless failure is secondary to a tachyarrhythmia that can be treated with propranolol).

NURSING CONSIDERATIONS
• Use cautiously in patients with renal impairment, nonallergic bronchospastic diseases, or hepatic disease and in those taking other antihypertensives. Because drug blocks some symptoms of hypoglycemia, use with caution in patients with diabetes mellitus. Also use cautiously in patients with thyrotoxicosis because drug may mask some signs of that disorder. Elderly patients may experience enhanced adverse reactions and may need dosage adjustment.
• Always check patient's apical pulse before giving drug. If you detect extremes in pulse rates, withhold drug

and call the doctor immediately.
• Double-check dose and route. I.V. doses are much smaller than oral doses.
• **I.V. use:** Give by direct injection into a large vessel or into the tubing of a free-flowing, compatible I.V. solution; continuous I.V. infusion generally is not recommended. Alternatively, dilute drug with 0.9% sodium chloride and give by intermittent infusion over 10 to 15 minutes in 0.1- to 0.2-mg increments. Drug is compatible with D_5W, 0.45% and 0.9% sodium chloride, and lactated Ringer's solution.
• Give consistently with meals. Food may increase absorption of propranolol.
• Monitor blood pressure, ECG, and heart rate and rhythm frequently, especially during I.V. administration. If the patient develops severe hypotension, notify the doctor; a vasopressor may be prescribed.
• Be aware that drug masks common signs of shock and hypoglycemia.
• *Don't discontinue drug before surgery for pheochromocytoma.* Before any surgical procedure, notify anesthesiologist that the patient is receiving propranolol.
• For overdose, give I.V. isoproterenol, I.V. atropine, or glucagon; refractory cases may require a pacemaker.
• Compliance may be improved by administering drug twice daily or as extended-release capsule. Check with the doctor.
• Caution the patient to continue taking this drug as prescribed, even when he is feeling well. Tell the patient not to discontinue the drug suddenly because this can exacerbate angina and MI.

verapamil
Apo-Verapt, Calan, Isoptin, Novo-Veramilt, Nu-Verapt

verapamil hydrochloride
Anpec‡, Calan, Calan SR, Cordilox‡,Cordilox SR‡, Isoptin, Isoptin SR, Veracaps SR‡, Verelan

Pregnancy Risk Category: C

HOW SUPPLIED
verapamil
Tablets: 40 mg, 80 mg, 120 mg
verapamil hydrochloride
Tablets: 40 mg‡, 80 mg‡, 120 mg‡, 160 mg‡
Tablets (extended-release): 120 mg, 180 mg, 240 mg
Capsules (extended-release): 120 mg, 160 mg‡, 180 mg, 240 mg
Injection: 2.5 mg/ml

ACTION
Not clearly defined. Verapamil is a calcium channel blocker that inhibits calcium ion influx across cardiac and smooth-muscle cells, thus decreasing myocardial contractility and oxygen demand; it also dilates coronary arteries and arterioles.

ONSET, PEAK, DURATION
Onset occurs within 1 to 2 hours with oral administration, within 1 to 5 minutes with I.V. administration. Serum levels peak within 1 to 2 hours (tablets), 7 to 9 hours (extended-release capsules), 5 to 7 hours (extended-release tablets), and immediately after I.V. administration. Effects persist 1 to 6 hours with I.V. form, about 8 to 10 hours with tablets, and about 24 hours with extended-release oral forms.

INDICATIONS & DOSAGE
Vasospastic angina (also called Prinzmetal's [variant] angina) and classic chronic, stable angina pectoris; chronic atrial fibrillation —
Adults: starting dose is 80 to 120 mg P.O. t.i.d. Dosage increased at weekly intervals as needed. Some patients may require up to 480 mg daily.
Supraventricular arrhythmias —

Adults: 0.075 to 0.15 mg/kg (5 to 10 mg) by I.V. push over 2 minutes with ECG and blood pressure monitoring. Repeat dose in 30 minutes if no response occurs.

Children under 1 year: 0.1 to 0.2 mg/kg as I.V. bolus over 2 minutes with continuous ECG monitoring. Repeat dose in 30 minutes if no response occurs.

Children 1 to 15 years: 0.1 to 0.3 mg/kg as I.V. bolus over 2 minutes.

Hypertension –

Adults: 240 mg extended-release tablet P.O. once daily in the morning. If response is not adequate, an additional ½ tablet in the evening or one tablet q 12 hours. Or, 80 mg immediate-release tablet t.i.d.

ADVERSE REACTIONS

CNS: dizziness, headache, fatigue.
CV: *transient hypotension, CHF,* bradycardia, AV block, *ventricular asystole,* peripheral edema.
GI: *constipation,* nausea.
Hepatic: elevated liver enzymes.

INTERACTIONS

Antihypertensives, quinidine: may result in hypotension. Monitor blood pressure.
Carbamazepine, digitalis glycosides: may increase serum levels of these drugs. Monitor the patient for toxicity.
Cyclosporine: may increase cyclosporine serum levels. Monitor cyclosporine levels.
Disopyramide, flecainide, propranolol (and other beta blockers, including ophthalmic timolol): may cause heart failure. Use together cautiously.
Lithium: may decrease serum lithium levels. Monitor closely.
Rifampin: may decrease oral bioavailability of verapamil. Monitor the patient for lack of effect.

CONTRAINDICATIONS

Contraindicated in patients with hypersensitivity to the drug; severe left ventricular dysfunction; cardiogenic shock; second- or third-degree AV block or sick sinus syndrome except in presence of functioning pacemaker; atrial flutter or fibrillation and accessory bypass tract syndrome; severe CHF (unless secondary to verapamil therapy); and severe hypotension. In addition, I.V. verapamil is contraindicated in patients receiving I.V. beta-adrenergic blocking agents and in those with ventricular tachycardia.

NURSING CONSIDERATIONS

• Use cautiously in elderly patients; in patients with increased intracranial pressure; and in patients with hepatic or renal disease.
• Although the drug should be taken with food, be aware that taking extended-release tablets with food may decrease rate and extent of absorption, but allows smaller fluctuations of peak and trough blood levels.
• Patients with severely compromised cardiac function or those receiving beta blockers should receive lower doses of verapamil. Monitor these patients closely.
• **I.V. use:** Give by direct injection into a vein or into the tubing of a free-flowing, compatible I.V. solution. Compatible solutions include D₅W, 0.45% and 0.9% sodium chloride, and Ringer's and lactated Ringer's solutions. Administer I.V. doses over at least 3 minutes to minimize the risk of adverse reactions.
• All patients receiving I.V. verapamil should be on a cardiac monitor. Monitor the R-R interval.
• Be aware that if verapamil is being used to terminate supraventricular tachycardia, the doctor may have the patient perform vagal maneuvers after receiving drug.
• Monitor blood pressure at the start of therapy and during dosage adjust-

ments. Assist the patient with ambulation because dizziness may occur.
• Notify the doctor if signs of CHF, such as swelling of hands and feet or shortness of breath, occur.
• Monitor liver function during prolonged treatment, as ordered.
• If the patient is kept on nitrate therapy during titration of oral verapamil dosage, urge continued compliance. Sublingual nitroglycerin, especially, may be taken as needed when anginal symptoms are acute.
• Encourage the patient to increase fluid and fiber intake to combat constipation. Administer a stool softener as ordered.

23

Antihypertensives

acebutolol
amlodipine besylate
(See Chapter 22, ANTIANGINALS.)
atenolol
benazepril hydrochloride
betaxolol hydrochloride
bisoprolol fumarate
captopril
carteolol
clonidine hydrochloride
diazoxide
diltiazem hydrochloride
(See Chapter 22, ANTIANGINALS.)
doxazosin mesylate
enalaprilat
enalapril maleate
felodipine
fosinopril sodium
guanabenz acetate
guanadrel sulfate
guanethidine monosulfate
guanfacine hydrochloride
hydralazine hydrochloride
isradipine
labetalol hydrochloride
lisinopril
losartan potassium
methyldopa
methyldopate hydrochloride
metoprolol succinate
metoprolol tartrate
minoxidil
nadolol
(See Chapter 22, ANTIANGINALS.)
nicardipine
(See Chapter 22, ANTIANGINALS.)
nifedipine
(See Chapter 22, ANTIANGINALS.)
nitroprusside sodium
penbutolol sulfate
phentolamine mesylate
pindolol
prazosin hydrochloride
propranolol hydrochloride
(See Chapter 22, ANTIANGINALS.)
quinapril hydrochloride

ramipril
rauwolfia serpentina
rescinnamine
reserpine
terazosin hydrochloride
timolol maleate
trimethaphan camsylate
verapamil hydrochloride
(See Chapter 22, ANTIANGINALS.)

COMBINATION PRODUCTS
ALDOCLOR-150: chlorothiazide 150 mg and methyldopa 250 mg.
ALDOCLOR-250: chlorothiazide 250 mg and methyldopa 250 mg.
ALDORIL-15: hydrochlorothiazide 15 mg and methyldopa 250 mg.
ALDORIL-25: hydrochlorothiazide 25 mg and methyldopa 250 mg.
ALDORIL D30: hydrochlorothiazide 30 mg and methyldopa 500 mg.
ALDORIL D50: hydrochlorothiazide 50 mg and methyldopa 500 mg.
APRESAZIDE 25/25: hydrochlorothiazide 25 mg and hydralazine hydrochloride 25 mg.
APRESAZIDE 50/50: hydrochlorothiazide 50 mg and hydralazine hydrochloride 50 mg.
APRESAZIDE 100/50: hydrochlorothiazide 50 mg and hydralazine hydrochloride 100 mg.
APRESODEX: hydrochlorothiazide 15 mg and hydralazine hydrochloride 25 mg.
APRESOLINE-ESIDRIX: hydrochlorothiazide 15 mg and hydralazine hydrochloride 25 mg.
CAM-AP-ES: hydrochlorothiazide 15 mg, hydralazine hydrochloride 25 mg, and reserpine 0.1 mg.
CAPOZIDE 25/15: hydrochlorothiazide 15 mg and captopril 25 mg.
CAPOZIDE 25/25: hydrochlorothiazide 25 mg and captopril 25 mg.

CAPOZIDE 50/15: hydrochlorothiazide 15 mg and captopril 50 mg.

CAPOZIDE 50/25: hydrochlorothiazide 25 mg and captopril 50 mg.

CHERAPAS: hydrochlorothiazide 15 mg, hydralazine hydrochloride 25 mg, and reserpine 0.1 mg.

COMBIPRES 0.1: chlorthalidone 15 mg and clonidine hydrochloride 0.1 mg.

COMBIPRES 0.2: chlorthalidone 15 mg and clonidine hydrochloride 0.2 mg.

CORZIDE: nadolol 40 mg or 80 mg and bendroflumethiazide 5 mg.

DEMI-REGROTON: chlorthalidone 25 mg and reserpine 0.125 mg.

DIUPRES-250: chlorothiazide 250 mg and reserpine 0.125 mg.

DIUPRES-500: chlorothiazide 500 mg and reserpine 0.125 mg.

DIURESE-R: trichlormethiazide 4 mg and reserpine 0.1 mg.

DIURIGEN WITH RESERPINE: chlorothiazide 250 mg and reserpine 0.125 mg.

DIUTENSEN-R: methyclothiazide 2.5 mg and reserpine 0.1 mg.

ESIMIL: hydrochlorothiazide 25 mg and guanethidine monosulfate 10 mg.

EXNA-R TABLETS: benzthiazide 50 mg and reserpine 0.125 mg.

H.H.R.: hydrochlorothiazide 15 mg, hydralazine hydrochloride 25 mg, and reserpine 0.1 mg.

HYDROMOX-R: quinethazone 50 mg and reserpine 0.125 mg.

HYDROPINE: hydroflumethiazide 25 mg and reserpine 0.125 mg.

HYDROPINE HP: hydroflumethiazide 50 mg and reserpine 0.125 mg.

HYDROPRES-25: hydrochlorothiazide 25 mg and reserpine 0.125 mg.

HYDRO-RESERP: hydrochlorothiazide 25 or 50 mg and reserpine 0.125 mg.

HYDRO-SERP: hydrochlorothiazide 25 or 50 mg and reserpine 0.125 mg.

HYDROSERPINE: hydrochlorothiazide 25 or 50 mg and reserpine 0.125 mg.

HYDROTENSIN-25 TABLETS: hydrochlorothiazide 25 mg and reserpine 0.125 mg.

HYZAAR: losartan 50 mg and hydrochlorothiazide 12.5 mg.

INDERIDE 40/25: propranolol hydrochloride 40 mg and hydrochlorothiazide 25 mg.

INDERIDE 80/25: propranolol hydrochloride 80 mg and hydrochlorothiazide 25 mg.

INDERIDE LA 80/50: propranolol hydrochloride 80 mg and hydrochlorothiazide 50 mg.

INDERIDE LA 120/50: propranolol hydrochloride 120 mg and hydrochlorothiazide 50 mg.

INDERIDE LA 160/50: propranolol hydrochloride 160 mg and hydrochlorothiazide 50 mg.

LOPRESSOR HCT 50/25: metoprolol tartrate 50 mg and hydrochlorothiazide 25 mg.

LOPRESSOR HCT 100/25: metoprolol tartrate 100 mg and hydrochlorothiazide 25 mg.

LOPRESSOR HCT 100/50: metoprolol tartrate 100 mg and hydrochlorothiazide 50 mg.

MAXZIDE: triamterene 75 mg and hydrochlorothiazide 50 mg.

METATENSIN TABLETS #2 or #4: trichlormethiazide 2 or 4 mg and reserpine 0.1 mg.

MINIZIDE 1: polythiazide 0.5 mg and prazosin hydrochloride 1 mg.

MINIZIDE 2: polythiazide 0.5 mg and prazosin hydrochloride 2 mg.

MINIZIDE 5: polythiazide 0.5 mg and prazosin hydrochloride 5 mg.

NAQUIVAL: trichlormethiazide 4 mg and reserpine 0.1 mg.

NORMOZIDE 100/25: labetalol hydrochloride 100 mg and hydrochlorothiazide 25 mg.

NORMOZIDE 200/25: labetalol hydrochloride 200 mg and hydrochlorothiazide 25 mg.

NORMOZIDE 300/25: labetalol hydrochloride 300 mg and hydrochlorothiazide 25 mg.

---

*Liquid form contains alcohol.
**May contain tartrazine.

Common reactions are in italics; ***life-threatening***, in bold italics.

PRINZIDE 10-12.5: lisinopril 10 mg and hydrochlorothiazide 12.5 mg.

PRINZIDE 20-12.5: lisinopril 20 mg and hydrochlorothiazide 12.5 mg.

PRINZIDE 20-25: lisinopril 20 mg and hydrochlorothiazide 25 mg.

RAUZIDE**: bendroflumethiazide 4 mg and powdered rauwolfia serpentina 50 mg.

REGROTON: chlorthalidone 50 mg and reserpine 0.25 mg.

RENESE-R: polythiazide 2 mg and reserpine 0.25 mg.

REZIDE: hydrochlorothiazide 15 mg, hydralazine hydrochloride 25 mg, and reserpine 0.1 mg.

R-HCTZ-H: hydrochlorothiazide 15 mg, hydralazine hydrochloride 25 mg, and reserpine 0.1 mg.

SALUTENSIN: hydroflumethiazide 50 mg and reserpine 0.125 mg.

SALUTENSIN DEMI: hydroflumethiazide 25 mg and reserpine 0.125 mg.

SER-A-GEN: hydrochlorothiazide 15 mg, hydralazine hydrochloride 25 mg, and reserpine 0.1 mg.

SERALAZIDE: hydrochlorothiazide 15 mg, hydralazine hydrochloride 25 mg, and reserpine 0.1 mg.

SER-AP-ES: hydrochlorothiazide 15 mg, reserpine 0.1 mg, and hydralazine hydrochloride 25 mg.

SERPASIL-APRESOLINE #1**: reserpine 0.1 mg and hydralazine hydrochloride 25 mg.

SERPASIL-APRESOLINE #2: reserpine 0.2 mg and hydralazine hydrochloride 50 mg.

SERPASIL-ESIDRIX #1: hydrochlorothiazide 25 mg and reserpine 0.1 mg (called Serpasil-Esidrix 25 in Canada).

SERPASIL ESIDRIX #2: hydrochlorothiazide 50 mg and reserpine 0.1 mg.

SERPAZIDE: hydrochlorothiazide 15 mg, hydralazine hydrochloride 25 mg, and reserpine 0.1 mg.

TENORETIC 50: atenolol 50 mg and chlorthalidone 25 mg.

TENORETIC 100: atenolol 100 mg and chlorthalidone 25 mg.

TIMOLIDE 10/25: timolol maleate 10 mg and hydrochlorothiazide 25 mg.

TRI-HYDROSERPINE: hydrochlorothiazide 15 mg, hydralazine hydrochloride 25 mg, and reserpine 0.1 mg.

UNIPRES: hydrochlorothiazide 15 mg, reserpine 0.1 mg, and hydralazine hydrochloride 25 mg.

VASERETIC: enalapril maleate 10 mg and hydrochlorothiazide 25 mg.

ZESTORETIC 20-12.5: lisinopril 20 mg and hydrochlorothiazide 12.5 mg

ZESTORETIC 20-25: lisinopril and hydrochlorothiazide 25 mg

ZIAC: bisoprolol fumarate 2.5 mg, 5 mg, or 10 mg and hydrochlorothiazide 6.5 mg.

---

acebutolol

Monitan†, Sectral

Pregnancy Risk Category: B

HOW SUPPLIED
Capsules: 200 mg, 400 mg

ACTION
Antihypertensive action is unknown. Possible mechanisms include reduced cardiac output, decreased sympathetic outflow to peripheral vasculature, and inhibition of renin release. Antiarrhythmic action decreases myocardial contractility and decreases heart rate. It has mild intrinsic sympathomimetic activity.

ONSET, PEAK, DURATION
Onset occurs within 1 to 1½ hours. Peak plasma levels of parent drug occur within 2½ hours; of active metabolite, in about 3½ hours. Effects persist up to 24 hours.

INDICATIONS & DOSAGE
Hypertension –
Adults: 400 mg P.O. either as a single daily dose or in divided doses b.i.d. Patients may receive as much as 1,200 mg daily.
Suppression of PVCs –

Adults: 400 mg P.O. daily divided b.i.d. Dosage increased to provide an adequate clinical response. Usual dosage is 600 to 1,200 mg daily.

In patients with impaired renal function, dosage is reduced.

Elderly patients may require lower dosage; dosage should not exceed 800 mg daily.

ADVERSE REACTIONS
CNS: *fatigue,* headache, dizziness, insomnia.
CV: chest pain, edema, bradycardia, *CHF,* hypotension.
GI: nausea, constipation, diarrhea, dyspepsia.
Respiratory: dyspnea, *bronchospasm.*
Skin: rash.
Other: fever, positive antinuclear antibody (ANA) test.

INTERACTIONS
Digitalis glycosides, diltiazem, verapamil: excessive bradycardia and increased depressant effect on myocardium. Use together cautiously.
Insulin, oral antidiabetic agents: can alter dosage requirements in previously stabilized diabetic patients. Observe the patient carefully.
NSAIDs: decreased antihypertensive effect. Monitor blood pressure and adjust dosage.

CONTRAINDICATIONS
Contraindicated in patients with persistently severe bradycardia, second- and third-degree heart block, overt cardiac failure, and cardiogenic shock.

NURSING CONSIDERATIONS
• Use cautiously in patients with cardiac failure, peripheral vascular disease, bronchospastic disease, and diabetes.
• Always check the patient's apical pulse before giving drug; if slower than 60 beats/minute, withhold drug and call the doctor. Also monitor blood pressure.
• Before surgery, notify the anesthesiologist that the patient is taking this drug.
• Be aware that acebutol may mask signs of hyperthyroidism.
• Advise the patient that abrupt discontinuation of drug can exacerbate angina and MI.

---

atenolol
Apo-Atenolol†, Noten‡, Nu-Atenol†, Tenormin

Pregnancy Risk Category: D

HOW SUPPLIED
Tablets: 25 mg, 50 mg, 100 mg
Injection: 5 mg/10 ml

ACTION
A beta-adrenergic blocker that selectively blocks $beta_1$-adrenergic receptors; decreases cardiac output, peripheral resistance, and cardiac oxygen consumption; and depresses renin secretion.

ONSET, PEAK, DURATION
Onset occurs 5 minutes after I.V. injection, 1 hour after oral administration. Peak effects occur 2 to 4 hours after oral dose or 5 minutes after direct I.V. injection. Effects persist less than 12 hours after I.V. dose or 24 hours after oral dose.

INDICATIONS & DOSAGE
Hypertension –
Adults: initially, 50 mg P.O. daily as a single dose. Dosage increased to 100 mg once daily after 7 to 14 days. Dosages > 100 mg are unlikely to produce further benefit. Dosage adjustment required in patients with creatinine clearance below 35 ml/minute.
Angina pectoris –
Adults: 50 mg P.O. once daily. Increased as needed to 100 mg daily af-

---

*Liquid form contains alcohol.   *Common* reactions are in italics; *life-threatening,* in bold italics.
**May contain tartrazine.

ter 7 days for optimal effect. Maximum dosage is 200 mg daily.
To reduce cardiovascular mortality and risk of reinfarction in patients with acute MI—
Adults: 5 mg I.V. over 5 minutes, followed by another 5 mg 10 minutes later. After an additional 10 minutes, 50 mg P.O., followed by 50 mg P.O. in 12 hours. Thereafter, 100 mg P.O. daily (as a single dose or 50 mg b.i.d.) for at least 7 days.

In patients with renal insufficiency: If creatinine clearance is 15 to 35 ml/minute, a maximum of 50 mg daily; if creatinine clearance is < 15 ml/minute, a maximum dosage of 50 mg daily. Hemodialysis patients require 25 to 50 mg after each dialysis session, but supervise closely because of the risk of hypotension.

ADVERSE REACTIONS
CNS: fatigue, lethargy.
CV: *bradycardia, hypotension, CHF,* intermittent claudication.
GI: nausea, vomiting, diarrhea.
Respiratory: dyspnea, *bronchospasm.*
Skin: rash.
Other: fever.

INTERACTIONS
Antihypertensives: enhanced hypotensive effect. Use together cautiously.
Digitalis glycosides, diltiazem, verapamil: excessive bradycardia and increased depressant effect on myocardium. Use together cautiously.
Insulin, oral antidiabetic agents: can alter dosage requirements in previously stabilized diabetic patients. Observe the patient carefully.

CONTRAINDICATIONS
Contraindicated in patients with sinus bradycardia, greater than first-degree heart block, overt cardiac failure, or cardiogenic shock.

NURSING CONSIDERATIONS
● Use cautiously in patients at risk for CHF and in patients with bronchospastic disease, diabetes, and hyperthyroidism.
● Always check the patient's apical pulse before giving drug; if slower than 60 beats/minute, withhold drug and call the doctor.
● **I.V. use:** Give by slow I.V. injection, not to exceed 1 mg/minute. I.V. doses may be mixed with D_5W, 0.9% sodium chloride, or dextrose and sodium chloride solutions. Solution is stable for 48 hours after mixing.
● Monitor blood pressure frequently.
● Caution the patient that abrupt discontinuation of drug can exacerbate angina and MI. Drug should be withdrawn gradually over a 2-week period.
● Once-daily dosing encourages patient compliance. Counsel patients to take drug at the same time every day.
● Tell female patient to notify doctor if pregnancy occurs. Drug will need to be discontinued.

---

benazepril hydrochloride
Lotensin

Pregnancy Risk Category: C (D in 2nd and 3rd trimesters)

HOW SUPPLIED
Tablets: 5 mg, 10 mg, 20 mg, 40 mg

ACTION
Benazepril and its active metabolite, benazeprilat, inhibit ACE, preventing conversion of angiotensin I to angiotensin II, a potent vasoconstrictor. Reduced formation of angiotensin II decreases peripheral arterial resistance, thus decreasing aldosterone secretion. This reduces sodium and water retention and lowers blood pressure. Benazepril also has antihypertensive activity in patients with low-renin hypertension.

ONSET, PEAK, DURATION
Onset occurs within 1 hour. Peak effects occur within 2 to 4 hours. Effects persist 24 hours.

INDICATIONS & DOSAGE
Hypertension –
Adults: In a patient not receiving a diuretic, 10 mg P.O. daily initially. Dosage titrated as needed and tolerated; most patients take 20 to 40 mg daily in one or two doses. For patient receiving a diuretic, 5 mg P.O. daily.

ADVERSE REACTIONS
CNS: headache, dizziness, lightheadedness, anxiety, amnesia, depression, insomnia, nervousness, neuralgia, neuropathy, paresthesia, somnolence.
CV: symptomatic hypotension, syncope, angina, arrhythmias, palpitations.
EENT: dysphagia, increased salivation.
GI: nausea, vomiting, abdominal pain, constipation, dyspepsia, gastritis.
Respiratory: dry, persistent, tickling, nonproductive cough; dyspnea.
Skin: hypersensitivity reactions, rash, dermatitis, pruritus, photosensitivity, purpura.
Other: angioedema, arthralgia, arthritis, edema, impotence, increased diaphoresis, myalgia, weight gain, asthenia, hyperkalemia.

INTERACTIONS
Diuretics, other antihypertensives: risk of excessive hypotension. Discontinue diuretic or lower dose of benazepril as needed.
Lithium: increased serum lithium levels and lithium toxicity. Avoid concomitant use.
Potassium-sparing diuretics, potassium supplements, sodium substitutes containing potassium: risk of hyperkalemia. Monitor closely.

CONTRAINDICATIONS
Contraindicated in patients with hypersensitivity to ACE inhibitors.

NURSING CONSIDERATIONS
• Use cautiously in patients with impaired hepatic or renal function.
• Monitor for hypotension. Excessive hypotension can occur when drug is given with diuretics. If possible, diuretic therapy should be discontinued 2 to 3 days before starting benazepril to decrease potential for excessive hypotensive response. If benazepril does not adequately control blood pressure, diuretic may be reinstituted with care.
• Measure blood pressure when drug levels are at peak (2 to 6 hours after administration) and at trough (just before a dose) to verify adequate blood pressure control.
• Assess renal and hepatic function before and periodically throughout therapy. Monitor serum potassium levels, as ordered.
• Know that other ACE inhibitors have been associated with agranulocytosis and neutropenia. Monitor CBC with differential counts before therapy, every 2 weeks for the first 3 months of therapy, and periodically thereafter.
• Instruct patients to take this drug on an empty stomach; meals, particularly those that are high in fat, can impair absorption.
• Tell patients to avoid sodium substitutes; these products may contain potassium, which can cause hyperkalemia in patients taking this drug.
• Light-headedness can occur, especially during the first few days of therapy. Tell patients to rise slowly to minimize this effect and to report symptoms to doctor. Patients who experience syncope should stop taking the drug and call the doctor immediately.
• Tell patients to use caution in hot weather and during exercise. Inadequate fluid intake, vomiting, diarrhea,

---

*Liquid form contains alcohol.   *Common* reactions are in italics; ***life-threatening,*** in bold italics.
**May contain tartrazine.

and excessive perspiration can lead to light-headedness and syncope.
• Advise patients to report any signs of infection, such as fever and sore throat. Also tell patients to call the doctor if any of the following signs or symptoms occur: easy bruising or bleeding; swelling of tongue, lips, face, eyes, mucous membranes, or extremities; difficulty swallowing or breathing; and hoarseness.
• Tell female patient to notify doctor if pregnancy occurs. Drug will need to be discontinued.

betaxolol hydrochloride
Kerlone

Pregnancy Risk Category: C

HOW SUPPLIED
Tablets: 10 mg, 20 mg

ACTION
Unknown. A selective beta$_1$-adrenergic blocking agent that decreases blood pressure, possibly by slowing heart rate and decreasing cardiac output.

ONSET, PEAK, DURATION
Onset occurs within 3 hours. Serum levels peak within 2 to 4 hours after a dose. Peak antihypertensive effects occur after 7 to 14 days of therapy. Effects persist 24 to 48 hours.

INDICATIONS & DOSAGE
Hypertension (used alone or with other antihypertensives) –
Adults: initially, 10 mg P.O. once daily. If necessary, 20 mg P.O. once daily if desired response not achieved in 7 to 14 days.

ADVERSE REACTIONS
CV: bradycardia, chest pain, hypotension, worsening of angina, peripheral vascular insufficiency, *CHF,* edema, syncope, postural hypotension, conduction disturbances.

CNS: dizziness, fatigue, headache, lethargy, anxiety.
GI: flatulence, constipation, nausea, diarrhea, vomiting, anorexia, dry mouth.
Respiratory: dyspnea, wheezing, *bronchospasm.*
Skin: rash.

INTERACTIONS
Calcium channel blockers: increased risk of hypotension, left ventricular failure, and AV conduction disturbances. Use I.V. calcium channel blockers with caution.
Catecholamine-depleting drugs, reserpine: may have an additive effect.
General anesthetics: increased hypotensive effects. Observe carefully for excessive hypotension or bradycardia or orthostatic hypotension.
Lidocaine: may increase lidocaine's effects.

CONTRAINDICATIONS
Contraindicated in patients with hypersensitivity to the drug, severe bradycardia, greater than first-degree heart block, cardiogenic shock, or uncontrolled CHF.

NURSING CONSIDERATIONS
• Use cautiously in patients with CHF controlled by digitalis glycosides and diuretics because these patients may exhibit signs of cardiac decompensation with beta-blocker therapy.
• Monitor patient's blood pressure closely.
• Monitor blood glucose levels regularly in patients with diabetes. Beta blockade may inhibit glycogenolysis as well as the signs and symptoms of hypoglycemia (such as tachycardia and blood pressure changes).
• Know that withdrawal of beta-blocker therapy before surgery is controversial. Some clinicians advocate withdrawal to prevent any impairment of cardiac responsiveness to reflex stimuli and decreased responsiveness

to administration of catecholamines. Advise the anesthesiologist that the patient is receiving a beta blocker so that isoproterenol or dobutamine is made readily available for reversal of drug's cardiac effects.

• Beta blockers may mask tachycardia associated with hyperthyroidism. In patients with suspected thyrotoxicosis, withdraw beta blocker gradually, as ordered, to avoid thyroid storm.

• Advise patients that abrupt discontinuation of drug may precipitate angina pectoris in patients with unrecognized coronary artery disease.

• Emphasize the importance of promptly reporting signs of CHF, including shortness of breath or difficulty breathing, unusually fast heartbeat, cough, or fatigue with exertion.

bisoprolol fumarate
Zebeta

Pregnancy Risk Category: C

HOW SUPPLIED
Tablets: 5 mg, 10 mg

ACTION
Not completely defined. Bisoprolol is a beta$_1$-selective blocking agent that decreases myocardial contractility, heart rate, and cardiac output; lowers blood pressure; and reduces myocardial oxygen consumption.

ONSET, PEAK, DURATION
Onset unknown. Peak effects occur within 2 to 4 hours. Effects last about 24 hours.

INDICATIONS & DOSAGE
Hypertension (used alone or in combination with other antihypertensives) –
Adults: initially, 5 mg P.O. once daily. If response is inadequate, increased to 10 mg once daily or to 20 mg P.O. daily if needed. Maximum recommended dosage is 20 mg daily.

For patients with renal or hepatic impairment, 2.5 mg P.O. daily initially. Subsequent dosage titration is done cautiously.

ADVERSE REACTIONS
CNS: asthenia, fatigue, dizziness, headache, hypoesthesia, vivid dreams, depression, insomnia.
CV: bradycardia, peripheral edema, chest pain.
EENT: pharyngitis, rhinitis, sinusitis.
GI: nausea, vomiting, diarrhea, dry mouth.
Respiratory: cough, dyspnea.
Other: sweating, arthralgia.

INTERACTIONS
NSAIDs: decreased antihypertensive effect. Monitor blood pressure and adjust dosage.

CONTRAINDICATIONS
Contraindicated in patients with hypersensitivity to the drug and in those with cardiogenic shock, overt cardiac failure, marked sinus bradycardia, or second- or third-degree AV block.

NURSING CONSIDERATIONS
• Use cautiously in patients with bronchospastic disease. In general, these patients should avoid beta-adrenergic blockers because blockade of pulmonary beta$_2$-receptors may result in worsening of symptoms. For patients who cannot tolerate or do not respond to other antihypertensives, bisoprolol is given in low doses, starting therapy at 2.5 mg P.O. daily. Know that bisoprolol blocks beta$_2$-receptors in higher doses (20 mg daily or more).

• Also use cautiously in patients with diabetes, peripheral vascular disease, or thyroid disease and in those with a history of heart failure.

• Monitor blood pressure frequently.

• Monitor blood glucose levels in diabetic patients closely. Beta blockers

---

*Liquid form contains alcohol.
**May contain tartrazine.

Common reactions are in italics; *life-threatening,* in bold italics.

may mask some of the manifestations of hypoglycemia, such as tachycardia. Nonselective beta blockers can potentiate insulin-induced hypoglycemia and delay the recovery of serum glucose levels. Because bisoprolol is a selective agent, this problem is minimal.

• Teach the patient about his disease and therapy. Explain the importance of taking drug as prescribed, even when he's feeling well. Advise the patient that abrupt discontinuation of this drug can exacerbate angina and precipitate MI. Drug must be withdrawn gradually over 1 to 2 weeks. Instruct the patient to call the doctor if unpleasant adverse reactions occur.

• Warn diabetic patients to closely monitor blood glucose levels.

• Tell the patient to check with the doctor or pharmacist before taking OTC medications.

---

captopril

Apo-Capto†, Capoten, Novo-Captopril†, Syn-Captopril†

Pregnancy Risk Category: C (D in 2nd and 3rd trimesters)

HOW SUPPLIED
Tablets: 12.5 mg, 25 mg, 50 mg, 100 mg

ACTION
Not clearly defined. Thought to inhibit ACE, preventing conversion of angiotensin I to angiotensin II, a potent vasoconstrictor. Reduced formation of angiotensin II decreases peripheral arterial resistance, thus decreasing aldosterone secretion. This reduces sodium and water retention and lowers blood pressure.

ONSET, PEAK, DURATION
Onset occurs in 15 to 60 minutes. Peak effects occur in 30 to 90 minutes. Effects persist 6 to 12 hours.

INDICATIONS & DOSAGE
Hypertension –
Adults: 25 mg P.O. b.i.d. or t.i.d. initially. If blood pressure isn't satisfactorily controlled in 1 to 2 weeks, dosage increased to 50 mg b.i.d. or t.i.d. If not satisfactorily controlled after another 1 to 2 weeks, expect a diuretic to be added to the regimen. If further blood pressure reduction is necessary, dosage may be raised to as high as 150 mg t.i.d. while continuing the diuretic. Maximum dosage is 450 mg daily.
CHF; to reduce risk of death and to slow development of heart failure after MI –
Adults: 6.25 to 12.5 mg P.O. t.i.d. initially. Gradually increased to 50 mg t.i.d. as needed. Maximum daily dosage is 450 mg.
Diabetic nephropathy –
Adults: 25 mg P.O. t.i.d.

ADVERSE REACTIONS
CNS: dizziness, fainting.
CV: *tachycardia, hypotension,* angina pectoris, ***CHF,*** pericarditis.
GI: anorexia, *dysgeusia.*
GU: *proteinuria, nephrotic syndrome, membranous glomerulopathy, renal failure* (in patients with preexisting renal disease or patients receiving high dosages), urinary frequency.
Hematologic: *leukopenia, agranulocytosis, pancytopenia.*
Hepatic: transient increase in hepatic enzymes.
Respiratory: *dry, persistent, tickling, nonproductive cough.*
Skin: *urticarial rash, maculopapular rash,* pruritus.
Other: fever, angioedema of face and extremities, hyperkalemia.

INTERACTIONS
Antacids: decreased captopril effect. Separate administration times.
Digitalis glycosides: may increase serum digoxin concentration by 15% to 30%.

Diuretics, other antihypertensives: risk of excessive hypotension. Diuretic may need to be discontinued or captopril dosage lowered.

Insulin, oral antidiabetic agents: risk of hypoglycemia when captopril therapy is initiated. Monitor closely.

Lithium: increased lithium levels and symptoms of toxicity may occur. Monitor patient closely.

NSAIDs: may reduce antihypertensive effect. Monitor blood pressure.

Potassium supplements, potassium-sparing diuretics: increased risk of hyperkalemia. Avoid these agents unless hypokalemic blood levels are confirmed.

CONTRAINDICATIONS
Contraindicated in patients with hypersensitivity to the drug or any other ACE inhibitor.

NURSING CONSIDERATIONS
• Use cautiously in patients with impaired renal function or serious autoimmune disease (particularly systemic lupus erythematosus) or in patients who have been exposed to other drugs known to affect WBC counts or immune response.
• Monitor the patient's blood pressure and pulse rate frequently.
• Be aware that elderly patients may be more sensitive to the drug's hypotensive effects.
• Monitor WBC and differential counts before starting treatment, every 2 weeks for the first 3 months of therapy, and periodically thereafter, as ordered.
• Instruct patients to take this medication 1 hour before meals; food in the GI tract may reduce absorption.
• Inform patient that light-headedness can occur, especially during the first few days of therapy. Tell patients to rise slowly to minimize this effect and to report symptoms to the doctor. Patients who experience syncope

should stop taking the drug and call the doctor immediately.
• Tell patients to use caution in hot weather and during exercise. Inadequate fluid intake, vomiting, diarrhea, and excessive perspiration can lead to light-headedness and syncope.
• Advise patients to report any signs of infection, such as fever and sore throat.
• Tell female patient to notify doctor if pregnancy occurs. Drug will need to be discontinued.

carteolol
Cartrol

Pregnancy Risk Category: C

HOW SUPPLIED
Tablets: 2.5 mg, 5 mg

ACTION
Unknown. Carteolol is a nonselective beta-adrenergic blocker with intrinsic sympathomimetic activity. Its antihypertensive effects are probably caused by decreased sympathetic outflow from the brain and decreased cardiac output. Carteolol does not have a consistent effect on renin output.

ONSET, PEAK, DURATION
Onset and duration unknown. Serum levels peak within 1 to 3 hours.

INDICATIONS & DOSAGE
Hypertension –
Adults: initially, 2.5 mg P.O. as a single daily dose. Gradually increased to 5 or 10 mg as a single daily dose as needed. Dosages that exceed 10 mg daily do not produce a greater response and may actually decrease response.

In patients with substantial renal failure: If creatinine clearance is >60 ml/minute administer drug at 24-hour intervals; 20 to 60 ml/minute, administer drug at 48-hour intervals; <20 ml/minute, at 72-hour intervals.

ADVERSE REACTIONS
CNS: lassitude, tiredness, fatigue, somnolence, *asthenia*.
CV: conduction disturbances.
Other: *muscle cramps.*

INTERACTIONS
Calcium channel blockers: increased risk of hypotension, left ventricular failure, and AV conduction disturbances. Use I.V. calcium antagonists with caution.
Catecholamine-depleting drugs, reserpine: may have an additive effect.
Digitalis glycosides: may produce additive effects on slowing AV node conduction. Avoid concomitant use.
General anesthetics: increased hypotensive effects. Observe carefully for excessive hypotension or bradycardia or orthostatic hypotension.
Insulin, oral antidiabetic agents: may alter hypoglycemic response. Adjust dosage as necessary.

CONTRAINDICATIONS
Contraindicated in patients with bronchial asthma, severe bradycardia, greater than first-degree heart block, cardiogenic shock, or uncontrolled CHF.

NURSING CONSIDERATIONS
• Use cautiously in patients with CHF controlled by digitalis glycosides and diuretics because these patients may exhibit signs of cardiac decompensation with beta-blocker therapy.
• Monitor blood pressure frequently.
• Know that beta blockade may inhibit glycogenolysis and the signs and symptoms of hypoglycemia (such as tachycardia and blood pressure changes). It may also attenuate insulin release. Monitor blood glucose levels frequently.
• Know that withdrawal of beta-blocker therapy before surgery is controversial. Some clinicians advocate withdrawal to prevent any impairment of cardiac responsiveness to reflex stimuli and decreased responsiveness to administration of catecholamines. However, the beta-blocking effects of carteolol may persist for weeks, and discontinuing drug before surgery may be impractical. Advise the anesthesiologist that the patient is receiving a beta blocker so that isoproterenol or dobutamine is made readily available for reversal of the drug's cardiac effects.
• Beta blockers may mask tachycardia associated with hyperthyroidism. In patients with suspected thyrotoxicosis, withdraw beta blocker therapy as ordered gradually to avoid thyroid storm.
• Be aware that patients with unrecognized coronary artery disease may exhibit signs of angina pectoris on withdrawal of drug. Monitor closely.
• Emphasize the importance of reporting signs of CHF, including shortness of breath or difficulty breathing, unusually fast heartbeat, cough, or fatigue with exertion.

---

clonidine hydrochloride
Catapres, Catapres-TTS, Dixarit†‡
Pregnancy Risk Category: C

HOW SUPPLIED
Tablets: 0.025 mg†‡, 0.1 mg, 0.2 mg, 0.3 mg
Transdermal: TTS-1 (releases 0.1 mg/24 hours), TTS-2 (releases 0.2 mg/24 hours), TTS-3 (releases 0.3 mg/24 hours)

ACTION
Unknown. Thought to inhibit the central vasomotor centers, thereby decreasing sympathetic outflow to the heart, kidneys, and peripheral vasculature; this results in decreased peripheral vascular resistance, decreased systolic and diastolic blood

pressure, and decreased heart rate.

ONSET, PEAK, DURATION
Onset occurs within 15 to 30 minutes after oral administration, 2 to 3 days after transdermal application. Peak effects occur within 1.5 to 2.5 hours after oral dose, about 2 to 3 days after transdermal application. Effects persist 6 to 8 hours after an oral dose; effects gradually decline over several days after transdermal system removal.

INDICATIONS & DOSAGE
Essential, renal, and malignant hypertension –
Adults: initially, 0.1 mg P.O. b.i.d. Then increased by 0.1 to 0.2 mg daily on a weekly basis. Usual dosage range is 0.2 to 0.8 mg daily in divided doses; infrequently, dosages as high as 2.4 mg daily are used.

Or, transdermal patch is applied to a nonhairy area of intact skin on the upper arm or torso, once every 7 days. Started with 0.1-mg system and titrated with another 0.1-mg system or larger system is used.

ADVERSE REACTIONS
CNS: *drowsiness, dizziness,* fatigue, sedation, nervousness, headache, vivid dreams.
CV: orthostatic hypotension, bradycardia, ***severe rebound hypertension.***
GI: *constipation, dry mouth,* nausea, vomiting.
GU: urine retention, impotence.
Skin: *pruritus, dermatitis* (with transdermal patch).
Other: transient glucose intolerance (with large doses).

INTERACTIONS
CNS depressants: enhanced CNS depression. Use together cautiously.
MAO inhibitors, tricyclic antidepressants: may decrease antihypertensive effect. Use together cautiously.
Propranolol, other beta blockers: par-adoxical hypertensive response. Monitor carefully.

CONTRAINDICATIONS
Contraindicated in patients with hypersensitivity to the drug. Transdermal form is contraindicated in patients with hypersensitivity to any component of the adhesive layer of the transdermal system.

NURSING CONSIDERATIONS
• Use cautiously in patients with severe coronary insufficiency, recent MI, cerebrovascular disease, chronic renal failure, or impaired liver function.
• Know that clonidine may be given to rapidly lower blood pressure in some hypertensive emergency situations.
• Monitor blood pressure and pulse rate frequently. Dosage is usually adjusted to patient's blood pressure and tolerance.
• Elderly patients may be more sensitive to drug's hypotensive effects.
• Observe for patient tolerance to drug's therapeutic effects, which may require increased dosage.
• Antihypertensive effects of transdermal clonidine may take 2 to 3 days to become apparent. Oral antihypertensive therapy may have to be continued in the interim.
• Remove transdermal patch before defibrillation to prevent arcing.
• When stopping therapy in patients receiving both clonidine and a beta blocker, gradually withdraw the beta blocker first to minimize adverse reactions, as ordered.
• Be aware that discontinuation of clonidine for surgery is not recommended.
• Advise the patient that abrupt discontinuation of drug may cause severe rebound hypertension. Reduce dosage gradually over 2 to 4 days as ordered.
• Tell patients to take their last dose immediately before retiring.

---

*Liquid form contains alcohol.   *Common* reactions are in italics; *life-threatening,* in bold italics.
**May contain tartrazine.

• Reassure the patient that the transdermal patch usually adheres despite showering and other routine daily activities. Instruct him on the use of the adhesive "overlay" to provide additional skin adherence if necessary. Also tell the patient to place the patch at a different site each week.
• Caution the patient that drug can cause drowsiness, but that tolerance to this adverse effect will develop.
• Inform the patient that orthostatic hypotension can be minimized by rising slowly and avoiding sudden position changes.

---

diazoxide
Hyperstat IV

Pregnancy Risk Category: C

HOW SUPPLIED
Injection: 300 mg/20 ml, 15 mg/ml

ACTION
Exact antihypertensive action unknown. Directly relaxes arteriolar smooth muscle and decreases peripheral vascular resistance.

ONSET, PEAK, DURATION
Onset occurs within 1 minute after I.V. bolus. Peak effects occur within 2 to 5 minutes after I.V. bolus. Effects persist 2 to 12 hours.

INDICATIONS & DOSAGE
Hypertensive crisis –
Adults and children: 1 to 3 mg/kg by I.V. bolus (up to a maximum of 150 mg) q 5 to 15 minutes until adequate response is seen. Repeat at 4- to 24-hour intervals as needed.

ADVERSE REACTIONS
CNS: *headache,* dizziness, lightheadedness, euphoria, cerebral ischemia.
CV: *sodium and water retention, orthostatic hypotension,* diaphoresis, flushing, warmth, angina, myocardial ischemia, arrhythmias, ECG changes.
GI: *nausea, vomiting,* abdominal discomfort.
Other: inflammation and pain resulting from extravasation, *hyperglycemia,* hyperuricemia.

INTERACTIONS
Antihypertensives, such as hydralazine: may cause severe hypotension. Use together cautiously.
Thiazide diuretics: may increase diazoxide's effects. Use together cautiously.

CONTRAINDICATIONS
Contraindicated in patients with hypersensitivity to the drug, other thiazides, or other sulfonamide-derived drugs. Also contraindicated in the treatment of compensatory hypertension (such as that associated with coarctation of the aorta or arteriovenous shunt).

NURSING CONSIDERATIONS
• Use cautiously in patients with impaired cerebral or cardiac function or uremia.
• **I.V. use:** Monitor blood pressure and ECG continuously. Place the patient in the supine position or in Trendelenburg's position during and for 1 hour after infusion. Notify the doctor immediately if severe hypotension develops. Keep norepinephrine available.
• Take care to avoid extravasation.
• Check the patient's standing blood pressure before discontinuing close monitoring for hypotension.
• Monitor the patient's fluid intake and output carefully. If fluid or sodium retention develops, the doctor may order diuretics.
• Weigh the patient daily and notify the doctor of any weight increase.
• Diazoxide may alter requirements for insulin, diet, or oral antidiabetic agents in previously controlled dia-

---

betic patients. Monitor blood glucose daily; watch closely for signs of severe hyperglycemia or hyperosmolar nonketotic syndrome. Insulin may be needed.
• Check the patient's uric acid levels frequently and report abnormalities to the doctor.
• Protect I.V. solutions from light. Darkened I.V. solutions of diazoxide are subpotent and should not be used.
• Inform the patient that orthostatic hypotension can be minimized by rising slowly and avoiding sudden position changes. Instruct the patient to remain in the supine position for 30 minutes after injection.

---

doxazosin mesylate
Cardura

Pregnancy Risk Category: C

HOW SUPPLIED
Tablets: 1 mg, 2 mg, 4 mg, 8 mg

ACTION
An alpha-adrenergic blocker that acts on the peripheral vasculature to produce vasodilation.

ONSET, PEAK, DURATION
Onset occurs in 1 to 2 hours. Peak antihypertensive effect occurs within 5 to 6 hours. Effects persist about 24 hours.

INDICATIONS & DOSAGE
Essential hypertension –
Adults: initially, 1 mg P.O. daily and determine effect on standing and supine blood pressure at 2 to 6 hours and 24 hours after dosing. If necessary, dose is increased to 2 mg daily. To minimize adverse reactions, dosage is titrated slowly (dosage typically increased only q 2 weeks). If necessary, dose increased to 4 mg daily, then 8 mg. Maximum daily dosage is 16 mg, but dosage that exceeds 4 mg daily is

associated with a greater incidence of adverse reactions.

ADVERSE REACTIONS
CNS: dizziness, vertigo, headache, somnolence, drowsiness, fatigue, malaise, syncope, paresthesia.
CV: *orthostatic hypotension,* hypotension, edema, palpitations, ***arrhythmias,*** tachycardia, peripheral ischemia.
GI: nausea, vomiting, diarrhea, constipation.
Skin: rash, pruritus.
Other: rhinitis, arthralgia, myalgia, muscle weakness.

INTERACTIONS
None significant.

CONTRAINDICATIONS
Contraindicated in patients with hypersensitivity to the drug and quinazoline derivatives (including prazosin and terazosin).

NURSING CONSIDERATIONS
• Use cautiously in patients with impaired hepatic function.
• Monitor blood pressure closely.
• If syncope occurs, place the patient in a recumbent position and treat supportively. A transient hypotensive response is not considered a contraindication to continued therapy.
• Advise patients taking doxazosin that they are susceptible to a "first-dose" effect similar to that produced by other alpha-adrenergic blockers—marked orthostatic hypotension accompanied by dizziness or syncope. Orthostatic hypotension is most common after first dose, but can also occur when therapy is interrupted for a few days and during dosage adjustment periods. Warn patients that dizziness or fainting may occur. Advise them to avoid driving and other hazardous activities or situations until drug's adverse CNS effects are known.

---

enalaprilat
Vasotec I.V.

enalapril maleate
Amprace‡, Renitec‡, Vasotec

Pregnancy Risk Category: C (D in 2nd and 3rd trimesters)

HOW SUPPLIED
Tablets: 2.5 mg, 5 mg, 10 mg, 20 mg
Injection: 1.25 mg/ml

ACTION
Unknown, but does inhibit ACE, preventing conversion of angiotensin I to angiotensin II, a potent vasoconstrictor. Reduced formation of angiotensin II decreases peripheral arterial resistance, thus decreasing aldosterone secretion.

ONSET, PEAK, DURATION
Onset occurs 15 minutes after I.V. injection, 1 hour after oral dose. Peak effects occur 1 to 4 hours after I.V. injection or 4 to 6 hours after oral dose. Effects persist about 6 hours after I.V. injection or 24 hours after oral dose.

INDICATIONS & DOSAGE
Hypertension –
Adults: for patient not receiving diuretics, initially 5 mg P.O. once daily, then adjusted according to response. Usual dosage range is 10 to 40 mg daily as a single dose or two divided doses. Alternatively, 1.25 mg I.V. infusion q 6 hours over 5 minutes. For patient on diuretics, initially 2.5 mg P.O. once daily. Alternatively, 0.625 mg I.V. over 5 minutes, repeated in 1 hour if needed, then followed by 1.25 mg I.V. q 6 hours.
To convert from I.V. therapy to oral therapy –
Adults: initially, 5 mg P.O. once daily; if patient was receiving 0.625 mg I.V. then 2.5 mg P.O. once daily. Dosage is adjusted to response.

To convert from oral therapy to I.V. therapy –
Adults: 1.25 mg I.V. over 5 minutes q 6 hours. Higher doses have not demonstrated greater efficacy.
Renal impairment or hyponatremia –
If serum creatinine is above 1.6 mg/dl or serum sodium is below 130 mEq/L, dosage is initiated at 2.5 mg P.O. daily and titrated slowly.

ADVERSE REACTIONS
CNS: *headache, dizziness, light-headedness, fatigue,* insomnia.
CV: *hypotension.*
GI: diarrhea, nausea.
GU: decreased renal function (in patients with bilateral renal artery stenosis or CHF).
Hematologic: *neutropenia, agranulocytosis.*
Respiratory: *dry, persistent, tickling, nonproductive cough.*
Skin: rash.
Other: *angioedema.*

INTERACTIONS
Insulin, oral antidiabetic agents: risk of hypoglycemia, especially at initiation of enalapril therapy. Monitor closely.
Lithium: lithium toxicity can occur. Monitor lithium levels.
NSAIDs: may reduce antihypertensive effect. Monitor blood pressure.
Potassium supplements, potassium-sparing diuretics: increased risk of hyperkalemia. Avoid these drugs unless hypokalemic blood levels are confirmed.

CONTRAINDICATIONS
Contraindicated in patients with hypersensitivity to the drug or history of angioedema related to previous treatment with an ACE inhibitor.

NURSING CONSIDERATIONS
• Use cautiously in patients with renal impairment.
• **I.V. use:** Inject drug slowly over at

---

least 5 minutes, or dilute in 50 ml of a compatible solution and infuse over 15 minutes. Compatible solutions include D₅W, 0.9% sodium chloride injection, dextrose 5% in lactated Ringer's injection, and dextrose 5% in 0.9% sodium chloride injection.

- Monitor blood pressure response to drug closely.
- Monitor CBC with differential counts before therapy, every 2 weeks for the first 3 months of therapy, and periodically thereafter.
- Diabetic patients, those with impaired renal function or CHF, and those receiving drugs that can increase serum potassium may develop hyperkalemia. Monitor potassium intake and serum potassium level.
- Advise the patient to report any signs or symptoms of angioedema, such as swelling of face, eyes, lips, or tongue or breathing difficulty. Angioedema (including laryngeal edema) may occur, especially after the first dose.
- Advise the patient to report any signs of infection, such as fever and sore throat.
- Advise the patient that light-headedness can occur, especially during the first few days of therapy. Tell the patient to rise slowly to minimize this effect and to report symptoms to the doctor. Patients who experience syncope should stop taking drug and call the doctor immediately.
- Tell the patient to use caution in hot weather and during exercise. Inadequate fluid intake, vomiting, diarrhea, and excessive perspiration can lead to light-headedness and syncope.
- Advise the patient to avoid sodium substitutes; these products may contain potassium, which can cause hyperkalemia in patients taking this drug.
- Tell female patient to notify doctor if pregnancy occurs. Drug will need to be discontinued.

felodipine
Agon‡, Agon SR‡, Plendil, Plendil ER‡, Renedil†

Pregnancy Risk Category: C

HOW SUPPLIED
Tablets: 5 mg‡
Tablets (extended-release): 5 mg, 10 mg

ACTION
Unknown. A dihydropyridine-derivative calcium channel blocker that prevents the entry of calcium ions into vascular smooth-muscle and cardiac cells; shows some selectivity for smooth muscle as compared with cardiac muscle.

ONSET, PEAK, DURATION
Onset occurs within 2 to 5 hours. Plasma levels peak within 2½ to 5 hours. Effects persist 24 hours.

INDICATIONS & DOSAGE
Hypertension –
Adults: initially, 5 mg P.O. daily. Dosage is adjusted according to patient response, generally at intervals not less than 2 weeks. Usual dose is 5 to 10 mg daily; maximum recommended dosage is 20 mg daily.

In elderly patients and patients with impaired hepatic function, 5 mg P.O. daily; dosage is adjusted as for adults. Maximum recommended dosage is 10 mg daily.

ADVERSE REACTIONS
CNS: headache, dizziness, paresthesia, asthenia.
CV: *peripheral edema,* chest pain, palpitations, increased heart rate.
EENT: rhinorrhea, pharyngitis.
GI: dyspepsia, abdominal pain, nausea, constipation, diarrhea.
Respiratory: upper respiratory infection, cough.
Skin: rash, *flushing.*

---

*Liquid form contains alcohol.   *Common* reactions are in italics; *life-threatening,* in bold italics.
**May contain tartrazine.

Other: muscle cramps, back pain, gingival hyperplasia.

INTERACTIONS
Anticonvulsants: decreased plasma concentration of felodipine. Avoid concomitant use.
Cimetidine: decreased clearance of felodipine. Use lower doses of felodipine.
Digoxin: decreased peak levels of digoxin, but total absorbed drug is unchanged. Clinical significance is unknown.
Metoprolol: may alter pharmacokinetics of metoprolol. No dosage adjustment appears necessary; monitor for adverse effects.

CONTRAINDICATIONS
Contraindicated in patients with hypersensitivity to the drug.

NURSING CONSIDERATIONS
• Use cautiously in patients with heart failure, particularly those receiving beta-adrenergic blockers, and in patients with impaired hepatic function because clearance of drug from the blood is dependent on the liver.
• Monitor blood pressure for response.
• Monitor patient for periperhal edema. Peripheral edema appears to be both dose- and age-dependent: it's more common in patients taking higher doses, especially those over age 60.
• Tell the patient to swallow tablets whole and not to crush or chew them.
• Teach patient to continue taking the drug even when he feels better; to watch his diet; and to check with the doctor or pharmacist before taking any other medications, including OTC drugs.
• Patients should be advised to observe good oral hygiene and to see a dentist regularly because use of drug

has been associated with mild gingival hyperplasia.

---

fosinopril sodium
Monopril

Pregnancy Risk Category: C in 1st trimester, D in 2nd and 3rd trimesters

HOW SUPPLIED
Tablets: 10 mg, 20 mg

ACTION
Antihypertensive action not clearly defined. Inhibits ACE, preventing conversion of angiotensin I to angiotensin II, a potent vasoconstrictor. Reduced formation of angiotensin II decreases peripheral arterial resistance, thus decreasing aldosterone secretion.

ONSET, PEAK, DURATION
Onset occurs within 1 hour. Serum levels peak in 2 to 6 hours. Effects persist about 24 hours.

INDICATIONS & DOSAGE
Hypertension –
Adults: initially, 10 mg P.O. daily. Dosage is adjusted based on blood pressure response at peak and trough levels. Usual dosage is 20 to 40 mg, up to 80 mg daily. Dosage is divided if needed.

ADVERSE REACTIONS
CNS: headache, dizziness, fatigue, light-headedness, syncope, memory disturbances, mood changes, paresthesia, sleep disturbance, drowsiness, weakness, *CVA.*
CV: chest pain, angina, *MI, hypertensive crisis,* rhythm disturbances, palpitations, hypotension, flushing, claudication, orthostatic hypotension.
EENT: tinnitus, vision disturbances, eye irritation, epistaxis, pharyngitis, sinusitis, rhinitis.
GI: nausea, vomiting, diarrhea, pan-

---

creatitis, hepatitis, dysphagia, dry mouth, abdominal distention, abdominal pain, flatulence, constipation, heartburn, appetite change, weight change.
GU: sexual dysfunction, decreased libido, urinary frequency, renal insufficiency.
Respiratory: *dry, persistent, tickling, nonproductive cough; bronchospasm;* laryngitis; hoarseness.
Skin: urticaria, rash, photosensitivity, pruritus.
Other: *angioedema,* fever, arthralgia, musculoskeletal pain, myalgia, jaundice, gout, hyperkalemia.

INTERACTIONS
Antacids: may impair absorption. Separate administration times by at least 2 hours.
Diuretics, other antihypertensives: risk of excessive hypotension. Diuretic may need to be discontinued or fosinopril dosage may need to be lowered.
Lithium: increased serum lithium levels and lithium toxicity. Avoid concomitant use.
Potassium-sparing diuretics, potassium supplements, sodium substitutes containing potassium: risk of hyperkalemia. Monitor during concomitant use.

CONTRAINDICATIONS
Contraindicated in patients with hypersensitivity to this drug or other ACE inhibitors and in breast-feeding patients.

NURSING CONSIDERATIONS
• Use cautiously in patients with impaired renal or hepatic function.
• Monitor blood pressure for effect.
• Monitor potassium intake and serum potassium level. Diabetic patients, those with impaired renal function, and those receiving drugs that can increase serum potassium may develop hyperkalemia.

• Other ACE inhibitors have been associated with agranulocytosis and neutropenia. Monitor CBC with differential counts before therapy, every 2 weeks for the first 3 months of therapy, and periodically thereafter, as ordered.
• Assess renal and hepatic function before and periodically throughout therapy.
• Tell the patient to avoid sodium substitutes; these products may contain potassium, which can cause hyperkalemia in patients taking this drug.
• Advise the patient to report any signs of infection, such as fever and sore throat.
• Also tell the patient to call the doctor if any of the following signs or symptoms occur: easy bruising or bleeding; swelling of tongue, lips, face, eyes, mucous membranes, or extremities; difficulty swallowing or breathing; and hoarseness.
• Tell patient to use caution in hot weather and during exercise. Inadequate fluid intake, vomiting, diarrhea, and excessive perspiration can lead to light-headedness and syncope.
• Tell female patient to notify doctor if pregnancy occurs. Drug will need to be discontinued.

guanabenz acetate
Wytensin

Pregnancy Risk Category: C

HOW SUPPLIED
Tablets: 4 mg, 8 mg

ACTION
Unknown. A centrally acting antihypertensive, its action is thought to be due to central alpha-adrenergic stimulation, which results in decreased sympathetic outflow to the heart, kidneys, and peripheral vasculature.

---

*Liquid form contains alcohol.   *Common* reactions are in italics; *life-threatening,* in bold italics.
**May contain tartrazine.

ONSET, PEAK, DURATION
Onset occurs within 1 hour. Peak effects occur within 2 to 5 hours. Effects persist about 12 hours.

INDICATIONS & DOSAGE
Hypertension –
Adults: initially, 4 mg P.O. b.i.d. Dosage increased in increments of 4 to 8 mg/day q 1 to 2 weeks. Maximum daily dosage is 32 mg b.i.d. To ensure adequate overnight blood pressure control, give last dose h.s.

ADVERSE REACTIONS
CNS: *drowsiness, sedation, dizziness, weakness,* headache, ataxia, depression.
CV: *severe rebound hypertension.*
GI: *dry mouth.*
GU: sexual dysfunction.

INTERACTIONS
CNS depressants: may cause increased sedation. Use together cautiously.
Tricyclic antidepressants, MAO inhibitors: may decrease antihypertensive effect.

CONTRAINDICATIONS
Contraindicated in patients with hypersensitivity to the drug.

NURSING CONSIDERATIONS
• Use cautiously in patients with severe coronary insufficiency, recent MI, cerebrovascular disease, or severe hepatic or renal failure. Also use cautiously in elderly patients.
• Caution the patient that abrupt discontinuation of drug may cause rebound hypertension.
• Monitor blood pressure for effects. Elderly patients may be more sensitive to drug's hypotensive effects.
• Advise the patient to avoid driving and other hazardous tasks that require alertness until drug's CNS effects are known.
• Inform the patient that orthostatic

hypotension can be minimized by rising slowly and avoiding sudden position changes. Dry mouth can be relieved with chewing gum, sour hard candy, or ice chips.
• Warn the patient that tolerance to alcohol or other CNS depressants may be diminished.

---

guanadrel sulfate
Hylorel

Pregnancy Risk Category: B

HOW SUPPLIED
Tablets: 10 mg, 25 mg

ACTION
Acts peripherally, inhibiting norepinephrine release and depleting norepinephrine stores in adrenergic nerve endings.

ONSET, PEAK, DURATION
Onset occurs in 2 hours. Peak effects occur within 4 to 6 hours. Effects persist 4 to 14 hours.

INDICATIONS & DOSAGE
Hypertension –
Adults: initially, 5 mg P.O. b.i.d. Dosage adjusted until blood pressure is controlled. Most patients require dosages of 20 to 75 mg/day, usually given b.i.d.; however, tolerance to hypotensive effect may necessitate upward titration of dosage to 100 to 400 mg daily in three to four divided doses.

In patients with renal impairment, dosage is reduced to 5 mg P.O. once daily if creatinine clearance is 30 to 60 ml/minute; if creatinine clearance is < 30 ml/minute, increase dosage interval to 48 hours. Dosage is adjusted every 7 to 14 days.

ADVERSE REACTIONS
CNS: *fatigue, dizziness,* drowsiness, faintness.
CV: *orthostatic hypotension,* edema.

GI: diarrhea, dry mouth.
GU: impotence, ejaculation disturbances.

INTERACTIONS
Amphetamines, ephedrine, methylphenidate, norepinephrine, phenothiazines, tricyclic antidepressants: may inhibit guanadrel's antihypertensive effect. Adjust dose accordingly.
Diuretics, other antihypertensives: hypotensive effect of guanadrel increased. Monitor blood pressure closely.
MAO inhibitors: antagonized hypotensive effects of guanadrel. Don't give guanadrel concurrently or within 1 week of MAO inhibitor therapy.

CONTRAINDICATIONS
Contraindicated in patients with hypersensitivity to the drug, known or suspected pheochromocytoma, or frank CHF.

NURSING CONSIDERATIONS
• Use cautiously in patients with regional vascular disease, bronchial asthma, or history of peptic ulcer disease.
• Monitor both supine and standing blood pressure, especially during dosage adjustment periods.
• Be aware that elderly patients may be more sensitive to drug's hypotensive effects.
• Know that guanadrel should be discontinued 48 to 72 hours before surgery to minimize risk of vascular collapse during anesthesia.
• Inform the patient that orthostatic hypotension can be minimized by rising slowly from a supine position and by avoiding sudden position changes. Dry mouth can be relieved with chewing gum, sour hard candy, or ice chips.
• Warn the patient to avoid strenuous exercise and hot showers; these may cause a hypotensive reaction. An ambient temperature that is too hot also

may potentiate the hypotensive effects of guanadrel.

guanethidine monosulfate
Apo-Guanethidine†, Ismelin
Pregnancy Risk Category: B

HOW SUPPLIED
Tablets: 10 mg, 25 mg

ACTION
An adrenergic neuron blocker that acts peripherally, inhibiting norepinephrine release and depleting norepinephrine stores in adrenergic nerve endings. This reduces arteriolar vasoconstriction.

ONSET, PEAK, DURATION
Onset unknown. Serum levels peak within 8 hours after single dose. Effects persist 3 to 4 days; blood pressure returns to pretreatment levels in 1 to 3 weeks.

INDICATIONS & DOSAGE
Moderate to severe hypertension and renal hypertension –
Adults: initially, 10 mg P.O. daily. Increase by 10 mg at weekly to monthly intervals, p.r.n. Usual dosage is 25 to 50 mg daily. Some patients may require up to 300 mg daily.

ADVERSE REACTIONS
CNS: *dizziness, weakness, syncope.*
CV: *orthostatic hypotension, bradycardia,* **CHF, arrhythmias.**
EENT: *nasal stuffiness.*
GI: *diarrhea,* dry mouth.
Other: *edema, weight gain, inhibition of ejaculation.*

INTERACTIONS
Ethanol, levodopa: may increase hypotensive effect of guanethidine. Use together cautiously.
Amphetamines, ephedrine, MAO inhibitors, methylphenidate, norepinephrine, phenothiazines, tricyclic

---

antidepressants: may inhibit guanethidine's antihypertensive effect. Adjust dose accordingly.

CONTRAINDICATIONS
Contraindicated in patients with pheochromocytoma, frank CHF, and hypersensitivity to guanethidine.

NURSING CONSIDERATIONS
• Use cautiously in patients with severe cardiac disease, recent MI, cerebrovascular disease, peptic ulceration, impaired renal function, or bronchial asthma and in those taking other antihypertensives.
• Monitor blood pressure for effect, especially during dosage adjustment periods.
• Elderly patients may be more sensitive to drug's hypotensive effects.
• Know that drug should be discontinued 2 to 3 weeks before elective surgery to reduce the possibility of vascular collapse and cardiac arrest during anesthesia.
• Know that if the patient develops diarrhea, the doctor may prescribe atropine or paregoric.
• Inform the patient that orthostatic hypotension can be minimized by rising slowly and avoiding sudden position changes. Dry mouth can be relieved with chewing gum, sour hard candy, or ice chips.
• Patients should receive instruction on a low-sodium diet. Monitor for possible weight gain and edema.
• Warn the patient to avoid strenuous exercise and hot showers; these may cause a hypotensive reaction. An ambient temperature that is too hot also may potentiate the hypotensive effects of guanethidine.

guanfacine hydrochloride
Tenex

Pregnancy Risk Category: B

HOW SUPPLIED
Tablets: 1 mg, 2 mg

ACTION
Unknown. Thought to be due to inhibition of the central vasomotor center, thereby decreasing sympathetic outflow to the heart, kidneys, and peripheral vasculature. This decreases blood pressure.

ONSET, PEAK, DURATION
Onset unknown. Serum levels peak in 1 to 4 hours. Effects persist 24 hours.

INDICATIONS & DOSAGE
Hypertension –
Adults: initially, 1 mg P.O. daily h.s. Dosage may be increased to 2 mg P.O. h.s. after 3 to 4 weeks, as needed. Dosage may be further increased to 3 mg P.O. h.s. after an additional 3 to 4 weeks, as needed. Average dosage is 1 to 3 mg daily.

ADVERSE REACTIONS
CNS: *drowsiness, dizziness,* fatigue, headache, insomnia.
CV: bradycardia, orthostatic hypotension, rebound hypertension.
GI: *constipation,* diarrhea, nausea, dry mouth.
Skin: dermatitis, pruritus.

INTERACTIONS
None significant.

CONTRAINDICATIONS
Contraindicated in patients with hypersensitivity to the drug.

NURSING CONSIDERATIONS
• Use cautiously in patients with severe coronary insufficiency, recent MI, cerebrovascular disease, or chronic renal or hepatic insufficiency.
• Monitor blood pressure frequently for effects.
• Be aware that the incidence and severity of adverse reactions increase with higher dosages.

• Know that guanfacine may be used alone or with a diuretic.
• Tell the patient not to discontinue therapy abruptly. Rebound hypertension is less common than with similar drugs, such as clonidine, but may occur.
• Because guanfacine causes drowsiness, advise the patient to avoid activities that require alertness until response to drug is established.

---

hydralazine hydrochloride
Alphapress‡, Apresoline**, Novo-Hylazin†

Pregnancy Risk Category: C

HOW SUPPLIED
Tablets: 10 mg, 25 mg, 50 mg, 100 mg
Injection: 20 mg/ml

ACTION
Unknown. A direct-acting vasodilator, its predominant effect relaxes arteriolar smooth muscle.

ONSET, PEAK, DURATION
Onset occurs within 5 minutes of I.V. injection, 20 to 30 minutes of oral dose, unknown after I.M. administration. Peak effects occur 15 to 30 minutes after I.V. administration or 1 to 2 hours after oral dose. Unknown after I.M. administration. Effects persist 3 to 8 hours.

INDICATIONS & DOSAGE
Essential hypertension (orally, alone or in combination with other antihypertensives); severe essential hypertension (parenterally, to lower blood pressure quickly) –
Adults: *oral* – initially, 10 mg P.O. q.i.d.; gradually increased to 50 mg q.i.d. as needed. Maximum recommended dosage is 200 mg daily, but some patients may require 300 to 400 mg daily.
I.V. – 10 to 20 mg given slowly and

repeated as necessary. Switched to oral antihypertensives as soon as possible.
I.M. – 10 to 50 mg, repeated as necessary. Switched to oral form as soon as possible.

ADVERSE REACTIONS
CNS: peripheral neuritis, *headache, dizziness.*
CV: orthostatic hypotension, *tachycardia,* arrhythmias, *angina, palpitations, sodium retention.*
GI: *nausea, vomiting, diarrhea, anorexia.*
Hematologic: neutropenia, leukopenia.
Skin: rash.
Other: *lupuslike syndrome* (especially with high doses), *weight gain.*

INTERACTIONS
Diazoxide, MAO inhibitors: may cause severe hypotension. Use together cautiously.

CONTRAINDICATIONS
Contraindicated in patients with hypersensitivity to the drug, coronary artery disease, or mitral valvular rheumatic heart disease.

NURSING CONSIDERATIONS
• Use cautiously in patients with suspected cardiac disease, CVA, or severe renal impairment and in those taking other antihypertensives.
• **I.V. use:** Give slowly and repeat as necessary, generally every 4 to 6 hours. Hydralazine will undergo color changes in most infusion solutions; these color changes do not indicate loss of potency. Compatible with 0.9% sodium chloride, Ringer's and lactated Ringer's solutions, and several other common I.V. solutions. Drug may undergo a reaction with dextrose. The manufacturer does not recommend mixing the drug in infusion solutions. Check with the phar-

---

*Liquid form contains alcohol.
**May contain tartrazine.
Common reactions are in italics; ***life-threatening,*** in bold italics.

macist for additional compatibility information.

• Monitor the patient's blood pressure, pulse rate, and body weight frequently. Some clinicians combine hydralazine therapy with diuretics and beta-adrenergic blockers to decrease sodium retention and tachycardia and to prevent anginal attacks.

• Be aware that elderly patients may be more sensitive to drug's hypotensive effects.

• Monitor CBC, lupus erythematosus cell preparation, and antinuclear antibody titer determination before therapy and periodically during long-term therapy, as ordered.

• Watch the patient closely for signs of lupuslike syndrome (sore throat, fever, muscle and joint aches, skin rash). Call the doctor immediately if any of these develop.

• Compliance may be improved by administering drug b.i.d. Check with the doctor.

• Instruct the patient to take oral form with meals to increase absorption.

• Inform the patient that orthostatic hypotension can be minimized by rising slowly and avoiding sudden position changes.

---

isradipine
DynaCirc

Pregnancy Risk Category: C

HOW SUPPLIED
Capsules: 2.5 mg, 5 mg

ACTION
Unknown. A calcium channel blocker that inhibits calcium ion influx across cardiac and smooth-muscle cells and is thought to decrease arteriolar resistance and blood pressure.

ONSET, PEAK, DURATION
Onset occurs within 20 minutes. Serum levels peak within 1½ hours. Effects persist more than 12 hours.

INDICATIONS & DOSAGE
Essential hypertension –
Adults: initially, 2.5 mg P.O. b.i.d., alone or with a thiazide diuretic. Dosage increased by gradual titration. If response is inadequate after first 2 to 4 weeks, dosage increased to 5 mg b.i.d., then increased at 5-mg daily intervals q 2 to 4 weeks to a maximum of 20 mg b.i.d.

ADVERSE REACTIONS
CNS: dizziness.
CV: edema, flushing, palpitations, tachycardia, orthostatic hypotension.
GI: nausea, diarrhea.
GU: frequent urination.
Respiratory: dyspnea.
Skin: rash.

INTERACTIONS
Fentanyl anesthesia: severe hypotension has been reported with concomitant use of a beta blocker and a calcium channel blocker.

CONTRAINDICATIONS
Contraindicated in patients with hypersensitivity to the drug.

NURSING CONSIDERATIONS
• Use cautiously in patients with CHF, especially if combined with a beta blocker.

• Monitor patient for adverse reactions. Like other calcium channel blockers, isradipine is known to cause symptomatic hypotension; however, syncope and severe dizziness have not been reported. Most adverse reactions are mild and transient and related to vasodilation (dizziness, edema, flushing, palpitations, and tachycardia).

• Monitor blood pressure closely.

• Before surgery, inform the anesthesiologist that the patient is taking a calcium channel blocker.

• Tell patients isradipine has some diuretic activity. Patients may note an increased need to void.

---

labetalol hydrochloride
Normodyne, Presolol‡, Trandate

Pregnancy Risk Category: C

HOW SUPPLIED
Tablets: 100 mg, 200 mg, 300 mg
Injection: 5 mg/ml

ACTION
Unknown. May be related to reduced peripheral vascular resistance as a result of alpha-adrenergic blockade.

ONSET, PEAK, DURATION
Onset occurs 2 to 5 minutes after I.V. administration, within 20 minutes after oral dose. Peak effects occur within 5 minutes of I.V. administration, 2 to 4 hours of oral dose. Effects persist 2 to 4 hours after I.V. dose and 12 to 24 hours after oral dose.

INDICATIONS & DOSAGE
Hypertension –
Adults: 100 mg P.O. b.i.d. with or without a diuretic. If needed, dosage is increased to 200 mg b.i.d. after 2 days. Further increases may be made q 2 to 3 days until optimum response is reached. Usual maintenance dosage is 200 to 400 mg b.i.d.
Severe hypertension and hypertensive emergencies –
Adults: 200 mg diluted in 160 ml of D$_5$W, infused at 2 mg/minute until satisfactory response is obtained, then infusion stopped. May be repeated q 6 to 12 hours.
  Alternatively, administered by repeated I.V. injection: Initially, 20 mg I.V. slowly over 2 minutes. Then repeat injections of 40 to 80 mg q 10 minutes until maximum dosage of 300 mg is reached, as needed.

ADVERSE REACTIONS
CNS: vivid dreams, fatigue, headache, transient scalp tingling.
CV: *orthostatic hypotension and diz-*

ziness, peripheral vascular disease, bradycardia.
EENT: nasal stuffiness.
GI: nausea, vomiting, diarrhea.
GU: sexual dysfunction, urine retention.
Respiratory: increased airway resistance.
Skin: rash.

INTERACTIONS
Cimetidine: may enhance labetalol's effect. Give together cautiously.
Halothane: additive hypotensive effect.
Insulin, oral antidiabetic agents: can alter dosage requirements in previously stabilized diabetic patients. Observe the patient carefully.

CONTRAINDICATIONS
Contraindicated in patients with bronchial asthma, overt cardiac failure, greater than first-degree heart block, cardiogenic shock, severe bradycardia, other conditions associated with severe and prolonged hypotension, and hypersensitivity to the drug.

NURSING CONSIDERATIONS
● Use cautiously in patients with CHF, hepatic failure, chronic bronchitis, emphysema, preexisting peripheral vascular disease, and pheochromocytoma.
● **I.V. use:** Administer labetalol injection with an infusion control device. Monitor blood pressure closely: every 5 minutes for 30 minutes, then every 30 minutes for 2 hours, then hourly for 6 hours. The patient should remain in a supine position for 3 hours after infusion.
● Be aware that sodium bicarbonate injection is incompatible with I.V. labetalol.
● Monitor blood pressure frequently. Know that drug masks common signs of shock.
● Be aware that when administered intravenously for hypertensive emer-

---

gencies, labetalol produces a rapid, predictable fall in blood pressure within 5 to 10 minutes.
• If dizziness occurs, ask doctor if patient may take a dose at bedtime or take smaller doses t.i.d. to help minimize this adverse reaction.
• Monitor blood glucose levels in diabetic patients closely because beta blockers may mask certain signs and symptoms of hypoglycemia.
• Tell the patient that abrupt discontinuation of therapy can exacerbate angina and precipitate MI.
• Dizziness is the most troublesome adverse reaction and tends to occur in early stages of treatment, in patients also receiving diuretics, and in those receiving higher dosages. Inform the patient that this can be minimized by rising slowly and avoiding sudden position changes.

lisinopril
Prinivil, Zestril

Pregnancy Risk Category: C (D in 2nd and 3rd trimesters)

HOW SUPPLIED
Tablets: 2.5 mg, 5 mg, 10 mg, 20 mg, 40 mg

ACTION
Unknown. Thought to result primarily from suppression of the renin-angiotensin-aldosterone system.

ONSET, PEAK, DURATION
Onset occurs within 1 hour. Plasma levels peak within 7 hours. Effects persist 24 hours.

INDICATIONS & DOSAGE
Hypertension –
Adults: initially, 10 mg P.O. daily for the patient not receiving a diuretic; 5 mg P.O. daily for the patient receiving a diuretic. Most patients are well controlled on 20 to 40 mg daily as a single dose.

Treatment adjunct in heart failure (with diuretics and digitalis) –
Adults: initially, 5 mg P.O. daily. Increased as needed to a maximum of 20 mg P.O. daily.

ADVERSE REACTIONS
CNS: *dizziness, headache, fatigue,* depression, somnolence, paresthesia.
CV: hypotension, *orthostatic hypotension,* chest pain.
EENT: *nasal congestion.*
GI: *diarrhea,* nausea, dyspepsia, dysgeusia.
GU: impotence.
Hematologic: neutropenia.
Respiratory: *dry, persistent, tickling, nonproductive cough.*
Skin: rash.
Other: *muscle cramps,* **angioedema,** decreased libido, hyperkalemia.

INTERACTIONS
Diuretics: excessive hypotension.
Indomethacin: attenuated hypotensive effect.
Insulin, oral antidiabetic agents: risk of hypoglycemia, especially at initiation of lisinopril therapy. Monitor closely.
Potassium-sparing diuretics, potassium supplements, potassium-containing sodium substitutes: possible hyperkalemia.
Thiazide diuretics: attenuation of potassium loss caused by thiazide diuretics. Discontinue diuretics 2 to 3 days before lisinopril therapy or reduce lisinopril dosage to 5 mg P.O. once daily, as ordered.

CONTRAINDICATIONS
Contraindicated in patients with hypersensitivity to ACE inhibitors or history of angioedema related to previous treatment with ACE inhibitor.

NURSING CONSIDERATIONS
• Use cautiously in patients with impaired renal function; dosage adjustment is required. Also use cautiously

in patients at risk for hyperkalemia (presence of renal insufficiency, presence of diabetes, or use of drugs that raise potassium levels).

• Monitor blood pressure frequently. Be aware that if drug does not adequately control blood pressure, diuretics may be added.

• Monitor WBC with differential counts before therapy, every 2 weeks for the first 3 months of therapy, and periodically thereafter.

• Angioedema (including laryngeal edema) may occur, especially after first dose. Advise the patient to report any signs or symptoms, such as swelling of face, eyes, lips, or tongue or breathing difficulty.

• Light-headedness can occur, especially during the first few days of therapy. Tell the patient to rise slowly to minimize this effect and to report symptoms to the doctor. Patients who experience syncope should stop taking drug and call the doctor immediately.

• Tell the patient not to discontinue drug suddenly, but to call the doctor, if unpleasant adverse reactions occur.

• Advise the patient to report any signs of infection, such as fever and sore throat.

• Tell female patient to notify doctor if pregnancy occurs. Drug will need to be discontinued.

losartan potassium
Cozaar

Pregnancy Risk Category: C (1st trimester), D (2nd and 3rd trimesters)

HOW SUPPLIED
Tablets: 25 mg, 50 mg

ACTION
An angiotensin II receptor antagonist that inhibits the vasoconstricting and aldosterone-secreting effects of angiotensin II by selectively blocking the binding of angiotensin II to its receptor sites that are found in many tissues, including vascular smooth muscle and adrenal glands.

ONSET, PEAK, DURATION
Onset and duration unknown. Serum levels peak in 1 hour for losartan and in 3 to 4 hours for its active metabolite. Although the effect of losartan is substantially present within one week, some studies have shown that maximal effect occurs within 3 to 6 weeks.

INDICATIONS & DOSAGE
Hypertension –
Adults: initially, 25 to 50 mg P.O. daily. Maximum daily dosage is 100 mg in one or two divided doses.

ADVERSE REACTIONS
CNS: dizziness, insomnia.
GI: diarrhea, dyspepsia.
Respiratory: nasal congestion, cough, upper respiratory tract infection, sinus disorder, sinusitis.
Musculoskeletal: muscle cramp, myalgia, back or leg pain.

INTERACTIONS
None significant.

CONTRAINDICATIONS
Contraindicated in patients with hypersensitivity to the drug.

NURSING CONSIDERATIONS
• Know that breast-feeding is not recommended during losartan therapy.

• Use cautiously in patients with impaired renal or hepatic function.

• Know that drugs that act directly on the renin-angiotensin system (such as losartan) can cause fetal and neonatal morbidity and death when administered to pregnant women. These problems have not been detected when exposure has been limited to the first trimester. If pregnancy is suspected, notify doctor because drug should probably be discontinued.

• Know that the lowest dosage (25

---

*Liquid form contains alcohol.   *Common* reactions are in italics; *life-threatening*, in bold italics.
**May contain tartrazine.

mg) should be used initially in patients with impaired hepatic function and in those who are intravascularly volume-depleted (such as those receiving diuretics).

• Be aware that losartan can be used alone or in combination with other antihypertensives.

• Be aware that if the antihypertensive effect measured by the serum trough level of the drug, using once-daily dosing, is inadequate, a twice-daily regimen using the same total daily dosage or an increase in dosage may give a more satisfactory response.

• Monitor the patient's blood pressure closely to evaluate effectiveness of therapy. Know that when losartan is used alone, the effect on blood pressure is notably less in black patients than in patients of other races.

• Monitor patients who also are taking diuretics for symptomatic hypotension.

• Regularly assess the patient's renal function (via serum creatinine and BUN levels), as ordered.

• Be aware that patients with severe CHF whose renal function depends on the angiotensin-aldosterone system have experienced acute renal failure during ACE inhibitor therapy. Manufacturer of losartan states that drug would be expected to do the same. Closely monitor patient, especially during the first few weeks of therapy.

• Tell the patient to avoid sodium substitutes; these products may contain potassium, which can cause hyperkalemia in patients taking losartan.

• Inform female patients of childbearing age about the consequences of second- and third-trimester exposure to losartan and instruct them to notify their doctor immediately if they suspect they have become pregnant.

methyldopa
Aldomet, Aldomet M‡, Apo-Methyldopa†, Dopamet†, Hydopa‡, Novomedopa†, Nu-Medopa†

methyldopate hydrochloride
Aldomet, Aldomet Ester Injection‡

Pregnancy Risk Category: B

HOW SUPPLIED
methyldopa
Tablets: 125 mg, 250 mg, 500 mg
Oral suspension: 250 mg/5 ml
methyldopate hydrochloride
Injection: 250 mg/5 ml

ACTION
Unknown. Thought to involve inhibition of the central vasomotor centers, thereby decreasing sympathetic outflow to the heart, kidneys, and peripheral vasculature.

ONSET, PEAK, DURATION
Onset unknown. Serum levels peak within 4 to 6 hours after I.V. or oral administration. Effects persist 12 to 24 hours after single oral dose, 24 to 48 hours after multiple oral doses, and 10 to 16 hours after I.V. administration.

INDICATIONS & DOSAGE
Hypertension, hypertensive crisis –
Adults: *oral* – initially, 250 mg P.O. b.i.d. to t.i.d. in first 48 hours. Then increased as needed q 2 days. May give entire daily dosage in the evening or h.s. Adjust dosages as needed if other antihypertensives are added to or deleted from therapy. Maintenance dosage is 500 mg to 2 g daily in two to four divided doses. Maximum recommended daily dosage is 3 g.
I.V. – 250 to 500 mg q 6 hours, diluted in D$_5$W and administered over 30 to 60 minutes. Maximum dosage is

---

1 g q 6 hours. Switch to oral antihypertensives as soon as possible.
Children: initially, 10 mg/kg P.O. daily in two to four divided doses; or 20 to 40 mg/kg I.V. daily in four divided doses. Increase dose daily until desired response occurs. Maximum daily dosage is 65 mg/kg or 3 g, whichever is least.

ADVERSE REACTIONS
CNS: *sedation,* headache, asthenia, weakness, dizziness, *decreased mental acuity,* involuntary choreoathetoid movements, psychic disturbances, depression, nightmares.
CV: bradycardia, *orthostatic hypotension,* aggravated angina, myocarditis, *edema.*
EENT: *nasal congestion.*
GI: nausea, vomiting, diarrhea, pancreatitis, *dry mouth*.
Hematologic: hemolytic anemia, reversible agranulocytosis, thrombocytopenia.
Hepatic: hepatic necrosis.
Other: gynecomastia, galactorrhea, skin rash, *drug-induced fever,* impotence, *weight gain*.

INTERACTIONS
Amphetamines, norepinephrine, phenothiazines, tricyclic antidepressants: possible hypertensive effects. Monitor carefully.
Levodopa: additive hypotensive effects may increase adverse CNS reactions.
Lithium: may increase lithium levels. Monitor for increased lithium levels.

CONTRAINDICATIONS
Contraindicated in patients with hypersensitivity to the drug or active hepatic disease (such as acute hepatitis) and active cirrhosis. Also contraindicated if previous methyldopa therapy has been associated with liver disorders.

NURSING CONSIDERATIONS
• Use cautiously in patients with history of impaired hepatic function and in breast-feeding patients.
• **I.V. use:** Observe for and report any involuntary choreoathetoid movements. The doctor may decide to discontinue drug if this occurs.
• Monitor patient's blood pressure regularly. Be aware that elderly patients are more likely to experience hypotension and sedation.
• After dialysis, monitor the patient for hypertension and notify doctor if necessary. The patient may need an extra dose of methyldopa.
• Monitor CBC with differential counts before therapy, every 2 weeks for the first 3 months of therapy, and periodically thereafter. Advise the patient to report any signs of infection, such as fever and sore throat.
• Patients who require blood transfusions should have direct and indirect Coombs' tests to prevent crossmatching problems.
• Monitor patient's Coombs' test results. In patients who have received this drug for several months, positive reaction to direct Coombs' test indicates hemolytic anemia.
• Tell the patient not to suddenly stop taking drug, but to contact the doctor, if unpleasant adverse reactions occur.
• Tell the patient to check his weight daily and notify the doctor of weight gain over 5 lb. Sodium and water retention may occur but can be relieved with diuretics.
• Warn the patient that drug may impair ability to perform tasks that require mental alertness, particularly at start of therapy. Once-daily dosage at bedtime will minimize daytime drowsiness.
• Inform the patient that orthostatic hypotension can be minimized by rising slowly and avoiding sudden position changes. Dry mouth can be relieved with chewing gum, sour hard candy, or ice chips.

---

*Liquid form contains alcohol.
**May contain tartrazine.
Common reactions are in italics; *life-threatening,* in bold italics.

• Tell the patient that urine may turn dark in toilet bowls treated with bleach.

---

metoprolol succinate
Toprol XL

metoprolol tartrate
Apo-Metoprolol†, Apo-Metoprolol (Type L)†, Betaloc†‡, Betaloc Durules†, Lopresor†, Lopresor SR†, Lopressor, Minax‡, Novometoprol†, Nu-Metop†

Pregnancy Risk Category: C

HOW SUPPLIED
metoprolol succinate
Tablets (extended-release): 50 mg, 100 mg, 200 mg
metoprolol tartrate
Tablets: 50 mg, 100 mg
Tablets (extended-release): 100 mg†, 200 mg†
Injection: 1 mg/ml in 5-ml ampules

ACTION
Unknown for antihypertensive action. A beta$_1$-selective blocking agent that decreases myocardial contractility, heart rate, and cardiac output; lowers blood pressure; and reduces myocardial oxygen consumption. Also depresses renin secretion.

ONSET, PEAK, DURATION
Onset occurs within 5 minutes of I.V. dose, 15 minutes of oral dose. Peak effects occur within 20 minutes of I.V. dose, 1 hour after regular-release tablet, or 6 to 12 hours after extended-release dosage forms. Effects persist 5 to 8 hours after I.V. dose, 6 to 12 hours after regular-release oral tablets, up to 24 hours after extended-release forms.

INDICATIONS & DOSAGE
Hypertension –
Adults: initially, 50 mg P.O. b.i.d. or 100 mg P.O. once daily, then up to 100 to 450 mg daily in two or three divided doses. Alternatively, 50 to 100 mg of extended-release tablets (tartrate) once daily. Dosage is adjusted as needed and tolerated at intervals of not less than 1 week to a maximum of 400 mg daily.
Early intervention in acute MI –
Adults: three 5-mg I.V. boluses q 2 minutes. Then, beginning 15 minutes after last dose, 25 to 50 mg P.O. q 6 hours for 48 hours. Maintenance dosage is 100 mg P.O. b.i.d. for at least 3 months and possibly for as long as 1 to 3 years.
Angina pectoris –
Adults: initially, 100 mg P.O. daily as a single dose or in two equally divided doses. Dosage increased at weekly intervals until an adequate response or a pronounced decrease in heart rate is seen. Daily dosage beyond 450 mg has not been studied. Alternatively, give 100 mg of extended-release tablets (tartrate) once daily. Dosage adjusted as needed and tolerated at intervals of not less than 1 week to a maximum of 400 mg daily.

ADVERSE REACTIONS
CNS: fatigue, lethargy, dizziness.
CV: *bradycardia, hypotension, CHF,* peripheral vascular disease.
GI: nausea, vomiting, diarrhea.
Respiratory: dyspnea, *bronchospasm.*
Skin: rash.
Other: fever, arthralgia.

INTERACTIONS
Barbiturates, rifampin: increased metabolism of metoprolol. Monitor for decreased effect.
Chlorpromazine, cimetidine, verapamil: decreased hepatic clearance. Monitor for greater beta-blocking effect.
Digitalis glycosides, diltiazem, verapamil: excessive bradycardia and increased depressant effect on myocardium. Use together cautiously.

Indomethacin: decreased antihypertensive effect. Monitor blood pressure and adjust dosage.
Insulin, oral antidiabetic agents: can alter dosage requirements in previously stabilized diabetic patients. Observe the patient carefully.

CONTRAINDICATIONS
Contraindicated in patients with hypersensitivity to the drug or other beta blockers. Also contraindicated in patients with sinus bradycardia, heart block greater than first-degree, cardiogenic shock, or overt cardiac failure when used to treat hypertension or angina. When used to treat MI, drug also is contraindicated in patients with heart rate less than 45 beats/minute, second- or third-degree heart block, PR interval equal to or greater than 0.24 seconds with first-degree heart block, systolic blood pressure less than 100 mm Hg, or moderate to severe cardiac failure.

NURSING CONSIDERATIONS
• Use cautiously in patients with heart failure, diabetes, or respiratory or hepatic disease.
• Always check the patient's apical pulse rate before giving drug. If it's slower than 60 beats/minute, withhold drug and call the doctor immediately.
• **I.V. use:** Give undiluted by direct injection. Although mixing with other drugs should be avoided, studies have shown that metoprolol is compatible when mixed with meperidine hydrochloride or morphine sulfate or when administered with alteplase infusions at a Y-site connection.
• Food may increase absorption of metoprolol. Give consistently with meals.
• Monitor blood glucose levels closely in diabetic patients because drug masks common signs of hypoglycemia.
• Monitor blood pressure frequently.

Know that metoprolol masks common signs of shock.
• Store drug at room temperature and protect from light. Discard solution if it's discolored or contains particles.
• Tell the patient that abrupt discontinuation of therapy can exacerbate angina and precipitate MI. Withdraw drug gradually over 1 to 2 weeks.

minoxidil
Loniten
Pregnancy Risk Category: C

HOW SUPPLIED
Tablets: 2.5 mg, 10 mg, 25 mg‡

ACTION
Unknown. The predominant effect produces direct arteriolar vasodilation.

ONSET, PEAK, DURATION
Onset occurs in about 30 minutes. Peak effects occur within 1 hour. Effects persist 2 to 5 days.

INDICATIONS & DOSAGE
Severe hypertension –
Adults: initially, 5 mg P.O. as a single dose. Effective dosage range is usually 10 to 40 mg daily. Maximum dosage is 100 mg daily.
Children under 12 years: 0.2 mg/kg P.O. (maximum 5 mg) as a single daily dose. Effective dosage range usually is 0.25 to 1 mg/kg daily. Maximum dosage is 50 mg.

ADVERSE REACTIONS
CV: *edema, tachycardia, pericardial effusion and tamponade,* **CHF,** ECG changes.
Skin: rash, **Stevens-Johnson syndrome.**
Other: *hypertrichosis* (elongation, thickening, and enhanced pigmentation of fine body hair), breast tenderness, weight gain.

---

*Liquid form contains alcohol.   *Common* reactions are in italics; *life-threatening,* in bold italics.
**May contain tartrazine.

INTERACTIONS
Guanethidine: severe orthostatic hypotension. Advise the patient to stand up slowly.

CONTRAINDICATIONS
Contraindicated in patients with pheochromocytoma or hypersensitivity to the drug.

NURSING CONSIDERATIONS
• Use cautiously in patients with impaired renal function and after acute MI.
• Closely monitor blood pressure and pulse at beginning of therapy.
• Know that elderly patients may be more sensitive to drug's hypotensive effects.
• Minoxidil is removed by hemodialysis. Be sure to administer dose after dialysis.
• Make sure the patient receives and reads the package insert prepared by the manufacturer that describes in layman's terms the drug and its adverse reactions. Also provide an oral explanation.
• Monitor fluid intake and urine output and check for weight gain and edema.
• Minoxidil usually is prescribed with a beta blocker to control tachycardia and a diuretic to counteract fluid retention. Make sure the patient understands the importance of compliance with total treatment regimen.
• Teach the patient how to take his own pulse and to report increases greater than 20 beats/minute to the doctor.
• Tell the patient not to suddenly stop taking the drug, but to call the doctor, if unpleasant adverse effects occur.
• Tell the patient to weigh himself at least weekly and to report weight gain over 5 lb.
• About 8 out of 10 patients will experience hypertrichosis within 3 to 6 weeks of beginning treatment. Unwanted hair can be controlled with a depilatory or shaving. Assure the patient that extra hair will disappear within 1 to 6 months of stopping minoxidil. Advise the patient, however, not to discontinue drug without the doctor's approval.

nitroprusside sodium
Nipride, Nitropress

Pregnancy Risk Category: C

HOW SUPPLIED
Injection: 50 mg/vial in 2-ml, 5-ml vials

ACTION
Relaxes both arteriolar and venous smooth muscle.

ONSET, PEAK, DURATION
Onset occurs within 1 minute. Peak effects are evident almost immediately. Effects dissipate within 10 minutes after infusion.

INDICATIONS & DOSAGE
To lower blood pressure quickly in hypertensive emergencies; to produce controlled hypotension during anesthesia; to reduce preload and afterload in cardiac pump failure or cardiogenic shock (may be used with or without dopamine) –
Adults: 50 mg vial diluted with 2 to 3 ml of D_5W and then added to 250, 500, or 1,000 ml of D_5W. Infused at 0.3 to 10 mcg/kg/minute. Average dose is 3 mcg/kg/minute. Maximum infusion rate is 10 mcg/kg/minute.

Patients taking other antihypertensives along with nitroprusside are extremely sensitive to nitroprusside. Dosage is adjusted accordingly.

ADVERSE REACTIONS
The following adverse reactions usually indicate overdose:
CNS: *headache, dizziness,* ataxia, loss of consciousness, ***coma,*** weak pulse, absent reflexes, widely dilated

pupils, *restlessness, muscle twitching, diaphoresis.*
CV: distant heart sounds, palpitations.
GI: *vomiting, nausea, abdominal pain.*
Respiratory: dyspnea, shallow breathing.
Skin: pink color.
Other: acidosis.

INTERACTIONS
Antihypertensives: may cause sensitivity to nitroprusside. Adjust dosage as ordered.
Ganglionic blocking agents, general anesthetics, negative inotropic agents, and other antihypertensives: Additive effects. Monitor blood pressure closely.

CONTRAINDICATIONS
Contraindicated in patients with hypersensitivity to the drug, compensatory hypertension (such as in arteriovenous shunt or coarctation of the aorta), inadequate cerebral circulation, congenital optic atrophy, or tobacco-induced amblyopia.

NURSING CONSIDERATIONS
• Use with extreme caution in patients with increased intracranial pressure. Use cautiously in patients with hypothyroidism, hepatic or renal disease, hyponatremia, or low vitamin B_{12} concentration.
• Obtain baseline vital signs before giving drug, and find out what parameters the doctor wants to achieve.
• Keep the patient in the supine position when initiating or titrating nitroprusside therapy.
• **I.V. use:** Don't use bacteriostatic water for injection or sterile sodium chloride solution for reconstitution.
• Because the drug is sensitive to light, wrap I.V. solution in foil; it's not necessary to wrap the tubing. Fresh solution should have faint brownish tint. Discard after 24 hours.

• Infuse with a infusion pump. Drug is best given via piggyback through a peripheral line with no other medication. Don't adjust rate of main I.V. line while drug is being infused. Even a small bolus of nitroprusside can cause severe hypotension.
• Check blood pressure every 5 minutes at start of infusion and every 15 minutes thereafter. If severe hypotension occurs, discontinue nitroprusside infusion—effects of drug quickly reverse. Notify the doctor. If possible, start an arterial pressure line. Regulate drug flow to specified level.
• Excessive doses or rapid infusion greater than 15 mcg/kg/minute can cause cyanide toxicity; therefore, check serum thiocyanate levels every 72 hours. Thiocyanate levels above 100 mcg/ml are associated with toxicity. Watch for signs of thiocyanate toxicity: profound hypotension, metabolic acidosis, dyspnea, headache, loss of consciousness, ataxia, and vomiting. If these occur, discontinue drug immediately and notify the doctor.

penbutolol sulfate
Levatol
Pregnancy Risk Category: C

HOW SUPPLIED
Tablets: 20 mg

ACTION
Unknown.

ONSET, PEAK, DURATION
Onset occurs within 1 hour. Peak effects occur within 1½ to 3 hours. Effects persist up to 24 hours.

INDICATIONS & DOSAGE
Mild to moderate hypertension—
Adults: 20 mg P.O. once daily. Usually given with other antihypertensives, such as thiazide diuretics.

---

*Liquid form contains alcohol.   *Common* reactions are in italics; *life-threatening*, in bold italics.
**May contain tartrazine.

ADVERSE REACTIONS

CNS: syncope, *dizziness,* vertigo, headache, fatigue, paresthesia, hypoesthesia or hyperesthesia, lethargy, anxiety, nervousness, diminished concentration, sleep disturbances, nightmares, bizarre or frequent dreams, sedation, changes in behavior, reversible mental depression, catatonia, hallucinations, alteration of time perception, memory loss, emotional lability, light-headedness.

CV: *bradycardia,* chest pain, *CHF,* asymptomatic hypotension, peripheral ischemia, worsening of angina or arterial insufficiency, peripheral vascular insufficiency, claudication, edema, *pulmonary edema,* vasodilation, symptomatic postural hypotension, tachycardia, palpitations, conduction disturbances, first-degree and third-degree heart block, intensification of AV block.

EENT: eye discomfort, pharyngitis.

GI: gastric pain, flatulence, nausea, constipation, heartburn, vomiting, taste alteration, dry mouth.

GU: impotence, nocturia, urine retention.

Respiratory: *laryngospasm,* respiratory distress, shortness of breath.

Skin: pallor, flushing, rash.

Other: hypersensitivity reactions, decreased libido, hyperglycemia, hypoglycemia.

INTERACTIONS

Clonidine: may cause paradoxical hypertension. Also, beta blockers may enhance rebound hypertension when clonidine is withdrawn.

Digoxin, diltiazem, verapamil: may produce additive depressant effects on AV node conduction. Monitor closely.

Insulin, oral antidiabetic agents: hypoglycemic response to these drugs may be altered. Monitor patient closely.

NSAIDs: may decrease antihypertensive effects.

Prazosin, terazosin: "first-dose" orthostatic hypotension seen with these drugs may be enhanced.

Sympathomimetics, including isoproterenol, dopamine, dobutamine, or norepinephrine: decreased hypotensive response.

Theophylline: may decrease bronchodilator effect.

CONTRAINDICATIONS

Contraindicated in patients with hypersensitivity to the drug or other beta blockers and in those with sinus bradycardia, cardiogenic shock, overt cardiac failure, greater than first-degree heart block, or chronic bronchitis.

NURSING CONSIDERATIONS

• Use cautiously in patients with CHF controlled by drug therapy and in those with a history of bronchospastic disease. Also use cautiously in diabetic patients because beta-adrenergic blockers may mask certain signs and symptoms of hypoglycemia.

• Always check the patient's apical pulse before giving drug. If you detect extremes in pulse rates, withhold drug and call the doctor immediately.

• Monitor blood pressure, ECG, and heart rate and rhythm frequently.

• Tell the patient to avoid abrupt discontinuation of therapy; sudden withdrawal of other beta blockers has precipitated angina and MI.

• Teach the patient the signs and symptoms of CHF (edema and pulmonary congestion). Advise him to contact the doctor if these symptoms occur.

---

phentolamine mesylate
Regitine, Rogitine†

Pregnancy Risk Category: C

HOW SUPPLIED

Injection: 5 mg/ml in 1-ml vials, 10 mg/ml‡

ACTION
An alpha-adrenergic blocker that competitively blocks the effects of catecholamines on alpha-adrenergic receptors.

ONSET, PEAK, DURATION
Unknown.

INDICATIONS & DOSAGE
To aid in diagnosis of pheochromocytoma; to control or prevent hypertension before or during pheochromocytomectomy –
Adults: I.V. diagnostic dose is 5 mg, with close monitoring of blood pressure.

Before surgical removal of tumor, 5 mg I.M. or I.V. During surgery, the patient may need 5 mg I.V.
Children: I.V. diagnostic dose is 1 mg with close monitoring of blood pressure.

Before surgical removal of tumor, 1 mg I.V. or I.M. During surgery, the patient may need 1 mg I.V.
Dermal necrosis and sloughing following I.V. extravasation of norepinephrine –
Adults and children: infiltrate area with 5 to 10 mg phentolamine in 10 ml 0.9% sodium chloride solution or give half the dosage through the infiltrated I.V. and the other half around the site. Must be done within 12 hours.

ADVERSE REACTIONS
CNS: *dizziness, weakness, flushing.*
CV: *hypotension,* **shock,** *arrhythmias,* palpitations, *tachycardia,* angina pectoris.
EENT: *nasal congestion.*
GI: *diarrhea,* abdominal pain, *nausea, vomiting,* hyperperistalsis.
Other: hypoglycemia.

INTERACTIONS
Epinephrine: excessive hypotension. Don't use together.
Narcotics, sedatives, rauwolfia alkaloids: false-positive test results for pheochromocytoma. Don't give 24 hours before phentolamine is given as a diagnostic test. Withdraw rauwolfia alkaloids at least 4 weeks before such testing.

CONTRAINDICATIONS
Contraindicated in patients with angina, coronary artery disease, MI or history of MI, and hypersensitivity to the drug.

NURSING CONSIDERATIONS
• Use cautiously in patients with gastritis or peptic ulcer.
• When drug is given as a diagnostic test for pheochromocytoma, check the patient's blood pressure first; also check blood pressure frequently during administration.
• Know that test is positive for pheochromocytoma if I.V. test dose causes severe hypotension.
• Don't administer epinephrine to treat phentolamine-induced hypotension because it may cause additional fall in blood pressure ("epinephrine reversal"). Use norepinephrine instead, as ordered.

---

pindolol
Barbloc‡, Novo-Pindol†, Syn-Pindolol†, Visken
Pregnancy Risk Category: B

HOW SUPPLIED
Tablets: 5 mg, 10 mg, 15 mg‡

ACTION
Unknown. Possible mechanisms include reduced cardiac output, decreased sympathetic outflow to peripheral vasculature, and inhibition of renin release by the kidneys.

ONSET, PEAK, DURATION
Onset unknown. Peak effect occurs in 1 to 2 hours. Effects persist for 24 hours.

INDICATIONS & DOSAGE
Hypertension –
Adults: initially, 5 mg P.O. b.i.d.
Dosage increased as needed and tolerated to a maximum of 60 mg daily.

ADVERSE REACTIONS
CNS: *insomnia, fatigue, dizziness, nervousness,* vivid dreams, hallucinations, lethargy.
CV: *edema,* bradycardia, *CHF,* peripheral vascular disease, hypotension.
EENT: visual disturbances.
GI: *nausea,* vomiting, diarrhea.
Respiratory: *increased airway resistance.*
Skin: rash.
Other: hypoglycemia without tachycardia, *muscle pain, joint pain.*

INTERACTIONS
Digitalis glycosides, diltiazem, verapamil: excessive bradycardia and additive depression of AV node. Use together cautiously.
Epinephrine: severe vasoconstriction. Monitor blood pressure and observe the patient carefully.
Indomethacin: decreased antihypertensive effect. Monitor blood pressure and adjust dosage.
Insulin, oral antidiabetic agents: can alter requirements for these drugs in previously stabilized diabetic patients. Monitor the patient for hypoglycemia.

CONTRAINDICATIONS
Contraindicated in patients with hypersensitivity to the drug, bronchial asthma, severe bradycardia, heart block greater than first degree, cardiogenic shock, or overt cardiac failure.

NURSING CONSIDERATIONS
● Use cautiously in patients with CHF, nonallergic bronchospastic disease, diabetes, hyperthyroidism, and impaired renal or hepatic function.
● Always check the patient's apical pulse rate before giving this drug. If you detect extremes in pulse rates, withhold medication and call the doctor immediately.
● Monitor blood pressure frequently and notify the doctor if severe hypotension occurs. A vasopressor may be required.
● Withdraw drug gradually (over 1 to 2 weeks) after long-term administration, as ordered.
● Monitor blood glucose levels in diabetic patients closely because drug masks certain signs and symptoms of hypoglycemia.
● Tell the patient that abrupt discontinuation of drug can exacerbate angina and precipitate MI.

prazosin hydrochloride
Minipress
Pregnancy Risk Category: C

HOW SUPPLIED
Capsules: 1 mg, 2 mg, 5 mg

ACTION
Unknown. Its alpha-adrenergic blocking activity is thought to account primarily for its effects.

ONSET, PEAK, DURATION
Onset occurs within 30 to 90 minutes. Peak effects occur in 2 to 4 hours, but maximal antihypertensive effect may not occur for 3 to 4 weeks after therapy begins. Effects persist about 7 to 10 hours.

INDICATIONS & DOSAGE
Mild to moderate hypertension, alone or in combination with a diuretic or other antihypertensive –
Adults: P.O. test dose is 1 mg h.s. to prevent "first-dose syncope." Initial dose is 1 mg P.O. t.i.d. Dosage increased slowly. Maximum daily dosage is 20 mg. Maintenance dosage is 6 to 15 mg daily in three divided doses. Some patients have required dosages

larger than this (up to 40 mg daily). If other antihypertensives or diuretics are added to this drug, prazosin is decreased to 1 to 2 mg t.i.d. and retitrated.

ADVERSE REACTIONS
CNS: *dizziness,* headache, drowsiness, weakness, *"first-dose syncope,"* depression.
CV: orthostatic hypotension, *palpitations.*
EENT: blurred vision.
GI: vomiting, diarrhea, abdominal cramps, constipation, *nausea,* dry mouth.
GU: priapism, impotence.

INTERACTIONS
Propranolol and other beta blockers: increased frequency of syncope with loss of consciousness. Advise the patient to sit or lie down if dizziness occurs.

CONTRAINDICATIONS
None known.

NURSING CONSIDERATIONS
• Use cautiously in patients receiving other antihypertensives.
• Monitor the patient's blood pressure and pulse rate frequently.
• Know that elderly patients may be more sensitive to drug's hypotensive effects.
• Be aware that if initial dose is greater than 1 mg, severe syncope with loss of consciousness may occur ("first-dose syncope"). Patients who experience dizziness should sit or lie down.
• Tell the patient not to suddenly stop taking this drug, but to call the doctor, if unpleasant adverse reactions occur.
• Advise the patient to minimize orthostatic hypotension by rising slowly and avoiding sudden position changes. Dry mouth can be relieved with chewing gum, sour hard candy, or ice chips.
• Compliance *may* be improved with twice-daily dosing. Suggest this dosing change with the doctor if you suspect compliance problems.

---

quinapril hydrochloride
Accupril, Asig‡

Pregnancy Risk Category: C (1st trimester), D (2nd and 3rd trimesters)

HOW SUPPLIED
Tablets: 5 mg, 10 mg, 20 mg, 40 mg

ACTION
Unknown, but thought to be related to inhibition of angiotensin I to angiotensin II, a potent vasoconstrictor. Reduced formation of angiotensin II decreases peripheral arterial resistance, thus decreasing aldosterone secretion.

ONSET, PEAK, DURATION
Onset occurs within 1 hour. Peak serum levels of quinapril are seen in 1 hour; quinaprilat, in 2 hours. Peak effects occur within 2 to 4 hours. Effects persist about 24 hours.

INDICATIONS & DOSAGE
Hypertension –
Adults: initially, 10 mg daily. Dosage adjusted based on patient response at intervals of about 2 weeks. Most patients are controlled at 20, 40, or 80 mg daily as a single dose or in two divided doses.
Heart failure –
Adults: initially, 5 mg P.O. b.i.d. if patient is receiving a diuretic and 10 mg P.O. b.i.d. if patient not receiving a diuretic. Dosage increased at weekly intervals. Usual effective dose is 20 to 40 mg b.i.d. in equally divided doses.

ADVERSE REACTIONS

CNS: somnolence, vertigo, light-headedness, syncope, nervousness, depression.

CV: palpitations, vasodilation, tachycardia, *hypertensive crisis,* angina, orthostatic hypotension, *rhythm disturbances.*

EENT: *cough,* dry throat.

GI: dry mouth, abdominal pain, constipation, hemorrhage.

Hepatic: elevated liver enzymes.

Respiratory: *dry, persistent, tickling, nonproductive cough.*

Skin: pruritus, *exfoliative dermatitis, photosensitivity.*

Other: *angioedema,* hyperkalemia, back pain, malaise, diaphoresis.

INTERACTIONS

Diuretics, other antihypertensives: risk of excessive hypotension. Discontinue diuretic or lower dose of quinapril as needed.

Lithium: increased serum lithium levels and lithium toxicity. Avoid concomitant use.

Potassium-sparing diuretics, potassium supplements, sodium substitutes containing potassium: risk of hyperkalemia. Monitor during concomitant use.

CONTRAINDICATIONS

Contraindicated in patients with hypersensitivity to ACE inhibitors or with a history of angioedema related to previous treatment with an ACE inhibitor.

NURSING CONSIDERATIONS

• Use cautiously in patients with impaired renal function.

• Assess renal and hepatic function before and periodically throughout therapy. Know that dosage adjustment is necessary for patients with renal impairment.

• Monitor blood pressure for effectiveness of therapy.

• Monitor serum potassium levels as ordered. Be aware that risk factors for the development of hyperkalemia include renal insufficiency, diabetes, and concomitant use of drugs that raise potassium level.

• Other ACE inhibitors have been associated with agranulocytosis and neutropenia. Monitor CBC with differential counts before therapy, every 2 weeks for the first 3 months of therapy, and periodically thereafter, as ordered.

• Advise the patient to report any signs of infection, such as fever and sore throat.

• Angioedema (including laryngeal edema) may occur, especially after the first dose. Advise the patient to report any signs or symptoms, such as swelling of face, eyes, lips, or tongue or breathing difficulty.

• Light-headedness can occur, especially during the first few days of therapy. Tell the patient to rise slowly to minimize effect and to report symptoms to the doctor. Patients who experience syncope should stop taking drug and call the doctor immediately.

• Inadequate fluid intake, vomiting, diarrhea, and excessive perspiration can lead to light-headedness and syncope. Tell the patient to use caution in hot weather and during exercise.

• Tell the patient to avoid sodium substitutes; these products may contain potassium, which can cause hyperkalemia in patients taking quinapril.

• Tell female patient to notify doctor if pregnancy occurs. Drug will need to be discontinued.

ramipril

Altace, Ramace‡, Tritace‡

Pregnancy Risk Category: C (1st trimester), D (2nd and 3rd trimesters)

HOW SUPPLIED

Capsules: 1.25 mg, 2.5 mg, 5 mg, 10 mg

ACTION
Unknown, but thought to be related to inhibition of angiotensin I to angiotensin II, a potent vasoconstrictor. Reduced formation of angiotensin II decreases peripheral arterial resistance, thus decreasing aldosterone secretion.

ONSET, PEAK, DURATION
Onset occurs within 1 to 2 hours. Peak serum levels of ramipril occur within 1 hour; of ramiprilat, in 3 hours. Peak effect occurs in 4 to 6.5 hours. Effects persist about 24 hours.

INDICATIONS & DOSAGE
Hypertension –
Adults: initially, 2.5 mg P.O. once daily for patients not receiving a diuretic, and 1.25 mg P.O. once daily for patients receiving a diuretic. Dosage increased as necessary based on patient response. Maintenance dosage is 2.5 to 20 mg daily as a single dose or in divided doses.

In patients with renal insufficiency: If creatinine clearance is < 40 ml/minute, 1.25 mg P.O. daily. Dosage is titrated gradually according to response. Maximum daily dosage is 5 mg.

ADVERSE REACTIONS
CNS: headache, dizziness, fatigue, asthenia, malaise, light-headedness, anxiety, amnesia, *seizures,* depression, insomnia, nervousness, neuralgia, neuropathy, paresthesia, somnolence, tremor, vertigo.
CV: orthostatic hypotension, syncope, angina, *arrhythmias,* chest pain, palpitations, *MI.*
EENT: epistaxis, dysphagia, increased salivation.
GI: nausea, vomiting, abdominal pain, anorexia, constipation, diarrhea, dyspepsia, dry mouth, taste disturbance, gastroenteritis.
GU: impotence.

Respiratory: *dry, persistent, tickling, nonproductive cough;* dyspnea.
Skin: hypersensitivity reactions, rash, dermatitis, pruritus, photosensitivity, purpura.
Other: *angioedema,* edema, hyperkalemia, increased diaphoresis, weight gain, arthralgia, arthritis, myalgia.

INTERACTIONS
Diuretics: excessive hypotension, especially at the start of therapy. Discontinue diuretic at least 3 days before therapy begins, increase sodium intake, or reduce starting dose of ramipril.
Insulin, oral antidiabetic agents: risk of hypoglycemia, especially at initiation of ramipril therapy. Monitor closely.
Lithium: increased serum lithium levels. Use together cautiously and monitor serum lithium levels.
Potassium-sparing diuretics, potassium supplements, sodium substitutes containing potassium: increased risk of hyperkalemia because ramipril attenuates potassium loss. Monitor plasma potassium levels closely.

CONTRAINDICATIONS
Contraindicated in patients with hypersensitivity to ACE inhibitors or a history of angioedema related to previous treatment with an ACE inhibitor.

NURSING CONSIDERATIONS
• Use cautiously in patients with renal impairment.
• Monitor blood pressure regularly for drug effectiveness.
• Closely assess renal function in patients during first few weeks of therapy. Regular assessment of renal function (serum creatinine and BUN levels) is advisable. Patients with severe CHF whose renal function depends on the angiotensin-aldosterone system have experienced acute renal failure

---

*Liquid form contains alcohol.   *Common* reactions are in italics; ***life-threatening,*** in bold italics.
**May contain tartrazine.

during ACE inhibitor therapy. Hypertensive patients with renal artery stenosis also may show signs of worsening renal function at start of therapy.

• Monitor CBC with differential counts before therapy, every 2 weeks for the first 3 months of therapy, and periodically thereafter. These effects may occur especially in patients with impaired renal function or collagen vascular diseases (systemic lupus erythematosus or scleroderma).

• Monitor serum potassium levels. Risk factors for the development of hyperkalemia include renal insufficiency, diabetes, and concomitant use of agents that raise potassium levels.

• Tell the patient to avoid abrupt discontinuation of therapy.

• Angioedema (including laryngeal edema) may occur, especially after the first dose. Advise the patient to report any signs or symptoms, such as swelling of face, eyes, lips, or tongue or breathing difficulty.

• Light-headedness can occur, especially during the first few days of therapy. Tell the patient to rise slowly to minimize this effect and to report symptoms to the doctor. Patients who experience syncope should stop taking drug and call the doctor immediately.

• Advise the patient to report any signs of infection, such as fever and sore throat.

• Tell the patient to avoid sodium substitutes; these products may contain potassium, which can cause hyperkalemia in patients taking ramipril.

• Tell female patient to notify doctor if pregnancy occurs. Drug will need to be discontinued.

---

rauwolfia serpentina
Raudixin**, Rauverid, Wolfina

Pregnancy Risk Category: C

HOW SUPPLIED
Tablets: 50 mg, 100 mg

ACTION
Unknown. Thought to be due to reduced cardiac output and possibly decreased peripheral resistance.

ONSET, PEAK, DURATION
Onset occurs in several days to 3 weeks. Peak effect is reached in 3 to 6 weeks. Effects persist for 1 to 6 weeks.

INDICATIONS & DOSAGE
Mild to moderate hypertension –
Adults: initially and for 1 to 3 weeks thereafter, 200 to 400 mg P.O. daily as a single dose or in two divided doses. Maintenance dosage is 50 to 300 mg daily.

ADVERSE REACTIONS
CNS: mental confusion, *depression, drowsiness, nervousness, paradoxical anxiety,* nightmares, sedation, headache, extrapyramidal symptoms.
CV: orthostatic hypotension, bradycardia, syncope.
EENT: *nasal congestion,* glaucoma.
GI: *hypersecretion of gastric acid, nausea, vomiting, dry mouth,* bleeding.
GU: impotence.
Skin: pruritus, rash.
Other: weight gain.

INTERACTIONS
Digitalis glycosides: rauwolfia may predispose patients to digitalis-induced arrhythmias. Use together cautiously.
MAO inhibitors: may cause excitability and hypertension. Use together cautiously.

CONTRAINDICATIONS
Contraindicated in patients with mental depression, active peptic ulcer disease or ulcerative colitis, hypersensitivity to the drug, and concurrent electroconvulsive therapy.

NURSING CONSIDERATIONS

• Use cautiously in patients with epilepsy, history of peptic ulcer, ulcerative colitis, or gallstones.
• Monitor blood pressure and pulse rate frequently.
• Tell patient that drug should be taken with meals.
• Tell the patient not to discontinue drug suddenly, but to call the doctor, if unpleasant adverse reactions occur.
• Warn the patient that drug can cause drowsiness. Patients should not drive or perform other activities that require alertness and good coordination until drug's CNS effects are known.
• Advise the patient to minimize orthostatic hypotension by rising slowly and avoiding sudden position changes. Dry mouth can be relieved with chewing gum, sour hard candy, or ice chips. Tell the patient to contact the doctor if relief is needed for nasal congestion.
• Tell the patient to weigh himself daily and notify the doctor of any weight gain over 5 lb.
• Advise the patient to have periodic eye examinations.
• Tell family to watch the patient closely for signs of mental depression. Warn patient to notify the doctor promptly if nightmares occur.

---

rescinnamine
Moderil

Pregnancy Risk Category: C

HOW SUPPLIED
Tablets: 0.25 mg, 0.5 mg

ACTION
Unknown. Thought to be due to reduced cardiac output and possibly decreased peripheral resistance.

ONSET, PEAK, DURATION
Unknown.

INDICATIONS & DOSAGE
Mild hypertension –
Adults: initially, 0.5 mg P.O. b.i.d. Maintenance dosage is 0.25 to 0.5 mg daily.

ADVERSE REACTIONS
CNS: mental confusion, *depression, drowsiness, nervousness, anxiety, nightmares,* sedation, parkinsonism.
CV: *orthostatic hypotension, bradycardia, syncope.*
EENT: *nasal congestion,* glaucoma.
GI: *hypersecretion of gastric acid, nausea, vomiting, dry mouth,* GI bleeding.
GU: impotence.
Skin: pruritus, rash.
Other: *weight gain.*

INTERACTIONS
Digitalis glycosides, quinidine: arrhythmias may occur. Monitor patient closely.
MAO inhibitors: may cause excitability and hypertension. Use together cautiously.

CONTRAINDICATIONS
Contraindicated in patients with mental depression, active peptic ulcer disease or ulcerative colitis, hypersensitivity to the drug, and concurrent electroconvulsive therapy.

NURSING CONSIDERATIONS
• Use cautiously in patients with history of peptic ulcer, ulcerative colitis, or gallstones.
• Monitor blood pressure and pulse rate frequently.
• Tell patient that drug should be taken with meals.
• Tell the patient not to discontinue drug suddenly, but to call the doctor, if unpleasant adverse reactions occur.
• Warn the patient that drug can cause drowsiness. Patients should not drive or perform other tasks that require alertness and coordination until drug's CNS effects are known.

---

*Liquid form contains alcohol.
**May contain tartrazine.

Common reactions are in italics; ***life-threatening***, in bold italics.

• Advise the patient to minimize orthostatic hypotension by rising slowly and avoiding sudden position changes. Dry mouth can be relieved with chewing gum, sour hard candy, or ice chips. Tell the patient to contact the doctor if relief is needed for nasal congestion.
• Tell the patient to weigh himself daily and to notify the doctor of any weight gain over 5 lb.
• Advise the patient to have periodic eye examinations.
• Tell family to watch the patient closely for signs of mental depression. Warn patient to notify the doctor promptly if nightmares occur.

reserpine
Novoreserpine†, Serpalan, Serpasil*

Pregnancy Risk Category: C

HOW SUPPLIED
Tablets: 0.1 mg, 0.25 mg, 1 mg

ACTION
Unknown. Thought to be due to reduced cardiac output and possibly decreased peripheral resistance.

ONSET, PEAK, DURATION
Onset occurs in several days to 3 weeks. Time to peak effect occurs in 3 to 6 weeks. Effects persist for 1 to 6 weeks.

INDICATIONS & DOSAGE
Mild to moderate essential hypertension –
Adults: 0.1 to 0.25 mg P.O. daily.
Children: 5 to 20 mcg/kg P.O. daily.

ADVERSE REACTIONS
CNS: mental confusion, *drowsiness, sedation, nervousness, paradoxical anxiety, nightmares, depression,* extrapyramidal symptoms.
CV: *orthostatic hypotension, bradycardia, syncope.*

EENT: *nasal congestion,* glaucoma.
GI: *hyperacidity, nausea, vomiting, dry mouth,* bleeding.
GU: *impotence.*
Skin: pruritus, rash.
Other: *weight gain.*

INTERACTIONS
Digitalis glycosides, quinidine: arrhythmias may occur. Monitor patient closely.
MAO inhibitors: may cause excitability and hypertension. Use together cautiously.

CONTRAINDICATIONS
Contraindicated in patients with hypersensitivity to the drug, mental depression, ulcerative colitis or peptic ulcer disease and in those receiving electroconvulsive therapy.

NURSING CONSIDERATIONS
• Use cautiously in patients with history of peptic ulcer, ulcerative colitis, or gallstones.
• Monitor blood pressure and pulse rate frequently.
• Tell patient that drug should be taken with meals.
• Tell the patient not to discontinue drug suddenly, but to call the doctor, if unpleasant adverse reactions occur.
• Warn the patient that drug can cause drowsiness. Patients should avoid hazardous activities that require alertness and coordination until drug's CNS effects are known.
• Advise the patient to minimize orthostatic hypotension by rising slowly and avoiding sudden position changes. Dry mouth can be relieved with chewing gum, sour hard candy, or ice chips. Tell the patient to contact the doctor if relief is needed for nasal congestion.
• Tell the patient to weigh himself daily and to notify the doctor of any weight gain over 5 lb.
• Advise the patient to have periodic eye examinations.

• Tell family to watch the patient closely for signs of mental depression. Warn patient to notify the doctor promptly if nightmares occur.

terazosin hydrochloride
Hytrin

Pregnancy Risk Category: C

HOW SUPPLIED
Tablets: 1 mg, 2 mg, 5 mg, 10 mg

ACTION
Decreases blood pressure by vasodilation produced in response to blockade of alpha$_1$-adrenergic receptors. Improves urine flow in patients with benign prostatic hyperplasia (BPH) by blocking alpha$_1$-adrenergic receptors in the smooth muscle of the bladder neck and prostate, thus relieving urethral pressure and reestablishing urine flow.

ONSET, PEAK, DURATION
Onset occurs within 15 minutes. Peak effects on blood pressure occur within 2 to 3 hours. Effects persist 24 hours.

INDICATIONS & DOSAGE
Hypertension –
Adults: initially, 1 mg P.O. h.s. Dosage increased gradually according to patient response. Usual dosage range is 1 to 5 mg daily. Maximum recommended dosage is 20 mg/day.
Symptomatic BPH –
Adults: initally, 1 mg P.O. h.s. Dosage increased in a stepwise fashion to 2 mg, 5 mg, or 10 mg once daily to achieve optimal response. Most patients require 10 mg daily for optimal response.

ADVERSE REACTIONS
CNS: asthenia, *dizziness,* headache, nervousness, paresthesia, somnolence.
CV: *palpitations,* postural hypotension, tachycardia, *peripheral edema.*

EENT: *nasal congestion,* sinusitis, blurred vision.
GI: *nausea.*
GU: impotence, decreased libido.
Respiratory: dyspnea.
Other: weight gain, back pain, muscle pain.

INTERACTIONS
Antihypertensives: excessive hypotension. Use together cautiously.

CONTRAINDICATIONS
Contraindicated in patients with hypersensitivity to the drug.

NURSING CONSIDERATIONS
• Monitor blood pressure frequently.
• Know that if terazosin is discontinued for several days, the patient will need to be retitrated using initial dosing regimen (1 mg P.O. h.s.).
• Tell the patient not to discontinue drug suddenly, but to call the doctor, if adverse reactions occur.
• Warn the patient to avoid hazardous activities that require mental alertness, such as driving or operating heavy machinery, for 12 hours after the first dose.

timolol maleate
Apo-Timol†, Blocadren

Pregnancy Risk Category: C

HOW SUPPLIED
Tablets: 5 mg, 10 mg, 20 mg

ACTION
Mechanism of antihypertensive action unknown. In MI, may decrease myocardial oxygen requirements. Prevents arterial dilation through beta blockade for migraine headache prophylaxis.

ONSET, PEAK, DURATION
Onset occurs in 15 to 30 minutes. Peak effects occur in 1 to 2 hours. Effects persist for 6 to 12 hours.

INDICATIONS & DOSAGE
Hypertension –
Adults: initially, 10 mg P.O. b.i.d.
Usual daily maintenance dosage is 20
to 40 mg. Maximum daily dosage is
60 mg. Allow at least 7 days to elapse
between increases in dosage.
*MI (long-term prophylaxis in patients
who have survived acute phase) –*
Adults: 10 mg P.O. b.i.d.
Migraine headache prophylaxis –
Adults: initially, 20 mg P.O. daily as
a single dose or in divided doses
b.i.d. Increase dosage as needed and
tolerated to maximum of 30 mg daily.
Discontinue treatment if no response
occurs after 6 to 8 weeks of therapy at
maximum dosage.

ADVERSE REACTIONS
CNS: fatigue, lethargy, vivid dreams.
CV: *bradycardia, hypotension, CHF,*
peripheral vascular disease.
GI: nausea, vomiting, diarrhea.
Respiratory: dyspnea, *broncho-
spasm, increased airway resistance.*
Skin: rash.
Other: fever.

INTERACTIONS
*Digitalis glycosides, diltiazem, verap-
amil:* excessive bradycardia and increased depressant effect on myocardium. Use together cautiously.
Indomethacin: decreased antihypertensive effect. Monitor blood pressure
and adjust dosage.
Insulin, oral antidiabetic agents: can
alter requirements for these drugs in
previously stabilized diabetic patients. Monitor the patient for hypoglycemia.

CONTRAINDICATIONS
Contraindicated in patients with bronchial asthma, severe COPD, sinus
bradycardia and heart block greater
than first-degree, cardiogenic shock,
overt CHF, or hypersensitivity to the
drug.

NURSING CONSIDERATIONS
● Use cautiously in patients with
compensated CHF; hepatic, renal, or
respiratory disease; diabetes; and hyperthyroidism.
● Always check the patient's apical
pulse rate before giving drug. If you
detect extremes in pulse rates, withhold drug and call the doctor immediately.
● Monitor blood pressure frequently.
● Monitor blood glucose levels in diabetic patients because drug can mask
certain signs and symptoms of hypoglycemia.
● Tell the patient that abrupt discontinuation of drug can exacerbate angina and precipitate MI. Dosage
should be reduced gradually over 1 to
2 weeks.

trimethaphan camsylate
Arfonad

Pregnancy Risk Category: D

HOW SUPPLIED
Injection: 50 mg/ml in 10-ml ampule,
250 mg/vial‡

ACTION
A ganglionic blocker that causes reduction in sympathetic tone and vasodilation.

ONSET, PEAK, DURATION
Onset and peak are immediate. Effects dissipate within 10 to 15 minutes of discontinuing drug.

INDICATIONS & DOSAGE
*To lower blood pressure quickly in hy-
pertensive emergencies; to control hypotension during surgery –*
Adults: 500 mg (10 ml) diluted in
500 ml D₅W to yield concentration of
1 mg/ml. I.V. drip started at 3 to 4
mg/minute and titrated to achieve desired hypotensive response. Range is
0.3 mg to 6 mg/minute.

ADVERSE REACTIONS
CNS: dilated pupils, *extreme weakness.*
CV: *severe orthostatic hypotension, tachycardia.*
GI: anorexia, *nausea, vomiting, dry mouth.*
GU: urine retention.
Respiratory: respiratory depression.
Skin: urticaria, itching.

INTERACTIONS
Anesthetics, diuretics, procainamide: increased hypotensive effect. Monitor the patient closely.
Neuromuscular blocking agents: potentiation of neuromuscular blocking action of the nondepolarized agents. Administer together with caution.

CONTRAINDICATIONS
Contraindicated in patients with uncorrected anemia, hypovolemia, hypovolemic shock, asphyxia, or uncorrected respiratory insufficiency.

NURSING CONSIDERATIONS
• Use with extreme caution in patients with arteriosclerosis; cardiac, hepatic, or renal disease; degenerative CNS disorders; Addison's disease; or diabetes mellitus. Also use cautiously in those receiving other antihypertensives or glucocorticoids. Also use with extreme caution in elderly or debilitated patients.
• **I.V. use:** Refrigerate before reconstitution and prepare solution just before use. Solution is stable for 24 hours after reconstitution.
• Use infusion pump to administer drug slowly and precisely.
• Place the patient in the supine position during drug administration. If necessary, elevate the head of the bed for maximal effect to avoid cerebral anoxia. Do not elevate bed more than 30 degrees.
• Monitor blood pressure and vital signs continuously.
• Watch closely for respiratory distress, especially if large doses are used. Large doses have caused apnea and respiratory arrest.
• If extreme hypotension occurs, discontinue drug and call the doctor. Use phenylephrine or mephentermine to counteract hypotension.
• Discontinue drug before wound closure in surgery as ordered to allow blood pressure to return to normal.

---

*Liquid form contains alcohol.   *Common* reactions are in italics; ***life-threatening,*** in bold italics.
**May contain tartrazine.

cholestyramine
clofibrate
colestipol hydrochloride
dextrothyroxine sodium
fluvastatin sodium
gemfibrozil
lovastatin
niacin
(See Chapter 91, VITAMINS AND MINERALS.)
pravastatin sodium
probucol
simvastatin

COMBINATION PRODUCTS
None.

---

cholestyramine
Questran**, Questran Light,
Questran Lite‡

Pregnancy Risk Category: NR

HOW SUPPLIED
Powder: 378-g cans, 9-g single-dose
packets. Each scoop of powder or single-dose packet contains 4 g of cholestyramine resin.

ACTION
A bile-acid sequestrant that combines
with bile acid to form an insoluble
compound that is excreted. The liver
must synthesize new bile acid from
cholesterol, which reduces low-density-lipoprotein cholesterol levels.

ONSET, PEAK, DURATION
Reduction of plasma cholesterol concentrations generally reduced within 1
to 2 weeks of therapy. After withdrawal of drug, cholesterol concentrations return to baseline in about 2 to 4
weeks.

INDICATIONS & DOSAGE
*Primary hyperlipidemia or pruritus
caused by partial bile obstruction; adjunct for reduction of elevated serum
cholesterol in patients with primary
hypercholesterolemia* —
Adults: 4 g once or twice daily. Maintenance dosage is 8 to 16 g daily.
Maximum daily dosage is 24 g.

ADVERSE REACTIONS
GI: *constipation,* fecal impaction,
hemorrhoids, *abdominal discomfort,*
flatulence, *nausea,* vomiting, steatorrhea.
Skin: *rash;* irritation of skin, tongue,
and perianal area.
Other: *vitamin A, D, and K deficiency resulting from decreased absorption;* hyperchloremic acidosis
with long-term use or very high dosage.

INTERACTIONS
*Acetaminophen, beta-adrenergic
blockers, corticosteroids, digitalis glycosides, fat-soluble vitamins (A, D, E,
and K), iron preparations, thiazide diuretics, thyroid hormones, warfarin
and other coumarin derivatives:* absorption may be substantially decreased by cholestyramine. Administer at least 2 hours apart.

CONTRAINDICATIONS
Contraindicated in patients with hypersensitivity to bile-acid sequestering resins and in those with complete
biliary obstruction.

NURSING CONSIDERATIONS
● Use cautiously in patients predisposed to constipation and in those
with conditions aggravated by constipation, such as severe, symptomatic
CAD.

• Monitor serum cholesterol and triglyceride levels regularly during therapy.

• Monitor serum levels of digitalis glycosides in patients receiving digitalis glycosides and cholestyramine concurrently. If cholestyramine therapy is discontinued, adjust dosage of digitalis glycosides as ordered to avoid toxicity.

• Monitor bowel habits. Encourage a diet high in fiber and fluids. If severe constipation develops, decrease dosage, add a stool softener, or discontinue drug, as ordered.

• Instruct the patient never to take drug in its dry form; esophageal irritation or severe constipation may result. Using a large glass, the patient should sprinkle the powder on the surface of preferred beverage; let the mixture stand a few minutes; then stir thoroughly. The best diluents are water, milk, and juice (especially pulpy fruit juice). Mixing with carbonated beverages may result in excess foaming. After drinking this preparation, the patient should swirl a small additional amount of liquid in the same glass and then drink it to ensure ingestion of the entire dose.

• Advise the patient to take all other drugs at least 1 hour before or 4 to 6 hours after cholestyramine to avoid blocking their absorption.

• Teach the patient about proper dietary management of serum lipids (restricting total fat and cholesterol intake), as well as measures to control other cardiac disease risk factors. When appropriate, recommend weight control, exercise, and smoking cessation programs.

• Be aware that long-term use may be associated with deficiency of vitamins A, D, E, and K and folic acid.

clofibrate
Arterioflexin‡, Atromid-S, Claripex†, Col‡, Novofibrate†

Pregnancy Risk Category: C

HOW SUPPLIED
Capsules: 500 mg

ACTION
Unknown. Seems to inhibit biosynthesis of cholesterol at an early stage.

ONSET, PEAK, DURATION
Plasma concentrations of very-low-density lipoprotein (VLDL) are reduced within 2 to 5 days. Time to peak effect occurs in 3 weeks with continued use. VLDL concentrations return to pretreatment levels within 3 weeks after drug is withdrawn.

INDICATIONS & DOSAGE
Hyperlipidemia –
Adults: 2 g P.O. daily in divided doses. Some patients may respond to lower doses as assessed by serum lipid monitoring.

ADVERSE REACTIONS
CNS: fatigue, weakness.
CV: *arrhythmias.*
GI: *nausea, diarrhea, vomiting,* stomatitis, *dyspepsia,* flatulence.
GU: impotence and decreased libido, *acute renal failure.*
Hematologic: leukopenia, anemia.
Hepatic: gallstones, *transient and reversible elevations of liver function tests.*
Skin: rash, urticaria, pruritus, dry skin and hair.
Other: myalgia and arthralgia, resembling a flulike syndrome; *weight gain; polyphagia;* fever.

INTERACTIONS
Furosemide, sulfonylureas: clofibrate may potentiate the clinical effects of these agents. Monitor the patient closely.

---

*Liquid form contains alcohol.
**May contain tartrazine.

Common reactions are in italics; **life-threatening,** in bold italics.

Lovastatin, pravastatin, simvastatin: risk of myositis, rhabdomyolysis, and renal failure. Avoid concomitant use.
Oral anticoagulants: clofibrate may potentiate the anticoagulant effects of warfarin or dicumarol. Decrease the anticoagulant dosage.
Oral contraceptives, rifampin: may antagonize clofibrate's lipid-lowering effect. Monitor serum lipids.
Probenecid: increased clofibrate effect. Monitor for toxicity.

CONTRAINDICATIONS
Contraindicated in patients with significant hepatic or renal dysfunction, primary biliary cirrhosis, or hypersensitivity to the drug and in pregnant or breast-feeding women.

NURSING CONSIDERATIONS
• Use cautiously in patients with peptic ulcer.
• Monitor serum cholesterol and triglyceride levels regularly during therapy.
• Monitor renal and hepatic function, blood counts, and serum electrolyte and blood glucose levels. If liver function tests show steady rise, expect discontinuation of clofibrate.
• Know that drug typically is discontinued if significant lipid lowering is not achieved within 3 months.
• Teach patients about proper dietary management of serum lipids (restricting total fat and cholesterol intake), as well as measures to control other cardiac disease risk factors. When appropriate, recommend weight control, exercise, and smoking cessation programs.
• Advise patients to report any flulike symptoms immediately because their occurrence may indicate rhabdomyolysis-induced renal failure.

colestipol hydrochloride
Colestid

Pregnancy Risk Category: NR

HOW SUPPLIED
Granules: 300 g and 500 g bottles, 5 g packets
Tablets: 1 g

ACTION
Combines with bile acid to form an insoluble compound that is excreted. The liver must synthesize new bile acid from cholesterol; this leads to reduced low-density-lipoprotein cholesterol levels.

ONSET, PEAK, DURATION
Reduced plasma cholesterol levels occur within 1 to 2 days. Antilipemic effects peak after about 1 month of therapy. Lipid levels return to pretreatment values within 1 month of discontinuing treatment.

INDICATIONS & DOSAGE
Primary hypercholesterolemia –
Adults: 5 to 30 g P.O. once daily or in divided doses.

ADVERSE REACTIONS
CNS: headache, dizziness.
GI: *constipation,* fecal impaction, hemorrhoids, abdominal discomfort, flatulence, nausea, vomiting, steatorrhea.
Skin: rash; irritation of tongue and perianal area.
Other: vitamin A, D, E, and K deficiency from decreased absorption; hyperchloremic acidosis with long-term use or high dosage.

INTERACTIONS
Oral antidiabetic agents: may antagonize response to colestipol. Monitor serum lipids.
Orally administered drugs: colestipol may decrease absorption. Separate administration times; give other drugs

at least 1 hour before or 4 hours after colestipol.

CONTRAINDICATIONS
Contraindicated in patients with hypersensitivity reactions to bile-acid sequestering resins.

NURSING CONSIDERATIONS
• Use cautiously in patients predisposed to constipation and in those with conditions aggravated by constipation, such as severe, symptomatic coronary artery disease.
• Monitor serum cholesterol and triglyceride levels regularly during therapy.
• Monitor bowel habits; if severe constipation develops, decrease dosage or add stool softener as ordered. Encourage a diet high in fiber and fluids.
• Monitor serum levels of digitalis glycosides in patients receiving digitalis glycosides and colestipol concurrently. If colestipol therapy is discontinued, adjust dosage of digitalis glycosides to avoid toxicity, as ordered.
• Instruct the patient never to take drug in its dry form; esophageal irritation or severe constipation may result.
• To prepare, instruct the patient to use a large glass containing water, milk, or juice (especially pulpy fruit juice). The patient should sprinkle the powder on the surface of the preferred beverage; let the mixture stand a few minutes; then stir thoroughly to obtain a uniform suspension. After drinking this preparation, the patient should swirl a small additional amount of liquid in the same glass and then drink it to ensure ingestion of the entire dose.
• To enhance palatability, mix and refrigerate the next daily dose the previous evening.
• Advise the patient to take all other drugs at least 1 hour before or 4 to 6 hours after colestipol to avoid blocking their absorption.

• Teach the patient about proper dietary management of serum lipids (restricting total fat and cholesterol intake), as well as measures to control other cardiac disease risk factors. When appropriate, recommend weight control, exercise, and smoking cessation programs.
• Inform patient that long-term use may be associated with deficiency of vitamins A, D, E, and K and folic acid. Instruct patient to report any unusual signs and symptoms.

---

dextrothyroxine sodium (d-thyroxine sodium)
Choloxin**

Pregnancy Risk Category: NR

HOW SUPPLIED
Tablets: 1 mg, 2 mg, 4 mg, 6 mg

ACTION
Unknown. Thought to accelerate hepatic catabolism of cholesterol and increase bile secretion to lower cholesterol levels.

ONSET, PEAK, DURATION
Onset unknown. Peak effects on serum lipids occur after 1 to 2 months of therapy. Effects persist for 1½ to 3 months.

INDICATIONS & DOSAGE
Hyperlipidemia in euthyroid patients, especially when cholesterol and triglyceride levels are elevated –
Adults: initially, 1 to 2 mg P.O. daily, increased by 1 to 2 mg daily at monthly intervals to a total of 4 to 8 mg daily.
Children: initially, 0.05 mg/kg P.O. daily, increased by 0.05 mg/kg daily at monthly intervals to a maximum of 4 mg daily. Alternatively, give 1.5 mg/m² P.O. daily, increased by 1.5 mg/m² daily at monthly intervals. Maximum daily dosage is 4 mg. The usual maintenance dosage is 0.1 mg/

---

*Liquid form contains alcohol.   *Common* reactions are in italics; *life-threatening,* in bold italics.
**May contain tartrazine.

kg or 3 mg/m² daily in euthyroid children.

ADVERSE REACTIONS
CNS: insomnia, nervousness, tremor, headache, tinnitus.
CV: palpitations, angina pectoris, *arrhythmias,* ischemic myocardial changes on ECG, *MI.*
EENT: visual disturbances, ptosis.
GI: nausea, vomiting, diarrhea, constipation, decreased appetite.
Other: *insomnia, weight loss, diaphoresis,* flushing, hyperthermia, hyperthyroidism, hair loss, menstrual irregularities.

INTERACTIONS
Digitalis glycosides: dextrothyroxine may enhance clinical effect. Use together cautiously.
Insulin, sulfonylureas: monitor for increased glucose levels.
Oral anticoagulants: dextrothyroxine may potentiate anticoagulant effect of warfarin or dicumarol.
Sympathomimetics, thyroid hormones: dextrothyroxine may precipitate arrhythmias or coronary insufficiency in patients with cardiac disease.

CONTRAINDICATIONS
Contraindicated in patients with advanced hepatic or renal disease or iodism. Also contraindicated in patients with organic heart disease; history of MI; arrhythmias; rheumatic heart disease; history of CHF or decompensation or borderline compensated cardiac status; and hypertension (other than mild, labile, systolic hypertension).

NURSING CONSIDERATIONS
• Use cautiously in patients with diabetes mellitus and impaired liver or kidney function.
• Monitor lipid levels regularly, as ordered.
• Observe the patient for signs of hyperthyroidism, such as nervousness,

insomnia, and weight loss. If these occur, decrease dosage or discontinue drug as ordered.
• Teach the patient about proper dietary management of serum lipids (restricting total fat and cholesterol intake), as well as measures to control other cardiac disease risk factors. When appropriate, recommend weight control, exercise, and smoking cessation programs.

---

fluvastatin sodium
Lescol
Pregnancy Risk Category: X

HOW SUPPLIED
Capsules: 20 mg, 40 mg

ACTION
Inhibits 3-hydroxy-3-methylglutaryl coenzyme A reductase. This enzyme is an early (and rate-limiting) step in the synthetic pathway of cholesterol.

ONSET, PEAK, DURATION
Unknown.

INDICATIONS & DOSAGE
Reduction of low-density lipoprotein and total cholesterol levels in patients with primary hypercholesterolemia (types IIa and IIb)—
Adults: initially, 20 mg P.O. h.s. Increase dosage as needed to a maximum of 40 mg daily.

ADVERSE REACTIONS
GI: dyspepsia, diarrhea, nausea.
Hematologic: thrombocytopenia, leukopenia, *hemolytic anemia.*
Respiratory: sinusitis.
Other: arthropathy, muscle pain, hypersensitivity reactions *(anaphylaxis, angioedema).*

INTERACTIONS
Cholestyramine, colestipol: may bind with fluvastatin in the GI tract and de-

crease absorption. Separate administration times by at least 4 hours.
Cimetidine, omeprazole, ranitidine: decreased fluvastatin metabolism. Monitor for enhanced effects.
Cyclosporine and other immunosuppressants, erythromycin, gemfibrozil, niacin: possible increased risk of polymyositis and rhabdomyolysis. Avoid concomitant use.
Digoxin: may alter digoxin pharmacokinetics. Monitor serum digoxin levels carefully.
Ethanol: increased risk of hepatotoxicity. Avoid concomitant use.
Rifampin: enhanced fluvastatin metabolism and decreased plasma levels. Monitor for lack of effect.

CONTRAINDICATIONS

Contraindicated in patients with hypersensitivity to the drug, and in those with active liver disease or conditions associated with unexplained persistent elevations of serum transaminase levels; in pregnant and breast-feeding women; and in women of childbearing age unless there is no risk of pregnancy.

NURSING CONSIDERATIONS

• Use cautiously in patients with severe renal impairment with history of liver disease or heavy alcohol ingestion.
• Know that fluvastatin should be initiated only after diet and other nonpharmacologic therapies have proven ineffective. The patient should be on a standard low-cholesterol diet during therapy.
• Be aware that liver function tests should be performed at the start of therapy and periodically thereafter.
• Watch for signs of myositis.
• Tell patient that drug may be taken without regard to meals; however, efficacy is enhanced if the drug is taken in the evening.
• Teach the patient about proper dietary management, weight control,

and exercise. Explain their importance in controlling elevated serum lipids levels.
• Warn the patient to restrict alcohol intake.
• Tell the patient to inform the doctor of any adverse reactions, particularly muscle aches and pains.

gemfibrozil
Lopid

Pregnancy Risk Category: C

HOW SUPPLIED
Tablets: 600 mg
Capsules: 300 mg

ACTION
Inhibits peripheral lipolysis and also reduces triglyceride synthesis in the liver. Lowers serum triglyceride levels and increases high-density-lipoprotein cholesterol levels.

ONSET, PEAK, DURATION
Onset occurs in 2 to 5 days. Peak effect occurs after 4 weeks of treatment. Duration unknown.

INDICATIONS & DOSAGE
Type IV and V hyperlipidemia unresponsive to diet and other drugs; reduction of risk of coronary heart disease in patients with type IIb hyperlipidemia who cannot tolerate or who are refractory to treatment with bile acid sequestrants or niacin—
Adults: 1,200 mg P.O. daily in two divided doses, 30 minutes before morning and evening meals. If no beneficial effect of drug is seen after 3 months of therapy, drug should be discontinued.

ADVERSE REACTIONS
CNS: blurred vision, headache, dizziness.
GI: *abdominal and epigastric pain, diarrhea, nausea,* vomiting, flatulence.

---

*Liquid form contains alcohol.
**May contain tartrazine.

Common reactions are in italics; *life-threatening,* in bold italics.

Hematologic: anemia, leukopenia.
Hepatic: bile duct obstruction, elevated liver enzymes.
Skin: rash, dermatitis, pruritus.
Other: painful extremities.

INTERACTIONS
Lovastatin: myopathy with rhabdomyolysis has been reported. Don't use together.
Oral anticoagulants: gemfibrozil may enhance the clinical effects of oral anticoagulants. Monitor the patient closely.

CONTRAINDICATIONS
Contraindicated in patients with hypersensitivity to the drug or hepatic or severe renal dysfunction (including primary biliary cirrhosis), and preexisting gallbladder disease.

NURSING CONSIDERATIONS
• Know that periodic CBCs and liver function tests should be performed during the first 12 months of therapy.
• Instruct the patient to take drug ½ hour before breakfast and dinner.
• Teach the patient about proper dietary management of serum lipids (restricting total fat and cholesterol intake), as well as measures to control other cardiac disease risk factors. When appropriate, recommend weight control, exercise, and smoking cessation programs.
• Because of possible dizziness and blurred vision, advise the patient to avoid driving or other potentially hazardous activities until drug's CNS effects are known.
• Tell the patient to observe bowel movements and to report any evidence of steatorrhea or other signs of bile duct obstruction.

---

lovastatin (mevinolin)
Mevacor
Pregnancy Risk Category: X

HOW SUPPLIED
Tablets: 10 mg, 20 mg, 40 mg

ACTION
Inhibits 3-hydroxy-3-methylglutaryl coenzyme A reductase. This enzyme is an early (and rate-limiting) step in the synthetic pathway of cholesterol.

ONSET, PEAK, DURATION
Onset unknown. Plasma levels peak within 2 to 6 hours after a dose. After withdrawal of continuous therapy, effects persist for 4 to 6 weeks.

INDICATIONS & DOSAGE
Reduction of low-density lipoprotein and total cholesterol levels in patients with primary hypercholesterolemia (types IIa and IIb) –
Adults: initially, 20 mg P.O. once daily with evening meal. For patients with severely elevated cholesterol levels (for example, over 300 mg/dl), initial dose is 40 mg. Recommended daily dosage range is 20 to 80 mg in single or divided doses.

ADVERSE REACTIONS
CNS: headache, dizziness, peripheral neuropathy.
EENT: blurred vision.
GI: constipation, diarrhea, dyspepsia, flatulence, abdominal pain or cramps, heartburn, dysgeusia, nausea.
Skin: rash, pruritus.
Other: muscle cramps, myalgia, myositis, *rhabdomyolysis*, elevated serum transaminase levels, abnormal liver test results.

INTERACTIONS
Cyclosporine or other immunosuppressants, erythromycin, gemfibrozil, niacin: possible increased risk of polymyositis and rhabdomyolysis. Maximum recommended lovastatin dosage is 20 mg daily; monitor the patient closely.

Ethanol: increased risk of hepatotoxicity. Avoid concomitant use.
Oral anticoagulants: lovastatin may enhance the clinical effects of oral anticoagulants. Monitor the patient closely.

CONTRAINDICATIONS
Contraindicated in patients with hypersensitivity to the drug and in those with active liver disease or conditions associated with unexplained persistent elevations of serum transaminase levels; in pregnant and breast-feeding patients; and in women of childbearing age unless there is no risk of pregnancy.

NURSING CONSIDERATIONS
• Use cautiously in patients who consume substantial quantities of alcohol or have a past history of liver disease.
• Know that lovastatin therapy should be initiated only after diet and other nonpharmacologic therapies have proved ineffective. The patient should be on a standard low-cholesterol diet during therapy.
• Be aware that liver function tests should be performed at the start of therapy and periodically thereafter.
• Instruct the patient to take lovastatin with the evening meal, when absorption is enhanced and cholesterol biosynthesis is greater.
• Teach the patient about proper dietary management of serum lipids (restricting total fat and cholesterol intake), as well as measures to control other cardiac disease risk factors. When appropriate, recommend weight control, exercise, and smoking cessation programs.
• Advise the patient to have periodic eye examinations; related compounds have caused cataracts in laboratory animals.
• Tell patient to store tablets at room temperature in a light-resistant container.
• Inform female patient that drug is contraindicated during pregnancy. Advise her to notify doctor immediately if pregnancy occurs.

pravastatin sodium (eptastatin)
Pravachol

Pregnancy Risk Category: X

HOW SUPPLIED
Tablets: 10 mg, 20 mg, 40 mg

ACTION
Inhibits 3-hydroxy-3-methylglutaryl coenzyme A reductase. This enzyme is an early (and rate-limiting) step in the synthetic pathway of cholesterol.

ONSET, PEAK, DURATION
Onset and duration are unknown. Plasma levels peak within 1 hour.

INDICATIONS & DOSAGE
Reduction of low-density lipoprotein and total cholesterol levels in patients with primary hypercholesterolemia (types IIa and IIb) –
Adults: initially, 10 or 20 mg P.O. daily h.s. Dosage adjusted q 4 weeks based on patient tolerance and response; maximum daily dosage is 40 mg. Most elderly patients respond to a daily dosage of 20 mg or less.

ADVERSE REACTIONS
CNS: headache, fatigue, dizziness.
CV: chest pain.
EENT: rhinitis.
GI: vomiting, diarrhea, heartburn, nausea.
Respiratory: cough.
Skin: rash.
Other: flulike symptoms, renal failure secondary to myoglobinuria, myositis, myopathy, localized muscle pain, myalgia, ***rhabdomyolysis.***

INTERACTIONS
Cholestyramine, colestipol: concomitant administration decreases plasma

---

*Liquid form contains alcohol.
**May contain tartrazine.

Common reactions are in italics; *life-threatening,* in bold italics.

levels of pravastatin. Administer pravastatin 1 hour before or 4 hours after these drugs.
Drugs that decrease levels or activity of endogenous steroids (such as cimetidine, ketoconazole, spironolactone): may increase risk of developing endocrine dysfunction. No intervention appears necessary; take complete drug history in patients who develop endocrine dysfunction.
Ethanol, hepatotoxic drugs: increased risk of hepatotoxicity. Avoid concomitant use.
Erythromycin, fibric acid derivatives (such as clofibrate or gemfibrozil), immunosuppressants (such as cyclosporine), high doses of niacin (nicotinic acid; 1 g or more daily): may increase the risk of rhabdomyolysis. Monitor the patient closely if concomitant use cannot be avoided.
Gemfibrozil: decreases protein-binding and urinary clearance of pravastatin. Avoid concomitant use.

CONTRAINDICATIONS
Contraindicated in patients with hypersensitivity to the drug and in those with active liver disease or conditions that have unexplained persistent elevations of serum transaminase levels; in pregnant and breast-feeding patients; and in women of childbearing age unless there is no risk of pregnancy.

NURSING CONSIDERATIONS
● Use cautiously in patients who consume large quantities of alcohol or have history of liver disease.
● Know that pravastatin therapy should be initiated only after diet and other nonpharmacologic therapies have proved ineffective. Patients should be on a standard low-cholesterol diet during therapy.
● Know that liver function tests should be performed at the start of therapy and periodically thereafter. A

liver biopsy may be performed if liver enzyme elevations persist.
● Be aware that dosage is adjusted about every 4 weeks. If cholesterol level falls below the target range, dosage may be reduced.
● Instruct the patient to take the recommended dosage in the evening, preferably at bedtime.
● Teach the patient about proper dietary management of serum lipids (restricting total fat and cholesterol intake), as well as measures to control other cardiac disease risk factors. When appropriate, recommend weight control, exercise, and smoking cessation programs.
● Inform female patient that drug is contraindicated during pregnancy. Advise her to notify doctor immediately if pregnancy occurs.

---

probucol
Lorelco, Lurselle‡

Pregnancy Risk Category: B

HOW SUPPLIED
Tablets: 250 mg, 500 mg

ACTION
Inhibits cholesterol transport from the intestine, prevents oxidation of low-density lipoprotein, and may decrease cholesterol synthesis. Appears to be more effective in patients with mild cholesterol elevations than in those with severe hypercholesterolemia.

ONSET, PEAK, DURATION
Onset and duration are unknown. Peak effect occurs after 20 to 50 days of therapy. Plasma levels gradually rise with continued therapy; peak levels occur after 3 to 4 months of treatment.

INDICATIONS & DOSAGE
Primary hypercholesterolemia (types IIa and IIb) –
Adults: 500 mg P.O. b.i.d. with

morning and evening meals. Do not exceed 1 g daily.

ADVERSE REACTIONS
CNS: headache, dizziness, insomnia.
CV: prolonged QT interval, arrhythmias.
GI: *diarrhea, flatulence, abdominal pain, nausea, vomiting.*
Hepatic: elevated liver enzymes.
Other: *hyperhidrosis,* fetid sweat, *angioedema.*

INTERACTIONS
Beta blockers, calcium channel blockers, class Ia antiarrhythmics, digitalis glycosides, phenothiazines, tricyclic antidepressants: increased risk of arrhythmias.

CONTRAINDICATIONS
Contraindicated in patients with hypersensitivity to the drug, recent or progressive myocardial damage, serious ventricular arrhythmias, abnormally long QT interval, or unexplained syncope or syncope of cardiovascular origin.

NURSING CONSIDERATIONS
• Obtain an ECG as ordered prior to initiation of therapy and repeat at appropriate intervals during therapy.
• Instruct the patient to take drug with food; effect is enhanced.
• Teach the patient about proper dietary management of serum lipids (restricting total fat and cholesterol intake), as well as measures to control other cardiac disease risk factors. When appropriate, recommend weight control, exercise, and smoking cessation programs.
• Because of drug's long half-life, advise women who wish to become pregnant to stop taking drug and use effective contraception for 6 months to delay pregnancy.

simvastatin (syvinolin)
Lipex‡, Zocor

Pregnancy Risk Category: X

HOW SUPPLIED
Tablets: 5 mg, 10 mg, 20 mg, 40 mg

ACTION
Inhibits 3-hydroxy-3-methylglutaryl coenzyme A reductase. This enzyme is an early (and rate-limiting) step in the synthetic pathway of cholesterol.

ONSET, PEAK, DURATION
Onset and duration unknown. Peak plasma levels occur in 1.3 to 2.4 hours. Peak antilipemic effects occur in 3 to 4 months.

INDICATIONS & DOSAGE
Reduction of low-density lipoprotein and total cholesterol levels in patients with primary hypercholesterolemia (types IIa and IIb) —
Adults: initially, 5 to 10 mg P.O. daily in the evening. Dosage adjusted q 4 weeks based on patient tolerance and response; maximum daily dosage is 40 mg.

ADVERSE REACTIONS
CNS: headache, asthenia.
GI: abdominal pain, constipation, diarrhea, dyspepsia, flatulence, nausea.
Hepatic: elevated liver enzymes.
Respiratory: cough.
Other: flulike symptoms, myositis, myopathy, *rhabdomyolysis.*

INTERACTIONS
Digoxin: simvastatin may elevate digoxin levels slightly. Closely monitor plasma digoxin levels at initiation of simvastatin therapy.
Drugs that decrease levels or activity of endogenous steroids (such as cimetidine, ketoconazole, spironolactone): may increase risk of developing endocrine dysfunction. No intervention ap-

pears necessary; take complete drug history in patients who develop endocrine dysfunction.

Ethanol, hepatotoxic drugs: increased risk of hepatotoxicity. Avoid concomitant use.

Erythromycin, fibric acid derivatives (such as clofibrate or gemfibrozil), immunosuppressants (such as cyclosporine), high doses of niacin (nicotinic acid; 1 g or more daily): may increase risk of rhabdomyolysis. Monitor the patient closely if concomitant use cannot be avoided. Limit daily dosage of simvastatin to 10 mg if the patient must take cyclosporine.

Warfarin: anticoagulant effect may be slightly enhanced. Monitor the patient's PT at start of therapy and during dosage adjustments.

CONTRAINDICATIONS
Contraindicated in patients with hypersensitivity to the drug and in those with active liver disease or conditions that have unexplained persistent elevations of serum transaminase; in pregnant and breast-feeding patients; and in women of childbearing age unless there is no risk of pregnancy.

NURSING CONSIDERATIONS
● Use cautiously in patients who consume substantial quantities of alcohol or have a history of liver disease.
● Know that simvastatin therapy is initiated only after diet and other non-pharmacologic therapies have proved ineffective. The patient should be on a standard low-cholesterol diet during therapy.
● Know that liver function tests should be performed at the start of therapy and periodically thereafter. A liver biopsy may be performed if enzyme elevations persist.
● Dosage may be adjusted about every 4 weeks. If the cholesterol level falls below the target range, dosage may be reduced.
● Instruct the patient to take simvas-

tatin with the evening meal; absorption is enhanced and cholesterol biosynthesis is greater.
● Teach the patient about proper dietary management of serum lipids (restricting total fat and cholesterol intake), as well as measures to control other cardiac disease risk factors. When appropriate, recommend weight control, exercise, and smoking cessation programs.
● Tell the patient to inform the doctor of any adverse reactions, particularly muscle aches and pains.
● Inform female patient that drug is contraindicated during pregnancy. Advise her to notify the doctor immediately if pregnancy occurs.

25

Miscellaneous cardiovascular drugs

alprostadil
dipyridamole
isoxsuprine hydrochloride
papaverine hydrochloride
pentoxifylline
ticlopidine hydrochloride
tolazoline hydrochloride

COMBINATION PRODUCTS
None.

---

alprostadil
Prostin VR Pediatric

HOW SUPPLIED
Injection: 500 mcg/ml

ACTION
A prostaglandin derivative that relaxes the smooth muscle of the ductus arteriosus.

ONSET, PEAK, DURATION
Onset occurs in 5 to 10 minutes. Peak levels occur within 20 minutes. Effects persist for 1 to 3 hours.

INDICATIONS & DOSAGE
Palliative therapy for temporary maintenance of patency of ductus arteriosus until surgery can be performed —
Infants: 0.05 to 0.1 mcg/kg/minute by I.V. infusion. When therapeutic response is achieved, infusion rate reduced to lowest dosage that will maintain response. Maximum dosage is 0.4 mcg/kg/minute. Alternatively, drug can be administered through umbilical artery catheter placed at ductal opening.

ADVERSE REACTIONS
CNS: *seizures.*
CV: bradycardia, hypotension, tachycardia.
GI: diarrhea.
Hematologic: ***disseminated intravascular coagulation.***
Other: ***apnea,*** *flushing, fever, sepsis.*

INTERACTIONS
None significant.

CONTRAINDICATIONS
None.

NURSING CONSIDERATIONS
• Know that a differential diagnosis should be made between respiratory distress syndrome and cyanotic heart disease before drug is administered. Drug should not be used in neonates with respiratory distress syndrome.
• Use cautiously in neonates with bleeding tendencies because drug inhibits platelet aggregation.
• Dilute drug before administering. Prepare fresh solution daily; discard solution after 24 hours.
• Do not use diluents that contain benzyl alcohol. Fatal toxic syndrome may occur.
• **I.V. use:** Know that this drug is not recommended for direct injection or intermittent infusion. Administer by continuous infusion using a constant-rate pump. Infuse through a large peripheral or central vein or through an umbilical artery catheter placed at the level of the ductus arteriosus. If flushing occurs from peripheral vasodilation, reposition catheter.
• Reduce infusion rate if fever or significant hypotension occurs.
• Keep respiratory support available.
• In infants with restricted pulmonary blood flow, measure drug's effectiveness by monitoring blood oxygenation. In infants with restricted systemic blood flow, measure drug's ef-

---

fectiveness by monitoring systemic blood pressure and blood pH.
• Monitor arterial pressure by umbilical artery catheter, auscultation, or Doppler transducer. Slow rate of infusion if arterial pressure falls significantly.
• If apnea and bradycardia (may reflect drug overdose) occur, stop infusion immediately.
• Keep in mind that CV and CNS adverse reactions are more frequent in infants weighing less than 2 kg and in those receiving infusions for longer than 48 hours.

dipyridamole
Apo-Dipyridamole†, Dipridacot, I.V. Persantine, Novodipiradol†, Persantin‡, Persantin 100‡, Persantine**

Pregnancy Risk Category: B

HOW SUPPLIED
Tablets: 25 mg, 50 mg, 75 mg
Injection: 10 mg/2 ml

ACTION
Unknown but may involve its ability to increase adenosine which is a coronary vasodilator and a platelet aggregation inhibitor.

ONSET, PEAK, DURATION
Onset and duration are unknown. Plasma levels peak 45 to 150 minutes after oral dose.

INDICATIONS & DOSAGE
Inhibition of platelet adhesion in prosthetic heart valves (in combination with warfarin or aspirin) –
Adults: 75 to 100 mg P.O. q.i.d.
Alternative to exercise in evaluation of coronary artery disease during thallium-201 myocardial perfusion scintigraphy –
Adults: 0.57 mg/kg as an I.V. infusion at a constant rate over 4 minutes (0.142 mg/kg/minute).

Acute coronary insufficiency‡ –
Adults: 10 mg I.V. or I.M.

ADVERSE REACTIONS
CNS: *headache, dizziness,* weakness.
CV: flushing, fainting, *hypotension; chest pain,* **ECG abnormalities,** *blood pressure lability, hypertension* (with I.V. infusion).
GI: *nausea,* vomiting, diarrhea.
Skin: rash, irritation (with undiluted injection).

INTERACTIONS
Heparin: monitor for increased bleeding.

CONTRAINDICATIONS
None known.

NURSING CONSIDERATIONS
• Use cautiously in patients with hypotension.
• If the patient develops GI distress, administer 1 hour before meals or with meals.
• **I.V. use:** If administering as a diagnostic agent, dilute in 0.45% or 0.9% sodium chloride or D₅W in at least a 1:2 ratio for a total volume of 20 to 50 ml. Inject thallium-201 within 5 minutes after completing the 4-minute dipyridamole infusion.
• Observe for adverse reactions, especially with large doses. Monitor blood pressure.
• Observe for signs of bleeding; note prolonged bleeding time (especially with large doses or long-term therapy).
• Know that dipyridamole's value as part of an antithrombotic regimen is controversial; using it may not provide significantly better results than using aspirin alone.

isoxsuprine hydrochloride
Duvadilan‡, Vasodilan

Pregnancy Risk Category: NR

HOW SUPPLIED
Tablets: 10 mg, 20 mg

ACTION
Produces peripheral vasodilation by a direct effect on vascular smooth muscle.

ONSET, PEAK, DURATION
Onset and duration unknown. Serum levels peak in 1 hour.

INDICATIONS & DOSAGE
Adjunct for relief of symptoms associated with cerebrovascular insufficiency, peripheral vascular diseases (such as arteriosclerosis obliterans, thromboangiitis obliterans, Raynaud's disease) –
Adults: 10 to 20 mg P.O. t.i.d. or q.i.d.

ADVERSE REACTIONS
CNS: trembling, nervousness, weakness.
CV: tachycardia, hypotension, chest pain.
GI: vomiting, abdominal distress, intestinal distention, nausea.
Skin: severe rash, flushing.

INTERACTIONS
None significant.

CONTRAINDICATIONS
Contraindicated in immediate postpartum period and in patients with arterial bleeding.

NURSING CONSIDERATIONS
• Use cautiously in patients with cardiovascular or cerebrovascular disease.
• Know that safe use during pregnancy and lactation has not been established, although drug has been used to inhibit contractions in premature labor.
• Discontinue drug if rash develops.
• To minimize the risk of orthostasis,

instruct the patient to avoid sudden position changes.

---

papaverine hydrochloride
Cerespan, Genabid, Pavabid, Pavabid HP Capsulets, Pavabid Plateau Caps, Pavacels, Pavagen, Pavarine Spancaps, Pavased, Pavatym, Paverolan Lanacaps
Pregnancy Risk Category: C

HOW SUPPLIED
Tablets: 60 mg, 100 mg, 200 mg, 300 mg
Tablets (timed-release): 200 mg
Capsules (timed-release): 150 mg
Injection: 30 mg/ml, 32.5 mg/ml†

ACTION
Has a direct, nonspecific relaxant effect on vascular, cardiac, and other smooth muscle.

ONSET, PEAK, DURATION
Onset is fairly rapid. Peak unknown. Persists for 12 hours after administration of timed-release form. Unknown for other forms of the drug.

INDICATIONS & DOSAGE
Relief from vascular spasm associated with acute MI (coronary occlusion), angina pectoris, peripheral and pulmonary embolism, peripheral vascular disease in which there is a vasospastic element or certain cerebral angiostatic states; and visceral spasm, as in ureteral, biliary, or gastrointestinal colic –
Adults: 75 to 300 mg P.O. one to five times daily, or 150- to 300-mg timed--release preparations q 8 to 12 hours; 30 to 120 mg I.M. or I.V. slowly over 1 to 2 minutes q 3 hours, as indicated.

ADVERSE REACTIONS
CNS: *headache,* depression.
CV: *increased heart rate, increased blood pressure* (with parenteral use), depressed AV and intraventricular

---

conduction, hypotension, *arrhythmias.*
GI: constipation, dry mouth, *nausea.*
Hepatic: *liver damage.*
Respiratory: increased depth of respiration, *apnea.*
Other: *diaphoresis, flushing,* malaise.

INTERACTIONS
Lactated Ringer's solution: precipitate forms when mixed with papaverine. Don't mix together.
Levodopa: papaverine may interfere with levodopa's therapeutic effects in patients with Parkinson's disease.

CONTRAINDICATIONS
I.V. use is contraindicated in patients with Parkinson's disease or complete AV block.

NURSING CONSIDERATIONS
• Use cautiously in patients with glaucoma.
• **I.V. use:** Give by direct injection over 1 to 2 minutes. Slow administration minimizes the risk of serious adverse reactions. Do not add to Lactated Ringer's Injection, because precipitation occurs.
• Be aware that it is most effective when given early in the course of a disorder.
• Know that the FDA has announced this drug may not be effective for disease states indicated.
• Monitor blood pressure and heart rate and rhythm, especially in patients with cardiac disease. Withhold dose and notify the doctor immediately if changes occur.
• Monitor for adverse hepatic reactions in patients receiving long-term therapy.
• Tell the patient to take medication regularly; long-term therapy is required.
• Advise the patient to avoid tasks that require mental alertness, such as

driving or operating heavy machinery, until drug's CNS effects are known.
• To minimize the risk of orthostatic hypotension, instruct the patient to avoid sudden posture changes.

pentoxifylline
Trental

Pregnancy Risk Category: C

HOW SUPPLIED
Tablets (extended-release): 400 mg

ACTION
Unknown. Improves capillary blood flow probably by increasing RBC flexibility and lowering blood viscosity.

ONSET, PEAK, DURATION
Onset and duration unknown. Serum levels peak within 2 to 4 hours but are not related to drug effect.

INDICATIONS & DOSAGE
Intermittent claudication caused by chronic occlusive vascular disease –
Adults: 400 mg P.O. t.i.d. with meals.

ADVERSE REACTIONS
CNS: headache, dizziness.
GI: dyspepsia, nausea, vomiting.

INTERACTIONS
Anticoagulants: increased anticoagulant effect. Adjust anticoagulant dosage as ordered.
Antihypertensives: increased hypotensive effect. Dosage adjustments may be necessary.

CONTRAINDICATIONS
Contraindicated in patients who are intolerant to methylxanthines, such as caffeine, theophylline, and theobromine, and in patients with recent cerebral or retinal hemorrhage.

NURSING CONSIDERATIONS
- Know that drug is useful in patients who are not good surgical candidates.
- Be aware that elderly patients may be more sensitive to drug's effects.
- Advise patients to take with meals to minimize GI upset.
- Instruct patients to swallow medication whole, without breaking, crushing, or chewing.
- Tell patients to report any GI or CNS adverse reactions; the doctor may reduce the dosage.
- Advise patients to avoid smoking because nicotine causes vasoconstriction that can worsen their condition.
- Tell patients not to discontinue drug during the first 8 weeks of therapy unless directed by their doctor.

---

ticlopidine hydrochloride
Ticlid

Pregnancy Risk Category: B

HOW SUPPLIED
Tablets: 250 mg

ACTION
Unknown. An antiplatelet agent that probably blocks adenosine diphosphate-induced platelet-fibrinogen and platelet-platelet binding.

ONSET, PEAK, DURATION
Onset occurs within 2 days. Serum levels peak in about 2 hours, although time to peak effect takes 8 to 11 days. Effects persist for 1 to 2 weeks.

INDICATIONS & DOSAGE
To reduce risk of thrombotic stroke in patients with history of stroke or who have experienced stroke precursors –
Adults: 250 mg P.O. b.i.d. with meals.

ADVERSE REACTIONS
CNS: dizziness, anorexia.
CV: vasculitis.

EENT: epistaxis, conjunctival hemorrhage.
GI: *diarrhea, nausea, dyspepsia,* vomiting, flatulence, *pain,* bleeding, light-colored stools.
GU: hematuria, **nephrotic syndrome,** dark-colored urine.
Hematologic: neutropenia, **pancytopenia, hemolytic anemia, immune thrombocytopenia.**
Hepatic: hepatitis, cholestatic jaundice.
Respiratory: *allergic pneumonitis.*
Skin: *rash,* purpura, pruritus, ecchymosis, maculopapular rash, urticaria, thrombocytopenic purpura, subcutaneous bleeding.
Other: hypersensitivity reactions, postoperative bleeding, systemic lupus erythematosus, **serum sickness,** arthropathy, myositis, **hyponatremia, increased serum cholesterol levels,** peripheral neuropathy.

INTERACTIONS
Antacids: decreased plasma ticlopidine levels. Separate administration times by at least 2 hours.
Aspirin: effects of aspirin on platelets potentiated. Avoid concomitant use.
Cimetidine: decreased clearance of ticlopidine and increased risk of toxicity. Avoid concomitant use.
Digoxin: slight decrease in serum digoxin levels. Monitor serum digoxin levels.
Theophylline: decreased theophylline clearance and risk of toxicity. Monitor closely and adjust theophylline dosage as ordered.

CONTRAINDICATIONS
Contraindicated in patients hypersensitive to the drug; in patients with hematopoietic disorders, such as neutropenia, thrombocytopenia, or disorders of hemostasis; in patients with active pathologic bleeding, such as peptic ulceration or active intracranial bleeding; and in those with severe hepatic impairment.

---

*Liquid form contains alcohol.   Common reactions are in italics; life-threatening, in bold italics.
**May contain tartrazine.

NURSING CONSIDERATIONS

• Use cautiously and with close monitoring of CBC and WBC differentials. Moderate to severe neutropenia and agranulocytosis have occurred in patients taking ticlopidine, usually within the first 3 weeks to 3 months of therapy.

• Monitor baseline liver function tests prior to therapy.

• Determine CBC and WBC differentials at the second week of therapy and repeat every 2 weeks until end of third month, as ordered. Frequency of tests are increased in patients showing signs of declining neutrophil count or if count is 30% less than baseline. After first 3 months of therapy, CBC and WBC differential determinations should be performed only in patients showing signs of infection.

• Monitor liver function tests and repeat whenever liver dysfunction is suspected. Monitor closely, especially during first 4 months of treatment.

• Know that thrombocytopenia has occurred rarely. Drug should be discontinued in patients having a platelet count of 80,000/mm³ or less, and doctor should be notified. If necessary, give methylprednisolone 20 mg I.V. to normalize bleeding time within 2 hours, as ordered. Know that platelet transfusions may also be used.

• Know that when used preoperatively, ticlopidine may decrease incidence of graft occlusion in patients receiving coronary artery bypass grafts and reduce severity of drop in platelet count in patients receiving extracorporeal hemoperfusion during open heart surgery.

• Tell patients to take drug with meals; this substantially increases bioavailability and improves GI tolerance.

• Tell patients to avoid aspirin and aspirin-containing products and to check with their doctor or pharmacist before taking any OTC medications.

• Explain to patients that drug will prolong the bleeding time and that any unusual or prolonged bleeding should be reported. Advise patients to tell dentists and other doctors that they are taking ticlopidine.

• Stress importance of regular blood tests. Because neutropenia can result in increased risk of infection, tell patients to immediately report any signs of infection, such as fever, chills, or sore throat.

• If ticlopidine is being substituted for a fibrinolytic or anticoagulant, tell patients to discontinue those drugs before starting ticlopidine therapy as ordered.

• Advise patients to discontinue drug 10 to 14 days before undergoing elective surgery, as ordered.

• Also tell patients to immediately report yellow skin or sclera, severe or persistent diarrhea, skin rashes, subcutaneous bleeding, light-colored stools, or dark urine.

tolazoline hydrochloride
Priscoline
Pregnancy Risk Category: C

HOW SUPPLIED
Injection: 25 mg/ml

ACTION
Direct-acting vasodilator. May have some alpha-receptor blocking effects.

ONSET, PEAK, DURATION
Onset occurs within 30 minutes. Peak and duration unknown.

INDICATIONS & DOSAGE
Persistent pulmonary hypertension of the newborn –
Neonates: initially, 1 to 2 mg/kg I.V. over 10 minutes, followed by infusion of 1 to 2 mg/kg/hour.

ADVERSE REACTIONS
CNS: weakness, paradoxical response in seriously damaged limbs, increased

pilomotor activity, tingling, chills, apprehension.
CV: *arrhythmias,* anginal pain, *hypertension, flushing,* transient postural vertigo, palpitations, *orthostatic hypotension.*
GI: *nausea, vomiting, diarrhea, epigastric discomfort, exacerbation of peptic ulcer.*
Hematologic: *agranulocytosis,* thrombocytopenia.
Respiratory: *pulmonary hemorrhage.*
Other: burning at injection site.

INTERACTIONS
Vasopressors (epinephrine, norepinephrine): may cause paradoxical fall in blood pressure.

CONTRAINDICATIONS
Contraindicated in neonates with hypersensitivity to the drug.

NURSING CONSIDERATIONS
• Use cautiously in patients with known or suspected mitral stenosis.
• **I.V. use:** Know that response to treatment of persistent pulmonary hypertension of the newborn should be evident within 30 minutes. Little information exists regarding infusions lasting longer than 48 hours.
• Place the patient in the supine position during infusion.
• To increase response, keep the patient warm during parenteral administration.
• Appearance of flushing usually indicates maximum tolerable dose.
• Monitor vital signs. Watch especially for blood pressure changes and arrhythmias.

---

*Liquid form contains alcohol.   *Common* reactions are in italics; *life-threatening,* in bold italics.
**May contain tartrazine.

26

Nonnarcotic analgesics and antipyretics

acetaminophen
aspirin
choline magnesium trisalicylate
choline salicylate
diflunisal
magnesium salicylate
salsalate
sodium salicylate

COMBINATION PRODUCTS

ALLEREST NO DROWSINESS TAB-LETS◇, COLDRINE◇, ORNEX NO DROWSINESS CAPLETS◇, SINUS RE-LIEF TABLETS, SINUTAB MAXIMUM STRENGTH WITHOUT DROWSI-NESS◇: acetaminophen 325 mg and pseudoephedrine hydrochloride 30 mg.

AMAPHEN, ANOQUAN, BUTACE, EN-DOLOR, ESGIC, FEMCET, FIORICET, ISOPAP, MEDIGESIC, REPAN, TEN-CET, TRIAD, TWO-DYNE: acetamino-phen 325 mg, caffeine 40 mg, and bu-talbital 50 mg.

ASCRIPTIN: aspirin 325 mg, magne-sium hydroxide 50 mg, aluminum hy-droxide 50 mg, and calcium carbonate 50 mg.◇

ASCRIPTIN A/D: aspirin 325 mg, magnesium hydroxide 75 mg, alumi-num hydroxide 75 mg, and calcium carbonate 75 mg.◇

AXOTAL: aspirin 650 mg and butalbi-tal 50 mg.

CAMA, ARTHRITIS STRENGTH: aspi-rin 500 mg, magnesium oxide 150 mg, and aluminum hydroxide 150 mg.

COPE: aspirin 421 mg, caffeine 32 mg, magnesium hydroxide 50 mg, and aluminum hydroxide 25 mg.

DOAN'S P.M. EXTRA STRENGTH ◇: magnesium salicylate 500 mg and di-phenhydramine 25 mg.

EXCEDRIN EXTRA STRENGTH◇: as-pirin 250 mg, acetaminophen 250 mg, and caffeine 65 mg.

EXCEDRIN P.M.◇: acetaminophen 500 mg and diphenhydramine citrate 38 mg.

FIORINAL, ISOLLYL IMPROVED, LANORINAL: aspirin 325 mg, caffeine 40 mg, and butalbital 50 mg.

LORTAB 2.5/500: acetaminophen 500 mg and hydrocodone bitartrate 2.5 mg.

LORTAB 5/500: acetaminophen 500 mg and hydrocodone bitartrate 5 mg.

LORTAB 7.5/500: acetaminophen 500 mg and hydrocodone bitartrate 7.5 mg.

MIDRIN: isometheptene mucate 65 mg, dichloralphenazone 100 mg, and acetaminophen 325 mg.

PAC TABLETS◇: aspirin 400 mg and caffeine 32 mg.

PHRENILIN: acetaminophen 325 mg and butalbital 50 mg.

PHRENILIN FORTE: acetaminophen 650 mg and butalbital 50 mg.

SINUS EXCEDRIN NO DROWSINESS◇: acetaminophen 500 mg and pseudo-ephedrine hydrochloride 30 mg.

SINUTAB◇: acetaminophen 325 mg, chlorpheniramine 2 mg, and pseudo-ephedrine hydrochloride 30 mg.

SINUTAB MAXIMUM STRENGTH◇: acetaminophen 500 mg, pseudo-ephedrine hydrochloride 30 mg, and chlorpheniramine maleate, 2 mg.

TECNAL†: aspirin 330 mg, caffeine 40 mg, and butalbital 50 mg.

VANQUISH◇: aspirin 227 mg, acet-aminophen 194 mg, caffeine 33 mg, aluminum hydroxide 25 mg, and magnesium hydroxide 50 mg.

VICODIN: acetaminophen 500 mg and hydrocodone bitartrate 5 mg.

VICODIN ES: acetaminophen 750 mg and hydrocodone bitartrate 7.5 mg.

---

†Available in Canada only.　　　‡Available in Australia only.　　　◇Available OTC.

acetaminophen
(APAP, paracetamol)

Abenol†◇; Aceta Elixir*◇; Acetaminophen Uniserts◇; Aceta Tablets◇; Actamin◇; Actamin Extra◇; Actimol†◇; Aminofen◇; Aminofen Max◇; Anacin-3◇; Anacin-3 Children's Elixir*◇; Anacin-3 Children's Tablets◇; Anacin-3 Extra Strength◇; Anacin-3 Infants'◇; Anacin-3 Maximum Strength Caplets◇; Apacet Capsules◇; Apacet Elixir*◇; Apacet Extra Strength Caplets◇; Apacet Extra Strength Tablets◇; Apacet Infants'◇; Apacet Regular Strength Tablets◇; Apo-Acetaminophen†◇; Arthritis Pain Formula Aspirin Free◇; Atasol Caplets†◇; Atasol Drops†◇; Atasol Elixir*†◇; Atasol Forte Caplets†◇; Atasol Forte Tablets†◇; Atasol Tablets†◇; Banesin◇; Dapa◇; Dapa XS◇; Datril XS; Dolanex*◇; Dorcol Children's Fever and Pain Reducer◇; Dymadon‡◇; Dymadon P‡◇; Exdol†◇; Exdol Strong†◇; Feverall, Children's‡; Feverall Junior Strength‡; Feverall Sprinkle Caps, Children's‡; Feverall Sprinkle Caps, Junior Strength‡; Genapap Children's Elixir◇; Genapap Children's Tablets◇; Genapap Extra Strength Caplets◇; Genapap Extra Strength Tablets◇; Genapap, Infants'◇; Genapap Regular Strength Tablets◇; Genebs Extra Strength Caplets◇; Genebs Regular Strength Tablets◇; Genebs X-Tra◇; Halenol Elixir*◇; Liquiprin Infants' Drops◇; Meda Cap◇; Myapap Elixir*◇; Myapap, Infants'◇; Neopap◇; Oraphen-PD◇; Panadol◇; Panadol, Children's◇; Panadol Extra Strength◇; Panadol, Infants'◇; Panadol Junior Strength Caplets◇; Panadol Maximum Strength Caplets◇; Panadol Maximum Strength Tablets◇; Panamax‡◇; Panex◇; Panex-500◇; Paralgin‡◇; Paraspen‡◇; Redutemp◇; Ridenol Caplets◇; Robigesic†◇; Rounox†◇; Setamol-500‡◇; Snaplets-FR◇; Stanback AF Extra Strength Powder; St. Joseph Aspirin-Free Fever Reducer for Children◇; Suppap-120◇; Suppap-325◇; Suppap-650◇; Tapanol Extra Strength Caplets◇; Tapanol Extra Strength Tablets◇; Tempra◇; Tempra Caplets◇; Tempra Chewable Tablets◇; Tempra Drops◇; Tempra D.S.◇; Tempra, Infants'◇; Tempra Syrup◇; Tenol◇; Tylenol Caplets◇; Tylenol Chewable Tablets◇; Tylenol Children's Elixir◇; Tylenol Children's Tablets◇; Tylenol Drops◇; Tylenol Elixir*◇; Tylenol Extended Relief◇; Tylenol Extra Strength Adult Liquid Pain Reliever◇; Tylenol Extra Strength Caplets◇; Tylenol Extra Strength Gelcaps◇; Tylenol Extra Strength Tablets◇; Tylenol Infants'◇; Tylenol Junior Strength Caplets◇; Tylenol Junior Strength Tablets◇; Tylenol Regular Strength Caplets◇; Tylenol Regular Strength Tablets◇; Tylenol Tablets◇; Ty-Pap◇; Ty-Pap, Infants'◇; Ty-Pap Syrup◇; Ty-Tab Caplets◇; Ty-Tab Capsules◇; Ty-Tab, Children's◇; Ty-Tab Tablets◇; Valorin◇; Valorin Extra◇

Pregnancy Risk Category: NR

HOW SUPPLIED
Tablets: 160 mg◇, 325 mg◇, 500 mg◇, 650 mg◇
Tablets (chewable): 80 mg◇, 160 mg◇
Caplets (extended-release): 650 mg
Capsules: 500 mg◇
Oral solution: 48 mg/ml◇, 100 mg/ml◇
Oral suspension: 120 mg/5 ml‡, 100 mg/ml◇, 160 mg/ml◇
Oral liquid: 160 mg/5 ml◇, 500 mg/15 ml◇
Elixir: 120 mg/5 ml, 130 mg/5 ml*◇, 160 mg/5 ml*◇, 325 mg/5 ml*◇

---

*Liquid form contains alcohol.   *Common* reactions are in italics; **life-threatening**, in bold italics.
**May contain tartrazine.

Granules: 80 mg/packet◊, 325 mg/
capful◊
Powder for solution: 1 g/packet
Sprinkles: 80 mg/capsule, 160 mg/
capsule
Tablets for solution: 325 mg
Suppositories: 120 mg◊, 125 mg◊,
300 mg◊, 325 mg◊, 650 mg◊
Wafers: 120 mg◊

ACTION
Unknown. Thought to produce analgesia by blocking generation of pain impulses, probably by inhibiting prostaglandin synthesis in the CNS or the synthesis or action of other substances that sensitize pain receptors to mechanical or chemical stimulation. It is thought to relieve fever by central action in the hypothalamic heat-regulating center.

ONSET, PEAK, DURATION
Onset unknown. Peak effects vary; average peak blood levels occur in 1 to 3 hours. Effects persist about 3 to 4 hours.

INDICATIONS & DOSAGE
Mild pain or fever –
Adults and children over 11 years:
325 to 650 mg P.O. q 4 to 6 hours; or 1 g P.O. t.i.d. or q.i.d., p.r.n. Alternatively, 2 extended-release caplets P.O. q 8 hours. Maximum dosage should not exceed 4 g daily. Dosage for long-term therapy should not exceed 2.6 g daily.
Children 11 years: 480 mg P.O. or rectally q 4 to 6 hours.
Children 9 to 10 years: 400 mg P.O. or rectally q 4 to 6 hours.
Children 6 to 8 years: 320 mg P.O. or rectally q 4 to 6 hours.
Children 4 to 5 years: 240 mg P.O. or rectally q 4 to 6 hours.
Children 2 to 3 years: 160 mg P.O. or rectally q 4 to 6 hours.
Children 12 to 23 months: 120 mg P.O. q 4 to 6 hours.

Children 4 to 11 months: 80 mg P.O. q 4 to 6 hours.
Children up to 3 months: 40 mg P.O. q 4 to 6 hours.

ADVERSE REACTIONS
Hematologic: hemolytic anemia, neutropenia, leukopenia, pancytopenia, thrombocytopenia (rare).
Hepatic: *severe liver damage with toxic doses,* jaundice.
Skin: rash, urticaria.
Other: hypoglycemia.

INTERACTIONS
Barbiturates, carbamazepine, hydantoins, rifampin, sulfinpyrazone: high doses or long-term use of these drugs may reduce the therapeutic effects and enhance the hepatotoxic effects of acetaminophen. Avoid concomitant use.
Caffeine: may enhance analgesic effects of acetaminophen.
Ethanol: increased risk of hepatic damage. Avoid concomitant use.
Warfarin: increased hypoprothrombinemic effects with long-term use with high doses of acetaminophen. Monitor PTs closely.
Zidovudine: may increase the incidence of bone marrow suppression because of impaired zidovudine metabolism. Monitor patient closely.

CONTRAINDICATIONS
None known.

NURSING CONSIDERATIONS
• Use cautiously in patients with history of chronic alcohol abuse because hepatotoxicity has occurred after therapeutic doses.
• Many OTC products contain acetaminophen; be aware of this when calculating total daily dosage.
• Liquid form is recommended for children and for all patients who have difficulty swallowing.
• Know that acetaminophen may interfere with certain laboratory tests

for urinary 5-hydroxyindoleacetic acid. It may also produce false-positive decreases in blood glucose levels in home monitoring systems.

• Tell parents to consult a doctor before giving this drug to children under 2 years.

• Tell patient this drug is only for short-term use. Tell patients to consult a doctor if administering to children for more than 5 days or adults for more than 10 days.

• Tell patient not to use for self-medication of marked fever (over 103.1° F [39.5° C]), fever persisting longer than 3 days, or recurrent fever unless directed by doctor.

• Warn patient that high doses or unsupervised long-term use can cause hepatic damage. Excessive ingestion of alcoholic beverages may increase the risk of hepatotoxicity.

• Tell patient who is breast-feeding acetaminophen is found in breast milk in low concentrations (less than 1% of dose). Breast-feeding patients may use it safely if therapy is short-term and does not exceed recommended doses.

aspirin (acetylsalicylic acid)

Ancasal†◇, Arthrinol†◇, Artria SR◇, ASA◇, ASA Enseals◇, Aspergum◇, Aspro‡, Astrin†◇, Bayer Aspirin◇, Bex‡, Coryphen†◇, Easprin◇, Ecotrin◇, Empirin◇, Entrophen†◇, Halfprin, Measurin◇, Norwich Aspirin Extra Strength◇, Novasen†◇, Riphen-10†◇, Sal-Adult†◇, Sal-Infant†◇, Solprin‡, Supasa†◇, Triaphen-10†◇, Vincent's Powders‡, Winsprin Capsules‡, ZORprin◇

Pregnancy Risk Category: C (D in 3rd trimester)

HOW SUPPLIED
Tablets◇: 325 mg, 500 mg, 600 mg, 650 mg

Tablets (chewable): 81 mg◇
Tablets (enteric-coated): 165 mg, 325 mg◇, 500 mg◇, 650 mg◇, 975 mg
Tablets (extended-release): 800 mg
Tablets (timed-release): 650 mg◇
Capsules: 325 mg◇, 500 mg◇
Powder: 500 mg
Chewing gum: 227.5 mg◇
Suppositories: 60 mg, 65 mg, 120 mg, 125 mg, 130 mg, 195 mg, 200 mg, 300 mg, 325 mg, 600 mg, 650 mg, 1.2 g

ACTION
Produces analgesia by blocking prostaglandin synthesis (peripheral action). Aspirin and other salicylates may prevent the lowering of the pain threshold that occurs when prostaglandins sensitize pain receptors to mechanical and chemical stimulation. Exerts its anti-inflammatory effect by inhibiting prostaglandin synthesis; also may inhibit the synthesis or action of other mediators of the inflammatory response. Relieves fever by acting on the hypothalamic heat-regulating center to cause peripheral vasodilation. This increases peripheral blood supply and promotes sweating, which leads to heat loss and to cooling by evaporation. In low doses, aspirin also appears to impede clotting by blocking prostaglandin synthesis, which prevents formation of the platelet-aggregating substance thromboxane A_2.

ONSET, PEAK, DURATION
Onset occurs 5 to 30 minutes after an oral, rapidly absorbed dose. With oral solution, serum aspirin levels peak in 15 to 40 minutes; peak serum levels of salicylate, its active metabolite, in ½ to 1 hour. With regular tablets, peak serum aspirin levels in 25 to 40 minutes; peak serum salicylate levels, in 1 to 2 hours. With buffered tablets, peak serum aspirin and salicylate levels occur in 1 to 2 hours. With extended-release tablets, peak aspirin levels occur

---

*Liquid form contains alcohol.
**May contain tartrazine.

Common reactions are in italics; ***life-threatening***, in bold italics.

in 1 to 2 hours; peak salicylate levels, in 3 to 4 hours. With enteric-coated tablets, peak aspirin and salicylate levels occur in 4 to 8 hours. With suppositories, peak aspirin and salicylate levels occur in 3 to 4 hours. Effects persist for 1 to 4 hours.

INDICATIONS & DOSAGE
Rheumatoid arthritis, osteoarthritis, or other polyarthritic or inflammatory conditions –
Adults: initially, 2.4 to 3.6 g P.O. daily in divided doses. Maintenance dosage is 3.6 to 5.4 g P.O. daily in divided doses.
Juvenile rheumatoid arthritis –
Children: weighing 25 kg or less, 60 to 90 mg/kg P.O. daily in divided doses; weighing more than 25 kg, 2.4 to 3.6 g P.O. daily in divided doses.
Mild pain or fever –
Adults and children over 11 years: 325 to 650 mg P.O. or P.R. q 4 hours, p.r.n.
Children 2 to 11 years: 1.5 g/m^2 or 65 mg/kg P.O. or P.R. daily in 4 to 6 divided doses.
Prevention of thrombosis –
Adults: 1.3 g P.O. daily in 2 to 4 divided doses.
Reduction of risk of heart attack in patients with previous MI or unstable angina –
Adults: 160 to 325 mg P.O. daily.
Kawasaki syndrome (mucocutaneous lymph node syndrome) –
Adults: 80 to 100 mg/kg P.O. daily in 4 divided doses during the febrile phase. Some patients may need up to 120 mg/kg. When fever subsides, dosage decreased to 3 to 8 mg/kg once daily, adjusted according to serum salicylate concentration.

ADVERSE REACTIONS
EENT: *tinnitus and hearing loss.*
GI: *nausea, vomiting, GI distress, occult bleeding.*
Hematologic: *prolonged bleeding time.*

Hepatic: abnormal liver function studies, hepatitis.
Skin: *rash,* bruising.
Other: hypersensitivity reactions, (*anaphylaxis,* asthma), *Reye's syndrome.*

INTERACTIONS
Ammonium chloride and other urine acidifiers: increased blood levels of aspirin products. Monitor for aspirin toxicity.
Antacids in high doses (and other urine alkalinizers): decreased levels of aspirin products. Monitor for decreased aspirin effect.
Beta blockers: decreased antihypertensive effect. Avoid long-term aspirin use if patient is taking antihypertensives.
Corticosteroids: enhanced salicylate elimination. Monitor for decreased salicylate effect.
Ethanol, NSAIDs, steroids: increased risk of GI bleeding. Avoid concomitant use.
Heparin, oral anticoagulants: increased risk of bleeding. Avoid using together if possible.
Methotrexate: increased risk of methotrexate toxicity. Avoid concomitant use.
NSAIDs, including diflunisal, fenoprofen, ibuprofen, indomethacin, piroxicam, meclofenamate, naproxen: altered pharmacokinetics of these agents, leading to lowered serum levels and decreased effectiveness. Avoid concomitant use.
Oral antidiabetic agents: increased hypoglycemic effect. Monitor closely.
Probenecid, sulfinpyrazone: decreased uricosuric effect. Avoid aspirin during therapy with these agents.

CONTRAINDICATIONS
Contraindicated in patients with hypersensitivity to the drug, G6PD deficiency, bleeding disorders such as hemophilia, von Willebrand's disease, or telangiectasia. Also contraindi-

---

cated in patients with NSAID-induced sensitivity reactions.

NURSING CONSIDERATIONS
• Use cautiously in patients with GI lesions, impaired renal function, hypoprothrombinemia, vitamin K deficiency, thrombocytopenia, thrombotic thrombocytopenic purpura, or severe hepatic impairment.
• Because of epidemiologic association with Reye's syndrome, the Centers for Disease Control and Prevention recommends not giving children or teenagers with chicken pox or influenza-like illness salicylates.
• Be aware that for inflammatory conditions, rheumatic fever, and thrombosis, aspirin is administered on a scheduled, rather than p.r.n., basis.
• Know that because enteric-coated and sustained release tablets are slowly absorbed, they are not suitable for rapid relief of acute pain, fever, or inflammation. They do cause less GI bleeding and may be more suited for long-term therapy, such as for the treatment of arthritis.
• For patients who cannot tolerate oral medications, ask doctor about the possibility of using aspirin rectal suppositories. Watch for rectal mucosal irritation or bleeding.
• Be aware that febrile, dehydrated children can develop toxicity rapidly.
• Monitor elderly patients closely because they may be more susceptible to aspirin's toxic effects.
• Monitor blood salicylate levels as indicated and ordered. Therapeutic blood salicylate level in arthritis is 10 to 30 mg/100 ml. Tinnitus may occur at plasma levels of 30 mg/100 ml and above, but this is not a reliable indicator of toxicity, especially in very young patients and those over age 60. With chronic therapy, mild toxicity may occur at plasma levels of 20 mg/100 ml.
• During prolonged therapy, hematocrit, hemoglobin level, PT, and renal function should be assessed periodically as ordered.
• Know that aspirin irreversibly inhibits platelet aggregation. It should be discontinued 5 to 7 days before elective surgery as ordered to allow time for the production and release of new platelets.
• To reduce adverse GI reactions, advise patients to take with food, milk, antacid, or large glass of water.
• For patients with swallowing difficulties, crush non-enteric-coated aspirin and dissolve in soft food or liquid. Administer liquid immediately after mixing because drug will break down rapidly.
• Tell patient aspirin tablets that have a strong vinegar-like odor should be discarded.
• Tell patients to consult a doctor if administering to children for more than 5 days or adults for more than 10 days.
• Advise patients receiving prolonged treatment with large doses of aspirin to watch for petechiae, bleeding gums, and signs of GI bleeding, and to maintain adequate fluid intake. Encourage the use of a soft-bristled toothbrush.
• Because of the many possible drug interactions involving aspirin, warn patients taking prescription drugs to check with a doctor or pharmacist before taking aspirin or OTC combination products containing aspirin.
• Inform female patient that aspirin should not be used during last trimester of pregnancy unless specifically directed to do so by a doctor.
• Caution parents to keep out of reach of children — aspirin is one of the leading causes of poisoning in children. Encourage the use of child-resistant containers.

---

*Liquid form contains alcohol.
**May contain tartrazine.

Common reactions are in italics; **life-threatening,** in bold italics.

choline magnesium trisalicylate (choline salicylate and magnesium salicylate)

Tricusal, Trilisate

Pregnancy Risk Category: C

HOW SUPPLIED

Tablets: 500 mg, 750 mg, 1,000 mg of salicylate
Solution: 500 mg of salicylate/5 ml

ACTION

Produces analgesia by blocking prostaglandin synthesis (peripheral action). Salicylates may prevent the lowering of the pain threshold that occurs when prostaglandins sensitize pain receptors to mechanical and chemical stimulation. Exerts its anti-inflammatory effect by inhibiting prostaglandin synthesis. Relieves fever by acting on the hypothalamic heat-regulating center to produce peripheral vasodilation. This increases peripheral blood supply and promotes sweating, which leads to heat loss and to cooling by evaporation.

ONSET, PEAK, DURATION

Onset and duration unknown. Serum levels peak within 1 to 2 hours.

INDICATIONS & DOSAGE

Rheumatoid arthritis and osteoarthritis or other polyarthritic or inflammatory conditions –
Adults: initially, 1.5 to 2.5 g P.O. daily as a single dose or in 2 or 3 divided doses. Dosage is adjusted according to patient response. Dosage range is 1 to 4.5 g daily.
Juvenile rheumatoid arthritis –
Children: 60 to 110 mg/kg/day in divided doses (q 6 to 8 hours).
Mild to moderate pain and fever –
Adults: 2 to 3 g P.O. daily in divided doses q 4 to 6 hours.
Children: 10 to 15 mg/kg/day q 4 hours, up to 60 to 80 mg/kg/day.

ADVERSE REACTIONS

EENT: tinnitus and hearing loss.
GI: GI distress.
Skin: rash.
Other: hypersensitivity reactions *(anaphylaxis)*.

INTERACTIONS

Ammonium chloride and other urine acidifiers: increased blood levels of salicylates. Monitor for salicylate toxicity.
Antacids in high doses (and other urine alkalinizers): decreased levels of salicylates. Monitor for decreased salicylate effect.
Corticosteroids: enhanced salicylate elimination. Monitor for decreased salicylate effect.
Ethanol, steroids, and other NSAIDs: enhanced risk of adverse GI effects.
Methotrexate: increased risk of methotrexate toxicity. Avoid concomitant use.
Oral anticoagulants: increased risk of bleeding. Use together cautiously.

CONTRAINDICATIONS

Contraindicated in patients hypersensitive to the drug. Also contraindicated in patients with hemophilia, bleeding ulcers, and hemorrhagic states.

NURSING CONSIDERATIONS

● Use cautiously in patients with renal insufficiency, hepatic impairment, peptic ulcer disease, and gastritis.
● Because of epidemiologic association with Reye's syndrome, the Centers for Disease Control and Prevention recommends not giving salicylates to children or teenagers with chicken pox or influenza-like illness.
● Be aware that febrile, dehydrated children can develop toxicity rapidly.
● Monitor serum salicylate levels in long-term therapy, as ordered. Therapeutic blood salicylate level in arthritis is 10 to 30 mg/100 ml. Tinnitus may occur at plasma levels of 30 mg/

100 ml and above, but this is not a reliable indicator of toxicity, especially in very young patients and those over age 60. With chronic therapy, mild toxicity may occur at plasma levels of 20 mg/100 ml.
• Periodically monitor hemoglobin level and PT in patients receiving long-term treatment with large doses.
• Know that this drug causes less GI distress than aspirin. If an antacid is needed, give it 2 hours after meals and choline magnesium trisalicylate before meals.
• Tell patients to take tablets with food or a full glass of water. Solution may be mixed with fruit juice, but not antacids.

---

choline salicylate
Arthropan, Teejel†*

Pregnancy Risk Category: NR

HOW SUPPLIED
Liquid: 870 mg/5 ml
Gel: 87 mg/g†*

ACTION
Produces analgesia by blocking prostaglandin synthesis (peripheral action). Salicylates may prevent the lowering of the pain threshold that occurs when prostaglandins sensitize pain receptors to mechanical and chemical stimulation. Exerts its anti-inflammatory effect by inhibiting prostaglandin synthesis. Relieves fever by acting on the hypothalamic heat-regulating center to produce peripheral vasodilation. This increases peripheral blood supply and promotes sweating, which leads to heat loss and to cooling by evaporation.

ONSET, PEAK, DURATION
Unknown.

INDICATIONS & DOSAGE
Rheumatoid arthritis, osteoarthritis, mild to moderate pain or fever –

Adults and children over 12 years: 1 teaspoonful (870 mg of choline salicylate) P.O. q 3 to 4 hours p.r.n. If tolerated and needed, dosage may be increased to 2 teaspoonsful. Not to exceed 6 teaspoonsful daily.
Relief of pain from inflamed gums –
Adults and children over 2 years: apply 1 cm of gel to affected area q 3 to 4 hours and h.s., p.r.n.

ADVERSE REACTIONS
EENT: *tinnitus* and hearing loss.
GI: nausea, vomiting, GI distress.
Skin: rash.
Other: hypersensitivity reactions (*anaphylaxis*).

INTERACTIONS
Ammonium chloride and other urine acidifiers: increased blood levels of salicylates. Monitor for salicylate toxicity.
Antacids in high doses and other urine alkalinizers: decreased levels of salicylates. Monitor for decreased salicylate effect.
Corticosteroids: enhanced salicylate elimination. Monitor for decreased salicylate effect.
Ethanol, other NSAIDs, steroids: enhanced risk of adverse GI reactions.
Methotrexate: increased risk of methotrexate toxicity. Avoid concomitant use.

CONTRAINDICATIONS
Contraindicated in patients with hypersensitivity to the drug. Also contraindicated in patients with hemophilia, bleeding ulcers, and hemorrhagic states.

NURSING CONSIDERATIONS
• Use cautiously in patients with impaired hepatic or renal function, hypoprothrombinemia, vitamin K deficiency, peptic ulcer disease, and gastritis, and in those with a known allergy to salicylates.
• Because of epidemiologic associa-

---

*Liquid form contains alcohol.
**May contain tartrazine.

Common reactions are in italics; ***life-threatening,*** in bold italics.

tion with Reye's syndrome, the Centers for Disease Control and Prevention recommends not giving salicylates to children or teenagers with chicken pox or influenza-like illness.
• Know that febrile, dehydrated children can develop toxicity rapidly.
• Monitor serum salicylate levels as ordered with patients on prolonged therapy. Therapeutic blood salicylate level in arthritis is 10 to 30 mg/100 ml. Tinnitus may occur at plasma levels of 30 mg/100 ml and above, but this is not a reliable indicator of toxicity, especially in very young patients and those over age 60. With chronic therapy, mild toxicity may occur at plasma levels of 20 mg/100 ml.
• Periodically monitor hemoglobin level and PT in patients receiving long-term treatment with large doses.
• Tell patients they may mix drug with water, fruit juice, or carbonated drinks, but not antacids.
• Inform patient that drug causes less GI distress than aspirin. If an antacid is needed, give it 2 hours after meals and choline salicylate before meals.

---

diflunisal
Dolobid

Pregnancy Risk Category: C

HOW SUPPLIED
Tablets: 250 mg, 500 mg

ACTION
Unknown. Probably related to inhibition of prostaglandin synthesis.

ONSET, PEAK, DURATION
Onset occurs in 1 hour for pain relief; unknown for anti-inflammatory action. Peak plasma levels and analgesic effects occur in 2 to 3 hours. Effects persist for pain relief 8 to 12 hours; unknown for anti-inflammatory effects.

INDICATIONS & DOSAGE
Mild to moderate pain, osteoarthritis, and rheumatoid arthritis –
Adults: 500 to 1,000 mg P.O. daily in two divided doses, usually q 12 hours. Maximum dosage is 1,500 mg daily.
Adults over 65: one-half the usual adult dose.

ADVERSE REACTIONS
CNS: *dizziness,* somnolence, insomnia, *headache,* fatigue.
EENT: *tinnitus, visual disturbances (rare).*
GI: *nausea, dyspepsia, GI pain, diarrhea,* vomiting, constipation, flatulence.
GU: renal impairment, hematuria, interstitial nephritis.
Skin: *rash,* pruritus, sweating, stomatitis, ***toxic epidermal necrolysis, Stevens-Johnson syndrome.***
Other: dry mucous membranes.

INTERACTIONS
Acetaminophen, hydrochlorothiazide, indomethacin: diflunisal may substantially increase blood levels, increasing the risk of toxicity. Avoid concomitant use.
Antacids, aspirin: decreased diflunisal blood levels. Monitor for possible decreased therapeutic effect.
Cyclosporine: diflunisal may enhance the nephrotoxicity of cyclosporine. Avoid concomitant use.
Methotrexate: diflunisal may enhance the toxicity of methotrexate. Avoid concomitant use.
Oral anticoagulants, thrombolytic agents: diflunisal may enhance pharmacologic effects of these agents. Use together cautiously.
Sulindac: diflunisal decreases blood levels of sulindac's active metabolite. Monitor for decreased pharmacologic effect.

CONTRAINDICATIONS
Contraindicated in patients with hypersensitivity to the drug, or for

---

whom acute asthmatic attacks, urticaria, or rhinitis are precipitated by aspirin or other NSAIDs.

NURSING CONSIDERATIONS
• Use cautiously in patients with GI bleeding, history of peptic ulcer disease, renal impairment, and compromised cardiac function, hypertension, or other conditions predisposing patient to fluid retention.
• Because of the epidemiologic association with Reye's syndrome, the Centers for Disease Control and Prevention recommends not giving salicylates to children and teenagers with chicken pox or influenza-like illness.
• Advise the patient to take with water, milk, or meals.

---

magnesium salicylate
Extra-Strength Doan's◇, Magan◇, Mobidin◇, Original Doan's◇

Pregnancy Risk Category: NR

HOW SUPPLIED
Tablets: 545 mg, 600 mg
Caplets: 325 mg◇, 500 mg◇

ACTION
Produces analgesia by blocking prostaglandin synthesis (peripheral action). Salicylates may prevent the lowering of the pain threshold that occurs when prostaglandins sensitize pain receptors to mechanical and chemical stimulation. Exerts its anti-inflammatory effect by inhibiting prostaglandin synthesis. Relieves fever by acting on the hypothalamic heat-regulating center to produce peripheral vasodilation. This increases peripheral blood supply and promotes sweating, which leads to heat loss and to cooling by evaporation.

ONSET, PEAK, DURATION
Onset and duration unknown. Blood levels peak within 1½ to 2 hours of a dose.

INDICATIONS & DOSAGE
Arthritis –
Adults: 545 mg to 1.2 g P.O. t.i.d. or q.i.d.
Mild pain or fever –
Adults and children older than 11 years of age: 300 to 600 mg P.O. q 4 hours, not to exceed 3.5 g/24 hours.

ADVERSE REACTIONS
EENT: *tinnitus and hearing loss.*
GI: *nausea, vomiting, GI distress.*
Hepatic: abnormal liver function studies, hepatitis.
Skin: *rash,* bruising.
Other: hypersensitivity reactions (**anaphylaxis,** asthma).

INTERACTIONS
Ammonium chloride and other urine acidifiers: increased blood levels of salicylates. Monitor for salicylate toxicity.
Antacids in high doses and other urine alkalinizers: decreased levels of salicylates. Monitor for decreased salicylate effect.
Corticosteroids: enhanced salicylate elimination. Monitor for decreased salicylate effect.
Ethanol, other NSAIDs, steroids: increased risk of GI bleeding. Avoid concomitant use.
Heparin, oral anticoagulants: increased risk of bleeding. Avoid using together if possible.
Methotrexate: increased risk of methotrexate toxicity. Avoid concomitant use.

CONTRAINDICATIONS
Contraindicated in patients with hypersensitivity to the drug, or severe chronic renal insufficiency because of risk of magnesium toxicity. Also contraindicated in patients with bleeding disorders, or aspirin hypersensitivity.

---

*Liquid form contains alcohol.   *Common* reactions are in italics; *life-threatening,* in bold italics.
**May contain tartrazine.

NURSING CONSIDERATIONS
• Use cautiously in patients with hypoprothrombinemia and vitamin K deficiency.
• Because of epidemiologic association with Reye's syndrome, the Centers for Disease Control and Prevention recommends not giving salicylates to children or teenagers with chicken pox or influenza-like illness.
• Know that febrile, dehydrated children can develop toxicity rapidly.
• Monitor serum salicylate levels when drug used long term, as ordered. Therapeutic blood salicylate level in arthritis is 10 to 30 mg/100 ml. Tinnitus may occur at plasma levels of 30 mg/100 ml and above, but this is not a reliable indicator of toxicity, especially in very young patients and those over age 60. With chronic therapy, mild toxicity may occur at plasma levels of 20 mg/100 ml.
• Monitor hemoglobin level and PT in patients receiving long-term treatment with large doses.
• To reduce adverse GI reactions, tell patients to take this drug with food, milk, antacid, or large glass of water.

salsalate (disalicylic acid, salicylsalicylic acid)
Amigesic, Argesic-SA, Arthra-G, Disalcid, Mono-Gesic, Salflex, Salgesic, Salsitab

Pregnancy Risk Category: C

HOW SUPPLIED
Tablets: 500 mg, 750 mg
Caplets: 750 mg
Capsules: 500 mg

ACTION
Salsalate is the salicylic ester of salicylic acid. Each molecule of salsalate is hydrolyzed to two molecules of salicylate in vivo. Produces analgesia by blocking prostaglandin synthesis (peripheral action). Salicylates prevent the lowering of the pain threshold that occurs when prostaglandins sensitize pain receptors to mechanical and chemical stimulation. Drug also has an ill-defined effect on the hypothalamus. Exact mechanism of its anti-inflammatory action is unknown.

ONSET, PEAK, DURATION
Onset and duration unknown. Plasma levels of salsalate peak within 1½ hours of an oral dose; of salicylate, within 2 to 4 hours.

INDICATIONS & DOSAGE
Arthritis –
Adults: 3 g P.O. daily in divided doses b.i.d. or t.i.d.

ADVERSE REACTIONS
EENT: *tinnitus and hearing loss.*
GI: *nausea, vomiting, GI distress,* occult bleeding (rare).
Hepatic: abnormal liver function studies, hepatitis.
Skin: *rash,* bruising.
Other: hypersensitivity reactions (***anaphylaxis***, asthma).

INTERACTIONS
Ammonium chloride and other urine acidifiers: increased blood levels of salicylates. Monitor for salicylate toxicity.
Antacids in high doses and other urine alkalinizers: decreased levels of salicylates. Monitor for decreased salicylate effect.
Corticosteroids: enhanced salicylate excretion. Monitor for decreased salicylate effect.
Ethanol, NSAIDs, steroids: increased risk of GI bleeding. Avoid concomitant use.
Methotrexate: increased risk of methotrexate toxicity. Avoid concomitant use.
Oral anticoagulants: possible increased risk of bleeding. Avoid using together if possible.

CONTRAINDICATIONS

Contraindicated in patients with salsalate hypersensitivity.

NURSING CONSIDERATIONS

• Use cautiously in patients with bleeding disorders, peptic ulcer disease or renal insufficiency. Also use cautiously in patients with hypoprothrombinemia, vitamin K deficiency, thrombocytopenia, thrombotic thrombocytopenic purpura, or severe hepatic impairment.
• Because of epidemiologic association with Reye's syndrome, the Centers for Disease Control and Prevention recommends not giving salicylates to children or teenagers with chicken pox or influenza-like illness.
• Monitor serum salicylate level as ordered. Therapeutic blood salicylate level in arthritis is 10 to 30 mg/100 ml. Tinnitus may occur at plasma levels of 30 mg/100 ml and above, but this is not a reliable indicator of toxicity, especially in very young patients and those over age 60. With long-term therapy, mild toxicity may occur at plasma levels of 20 mg/100 ml.
• In patients on long-term therapy, obtain hemoglobin and PT tests periodically.
• To reduce adverse GI reactions, tell patients to take this drug with food, milk, antacid, or large glass of water.
• Advise patients receiving long-term treatment with large doses to watch for petechiae, bleeding gums, and signs of GI bleeding, and to maintain adequate fluid intake. Encourage the use of a soft-bristled toothbrush.

---

sodium salicylate

Pregnancy Risk Category: NR

HOW SUPPLIED

Tablets (enteric-coated): 325 mg◇,
650 mg◇
Injection: 100 mg/ml

ACTION

Produces analgesia by blocking prostaglandin synthesis (peripheral action). Salicylates may prevent the lowering of the pain threshold that occurs when prostaglandins sensitize pain receptors to mechanical and chemical stimulation. Exact anti-inflammatory action unknown although it is thought to exert its anti-inflammatory effect by inhibiting prostaglandin synthesis; also may inhibit the synthesis or action of other mediators of the inflammatory response. Relieves fever by acting on the hypothalamic heat-regulating center to produce peripheral vasodilation. This increases peripheral blood supply and promotes sweating, which leads to heat loss and to cooling by evaporation.

ONSET, PEAK, DURATION

Unset and duration unknown. Plasma levels peak within 6 hours of oral administration.

INDICATIONS & DOSAGE

Minor pain or fever –
Adults and children older than 11 years: 325 to 650 mg P.O. q 4 hours, p.r.n. Maximum dosage is 1 g daily. Alternatively, 500 mg I.V. not to exceed 1 g daily except in rheumatic fever in which single daily I.V. infusions of up to 10 g have been given.
Children 2 to 11 years: 25 to 50 mg/kg daily or 1.5 g/m² daily, administered in 4 to 6 divided doses.
Rheumatoid arthritis, osteoarthritis, and other polyarthritic or inflammatory conditions –
Adults: 3.6 to 5.4 g P.O. daily in divided doses.

ADVERSE REACTIONS

EENT: *tinnitus, hearing loss.*
GI: *nausea, vomiting, GI distress.*
Hepatic: abnormal liver function studies, hepatitis.
Skin: *rash.*

---

*Liquid form contains alcohol.
**May contain tartrazine.

Common reactions are in italics; **life-threatening**, in bold italics.

Other: hypersensitivity reactions (*anaphylaxis*, asthma).

INTERACTIONS

Ammonium chloride and other urine acidifiers: increased blood levels of salicylates. Monitor for salicylate toxicity.

Antacids in large doses and other urine alkalinizers: decreased levels of salicylates. Monitor for decreased salicylate effect.

Corticosteroids: enhanced salicylate elimination. Monitor for decreased salicylate effect.

Ethanol, other NSAIDs, steroids: increased risk of GI distress. Avoid concomitant use.

Methotrexate: increased risk of methotrexate toxicity. Avoid concomitant use.

Oral anticoagulants: increased risk of bleeding. Avoid using together if possible.

CONTRAINDICATIONS

Contraindicated in patients with GI ulcer, GI bleeding, or aspirin hypersensitivity.

NURSING CONSIDERATIONS

● Use cautiously in patients with hypoprothrombinemia, vitamin K deficiency, or bleeding disorders and in asthmatic patients with nasal polyps (may cause severe bronchospasm). Also use cautiously in patients with CHF or hypertension because of increased sodium load.

● Because of epidemiologic association with Reye's syndrome, the Centers for Disease Control and Prevention recommends not giving salicylates to children or teenagers with chicken pox or influenza-like illness.

● **I.V. use:** Dilute drug in 1 liter of 0.9% sodium chloride or lactated Ringer's solution and infuse over 4 to 8 hours. Avoid extravasation because the drug is highly irritating to local tissues. Rapid infusion may cause thrombophlebitis.

● Administer oral drug with food, milk, antacid, or large glass of water.

● Know that febrile, dehydrated children can develop toxicity rapidly.

● Monitor serum salicylate levels as ordered in long-term therapy. Therapeutic salicylate level in arthritis is 10 to 30 mg/100 ml. Tinnitus may occur at plasma levels of 30 mg/100 ml and above, but this is not a reliable indicator of toxicity, especially in very young patients and in those over age 60. With long-term therapy, mild toxicity may occur at plasma levels of 20 mg/100 ml.

● In patients on long-term therapy, monitor hemoglobin level and PT periodically as ordered.

● To reduce adverse GI reactions, tell patients to take this drug with food, milk, antacid, or large glass of water.

● Advise patients receiving long-term treatment with large doses to watch for petechiae, bleeding gums, and signs of GI bleeding, and to maintain adequate fluid intake.

27

Nonsteroidal anti-inflammatory drugs

diclofenac sodium
diclofenac potassium
etodolac
fenoprofen calcium
flurbiprofen
ibuprofen
indomethacin
indomethacin sodium trihydrate
ketoprofen
ketorolac tromethamine
meclofenamate
mefenamic acid
nabumetone
naproxen
naproxen sodium
oxaprozin
piroxicam
sulindac
tolmetin sodium

COMBINATION PRODUCTS

ADVIL COLD AND SINUS◇, DRISTAN SINUS CAPLETS◇: pseudoephedrine hydrochloride 30 mg and ibuprofen 200 mg.

---

diclofenac sodium
Fenac‡, Voltaren, Voltaren SR†

diclofenac potassium
Cataflam

Pregnancy Risk Category: B

HOW SUPPLIED
Tablets: 50 mg
Tablets (enteric-coated): 25 mg, 50 mg, 75 mg
Tablets (slow-release): 100 mg†
Suppositories: 50 mg†, 100 mg†

ACTION
Unknown. Produces anti-inflammatory, analgesic, and antipyretic effects, possibly by inhibiting prostaglandin synthesis.

ONSET, PEAK, DURATION
Onset occurs in 30 minutes. Plasma levels peak within 2 to 3 hours of oral administration of enteric-coated tablets; unknown for regular tablets. Analgesic effects persist for up to 8 hours.

INDICATIONS AND DOSAGE
Ankylosing spondylitis –
Adults: 25 mg P.O. q.i.d. (and h.s. as needed)
Osteoarthritis –
Adults: 50 mg P.O. b.i.d. or t.i.d., or 75 mg P.O. b.i.d. (diclofenac sodium only)
Rheumatoid arthritis –
Adults: 50 mg P.O. t.i.d. or q.i.d. Alternatively, 75 mg P.O. b.i.d. (diclofenac sodium only) or 50 to 100 mg P.R. (where available) h.s. as a substitute for the last oral dose of the day. Not to exceed 225 mg daily.
Analgesia and primary dysmenorrhea –
Adults: 50 mg P.O. t.i.d. (diclofenac potassium only).

ADVERSE REACTIONS
CNS: anxiety, depression, dizziness, drowsiness, insomnia, irritability, myoclonus, migraine, *headache.*
CV: *CHF,* hypertension, edema, fluid retention.
EENT: *tinnitus,* laryngeal edema, swelling of the lips and tongue, blurred vision, eye pain, night blindness.
GI: *abdominal pain or cramps, constipation, diarrhea, indigestion, nausea,* abdominal distention, flatulence, peptic ulceration, ***bleeding,*** melena, bloody diarrhea, appetite change, colitis.
GU: azotemia, proteinuria, acute renal failure, oliguria, interstitial ne-

---

phritis, papillary necrosis, *nephrotic syndrome,* fluid retention.
Hepatic: elevated liver enzymes, jaundice, hepatitis, *hepatotoxicity.*
Respiratory: asthma.
Skin: rash, pruritus, urticaria, eczema, dermatitis, alopecia, photosensitivity, bullous eruption, *Stevens-Johnson syndrome (rare),* allergic purpura.
Other: *anaphylaxis; anaphylactoid reactions;* angioedema; back, leg, or joint pain; hypoglycemia; hyperglycemia.

INTERACTIONS
Anticoagulants (including warfarin): possible increased incidence of bleeding. Monitor patient closely.
Aspirin: concomitant use not recommended by manufacturer.
Cyclosporine, digoxin, lithium, methotrexate: diclofenac may reduce renal clearance of these drugs and increase risk of toxicity. Monitor patient closely.
Diuretics: decreased effectiveness of diuretics.
Insulin, oral antidiabetic agents: diclofenac may alter requirements for antidiabetic agents. Monitor patient closely.
Potassium-sparing diuretics: enhanced potassium retention and increased serum potassium levels.

CONTRAINDICATIONS
Contraindicated in patients with hypersensitivity to this drug, hepatic porphyria and in patients with a history of asthma, urticaria, or other allergic reactions after taking aspirin or other NSAIDs. Not recommended for use during late pregnancy or breastfeeding.

NURSING CONSIDERATIONS
• Use cautiously in patients with a history of peptic ulcer disease, hepatic dysfunction, cardiac disease, hypertension, conditions associated with fluid retention, or impaired renal function.
• Because NSAIDs impair the synthesis of renal prostaglandins, they can decrease renal blood flow and lead to reversible renal impairment, especially in patients with preexisting renal failure, liver dysfunction, or heart failure; in elderly patients; and in those taking diuretics. Monitor these patients closely.
• Elevations of liver tests may occur during therapy. Monitor serum transaminase, especially ALT levels, periodically in patients undergoing long-term therapy as ordered. Know that the first serum transaminase measurement should be no later than 8 weeks after initiation of therapy.
• Be aware that because of their antipyretic and anti-inflammatory actions, NSAIDs may mask the signs and symptoms of infection.
• To minimize GI distress, tell patients to take diclofenac with milk or meals.
• Instruct patient not to crush, break, or chew enteric-coated tablets.
• Serious GI toxicity, including peptic ulceration and bleeding, can occur in patients taking NSAIDs despite the absence of GI symptoms. Teach patients the signs and symptoms of GI bleeding, and tell them to contact the doctor immediately if any of these occurs.
• Teach patients the signs and symptoms of hepatotoxicity, including nausea, fatigue, lethargy, pruritus, jaundice, right upper quadrant tenderness, and flulike symptoms. Tell them to contact doctor immediately if these symptoms appear.
• Tell patient that use during last trimester of pregnancy should be avoided.

etodolac (ultradol)
Lodine

Pregnancy Risk Category: C

HOW SUPPLIED
Capsules: 200 mg, 300 mg
Tablets: 400 mg

ACTION
Unknown, but believed related to inhibition of prostaglandin biosynthesis.

ONSET, PEAK, DURATION
Onset occurs within 30 minutes. Plasma levels peak within 1 to 2 hours. Analgesic effects persist 4 to 12 hours.

INDICATIONS & DOSAGE
Acute and chronic management of osteoarthritis and pain –
Adults: 200 to 400 mg P.O. q 6 to 8 hours p.r.n., not to exceed 1,200 mg daily. For patients weighing 132 lb (60 kg) or under, total daily dose should not exceed 20 mg/kg.

ADVERSE REACTIONS
CNS: *asthenia, malaise, dizziness,* depression, drowsiness, nervousness, insomnia, headache.
CV: anemia, hypertension, *CHF,* flushing, palpitations, edema, fluid retention.
EENT: blurred vision, tinnitus, photophobia, dry mouth.
GI: *dyspepsia, flatulence, abdominal pain, diarrhea, nausea,* constipation, gastritis, melena, vomiting, anorexia, peptic ulceration with or without bleeding or perforation, ulcerative stomatitis, thirst.
GU: dysuria, urinary frequency, *renal failure.*
Hematologic: anemia (rare), leukopenia, thrombocytopenia.
Hepatic: hepatitis.
Respiratory: asthma.

Skin: pruritus, rash, photosensitivity, *Stevens-Johnson syndrome.*
Other: chills, fever, weight gain, edema.

INTERACTIONS
Antacids: may decrease peak levels of the drug. Monitor for decreased effect of etodolac.
Aspirin: reduced protein-binding of etodolac without altering its clearance. Clinical significance unknown. Recommend avoiding concomitant use.
Cyclosporine: impaired elimination and increased risk of nephrotoxicity. Avoid concomitant use.
Digoxin, lithium, methotrexate: etodolac may impair elimination of these drugs, resulting in increased levels and risk of toxicity. Monitor blood levels.
Warfarin: etodolac decreases the protein-binding of warfarin but does not change its clearance. Although no dosage adjustment is necessary, monitor PT closely and watch for bleeding.

CONTRAINDICATIONS
Contraindicated in patients with hypersensitivity to the drug and in those with a history of aspirin- or NSAID-induced asthma, rhinitis, urticaria, or other allergic reactions.

NURSING CONSIDERATIONS
• Use cautiously in patients with a history of GI bleeding, ulceration, and perforation and renal or hepatic impairment.
• Because NSAIDs impair the synthesis of renal prostaglandins, they can decrease renal blood flow and lead to reversible renal impairment, especially in patients with preexisting renal failure, liver dysfunction, or heart failure; in elderly patients; and in those taking diuretics. Monitor these patients closely during therapy.
• Know that etodolac appears to

---

*Liquid form contains alcohol.   *Common* reactions are in italics; *life-threatening,* in bold italics.
**May contain tartrazine.

cause fewer GI problems than most NSAIDS. Minimal GI blood loss has been reported at dosages up to 1,200 mg daily.
• Know that metabolites of etodolac may cause a false-positive test for urinary bilirubin, decreased serum uric acid levels, and borderline elevations of one or more liver function tests.
• To minimize GI discomfort, tell patients to take etodolac with milk or meals.
• Serious GI toxicity, including peptic ulceration and bleeding, can occur in patients taking NSAIDs despite the absence of GI symptoms. Teach patients the signs and symptoms of GI bleeding, and tell them to contact the doctor immediately if any of these occurs.
• This drug has been associated with photosensitivity reactions. Advise patients to use a sunblock, wear protective clothing, and avoid prolonged exposure to sunlight.
• Tell patient that use during last trimester of pregnancy should be avoided.

fenoprofen calcium
Nalfon, Nalfon-200

Pregnancy Risk Category: NR

HOW SUPPLIED
Tablets: 600 mg
Capsules: 200 mg, 300 mg

ACTION
Unknown. Produces anti-inflammatory, analgesic, and antipyretic effects, possibly by inhibiting prostaglandin synthesis.

ONSET, PEAK, DURATION
Onset occurs within 15 to 30 minutes. Plasma levels peak in about 2 hours. Analgesic effects persist 4 to 6 hours.

INDICATIONS & DOSAGE
Rheumatoid arthritis and osteoarthritis –
Adults: 300 to 600 mg P.O. t.i.d. or q.i.d. Maximum dosage is 3.2 g daily.
Mild to moderate pain –
Adults: 200 mg P.O. q 4 to 6 hours, p.r.n.

ADVERSE REACTIONS
CNS: *headache,* drowsiness, dizziness, *somnolence.*
CV: peripheral edema.
EENT: auditory abnormalities.
GI: *epigastric distress, nausea, GI bleeding,* vomiting, occult blood loss, peptic ulceration, constipation, anorexia.
GU: oliguria, azotemia, interstitial nephritis, proteinuria, reversible renal failure.
Hematologic: prolonged bleeding time, anemia, *aplastic anemia, agranulocytosis,* thrombocytopenia.
Hepatic: elevated enzymes, hepatitis.
Respiratory: pulmonary infiltrates.
Skin: *pruritus,* rash, urticaria, *toxic epidermal necrolysis.*

INTERACTIONS
Aspirin: decreased fenoprofen half-life; may increase GI toxicity. Avoid concomitant use.
Diuretics: decreased diuretic effectiveness. Monitor closely.
Ethanol, corticosteroids: increased risk of adverse GI reactions. Avoid concomitant use.
Oral anticoagulants, sulfonylureas: fenoprofen enhances pharmacologic effects of these drugs. Use together cautiously.
Phenobarbital: enhanced metabolism of fenoprofen. Monitor for lack of fenoprofen effectiveness.

CONTRAINDICATIONS
Contraindicated in patients with hypersensitivity to this drug, significantly impaired renal function, or his-

tory of aspirin- or NSAID-induced asthma, rhinitis, or urticaria. Also contraindicated in pregnancy.

NURSING CONSIDERATIONS
• Use cautiously in elderly patients; in patients with history of serious GI events or peptic ulcer disease, compromised cardiac function or hypertension.
• Because NSAIDs impair the synthesis of renal prostaglandins, they can decrease renal blood flow and lead to reversible renal impairment, especially in patients with preexisting renal failure, liver dysfunction, or heart failure; in elderly patients; and in those taking diuretics. Monitor these patients closely during therapy.
• Be aware that safety has not been established for pregnancy. Administration to pregnant patients is not recommended.
• Know that because of their antipyretic and anti-inflammatory actions, NSAIDs may mask the signs and symptoms of infection.
• Be aware that renal, hepatic, ocular, and auditory function should be checked periodically in long-term therapy. Drug is stopped if abnormalities occur.
• Be aware that fenoprofen may cause false elevations in free and total serum triiodothyronine (T_3) levels as measured by the Amerlex-T assay. Fenoprofen or its metabolite may cross-react with the antibody used in the Amerlex-M assay. Limited data suggest that drug may alter free and total T_3 concentrations determined by the Corning method.
• Tell patients to take this drug 30 minutes before or 2 hours after meals. If adverse GI reactions occur, drug may be taken with milk or meals.
• Tell patients that full therapeutic effect for arthritis may be delayed for 2 to 4 weeks.
• Because fenoprofen may cause somnolence, warn patients to avoid driv-ing and other hazardous activities that require alertness until adverse CNS effects of the drug are known.
• Serious GI toxicity, including peptic ulceration and bleeding, can occur in patients taking NSAIDs despite the absence of GI symptoms. Teach patients the signs and symptoms of GI bleeding, and tell them to contact the doctor immediately if any occurs.

---

flurbiprofen
Ansaid, Apo-Flurbiprofen†, Froben†, Froben SR†

Pregnancy Risk Category: B

HOW SUPPLIED
Tablets: 50 mg, 100 mg
Capsules (extended-release)†: 200 mg

ACTION
Unknown. Possibly inhibits prostaglandin synthesis.

ONSET, PEAK, DURATION
Onset and duration unknown. Serum levels peak about 2 hours after a dose.

INDICATIONS AND DOSAGE
Rheumatoid arthritis and osteoarthritis –
Adults: 200 to 300 mg P.O. daily, divided b.i.d. to q.i.d. Where available, patients maintained on 200 mg daily may switch to one 200-mg extended-release capsule P.O. daily, taken in the evening after food.

ADVERSE REACTIONS
CNS: *headache,* anxiety, insomnia, increased reflexes, tremors, amnesia, asthenia, drowsiness, malaise, depression, *dizziness.*
CV: *edema, CHF,* hypertension, vasodilation.
EENT: rhinitis, tinnitus, visual changes.
GI: *dyspepsia, diarrhea, abdominal pain, nausea,* constipation, ***bleeding,*** flatulence, vomiting.

---

*Liquid form contains alcohol.
**May contain tartrazine.

Common reactions are in italics; ***life-threatening,*** in bold italics.

GU: *symptoms suggesting urinary tract infection,* nephrotoxicity.
Hematologic: thrombocytopenia, neutropenia, anemia, *aplastic anemia.*
Hepatic: elevated liver enzymes, jaundice.
Respiratory: asthma.
Skin: rash.
Other: weight changes.

INTERACTIONS
Aspirin: decreased flurbiprofen levels. Concomitant use is not recommended.
Diuretics: possible decreased diuretic effect. Monitor patient closely.
Methotrexate: increased risk of methotrexate toxicity. Monitor closely.
Oral anticoagulants: increased bleeding tendencies. Monitor patient closely.

CONTRAINDICATIONS
Contraindicated in patients with hypersensitivity to the drug, or history of aspirin- or NSAID-induced asthma, urticaria, or other allergic-type reactions.

NURSING CONSIDERATIONS
• Use cautiously in patients with a history of peptic ulcer disease, hepatic dysfunction, cardiac disease, or other conditions associated with fluid retention or impaired renal function.
• Be aware that elderly or debilitated patients and those patients with hepatic or renal dysfunction should be closely monitored and probably should receive lower doses. These patients may be at risk for renal toxicity, jaundice, or toxic hepatitis. Periodically monitor renal and hepatic function as ordered.
• Because NSAIDs impair the synthesis of renal prostaglandins, they can decrease renal blood flow and lead to reversible renal impairment, especially in patients with preexisting renal failure, liver dysfunction, or heart failure; in elderly patients; and in those taking diuretics. Monitor these patients closely during therapy.
• Know that patients receiving long-term therapy should have periodic liver function studies, eye examinations, and hematocrit determinations.
• Know that use during pregnancy is not recommended in last trimester.
• Tell patients to take drug with food, milk, or antacid if GI upset occurs.
• Tell patients taking extended-release capsules to swallow them whole; do not crush, chew, or break open the capsules.
• Advise patients to avoid hazardous activities that require mental alertness until CNS effects are known.
• Serious GI toxicity, including peptic ulceration and bleeding, can occur in patients taking NSAIDs despite the absence of GI symptoms. Teach patients the signs and symptoms of GI bleeding, and tell them to contact the doctor immediately if any of these occurs.

---

ibuprofen

Aches-N-Pain◊, ACT-3‡, Advil◊, Amersol†, Apo-Ibuprofen†, Brufen‡, Children's Advil, Excedrin-IB Caplets◊, Excedrin-IB Tablets◊, Genpril Caplets◊,Genpril Tablets◊, Haltran◊, Ibu-Cream‡, Ibuprin◊, Ibuprohm Caplets◊, Ibuprohm Tablets◊, Ibu-Tab◊, Inflam‡, Medipren Caplets◊, Medipren Tablets◊, Midol-200◊, Motrin, Motrin IB Caplets◊, Motrin IB Tablets◊, Novoprofen†, Nuprin Caplets◊, Nuprin Tablets◊, Nurofen‡, Pamprin-IB, PediaProfen, Rafen‡, Rufen, Saleto-200, Saleto-400, Saleto-600, Saleto-800, Trendar◊

Pregnancy Risk Category: NR

---

†Available in Canada only.   ‡Available in Australia only.   ◊Available OTC.

HOW SUPPLIED
Tablets: 200 mg◇, 300 mg, 400 mg, 600 mg, 800 mg
Caplets: 200 mg◇
Oral suspension: 100 mg/5 ml
Topical cream: 10%

ACTION
Unknown. Produces anti-inflammatory, analgesic, and antipyretic effects, possibly by inhibiting prostaglandin synthesis.

ONSET, PEAK, DURATION
Analgesic and antipyretic effects, within 30 minutes; antirheumatic effects, within 7 days. Plasma levels peak 2 to 4 hours after oral dose. Effects persist 4 hours or more.

INDICATIONS & DOSAGE
Rheumatoid or osteoarthritis, arthritis –
Adults: 300 to 800 mg P.O. t.i.d. or q.i.d. not to exceed 3.2 g/day.
Mild to moderate pain, dysmenorrhea –
Adults: 400 mg P.O. q 4 to 6 hours p.r.n.
Fever –
Adults: 200 to 400 mg P.O. q 4 to 6 hours. Do not exceed 1.2 g daily or give longer than 3 days.
Children 6 months to 12 years: if fever is below 102.5° F (39.2° C), the recommended dose is 5 mg/kg P.O. q 6 to 8 hours. Treat higher fevers with 10 mg/kg q 6 to 8 hours. Do not exceed 40 mg/kg daily.
External treatment of joint pain; swelling of tissues adjacent to joints†–
Adults: apply a 4- to 10-cm strip of cream to the skin and massage briskly. Apply t.i.d.

ADVERSE REACTIONS
CNS: *headache, drowsiness, dizziness,* cognitive dysfunction, aseptic meningitis.
CV: *peripheral edema,* hypertension, ***CHF.***
EENT: visual disturbances, *tinnitus.*
GI: *epigastric distress, nausea, occult blood loss, peptic ulceration.*
GU: reversible renal failure.
Hematologic: prolonged bleeding time, anemia, neutropenia, pancytopenia, thrombocytopenia, aplastic anemia, leukopenia, agranulocytosis.
Hepatic: elevated enzymes.
Respiratory: ***bronchospasm.***
Skin: pruritus, *rash,* urticaria, photosensitivity, ***Stevens-Johnson syndrome.***
Other: edema.

INTERACTIONS
Antihypertensives, furosemide, thiazide diuretics: ibuprofen may decrease the effectiveness of diuretics or antihypertensives.
Aspirin: may decrease serum levels of ibuprofen. Avoid concomitant use.
Aspirin, corticosteroids, ethanol: increased risk of adverse GI reactions. Avoid concomitant use.
Lithium, oral anticoagulants: ibuprofen may increase plasma levels or effects of these drug. Monitor for toxicity.

CONTRAINDICATIONS
Contraindicated in patients with hypersensitivity to this drug, or who have the syndrome of nasal polyps, angioedema, and bronchospastic reactivity to aspirin or other NSAIDs.

NURSING CONSIDERATIONS
• Use cautiously in patients with GI disorders, history of peptic ulcer disease, hepatic or renal disease, cardiac decompensation, hypertension, known intrinsic coagulation defects.
• Know that use during pregnancy is not recommended.
• Check renal and hepatic function periodically in patients on long-term therapy. Stop drug if abnormalities occur and notify doctor.

*Liquid form contains alcohol.   *Common* reactions are in italics; ***life-threatening,*** in bold italics.
**May contain tartrazine.

• Be aware that because of their anti-pyretic and anti-inflammatory actions, NSAIDs may mask the signs and symptoms of infection.

• To reduce adverse GI reactions, tell patient to take with meals or milk.

• Drug is available OTC in several brands (200 mg). Instruct the patient to not exceed 1.2 g daily, give to children under age 12, or self-medicate for extended periods without consulting the doctor.

• Tell patients that full therapeutic effect for arthritis may be delayed for 2 to 4 weeks. Although analgesic effect occurs at low dosage levels, anti-inflammatory effect does not occur at dosages below 400 mg q.i.d.

• Caution patients that concomitant use with aspirin, alcohol, or corticosteroids may increase the risk of GI adverse reactions.

• Serious GI toxicity, including peptic ulceration and bleeding, can occur in patients taking NSAIDs despite the absence of GI symptoms. Teach patients the signs and symptoms of GI bleeding, and tell them to contact the doctor immediately if any occurs.

indomethacin
Apo-Indomethacin†, Arthrexin‡, Indameth, Indochron E-R, Indocid†‡, Indocid SR†, Indocin, Indocin SR, Novomethacin†, Rheumacin‡

indomethacin sodium trihydrate
Apo-Indomethacin†, Indameth, Indocid PDA†, Indocin I.V., Novomethacin†

Pregnancy Risk Category: NR

HOW SUPPLIED
indomethacin
Capsules: 25 mg, 50 mg
Capsules (sustained-release): 75 mg
Oral suspension: 25 mg/5 ml
Suppositories: 50 mg

indomethacin sodium trihydrate
Injection: 1-mg vials

ACTION
Unknown. Produces anti-inflammatory, analgesic, and antipyretic effects, possibly by inhibiting prostaglandin synthesis.

ONSET, PEAK, DURATION
Onset occurs within 2 to 4 hours. Serum levels peak within 1 to 2 hours after a dose of immediate-release capsules or oral suspension, within 2 to 4 hours of a sustained-release capsule, or immediately following an I.V. injection. Peak antirheumatic effects occur after 1 to 2 weeks of therapy. Analgesic effects persist 4 to 6 hours.

INDICATIONS & DOSAGE
Moderate to severe rheumatoid or osteoarthritis, ankylosing spondylitis –
Adults: 25 mg P.O. or P.R. b.i.d. or t.i.d. with food or antacids; increased dosage by 25 mg or 50 mg daily q 7 days up to 200 mg daily. Alternatively, sustained-release capsules (75 mg): 75 mg P.O. to start, in the morning or h.s., followed, if necessary, by 75 mg b.i.d.
Acute gouty arthritis –
Adults: 50 mg P.O. t.i.d. Dose reduced as soon as possible; then discontinued. Sustained-release capsules shouldn't be used for this condition.
Acute painful shoulders (bursitis and/or tendinitis) –
Adults: 75 to 150 mg P.O. daily t.i.d. or q.i.d. for 7 to 14 days.
To close a hemodynamically significant patent ductus arteriosus in premature infants (I.V. form only) –
Neonates under 48 hours: 0.2 mg/kg I.V. followed by two doses of 0.1 mg/kg at 12- to 24-hour intervals.
Neonates 2 to 7 days: 0.2 mg/kg I.V. followed by two doses of 0.2 mg/kg at 12- to 24-hour intervals.
Neonates over 7 days: 0.2 mg/kg I.V.

---

†Available in Canada only.   ‡Available in Australia only.   ◇Available OTC.

followed by two doses of 0.25 mg/kg at 12- to 24-hour intervals.

ADVERSE REACTIONS
Oral and rectal form:
CNS: *headache, dizziness,* depression, drowsiness, confusion, peripheral neuropathy, *seizures,* psychic disturbances, syncope, *vertigo.*
CV: hypertension, *edema, CHF.*
EENT: blurred vision, corneal and retinal damage, hearing loss, tinnitus.
GI: *nausea, vomiting,* anorexia, *diarrhea, peptic ulceration,* **GI bleeding,** pancreatitis.
GU: hematuria, *acute renal failure.*
Hematologic: *hemolytic anemia, aplastic anemia, agranulocytosis,* leukopenia, thrombocytopenic purpura, iron deficiency anemia.
Hepatic: elevated enzymes.
Skin: pruritus, urticaria, *Stevens-Johnson syndrome.*
Other: hypersensitivity (rash, respiratory distress, *anaphylaxis, angioedema),* hyperkalemia.
I.V. form:
GI: *bleeding,* vomiting.
GU: *renal dysfunction, azotemia.*
Hematologic: decreased platelet aggregation.
Other: *hyponatremia, hyperkalemia, hypoglycemia,* hypersensitivity (rash, respiratory distress, *anaphylaxis, angioedema).*

INTERACTIONS
Aminoglycosides, cyclosporine, methotrexate: indomethacin may enhance the toxicity of these agents. Avoid concomitant use.
Antihypertensive agents: reduced antihypertensive effect. Monitor closely.
Aspirin: decreased blood levels of indomethacin. Avoid concomitant use.
Corticosteroids, ethanol: increased risk of GI toxicity. Don't use together.
Diflunisal, probenecid: decreased indomethacin excretion; watch for increased incidence of indomethacin adverse reactions.
Digoxin: indomethacin may prolong the half-life of digoxin. Use together cautiously.
Dipyridamole: enhanced fluid retention. Avoid concomitant use.
Furosemide, thiazide diuretics: impaired response to both drugs. Avoid using together if possible.
Lithium: increased plasma lithium levels. Monitor for toxicity.
Triamterene: possible nephrotoxicity. Monitor closely.

CONTRAINDICATIONS
Contraindicated in patients with hypersensitivity to this drug, or history of aspirin- or NSAID-induced asthma, rhinitis, or urticaria; pregnancy, or lactation. Also contraindicated in infants with untreated infection, active bleeding, coagulation defects or thrombocytopenia, congenital heart disease in whom patency of the ductus arteriosus is necessary for satisfactory pulmonary or systemic blood flow, necrotizing enterocolitis, or impaired renal function. Suppositories are contraindicated in patients with a history of proctitis or recent rectal bleeding.

NURSING CONSIDERATIONS
• Use cautiously in patients with epilepsy, parkinsonism, hepatic or renal disease, cardiovascular disease, infection, and mental illness or depression. Also use cautiously in elderly patients and patients with history of GI disease.
• Be aware that because of its high incidence of adverse effects during chronic use, indomethacin should not be used routinely as an analgesic or antipyretic.
• Know that use during pregnancy is not recommended.
• Administer oral dosage with food, milk, or antacid if GI upset occurs.
• **I.V. use:** Reconstitute powder for injection with sterile water for injection or 0.9% sodium chloride. For

---

*Liquid form contains alcohol.   *Common* reactions are in italics; *life-threatening,* in bold italics.
**May contain tartrazine.

each 1-mg vial, add 1 ml of diluent for a solution containing 1 mg/ml; add 2 ml of diluent to yield a solution containing 0.5 mg/ml. Give by direct injection over 5 to 10 seconds.

• Use only preservative-free diluents to prepare I.V. injection. Never use diluents containing benzyl alcohol because this has been associated with a fatal gasping syndrome in neonates. Because the injection contains no preservatives, reconstitute immediately before administration, and discard any unused solution.

• Don't administer second or third scheduled I.V. dose if anuria or marked oliguria is evident; instead notify physician.

• Be aware that if ductus arteriosus reopens, a second course of one to three doses may be given. If ineffective, surgery may be necessary.

• Monitor carefully for bleeding and for reduced urine output with I.V. administration. Discontinue drug and notify the doctor if either occurs.

• Monitor for bleeding in patients receiving anticoagulants, patients with coagulation defects, and neonates.

• Because NSAIDs impair the synthesis of renal prostaglandins, they can decrease renal blood flow and lead to reversible renal impairment, especially in patients with preexisting renal failure, liver dysfunction, or heart failure; in elderly patients; and in those taking diuretics. Monitor these patients closely during therapy.

• Causes sodium retention; monitor for weight gain (especially in elderly patients) and increased blood pressure in patients with hypertension.

• Be aware that adverse CNS reactions are more common and serious in elderly patients.

• Know that because of their antipyretic and anti-inflammatory actions, NSAIDs may mask the signs and symptoms of infection.

• Indomethacin may enhance the hypothalamic-pituitary-adrenal axis response to the dexamethasone suppression test. Inform clinical laboratory personnel that the patient is taking indomethacin.

• Tell patients to take oral form of this drug with food, milk, or antacid if GI upset occurs.

• Alert patient that concomitant use of oral form with aspirin, alcohol, or corticosteroids may increase the risk of adverse GI reactions.

• Serious GI toxicity, including peptic ulceration and bleeding, can occur in patients taking oral NSAIDs despite the absence of GI symptoms. Teach patients the signs and symptoms of GI bleeding, and tell them to contact the doctor immediately if any of these occurs.

• Tell patients to notify the doctor immediately if any visual or hearing changes occurs. Patients on long-term oral therapy should have regular eye examinations, hearing tests, CBC, and renal function tests to monitor for toxicity.

ketoprofen
Apo-Keto†, Apo-Keto-E†, Novo-Keto-EC†, Orudis, Orudis E†, Orudis SR†‡, Oruvail, Rhodis†, Rhodis-E†, Rhodis-EC†

Pregnancy Risk Category: NR

HOW SUPPLIED
Tablets (sustained-release): 200 mg†
Tablets (enteric-coated): 50 mg†, 100 mg†
Capsules (extended-release): 200 mg
Capsules: 25 mg, 50 mg, 75 mg
Suppositories: 100 mg†

ACTION
Unknown. Produces anti-inflammatory, analgesic, and antipyretic effects, possibly by inhibiting prostaglandin synthesis.

ONSET, PEAK, DURATION
Analgesic onset occurs in 1 to 2 hours; unknown for arthritis. Serum levels peak ½ to 2 hours. Effects persist for 3 to 4 hours when used for analgesia; unknown for arthritis.

INDICATIONS & DOSAGE
Rheumatoid arthritis and osteoarthritis –
Adults: 75 mg t.i.d. or 50 mg q.i.d. or 200 mg as a sustained- release tablet once daily. Maximum dosage is 300 mg/day.

Alternatively, where suppository is available, 100 mg P.R. b.i.d.; or 1 suppository h.s. (in conjunction with oral ketoprofen during the day).
Mild to moderate pain; dysmenorrhea –
Adults: 25 to 50 mg P.O. q 6 to 8 hours p.r.n.

ADVERSE REACTIONS
CNS: *headache,* dizziness, *CNS excitation* or depression.
EENT: tinnitus, visual disturbances.
GI: *nausea, abdominal pain, diarrhea, constipation, flatulence, peptic ulceration,* anorexia, vomiting, stomatitis.
GU: *nephrotoxicity, elevated BUN.*
Hematologic: prolonged bleeding time, thrombocytopenia, *agranulocytosis.*
Hepatic: elevated liver enzymes.
Respiratory: dyspnea, *bronchospasm, laryngeal edema.*
Skin: rash, photosensitivity, *exfoliative dermatitis.*

INTERACTIONS
Aspirin, corticosteroids, ethanol: increased risk of adverse GI reactions. Avoid concomitant use.
Aspirin, probenecid: increased plasma levels of ketoprofen. Avoid concomitant use.
Hydrochlorothiazide, other diuretics: decreased diuretic effectiveness. Monitor for lack of effect.
Lithium, methotrexate: increased levels of these drugs, leading to toxicity. Monitor closely.
Oral anticoagulants: increased risk of bleeding. Monitor closely.

CONTRAINDICATIONS
Contraindicated in patients with hypersensitivity to this drug, or history of aspirin- or NSAID-induced asthma, urticaria, or other allergic-type reactions.

NURSING CONSIDERATIONS
• Use cautiously in patients with history of peptic ulcer disease, renal dysfunction, hypertension, heart failure, or fluid retention.
• Know that use during third trimester of pregnancy should be avoided.
• Know that the sustained-release dosage form is not recommended for patients in acute pain.
• Because NSAIDs impair the synthesis of renal prostaglandins, they can decrease renal blood flow and lead to reversible renal impairment, especially in patients with preexisting renal failure, liver dysfunction, or heart failure; in elderly patients; and in those taking diuretics. Monitor these patients closely during therapy.
• Check renal and hepatic function every 6 months or as indicated and ordered during long-term therapy.
• Be aware that NSAIDs may mask the signs and symptoms of infection because of their antipyretic and anti-inflammatory actions.
• Inform laboratory personnel that patient is taking indomethacin. Ketoprofen may interfere with some laboratory determinations of blood glucose and serum iron levels, depending on the testing method used.
• Tell patients to take drug 30 minutes before or 2 hours after meals. If adverse GI reactions occur, patients may take the drug with milk or meals.
• Tell patients that full therapeutic effect may be delayed for 2 to 4 weeks.

---

*Liquid form contains alcohol.
**May contain tartrazine.

Common reactions are in italics; *life-threatening,* in bold italics.

• Tell patients to report visual or auditory adverse reactions immediately.

• Serious GI toxicity, including peptic ulceration and bleeding, can occur in patients taking NSAIDs despite the absence of GI symptoms. Teach patients the signs and symptoms of GI bleeding, and tell them to contact the doctor immediately if any of these occurs.

• Alert patient that concomitant use with aspirin, alcohol, or corticosteroids may increase the risk of adverse GI reactions.

• This drug has been associated with photosensitivity reactions. Advise patients to use a sunblock, wear protective clothing, and avoid prolonged exposure to sunlight.

ketorolac tromethamine
Toradol

Pregnancy Risk Category: C

HOW SUPPLIED
Tablets: 10 mg
Injection: 15 mg, 30 mg, 60 mg

ACTION
Unknown. Thought to inhibit prostaglandin synthesis.

ONSET, PEAK, DURATION
Onset immediate with I.V. administration; within 10 minutes of an I.M. injection; 30 to 60 minutes after oral dose. Plasma levels peak in 30 minutes to 1 hour after either oral or I.M. administration; immediate after I.V. injection. Analgesic effects persist up to 6 to 8 hours.

INDICATIONS & DOSAGE
Short-term management of pain –
Adults: initially, give 30 or 60 mg I.M. as a loading dose, followed by half of the loading dose (15 or 30 mg) I.M. q 6 hours on a regular schedule or p.r.n. (up to 5 days). Subsequent dosage should be based on patient response.

Alternatively, the drug may be used orally on a short-term basis (up to 15 days); 10 mg P.O. q 4 to 6 hours p.r.n.

ADVERSE REACTIONS
CNS: *drowsiness, sedation,* dizziness, *headache,* sweating.
CV: edema, hypertension, palpitations, arrhythmias.
GI: *nausea, dyspepsia, GI pain,* diarrhea, peptic ulceration.
Hematologic: decreased platelet adhesion, pupura.
Other: hyperkalemia, pain at injection site.

INTERACTIONS
Antihypertensives, diuretics: decreased effectiveness. Monitor closely.
Lithium: increased lithium levels. Monitor closely.
Methotrexate: decreased methotrexate clearance and increased toxicity. Don't use together.
Salicylates, warfarin: ketorolac may increase the levels of free (unbound) salicylates or warfarin in the blood. Clinical significance is unknown.

CONTRAINDICATIONS
Contraindicated in patients with hypersensitivity to this drug, or history of the syndrome of nasal polyps, angioedema, bronchospastic reactivity or other allergic manifestations to aspirin or other NSAIDS.

NURSING CONSIDERATIONS
• Use cautiously in patients with hepatic or renal impairment; history of serious GI events or peptic ulcer disease; or cardiac decompensation, hypertension, or coagulation disorders. Also use cautiously during perioperative period.

• Trace amounts of ketorolac have been detected in breast milk. Use with caution in breast-feeding patients.

• Know that lower initial doses should be used in patients who are over age 65 or who weigh less than 110 lb (50 kg).

• I.M. administration may cause pain at the injection site. Holding pressure over the site for 15 to 30 seconds after the injection may minimize local effects.

• When switching patients from injectable to oral ketorolac, be aware that a total dosage of 120 mg of drug on the day of transition should not be exceeded, including a maximum of 40 mg P.O.

• Be aware that this drug is intended solely for short-term management of pain. The incidence and severity of adverse reactions should be less than that observed in patients taking NSAIDs on a chronic basis.

• Carefully observe patients with coagulopathies and those who are taking anticoagulants. Ketorolac inhibits platelet aggregation and can prolong bleeding time. This effect will disappear within 48 hours of discontinuing the drug. It will not alter platelet count, PTT, or PT.

• Be aware that NSAIDs may mask the signs and symptoms of infection because of their antipyretic and anti-inflammatory actions.

• Serious GI toxicity, including peptic ulceration and bleeding, can occur in patients taking NSAIDs despite the absence of GI symptoms. Teach patients the signs and symptoms of GI bleeding, and tell them to notify the doctor immediately if any occurs.

---

meclofenamate
Meclomen

Pregnancy Risk Category: NR

HOW SUPPLIED
Capsules: 50 mg, 100 mg

ACTION
Unknown. Produces anti-inflammatory, analgesic, and antipyretic effects, possibly by inhibiting prostaglandin synthesis.

ONSET, PEAK, DURATION
Onset occurs within 30 minutes for analgesic effects; antirheumatic effects, within a few days of therapy. Plasma levels peak in ½ to 1 hour; peak antirheumatic activity occurs after 2 to 3 weeks of therapy. Duration unknown.

INDICATIONS & DOSAGE
Rheumatoid arthritis and osteoarthritis –
Adults: 200 to 400 mg/day P.O. in three or four equally divided doses.
Mild to moderate pain –
Adults: 50 to 100 mg P.O. q 4 to 6 hours. Maximum dosage is 400 mg/day.
Dysmenorrhea or menorrhagia –
Adults: 100 mg P.O. t.i.d.

ADVERSE REACTIONS
CNS: fatigue, malaise, insomnia, *dizziness,* nervousness, *headache.*
CV: edema.
EENT: blurred vision, eye irritation.
GI: *abdominal pain, flatulence, peptic ulceration,* nausea, vomiting, *diarrhea,* hemorrhage.
GU: dysuria, hematuria, nephrotoxicity.
Hematologic: leukopenia, thrombocytopenia, *agranulocytosis, aplastic anemia.*
Hepatic: *hepatotoxicity.*
Skin: rash, urticaria.

INTERACTIONS
Antihypertensives, diuretics: decreased effectiveness. Monitor closely.
Aspirin: decreased plasma levels of meclofenamate.
Corticosteroids, ethanol, other

NSAIDS: increased risk of GI adverse reactions. Avoid concomitant use.
Oral anticoagulants: enhanced anticoagulant effect. Monitor for toxicity.

CONTRAINDICATIONS
Contraindicated in patients with hypersensitivity to the drug or with a history of aspirin- or NSAID-induced bronchospasm, uritcaria, or rhinitis.

NURSING CONSIDERATIONS
• Use cautiously in patients with hepatic or renal disease, cardiovascular disease, blood dyscrasia, and in those with a history of peptic ulcer disease; and in elderly patients, who are more likely to experience adverse reactions.
• Know that use during pregnancy is not recommended, especially during 1st and 3rd trimesters.
• Because NSAIDs impair the synthesis of renal prostaglandins, they can decrease renal blood flow and lead to reversible renal impairment, especially in patients with preexisting renal failure, liver dysfunction, or heart failure; in elderly patients; and in those taking diuretics. Monitor these patients closely during therapy.
• Know that NSAIDs may mask the signs and symptoms of infection because of their anti-inflammatory and antipyretic actions.
• Be aware that CBC and renal and hepatic function should be assessed every 6 months or as indicated in patients receiving long term therapy.
• Know that false-positive reactions for urine bilirubin using the diazo tablet test have been reported.
• Tell patients to take this drug with food to minimize adverse GI reactions.
• Tell patients to stop drug and contact the doctor immediately if rash, visual disturbances, or diarrhea develops.
• Caution patients that concomitant use with other NSAIDs, alcohol, or corticosteroids may increase the risk of GI adverse reactions.
• Advise patients to avoid driving or other hazardous activities that require mental alertness until CNS effects are known.
• Serious GI toxicity, including peptic ulceration and bleeding, can occur in patients taking NSAIDs despite the absence of GI symptoms. Teach patients the signs and symptoms of GI bleeding, and tell them to contact the doctor immediately if any of these occurs.

mefenamic acid
Mefic‡, Ponstan†, Ponstel
Pregnancy Risk Category: C

HOW SUPPLIED
Capsules: 250 mg

ACTION
Unknown. Produces anti-inflammatory, analgesic, and antipyretic effects, possibly by inhibiting prostaglandin synthesis.

ONSET, PEAK, DURATION
Onset and duration unknown. Serum levels peak 2 to 4 hours after a dose.

INDICATIONS & DOSAGE
Mild to moderate pain, dysmenorrhea –
Adults and children over 14 years: Initially, 500 mg P.O.; then 250 mg q 6 hours, p.r.n. Maximum therapy 1 week.

ADVERSE REACTIONS
CNS: drowsiness, dizziness, nervousness, headache.
CV: edema.
EENT: blurred vision, eye irritation.
GI: nausea, vomiting, *diarrhea, peptic ulceration, pancreatitis,* hemorrhage.
GU: dysuria, hematuria, nephrotoxicity.

Hematologic: leukopenia, thrombocytopenia, *agranulocytosis, aplastic anemia, hemolytic anemia.*
Hepatic: *hepatotoxicity.*
Skin: rash, urticaria.

INTERACTIONS

Antihypertensives, diuretics: decreased effect. Monitor closely.
Aspirin, corticosteroids, ethanol: increased risk of GI adverse reactions. Avoid concomitant use.
Oral anticoagulants, sulfonylureas, and other drugs that are highly protein-bound: increased risk of toxicity.

CONTRAINDICATIONS

Contraindicated in patients with hypersensitivity to the drug; history of aspirin- or NSAID-induced bronchospasm, allergic rhinitis, or urticaria; GI ulceration or inflammation; or renal disease.

NURSING CONSIDERATIONS

• Use cautiously in patients with hepatic disease, cardiovascular disease, and in those with a history of peptic ulcer disease.
• Know that use during 3rd trimester of pregnancy is not recommended.
• Be aware that mefenamic acid should not be administered for more than 1 week at a time because of increased risk of toxicity.
• Severe hemolytic anemia may occur with prolonged use. Monitor CBC every 4 to 6 months as ordered or as indicated.
• Because NSAIDs impair the synthesis of renal prostaglandins, they can decrease renal blood flow and lead to reversible renal impairment, especially in patients with preexisting renal failure, liver dysfunction, or heart failure; in elderly patients; and in those taking diuretics. Monitor these patients closely during therapy.
• Know that NSAIDs may mask the signs and symptoms of infection be-

cause of their anti-inflammatory and antipyretic actions.
• Note that false-positive reactions for urine bilirubin using the diazo tablet test have been reported.
• Tell patients to take this drug with food to minimize adverse GI reactions.
• Warn patient against hazardous activities that require alertness until CNS effects are known.
• Tell patients to stop drug and contact the doctor immediately if rash, visual disturbances, or diarrhea develops.
• Caution patients that concomitant use with aspirin, alcohol, or corticosteroids may increase the risk of GI adverse reactions.
• Serious GI toxicity, including peptic ulceration and bleeding, can occur in patients taking NSAIDs despite the absence of GI symptoms. Teach patients the signs and symptoms of GI bleeding, and tell them to contact the doctor immediately if any of those occurs.

nabumetone
Relafen

Pregnancy Risk Category: C

HOW SUPPLIED
Tablets: 500 mg, 750 mg

ACTION
Unknown. Probably acts by inhibiting prostaglandin synthesis.

ONSET, PEAK, DURATION
Onset and duration unknown. Plasma levels peak 2 to 4 hours after a dose.

INDICATIONS & DOSAGE
Rheumatoid arthritis or osteoarthritis –
Adults: initially, 1,000 mg P.O. daily as a single dose or in divided doses b.i.d. Maximum daily dosage is 2,000 mg.

ADVERSE REACTIONS
CNS: *dizziness, headache,* fatigue, increased sweating, insomnia, nervousness, somnolence.
CV: *vasculitis.*
EENT: *tinnitus.*
GI: *diarrhea, dyspepsia, abdominal pain, constipation, flatulence, nausea,* dry mouth, gastritis, stomatitis, vomiting, ***bleeding,*** ulceration.
Respiratory: dyspnea, pneumonitis.
Skin: *pruritus, rash.*
Other: *edema.*

INTERACTIONS
Diuretics: NSAIDs may decrease diuretic effectiveness. Monitor patients closely during therapy.
Drugs that are highly bound to plasma proteins (such as warfarin): increased risk of adverse effects from displacement of drug by nabumetone. Use cautiously.
Ethanol: associated with an increased risk of additive GI toxicity. Concomitant use should be avoided.

CONTRAINDICATIONS
Contraindicated in patients with hypersensitivity reactions, or history of aspirin- or NSAID-induced asthma, urticaria, or other allergic-type reactions.

NURSING CONSIDERATIONS
• Use cautiously in patients with renal or hepatic impairment; CHF, hypertension, or other conditions that may predispose the patient to fluid retention; and in patients with a history of peptic ulcer disease.
• Know that use during 3rd trimester of pregnancy is not recommended.
• Because NSAIDs impair the synthesis of renal prostaglandins, they can decrease renal blood flow and lead to reversible renal impairment, especially in patients with preexisting renal failure, liver dysfunction, or heart failure; in elderly patients; and

in those taking diuretics. Monitor these patients closely during therapy.
• During long-term therapy, periodically monitor renal and liver function, CBC, and hematocrit as ordered; assess these patients for signs and symptoms of GI bleeding.
• Instruct patients to take this drug with food, milk, or antacids. Nabumetone is absorbed more rapidly when administered with food or milk.
• Advise patients to limit alcohol intake because of additive GI toxicity risk.
• Serious GI toxicity, including peptic ulceration and bleeding, can occur in patients taking NSAIDs despite the absence of GI symptoms. Teach patients the signs and symptoms of GI bleeding and tell them to contact the doctor immediately if any occurs.

---

naproxen
Apo-Naproxen†, Inza-250‡, Inza-500‡, Naprosyn, Naprosyn-E†, Naprosyn SR†‡, Naxen†‡, Novonaprox†, Nu-Naprox†

naproxen sodium
Aleve◊, Anaprox, Anaprox DS, Apo-Napro-Na†, Naprogesic‡, Novonaprox Sodium†, Synflex†

Pregnancy Risk Category: NR

HOW SUPPLIED
naproxen
Tablets: 250 mg, 375 mg, 500 mg
Tablets (extended-release)†: 750 mg, 1,000 mg
Oral suspension: 125 mg/5 ml
Suppositories: 500 mg‡
naproxen sodium
Tablets (film-coated): 220 mg◊, 275 mg, 550 mg
  Note: 275 mg of naproxen sodium = 250 mg of naproxen

ACTION
Unknown. Produces anti-inflammatory, analgesic, and antipyretic ef-

---

fects, possibly by inhibiting prostaglandin synthesis.

ONSET, PEAK, DURATION

Onset of analgesic effect, within 1 hour; antirheumatic effect, within 14 days. Peak serum levels after administration of naproxen sodium occur within 1 to 2 hours; peak levels after naproxen (base) occur in 2 to 4 hours. Analgesic effects persist about 7 hours.

INDICATIONS & DOSAGE

Rheumatoid arthritis, osteoarthritis, ankylosing spondylitis –
Adults: 250 to 500 mg P.O. b.i.d. Alternatively, where suppository is available, give 500 mg P.R. h.s. with oral naproxen during the day. Maximum dosage is 1,500 mg daily.
Juvenile arthritis –
Children: 10 mg/kg P.O. in 2 divided doses.
Acute gout –
Adults: 750 mg P.O., followed by 250 mg q 8 hours until attack subsides.
Mild to moderate pain, primary dysmenorrhea (naproxen sodium), acute tendinitis and bursitis –
Adults: 500 mg. P.O., followed by 250 mg q 6 to 8 hours p.r.n.

ADVERSE REACTIONS

CNS: *headache, drowsiness, dizziness,* tinnitus, cognitive dysfunction, aseptic meningitis.
CV: *peripheral edema,* palpitations, digital vasculitis.
EENT: visual disturbances, *tinnitus.*
GI: *epigastric distress, occult blood loss, nausea,* **peptic ulceration.**
GU: nephrotoxicity.
Hematologic: prolonged bleeding time, ***agranulocytosis,*** neutropenia.
Hepatic: elevated liver enzymes.
Respiratory: dyspnea.
Skin: *pruritus, rash,* urticaria.
Other: hyperkalemia.

INTERACTIONS

Antihypertensives, diuretics: decreased effect of these drugs. Monitor closely.
Aspirin, corticosteroids, ethanol: increased risk of adverse GI reactions. Avoid concomitant use.
Methotrexate: increased risk of toxicity. Monitor closely.
Oral anticoagulants, sulfonylureas, and drugs that are highly protein-bound: increased risk of toxicity. Monitor closely.
Probenecid: decreased elimination of naproxen. Monitor for toxicity.

CONTRAINDICATIONS

Contraindicated in patients with hypersensitivity to this drug or with the syndrome of asthma, rhinitis, and nasal polyps.

NURSING CONSIDERATIONS

• Use cautiously in elderly patients and in patients with renal disease, cardiovascular disease, GI disorders, hepatic disease, or a history of peptic ulcer disease.
• Know that use during last trimester of pregnancy should be avoided.
• Because NSAIDs impair the synthesis of renal prostaglandins, they can decrease renal blood flow and lead to reversible renal impairment, especially in patients with preexisting renal failure, liver dysfunction, or heart failure; in elderly patients; and in those taking diuretics. Monitor these patients closely during therapy.
• Monitor CBC and renal and hepatic function every 4 to 6 months or as indicated and ordered during long-term therapy.
• Be aware that because of their antipyretic and anti-inflammatory actions, NSAIDs may mask the signs and symptoms of infection.
• Inform clinical laboratory personnel that patient is taking naproxen. Naproxen may interfere with certain urinary assays of 5-hydroxyindoleace-

---

*Liquid form contains alcohol.
**May contain tartrazine.
Common reactions are in italics; ***life-threatening,*** in bold italics.

tic acid and may cause false elevations of urinary 17-ketosteroid concentrations.
• Advise patients to take drug with food or milk to minimize GI upset. A full glass of water or other liquid should be taken with each dose.
• Tell patients taking prescription doses of naproxen for arthritis that full therapeutic effect may be delayed 2 to 4 weeks.
• Warn patients against taking both naproxen and naproxen sodium at the same time because both circulate in the blood as the naproxen anion.
• Serious GI toxicity, including peptic ulceration and bleeding, can occur in patients taking NSAIDs despite the absence of GI symptoms. Teach patients the signs and symptoms of GI bleeding and tell them to contact the doctor immediately if any of these occurs.
• Caution patients that concomitant use with aspirin, alcohol, or corticosteroids may increase the risk of adverse GI reactions.
• Advise patient to have periodic eye examinations.

oxaprozin
Daypro
Pregnancy Risk Category: C

HOW SUPPLIED
Caplets: 600 mg

ACTION
Unknown. Produces anti-inflammatory, analgesic, and antipyretic effects, possibly by inhibiting prostaglandin synthesis.

ONSET, PEAK, DURATION
Onset and duration unknown. Serum levels peak 3 to 5 hours after a dose.

INDICATIONS & DOSAGE
Osteoarthritis or rheumatoid arthritis –

Adults: initially, 1,200 mg P.O. daily. Then, individualized to the smallest effective dosage to minimize adverse reactions. Smaller patients or those with mild symptoms may require only 600 mg daily. Maximum is 1,800 mg or 26 mg/kg, whichever is lower, in divided doses.

ADVERSE REACTIONS
CNS: depression, sedation, somnolence, confusion, sleep disturbances.
EENT: tinnitus, visual disturbances.
GI: *nausea, dyspepsia, diarrhea, constipation,* abdominal pain or distress, anorexia, flatulence, vomiting, *hemorrhage.*
GU: dysuria, urinary frequency.
Hepatic: elevated liver function test results (with chronic use); severe hepatic dysfunction (rare).
Skin: *rash,* photosensitivity.

INTERACTIONS
Antihypertensives, diuretics: decreased effect. Monitor closely and adjust dosage as ordered.
Aspirin, corticosteroids, ethanol: increased risk of adverse GI reactions. Avoid concomitant use.
Aspirin: oxaprozin displaces salicylates from plasma protein-binding sites, increasing risk of salicylate toxicity. Avoid concomitant use.
Methotrexate: increased risk of methotrexate toxicity. Avoid concomitant use.
Oral anticoagulants: although problems haven't been reported, there is an increased risk of bleeding. Use together cautiously.

CONTRAINDICATIONS
Contraindicated in patients with hypersensitivity to this drug or with the syndrome of nasal polyps, angioedema, and bronchospastic reactivity to aspirin or other NSAIDs.

NURSING CONSIDERATIONS

• Use cautiously in patients with a history of peptic ulcer disease, hepatic or renal dysfunction, hypertension, cardiovascular disease, or conditions predisposing patient to fluid retention.

• Because renal prostaglandins play a role in the maintenance of renal perfusion, patients with preexisting conditions leading to a reduction in renal blood flow may experience renal toxicity with NSAID therapy. Those at greatest risk are elderly patients, patients taking diuretics, and those with impaired renal, hepatic, or cardiac function. Closely monitor renal function in these patients, and discontinue NSAID therapy if problems develop.

• Elevations of liver function tests can occur after chronic use. These abnormal findings may persist, worsen, or resolve with continued therapy. Rarely, patients may progress to severe hepatic dysfunction. Periodically monitor liver function tests in patients receiving long-term therapy, and closely monitor patients with abnormal test results.

• Be aware that because of their antipyretic and anti-inflammatory actions, NSAIDs may mask the signs and symptoms of infection.

• Tell patients to take this drug 30 minutes before or 2 hours after meals. If adverse GI reactions occur, drug may be taken with milk or meals.

• Tell patients that full therapeutic effects may be delayed for 2 to 4 weeks.

• Tell patients to report visual or auditory adverse reactions immediately.

• Serious GI toxicity, including peptic ulceration and bleeding, can occur in patients taking NSAIDs despite the absence of GI symptoms. Teach patients the signs and symptoms of GI bleeding and tell them to contact the doctor immediately if any occurs.

• This drug has been associated with photosensitivity reactions. Advise patients to use a sunblock, wear protective clothing, and avoid prolonged exposure to sunlight.

---

piroxicam
Apo-Piroxicam†, Feldene, Novopirocam†

Pregnancy Risk Category: NR

HOW SUPPLIED
Capsules: 10 mg, 20 mg

ACTION
Unknown. Produces anti-inflammatory, analgesic, and antipyretic effects, possibly by inhibiting prostaglandin synthesis.

ONSET, PEAK, DURATION
Onset occurs within 15 to 30 minutes for analgesia; antirheumatic action, 7 to 12 days. Serum levels peak in 3 to 5 hours; peak rheumatic action occurs after 2 to 3 weeks of therapy. Analgesic effects persist for about 24 hours.

INDICATIONS & DOSAGE
Osteoarthritis and rheumatoid arthritis —
Adults: 20 mg P.O. daily. If desired, the dosage may be divided b.i.d.

ADVERSE REACTIONS
CNS: headache, drowsiness, dizziness, paresthesia, somnolence.
CV: peripheral edema.
EENT: auditory disturbances.
GI: *epigastric distress, nausea, occult blood loss,* **peptic ulceration, severe GI bleeding.**
GU: **nephrotoxicity,** elevated BUN level.
Hematologic: prolonged bleeding time, anemia, leukopenia, **aplastic anemia, agranulocytosis.**
Hepatic: elevated liver enzymes.
Skin: pruritus, rash, urticaria, *photosensitivity.*
Other: hyperkalemia, acidosis, dilutional hypernatremia.

INTERACTIONS

Aspirin, corticosteroids, ethanol: increased risk of GI toxicity. Decreased plasma levels of piroxicam. Avoid concomitant use.

Lithium: increased plasma lithium levels. Monitor for toxicity.

Oral anticoagulants: enhanced risk of bleeding. Monitor patient closely.

Oral antidiabetic agents: enhanced antidiabetic effects. Monitor patient closely.

CONTRAINDICATIONS

Contraindicated in patients with hypersensitivity to this drug or with bronchospasm or angioedema precipitated by aspirin or NSAIDs and in pregnancy or lactation.

NURSING CONSIDERATIONS

• Use cautiously in elderly patients and in patients with GI disorders, history of renal or peptic ulcer disease, cardiac disease, hypertension, or conditions predisposing to fluid retention.

• Because NSAIDs impair the synthesis of renal prostaglandins, they can decrease renal blood flow and lead to reversible renal impairment, especially in patients with preexisting renal failure, liver dysfunction, or heart failure; in elderly patients; and in those taking diuretics. Monitor these patients closely during therapy.

• Check renal, hepatic, and auditory function and CBC periodically during prolonged therapy. Discontinue drug if abnormalities occur and notify physician.

• Be aware that NSAIDs may mask the signs and symptoms of infection because of their antipyretic and anti-inflammatory actions.

• Tell patients to take this drug with milk, antacids, or meals if GI adverse reactions occur.

• Tell patients that full therapeutic effects may be delayed for 2 to 4 weeks.

• Serious GI toxicity, including peptic ulceration and bleeding, can occur in patients taking NSAIDs despite the absence of GI symptoms. Teach patients the signs and symptoms of GI bleeding and tell them to contact the doctor immediately if any of these occurs.

• Advise patients to use a sunblock, wear protective clothing, and avoid prolonged exposure to sunlight. Causes adverse skin reactions more often than other drugs in its class. Photosensitivity reactions are the most common.

sulindac

Aclin‡, Apo-Sulin†, Clinoril, Novo-Sundac†

Pregnancy Risk Category: NR

HOW SUPPLIED

Tablets: 100 mg‡, 150 mg, 200 mg

ACTION

Unknown. Produces anti-inflammatory, analgesic, and antipyretic effects, possibly by inhibiting prostaglandin synthesis.

ONSET, PEAK, DURATION

Onset and duration unknown. Plasma levels peak 2 to 4 hours after a dose; peak antirheumatic effects occur in 2 to 3 weeks.

INDICATIONS & DOSAGE

Osteoarthritis, rheumatoid arthritis, ankylosing spondylitis –

Adults: initially, 150 mg P.O. b.i.d.; increased to 200 mg b.i.d. as needed.

Acute subacromial bursitis or supraspinatus tendinitis, acute gouty arthritis –

Adults: 200 mg P.O. b.i.d. for 7 to 14 days. Dose reduced as symptoms subside.

ADVERSE REACTIONS

CNS: dizziness, headache, nervousness, delerium, psychosis, neuropa-

thy, hallucinations, aseptic meningitis.
CV: hypertension.
EENT: tinnitus, transient visual disturbances.
GI: *epigastric distress,* **peptic ulceration, pancreatitis,** occult blood loss, nausea.
GU: interstitial nephritis, **nephrotic syndrome, renal failure.**
Hematologic: prolonged bleeding time, **aplastic anemia,** thrombocytopenia, neutropenia.
Hepatic: elevated liver enzymes.
Skin: *rash,* pruritus, **Stevens-Johnson syndrome**
Other: edema, drug fever, **anaphylaxis.**

INTERACTIONS

Anticoagulants: increased risk of bleeding. Monitor PT closely.
Aspirin: decreased sulindac plasma concentration and increased risk of GI adverse reactions. Concomitant use not recommended.
Cyclosporine: increased nephrotoxicity of cyclosporine. Avoid concomitant use.
Diflunisal, dimethyl sulfoxide: decreased metabolism of sulindac to its active metabolite, reducing its effectiveness. Don't use together.
Methotrexate: increased methotrexate toxicity. Avoid concomitant use.
Probenecid: increased plasma levels of sulindac and its active metabolite. Monitor for toxicity.
Sulfonamides, sulfonylureas, other highly protein-bound drugs: possible displacement of these drugs from plasma protein-binding sites, leading to increased toxicity. Monitor closely.

CONTRAINDICATIONS

Contraindicated in patients with hypersensitivity to this drug or in whom acute asthmatic attacks, urticaria, or rhinitis is precipitated by aspirin or NSAIDs.

NURSING CONSIDERATIONS

• Use cautiously in patients with a history of ulcers and GI bleeding, renal dysfunction, compromised cardiac function, or hypertension, or conditions predisposing to fluid retention.
• Know that use during pregnancy is not recommended.
• Periodically monitor hepatic and renal function and CBC in patients receiving long-term therapy as ordered.
• Be aware that because of their antipyretic and anti-inflammatory actions, NSAIDs may mask the signs and symptoms of infection.
• Tell patients to take this drug with food, milk, or antacids to reduce adverse GI reactions.
• Advise patients to avoid driving or other hazardous activities that require mental alertness until CNS effects are known.
• Serious GI toxicity, including peptic ulceration and bleeding, can occur in patients taking NSAIDs despite the absence of GI symptoms. Teach patients the signs and symptoms of GI bleeding and tell them to contact the doctor immediately if any of these occurs.
• Tell patients to notify the doctor immediately if easy bruising or prolonged bleeding occurs.
• Instruct patients to report edema and have blood pressure checked monthly. Drug causes sodium retention but is thought to have less effect on the kidneys than other NSAIDs.
• Patients should notify the doctor and have complete eye examinations if any visual disturbances occur.

tolmetin sodium
Tolectin-200, Tolectin-400, Tolectin-600, Tolectin DS

Pregnancy Risk Category: C

HOW SUPPLIED
Tablets: 200 mg, 600 mg
Capsules: 400 mg

---

*Liquid form contains alcohol.
**May contain tartrazine.

Common reactions are in italics; ***life-threatening,*** in bold italics.

ACTION

Unknown. Produces anti-inflammatory, analgesic, and antipyretic effects, possibly by inhibiting prostaglandin synthesis.

ONSET, PEAK, DURATION

Onset and duration unknown. Serum levels peak in 30 minutes to 1 hour; peak antirheumatic effect occurs after 1 to 2 weeks.

INDICATIONS & DOSAGE

Rheumatoid arthritis, osteoarthritis, juvenile rheumatoid arthritis –
Adults: 400 mg P.O. t.i.d. Maximum daily dosage is 1.8 g.
Children 2 years or over: initially, 20 mg/kg/day P.O. in divided doses, followed by maintenance dosage of 15 to 30 mg/kg P.O. daily in divided doses.

ADVERSE REACTIONS

CNS: *headache,* dizziness, drowsiness.
EENT: tinnitus, visual disturbances.
GI: *epigastric distress, peptic ulceration,* occult blood loss, nausea.
GU: *nephrotoxicity,* pseudoproteinuria.
Hematologic: prolonged bleeding time, granulocytopenia, thrombocytopenia, *agranulocytosis.*
Skin: rash, urticaria, pruritus.
Other: sodium retention, edema, *anaphylaxis, weight gain.*

INTERACTIONS

Aspirin: increased tolmetin levels. Avoid concurrent use.
Ethanol: increased risk of GI toxicity. Avoid concomitant use.
Methotrexate: increased risk of methotrexate toxicity. Monitor patient closely.
Oral anticoagulants: increased risk of bleeding. Monitor patient closely.

CONTRAINDICATIONS

Contraindicated in patients with hypersensitivity to this drug or in whom acute asthmatic attacks, urticaria, or rhinitis is precipitated by aspirin or NSAIDs as well as in lactation.

NURSING CONSIDERATIONS

• Use cautiously in patients with cardiac and renal disease, GI bleeding, history of peptic ulcer disease, hypertension, and conditions predisposing to fluid retention.
• Because NSAIDs impair the synthesis of renal prostaglandins, they can decrease renal blood flow and lead to reversible renal impairment, especially in patients with preexisting renal failure, liver dysfunction, or heart failure; in elderly patients; and in those taking diuretics. Monitor these patients closely during therapy.
• Know that NSAIDs may mask the signs and symptoms of infection because of their antipyretic and anti-inflammatory actions.
• Be aware that tolmetin may interfere with certain tests for urinary proteins; it does not interfere with dye-impregnated reagent strips.
• Tell patients to take this drug with food, milk, or antacids to reduce adverse GI reactions.
• Tell patients that therapeutic effect begins within 1 week, but full effect may be delayed 2 to 4 weeks.
• Advise patients to avoid driving or other hazardous activities that require mental alertness until the CNS effects of the drug are known.
• Serious GI toxicity, including peptic ulceration and bleeding, can occur in patients taking NSAIDs despite the absence of GI symptoms. Teach patients the signs and symptoms of GI bleeding and tell them to contact the doctor immediately if any occurs.
• Tell patients to notify the doctor immediately if any visual or hearing change occurs. During prolonged therapy, patients should have regular eye examinations, hearing tests, CBCs, and renal function tests to monitor for toxicity.

Narcotic and opioid analgesics

alfentanil hydrochloride
buprenorphine hydrochloride
butorphanol tartrate
codeine phosphate
codeine sulfate
dezocine
fentanyl citrate
fentanyl transdermal system
fentanyl transmucosal
hydromorphone hydrochloride
meperidine hydrochloride
methadone hydrochloride
morphine hydrochloride
morphine sulfate
morphine tartrate
nalbuphine hydrochloride
oxycodone hydrochloride
oxycodone pectinate
oxymorphone hydrochloride
pentazocine hydrochloride
pentazocine hydrochloride and
  naloxone hydrochloride
pentazocine lactate
propoxyphene hydrochloride
propoxyphene napsylate
sufentanil citrate
tramadol hydrochloride

COMBINATION PRODUCTS

222†: aspirin 375 mg, codeine phosphate 8 mg, and caffeine citrate 30 mg.

222 FORTE†: aspirin 500 mg, codeine phosphate 8 mg, and caffeine citrate 30 mg.

282†: aspirin 375 mg, codeine phosphate 15 mg, and caffeine citrate 30 mg.

292†: aspirin 375 mg, codeine phosphate 30 mg, and caffeine citrate 30 mg.

293†: aspirin 375 mg, codeine phosphate 30 mg, codeine phosphate (slow-release) 30 mg, and caffeine citrate 30 mg.

692†: aspirin 375 mg, propoxyphene

hydrochloride 65 mg, and caffeine 30 mg.

A.C.&C.†: aspirin 375 mg, codeine phosphate 8 mg, and caffeine 30 mg.

ACETA WITH CODEINE, EMPRACET-30†, EMTEC-30† : acetaminophen 300 mg and codeine phosphate 30 mg.

ANACIN WITH CODEINE†: aspirin 325 mg, codeine phosphate 8 mg, and caffeine 32 mg.

ANCASAL 8†, C2 WITH CODEINE†: aspirin 375 mg, codeine phosphate 8 mg, and caffeine 15 mg.

ANCASAL 15†: aspirin 375 mg, codeine phosphate 15 mg, and caffeine 15 mg.

ANCASAL 30†: aspirin 375 mg, codeine phosphate 30 mg, and caffeine 15 mg.

BUFF-A-COMP NO. 3: aspirin 325 mg, codeine phosphate 30 mg, caffeine 40 mg, and butalbital 50 mg.

CAPITAL WITH CODEINE, MYAPAP WITH CODEINE*, TYLENOL WITH CODEINE ELIXIR*, TY-PAP WITH CODEINE ELIXIR*: acetaminophen 120 mg and codeine phosphate 12 mg/5 ml.

DARVOCET-N 50: acetaminophen 325 mg and propoxyphene napsylate 50 mg.

DARVOCET-N 100, DOXAPAP-N, PROPACET 100: acetaminophen 650 mg and propoxyphene napsylate 100 mg.

DARVON COMPOUND†: aspirin 325 mg, propoxyphene hydrochloride 32 mg, and caffeine 32.4 mg.

DARVON COMPOUND-65: aspirin 389 mg, propoxyphene hydrochloride 65 mg, and caffeine 32.4 mg.

DARVON-N COMPOUND†: aspirin 375 mg, propoxyphene napsylate 100 mg, and caffeine 30 mg.

DARVON-N WITH A.S.A.†: aspirin

---

*Liquid form contains alcohol.
**May contain tartrazine.

Common reactions are in italics; ***life-threatening***, in bold italics.

325 mg and propoxyphene napsylate 100 mg.

DARVON WITH A.S.A.†: aspirin 325 mg and propxyphene hydrochloride 65 mg.

DOLENE-AP-65, D-REX-65, E-LOR, GENAGESIC, PRO POX WITH APAP, WYGESIC: acetaminophen 650 mg and propoxyphene hydrochloride 65 mg.

EMPIRIN WITH CODEINE NO. 2: aspirin 325 mg and codeine phosphate 15 mg.

EMPIRIN WITH CODEINE NO. 3: aspirin 325 mg and codeine phosphate 30 mg.

EMPIRIN WITH CODEINE NO. 4: aspirin 325 mg and codeine phosphate 60 mg.

EMPRACET-60†: acetaminophen 300 mg and codeine phosphate 60 mg.

ENDOCAN†, OXYCODAN†, PERCODAN†: aspirin 325 mg and oxycodone hydrochloride 5 mg.

ENDOCET†, OXYCOCET†, PERCOCET, ROXICET: acetaminophen 325 mg and oxycodone hydrochloride 5 mg.

FIORICET WITH CODEINE: acetaminophen 325 mg, butalbital 50 mg, caffeine 40 mg, and codeine phosphate 30 mg.

FIORINAL WITH CODEINE: aspirin 325 mg, butalbital 50 mg, caffeine 40 mg, and codeine 30 mg.

INNOVAR INJECTION: droperidol 2.5 mg and fentanyl citrate 0.05 mg/ml.

LENOLTEC WITH CODEINE NO. 1†, NOVOGESIC C8†: acetaminophen 300 mg, codeine phosphate 8 mg, and caffeine 15 mg.

LORCET 10/650: acetaminophen 650 mg and hydrocodone bitartrate 10mg.

LORTAB 5/500: acetaminophen 500 mg and hydrocodone bitartrate 5 mg.

PERCODAN-DEMI: aspirin 325 mg, oxycodone hydrochloride 2.25 mg, and oxycodone terephthalate 0.19 mg.

PERCODAN-DEMI†: aspirin 325 mg and oxycodone hydrochloride 2.5 mg.

PERCODAN, ROXIPRIN: aspirin 325 mg, oxycodone hydrochloride 4.5 mg, and oxycodone terephthalate 0.38 mg.

PHENAPHEN-650 WITH CODEINE: acetaminophen 650 mg and codeine phosphate 30 mg.

ROUNOX AND CODEINE 15†: acetaminophen 325 mg and codeine phosphate 15 mg.

ROUNOX AND CODEINE 30†: acetaminophen 325 mg and codeine phosphate 30 mg.

ROUNOX AND CODEINE 60†: acetaminophen 325 mg and codeine phosphate 60 mg.

ROXICET 5/500: acetaminophen 500 mg and oxycodone hydrochloride 5 mg.

ROXICET ORAL SOLUTION*: acetaminophen 325 mg and oxycodone hydrochloride 5 mg/5 ml.

TALACEN: acetaminophen 650 mg and pentazocine hydrochloride 25 mg.

TALWIN COMPOUND: aspirin 325 mg and pentazocine hydrochloride 12.5 mg.

TYLENOL WITH CODEINE NO. 1: acetaminophen 300 mg and codeine phosphate 7.5 mg.

TYLENOL WITH CODEINE NO. 2: acetaminophen 300 mg and codeine phosphate 15 mg.

TYLENOL WITH CODEINE NO. 3: acetaminophen 300 mg and codeine phosphate 30 mg.

TYLENOL WITH CODEINE NO. 4: acetaminophen 300 mg and codeine phosphate 60 mg.

TYLOX: acetaminophen 500 mg and oxycodone hydrochloride 5 mg.

---

alfentanil hydrochloride

Alfenta

Controlled Substance Schedule II

Pregnancy Risk Category: C

HOW SUPPLIED

Injection: 500 mcg/ml

ACTION

Binds with opiate receptors in the CNS, altering both perception of and emotional response to pain through an unknown mechanism.

ONSET, PEAK, DURATION

Onset within 1 minute. Serum levels peak within 1.5 to 2 minutes. Effects persist 5 to 10 minutes.

INDICATIONS & DOSAGE

Adjunct to general anesthetic –
Adults: initially, 8 to 50 mcg/kg I.V.; then increments of 3 to 15 mcg/kg I.V. q 5 to 20 minutes.
As a primary anesthetic –
Adults: initially, 130 to 245 mcg/kg I.V.; then 0.5 to 1.5 mcg/kg/minute I.V.

In elderly and debilitated patients: dosage should be reduced.

ADVERSE REACTIONS

CNS: blurred vision, agitation, anxiety, headache, confusion.
CV: hypotension, hypertension, bradycardia, tachycardia, palpitations, headache, orthostatic hypotension.
GI: nausea, vomiting.
Respiratory: *chest wall rigidity, bronchospasm, respiratory depression,* hypercapnia.
Skin: itching.
Other: intraoperative muscle movement.

INTERACTIONS

CNS depressants, ethanol: additive effects. Use together cautiously.

CONTRAINDICATIONS

Contraindicated in patients with hypersensitivity to this drug.

NURSING CONSIDERATIONS

• Use cautiously in patients with head injury, pulmonary disease, decreased respiratory reserve, or hepatic or renal impairment.

• Be aware drug should be administered only by persons specifically trained in the use of I.V. anesthetics.

• **I.V. use:** Compatible with D_5W, D_5W in lactated Ringer's solution, and 0.9% sodium chloride. Most clinicians use infusions containing 25 to 80 mcg/ml.

• Discontinue infusion at least 10 to 15 minutes before the end of surgery.

• To administer small volumes of alfentanil accurately, use a tuberculin syringe.

• Keep narcotic antagonist (naloxone) and resuscitation equipment available when giving drug I.V.

• Periodically monitor postoperative vital signs and bladder function. Because drug decreases both rate and depth of respirations, monitoring of arterial oxygen saturation may aid in assessing respiratory depression.

---

buprenorphine hydrochloride

Buprenex, Temgesic Injection‡
Controlled Substance Schedule V

Pregnancy Risk Category: C

HOW SUPPLIED

Injection: 0.324 mg (equivalent to 0.3 mg base/ml).

ACTION

Binds with opiate receptors in the CNS, altering both perception of and emotional response to pain through an unknown mechanism.

ONSET, PEAK, DURATION

Onset occurs within 15 minutes. Analgesic effects peak within 1 hour. Effects persist about 6 hours.

INDICATIONS & DOSAGE

Moderate to severe pain –
Adults and children 13 years of age and over: 0.3 mg I.M. or slow I.V. q 6 hours, p.r.n. or around the clock; dosage repeated (up to 0.3 mg) if re-

---

quired, 30 to 60 minutes after initial dose.

Children 2 to 12: 2 to 6 mcg/kg I.M. or I.V. q 4 to 6 hours.

ADVERSE REACTIONS
CNS: *dizziness, sedation, headache,* confusion, nervousness, euphoria, increased intracranial pressure.
CV: *hypotension,* bradycardia, tachycardia, hypertension.
EENT: *miosis,* blurred vision.
GI: *nausea,* vomiting, constipation.
GU: urine retention.
Respiratory: *respiratory depression,* hypoventilation.
Skin: pruritus, *sweating.*

INTERACTIONS
CNS depressants, ethanol, MAO inhibitors: additive effects. Use together cautiously.
Narcotic analgesics: possible decreased analgesic effect. Avoid concomitant use.

CONTRAINDICATIONS
Contraindicated in patients with hypersensitivity to this drug.

NURSING CONSIDERATIONS
• Use cautiously in elderly or debilitated patients or patients with head injury, intracranial lesions, and increased intracranial pressure; severe respiratory, liver, or kidney impairment; CNS depression or coma; thyroid irregularities; adrenal insufficiency; and prostatic hyperplasia, urethral stricture, acute alcholism, delirum tremens, or kyphoscoliosis.
• **I.V. use:** Give by direct I.V. injection, slowly into a vein or through the tubing of a free-flowing, compatible I.V. solution over not less than 2 minutes.
• S.C. administration not recommended.
• Be aware that buprenorphine 0.3 mg is equal to 10 mg of morphine and 75 mg of meperidine in analgesic po-

tency. Has longer duration of action than morphine or meperidine.
• Caution ambulatory patients about getting out of bed or walking.
• Know that naloxone will not completely reverse the respiratory depression caused by buprenorphine overdose; an overdose may necessitate mechanical ventilation. Larger than customary doses of naloxone (more than 0.4 mg) and doxapram also may be ordered.
• Be aware that drug's narcotic antagonist properties may precipitate withdrawal syndrome in narcotic-dependent patients.
• When drug is used postoperatively, encourage patient turning, coughing, and deep breathing to prevent atelectasis.
• Know that if dependence occurs, withdrawal symptoms may appear up to 14 days after drug is stopped.

---

butorphanol tartrate
Stadol, Stadol NS

Pregnancy Risk Category: C

HOW SUPPLIED
Injection: 1 mg/ml, 2 mg/ml
Nasal spray: 10 mg/ml

ACTION
Binds with opiate receptors in the CNS, altering both perception of and emotional response to pain through an unknown mechanism.

ONSET, PEAK, DURATION
Onset occurs within 2 to 3 minutes after an I.V. injection; within 10 to 30 minutes after I.M. injection; within 15 minutes of nasal use. Analgesic effects peak within 30 minutes to 1 hour of I.M. or I.V. use, within 1 to 2 hours of nasal use. Analgesic effects persist 3 to 4 hours after I.M. use, 2 to 4 hours after I.V. use, or 4 to 5 hours after nasal administration.

INDICATIONS & DOSAGE

Moderate to severe pain —
Adults: 1 to 4 mg I.M. q 3 to 4 hours, p.r.n. or around the clock; or 0.5 to 2 mg I.V. q 3 to 4 hours, p.r.n. or around the clock. Not to exceed 4 mg per dose. Alternatively, 1 mg by nasal spray q 3 to 4 hours (1 spray in one nostril); repeated in 60 to 90 minutes if pain relief is inadequate.
Labor for patients at full term and in early labor —
Adults: 1 to 2 mg I.V. or I.M., repeated after 4 hours as needed.
Preoperative anesthesia or preanesthesia —
Adults: 2 mg. I.M. 60 to 90 minutes before surgery.
Adjunct to balanced anesthesia —
Adults: 2 mg I.V. shortly before induction or 0.5 to 1.0 mg I.V. in increments during anesthesia.

ADVERSE REACTIONS

CNS: *sedation, headache, vertigo, floating sensation,* lethargy, *confusion,* nervousness, unusual dreams, agitation, euphoria, hallucinations, flushing, increased intracranial pressure.
CV: palpitations, fluctuation in blood pressure.
EENT: diplopia, blurred vision, *nasal congestion* (with nasal spray), *dry mouth.*
GI: *nausea, vomiting, constipation.*
Respiratory: *respiratory depression.*
Skin: rash, hives, *clamminess, excessive sweating.*

INTERACTIONS

CNS depressants, ethanol: additive effects. Use together cautiously.
Narcotic analgesics: possible decreased analgesic effect. Avoid concomitant use.

CONTRAINDICATIONS

Contraindicated in patients with narcotic addiction; may precipitate withdrawal syndrome. Also contraindicated in patient with hypersensitivity to the drug or to the preservative, benzethonium chloride.

NURSING CONSIDERATIONS

● Use cautiously in patients with head injury, increased intracranial pressure, acute MI, ventricular dysfunction, coronary insufficiency, respiratory disease or depression, and renal or hepatic dysfunction. Also administer cautiously to patients who have recently received repeated doses of narcotic analgesic medication.
● **I.V. use:** Give by direct injection into a vein or into the tubing of a free-flowing I.V. solution. Compatible solutions include D_5W and 0.9% sodium chloride.
● S.C. route not recommended.
● Know that respiratory depression apparently does not increase with larger dosage.
● Be aware that psychological and physical addiction may occur.
● Periodically monitor postoperative vital signs and bladder function. Because drug decreases both rate and depth of respirations, monitoring of arterial oxygen saturation may aid in assessing respiratory depression.
● Caution ambulatory patients about getting out of bed or walking. Warn outpatients to avoid driving and other potentially hazardous activities that require mental alertness until drug's CNS effects are known.

---

codeine phosphate
Paveral†

codeine sulfate

Controlled Substance Schedule II
Pregnancy Risk Category: C

HOW SUPPLIED
codeine phosphate
Oral solution: 15 mg/5 ml, 10 mg/ml†
Injection: 30 mg/ml, 60 mg/ml

---

*Liquid form contains alcohol.   Common reactions are in italics; **life-threatening**, in bold italics.
**May contain tartrazine.

Soluble tablets: 30 mg, 60 mg
codeine sulfate
Tablets: 15 mg, 30 mg, 60 mg

ACTION
Binds with opiate receptors in the CNS, altering both perception of and emotional response to pain through an unknown mechanism. Also suppresses the cough reflex by direct action on the cough center in the medulla.

ONSET, PEAK, DURATION
Onset occurs immediately with I.V. administration, 10 to 30 minutes after I.M. or S.C. injection, 30 to 45 minutes after oral use. Peak effects occur immediately after I.V. administration, within 30 minutes to 1 hour after I.M. injection, unknown after S.C. administration, and 1 to 2 hours after oral administration. Effects persist 4 to 6 hours.

INDICATIONS & DOSAGE
Mild to moderate pain –
Adults: 15 to 60 mg P.O. or 15 to 60 mg (phosphate) S.C., I.M., or I.V. q 4 to 6 hours, p.r.n.
Children over age 1: 0.5 mg/kg P.O., S.C., or I.M. q 4 hours, p.r.n.
Nonproductive cough –
Adults: 10 to 20 mg P.O. q 4 to 6 hours. Maximum dosage is 120 mg/ 24 hours.
Children 6 to 12 years: 5 to 10 mg P.O. q 4 to 6 hours. Maximum dosage is 60 mg/24 hours.
Children 2 to 6 years: 2.5 to 5 mg P.O. q 6 hours. Do not exceed 30 mg in 24 hours.

ADVERSE REACTIONS
CNS: *sedation, clouded sensorium, euphoria,* dizziness, *seizures* (with large doses).
CV: *hypotension,* bradycardia.
GI: *nausea, vomiting, constipation, dry mouth,* ileus.
GU: *urine retention.*

Respiratory: *respiratory depression.*
Skin: pruritus, flushing.
Other: physical dependence.

INTERACTIONS
CNS depressants, ethanol, general anesthetics, hypnotics, MAO inhibitors, other narcotic analgesics, sedatives, tranquilizers, tricyclic antidepressants: additive effects. Use together with extreme caution. Monitor patient response.

CONTRAINDICATIONS
Contraindicated in patients with hypersensitivity to this drug.

NURSING CONSIDERATIONS
• Use with extreme caution in patients with head injury, increased intracranial pressure, increased CSF pressure, hepatic or renal disease, hypothyroidism, Addison's disease, acute alcoholism, seizures, severe CNS depression, bronchial asthma, COPD, respiratory depression, and shock. Also use with extreme caution in elderly or debilitated patients.
• **I.V. use:** Give by direct injection into a large vein. Administer very slowly. Don't mix with other solutions because codeine phosphate is incompatible with many drugs.
• Don't administer discolored injection solution.
• Know that codeine and aspirin or acetaminophen are often prescribed together to provide enhanced pain relief.
• For full analgesic effect, administer drug before patient has intense pain.
• Be aware that drug is an antitussive and should not be used when cough is a valuable diagnostic sign or is beneficial (as after thoracic surgery).
• Monitor cough type and frequency.
• Monitor respiratory and circulatory status.
• Be aware that codeine's abuse potential is much lower than morphine's.
• To mimimize GI distress caused by

oral administration, advise patients to take this drug with milk or meals.
• Caution ambulatory patients about getting out of bed or walking. Warn outpatients to avoid driving and other potentially hazardous activities that require mental alertness until drug's CNS effects are known.
• Opiates may cause constipation. Assess bowel function and need for stool softeners or laxatives. Constipating effect makes codeine useful in the treatment of diarrhea.

---

dezocine
Dalgan

Pregnancy Risk Category: C

HOW SUPPLIED
Injection: 5 mg/ml, 10 mg/ml, 15 mg/ml

ACTION
Unknown. A synthetic opioid agonist-antagonist that produces postoperative analgesia qualitatively similar to morphine.

ONSET, PEAK, DURATION
Onset occurs within 15 minutes of I.V. injection, 30 minutes of I.M. injection. Peak effects occur within ½ to 2½ hours. Duration unknown.

INDICATIONS & DOSAGE
Management of moderate to severe pain –
Adults: 5 to 20 mg I.M. q 3 to 6 hours or 2.5 to 10 mg I.V. q 2 to 4 hours. Maximum recommended single I.M. dose is 20 mg, with a maximum daily dosage of 120 mg. Maximum dosage for I.V. use has not been determined.

ADVERSE REACTIONS
CNS: *sedation, dizziness, vertigo,* anxiety, mood disorders, sleep disturbances, headache, slurred speech, sweating, chills, flushing, pallor.
CV: edema, hypotension, irregular heartbeat, hypertension, chest pain, thrombophlebitis.
EENT: dry mouth.
GI: *nausea, vomiting,* constipation, diarrhea, abdominal distress.
Hematologic: low hemoglobin.
Respiratory: *respiratory depression.*
Skin: rash, pruritus, *irritation at injection site.*

INTERACTIONS
CNS depressants, ethanol: may increase risk of CNS depression.
Opiates: opioid-dependent patients may experience withdrawal symptoms after receiving dezocine. May increase risk of CNS depression.

CONTRAINDICATIONS
Contraindicated in patients with hypersensitivity to the drug and in patients physically dependent on narcotics.

NURSING CONSIDERATIONS
• Use with extreme caution in patients with head injury because drug's CNS depressant effects may obscure clinical signs. Related drugs have caused elevations of CSF pressure in patients with head injury.
• Use cautiously and in lower doses in patients with chronic respiratory disease and in patients undergoing biliary surgery. Related drugs have caused significant increases in pressure within the common bile duct.
• Like other potent analgesics, dezocine should be administered with caution to elderly patients and patients who have recently received substantial amounts of narcotic medication.
• Use cautiously in patients with renal or hepatic failure. Expect dosages to be lower because of increased elimination half-life in these patients.
• Because it is not known if dezocine is excreted in breast milk, breast-feeding is not recommended.
• Use of dezocine is not recom-

mended in patients who are opioid-dependent because it may precipitate withdrawal syndrome. Also not recommended for patients with chronic pain because of limited clinical experience and because drug can precipitate withdrawal syndrome in patients with substantial tolerance to opiates.
• Dezocine produces a dose-dependent respiratory depression similar to that of morphine. Use only in clinical settings where adequate respiratory support and an opiate antagonist (naloxone) is available to reverse respiratory depression.
• **I.V. use:** Give by direct injection into a large vein. Avoid mixing with other drugs because there is little information regarding drug and solution compatibility. Infuse over at least 5 minutes. The injection contains sulfite preservatives, which may cause allergic reactions in certain sensitive patients.
• Be aware that plasma concentrations higher than 45 ng/ml are associated with an increased incidence of adverse reactions.
• Caution ambulatory patients about getting out of bed or walking. Warn outpatients to avoid driving and other potentially hazardous activities that require mental alertness until drug's CNS effects are known.

fentanyl citrate
Sublimaze

fentanyl transdermal system
Duragesic-25, Duragesic-50, Duragesic-75, Duragesic-100

fentanyl transmucosal
Fentanyl Oralet
Controlled Substance Schedule II

Pregnancy Risk Category: C

HOW SUPPLIED
Injection: 50 mcg/ml
Transdermal system: patches designed to release 25 mcg, 50 mcg, 75 mcg, or 100 mcg of fentanyl per hour.
Transmucosal: 200 mcg, 300 mcg, 400 mcg

ACTION
Unknown. Binds with opiate receptors in the CNS, altering both perception of and emotional response to pain through an unknown mechanism.

ONSET, PEAK, DURATION
Onset within 1 to 2 minutes with I.V. administration; within 7 to 15 minutes of I.M. injection; within 5 to 15 minutes of transmucosal use; onset after transdermal use may take 12 to 24 hours. Peak effect after I.V. use occurs in 3 to 5 minutes; after I.M. or transmucosal use, 20 to 30 minutes; after trandermal use, 1 to 3 days. Effects persist ½ to 1 hour after I.V. use or 1 to 2 hours after I.M. use; variable with transdermal system; not clearly defined with transmucosal use.

INDICATIONS & DOSAGE
Adjunct to general anesthetic –
Adults: for low-dose therapy, 2 mcg/kg I.V. For moderate-dose therapy, 2 to 20 mcg I.V.; then 25 to 100 mcg I.V. p.r.n. For high-dose therapy, 20 to 50 mcg I.V.; then 25 mcg to one-half the initial loading dose I.V. p.r.n.
Adjunct to regional anesthesia –
Adults: 0.05 to 0.1 mg I.M. or slowly I.V. q 1 to 2 hours p.r.n.
Postoperatively –
Adults: 0.05 to 0.1 mg I.M. q 1 to 2 hours p.r.n.
Preoperatively –
Adults: 0.05 to 0.1 mg I.M. 30 to 60 minutes before surgery. Alternatively, 5 mcg/kg dispensed as oralet unit, 20 to 40 minutes prior to need of desired effects.
Management of chronic pain –
Adults: one transdermal system ap-

plied to a portion of the upper torso on an area of skin that is not irritated and has not been irradiated. Therapy initiated with the 25-mcg/hour system; dosage adjusted as needed and tolerated. Each system may be worn for 72 hours.

ADVERSE REACTIONS
CNS: *sedation, somnolence, clouded sensorium, euphoria,* dizziness, *seizures* (with large doses).
CV: *hypotension,* bradycardia.
GI: nausea, vomiting, *constipation,* ileus.
GU: *urine retention.*
Respiratory: *respiratory depression.*
Skin: reaction at application site (erythema, papules, edema), *pruritus.*
Other: muscle rigidity, physical dependence.

INTERACTIONS
CNS depressants, ethanol, general anesthetics, hyponotics, MAO inhibitors, other narcotic analgesics, sedatives, tricyclic antidepressants: additive effects. Use together with extreme caution. Fentanyl dose should be reduced by one-quarter to one-third. Also give above drugs in reduced dosages.

CONTRAINDICATIONS
Contraindicated in patients with known intolerance of the drug.

NURSING CONSIDERATIONS
• Use with caution in patients with head injury, increased CSF pressure, COPD, decreased respiratory reserve, potentially compromised respirations, hepatic or renal disease, and cardiac bradyarrhythmias. Also use with caution in elderly or debilitated patients.
• Keep narcotic antagonist (naloxone) and resuscitation equipment available when giving drug intravenously.
• For better analgesic effect, administer drug before patient has intense pain.
• Be aware that high doses can pro-

duce muscle rigidity, which can be reversed with neuromuscular blockers; however, patient must be artificially ventilated.
• Monitor circulatory and respiratory status and urinary function carefully. Drug may cause respiratory depression, hypotension, urine retention, nausea, vomiting, ileus, or altered level of consciousness without regard to route of administration.
• Periodically monitor postoperative vital signs and bladder function. Because drug decreases both rate and depth of respirations, monitoring of arterial oxygen saturation (SaO_2) may help assess respiratory depression. Immediately report respiratory rate below 12 breaths/minute, decreased respiratory volume, or decreased SaO_2.
• When drug is used postoperatively, encourage patient turning, coughing, and deep breathing to prevent atelectasis.
I.V. form:
• Know that only staff trained in administration of I.V. anesthetics and management their potential adverse effects should administer I.V. fentanyl.
• Be aware that drug often used I.V. with droperidol to produce neuroleptanalgesia.
Transmucosal form:
• Remove foil overwrap of fentanyl oralet just prior to administration.
• Instruct patient to place the fentanyl oralet in mouth and suck (not chew) it.
• Remove fentanyl oralet unit using the handle after it has been consumed, patient shows adequate effect, or patient shows signs of respiratory depression. Place any remaining portion in the plastic overwrap provided and dispose accordingly for Schedule II drugs.
Transdermal form:
• Know that transdermal fentanyl is

---

*Liquid form contains alcohol.   *Common* reactions are in italics; *life-threatening,* in bold italics.
**May contain tartrazine.

not recommended for postoperative pain.

• Dosage equivalent charts are available to calculate the fentanyl transdermal dose based on the daily morphine intake – for example, for every 90 mg of oral morphine or 15 mg of I.M. morphine per 24 hours, 25 mcg/hour of transdermal fentanyl is required. Some patients will require alternative means of opiate administration when the dosage exceeds 300 mcg/hour.

• Be aware that dosage adjustments in patients using the transdermal system should be made gradually. Reaching steady-state levels of a new dosage may take up to 6 days; delay dosage adjustment until after at least two applications.

• Monitor patients who develop adverse reactions to the transdermal system for at least 12 hours after removal. Serum levels of fentanyl drop gradually and may take as long as 17 hours to decline by 50%.

• Most patients experience good control of pain for 3 days while wearing the transdermal system, but a few may need a new application after 48 hours. Because serum fentanyl concentration rises for the first 24 hours after application, analgesic effect cannot be evaluated for the first day. Be sure the patient has adequate supplemental analgesic to prevent breakthrough pain.

• When reducing opiate therapy or switching to a different analgesic, know the transdermal system should be withdrawn gradually. Because fentanyl's serum level drops gradually after removal, give half of the equianalgesic dose of the new analgesic 12 to 18 hours after removal as ordered.

• Teach patients proper application of the transdermal patch. Clip hair at the application site, but do not use a razor, which may irritate the skin. Wash area with clear water if necessary, but not with soaps, oils, lotions, alcohol, or other substances that may irritate

the skin or prevent adhesion. Dry the area completely before application.

• Tell patient to remove the transdermal system from the package just before applying. Hold in place for 10 to 20 seconds, and be sure the edges of the patch adhere to the patient's skin.

• Teach patients to dispose of the transdermal patch by folding so the adhesive side adheres to itself and then flushing it down the toilet.

• Tell patient if another patch is needed after 72 hours, apply to a new site.

• Inform patient that heat from fever or environment may increase transdermal delivery and cause toxicity requiring dosage adjustment. Instruct patient to notify doctor if fever occurs or if patient will be spending time in a hot climate region.

---

hydromorphone hydrochloride (dihydromorphinone hydrochloride)
Dilaudid, Dilaudid-HP
Controlled Substance Schedule II

Pregnancy Risk Category: C

HOW SUPPLIED
Tablets: 1 mg, 2 mg, 3 mg, 4 mg
Injection: 1 mg/ml, 2 mg/ml, 3 mg/ml, 4 mg/ml, 10 mg/ml
Suppositories: 3 mg
Syrup: 1mg/5 ml

ACTION
Binds with opiate receptors in the CNS, altering both perception of and emotional response to pain through an unknown mechanism. Also suppresses the cough reflex by direct action on the cough center in the medulla.

ONSET, PEAK, DURATION
Onset occurs 10 to 15 minutes after I.V. injection, about 15 minutes after S.C. or I.M. administration, about 30

minutes after oral dose. Peak effects occur 15 to 30 minutes after I.V. injection, 30 to 60 minutes after I.M. injection, 30 to 90 minutes after S.C. administration, 1½ to 2 hours after oral administration. Effects persist about 2 to 3 hours after I.V. injection, 4 to 5 hours after I.M. injection, 4 hours after S.C. or oral administration.

INDICATIONS & DOSAGE
Moderate to severe pain –
Adults: 2 to 4 mg P.O. q 4 to 6 hours, p.r.n.; or 2 to 4 mg I.M., S.C., or I.V. (slowly over at least 2 to 3 minutes) q 4 to 6 hours p.r.n.; or 3 mg rectal suppository q 6 to 8 hours p.r.n.
Cough –
Adults: 1 teaspoon (5 ml) P.O. q 3 to 4 hours p.r.n.

ADVERSE REACTIONS
CNS: *sedation, somnolence, clouded sensorium,* dizziness, *euphoria,* **seizures** (with large doses).
CV: *hypotension,* bradycardia.
EENT: blurred vision, diplopia, nystagmus.
GI: *nausea, vomiting, constipation,* ileus.
GU: *urine retention.*
Respiratory: *respiratory depression, bronchospasm.*
Other: induration with repeated S.C. injections, physical dependence.

INTERACTIONS
CNS depressants, ethanol, general anesthetics, hypnotics, MAO inhibitors, other narcotic analgesics, sedatives, tranquilizers, tricyclic antidepressants: additive effects. Use together with extreme caution. Reduce hydromorphone dose and monitor patient response.

CONTRAINDICATIONS
Contraindicated in patients with hypersensitivity to this drug, intracranial lesions associated with increased intracranial pressure, and whenever ventilator function is depressed such as in status asthmaticus, COPD, cor pulmonale, emphysema, and kryphoscoliosis.

NURSING CONSIDERATIONS
• Use with extreme caution in patients with hepatic or renal disease, hypothyroidism, Addison's disease, prostatic hypertrophy, or urethral stricture. Also use with caution in elderly or debilitated patients.
• For better analgesic effect, give this drug before patient has intense pain.
• Dilaudid-HP, a highly concentrated form (10 mg/ml), may be administered in smaller volumes to prevent the discomfort associated with large-volume I.M. or S.C. injections. Check dosage carefully.
• Rotate injection sites to avoid induration with S.C. injection.
• **I.V. use:** Give by direct injection over no less than 2 minutes. For infusion, drug may be mixed in D_5W, 0.9% sodium chloride, dextrose 5% in 0.9% sodium chloride, dextrose 5% in 0.45% sodium chloride, or Ringer's or lactated Ringer's solutions.
• Respiratory depression and hypotension can occur with I.V. administration. Give very slowly and monitor constantly. Keep resuscitation equipment available.
• Monitor respiratory and circulatory status and bowel function.
• Keep narcotic antagonist (naloxone) available.
• Be aware that drug may worsen or mask gallbladder pain.
• Be aware drug is a commonly abused narcotic.
• When drug is used postoperatively, encourage patient turning, coughing, and deep breathing to avoid atelectasis.
• Caution ambulatory patients about getting out of bed or walking. Warn outpatients to avoid driving and other

*Liquid form contains alcohol.   *Common* reactions are in italics; *life-threatening,* in bold italics.
**May contain tartrazine.

potentially hazardous activities that require mental alertness until drug's CNS effects are known.

---

meperidine hydrochloride (pethidine hydrochloride)
Demerol
Controlled Substance Schedule II

Pregnancy Risk Category: NR

HOW SUPPLIED
Tablets: 50 mg, 100 mg
Syrup: 50 mg/ml
Injection: 10 mg/ml, 25 mg/ml, 50 mg/ml, 75 mg/ml, 100 mg/ml

ACTION
Binds with opiate receptors in the CNS, altering both perception of and emotional response to pain through an unknown mechanism.

ONSET, PEAK, DURATION
Onset occurs about 1 minute following I.V. administration, 10 to 15 minutes after S.C. or I.M. injection, about 15 minutes after oral administration. Peak effect occurs within 5 to 7 minutes after I.V. injection, 30 to 50 minutes after I.M. or S.C. injection, and 60 to 90 minutes after oral administration. Effects persist 2 to 4 hours for all routes of administration.

INDICATIONS & DOSAGE
Moderate to severe pain –
Adults: 50 to 150 mg P.O., I.M., or S.C. q 3 to 4 hours, p.r.n.; or 15 to 35 mg/hour by continuous I.V. infusion.
Children: 1.1 to 1.76 mg/kg P.O., I.M., or S.C. q 3 to 4 hours. Maximum dosage is 100 mg q 4 hours, p.r.n..
Preoperatively –
Adults: 50 to 100 mg I.M. or S.C. 30 to 90 minutes before surgery.
Children: 1 to 2.2 mg/kg I.M. or S.C. up to the adult dose 30 to 90 minutes before surgery.
Adjunct to anesthesia –

Adults: Repeated slow I.V. injections of fractional doses (i.e. 10 mg/ml); alternatively, continuous I.V. infusion of a more dilute solution (i.e. 1 mg/ml) titrated to needs of patient.
Obstetrical analgesia –
Adults: 50 to 100 mg I.M. or S.C. when pain becomes regular, repeated at 1- to 3-hour intervals.

ADVERSE REACTIONS
CNS: *sedation, somnolence, clouded sensorium, euphoria,* paradoxical excitement, tremor, dizziness, *seizures* (with large doses).
CV: *hypotension,* bradycardia, tachycardia.
GI: *nausea, vomiting, constipation,* ileus.
GU: *urine retention.*
Respiratory: *respiratory depression.*
Skin: pain at injection site, local tissue irritation and induration after S.C. injection; phlebitis after I.V. use.
Other: physical dependence, muscle twitching.

INTERACTIONS
Aminophylline, barbiturates, heparin, methicillin, morphine sulfate, phenytoin, sodium bicarbonate, sulfonamides: incompatible when mixed in the same I.V. container.
CNS depressants, ethanol, general anesthetics, hypnotics, other narcotic analgesics, phenothiazines, sedatives, tricyclic antidepressants: possible respiratory depression, hypotension, profound sedation, or coma. Use together with extreme caution. Reduce meperidine dosage.
MAO inhibitors: increased CNS excitation or depression that can be severe or fatal. Don't use together.
Phenytoin: decreased blood levels of meperidine. Monitor for decreased analgesia.

CONTRAINDICATIONS
Contraindicated in patients with hypersensitivity to this drug and in pa-

---

tients who have received MAO inhibitors within past 14 days.

NURSING CONSIDERATIONS
● Use with extreme caution in patients with increased intracranial pressure, head injury, asthma, and other respiratory conditions; in supraventricular tachycardias, seizures, acute abdominal conditions, hepatic or renal disease, hypothyroidism, Addison's disease, urethral stricture, and prostatic hyperplasia; and in elderly or debilitated patients.
● May be used in some patients allergic to morphine.
● **I.V. use:** Give slowly by direct I.V. injection. Meperidine also may be given by slow continuous I.V. infusion. Drug is compatible with most I.V. solutions, including D_5W, 0.9% sodium chloride, and Ringer's or lactated Ringer's solutions.
● Keep narcotic antagonist (naloxone) available when giving this drug I.V.
● S.C. injection is not recommended because it is very painful.
● Oral dose is less than half as effective as parenteral dose. Give I.M. if possible. When changing from parenteral to oral route, know that dosage should be increased.
● Syrup has local anesthetic effect. Give with full glass of water.
● Meperidine and its active metabolite normeperidine accumulate in the body. Monitor for increased toxic effect, especially in patients with impaired renal function.
● Because meperidine toxicity often appears after several days of treatment, this drug is not recommended for treatment of chronic pain.
● Monitor respirations of neonates exposed to drug during labor. Have resuscitation equipment and naloxone available.
● Monitor respiratory and cardiovascular status carefully. Don't give if respirations are below 12 breaths/minute, if respiratory rate or depth is

decreased, or if change in pupils is noted.
● Watch for withdrawal symptoms if drug is discontinued abruptly after long-term use.
● Monitor bladder function in postoperative patients.
● Monitor bowel function. Patient may need a laxative or stool softener.
● When drug is used postoperatively, encourage patient turning, coughing, and deep breathing and use of an incentive spirometer to prevent atelectasis.
● Caution ambulatory patients about getting out of bed or walking. Warn outpatients to avoid driving and other potentially hazardous activities that require mental alertness until drug's CNS effects are known.

methadone hydrochloride
Dolophine, Methadose, Physeptone‡
Controlled Substance Schedule II

Pregnancy Risk Category: NR

HOW SUPPLIED
Tablets: 5 mg, 10 mg
Dispersible tablets (for methadone maintenance therapy): 40 mg
Oral solution: 5 mg/5 ml, 10 mg/5 ml, 10 mg/ml (concentrate)
Injection: 10 mg/ml

ACTION
Binds with opiate receptors at many sites in the CNS (brain, brain stem, and spinal cord), altering both perception of and emotional response to pain through an unknown mechanism.

ONSET, PEAK, DURATION
Onset occurs immediately after I.V. administration, 10 to 20 minutes after I.M. injection, 30 to 60 minutes after oral administration. Peak effects occur within 15 to 30 minutes after I.V injection, 1 to 2 hours after I.M. injection, 1½ to 2 hours after oral ad-

---

ministration. Effects persist 3 to 4 hours after I.V. use, 4 to 5 hours after I.M. use, 4 to 6 hours after oral use.

INDICATIONS & DOSAGE
Severe pain –
Adults: 2.5 to 10 mg P.O., I.M., or S.C. q 3 to 4 hours, p.r.n.
Narcotic withdrawal syndrome –
Adults: 15 to 40 mg P.O. daily (highly individualized). Maintenance dosage is 20 to 120 mg P.O. daily. Dosage adjusted as needed. Daily dosages greater than 120 mg require special state and federal approval.

ADVERSE REACTIONS
CNS: *sedation, somnolence, clouded sensorium, euphoria,* dizziness, choreic movements, *seizures* (with large doses).
CV: *hypotension,* bradycardia.
EENT: visual disturbances.
GI: *nausea, vomiting, constipation,* ileus.
GU: *urine retention,* decreased libido.
Respiratory: *respiratory depression.*
Skin: pain at injection site, tissue irritation, induration following S.C. injection, diaphoresis.
Other: physical dependence.

INTERACTIONS
Ammonium chloride and other urine acidifiers, phenytoin: may reduce methadone effect. Monitor for decreased pain control.
CNS depressants, ethanol, general anesthetics, hypnotics, MAO inhibitors, sedatives, tranquilizers, tricyclic antidepressants: possible respiratory depression, hypotension, profound sedation, or coma. Use together with extreme caution. Monitor patient response.
Rifampin: withdrawal symptoms; reduced blood levels of methadone. Use together cautiously.

CONTRAINDICATIONS
Contraindicated in patients with hypersensitivity to this drug.

NURSING CONSIDERATIONS
• Use with extreme caution in patients with acute abdominal conditions, severe hepatic or renal impairment, hypothyroidism, Addison's disease, prostatic hyperplasia, urethral stricture, head injury, increased intracranial pressure, asthma, and other respiratory conditions. Also use with caution in elderly or debilitated patients.
• Oral liquid form legally required in maintenance programs. Completely dissolve tablets in 120 ml of orange juice or powdered citrus drink.
• For parenteral use, I.M. injection is preferred. Rotate injection sites.
• **I.V. use:** Dilute to a maximum concentration of 10 mg/ml using 0.9% sodium chloride. Give slowly by direct injection. Alternatively, dilute to 1 mg/ml and give as a slow I.V. infusion (15 to 35 mg/hour).
• Know that oral dose is half as potent as injected dose.
• Know that an around-the-clock regimen is necessary to manage severe, chronic pain.
• Monitor patient closely; has cumulative effect; marked sedation can occur after repeated doses.
• Monitor circulatory and respiratory status and bladder and bowel function. Patient may need a laxative.
• Be aware that patient treated for narcotic withdrawal syndrome usually will require an additional analgesic if pain control is necessary.
• Be aware that when used as an adjunct in the treatment of narcotic addiction (maintenance), withdrawal usually will be delayed and mild.
• Caution ambulatory patients about getting out of bed or walking. Warn outpatients to avoid driving and other potentially hazardous activities that

---

require mental alertness until drug's CNS effects are known.

morphine hydrochloride
Morphitec†, M.O.S.†, M.O.S.-S.R.†

morphine sulfate
Astramorph PF, Duramorph, Duramorph PF, Epimorph†, Infumorph 200, Infumorph 500, Morphine H.P.†, MS Contin, MSIR, Oramorph SR, RMS Uniserts, Roxanol, Roxanol 100, Roxanol Rescudose, Roxanol SR, Roxanol UD, Statex†

Controlled Substance Schedule II

morphine tartrate‡

Pregnancy Risk Category: C

HOW SUPPLIED
morphine hydrochloride
Tablets: 10 mg†, 20 mg†, 40 mg†, 60 mg†
Tablets (extended-release): 30 mg†, 60 mg†
Oral solution†: 1 mg/ml, 5 mg/ml, 10 mg/ml, 20 mg/ml, 50 mg/ml
Syrup: 1 mg/ml†, 5 mg/ml†, 10 mg/ml†, 20 mg/ml†, 50 mg/ml†
Suppositories: 10 mg†, 20 mg†, 30 mg†
morphine sulfate
Tablets: 15 mg, 30 mg
Tablets (extended-release): 15 mg, 30 mg, 60 mg, 100 mg
Soluble tablets: 10 mg, 15 mg, 30 mg
Oral solution: 10 mg/5 ml, 20 mg/5 ml, 20 mg/ml (concentrate)
Syrup: 1 mg/ml, 5 mg/ml
Injection (with preservative): 500 mcg/ml, 1 mg/ml, 2 mg/ml, 3 mg/ml, 4 mg/ml, 5 mg/ml, 8 mg/ml, 10 mg/ml, 15 mg/ml, 25 mg/ml, 50 mg/ml
Injection (without preservative): 500 mcg/ml, 1 mg/ml, 10 mg/ml, 25 mg/ml
Suppositories: 5 mg, 10 mg, 20 mg, 30 mg

morphine tartrate
Injection: 80 mg/ml‡

ACTION
Binds with opiate receptors in the CNS, altering both perception of and emotional response to pain through an unknown mechanism.

ONSET, PEAK, DURATION
Onset occurs within 1 hour after oral dose, 20 to 60 minutes after rectal dose, 10 to 30 minutes after S.C. or I.M. dose, less than 5 minutes after I.V. dose, 15 to 60 minutes after epidural or intrathecal dose. Peak analgesic effect is 1 to 2 hours after oral dose, 20 to 60 minutes after rectal dose, 50 to 90 minutes after S.C. dose, 30 to 60 minutes after I.M. dose, 20 minutes after direct I.V. injection, 15 to 60 minutes after epidural injection. Effects persist 4 to 5 hours after immediate-release oral forms, 8 to 12 hours after extended-release oral forms, 4 to 5 hours after rectal, S.C., I.M., or I.V. dose, up to 24 hours after intrathecal or epidural dose.

INDICATIONS & DOSAGE
Severe pain –
Adults: 5 to 20 mg S.C. or I.M. or 2.5 to 15 mg I.V. q 4 hours p.r.n.; or 10 to 30 mg P.O. or 10 to 20 mg rectally q 4 hours, p.r.n. When given by continuous I.V. infusion, a loading dose of 15 mg I.V. may be followed by a continuous infusion of 0.8 to 10 mg/hour. 15 to 30 mg controlled-release tablets P.O. q 12 hours may also be administered. As an epidural injection, 5 mg by epidural catheter, then if adequate pain relief not obtained within 1 hour, additional doses of 1 to 2 mg given at intervals sufficient to assess efficacy. Maximum total epidural dose should not exceed 10 mg.
Children: 0.1 to 0.2 mg/kg S.C. or I.M. q 4 hours. Maximum single dose is 15 mg.

---

*Liquid form contains alcohol.
**May contain tartrazine.

Common reactions are in italics; ***life-threatening***, in bold italics.

ADVERSE REACTIONS

CNS: *sedation, somnolence, clouded sensorium, euphoria, seizures* (with large doses), dizziness, *nightmares* (with long-acting oral forms).
CV: *hypotension,* bradycardia.
GI: *nausea, vomiting, constipation,* ileus.
GU: *urine retention.*
Hematologic: thrombocytopenia.
Respiratory: *respiratory depression.*
Skin: pruritus and skin flushing (with epidural administration).
Other: *physical dependence.*

INTERACTIONS

CNS depressants, ethanol, general anesthetics, hypnotics, MAO inhibitors, other narcotic analgesics, sedatives, tranquilizers, tricyclic antidepressants: possible respiratory depression, hypotension, profound sedation, or coma. Use together with extreme caution. Reduce morphine dosage and monitor patient response.

CONTRAINDICATIONS

Contraindicated in patients with hypersensitivity to this drug or conditions that would preclude administration of opioids by I.V. route (acute bronchial asthma or upper airway obstruction).

NURSING CONSIDERATIONS

• Use with extreme caution in patients with head injury, increased intracranial pressure, seizures, chronic pulmonary disease, prostatic hyperplasia, severe hepatic or renal disease, acute abdominal conditions, hypothyroidism, Addison's disease, and urethral stricture. Also use with extreme caution in elderly or debilitated patients.
• Keep narcotic antagonist (naloxone) and resuscitation equipment available.
• **I.V. use:** When given by direct injection, 2.5 to 15 mg may be diluted in 4 or 5 ml of sterile water for injection and given over 4 to 5 minutes. Alternatively, the drug may be mixed with D_5W to a concentration of 0.1 to 1 mg/ml and administered by a continuous infusion device. Morphine sulfate is compatible with most common I.V. solutions.
• Oral solutions of various concentrations are available as well as an intensified oral solution (20 mg/ml). Carefully note the strength administered.
• Do not crush or break extended-release tablets.
• S.L. administration may be ordered. Measure oral solution with tuberculin syringe. Administer dose a few drops at a time to allow maximal S.L. absorption and minimize swallowing.
• Refrigeration of rectal suppository is not necessary. In some patients, rectal and oral absorption may not be equivalent.
• Preservative-free preparations are available for epidural and intrathecal administration.
• When given epidurally, monitor closely for respiratory depression up to 24 hours after the injection. Check respiratory rate and depth every 30 to 60 minutes for 24 hours.
• Know that morphine is the drug of choice in relieving pain of MI. May cause transient decrease in blood pressure.
• Be aware that an around-the-clock regimen best manages severe, chronic pain.
• When drug is used postoperatively, encourage patient turning, coughing, and deep breathing and use of incentive spirometer to prevent atelectasis.
• Be aware morphine may worsen or mask gallbladder pain.
• Monitor circulatory, respiratory, bladder, and bowel functions carefully. Drug may cause respiratory depression, hypotension, urine retention, nausea, vomiting, ileus, or altered level of consciousness regardless of the route used. Withhold dose

and notify doctor if respirations are below 12 breaths/minute.
• Constipation is often severe with maintenance dosage. Ensure that stool softener or other laxative is ordered.
• Caution ambulatory patients about getting out of bed or walking. Warn outpatients to avoid driving and other potentially hazardous activities that require mental alertness until drug's adverse CNS effects are known.

---

nalbuphine hydrochloride
Nubain

Pregnancy Risk Category: NR

HOW SUPPLIED
Injection: 10 mg/ml, 20 mg/ml

ACTION
Binds with opiate receptors in the CNS, altering both perception of and emotional response to pain through an unknown mechanism.

ONSET, PEAK, DURATION
Onset occurs 2 to 3 minutes after I.V. administration, within 15 minutes of S.C. or I. M. injection. Peak effects occur within 30 minutes of I.V. administration, 60 minutes of I.M. injection. Effects persist 3 to 4 hours after I.V. use, 3 to 6 hours after S.C. or I.M. injection.

INDICATIONS & DOSAGE
Moderate to severe pain –
Adults: For an average (70 kg) person, give 10 to 20 mg S.C., I.M., or I.V. q 3 to 6 hours, p.r.n. Maximum daily dosage is 160 mg.
Adjunct to balanced anesthesia –
Adults: 0.3 mg/kg to 3.0 mg/kg I.V. over 10 to 15 minutes followed by maintenance doses of 0.25 to 0.50 mg/kg in single I.V. doses p.r.n.

ADVERSE REACTIONS
CNS: *headache, sedation, dizziness, vertigo,* nervousness, depression, restlessness, crying, euphoria, hostility, unusual dreams, confusion, hallucinations, speech difficulty, delusions.
CV: hypertension, hypotension, tachycardia, bradycardia.
EENT: blurred vision, *dry mouth.*
GI: cramps, dyspepsia, bitter taste, *nausea, vomiting,* constipation.
GU: urinary urgency.
Skin: itching; burning; urticaria; *sweaty, clammy feeling.*
Respiratory: *respiratory depression, pulmonary edema.*

INTERACTIONS
CNS depressants, ethanol, general anesthetics, hypnotics, MAO inhibitors, sedatives, tranquilizers, tricyclic antidepressants: possible respiratory depression, hypertension, profound sedation, or coma. Use together with extreme caution. Monitor patient response.
Narcotic analgesics: possible decreased analgesic effect. Avoid concomitant use.

CONTRAINDICATIONS
Contraindicated in patients with hypersensitivity to the drug.

NURSING CONSIDERATIONS
• Use cautiously in patients with history of drug abuse or in patients with emotional instability, head injury, increased intracranial pressure, impaired ventilation, MI accompanied by nausea and vomiting, upcoming biliary surgery, and hepatic or renal disease.
• Respiratory depression can be reversed with naloxone. Keep resuscitation equipment available, particularly when administering intravenously.
• Acts as a narcotic antagonist; may precipitate withdrawal syndrome. For patients who have chronically received opiates, administer 25% of the usual dose initially as ordered. Observe for signs of withdrawal.
• **I.V. use:** Inject slowly over at least

---

*Liquid form contains alcohol.   *Common* reactions are in italics; **life-threatening,** in bold italics.
**May contain tartrazine.

2 to 3 minutes into a vein or into an I.V. line containing a compatible, free-flowing I.V. solution, such as D₅W, 0.9% sodium chloride, or lactated Ringer's solution.

- Causes respiratory depression, which at 10 mg is equal to the respiratory depression produced by 10 mg of morphine.
- Monitor circulatory and respiratory status and bladder and bowel function. Withhold dose and notify doctor if respirations are shallow or rate is below 12 breaths/minute.
- Constipation is often severe with maintenance therapy. Make sure stool softener or other laxative is ordered.
- Know that psychological and physical dependence may occur with prolonged use.
- Caution ambulatory patients about getting out of bed or walking. Warn outpatients to avoid driving and other potentially hazardous activities that require mental alertness until drug's CNS effects are known.

---

oxycodone hydrochloride
Endone‡, Roxicodone, Roxicodone Intensol, Supeudol†
Controlled Substance Schedule II

oxycodone pectinate
Proladone‡

Pregnancy Risk Category: NR

HOW SUPPLIED
oxycodone hydrochloride
Tablets: 5 mg
Oral solution: 5 mg/5 ml, 20 mg/ml (concentrate)
Suppositories: 10 mg, 20 mg
oxycodone pectinate
Suppositories: 30 mg‡

ACTION
Binds with opiate receptors in the CNS, altering both perception of and emotional response to pain through an unknown mechanism.

ONSET, PEAK, DURATION
Onset occurs in 10 to 15 minutes. Peak effects occur within 1 hour. Effects persist 3 to 6 hours.

INDICATIONS & DOSAGE
Moderate to severe pain –
Adults: 5 mg P.O. q 6 hours, p.r.n. Alternatively, 1 to 3 suppositories P.R. daily, p.r.n.
Children 6 to 12 years: 0.61 mg of combined salts P.O. q 6 hours, p.r.n.
Children 12 years and older: 1.22 mg of combined salts P.O. q 6 hours, p.r.n.

ADVERSE REACTIONS
CNS: *sedation, somnolence, clouded sensorium, euphoria,* dizziness, *seizures* (with large doses).
CV: *hypotension,* bradycardia.
GI: *nausea, vomiting, constipation,* ileus.
GU: *urine retention.*
Respiratory: *respiratory depression.*
Other: physical dependence.

INTERACTIONS
Anticoagulants: oxycodone hydrochloride products containing aspirin may increase anticoagulant effect. Monitor clotting times. Use together cautiously.
CNS depressants, ethanol, general anesthetics, hypnotics, MAO inhibitors, other narcotic analgesics, sedatives, tranquilizers, tricyclic antidepressants: additive effects. Use together with extreme caution. Reduce oxycodone dose and monitor patient response.

CONTRAINDICATIONS
Contraindicated in patients with hypersensitivity to this drug.

NURSING CONSIDERATIONS
- Use with extreme caution in patients with head injury, increased intracranial pressure, seizures, asthma, COPD, prostatic hypertrophy, severe

---

hepatic or renal disease, acute abdominal conditions, urethral stricture, hypothyroidism, Addison's disease, and arrhythmias. Also use with extreme caution in elderly or debilitated patients.

• For full analgesic effect, administer drug before patient has intense pain.

• To minimize GI upset, administer drug after meals or with milk.

• Be aware that single-agent oxycodone solution or tablets are especially good for patients who shouldn't take aspirin or acetaminophen.

• Monitor circulatory and respiratory status. Withhold dose and notify doctor if respirations are shallow or if respiratory rate falls below 12 breaths/minute.

• Monitor patient's bladder and bowel patterns. Patient may require a laxative because drug has a constipating effect.

• Caution ambulatory patients about getting out of bed or walking. Warn outpatients to avoid driving and other potentially hazardous activities that require mental alertness until drug's CNS effects are known.

oxymorphone hydrochloride
Numorphan, Numorphan H.P.
Controlled Substance Schedule II

Pregnancy Risk Category: NR

HOW SUPPLIED
Injection: 1 mg/ml, 1.5 mg/ml
Suppositories: 5 mg

ACTION
Binds with opiate receptors in the CNS, altering both perception of and emotional response to pain through an unknown mechanism.

ONSET, PEAK, DURATION
Onset occurs within 5 to 10 minutes after I.V. use, 10 to 15 minutes after I.M. use, 10 to 20 minutes after S.C.

use, 15 to 30 minutes after rectal use. Peak effects occur within 15 to 30 minutes after I.V. use, 30 to 90 minutes after I.M. use, 60 to 90 minutes after S.C. use, 2 hours after rectal use. Effects persist 3 to 4 hours after I.V. use; 3 to 6 hours after I.M., S.C., or rectal use.

INDICATIONS & DOSAGE
Moderate to severe pain –
Adults: 1 to 1.5 mg I.M. or S.C. q 4 to 6 hours, p.r.n.; or 0.5 mg I.V. q 4 to 6 hours, p.r.n.; or 5 mg P.R. q 4 to 6 hours, p.r.n.

ADVERSE REACTIONS
CNS: *sedation, somnolence, clouded sensorium, euphoria,* dizziness, *seizures* (with large doses).
CV: *hypotension,* bradycardia.
GI: *nausea, vomiting, constipation,* ileus.
GU: *urine retention.*
Respiratory: *respiratory depression.*
Other: physical dependence.

INTERACTIONS
CNS depressants, ethanol, general anesthetics, MAO inhibitors, tricyclic antidepressants: additive effects. Use together with extreme caution.

CONTRAINDICATIONS
Contraindicated in patients with hypersensitivity to this drug.

NURSING CONSIDERATIONS
• Use with extreme caution in patients with head injury, increased intracranial pressure, seizures, asthma, COPD, acute abdominal conditions, prostatic hyperplasia, severe hepatic or renal disease, urethral stricture, respiratory depression, hypothyroidism, Addison's disease, and arrhythmias. Also use with extreme caution in elderly or debilitated patients.

• Keep narcotic antagonist (naloxone) and resuscitation equipment available.

• Know that drug is not intended for

---

*Liquid form contains alcohol.
**May contain tartrazine.
Common reactions are in italics; *life-threatening*, in bold italics.

mild to moderate pain. May worsen gallbladder pain.
• For better analgesic effect, administer drug before patient has intense pain.
• **I.V. use:** Give by direct I.V. injection. If necessary, drug may be diluted in 0.9% sodium chloride.
• Monitor cardiovascular and respiratory status. Withhold dose and notify doctor if respirations decrease or rate is below 12 breaths/minute.
• Monitor patient's bladder and bowel function. Patient may need laxative.
• When drug is used postoperatively, encourage patient turning, coughing, and deep breathing and use of incentive spirometer to avoid atelectasis.
• Caution ambulatory patients about getting out of bed or walking. Warn outpatients to avoid driving and other potentially hazardous activities that require mental alertness until drug's CNS effects are known.

pentazocine hydrochloride
Fortral†‡, Talwin†

pentazocine hydrochloride and naloxone hydrochloride
Talwin Nx
Controlled Substance Schedule IV

pentazocine lactate
Fortral‡, Talwin
Controlled Substance Schedule IV

Pregnancy Risk Category: NR

HOW SUPPLIED
pentazocine hydrochloride
Tablets: 25 mg‡, 50 mg†‡
pentazocine hydrochloride and naloxone hydrochloride
Tablets: 50 mg pentazocine hydrochloride and 500 mcg naloxone hydrochloride
pentazocine lactate
Injection: 30 mg/ml

ACTION
Binds with opiate receptors at many sites in the CNS, altering both perception of and emotional response to pain through an unknown mechanism.

ONSET, PEAK, DURATION
Onset occurs within 2 to 3 minutes after I.V. use, 15 to 20 minutes after I.M. or S.C. use, 15 to 30 minutes after oral use. Peak effects occur within 15 to 30 minutes after I.V. use, 30 to 60 minutes after I.M. or S.C. use, 60 to 90 minutes after oral use. Effects persist 2 to 3 hours after parenteral use, 2 to 3 hours after oral use.

INDICATIONS & DOSAGE
Moderate to severe pain –
Adults: 50 to 100 mg P.O. q 3 to 4 hours, p.r.n. Maximum oral dosage is 600 mg/day. Alternatively, 30 mg I.M., I.V., or S.C. q 3 to 4 hours, p.r.n. Maximum parenteral dosage is 360 mg/day. Single doses above 30 mg I.V. or 60 mg I.M. or S.C. are not recommended.
Labor –
Adults: 30 mg I.M. or 20 mg I.V. q 2 to 3 hours when contractions become regular.

ADVERSE REACTIONS
CNS: *sedation,* visual disturbances, hallucinations, drowsiness, *dizziness, light-headedness,* confusion, *euphoria,* headache, psychotomimetic effects.
CV: hypotension.
EENT: dry mouth, dysgeusia.
GI: *nausea, vomiting,* constipation.
GU: urine retention.
Respiratory: *respiratory depression.*
Skin: induration, nodules, sloughing, and sclerosis of injection site.
Other: hypersensitivity reactions *(anaphylaxis)*, physical and psychological dependence.

INTERACTIONS
CNS depressants, ethanol: additive effects. Use together cautiously.
Narcotic analgesics: possible decreased analgesic effect. Avoid concomitant use.

CONTRAINDICATIONS
Contraindicated in patients with hypersensitivity to the drug, or any product component. Not recommended for children under 12 years.

NURSING CONSIDERATIONS
• Use cautiously in patients with hepatic or renal disease, acute MI, head injury, increased intracranial pressure, and respiratory depression.
• Have naloxone readily available. Respiratory depression can be reversed with naloxone.
• **I.V. use:** Give by direct I.V. injection. Administer slowly. Do not mix in same syringe with aminophylline, barbiturates, or other alkaline substances.
• When giving by S.C. or I.M. injection, rotate injection sites to minimize tissue irritation. If possible, avoid giving by S.C.route.
• Know that drug possesses narcotic antagonist properties. May precipitate withdrawal syndrome in narcotic-dependent patients.
• Be aware that psychological and physical dependence may occur with prolonged use.
• Know that Talwin Nx, the oral pentazocine available in the U.S., contains the narcotic antagonist naloxone. This prevents illicit I.V. use.
• Know that pentazocine may interfere with certain laboratory tests for urinary 17-hydroxycorticosteroids.
• Caution ambulatory patients about getting out of bed or walking. Warn outpatients to avoid driving and other potentially hazardous activities that require mental alertness until drug's CNS effects are known.

propoxyphene hydrochloride (dextropropoxyphene hydrochloride)
Darvon, Dolene, Novopropoxyn†, 642†

propoxyphene napsylate (dextropropoxyphene napsylate)
Darvon-N, Doloxene‡, Doloxene Co‡
Controlled Substance Schedule IV

Pregnancy Risk Category: C

HOW SUPPLIED
propoxyphene hydrochloride
Capsules: 32 mg, 65 mg
propoxyphene napsylate
Tablets: 100 mg
Oral suspension: 10 mg/ml

ACTION
Binds with opiate receptors in the CNS, altering both perception of and emotional response to pain through an unknown mechanism.

ONSET, PEAK, DURATION
Onset occurs within 15 to 60 minutes. Plasma levels peak in 2 to 2½ hours. Effects persist 4 to 6 hours.

INDICATIONS & DOSAGE
Mild to moderate pain—
Adults: 65 mg (hydrochloride) P.O. q 4 hours p.r.n. Maximum dosage is 390 mg/day.
Mild to moderate pain—
Adults: 100 mg (napsylate) P.O. q 4 hours p.r.n. Maximum dosage is 600 mg/day.

ADVERSE REACTIONS
CNS: *dizziness,* headache, *sedation,* euphoria, paradoxical excitement, insomnia.
GI: *nausea, vomiting,* constipation.
Respiratory: *respiratory depression.*

Other: psychological and physical dependence.

INTERACTIONS
Carbamazepine: may increase carbamazepine levels. Monitor closely.
CNS depressants, ethanol: additive effects. Use together cautiously.
Warfarin: increased anticoagulant effect. Monitor PT.

CONTRAINDICATIONS
Contraindicated in patients with hypersensitivity to this drug.

NURSING CONSIDERATIONS
• Use cautiously in patients with hepatic or renal disease, emotional instability, or history of drug or alcohol abuse.
• Remember that 65 mg of propoxyphene hydrochloride equals 100 mg of propoxyphene napsylate.
• Know that drug can be considered a mild narcotic analgesic, but pain relief is equivalent to that provided by aspirin. Tolerance and physical dependence have been observed. Typically used with aspirin or acetaminophen to maximize analgesia.
• Be aware that drug may cause false decreases in urinary steroid excretion tests.
• To minimize GI upset, advise patient to take drug with food or milk.
• Warn patient not to exceed recommended dosage. Respiratory depression, hypotension, profound sedation, and coma may result if used in excessive doses or with other CNS depressants. Studies have shown that propoxyphene-containing products alone or in combination with other drugs are a major cause of drug-related overdose and death.
• Advise patient to limit alcohol intake when taking this drug.
• Caution ambulatory patients about getting out of bed or walking. Warn outpatients to avoid driving and other hazardous activities that require mental alertness until drug's CNS effects are known.

sufentanil citrate
Sufenta
Controlled Substance Schedule II
Pregnancy Risk Category: C

HOW SUPPLIED
Injection: 50 mcg/ml

ACTION
Binds with opiate receptors in the CNS, altering both perception of and emotional response to pain through an unknown mechanism.

ONSET, PEAK, DURATION
Onset and peak occur within 1 minute for analgesic effects. Time to loss of consciousness dependent on rate of administration, generally within 1 to 2 minutes. Analgesic effects persist for 5 minutes. Time to awakening is 0.7 to 2.9 hours following average dose.

INDICATIONS & DOSAGE
Adjunct to general anesthetic –
Adults: 1 to 8 mcg/kg I.V. administered with nitrous oxide and oxygen.
As a primary anesthetic –
Adults: 8 to 30 mcg/kg I.V. administered with 100% oxygen and a muscle relaxant.

ADVERSE REACTIONS
CNS: chills, *seizures.*
CV: *hypotension,* hypertension, *bradycardia,* tachycardia.
GI: nausea, vomiting.
Respiratory: *chest wall rigidity, respiratory depression.*
Skin: itching.
Other: intraoperative muscle movement.

INTERACTIONS
CNS depressants, ethanol: additive effects. Use together cautiously.

CONTRAINDICATIONS
Contraindicated in patients with hypersensitivity to this drug.

NURSING CONSIDERATIONS
• Use with extreme caution in patients with head injury; in those with pulmonary, hepatic, or renal disease; in those with decreased respiratory reserve; and in elderly or debilitated patients.
• Should be administered only by persons specifically trained in the use of I.V. anesthetics.
• Be aware that reduced dosage is required for elderly and debilitated patients.
• For obese patients who exceed 20% of their ideal body weight, dosage calculations should be based upon an estimate of ideal weight.
• When used at doses over 8 mcg/kg, postoperative mechanical ventilation and observation are essential because of prolonged respiratory depression.
• Keep narcotic antagonist (naloxone) and resuscitation equipment available.
• **I.V. use:** Give by direct I.V. injection. Although the drug has been given by intermittent I.V. infusion, drug compatibility and stability in I.V. solutions have not been fully investigated.
• Because drug decreases both rate and depth of respirations, monitoring of arterial oxygen saturation may aid in assessing respiratory depression. Notify the doctor if respirations decrease or rate falls below 12 breaths/minute.
• Monitor respirations of neonates exposed to the drug during labor.
• Know that high doses can produce muscle rigidity reversible by neuromuscular blockers; however, patient must be artificially ventilated.
• Monitor postoperative vital signs frequently, including circulatory and respiratory status and urinary function. Drug may cause respiratory depression, hypotension, urine retention, nausea, vomiting, ileus, or altered level of consciousness. Encourage turning, coughing, and deep breathing to prevent atelectasis.

---

tramadol hydrochloride
Ultram

Pregnancy Risk Category: C

HOW SUPPLIED
Tablets: 50 mg

ACTION
Unknown. A centrally acting synthetic analgesic compound not chemically related to opiates that is thought to bind to opioid receptors and inhibit reuptake of norepinephrine and serotonin.

ONSET, PEAK, DURATION
Onset and duration unknown. Serum levels peak in about 2 hours.

INDICATIONS & DOSAGE
Moderate to moderately severe pain –
Adults: 50 to 100 mg P.O. q 4 to 6 hours, p.r.n. Maximum dosage is 400 mg daily.

ADVERSE REACTIONS
CNS: *dizziness, vertigo, headache, somnolence,* CNS stimulation, asthenia, anxiety, confusion, coordination disturbance, euphoria, nervousness, sleep disorder.
CV: vasodilation.
EENT: visual disturbances.
GI: *nausea, constipation, vomiting,* dyspepsia, dry mouth, diarrhea, abdominal pain, anorexia, flatulence.
GU: urine retention, urinary frequency, menopausal symptoms.
Skin: pruritus, sweating, rash.
Other: malaise, hypertonia.

INTERACTIONS
Carbamazepine: increased tramadol metabolism. Patients receiving chronic carbamazepine therapy at a

---

*Liquid form contains alcohol. *Common* reactions are in italics; ***life-threatening,*** in bold italics.
**May contain tartrazine.

dosage of up to 800 mg daily may require up to twice the recommended dose of tramadol.

CNS depressants: additive effects. Use together with caution. Dosage of tramadol may need to be reduced.

MAO inhibitors, neuroleptics: increased risk of seizures. Monitor closely.

CONTRAINDICATIONS
Contraindicated in patients with hypersensitivity to drug or with acute intoxication from alcohol, hypnotics, centrally acting analgesics, opioids, or psychotropic drugs.

NURSING CONSIDERATIONS
• Use cautiously in patients at risk for seizures or respiratory depression; in patients with increased intracranial pressure or head injury, acute abdominal conditions, or renal or hepatic impairment; and in patients physically dependent on opioids.
• Monitor CV and respiratory status. Withhold dose and notify doctor if respirations decrease or rate is below 12 breaths/minute.
• Monitor bowel and bladder function. Because constipation is a common adverse effect, anticipate the need for laxative therapy.
• For better analgesic effect, drug should be given before onset of intense pain.
• Closely monitor patients at risk for seizures. Drug has been reported to reduce seizure threshold.
• Monitor patient for drug dependence. Tramadol can produce dependence similar to that of codeine or dextropropoxyphene and thus has the potential to be abused.
• Instruct patient to take drug only as prescribed and not to increase dosage or dosage interval unless instructed by doctor.
• Caution ambulatory patients to be careful when getting out of bed and walking. Warn outpatients to avoid driving and other potentially hazardous activities that require mental alertness until drug's CNS effects are known.
• Advise patient to check with doctor before taking OTC medications; drug interactions can occur.

amobarbital
amobarbital sodium
aprobarbital
butabarbital sodium
chloral hydrate
estazolam
ethchlorvynol
flurazepam hydrochloride
pentobarbital
pentobarbital sodium
phenobarbital sodium
  (See Chapter 30, ANTICONVULSANTS.)
quazepam
secobarbital sodium
temazepam
triazolam
zolpidem tartrate

COMBINATION PRODUCTS
TRI-BARBS CAPSULES: phenobarbital
32 mg, butabarbital sodium 32 mg,
and secobarbital sodium 32 mg.
TUINAL 50 MG PULVULES: amobarbital sodium 25 mg and secobarbital
sodium 25 mg.
TUINAL 100 MG PULVULES: amobarbital sodium 50 mg and secobarbital
sodium 50 mg.
TUINAL 200 MG PULVULES: amobarbital sodium 100 mg and secobarbital
sodium 100 mg.

---

amobarbital
Amytal

amobarbital sodium
Amytal Sodium

Controlled Substance Schedule II
Pregnancy Risk Category: D

HOW SUPPLIED
amobarbital
Tablets: 30 mg
amobarbital sodium
Capsules: 200 mg

Powder for injection: 250 mg, 500 mg

ACTION
Unknown. A barbiturate that probably
interferes with transmission of impulses from the thalamus to the cortex
of the brain.

ONSET, PEAK, DURATION
Onset occurs in 60 minutes. Peak unknown. Effects persist 10 to 12 hours.

INDICATIONS & DOSAGE
Sedation –
Adults: usually 30 to 50 mg P.O.
b.i.d. or t.i.d.
Children: 2 mg/kg or 70 mg/m^2 P.O.
daily in four equally divided doses.
Insomnia –
Adults: 65 to 200 mg P.O. or deep
I.M. h.s. I.M. dose not to exceed 500
mg; I.M. injection not to exceed 5 ml
in any one site.
Children: 2 to 3 mg/kg I.M. h.s.
Preanesthetic sedation –
Adults: 200 mg P.O. or I.M. 1 to 2
hours before surgery.
Labor –
Adults: 200 to 400 mg P.O. followed
by 200 to 400 mg at 1 to 3 hour inter-
vals up to a maximum dose of 1 g.
*Manic reactions, as an adjunct in psy-
chotherapy, anticonvulsant –*
Adults and children over 6 years: 65
to 500 mg slow I.V.; not to exceed 100
mg/minute. Maximum dosage is 1 g.

ADVERSE REACTIONS
CV: bradycardia, hypotension, syn-
cope.
CNS: *drowsiness, lethargy, hangover,*
paradoxical excitement.
GI: nausea, vomiting.
Hematologic: exacerbation of por-
phyria.
Respiratory: respiratory depression.

---

*Liquid form contains alcohol.
**May contain tartrazine.

Common reactions are in italics; ***life-threatening,*** in bold italics.

Skin: rash; urticaria; *Stevens-Johnson syndrome;* pain, irritation, sterile abscess at injection site.
Other: angioedema.

INTERACTIONS

Chloramphenicol, MAO inhibitors, valproic acid: inhibit metabolism of barbiturates; may cause prolonged CNS depression. Reduce barbiturate dosage.
Corticosteroids, digitoxin, doxycycline, estrogens and oral contraceptives, oral anticoagulants, tricyclic antidepressants: amobarbital may enhance the metabolism of these drugs. Monitor for decreased effect.
Ethanol or other CNS depressants, including narcotic analgesics: excessive CNS and respiratory depression. Use together cautiously.
Griseofulvin: decreased absorption of griseofulvin.
Rifampin: may decrease barbiturate levels. Monitor for decreased effect.

CONTRAINDICATIONS

Contraindicated in patients with bronchopneumonia or other severe pulmonary insufficiency or hypersensitivity to barbiturates, or porphyria.

NURSING CONSIDERATIONS

• Use cautiously in patients with acute or chronic pain, suicidal tendencies, depression, history of drug abuse, or hepatic or renal impairment. Use parenteral form cautiously in patients with blood pressure alterations or pulmonary or cardiovascular disease.
• Elderly patients are more sensitive to the drug's adverse CNS effects. Assess mental status before and after initiating therapy.
• To minimize deterioration, use injection solution within 30 minutes after opening container. Don't use cloudy or precipitated solution. Don't shake solution; mix with sterile water only.

• **I.V. use:** Know that I.V. injection is reserved for emergency treatment. Close supervision required. Administer slowly intravenously; do not exceed 100 mg/minute.
• I.V. administration of barbiturates may cause severe respiratory depression, laryngospasm, or hypotension. Have emergency resuscitation equipment available.
• Assess patency of I.V. site before and during administration. Local tissue reactions and injection site pain have been noted with I.V. use.
• Administer I.M. injection deeply. Superficial injection may cause pain, sterile abscess, and sloughing.
• Take precautions to prevent hoarding or self-overdosing by patients who are depressed, suicidal, or drug-dependent or who have a history of drug abuse.
• Be aware long-term use not recommended; drug loses its efficacy in promoting sleep after 14 days of continued use.
• Monitor patient for skin changes. Skin eruptions may precede potentially fatal reactions to barbiturate therapy. Discontinue drug when skin reactions occur and notify doctor. In some patients, high fever, stomatitis, headache, or rhinitis may precede skin reactions.
• Watch for signs of barbiturate toxicity: coma, pupillary constriction, cyanosis, clammy skin, and hypotension. Overdose can be fatal.
• Inform patient that morning "hangover" common after hypnotic dose, which also suppresses REM sleep. Patients may experience increased dreaming after drug is discontinued.
• Caution patients about performing activities that require mental alertness or physical coordination. For inpatients, supervise walking and raise bed rails, particularly for elderly patients.
• Tell patients using oral contraceptives that they should consider alter-

---

nate birth control methods because drug may enhance contraceptive hormone metabolism and decrease its effect.

aprobarbital
Alurate*
Controlled Substance Schedule III
Pregnancy Risk Category: D

HOW SUPPLIED
Elixir: 40 mg/5 ml

ACTION
Unknown. A barbiturate that probably interferes with transmission of impulses from the thalamus to the cortex of the brain.

ONSET, PEAK, DURATION
Onset occurs within 45 to 60 minutes. Peak levels occur within 3 hours. Effects persist 6 to 8 hours.

INDICATIONS & DOSAGE
Sedation –
Adults: 40 mg P.O. t.i.d.
Insomnia –
Adults: 40 to 160 mg P.O. h.s.

ADVERSE REACTIONS
CNS: *drowsiness, lethargy, hangover,* paradoxical excitement in elderly patients.
GI: nausea, vomiting.
Hematologic: exacerbation of porphyria.
Respiratory: *respiratory depression.*
Skin: rash, urticaria, *Stevens-Johnson syndrome.*
Other: *angioedema.*

INTERACTIONS
Chloramphenicol, MAO inhibitors, valproic acid: inhibit metabolism of barbiturates; may cause prolonged CNS depression. Reduce barbiturate dosage.
Corticosteroids, digitoxin, doxycycline, estrogens and oral contracep- *tives, oral anticoagulants, tricyclic antidepressants:* aprobarbital may enhance the metabolism of these drugs. Monitor for decreased effectiveness.
Ethanol or other CNS depressants, including narcotic analgesics: excessive CNS and respiratory depression. Use together cautiously.
Griseofulvin: decreased absorption of griseofulvin.
Rifampin: may decrease barbiturate levels. Monitor for decreased effect.

CONTRAINDICATIONS
Contraindicated in patients with hypersensitivity to barbiturates, bronchopneumonia or other severe pulmonary insufficiency, or porphyria.

NURSING CONSIDERATIONS
• Use cautiously in patients with acute or chronic pain, suicidal tendencies, depression, history of drug abuse, or hepatic or renal impairment.
• Take precautions to prevent hoarding or self-overdosing by patients who are depressed, suicidal, or drug-dependent or who have a history of drug abuse.
• Be aware that long-term use is not recommended; drug loses its efficacy in promoting sleep after 14 days of continued use.
• Watch for signs of barbiturate toxicity: coma, pupillary constriction, cyanosis, clammy skin, and hypotension. Overdose can be fatal.
• Assess patient's skin. Skin eruptions may precede potentially fatal reactions to barbiturate therapy. Discontinue drug when skin reactions occur. In some patients, high fever, stomatitis, headache, or rhinitis may precede skin reactions.
• Inform patient that morning "hangover" common after hypnotic dose, which also suppresses REM sleep. Patients may experience increased dreaming after drug is discontinued.
• Caution patients about performing

---

*Liquid form contains alcohol.   *Common* reactions are in italics; *life-threatening,* in bold italics.
**May contain tartrazine.

activities that require mental alertness or physical coordination. For inpatients, supervise walking and raise bed rails, particularly for elderly patients.
• Tell patients using oral contraceptives that she should consider alternate birth control methods because drug may enhance contraceptive hormone metabolism and decrease its effect.

---

butabarbital sodium (butabarbitone sodium)
Butalan*, Butisol* **, Saneryl‡, Sarisol #2* **
Controlled Substance Schedule III

Pregnancy Risk Category: D

HOW SUPPLIED
Tablets: 15 mg, 30 mg, 50 mg, 100 mg
Elixir: 30 mg/5 ml, 33.3 mg/5 ml

ACTION
Unknown. A barbiturate that probably interferes with transmission of impulses from the thalamus to the cortex of the brain.

ONSET, PEAK, DURATION
Onset occurs in 45 to 60 minutes. Peak levels occur within 3 hours. Effects persist 6 to 8 hours.

INDICATIONS & DOSAGE
Sedation –
Adults: 15 to 30 mg P.O. t.i.d. or q.i.d.
Children: 6 mg/kg or 180 mg/m² P.O. divided t.i.d. Dosage range is 7.5 to 30 mg P.O. t.i.d.
Preoperatively –
Adults: 50 to 100 mg P.O. 60 to 90 minutes before surgery.
Children: 2 to 6 mg/kg P.O. (not to exceed 100 mg) 60 to 90 minutes before surgery.
Insomnia –
Adults: 50 to 100 mg P.O. h.s.

ADVERSE REACTIONS
CNS: *drowsiness, lethargy, hangover,* paradoxical excitement in elderly patients.
GI: nausea, vomiting.
Hematologic: exacerbation of porphyria.
Respiratory: *respiratory depression.*
Skin: rash, urticaria, *Stevens-Johnson syndrome.*
Other: *angioedema.*

INTERACTIONS
Chloramphenicol, MAO inhibitors, valproic acid: inhibited metabolism of barbiturates; may cause prolonged CNS depression. Reduce barbiturate dosage.
Corticosteroids, digitoxin, doxycycline, estrogens and oral contraceptives, oral anticoagulants, tricyclic antidepressants: barbiturates may enhance the metabolism of these drugs. Monitor for decreased effectiveness.
Ethanol or other CNS depressants, including narcotic analgesics: excessive CNS and respiratory depression. Use together cautiously.
Griseofulvin: decreased absorption of griseofulvin.
Rifampin: may decrease barbiturate levels. Monitor for decreased effect.

CONTRAINDICATIONS
Contraindicated in patients with bronchopneumonia, or other severe pulmonary insufficiency, hypersensitivity to barbiturates, or porphyria.

NURSING CONSIDERATIONS
• Use cautiously in patients with acute or chronic pain, depression, suicidal tendencies, history of drug abuse, or hepatic or renal impairment.
• Elderly patients are more sensitive to drug's adverse CNS reactions. Assess mental status before and after initiating therapy.
• Take precautions to prevent hoarding or self-overdosing by patients who

---

are depressed, suicidal, or drug-dependent or who have a history of drug abuse.

• Watch for signs of barbiturate toxicity: coma, pupillary constriction, cyanosis, clammy skin, and hypotension. Overdose can be fatal.

• Discontinue drug when skin reactions occur because skin eruptions may precede potentially fatal reactions to barbiturate therapy. In some patients, high fever, stomatitis, headache, or rhinitis may precede skin reactions.

• Long-term use is not recommended; drug loses its efficacy in promoting sleep after 14 days. A drug-free interval of at least 1 week is advised if continued treatment is appropriate. Long-term high dosage may cause drug dependence, and patients may experience withdrawal symptoms if drug is suddenly stopped. Withdraw barbiturates gradually.

• Inform patient morning "hangover" common after hypnotic dose. Hypnotic doses suppress REM sleep. Patients may experience increased dreaming after drug is discontinued.

• Caution patients about performing activities that require mental alertness or physical coordination. For inpatients, supervise walking and raise bed rails, particularly for elderly patients.

• Tell patients using oral contraceptives that she should consider alternate birth control methods because drug may enhance contraceptive hormone metabolism and decrease its effect.

---

chloral hydrate
Aquachloral Supprettes, Dormel‡, Noctec, Novo-Chlorhydrate†
Controlled Substance Schedule IV

Pregnancy Risk Category: C

HOW SUPPLIED
Capsules: 250 mg, 500 mg
Syrup: 250 mg/5 ml, 500 mg/5 ml
Suppositories: 324 mg, 500 mg, 648 mg

ACTION
Unknown. Sedative effects may be caused by its primary metabolite, trichloroethanol.

ONSET, PEAK, DURATION
Onset occurs within 30 minutes. Peak unknown. Effects persist 4 to 8 hours.

INDICATIONS & DOSAGE
Sedation –
Adults: 250 mg P.O. or P.R. t.i.d. after meals.
Children: 8.3 mg/kg or 250 mg/m^2 P.O. or P.R. t.i.d. Maximum daily dosage is 500 mg t.i.d.
Insomnia –
Adults: 500 mg to 1 g P.O. or P.R. 15 to 30 minutes before bedtime.
Children: 50 mg/kg or 1.5 g/m^2 P.O. or P.R. 15 to 30 minutes before bedtime. Maximum single dose is 1 g.
Preoperatively –
Adults: 500 mg to 1 g P.O. or P.R. 30 minutes before surgery.
Premedication for EEG –
Children: 20 to 25 mg/kg P.O. or P.R.
Management of alcohol withdrawal symptoms –
Adults: 500 mg to 1 g P.O. or P.R. q 6 hours p.r.n., not to exceed 2 g daily.

ADVERSE REACTIONS
CNS: hangover, drowsiness, nightmares, dizziness, ataxia, paradoxical excitement.
GI: *nausea, vomiting, diarrhea,* flatulence.
Hematologic: eosinophilia, leukopenia.
Skin: hypersensitivity reactions.

---

*Liquid form contains alcohol.
**May contain tartrazine.
Common reactions are in italics; **life-threatening,** in bold italics.

INTERACTIONS

Alkaline solutions: incompatible with aqueous solutions of chloral hydrate. Don't mix together.

Ethanol or other CNS depressants, including narcotic analgesics: excessive CNS depression or vasodilation reaction. Use together cautiously.

Furosemide I.V.: sweating, flushes, variable blood pressure, and uneasiness. Use together cautiously or use a different hypnotic drug.

Oral anticoagulants: increased risk of bleeding. Monitor patient closely.

Phenytoin: decreased phenytoin levels. Monitor closely.

CONTRAINDICATIONS

Contraindicated in patients with hepatic or renal impairment and in those with hypersensitivity to chloral hydrate. Oral administration contraindicated in patients with gastric disorders.

NURSING CONSIDERATIONS

• Use with extreme caution in patients with severe cardiac disease. Use cautiously in patients with mental depression, suicidal tendencies, or history of drug abuse.

• Note two strengths of oral liquid form. Double-check dose, especially when administering to children. Fatal overdoses have occurred.

• To minimize unpleasant taste and stomach irritation, dilute or administer with liquid. Drug should be taken after meals.

• Take precautions to prevent hoarding or self-overdosing by patients who are depressed, suicidal, or drug-dependent or who have a history of drug abuse.

• Be aware that long-term use is not recommended; drug loses its efficacy in promoting sleep after 14 days of continued use. Long-term use may cause drug dependence, and patient may experience withdrawal symptoms if drug is suddenly stopped.

• Monitor BUN levels as ordered. Large dosage may raise BUN levels.

• May interfere with fluorometric tests for urine catecholamines and Reddy-Jenkins-Thorn test for urine 17-hydroxycorticosteroids. Do not administer drug for 48 hours before fluorometric test as ordered. May also cause false-positive tests for urine glucose when using copper sulfate tests. Use glucose enzymatic tests instead.

• Caution patients about performing activities that require mental alertness or physical coordination. For inpatients, supervise walking and raise bed rails, particularly for elderly patients.

• Tell patient to store in dark container; store suppositories in refrigerator.

---

estazolam

ProSom

Controlled Substance Schedule IV

Pregnancy Risk Category: X

HOW SUPPLIED

Tablets: 1 mg, 2 mg

ACTION

Unknown. Thought to act on the limbic system and thalamus of the CNS by binding to specific benzodiazepine receptors.

ONSET, PEAK, DURATION

Onset and duration unknown. Serum levels peak in 1 to 3 hours.

INDICATIONS & DOSAGE

Insomnia –

Adults: 1 mg P.O. h.s. Some patients may require 2 mg.

Elderly patients: 1 mg P.O. h.s. Use higher doses with extreme care. Frail elderly or debilitated patients may take 0.5 mg, but this low dose may be only marginally effective.

ADVERSE REACTIONS
CNS: fatigue, dizziness, *daytime drowsiness, somnolence, asthenia, hypokinesia,* headache.
GI: dyspepsia.

INTERACTIONS
Cigarette smoking, rifampin: may increase metabolism and clearance and decrease plasma half-life. Monitor for decreased effectiveness.
Cimetidine, disulfiram, isoniazid, oral contraceptives: may impair the metabolism and clearance of benzodiazepines and prolong their plasma half-life. Monitor for increased CNS depression.
CNS depressants, including antihistamines, opiate analgesics, and other benzodiazepines; ethanol: increased CNS depression. Avoid concomitant use.
Theophylline: pharmacologic antagonism. Monitor for decreased effectiveness.

CONTRAINDICATIONS
Contraindicated in pregnant patients or patients with hypersensitivity to drug.

NURSING CONSIDERATIONS
• Use cautiously in patients with hepatic, renal, or pulmonary disease; depression, or suicidal tendencies.
• Liver and renal function and CBC should be checked before and periodically during long-term therapy as ordered.
• Take precautions to prevent hoarding by depressed, suicidal, or drug-dependent patients or those who have a history of drug abuse.
• Be aware that patients who receive prolonged treatment with benzodiazepines may experience withdrawal symptoms if the drug is suddenly discontinued (possibly after 6 weeks of continuous therapy).
• Tell patients not to increase dosage of the drug but to inform the doctor if

they feel that the drug is no longer effective.
• Caution patients about performing activities that require mental alertness or physical coordination. For inpatients, supervise walking and raise bed rails, particularly for elderly patients.
• Warn patients that additive depressant effects can occur if alcohol is consumed while taking this drug or within 24 hours after taking drug.
• Tell patient using oral contraceptives that she should consider alternate birth control methods when taking this drug because drug may enhance contraceptive hormone metabolism and decrease its effect.

---

ethchlorvynol
Placidyl**
Controlled Substance Schedule IV
Pregnancy Risk Category: C

HOW SUPPLIED
Capsules: 200 mg, 500 mg, 750 mg**

ACTION
Unknown; pharmacologic effects are similar to those produced by barbiturates.

ONSET, PEAK, DURATION
Onset occurs within 30 minutes to 1 hour. Plasma levels peak within 1 to 2 hours. Effects persist about 5 hours.

INDICATIONS & DOSAGE
Insomnia –
Adults: 500 mg to 1 g P.O. h.s. An additional 200 mg dose P.O. if awakened in early morning.

ADVERSE REACTIONS
CNS: facial numbness, drowsiness, fatigue, nightmares, dizziness, residual sedation, hangover, muscular weakness, syncope, ataxia.
CV: hypotension.

EENT: unpleasant aftertaste, blurred vision.
GI: distress, nausea, vomiting.
Hematologic: thrombocytopenia, exacerbation of porphyria.
Skin: rashes, urticaria.

INTERACTIONS
Ethanol or other CNS depressants, including MAO inhibitors, narcotic analgesics, and tricyclic antidepressants: excessive CNS depression. Use together cautiously.
Oral anticoagulants: ethchlorvynol may enhance the metabolism of coumarin derivatives, decreasing their effectiveness. Monitor closely.

CONTRAINDICATIONS
Contraindicated in patients with hypersensitivity to this drug and in those with porphyria.

NURSING CONSIDERATIONS
• Use cautiously in patients with hepatic or renal impairment, in elderly or debilitated patients, mental depression, and in those with suicidal tendencies.
• Minimize transient dizziness or ataxia, which is caused by rapid absorption, by giving this drug with milk or food.
• Take precautions to prevent hoarding or self-overdosing by patients who are depressed, suicidal, or drug-dependent or who have a history of drug abuse. Overdose is difficult to treat and is associated with high mortality.
• Monitor patient for allergic reactions. The 750-mg strength contains tartrazine dye, which may cause allergic reactions in susceptible patients.
• Watch for signs of toxicity, such as poor muscle coordination, confusion, hypothermia, speech or vision disturbances, tremor, and weakness.
• Be aware that drug is effective for short-term use only; treatment period should not exceed 1 week.

• Know that slight darkening of liquid from exposure to air and light doesn't affect safety or potency, but store in tight, light-resistant container to avoid possible deterioration.
• Caution patients about performing activities that require mental alertness or physical coordination. For inpatients, supervise walking and raise bed rails, particularly for elderly patients.

flurazepam hydrochloride
Apo-Flurazepam†, Dalmane, Novoflupam†
Controlled Substance Schedule IV
Pregnancy Risk Category: NR

HOW SUPPLIED
Capsules: 15 mg, 30 mg

ACTION
Unknown. A benzodiazepine that is thought to act on the limbic system, thalamus, and hypothalamus of the CNS to produce hypnotic effects.

ONSET, PEAK, DURATION
Onset and duration unknown. Peak effects occur in ½ to 1 hour.

INDICATIONS & DOSAGE
Insomnia –
Adults: 15 to 30 mg P.O. h.s. Dose repeated once as needed.

ADVERSE REACTIONS
CNS: *daytime sedation, dizziness, drowsiness, disturbed coordination,* lethargy, confusion, *headache.*
GI: nausea, vomiting, heartburn.
Hepatic: elevated liver enzymes.
Other: physical or psychological dependence.

INTERACTIONS
Cigarette smoking, rifampin: enhanced metabolism of benzodiazepines. Monitor for decreased effectiveness.

Cimetidine: increased sedation. Monitor carefully.

Disulfiram, isoniazid, oral contraceptives: decreased metabolism of benzodiazepines, leading to toxicity. Monitor closely.

Ethanol or other CNS depressants, including narcotic analgesics: excessive CNS depression. Use together cautiously.

Phenytoin: increased phenytoin levels. Monitor for toxicity.

CONTRAINDICATIONS
Contraindicated in patients with hypersensitivity to the drug and during pregnancy.

NURSING CONSIDERATIONS
• Use cautiously in patients with impaired hepatic or renal function, chronic pulmonary insufficiency, mental depression, suicidal tendencies, or history of drug abuse.

• Check hepatic and renal function and CBC before and periodically during long-term therapy. May cause elevations in certain liver function tests (AST, ALT, total and direct bilirubin, and alkaline phosphatase).

• Assess mental status before initiating therapy. Elderly patients are more sensitive to the drug's adverse CNS reactions.

• Take precautions to prevent hoarding or self-overdosing by patients who are depressed, suicidal, or drug-dependent or who have a history of drug abuse.

• Be aware physical and psychological dependence is possible with long-term use.

• Advise patients that this drug is more effective on second, third, and fourth nights of use because active metabolite accumulates. Encourage them to continue drug, even if it doesn't relieve insomnia the first night.

• Caution patients about performing activities that require mental alertness or physical coordination. For inpatients, supervise walking and raise bed rails, particularly for elderly patients.

---

pentobarbital (pentobarbitone)
Nembutal* **

pentobarbital sodium
Carbrital‡, Nembutal Sodium*, Nova Rectal†, Novopentobarb†
Controlled Substance Schedule II

Pregnancy Risk Category: D

HOW SUPPLIED
pentobarbital
Elixir: 18.2 mg/5 ml
pentobarbital sodium
Capsules: 50 mg, 100 mg
Injection: 50 mg/ml
Suppositories: 30 mg, 60 mg, 120 mg, 200 mg

ACTION
Unknown. Probably interferes with transmission of impulses from the thalamus to the cortex of the brain. A barbiturate.

ONSET, PEAK, DURATION
Onset occurs immediately after I.V. administration, within 10 to 25 minutes after I.M. administration, within 15 minutes after oral or rectal administration. Serum levels peak immediately after I.V. administration, 30 to 60 minutes with oral dose, unknown for I.M. or rectal routes. Effects persist 1 to 4 hours following oral or rectal administration, 15 minutes following I.V. administration, unknown for I.M. administration.

INDICATIONS & DOSAGE
Sedation –
Adults: 20 to 40 mg P.O. b.i.d., t.i.d., or q.i.d.
Children: 2 to 6 mg/kg daily P.O. in

---

*Liquid form contains alcohol.   *Common* reactions are in italics; *life-threatening,* in bold italics.
**May contain tartrazine.

3 divided doses. Maximum daily dosage is 100 mg.
Insomnia –
Adults: 100 mg P.O. h.s. or 150 to 200 mg deep I.M.; 100 mg initially I.V., then additional doses up to 500 mg; 120 or 200 mg rectally.
Children: 2 to 6 mg/kg I.M. Maximum dosage is 100 mg. Rectal doses are: 2 months to 1 year, 30 mg; 1 to 4 years, 30 or 60 mg; 5 to 11 years, 60 mg; 12 to 14 years, 60 or 120 mg.
Preoperative sedation –
Adults: 150 to 200 mg I.M.
Children: 5 mg/kg P.O. or I.M. if 10 or older; 5 mg/kg I.M. or rectally if younger than 10.

ADVERSE REACTIONS
CNS: *drowsiness, lethargy, hangover,* paradoxical excitement in elderly patients.
GI: nausea, vomiting.
Hematologic: exacerbation of porphyria.
Skin: rash, urticaria, *Stevens-Johnson syndrome.*
Other: *angioedema.*

INTERACTIONS
Corticosteroids, doxycycline, estrogens and oral contraceptives, oral anticoagulants: pentobarbital may enhance the metabolism of these drugs. Monitor for decreased effect.
Ethanol or other CNS depressants, including narcotic analgesics: excessive CNS and respiratory depression. Use together cautiously.
Griseofulvin: decreased absorption of griseofulvin.
MAO inhibitors: inhibited metabolism of barbiturates; may cause prolonged CNS depression. Reduce barbiturate dosage.
Rifampin: may decrease barbiturate levels. Monitor for decreased effect.

CONTRAINDICATIONS
Contraindicated in patients with hypersensitivity to barbiturates, or porphyria.

NURSING CONSIDERATIONS
• Use cautiously in patients with acute or chronic pain, mental depression, suicidal tendencies, history of drug abuse, or hepatic impairment. Also administer cautiously to elderly or debilitated patients.
• Assess mental status before initiating therapy and use reduced doses as ordered. Elderly patients are more sensitive to the drug's adverse CNS effects.
• **I.V. use:** I.V. administration of barbiturates may cause severe respiratory depression, laryngospasm, or hypotension. Have emergency resuscitation equipment available.
• To minimize deterioration, use I.V injection solution within 30 minutes after opening container. Don't use cloudy solution.
• Reserve I.V. injection for emergency treatment, which should be given under close supervision. Administer slowly at a rate not exceeding 50 mg/minute.
• Parenteral solution is alkaline. Local tissue reactions and injection site pain have followed I.V. use. Avoid extravasation. Assess patency of I.V. site before and during administration.
• Do not mix in syringe or in I.V. solutions or in lines with other drugs.
• Administer I.M. injection deeply. Superficial injection may cause pain, sterile abscess, and sloughing.
• To ensure accurate dosage, don't divide suppositories.
• Take precautions to prevent hoarding or self-overdosing by patients who are depressed, suicidal, or drug-dependent or who have a history of drug abuse.
• Watch for signs of barbiturate toxicity: coma, pupillary constriction, cya-

---

nosis, clammy skin, and hypotension. Overdose can be fatal.

• Inspect patient's skin. Skin eruptions may precede potentially fatal reactions to barbiturate therapy. Discontinue drug when skin reactions occur and call doctor. In some patients, high fever, stomatitis, headache, or rhinitis may precede skin reactions.

• Know that pentobarbital has no analgesic effect and may cause restlessness or delirium in patients with pain. erile abscess, and sloughing.

• Be aware that long-term use is not recommended; drug loses its efficacy in promoting sleep after 14 days of continued use. Long-term high dosage may cause drug dependence, and patient may experience withdrawal symptoms if drug is suddenly discontinued. Withdraw barbiturates gradually.

• Caution patients about performing activities that require mental alertness or physical coordination. For inpatients, supervise walking and raise bed rails, particularly for elderly patients.

• Inform patient that morning "hangover" is common after hypnotic dose, which suppresses REM sleep. Patient may experience increased dreaming after drug is discontinued.

• Tell patients who use oral contraceptives that she should consider alternate birth control methods because drug may enhance contraceptive hormone metabolism and decrease its effect.

quazepam
Doral
Controlled Substance Schedule IV
Pregnancy Risk Category: X

HOW SUPPLIED
Tablets: 7.5 mg, 15 mg

ACTION
Unknown although drug acts on the limbic system and thalamus of the CNS by binding to specific benzodiazepine receptors.

ONSET, PEAK, DURATION
Onset and duration unknown. Plasma levels peak in about 2 hours.

INDICATIONS & DOSAGE
Insomnia –
Adults: 15 mg P.O. h.s. Some patients may respond to lower dosages. Dosage decreased in elderly patients after 2 days of therapy if possible.

ADVERSE REACTIONS
CNS: *fatigue, dizziness, daytime drowsiness, headache.*

INTERACTIONS
Anticonvulsants, antihistamines, ethanol, psychotropic drugs, and other drugs which produce CNS depression: additive CNS depressant effects. Avoid concomitant use.

CONTRAINDICATIONS
Contraindicated in patients with hypersensitivity to this drug or other benzodiazepines, in pregnant patients, and in patients with suspected or established sleep apnea.

NURSING CONSIDERATIONS
• Use cautiously in patients with hepatic, renal, or respiratory disease, depression, and in elderly patients.
• Take precautions to prevent hoarding or self-overdosing by patients who are depressed, suicidal, or drug-dependent or who have a history of drug abuse.
• Be aware patients on long-term therapy with benzodiazepines may experience withdrawal symptoms if the drug is suddenly withdrawn (possibly after 6 weeks of continuous therapy).
• Caution patients about performing activities that require mental alertness

---

*Liquid form contains alcohol.   *Common* reactions are in italics; ***life-threatening,*** in bold italics.
**May contain tartrazine.

or physical coordination. For inpatients, supervise walking and raise bed rails, particularly for elderly patients.

• Warn patients not to increase the drug dosage but to inform the doctor if they feel lack of effectiveness.

• Warn patients about the possible additive depressant effects that can occur if alcohol is consumed within 24 hours of quazepam.

---

secobarbital sodium
Novosecobarb†, Seconal Sodium
Controlled Substance Schedule II

Pregnancy Risk Category: D

HOW SUPPLIED
Capsules: 50 mg, 100 mg
Injection: 50 mg/ml

ACTION
Unknown. Probably interferes with transmission of impulses from the thalamus to the cortex of the brain. A barbiturate.

ONSET, PEAK, DURATION
Onset occurs within 15 minutes with oral dose, almost immediate with I.V. dose, unknown for I.M. administration. Serum levels peak 1 to 3 minutes with I.V. administration, 7 to 10 minutes with I.M. administration, and 15 to 30 minutes with oral dose. Effects persist for 1 to 4 hours for oral dose, 15 minutes for I.V. dose, unknown for I.M. dose.

INDICATIONS & DOSAGE
Preoperative sedation–
Adults: 100 to 300 mg P.O. 1 to 2 hours before surgery.
Children: 50 to 100 mg P.O. 1 to 2 hours before surgery. Maximum single dose is 100 mg.
Insomnia–
Adults: 100 to 200 mg P.O. or I.M.
Children: 3 to 5 mg/kg I.M. or 125 mg/m², not to exceed 100 mg, with no more than 5 ml injected in any one site.
Acute tetanus seizure–
Adults and children: 5.5 mg/kg I.M. or slow I.V., repeated q 3 to 4 hours, if needed; I.V. injection rate not to exceed 50 mg/15 seconds.
Status epilepticus–
Children: 15 to 20 mg/kg I.V. over 15 minutes.

ADVERSE REACTIONS
CNS: *drowsiness, lethargy, hangover,* paradoxical excitement in elderly patients.
CV: hypotension (with I.V. use).
GI: nausea, vomiting.
Hematologic: exacerbation of porphyria.
Respiratory: *respiratory depression.*
Skin: rash, urticaria, **Stevens-Johnson syndrome,** tissue reactions and injection-site pain.
Other: *angioedema.*

INTERACTIONS
Chloramphenicol, MAO inhibitors, valproic acid: inhibited metabolism of barbiturates; may cause prolonged CNS depression. Reduce barbiturate dosage.
Corticosteroids, digitoxin, doxycycline, estrogens and oral contraceptives, oral anticoagulants, tricyclic antidepressants: secobarbital may enhance the metabolism of these drugs. Monitor for decreased effect.
Ethanol or other CNS depressants, including narcotic analgesics: excessive CNS and respiratory depression. Use together cautiously.
Griseofulvin: decreased absorption of griseofulvin.
Lactated Ringer's solution, acidic solutions: incompatible with I.V. form of drug. Don't mix.
Rifampin: may decrease barbiturate levels. Monitor for decreased effect.

CONTRAINDICATIONS

Contraindicated in patients with marked liver impairment, respiratory disease in which dyspnea or obstruction is evident, hypersensitivity to barbiturates, or porphyria.

NURSING CONSIDERATIONS

• Use cautiously in patients with acute or chronic pain, depression, suicidal tendencies, history of drug abuse, or hepatic impairment.

• Assess mental status before initiating therapy. Elderly patients are more sensitive to the drug's adverse CNS effects.

• **I.V. use:** Know that I.V. injection is reserved for emergency treatment and given under close supervision by direct injection, and administered slowly at a rate not exceeding 50 mg/ 15 seconds. May be administered as supplied or diluted.

• Local tissue reactions and injection-site pain have been noted with I.V. use. Assess patency of I.V. site before and during administration.

• I.V. administration of barbiturates may cause severe respiratory depression, laryngospasm, or hypotension. Have emergency resuscitation equipment readily available.

• Know that secobarbital sodium injection is not compatible with lactated Ringer's solution, but is compatible with Ringer's solution, sterile water for injection, and 0.9% sodium chloride. Don't mix with acidic solutions.

• Use injection solution within 30 minutes after opening container to minimize deterioration. Don't use cloudy solution.

• Give I.M. injection deeply. Superficial injection may cause pain, sterile abscess, and sloughing.

• Take precautions to prevent hoarding or self-overdosing by patients who are depressed, suicidal, or drug-dependent or who have a history of drug abuse.

• Watch for signs of barbiturate toxicity: coma, pupillary constriction, cyanosis, clammy skin, and hypotension. Overdose can be fatal.

• Inspect patient's skin. Skin eruptions may precede potentially fatal reactions to barbiturate therapy. Discontinue drug when skin reactions occur and notify physician. In some patients, high fever, stomatitis, headache, or rhinitis may precede skin reactions.

• Be aware that long-term use is not recommended; drug loses its efficacy in promoting sleep after 14 days of continued use.

• Caution patients about performing activities that require mental alertness or physical coordination. For inpatients, supervise walking and raise bed rails, particularly for elderly patients.

• Inform patient morning "hangover" is common after hypnotic dose, which suppresses REM sleep. Patient may experience increased dreaming after drug is discontinued.

• Tell patients who use oral contraceptives that she should consider alternate birth control methods because drug may enhance contraceptive hormone metabolism and decrease its effect.

temazepam

Euhypnos 10‡, Euhypnos 20‡, Normison‡, Restoril, Temaze‡
Controlled Substance Schedule IV

Pregnancy Risk Category: X

HOW SUPPLIED

Capsules: 10 mg‡, 15 mg, 20 mg‡, 30 mg

ACTION

Unknown. A benzodiazepine that probably acts on the limbic system, thalamus, and hypothalamus of the CNS to produce hypnotic effects.

---

*Liquid form contains alcohol.   *Common* reactions are in italics; *life-threatening*, in bold italics.
**May contain tartrazine.

ONSET, PEAK, DURATION
Onset and duration unknown. Serum levels peak in 1 to 2 hours.

INDICATIONS & DOSAGE
Insomnia –
Adults: 7.5 to 30 mg P.O. h.s.
Adults over 65 years: 7.5 mg P.O. h.s.

ADVERSE REACTIONS
CNS: *drowsiness, dizziness, lethargy,* disturbed coordination, daytime sedation, confusion.
GI: anorexia, diarrhea.

INTERACTIONS
Ethanol or other CNS depressants, including narcotic analgesics: increased CNS depression. Use together cautiously.

CONTRAINDICATIONS
Contraindicated in patients with hypersensitivity to this drug or other benzodiazepines and during pregnancy.

NURSING CONSIDERATIONS
• Use cautiously in patients with chronic pulmonary insufficiency, impaired hepatic or renal function, severe or latent mental depression, suicidal tendencies, and history of drug abuse.
• Assess mental status before initiating therapy. Elderly patients are more sensitive to the drug's adverse CNS effects.
• Take precautions to prevent hoarding or self-overdosing by patients who are depressed, suicidal, or drug-dependent or who have a history of drug abuse.
• Caution patients about performing activities that require mental alertness or physical coordination. For inpatients, supervise walking and raise bed rails, particularly for elderly patients.
• Know that drug may cause less residual sedation ("hangover") than flurazepam and diazepam. Relatively short-acting.
• Tell patients that onset of the drug's effects may take as long as 2 to 2 ½ hours.

---

triazolam
Apo-Triazo†, Halcion, Novo-Triolam†, Nu-Triazo†
Controlled Substance Schedule IV
Pregnancy Risk Category: X

HOW SUPPLIED
Tablets: 0.125 mg, 0.25 mg

ACTION
Unknown. A benzodiazepine that probably acts on the limbic system, thalamus, and hypothalamus of the CNS to produce hypnotic effects.

ONSET, PEAK, DURATION
Onset and duration unknown. Serum levels peak in 1 to 2 hours.

INDICATIONS & DOSAGE
Insomnia –
Adults: 0.125 to 0.5 mg P.O. h.s.
Adults over 65: 0.125 mg P.O. h.s.; increased, as needed, to 0.25 mg P.O. h.s.

ADVERSE REACTIONS
CNS: *drowsiness, dizziness, headache,* rebound insomnia, amnesia, light-headedness, lack of coordination, mental confusion, depression.
GI: nausea, vomiting.
Other: physical or psychological abuse.

INTERACTIONS
Cimetidine, erythromycin: may cause prolonged triazolam blood levels. Monitor for increased sedation.
Ethanol or other CNS depressants, including narcotic analgesics: excessive CNS depression. Use together cautiously.

CONTRAINDICATIONS
Contraindicated in patients with hypersensitivity to benzodiazepines and in pregnancy.

NURSING CONSIDERATIONS
• Use cautiously in patients with impaired hepatic or renal function, chronic pulmonary insufficiency, sleep apnea, mental depression, suicidal tendencies, or history of drug abuse.
• Assess mental status before initiating therapy. Elderly patients are more sensitive to the drug's CNS effects.
• Take precautions to prevent hoarding or self-overdosing by patients who are depressed, suicidal, or drug-dependent or who have a history of drug abuse.
• Warn patients not to take more than the prescribed amount because overdose can occur at a total daily dose of 2 mg (or four times the highest recommended amount).
• Caution patients about performing activities that require mental alertness or physical coordination. For inpatients, supervise walking and raise bed rails, particularly for elderly patients.
• Inform patient it is very short-acting and therefore has less tendency to cause morning drowsiness.
• Tell patients that rebound insomnia may develop for one or two nights after stopping therapy.

---

zolpidem tartrate
Ambien
Controlled Substance Schedule IV

Pregnancy Risk Category: B

HOW SUPPLIED
Tablets: 5 mg, 10 mg

ACTION
Although zolpidem interacts with one of three identified GABA-benzodiazepine (gamma-aminobutyric acid-

benzodiazepine) receptor complexes, it's not a benzodiazepine. It exhibits hypnotic activity, but no muscle relaxant or anticonvulsant properties.

ONSET, PEAK, DURATION
Onset rapid. Serum levels peak within ½ to 2 hours. Duration unknown.

INDICATIONS & DOSAGE
Short-term management of insomnia –
Adults: 10 mg P.O. immediately before bedtime.
   In elderly or debilitated patients and in patients with hepatic insufficiency: 5 mg P.O. immediately before bedtime. Maximum daily dosage is 10 mg.

ADVERSE REACTIONS
CNS: daytime drowsiness, light-headedness, abnormal dreams, amnesia, dizziness, headache, hangover effect, sleep disorder.
CV: palpitations.
EENT: sinusitis, pharyngitis, dry mouth.
GI: nausea, vomiting, diarrhea.
Skin: rash.
Other: back or chest pain, flulike-symptoms, hypersensitivity reactions.

INTERACTIONS
Ethanol or other CNS depressants: enhanced CNS depression. Avoid concomitant use.

CONTRAINDICATIONS
None known.

NURSING CONSIDERATIONS
• Use cautiously in patients with diseases or conditions that could affect metabolism or hemodynamic responses and in those with compromised respiratory status because hypnotics may depress respiratory drive. Also use cautiously in patients with depression or a history of alcohol or drug abuse.
• Be aware that hypnotics should be

---

*Liquid form contains alcohol.   *Common* reactions are in italics; *life-threatening,* in bold italics.
**May contain tartrazine.

used only for short-term management of insomnia, usually 7 to 10 days. Persistent insomnia may indicate a primary psychiatric or medical disorder.

• Know that because most adverse reactions are dose-related, the smallest effective dose should be used in all patients, especially in elderly and debilitated patients.

• Take precautions to prevent hoarding or self-overdosing by patients who are depressed, suicidal, or drug-dependent or who have a history of drug abuse.

• For faster sleep onset, instruct patients not to take drug with or immediately after meals. Food decreases drug's absorption.

• Caution patients about performing activities that require mental alertness or physical coordination. For inpatients, supervise walking and raise bed rails, particularly for elderly patients.

acetazolamide sodium
(See Chapter 62, DIURETICS.)
carbamazepine
clonazepam
clorazepate dipotasium
(See Chapter 32, ANTIANXIETY AGENTS.)
diazepam
(See Chapter 32, ANTIANXIETY AGENTS.)
ethosuximide
ethotoin
felbamate
gabapentin
lamotrigine
magnesium sulfate
mephenytoin
mephobarbital
methsuximide
phenacemide
phenobarbital
phenobarbital sodium
phensuximide
phenytoin
phenytoin sodium
phenytoin sodium (extended)
primidone
trimethadione
valproate sodium
valproic acid
divalproex sodium

COMBINATION PRODUCTS
DILANTIN WITH PHENOBARBITAL KAPSEALS: phenytoin sodium 100 mg and phenobarbital 16 mg; phenytoin sodium 100 mg and phenobarbital 32 mg.

carbamazepine
Apo-Carbamazepine†, Epitol, Mazepine†, Novocarbamaz†, PMS-Carbamazepine†, Tegretol, Tegretol Chewable Tablets, Tegretol CR†, Teril‡

Pregnancy Risk Category: C

HOW SUPPLIED
Tablets: 200 mg
Tablets (chewable): 100 mg
Tablets (extended-release)†: 200 mg, 400 mg
Oral suspension: 100 mg/5 ml

ACTION
Unknown. Thought to stabilize neuronal membranes and limits seizure activity by either increasing efflux or decreasing influx of sodium ions across cell membranes in the motor cortex during generation of nerve impulses.

ONSET, PEAK, DURATION
Onset occurs in trigeminal neuralgia, 8 to 72 hours; anticonvulsant effect, hours to days. Serum levels peak in 1 ½ hours after oral suspension, 4 to 12 hours after tablets. Duration unknown.

INDICATIONS & DOSAGE
Generalized tonic-clonic and complex partial seizures, mixed seizure patterns –
Adults and children over 12 years: initially, 200 mg P.O. b.i.d. for tablets or 1 teaspoon of suspension P.O. q.i.d. May be increased at weekly intervals by 200 mg P.O. daily, in divided doses at 6- to 8-hour intervals. Adjusted to minimum effective level when control is achieved. Maximum daily dosage is 1 g/day in children ages 12 to 15, or 1.2 g/day in patients over age 15.
Children under 12 years: initially, 100 mg P.O. b.i.d. or ½ teaspoon of suspension P.O. q.i.d. Increased at weekly intervals by 100 mg P.O. daily. Maximum daily dosage is1 g/day.

---

*Liquid form contains alcohol.
**May contain tartrazine.

Common reactions are in italics; *life-threatening,* in bold italics.

Trigeminal neuralgia –
Adults: initially, 100 mg P.O. b.i.d. or ½ teaspoon of suspension q.i.d. with meals. Increased by 100 mg q 12 hours for tablets or ½ teaspoon of suspension q.i.d. until pain is relieved. Maximum daily dosage is 1.2 g/day. Maintenance dosage is 200 to 400 mg P.O. b.i.d.

ADVERSE REACTIONS
CNS: *dizziness, vertigo, drowsiness,* fatigue, *ataxia,* **worsening of seizures** (usually in patients with mixed seizure disorders, including atypical absence seizures).
CV: *CHF,* hypertension, hypotension, aggravation of coronary artery disease.
EENT: conjunctivitis, dry mouth and pharynx, blurred vision, diplopia, nystagmus.
GI: *nausea, vomiting,* abdominal pain, diarrhea, anorexia, stomatitis, glossitis.
GU: urinary frequency, urine retention, impotence, albuminuria, glycosuria, elevated BUN.
Hematologic: *aplastic anemia, agranulocytosis,* eosinophilia, leukocytosis, *thrombocytopenia.*
Hepatic: abnormal liver function test results, *hepatitis.*
Respiratory: pulmonary hypersensitivity.
Skin: rash, urticaria, erythema multiforme, *Stevens-Johnson syndrome.*
Other: excessive sweating, fever, chills, water intoxication.

INTERACTIONS
Cimetidine, danazol, diltiazem, macrolides (such as erythromycin), isoniazid, propoxyphene, valproic acid, verapamil: may increase carbamazepine blood levels. Use cautiously.
Lithium: increased CNS toxicity of lithium. Avoid concomitant use.
MAO inhibitors: increased depressant and anticholinergic effects. Don't use together.

Oral contraceptives, doxycycline, haloperidol, phenytoin, theophylline, warfarin: carbamazepine may decrease blood levels of these drugs. Monitor for decreased effect.
Phenobarbital, phenytoin, primidone: may decrease carbamazepine levels. Monitor for decreased effect.

CONTRAINDICATIONS
Contraindicated in patients with history of previous bone marrow suppression or hypersensitivity to carbamazepine or tricyclic antidepressants and in patients who have taken an MAO inhibitor within 14 days of therapy.

NURSING CONSIDERATIONS
• Use cautiously in patients with mixed seizure disorders because they may experience an increased incidence of seizures (usually atypical absence or generalized seizures).
• Obtain baseline determinations of urinalysis, BUN level, liver function, CBC, platelet and reticulocyte counts, and serum iron level as ordered. Monitor periodically thereafter.
• Shake oral suspension well before measuring dose.
• When administering by nasogastric tube, mix dose with an equal volume of water, 0.9% sodium chloride, or D_5W. Flush tube with 100 ml of diluent after administering dose.
• Never discontinue suddenly when treating seizures or status epilepticus. Notify doctor immediately if adverse reactions occur.
• Know that adverse reactions may be minimized by increasing dosage gradually.
• Therapeutic carbamazepine blood level is 4 to 12 mcg/ml. Monitor blood levels and effects closely. Ask the patient when last dose of medication was taken to approximately evaluate blood levels.
• When managing seizures, institute appropriate precautions.

†Available in Canada only.   ‡Available in Australia only.   ◊Available OTC.

- Observe for signs of anorexia or subtle appetite changes, which may indicate excessive blood levels.
- Tell patient to take carbamazepine with food to minimize GI distress.
- Tell patients to keep tablets in their original container, tightly closed, and away from moisture. Some formulations may harden when exposed to excess moisture, resulting in decreased bioavailability and loss of seizure control.
- Inform patient that when used for trigeminal neuralgia, an attempt to decrease dosage or withdraw drug is usually done every 3 months.
- Tell patients to notify the doctor immediately if fever, sore throat, mouth ulcers, or easy bruising or bleeding occurs.
- Tell patient drug may cause mild to moderate dizziness and drowsiness when first taken. Advise him to avoid hazardous activities until effects disappear. Effect usually disappears within 3 to 4 days.
- Advise patient that periodic eye examinations are recommended.

---

clonazepam
Klonopin
Controlled Substance Schedule IV
Pregnancy Risk Category: NR

HOW SUPPLIED
Tablets: 0.5 mg, 1 mg, 2 mg
Drops: 2.5 mg/ml‡
Injection: 1 mg/ml‡

ACTION
Unknown. A benzodiazepine that probably acts by facilitating the effects of the inhibitory neurotransmitter gamma-aminobutyric acid (GABA).

ONSET, PEAK, DURATION
Onset and duration unknown. Serum levels peak in 1 to 2 hours, although peak concentrations may not be achieved for 4 to 8 hours.

INDICATIONS & DOSAGE
Lennox-Gastaut syndrome; atypical absence seizures; akinetic and myoclonic seizures –
Adults: initially, not to exceed 1.5 mg P.O. daily in three divided doses. May be increased by 0.5 to 1 mg q 3 days until seizures are controlled. If given in unequal doses, the largest dose given h.s. Maximum recommended daily dosage is 20 mg.
Children up to 10 years or 30 kg: initially, 0.01 to 0.03 mg/kg P.O. daily (not to exceed 0.05 mg/kg daily), in 2 or 3 divided doses. Increased by 0.25 to 0.5 mg q third day to a maximum maintenance dosage of 0.1 to 0.2 mg/kg daily as needed.
Status epilepticus (where parenteral form is available) –
Adults: 1 mg by slow I.V. infusion.
Children: 0.5 mg by slow I.V. infusion.

ADVERSE REACTIONS
CNS: *drowsiness, ataxia, behavioral disturbances* (especially in children), slurred speech, tremor, confusion, psychosis, agitation.
EENT: *increased salivation,* diplopia, nystagmus, abnormal eye movements, sore gums.
GI: constipation, gastritis, change in appetite, nausea, abnormal thirst.
GU: dysuria, enuresis, nocturia, urine retention.
Hematologic: leukopenia, thrombocytopenia, eosinophilia.
Respiratory: *respiratory depression.*
Skin: rash.

INTERACTIONS
Ethanol or other CNS depressants: increased CNS depression. Monitor closely.

---

*Liquid form contains alcohol.
**May contain tartrazine.

Common reactions are in italics; ***life-threatening***, in bold italics.

CONTRAINDICATIONS

Contraindicated in patients with significant hepatic disease; in those with sensitivity to benzodiazepines; or in patients with acute angle-closure glaucoma.

NURSING CONSIDERATIONS

• Use cautiously in patients with mixed type of seizure because drug may precipitate generalized tonic-clonic seizures. Also use cautiously in children and in patients with chronic respiratory disease, or open-angle glaucoma.
• **I.V. use‡:** Give slowly by direct injection or by slow I.V. infusion. Drug may be diluted with D_5W, dextrose 2.5% in water, 0.9% sodium chloride, or 0.45% sodium chloride.
• Mix solutions in glass bottles because the drug binds to polyvinyl chloride (PVC) plastics. If PVC infusion bags are used, administer immediately and infuse at a rate of 60 ml/ hour or greater.
• Never withdraw suddenly because seizures may worsen. Call the doctor at once if adverse reactions develop.
• Monitor blood levels. Therapeutic blood level is 20 to 80 ng/ml.
• Assess elderly patient's response closely. Elderly patients are more sensitive to the drug's CNS effects.
• Monitor patient for oversedation.
• Monitor CBCs and liver function tests as ordered.
• Know that withdrawal symptoms are similar to those of barbiturates.
• Advise patients to avoid driving or other potentially hazardous activities that require mental alertness until drug's CNS effects are known.
• Instruct parents to monitor child's school performance because clonazepam may interfere with attentiveness in school.
• Instruct patient and parents never to stop drug abruptly because seizures may occur.

ethosuximide

Zarontin

Pregnancy Risk Category: NR

HOW SUPPLIED

Capsules: 250 mg
Syrup: 250 mg/5 ml

ACTION

Not clearly defined. A succinimide derivative that probably increases seizure threshold. Reduces the paroxysmal spike-and-wave pattern of absence seizures by depressing nerve transmission in the motor cortex.

ONSET, PEAK, DURATION

Onset and duration unknown. Peak effect occurs in 3 to 7 hours.

INDICATIONS & DOSAGE

Absence seizures –
Adults and children 6 years and older: 500 mg P.O. daily. Optimal dose is 20 mg/kg/day.
Children 3 to 6 years: 250 mg P.O. daily. Optimal dose is 20 mg/kg/day.

ADVERSE REACTIONS

CNS: *drowsiness, headache, fatigue, dizziness, ataxia, irritability, hiccups, euphoria, lethargy, depression, psychosis.*
EENT: myopia, tongue swelling, gum hypertrophy.
GI: *nausea, vomiting, diarrhea, weight loss, cramps, anorexia, epigastric and abdominal pain.*
GU: vaginal bleeding, urinary frequency.
Hematologic: leukopenia, eosinophilia, *agranulocytosis,* pancytopenia, *aplastic anemia.*
Skin: urticaria, pruritic and erythematous rashes, hirsutism.

INTERACTIONS

None significant.

CONTRAINDICATIONS

Contraindicated in patients with hypersensitivity to succinimide derivatives.

NURSING CONSIDERATIONS

• Use with extreme caution in patients with hepatic or renal disease.
• Be aware that ethosuximide is currently the drug of choice for treating absence seizures.
• Never withdraw drug suddenly. Abrupt withdrawal may precipitate absence seizures. Call doctor immediately if adverse reactions develop.
• Monitor blood levels. Therapeutic blood levels are 40 to 80 mcg/ml.
• Obtain CBC every 3 to 6 months as ordered.
• Know that drug may increase frequency of generalized tonic-clonic seizures when used alone in patients who have mixed types of seizures.
• Know that drug may cause positive direct Coombs' test.
• Advise patients to take ethosuximide with food to minimize GI distress.
• Advise patients to avoid driving or other potentially hazardous activities that require mental alertness until drug's CNS effects are known.
• Warn patient and parents not to stop drug abruptly.

---

ethotoin
Peganone

Pregnancy Risk Category: C

HOW SUPPLIED
Tablets: 250 mg, 500 mg

ACTION
Unknown. A hydantoin derivative that probably stabilizes neuronal membranes and limits seizure activity by either increasing efflux or decreasing influx of sodium ions across cell membranes in the motor cortex during generation of nerve impulses.

ONSET, PEAK, DURATION
Unknown.

INDICATIONS & DOSAGE
Tonic-clonic (grand mal) or complex partial (psychomotor) seizures –
Adults: initially, up to 1 g P.O. daily in divided doses. Increased slowly over several days to 3 g daily in divided doses as needed.
Children: initially, up to 750 mg P.O. daily in divided doses. Increased up to 1 g daily in divided doses as needed. Rarely, 2 to 3 g daily may be required.

ADVERSE REACTIONS
CNS: fatigue, insomnia, dizziness, headache, numbness, slurred speech, ataxia.
CV: chest pain.
EENT: diplopia, nystagmus, gingival hyperplasia (rare).
GI: *nausea, vomiting, diarrhea.*
Hematologic: thrombocytopenia, leukopenia, ***agranulocytosis, pancytopenia,*** megaloblastic anemia.
Skin: rash.
Other: fever, lymphadenopathy.

INTERACTIONS
Antihistamines, chloramphenicol, cimetidine, diazepam, disulfiram, isoniazid, phenylbutazone, salicylates, sulfamethizole, valproate: increased ethotoin activity and toxicity; monitor closely.
Diazoxide: decreased ethotoin activity. Monitor closely.
Ethanol (with chronic use), folic acid: decreased ethotoin activity; monitor closely.
Phenacemide: paranoia. Use together cautiously.

CONTRAINDICATIONS
Contraindicated in patients with hydantoin hypersensitivity and in those with hepatic or hematologic disorders.

---

*Liquid form contains alcohol.   *Common* reactions are in italics; *life-threatening,* in bold italics.
**May contain tartrazine.

NURSING CONSIDERATIONS
• Know that ethotoin is the hydantoin derivative of choice for young adults prone to gingival hyperplasia caused by phenytoin. Otherwise, it is used infrequently to treat epilepsy.
• Never withdraw drug suddenly because seizures may worsen. Call the doctor at once if adverse reactions develop.
• Monitor CBC and urinalysis when therapy starts and periodically thereafter as ordered. Also, periodically monitor liver function test results during long-term use.
• Monitor blood levels. Therapeutic blood levels are 15 to 50 mcg/ml.
• Notify doctor if lymphadenopathy or lupuslike syndrome (fever, bruising, and sore throat) develops.
• Tell patients to take drug after meals. Schedule doses as evenly as possible over 24 hours.
• Advise patients to avoid driving or other potentially hazardous activities that require mental alertness until drug's CNS effects are known.
• Caution patients that heavy alcohol use may diminish drug's benefits.
• Warn patient and parents never to stop drug therapy abruptly.

---

felbamate
Felbatol

Pregnancy Risk Category: C

HOW SUPPLIED
Tablets: 400 mg, 600 mg
Oral suspension: 600 mg/5 ml

ACTION
Unknown. A dicarbamate anticonvulsant that may act by elevating the seizure threshold or preventing the spread of seizure activity.

ONSET, PEAK, DURATION
Onset and duration unknown. Serum levels peak in 1 to 6 hours.

INDICATIONS & DOSAGE
Refractory partial seizures in adults with epilepsy; Lennox-Gastaut syndrome in chidlren –
Adults and children ages 14 and older: when used as the sole treatment, initially 1,200 mg P.O. daily in 3 or 4 divided doses. Dosage titrated in 600-mg increments every 2 weeks to 2,400 mg daily and finally to 3,600 mg daily if needed and tolerated.

When used as adjunctive therapy in patients taking other anticonvulsant drugs, felbamate therapy initiated at 1,200 mg P.O. daily in 3 or 4 divided doses while the dosage of carbamazepine, phenytoin, or valproic acid is reduced by 20%. Felbamate dosage is increased by 1,200 mg daily in divided doses at weekly intervals to a maximum of 3,600 mg daily; concomitant reductions in the dosage of other anticonvulsants may be necessary.
To switch to felbamate monotherapy from other anticonvulsants –
Adults and children ages 14 and over: initially, 1,200 mg P.O. daily in 3 or 4 divided doses while the dosage of concurrent anticonvulsants is reduced by one-third. During the second week of treatment, felbamate dosage increased to 2,400 mg daily in 3 or 4 divided doses while the dosage of the other anticonvulsant is cut by another one-third. The dosage of felbamate is increased to 3,600 mg daily in divided doses by the third week, and the dosage of other anticonvulsants continued to be reduced as needed and tolerated.
Children ages 2 to 14: felbamate therapy initiated at 15 mg/kg/day in divided doses 3 or 4 times a day while the dosage of carbamazepine, phenytoin, or valproic acid is reduced by 20%. Felbamate dosage increased by 15 mg/kg/day in 3 or 4 divided doses in weekly intervals to a maximum of 45 mg/day. Dosage reduction of other

---

anticonvulsants is done as needed to minimize adverse effects.

ADVERSE REACTIONS
CNS: *insomnia, headache, fatigue,* anxiety.
EENT: blurred or double vision, otitis media, *rhinitis.*
GI: *dyspepsia, vomiting, constipation, diarrhea.*
GU: urinary tract infection.
Hematologic: *aplastic anemia.*
Hepatic: *acute liver failure.*
Skin: acne, rash.
Other: increased ALT, *upper respiratory infection,* hypophosphatemia, weight loss, facial edema.

INTERACTIONS
Carbamazepine: decreased steady-state levels of carbamazepine and increased levels of its active metabolite; increased felbamate clearance, resulting in decreased plasma levels. Use together cautiously.
Phenytoin, valproic acid: increased steady-state levels of phenytoin or valproic acid; increased felbamate clearance, reducing its blood levels. Use together cautiously.

CONTRAINDICATIONS
Contraindicated in patients hypersensitive to the drug or to other carbamates or history of previous bone marrow depression.

NURSING CONSIDERATIONS
• Know that because of the higher than expected rate of aplastic anemia, it is recommended that use of felbamate be suspended unless the patient's well-being is judged dependent upon continued treatment. FDA recommends that felbamate be used as second-line therapy only.
• Institute appropriate seizure precautions.
• Check to ensure a full hematologic evaluation has been performed before therapy begins.

• Shake oral suspension well before measuring dose.
• Know that food does not interfere with absorption of felbamate's tablet form; food's effects on the suspension are unknown.
• When added to other anticonvulsants, monitor blood levels of these drugs and patient response closely because felbamate can alter pharmacokinetics of carbamazepine, phenytoin, and valproic acid. Ask the patient when last dose of medication was taken to approximately evaluate blood levels. When used alone, routine monitoring of felbamate blood levels is not necessary.
• Discontinue other anticonvulsants slowly as ordered because of a possible increase in the frequency of seizures.
• Monitor CBC and platelets as ordered frequently during therapy and for a significant time after drug is discontinued.
• Warn patients to avoid hazardous activities that require alertness and good psychomotor coordination until drug's CNS effects are known.
• Photosensitivity may occur. Warn patients to use a sunscreen.

---

gabapentin
Neurontin

Pregnancy Risk Category: C

HOW SUPPLIED
Capsules: 100 mg, 300 mg, 400 mg

ACTION
Unknown. Although structurally related to gamma-amino butyric acid (GABA), the drug doesn't interact with GABA receptors and isn't converted metabolically into GABA or a GABA agonist.

ONSET, PEAK, DURATION
Unknown.

INDICATIONS & DOSAGE
Adjunctive treatment of partial seizures with and without secondary generalization in adults with epilepsy –
Adults: initially 300 mg P.O. h.s. on day 1; 300 mg P.O. b.i.d. on day 2; then 300 mg P.O. t.i.d. on day 3. Dosage increased as needed and tolerated to 1,800 mg daily in divided doses. Dosages up to 3,600 mg daily have been well tolerated.

In patients with renal failure: if creatinine clearance is > 60 ml/minute, 400 mg P.O. t.i.d.; if creatinine clearance is 30 to 60 ml/minute, 300 mg P.O. b.i.d.; if creatinine clearance is 15 to 30 ml/minute, 300 mg P.O. daily; if creatinine clearance is < 15 ml/minute, 300 mg P.O. every other day. Patients on dialysis should receive a loading dose of 300 to 400 mg P.O.; then 200 mg to 300 mg P.O. following every 4 hours of hemodialysis.

ADVERSE REACTIONS
CNS: *somnolence, dizziness, ataxia, fatigue, nystagmus, tremor,* nervousness, dysarthria, amnesia, depression, abnormal thinking, twitching, abnormal coordination.
CV: peripheral edema, vasodilation.
EENT: *diplopia, rhinitis,* pharyngitis, dry throat, coughing, *amblyopia.*
GI: nausea, vomiting, dyspepsia, dry mouth, constipation.
GU: impotence.
Hematologic: leukopenia, decreased WBC count.
Skin: pruritus, abrasion.
Other: dental abnormalities, increased appetite, weight gain, back pain, myalgia, fractures.

INTERACTIONS
Antacids: decreased absorption of gabapentin. Separate administration times by at least 2 hours.

CONTRAINDICATIONS
Contraindicated in patients hypersensitive to the drug.

NURSING CONSIDERATIONS
• Give the first dose at bedtime to minimize drowsiness, dizziness, fatigue, and ataxia.
• If gabapentin therapy is discontinued or alternative medication is substituted, do so gradually over at least 1 week as ordered to minimize risk of precipitating seizures. Do not suddenly withdraw other anticonvulsants in patients starting gabapentin therapy.
• Know that routine monitoring of plasma levels of gabapentin is not necessary. The drug does not appear to alter plasma levels of other anticonvulsants.
• Know that it may cause false-positive tests for urine protein when the Ames-N-Multistix SG dipstick test is used.
• Tell patients to take the drug without regard to meals.
• Warn patients to avoid driving or operating heavy machinery until drug's CNS effects are known.

lamotrigine
Lamictal
Pregnancy Risk Category: C

HOW SUPPLIED
Tablets: 25 mg, 100 mg, 150 mg, 200 mg

ACTION
Unknown. May cause inhibited release of glutamate and aspartate, excitatory neurotransmitters, in the brain. This may occur by way of an action at voltage-sensitive sodium channels.

ONSET, PEAK, DURATION
Onset and duration unknown. Serum levels peak in 1.4 to 4.8 hours after administration.

INDICATIONS & DOSAGE
Adjunct therapy in treatment of partial seizures caused by epilepsy –
Adults: 50 mg P.O. daily for 2 weeks, followed by 100 mg daily in two divided doses for 2 weeks. Thereafter, usual maintenance dosage is 300 to 500 mg P.O. daily in two divided doses. For patients also taking valproic acid, 25 mg P.O. every other day for 2 weeks, followed by 25 mg P.O. daily for 2 weeks. Thereafter, no more than 150 mg P.O. daily in two divided doses.

ADVERSE REACTIONS
CNS: *dizziness, headache, ataxia, somnolence,* incoordination, insomnia, tremor, depression, anxiety, convulsions, irritability, speech disorder, decreased memory, aggravated reaction, concentration disturbance, sleep disorder, emotional lability, vertigo, mind racing.
CV: palpitations.
EENT: *diplopia, blurred vision,* vision abnormality, nystagmus.
GI: *nausea, vomiting,* diarrhea, dyspepsia, abdominal pain, constipation, tooth disorder, anorexia, dry mouth.
Respiratory: rhinitis, pharyngitis, cough, dyspnea.
Skin: rash, pruritus, hot flashes, alopecia, acne.
Other: dysarthria, muscle spasm, flulike syndrome, fever, infection, neck pain, malaise, chills, dysmenorrhea, vaginitis, amenorrhea.

INTERACTIONS
Carbamazepine, phenobarbital, phenytoin, primidone: decreased lamotrigine's steady-state concentrations. Monitor patient closely.
Folate inhibitors (such as cotrimoxazole, methotrexate): lamotrigine inhibits dihydrofolate reductase, an enzyme involved in folic acid synthesis. May have an additive effect. Monitor patient closely.
Valproic acid: decreases lamotrigine's clearance, which increases the drug's steady-state concentrations. Monitor patient closely for toxicity.

CONTRAINDICATIONS
Contraindicated in patients with hypersensitivity to the drug.

NURSING CONSIDERATIONS
• Use cautiously in patients with renal, hepatic, or cardiac impairment.
• Know that drug should not be discontinued abruptly because of the possibility of increased seizure frequency. Instead, drug should be tapered over at least 2 weeks.
• Be aware that lamotrigine dose should be lowered if drug is added to a multidrug regimen that includes valproate.
• Know that a lowered maintenance dosage should be used in a patient with severe renal impairment.
• Be aware that patients should be evaluated for reduction in the frequency and duration of seizures. Periodic evaluation of adjunct anticonvulsant's serum levels should be checked, as ordered.
• Inform patient that lamotrigine may cause a rash, especially in the first 6 weeks of therapy. Combination therapy of valproic acid and lamotrigine appears to be more likely to precipitate a serious rash. Although rash may resolve with continued therapy, tell patient to report it promptly to the doctor because it could be serious enough to warrant drug discontinuation.
• Warn patient not to engage in hazardous activity until drug's CNS effects are known.

---

magnesium sulfate
Pregnancy Risk Category: A

---

*Liquid form contains alcohol.
**May contain tartrazine.

Common reactions are in italics; ***life-threatening,*** in bold italics.

HOW SUPPLIED
Injection: 4%, 8%, 10%, 12.5%, 25%, 50%
Injection solution: 1% in 5% dextrose, 2% in 5% dextrose

ACTION
Unknown. May decrease acetylcholine released by nerve impulses, but its anticonvulsant mechanism is unknown.

ONSET, PEAK, DURATION
Onset occurs 1 to 2 minutes after I.V. use; 1 hour after I.M. injection. Serum levels peak almost immediately after I.V. administration, unknown after I.M. administration. Effects persist about 30 minutes after I.V. administration, 3 to 4 hours after I.M. injection.

INDICATIONS & DOSAGE
Prevention or control of seizures in preeclampsia or eclampsia –
Women: initially, 4 g I.V. in 250 ml D₅W and 4 to 5 g deep I.M. each buttock; then 4 to 5 g deep I.M. into alternate buttock q 4 hours, p.r.n. Alternatively, 4 g I.V. loading dose, followed by 1 to 2 g hourly as I.V. infusion.
Hypomagnesemia –
Adults: 1 g I.M. q 6 hours for 4 doses for mild deficiency; up to 250 mg/kg I.M. over 4 hour period for severe deficiency.
Seizures, hypertension, and encephalopathy associated with acute nephritis in children –
Children: 0.2 ml/kg of 50% solution I.M. q 4 to 6 hours, p.r.n. For severe symptoms, 100 to 200 mg/kg I.V. very slowly over 1 hour with one-half of the dose administered in first 15 to 20 minutes.. Dosage titrated according to blood magnesium levels and seizure response.
Management of paroxysmal atrial tachycardia –
Adults: 3 to 4 g I.V. over 30 seconds.

Management of life-threatening ventricular arrhythmias, such as sustained ventricular tachycardia or torsades de pointes –
Adults: 2 to 6 g I.V. over several minutes, followed by a continuous infusion of 3 to 20 mg/minute for 5 to 48 hours. Dosage and duration of therapy depend on patient response and serum magnesium levels.

ADVERSE REACTIONS
CNS: drowsiness, *depressed reflexes,* flaccid paralysis, hypothermia.
CV: *hypotension, flushing,* **circulatory collapse,** depressed cardiac function, **heart block.**
Other: diaphoresis, *respiratory paralysis,* hypocalcemia.

INTERACTIONS
Anesthetics, CNS depressants: may cause additive CNS depression. Use cautiously.
Digitalis: concomitant use may exacerbate arrhythmias. Use together cautiously.
Neuromuscular blocking agents: may cause increased neuromuscular blockade. Use cautiously.

CONTRAINDICATIONS
Parenteral administration of drug contraindicated in patients with heart block or myocardial damage.

NURSING CONSIDERATIONS
● Use cautiously in patients with impaired renal function. Also use cautiously in women who are in labor.
● If used to treat seizures, institute appropriate seizure precautions.
● **I.V. use:** If necessary, dilute to a maximum concentration of 20%. Infuse no faster than 150 mg/minute (1.5 ml/minute of a 10% solution or 0.75 ml/minute of a 20% solution). Drug is compatible with D₅W.
● Maximum infusion rate is 150 mg/minute. Rapid drip will induce uncomfortable feeling of heat.

• Monitor vital signs every 15 minutes when giving drug intravenously.
• Watch for respiratory depression and signs of heart block. Respirations should be approximately 16 breaths/minute before each dose.
• Keep I.V. calcium gluconate available to reverse magnesium intoxication; however, use cautiously in patients undergoing digitalization because of danger of arrhythmias.
• Check blood magnesium levels after repeated doses. Disappearance of knee-jerk and patellar reflexes is a sign of pending magnesium toxicity.
• Signs of hypermagnesemia begin to appear at blood levels of 4 mEq/liter.
• Monitor fluid intake and output. Urine output should be 100 ml or more in 4-hour period before each dose.
• Observe neonates for signs of magnesium toxicity, including neuromuscular or respiratory depression, when giving I.V. form of drug to toxemic mothers within 24 hours before delivery.

mephenytoin
Mesantoin

Pregnancy Risk Category: C

HOW SUPPLIED
Tablets: 100 mg

ACTION
Unknown. A hydantoin derivative that probably stabilizes neuronal membranes and limits seizure activity by either increasing efflux or decreasing influx of sodium ions across cell membranes in the motor cortex during generation of nerve impulses.

ONSET, PEAK, DURATION
Onset and duration unknown. Serum levels peak in 45 minutes to 4 hours.

INDICATIONS & DOSAGE
Tonic-clonic, simple partial, and complex partial seizures in patients refractory to less toxic anticonvulsants –
Adults: 50 to 100 mg P.O. daily. Increased by 50 to 100 mg at weekly intervals. Maintenance dosage ranges from 200 to 800 mg daily in 3 equally divided doses.
Children: initially, 50 to 100 mg P.O. daily. Increased by 50 to 100 mg at weekly intervals. Maintenance dosage ranges from 100 to 400 mg or 100 to 450 mg/m² daily in 3 equally divided doses.

ADVERSE REACTIONS
CNS: ataxia, *drowsiness,* fatigue, irritability, choreiform movements, depression, tremor, sleeplessness, dizziness (usually transient).
EENT: conjunctivitis, diplopia, nystagmus, gingival hyperplasia (with prolonged use).
GI: nausea and vomiting (with prolonged use).
Hematologic: *leukopenia, neutropenia, agranulocytosis, thrombocytopenia, pancytopenia,* eosinophilia.
Skin: *rashes, exfoliative dermatitis,* hypertrichosis, photosensitivity.
Other: edema, dysarthria, lymphadenopathy, polyarthropathy, *pulmonary fibrosis.*

INTERACTIONS
Antihistamines, chloramphenicol, cimetidine, diazepam, disulfiram, isoniazid, phenylbutazone, salicylates, sulfamethizole, valproate: increased mephenytoin activity and toxicity; monitor closely.
Diazoxide: decreased mephenytoin activity. Monitor closely.
Ethanol (with chronic use), folic acid: decreased mephenytoin activity; monitor closely.

---

*Liquid form contains alcohol.   *Common* reactions are in italics; *life-threatening,* in bold italics.
**May contain tartrazine.

CONTRAINDICATIONS
Contraindicated in patients with hydantoin hypersensitivity.

NURSING CONSIDERATIONS
• Use cautiously in patients receiving other hydantoin derivatives.
• Periodically monitor liver function studies with long-term use. Check CBC and platelet count before therapy and periodically thereafter as ordered. Alert doctor if neutrophil count becomes less than $1,600/mm^3$.
• Know that potentially life-threatening blood dyscrasias limit this drug's usefulness.
• Never withdraw drug suddenly because seizures may worsen. Call the doctor if adverse reactions develop.
• Monitor blood levels. Therapeutic blood level of mephenytoin and its active metabolite is 25 to 40 mcg/ml.
• Tell patients to notify the doctor if fever, sore throat, bleeding, or rash occurs.
• Advise patients to avoid driving or other hazardous activities that require mental alertness until drug's CNS effects are known.
• Caution patients that heavy alcohol use may diminish drug's benefits.
• This drug has been associated with photosensitivity reactions. Advise patients to use a sunblock, wear protective clothing, and avoid prolonged exposure to sunlight.
• Warn patient and parents never to stop drug abruptly.

---

mephobarbital
Mebaral
Controlled Substance Schedule IV
Pregnancy Risk Category: D

HOW SUPPLIED
Tablets: 32 mg, 50 mg, 100 mg

ACTION
Unknown. A barbiturate that probably depresses monosynaptic and polysyn-aptic transmission in the CNS and increases the threshold for seizure activity in the motor cortex. Some activity comes from phenobarbital, an active metabolite. A barbiturate.

ONSET, PEAK, DURATION
Onset occurs in 60 minutes or longer. Peak unknown. Effects persist for 10 to 12 hours.

INDICATIONS & DOSAGE
Generalized tonic-clonic or absence seizures –
Adults: 400 to 600 mg P.O. once daily or in divided doses.
Children under 5 years: 16 to 32 mg P.O. t.i.d. or q.i.d.
Children 5 and over: 32 to 64 mg P.O. t.i.d. or q.i.d.
Relief of anxiety, tension, and apprehension –
Adults: 32 to 100 mg P.O. t.i.d. or q.i.d.
Children: 1.6 to 3 mg P.O. t.i.d. or q.i.d.

ADVERSE REACTIONS
CNS: *dizziness,* headache, *hangover,* confusion, paradoxical excitation, exacerbation of existing pain, drowsiness.
CV: hypotension, bradycardia.
GI: nausea, vomiting, epigastric pain.
Hematologic: megaloblastic anemia, *agranulocytosis,* thrombocytopenia, enhanced porphyria.
Respiratory: *respiratory depression.*
Skin: urticaria, morbilliform rash, blisters, purpura, *erythema multiforme.*
Other: allergic reactions (facial edema).

INTERACTIONS
Chloramphenicol, MAO inhibitors, valproic acid: potentiated barbiturate effect. Monitor patient for increased CNS and respiratory depression.
Corticosteroids, digitoxin, doxycy-

cline, estrogens and oral contraceptives, oral anticoagulants, tricyclic antidepressants: mephobarbital may enhance the metabolism of these drugs. Monitor for decreased effect.
Ethanol or other CNS depressants, including narcotic analgesics: excessive CNS depression. Use cautiously.
Griseofulvin: decreased absorption of griseofulvin.
Rifampin: may decrease barbiturate levels. Monitor for decreased effect.

CONTRAINDICATIONS
Contraindicated in patients with barbiturate hypersensitivity or porphyria.

NURSING CONSIDERATIONS
• Use cautiously in patients with acute or chronic pain, depression, suicidal tendencies, or history of drug abuse; hepatic, renal, cardiac, or respiratory function impairment; myasthenia gravis; or myxedema. Also use cautiously in elderly or debilitated patients.
• Know that dosage should be reduced in elderly or debilitated patients because these patients may be more sensitive to barbiturates. Dosage also should be reduced for patients with impaired renal or hepatic disease.
• Never withdraw drug suddenly because seizures may worsen. Call the doctor at once if adverse reactions develop.
• Monitor phenobarbital blood levels. Therapeutic blood levels of phenobarbital are 15 to 40 mcg/ml.
• Periodically monitor CBC and BUN and creatinine levels.
• Advise patients to avoid driving or drug's other potentially hazardous activities that require mental alertness until drug's CNS effects are known.
• Advise adults with nighttime seizures to take total or largest dose at night after checking with physician.
• Warn patient and parents never to stop drug abruptly.

• Instruct patient to store in light-resistant container.
• Inform patients who use oral contraceptives that she should consider alternate birth control methods because drug may enhance contraceptive hormone metabolism and decrease its effectiveness.
• Tell patient drug suppresses REM sleep. When drug is discontinued, patient may experience increased dreaming.

---

methsuximide (mesuximide)
Celontin

Pregnancy Risk Category: NR

HOW SUPPLIED
Capsules: 150 mg, 300 mg

ACTION
Unknown. A succinimide that probably increases seizure threshold. Reduces the paroxysmal spike-and-wave pattern of absence seizures by depressing nerve transmission in the motor cortex. A succinimide derivative.

ONSET, PEAK, DURATION
Onset and duration unknown. Serum levels peak in 1 to 4 hours.

INDICATIONS & DOSAGE
Refractory absence seizures –
Adults and children: initially, 300 mg P.O. daily. Increased by 300 mg daily at weekly intervals as needed. Maximum daily dosage is 1.2 g in divided doses.

ADVERSE REACTIONS
CNS: *drowsiness, ataxia, dizziness,* irritability, nervousness, headache, insomnia, confusion, depression, aggressiveness.
EENT: blurred vision, photophobia, periorbital edema.
GI: *nausea, vomiting, anorexia,* diar-

---

rhea, weight loss, abdominal or epigastric pain.
Hematologic: eosinophilia, *aplastic anemia, leukopenia,* monocytosis, *pancytopenia.*
Skin: urticaria, pruritic and erythematous rashes.

INTERACTIONS
None significant.

CONTRAINDICATIONS
Contraindicated in patients with hypersensitivity to succinimide derivatives.

NURSING CONSIDERATIONS
• Use with extreme caution in patients with hepatic or renal dysfunction.
• Never change or withdraw drug suddenly. Abrupt withdrawal may precipitate absence seizures. Call the doctor immediately if adverse reactions develop.
• Check CBC, urinalysis, and liver function tests periodically as ordered.
• Monitor blood levels closely. Therapeutic serum level is 10 to 40 mcg/ml.
• Advise patients to avoid driving or other hazardous activities that require mental alertness until drug's CNS effects are known.
• Tell patients to call the doctor promptly if lupuslike syndrome develops.
• Warn patient and parents never to stop drug abruptly.
• Caution patients that this drug may color urine pink or brown.

---

phenacemide
(phenacetylcarbamide)
Phenurone

Pregnancy Risk Category: D

HOW SUPPLIED
Tablets: 500 mg

ACTION
Unknown. A hydantoin derivative that probably stabilizes neuronal membranes and limits seizure activity by either increasing efflux or decreasing influx of sodium ions across cell membranes in the motor cortex during generation of nerve impulses. Hydantoin derivative.

ONSET, PEAK, DURATION
Onset unknown. Serum levels peak 1 to 2 hours after a dose. Effects persist for 5 hours.

INDICATIONS & DOSAGE
Severe epilepsy (particularly mixed forms of complex partial seizures) refractory to other drugs –
Adults: 500 mg P.O. t.i.d. Increased by 500 mg P.O. daily at weekly intervals up to a maximum of 5 g daily.
Children 5 to 10 years: 250 mg P.O. t.i.d. Increased by 250 mg daily at weekly intervals, up to a maximum of 2.5 g daily.

ADVERSE REACTIONS
CNS: *drowsiness,* dizziness, insomnia, headache, paresthesia, *depression, suicidal tendencies,* aggressiveness.
GI: *anorexia,* weight loss.
GU: nephritis with marked albuminuria.
Hematologic: *aplastic anemia, agranulocytosis,* leukopenia.
Hepatic: hepatitis, jaundice.
Skin: rashes.

INTERACTIONS
Ethotoin: causes paranoia. Use together cautiously.
Other anticonvulsants: enhanced risk of toxicity.

CONTRAINDICATIONS
Contraindicated in patients with hypersensitivity or severe blood dyscrasias and in patients achieving satisfac-

---

tory seizure control with other anti-convulsants.

NURSING CONSIDERATIONS
• Use cautiously in patients with hepatic dysfunction, history of personality disturbances, or allergies to other anticonvulsants.
• Know that drug is extremely toxic.
• Check liver function tests, CBCs, and urinalyses before and at monthly intervals during therapy as ordered.
• Notify the doctor if the patient develops jaundice or other signs of hepatitis, abnormal urinary findings, or WBC count below 4,000/mm^3.
• When phenacemide replaces another anticonvulsant, increase phenacemide dosage slowly while slowly decreasing the dosage of the drug being discontinued as ordered to maintain adequate seizure control.
• Never withdraw drug suddenly. Call the doctor at once if adverse reactions develop.
• Tell patients to report sore throat, easy bruising, bleeding, or fever to the doctor immediately.
• Warn patients to avoid activities that require alertness or good psychomotor coordination until drug's CNS effects are known.
• Warn patients and parents never to stop drug abruptly.
• Tell the patient's family to watch for personality or psychological changes and report them to the doctor at once.

phenobarbital
(phenobarbitone)
Ancalixir†, Barbita, Solfoton

phenobarbital sodium
(phenobarbitone sodium)
Luminal Sodium

Controlled Substance Schedule IV
Pregnancy Risk Category: D

HOW SUPPLIED
Tablets: 15 mg, 16 mg, 30 mg, 32 mg, 60 mg, 65 mg, 100 mg
Capsules: 16 mg
Elixir*: 15 mg/5 ml, 20 mg/5 ml
Injection: 30 mg/ml, 60 mg/ml, 65 mg/ml, 130 mg/ml

ACTION
Unknown. A barbiturate that probably depresses monosynaptic and polysynaptic transmission in the CNS and increases the threshold for seizure activity in the motor cortex. As a sedative, probably interferes with transmission of impulses from the thalamus to the cortex of the brain.

ONSET, PEAK, DURATION
Onset occurs in 60 minutes or longer. Peak concentration levels are reached in 8 to 12 hours. Effects persist for as long as 10 to 12 hours.

INDICATIONS & DOSAGE
All forms of epilepsy, febrile seizures in children –
Adults: 60 to 200 mg P.O. daily, in divided dose t.i.d. or as single dose h.s.
Children: 3 to 6 mg/kg P.O. daily, usually divided q 12 hours. It can, however, be administered once daily, usually h.s.
Status epilepticus –
Adults: 200 to 600 mg I.V.
Children: 100 to 400 mg I.V. Do not exceed 50 mg/minute.
Sedation –
Adults: 30 to 120 mg P.O. daily in two or three divided doses.
Children: 3 to 5 mg/kg P.O. daily in divided doses t.i.d.
Insomnia –
Adults: 100 to 200 mg P.O. or I.M. h.s.
Preoperative sedation –
Adults: 100 to 200 mg I.M. 60 to 90 minutes before surgery.
Children: 16 to 100 mg I.M. 60 to 90 minutes before surgery.

---

*Liquid form contains alcohol.   *Common* reactions are in italics; *life-threatening*, in bold italics.
**May contain tartrazine.

ADVERSE REACTIONS
CNS: *drowsiness, lethargy, hangover,* paradoxical excitement in elderly patients.
CV: bradycardia, hypotension.
GI: nausea, vomiting.
Hematologic: exacerbation of porphyria.
Respiratory: *respiratory depression.*
Skin: rash, *erythema multiforme, Stevens-Johnson syndrome,* urticaria; pain, swelling, thrombophlebitis, necrosis, nerve injury at injection site.
Other: *angioedema.*

INTERACTIONS
Chloramphenicol, MAO inhibitors, valproic acid: potentiated barbiturate effect. Monitor patient for increased CNS and respiratory depression.
Corticosteroids, digitoxin, doxycycline, estrogens and oral contraceptives, oral anticoagulants, tricyclic antidepressants: phenobarbital may enhance the metabolism of these drugs. Monitor for decreased effect.
Diazepam: increased effects of both drugs. Use together cautiously.
Ethanol or other CNS depressants, including narcotic analgesics: excessive CNS depression. Use cautiously.
Griseofulvin: decreased absorption of griseofulvin.
Mephobarbital, primidone: excessive phenobarbital blood levels; monitor closely.
Rifampin: may decrease barbiturate levels. Monitor for decreased effect.
Valproic acid: increased phenobarbital levels. Monitor for toxicity.

CONTRAINDICATIONS
Contraindicated in patients with barbiturate hypersensitivity, history of manifest or latent porphyria, hepatic dysfunction, respiratory disease with dyspnea or obstruction, and nephritis.

NURSING CONSIDERATIONS
• Use cautiously in patients with acute or chronic pain, depression, suicidal tendencies, history of drug abuse, blood pressure alterations, cardiovascular disease, shock, uremia, and in elderly or debilitated patients.
• **I.V. use:** Know that I.V. injection is reserved for emergency treatment and give slowly under close supervision. Monitor respirations closely. When administering, do not give more than 60 mg/minute. Have resuscitation equipment available.
• Do not mix parenteral form with acidic solutions; precipitation may result.
• Do not use injectable solution if it contains a precipitate.
• Give I.M. injection deeply. Superficial injection may cause pain, sterile abscess, and tissue sloughing.
• Know that elderly patients are more sensitive to the drug's effects. Monitor closely.
• Watch for signs of barbiturate toxicity: coma, asthmatic breathing, cyanosis, clammy skin, and hypotension. Overdose can be fatal.
• Monitor blood levels closely. Therapeutic blood levels are 15 to 40 mcg/ ml.
• Don't stop drug abruptly because seizures may worsen. Call the doctor immediately if adverse reactions develop.
• Make sure patients are aware that phenobarbital is available in different milligram strengths and sizes. Advise patient to check prescription and refills closely.
• Inform patient that full therapeutic effects not seen for 2 to 3 weeks, except when loading dose is used.
• Advise patients to avoid driving or other potentially hazardous activities that require mental alertness until drug's CNS effects are known.
• Warn patient and parents not to discontinue drug abruptly.
• Tell patients using oral contraceptives that she should consider alternate birth control methods because drug may enhance contraceptive hor-

mone metabolism and decrease its effect.

phensuximide
Milontin

Pregnancy Risk Category: NR

HOW SUPPLIED
Capsules: 500 mg

ACTION
Unknown. A succinimide that probably increases seizure threshold. Reduces the paroxysmal spike-and-wave pattern of absence seizures by depressing nerve transmission in the motor cortex. A succinimide derivative.

ONSET, PEAK, DURATION
Onset and duration unknown. Serum levels peak in 1 to 4 hours.

INDICATIONS & DOSAGE
Absence seizures –
Adults and children: 500 mg to 1 g P.O. b.i.d. or t.i.d.

ADVERSE REACTIONS
CNS: muscular weakness, *drowsiness,* dizziness, ataxia, headache.
GI: *nausea, vomiting,* anorexia.
GU: urinary frequency, renal damage, hematuria.
Hematologic: transient leukopenia, *aplastic anemia, pancytopenia, agranulocytosis.*
Skin: pruritus, eruptions, erythema.
Other: lupuslike syndrome.

INTERACTIONS
None significant.

CONTRAINDICATIONS
Contraindicated in patients with hypersensitivity to succinimide derivatives.

NURSING CONSIDERATIONS
• Use with extreme caution in patients with hepatic or renal disease.
• Monitor blood levels as ordered. Therapeutic blood level is 40 to 80 mcg/ml.
• Check CBC every 3 to 4 months; urinalysis and liver function tests every 6 months as ordered.
• Never withdraw drug suddenly. Abrupt withdrawal may precipitate absence seizures. Call the doctor immediately if adverse reactions develop.
• Advise patients to avoid driving or other potentially hazardous activities that require mental alertness until drug's CNS effects are known.
• Warn patient and parents not to stop drug therapy suddenly.
• Tell patients to report lupuslike symptoms immediately.
• Caution patients that this drug may color urine pink, red, or reddish brown.

phenytoin
(diphenylhydantoin)
Dilantin, Dilantin-30 Pediatric, Dilantin-125, Dilantin Infatabs

phenytoin sodium
Dilantin, Phenytex

phenytoin sodium
(extended)
Dilantin Kapseals

Pregnancy Risk Category: NR

HOW SUPPLIED
phenytoin
Tablets (chewable): 50 mg
Oral suspension: 30 mg/5 ml, 125 mg/5 ml
phenytoin sodium
Capsules: 30 mg (27.6-mg base), 100 mg (92-mg base)
Injection: 50 mg/ml (46-mg base)

---

*Liquid form contains alcohol.   *Common* reactions are in italics; *life-threatening,* in bold italics.
**May contain tartrazine.

phenytoin sodium (extended)
Capsules: 30 mg (27.6-mg base), 100 mg (92-mg base)

ACTION
Unknown. A hydantoin derivative that probably stabilizes neuronal membranes and limits seizure activity by either increasing efflux or decreasing influx of sodium ions across cell membranes in the motor cortex during generation of nerve impulses.

ONSET, PEAK, DURATION
Onset immediate with I.V. administration, unknown for other routes. Peak levels occur 1 to 2 hours after I.V. injection, 1½ to 3 hours after tablets or oral solution, 4 to 12 hours after extended capsules. Duration unknown.

INDICATIONS & DOSAGE
Control of tonic-clonic (grand mal) and complex partial (temporal lobe) seizures –
Adults: highly individualized. Initially, 100 mg P.O. t.i.d., increased in increments of 100 mg P.O. every 2 to 4 weeks until desired response is obtained. Usual range is 300 to 600 mg daily. If patient stabilized with extended-release capsules, once-daily dosing with 300 mg extended-release capsules possible as an alternative.
Children: 5 mg/kg or 250 mg/m² P.O. daily b.i.d. or t.i.d. Maximum daily dosage is 300 mg.
For patient requiring a loading dose –
Adults: initially, 1 g P.O. daily divided into 3 doses and administered at 2-hour intervals. Alternatively, 10 to 15 mg/kg I.V. at a rate not exceeding 50 mg/minute. Normal maintenance dosage instituted 24 hours later.
Children: 5 mg/kg/day P.O. in 2 or 3 equally divided doses with subsequent dosage individualized to a maximum of 300 mg daily.
Prevention and treatment of seizures occurring during neurosurgery –
Adults: 100 to 200 mg I.M. q 4 hours during surgery and continued during the postoperative period.
Status epilepticus –
Adults: loading dose of 10 to 15 mg/kg I.V. (1 to 1.5 g may be needed) at a rate not exceeding 50 mg/minute followed by maintenance doses of 100 mg P.O. or I.V. q 6 to 8 hours.
Children: loading dose of 15 to 20 mg/kg I.V., at a rate not exceeding 1 to 3 mg/kg/min followed by highly individualized maintenance dosages.

ADVERSE REACTIONS
CNS: *ataxia, slurred speech, confusion,* dizziness, insomnia, nervousness, twitching, headache.
CV: hypotension, *ventricular fibrillation.*
EENT: *nystagmus, diplopia,* blurred vision, *gingival hyperplasia* (especially in children).
GI: *nausea, vomiting.*
Hematologic: *thrombocytopenia, leukopenia, agranulocytosis, pancytopenia,* macrocythemia, megaloblastic anemia.
Hepatic: *toxic hepatitis.*
Skin: scarlatiniform or morbilliform rash; bullous, *exfoliative,* or purpuric dermatitis; *Stevens-Johnson syndrome;* lupus erythematosus; *hirsutism; toxic epidermal necrolysis;* photosensitivity; pain, necrosis, and inflammation at injection site; discoloration of skin ("purple glove syndrome") if given by I.V. push in back of hand.
Other: periarteritis nodosa, lymphadenopathy, hyperglycemia, osteomalacia, hypertrichosis.

INTERACTIONS
Amiodarone, antihistamines, chloramphenicol, cimetidine, cycloserine, diazepam, disulfiram, influenza vaccine, isoniazid, phenylbutazone, salicylates, sulfamethizole, valproate: monitor for increased phenytoin activity and toxicity.

Dexamethasone, diazoxide, ethanol (with chronic use), folic acid: decreased phenytoin activity; monitor closely.

Oral tube feedings with Osmolite or Isocal: may interfere with absorption of oral phenytoin. Schedule feedings as far as possible from drug administration.

CONTRAINDICATIONS

Contraindicated in patients with hydantoin hypersensitivity, sinus bradycardia, SA block, second- or third-degree AV block, or Adams-Stokes syndrome.

NURSING CONSIDERATIONS

• Use cautiously in patients with hepatic dysfunction, hypotension, myocardial insufficiency, diabetes, and respiratory depression; in elderly or debilitated patients; and in patients receiving other hydantoin derivatives.

• Be aware elderly patients tend to metabolize phenytoin slowly and may require lower dosages.

• Know that phenytoin requirements usually increase during pregnancy.

• Suspension available as 30 mg/5 ml or 125 mg/5 ml. Read label carefully.

• Know that therapy with phenytoin may cause altered laboratory test results, including reduced serum protein-bound iodine and free thyroxine levels without clinical signs of hypothyroidism; a slight decrease in urinary 17-hydroxysteroid and 17-ketosteroid levels; increased urine 6-ß hydroxycortisol excretion and serum levels of alkaline phosphatase or γ-glutamyltransferase; and decreased values for dexamethasone suppression or metyrapone tests.

• Shake suspension well before each dose.

• Use only clear solution for injection. A slight yellow color is acceptable. Don't refrigerate.

• **I.V. use:** Administer slowly (50 mg/ minute) as I.V. bolus. If giving as an infusion, don't mix drug with D$_5$W because it will precipitate. Clear I.V. tubing first with 0.9% sodium chloride solution. Never use cloudy solution. May mix with 0.9% sodium chloride solution if necessary and give as an infusion over 30 to 60 minutes when possible. Infusion must begin within 1 hour after preparation and should run through an in-line filter. Discard 4 hours after preparation.

• Check patency of I.V. catheter before administering. Extravasation has caused severe local tissue damage.

• Avoid administering phenytoin by I.V. push into veins on the back of the hand to avoid discoloration known as purple glove syndrome. Inject into larger veins or central venous catheter if available.

• Check vital signs, blood pressure, and ECG during I.V. administration.

• Do not give I.M. unless dosage adjustments are made. Drug may precipitate at injection site, cause pain, and be erratically absorbed.

• Divided doses given with or after meals may decrease adverse GI reactions.

• Be aware that drug should be discontinued if rash appears. If rash is scarlatiniform or morbilliform, drug may be resumed after rash clears. If rash reappears, therapy should be discontinued. If rash is exfoliative, purpuric, or bullous, drug will not be resumed.

• Don't withdraw drug suddenly because seizures may worsen. Call the doctor at once if adverse reactions develop.

• Monitor blood levels as ordered. Therapeutic phenytoin blood level is 10 to 20 mcg/ml.

• Monitor CBC and serum calcium level every 6 months, and periodically monitor hepatic function as ordered. If megaloblastic anemia is evident, the doctor may order folic acid and vitamin B$_{12}$.

---

*Liquid form contains alcohol.
**May contain tartrazine.

Common reactions are in italics; *life-threatening,* in bold italics.

- If using to treat seizures, take appropriate precautions.
- Mononucleosis may decrease phenytoin levels. Monitor for increased seizure activity.
- Advise patients to avoid driving or other potentially hazardous activities that require mental alertness until drug's CNS effects are known.
- Advise patient not to change brands or dosage forms once stabilized on therapy.
- Dilantin capsules is the only oral form that can be given once daily. Toxic levels may result if any other brand or form is given once daily. Dilantin brand tablets and oral suspension should not be taken once daily.
- Warn patient and parents not to stop drug abruptly.
- Stress importance of good oral hygiene and regular dental examinations. Gingivectomy may be necessary periodically if dental hygiene is poor.
- Caution patients that this drug may color urine pink, red, or reddish brown.
- Inform patient heavy alcohol use may diminish drug's benefits.

primidone

Apo-Primidone†, Mysoline, PMS-Primidone†, Sertan†

Pregnancy Risk Category: NR

HOW SUPPLIED
Tablets: 50 mg, 250 mg
Oral suspension: 250 mg/5 ml

ACTION
Unknown, but some activity may be caused by phenylethylmalonamide (PEMA) and phenobarbital, which are active metabolites.

ONSET, PEAK, DURATION
Onset and duration unknown. Serum levels peak in 3 to 4 hours.

INDICATIONS & DOSAGE
Tonic-clonic, complex partial, and simple partial seizures –
Adults and children 8 years and over: initially, 100 to 125 mg P.O. h.s. on days 1 to 3; then 100 to 125 mg P.O. b.i.d. on days 4 to 6; then 100 to 125 mg P.O. on days 7 to 9; followed by maintenance dosage of 250 mg P.O. t.i.d. Maintenance dosage increased to 250 mg q.i.d. if needed.
Children under 8 years: initially, 50 mg P.O. h.s., then 50 mg P.O. b.i.d., then 100 mg P.O. b.i.d. followed by maintenance dosage of 125 to 250 mg P.O. t.i.d.

ADVERSE REACTIONS
CNS: *drowsiness, ataxia,* emotional disturbances, vertigo, hyperirritability, fatigue.
EENT: *diplopia,* nystagmus, edema of the eyelids.
GI: anorexia, *nausea, vomiting,* thirst.
GU: impotence, polyuria.
Hematologic: leukopenia, eosinophilia.
Respiratory: *respiratory depression.*
Skin: morbilliform rash, alopecia.
Other: edema.

INTERACTIONS
Carbamazepine: increased primidone levels. Observe for toxicity.
Phenytoin: stimulated conversion of primidone to phenobarbital. Observe for increased phenobarbital effect.

CONTRAINDICATIONS
Contraindicated in patients with phenobarbital hypersensitivity or porphyria.

NURSING CONSIDERATIONS
- Shake liquid suspension well.
- Don't withdraw drug suddenly because seizures may worsen. Call the doctor immediately if adverse reactions develop.

• Monitor blood levels as ordered. Therapeutic blood level of primidone is 5 to 12 mcg/ml. Therapeutic blood level of phenobarbital is 15 to 40 mcg/ml.
• Monitor CBC and routine blood chemistry every 6 months, as ordered.
• Advise patients to avoid driving or other potentially hazardous activities that require mental alertness until drug's CNS effects are known.
• Warn patient and parents not to stop drug therapy suddenly.
• Tell patient full therapeutic response may take 2 weeks or more.

trimethadione
Tridione, Tridione Dulcets

Pregnancy Risk Category: NR

HOW SUPPLIED
Capsules: 300 mg
Tablets (chewable): 150 mg
Oral solution: 200 mg/5 ml

ACTION
Raises the threshold for cortical seizure but does not modify seizure pattern. Decreases projection of focal activity and reduces both repetitive spinal-cord transmission and spike-and-wave patterns of absence (petit mal) seizures. An oxazolidinedione derivative.

ONSET, PEAK, DURATION
Unknown.

INDICATIONS & DOSAGE
Refractory absence seizures –
Adults and children over 13 years: initially, 300 mg P.O. t.i.d. May increase by 300 mg P.O. daily at weekly intervals to a maximum of 600 mg P.O. q.i.d.
Children: 13 mg/kg P.O. t.i.d. or 335 mg/m² P.O. t.i.d.; alternatively, give according to age.

Children under 2 years: 100 mg P.O. t.i.d.
Children 2 to 6 years: 200 mg P.O. t.i.d.
Children 6 to 13 years: 300 mg P.O. t.i.d.

ADVERSE REACTIONS
CNS: *drowsiness,* fatigue, *malaise,* insomnia, dizziness, headache, paresthesia, irritability.
CV: hypertension, hypotension.
EENT: *day blindness (hemeralopia),* diplopia, photophobia, epistaxis, retinal hemorrhage.
GI: nausea, vomiting, anorexia, abdominal pain, bleeding gums.
GU: nephrosis, albuminuria, vaginal bleeding.
Hematologic: *neutropenia, leukopenia,* eosinophilia, *thrombocytopenia, pancytopenia, agranulocytosis, hypoplastic and aplastic anemia.*
Hepatic: abnormal liver function test results.
Skin: acneiform and morbilliform rash, *exfoliative dermatitis, erythema multiforme,* petechiae, alopecia, photosensitivity.
Other: lymphadenopathy, lupuslike syndrome, myasthenic syndrome.

INTERACTIONS
None significant.

CONTRAINDICATIONS
Contraindicated in patients with paramethadione and trimethadione hypersensitivity, severe blood dyscrasia, or hepatic dysfunction.

NURSING CONSIDERATIONS
• Use with extreme caution in patients with retinal and optic nerve diseases.
• Check CBC, hepatic function, and urinalysis before starting therapy and monthly thereafter as ordered. Notify doctor if neutrophil count falls below 2,500/mm³ because drug should be stopped.

---

*Liquid form contains alcohol.   *Common* reactions are in italics; *life-threatening,* in bold italics.
**May contain tartrazine.

- Watch for impending toxicity; may precipitate tonic-clonic seizure.
- Notify doctor if scotomata or rash develops; drug should be discontinued.
- Don't withdraw drug suddenly. Abrupt withdrawal may precipitate absence seizures. Call doctor immediately if adverse reactions develop.
- Warn patients to report skin rash, alopecia, sore throat, fever, bruises, or epistaxis to the doctor immediately.
- Advise patients to avoid driving or other potentially hazardous activities that require mental alertness until drug's CNS effects are known.
- Warn patient and parents not to stop drug therapy abruptly.
- Advise patients to use a sunblock, wear protective clothing, and avoid prolonged exposure to sunlight.
- Suggest sunglasses if bright light blurs the patient's vision. Tell patient to notify the doctor if this occurs.

---

valproate sodium
Depakene Syrup, Epilim‡, Myproic Acid Syrup

valproic acid
Depakene, Myproic Acid

divalproex sodium
Depakote, Depakote Sprinkle, Epival†, Valcote‡

Pregnancy Risk Category: D

HOW SUPPLIED
valproate sodium
Syrup: 250 mg/ml
valproic acid
Tablets (enteric-coated): 200 mg‡, 500 mg‡
Crushable tablets: 100 mg‡
Capsules: 250 mg
Syrup: 200 mg/5 ml‡
divalproex sodium
Capsules (delayed-release): 125 mg
Tablets (enteric-coated): 125 mg, 250 mg, 500 mg

ACTION
Unknown. Probably increases brain levels of gamma-aminobutyric acid, which transmits inhibitory nerve impulses in the CNS.

ONSET, PEAK, DURATION
Onset and duration unknown. Serum levels peak within 1 to 4 hours after capsules or syrup; 3 to 4 hours after tablets and delayed-release capsules.

INDICATIONS & DOSAGE
Simple and complex absence seizures, mixed seizure types (including absence seizures) –
Adults and children: initially, 15 mg/kg P.O. daily; then increased by 5 to 10 mg/kg daily at weekly intervals up to maximum of 60 mg/kg daily. When dosage exceeds 250 mg daily, drug should be equally divided into 2 or more divided doses.

ADVERSE REACTIONS
Because drug usually is used in combination with other anticonvulsants, adverse reactions reported may not be caused by valproic acid alone.
CNS: *sedation,* emotional upset, depression, psychosis, aggressiveness, hyperactivity, behavioral deterioration, muscle weakness, tremor.
EENT: stomatitis.
GI: *nausea, vomiting, indigestion,* diarrhea, abdominal cramps, constipation, increased appetite and weight gain, anorexia, *pancreatitis. (Note:* lower incidence of GI effects occur with divalproex sodium.)
Hematologic: inhibited platelet aggregation, thrombocytopenia, increased bleeding time.
Hepatic: *elevated liver enzymes, toxic hepatitis.*
Other: alopecia, elevated serum ammonia level.

INTERACTIONS
Aspirin, chlorpromazine, cimetidine: May cause valproic acid toxicity. Use

---

together cautiously and monitor blood levels.

Ethanol: excessive CNS depression. Avoid concomitant use.

Phenobarbital: increased phenobarbital levels.

Phenytoin: increased or decreased phenytoin levels.

CONTRAINDICATIONS
Contraindicated in patients with hypersensitivity.

NURSING CONSIDERATIONS
• Use with extreme caution in patients with history of hepatic dysfunction.

• Monitor liver function studies, platelet counts, and PT before starting drug and periodically thereafter as ordered.

• Don't administer syrup to patients who need sodium restriction. Check with the doctor.

• Never withdraw the drug suddenly because sudden withdrawal may worsen seizures. Call the doctor at once if adverse reactions develop.

• Be aware serious or fatal hepatotoxicity may follow nonspecific symptoms, such as malaise, fever, and lethargy. Notify doctor at once as drug will need to be discontinued in the presence of suspected or apparent substantial hepatic dysfunction.

• Know that patients at high risk for developing hepatotoxicity include congenital metabolic disoders, mental retardation, children under 2, presence of organic brain disease, and in those taking multiple anticonvulsants.

• Notify doctor if tremors occur. May need to reduce dosage if tremors occur.

• Monitor blood levels as ordered. Therapeutic blood level is 50 to 100 mcg/ml.

• Know that drug may produce false-positive test results for ketones in urine.

• To reduce adverse GI effects, tell patient this drug may be taken with food or milk.

• Advise patients not to chew capsules; irritation of mouth and throat may result.

• Tell patient and parents syrup shouldn't be mixed with carbonated beverages; may be irritating to mouth and throat.

• Tell patient and parents to keep out of children's reach.

• Warn patient and parents not to stop drug therapy abruptly.

• Advise patients to avoid driving or other potentially hazardous activities that require mental alertness until drug's CNS effects are known.

---

*Liquid form contains alcohol.   *Common* reactions are in italics; ***life-threatening***, in bold italics.
**May contain tartrazine.

amitriptyline hydrochloride *Elavil*
amitriptyline pamoate
amoxapine
bupropion hydrochloride
clomipramine hydrochloride
desipramine hydrochloride
doxepin hydrochloride
fluoxetine hydrochloride
imipramine hydrochloride
imipramine pamoate
isocarboxazid
maprotiline hydrochloride
nefazodone hydrochloride
nortriptyline hydrochloride
paroxetine hydrochloride
phenelzine sulfate
protriptyline hydrochloride
sertraline hydrochloride
tranylcypromine sulfate
trazodone hydrochloride
trimipramine maleate
venlafaxine hydrochloride

COMBINATION PRODUCTS
ETRAFON: perphenazine 2 mg and
amitriptyline hydrochloride 25 mg.
ETRAFON 2-10: perphenazine 2 mg
and amitriptyline hydrochloride 10
mg.
ETRAFON-A: perphenazine 4 mg and
amitriptyline hydrochloride 10 mg.
ETRAFON-FORTE: perphenazine 4 mg
and amitriptyline hydrochloride 25
mg.
LIMBITROL DS: chlordiazepoxide 10
mg and amitriptyline hydrochloride
25 mg.
TRIAVIL 2-10, TRIAVIL 4-10, TRIA-
VIL 2-25, TRIAVIL 4-25 are products
identical to the Etrafon products
listed above. Triavil is also available
as TRIAVIL 4-50 (perphenazine 4 mg
and amitriptyline hydrochloride 50
mg).

amitriptyline hydrochloride
Apo-Amitriptyline†, Elavil, Emitrip,
Endep, Enovil, Levate†,
Novotriptyn†, PMS-Amitriptyline,
Tryptanol‡

amitriptyline pamoate
Elavil†

Pregnancy Risk Category: NR

HOW SUPPLIED
amitriptyline hydrochloride
Tablets: 10 mg, 25 mg, 50 mg, 75 mg,
100 mg, 150 mg
Injection: 10 mg/ml
amitriptyline pamoate
Syrup: 10 mg/5 ml

ACTION
Unknown but a tricyclic antidepressant (TCA) increases the amount of
norepinephrine, serotonin, or both in
the CNS by blocking their reuptake by
the presynaptic neurons.

ONSET, PEAK, DURATION
Onset unknown although thought to
take several weeks. Serum levels peak
in 2 to 12 hours. Duration unknown.

INDICATIONS & DOSAGE
Depression –
Adults: 50 to 100 mg P.O. h.s., increasing to 150 mg daily; maximum
dosage is 300 mg daily, if needed. Or
20 to 30 mg I.M. q.i.d.
Elderly patients and adolescents: 10
mg P.O. t.i.d. and 20 mg h.s. daily.

ADVERSE REACTIONS
CNS: *drowsiness, dizziness,* excitation, tremors, weakness, confusion,
headache, nervousness, EEG alterations, *seizures,* extrapyramidal reactions.

CV: *orthostatic hypotension, tachycardia, ECG changes,* hypertension.
EENT: *blurred vision,* tinnitus, mydriasis.
GI: *dry mouth, constipation,* nausea, vomiting, anorexia, paralytic ileus.
GU: *urine retention.*
Skin: rash, urticaria, photosensitivity.
Other: *diaphoresis,* hypersensitivity reaction.
After abrupt withdrawal of long-term therapy: nausea, headache, malaise (does not indicate addiction).

INTERACTIONS
Barbiturates, CNS depressants, ethanol: enhanced CNS depression. Avoid concomitant use.
Cimetidine, methylphenidate: increased TCA blood levels. Monitor for enhanced antidepressant effect.
Epinephrine, norepinephrine: increased hypertensive effect. Use with caution.
MAO inhibitors: may cause severe excitation, hyperpyrexia, or seizures, usually with high dosage. Use with caution.

CONTRAINDICATIONS
Contraindicated during acute recovery phase of MI, in patients with hypersensitivity, and in patients who have received an MAO inhibitor within the past 14 days.

NURSING CONSIDERATIONS
• Use cautiously in patients with history of seizures, urine retention, angle-closure glaucoma, or increased intraocular pressure; in those with hyperthyroidism, CV disease, diabetes, or impaired liver function; and in those receiving thyroid medications.
• Amitriptyline has strong anticholinergic effects and is one of the most sedating TCAs. Be aware that anticholinergic effects have a rapid onset even though therapeutic effect is delayed for weeks.

• If signs of psychosis occur or increase, expect doctor to reduce dosage. Record mood changes. Monitor patients for suicidal tendencies, and allow them only a minimum supply of the drug.
• Because hypertensive episodes have occurred during surgery in patients receiving TCAs, be aware drug should be gradually discontinued several days before surgery.
• Do not withdraw drug abruptly.
• Check for urine retention and constipation. Increase fluids and suggest stool softener or high-fiber diet as needed.
• Advise patients to take full dose h.s., but warn them of possible morning orthostatic hypotension.
• Tell patients to avoid alcohol while taking this drug.
• Warn patients to avoid activities that require alertness and good psychomotor coordination until CNS effects of drug are known. Drowsiness and dizziness usually subside after a few weeks.
• Advise patients to consult their doctors before taking any other prescription or OTC medications.
• Tell patient dry mouth may be relieved with sugarless hard candy or gum. Saliva substitutes may be necessary.
• To prevent photosensitivity reactions, advise patients to use a sunblock, wear protective clothing, and avoid prolonged exposure to strong sunlight.
• Warn patient not to stop drug therapy rapidly.

---

amoxapine
Asendin
Pregnancy Risk Category: C

HOW SUPPLIED
Tablets: 25 mg, 50 mg, 100 mg, 150 mg

---

*Liquid form contains alcohol.
**May contain tartrazine.
Common reactions are in italics; **life-threatening,** in bold italics.

ACTION
Unknown but a tricyclic antidepressant (TCA) that increases the amount of norepinephrine, serotonin, or both in the CNS by blocking their reuptake by the presynaptic neurons.

ONSET, PEAK, DURATION
Onset thought to occur in 2 to 4 weeks. Serum levels peak in about 90 minutes. Duration unknown.

INDICATIONS & DOSAGE
Depression –
Adults: initially, 50 mg P.O. b.i.d. or t.i.d. Increased to 100 mg b.i.d. or t.i.d. on third day of treatment if tolerated. Increases above 300 mg daily are made only if 300 mg daily has been ineffective during a trial period of at least 2 weeks. When effective dosage is established, entire dosage (not to exceed 300 mg) may be given h.s.

ADVERSE REACTIONS
CNS: *drowsiness, dizziness,* excitation, tremors, weakness, confusion, headache, nervousness, *tardive dyskinesia* (especially in elderly women); EEG changes, *seizures,* extrapyramidal reactions (rare), *neuroleptic malignant syndrome* (high fever, tachycardia, tachypnea, profuse diaphoresis).
CV: *orthostatic hypotension, tachycardia, ECG changes,* hypertension.
EENT: *blurred vision,* tinnitus, mydriasis.
GI: *dry mouth, constipation,* nausea, vomiting, anorexia, paralytic ileus.
GU: *urine retention, acute renal failure* (with overdose).
Skin: rash, urticaria, photosensitivity.
Other: *diaphoresis,* weight gain and craving for sweets, hypersensitivity reaction.
After abrupt withdrawal of long-term therapy: nausea, headache, malaise (does not indicate addiction).

INTERACTIONS
Barbiturates: decreased TCA blood levels. Monitor for decreased antidepressant effect.
Cimetidine, methylphenidate, oral contraceptives: may increase amoxapine serum levels. Monitor for increased adverse effects.
Clonidine, epinephrine, norepinephrine: increased hypertensive effect. Use with caution.
CNS depressants, ethanol: enhanced CNS depression. Avoid concomitant use.
MAO inhibitors: may cause severe excitation, hyperpyrexia, or seizures, usually with high dosage. Use with caution.

CONTRAINDICATIONS
Contraindicated in patients with hypersensitivity, during acute recovery phase of MI, and in patients who have received an MAO inhibitor within the past 14 days.

NURSING CONSIDERATIONS
• Use cautiously in patients with history of urine retention, angle-closure glaucoma, or increased intraocular pressure, as well as patients with CV disease. Use with extreme caution in patients with history of convulsive disorders or those with overt or latent seizure disorders.
• Be aware that dosage should be reduced in elderly or debilitated persons and adolescents.
• Do not withdraw drug abruptly.
• Because hypertensive episodes have occurred during surgery in patients receiving TCAs, be aware that drug should be gradually discontinued several days before surgery.
• Expect delay of 2 weeks or more before noticeable effect. Full effect may take 4 weeks or more. However, know that adverse anticholinergic effects can occur rapidly.
• If signs of psychosis occur or increase, expect doctor to reduce dos-

age. Record mood changes. Monitor patients for suicidal tendencies, and allow them only a minimum supply of the drug.

• Monitor for signs and symptoms of tardive dyskinesia, especially in elderly women.

• Amoxapine therapy has been associated with neuroleptic malignant syndrome, a rare but life-threatening syndrome usually seen with phenothiazines. Discontinue drug immediately and institute appropriate therapy if symptoms occur.

• Relieve dry mouth with sugarless hard candy or gum. Saliva substitutes may be necessary.

• Check for urine retention and constipation. Increase fluids to lessen constipation. Suggest stool softener or high-fiber diet, if needed.

• Whenever possible, tell patient to take full dose at bedtime.

• Warn patient not to stop drug therapy abruptly.

• Warn patient to avoid activities that require alertness and good psychomotor coordination until CNS effects of the drug are known. Drowsiness and dizziness usually subside after first few weeks.

• Some patients may experience photosensitivity reactions. Advise the patient to use a sunblock, wear protective clothing, and avoid prolonged exposure to strong sunlight.

---

bupropion hydrochloride
Wellbutrin

Pregnancy Risk Category: B

HOW SUPPLIED
Tablets: 75 mg, 100 mg

ACTION
Unknown. Bupropion is not a tricyclic antidepressant, does not inhibit MAO, and is a weak inhibitor of norepinephrine, dopamine, and serotonin reuptake.

ONSET, PEAK, DURATION
Onset occurs in 1 to 3 weeks. Serum levels peak within 2 hours. Duration unknown.

INDICATIONS & DOSAGE
Depression –
Adults: initially, 100 mg P.O. b.i.d. Dosage increased after 3 days to 100 mg P.O. t.i.d. if needed. If no response occurs after several weeks of therapy, dosage increased to 150 mg t.i.d.

ADVERSE REACTIONS
CNS: *headache,* akathisia, *seizures, agitation,* anxiety, *confusion,* delusions, euphoria, hostility, impaired sleep quality, insomnia, sedation, sensory disturbance, tremor.
CV: *arrhythmias,* hypertension, hypotension, palpitations, syncope, tachycardia.
EENT: auditory disturbance, blurred vision.
GI: dry mouth, taste disturbance, increased appetite, constipation, dyspepsia, nausea, vomiting.
GU: impotence, menstrual complaints, urinary frequency, decreased libido.
Skin: pruritus, rash, cutaneous temperature disturbance.
Other: arthritis, fever and chills, diaphoresis.

INTERACTIONS
Ethanol, levodopa, phenothiazines, MAO inhibitors, or tricyclic antidepressants; recent and rapid withdrawal of benzodiazepines: increased risk of adverse reactions, including seizures.

CONTRAINDICATIONS
Contraindicated in patients who are hypersensitive to the drug, who have taken MAO inhibitors within the previous 14 days, and in patients with seizure disorders. Also contraindicated in patients with a history of bu-

---

*Liquid form contains alcohol.   *Common* reactions are in italics; ***life-threatening,*** in bold italics.
**May contain tartrazine.

limia or anorexia nervosa because of a higher incidence of seizures.

NURSING CONSIDERATIONS

• Use cautiously in patients with recent history of MI or unstable heart disease, as well as impaired renal or hepatic impairment.
• Know that many patients experience a period of increased restlessness, especially at initiation of therapy. This may include agitation, insomnia, and anxiety.
• Risk of seizure may be minimized by not exceeding 450 mg/day and by administering daily dosage in three to four equally divided doses. Be aware that patients who experience seizures often have predisposing factors, including history of head trauma or prior seizures, or CNS tumors, or they may be taking a drug that lowers the seizure disorder.
• Monitor patients with history of bipolar disorders closely. Antidepressants can cause manic episodes during the depressed phase of bipolar disorder.
• From 28% to 30% of patients taking this drug may experience a weight loss of 5 lb or more. Consider this if weight loss is a major factor in the patient's depressive illness.
• Advise patients to take the drug as scheduled, and to take each day's dosage in three divided doses to minimize the risk of seizures.
• Tell patients to avoid alcohol while taking this drug, because it may contribute to the development of seizures.
• Advise patients to avoid hazardous activities that require alertness and good psychomotor coordination until CNS effects of the drug are known.
• Advise patients to consult their doctor before taking any other prescription or OTC medications.

clomipramine hydrochloride
Anafranil

Pregnancy Risk Category: C

HOW SUPPLIED
Capsules: 25 mg, 50 mg, 75 mg

ACTION
Unknown but a tricyclic antidepressant (TCA) that selectively inhibits reuptake of serotonin.

ONSET, PEAK, DURATION
Unknown although onset is thought to take 2 weeks or longer.

INDICATIONS & DOSAGE
Obsessive-compulsive disorder –
Adults: initially, 25 mg P.O. daily in divided doses with meals, gradually increased to 100 mg daily during first 2 weeks. Thereafter, increased to maximum dosage of 250 mg daily in divided doses with meals as needed. After titration, total daily dosage may be given h.s.
Children and adolescents: initially, 25 mg P.O. daily in divided doses with meals, gradually increased to daily maximum of 3 mg/kg or 100 mg P.O., whichever is smaller. Maximum daily dosage is 3 mg/kg or 200 mg, whichever is smaller; may be given h.s. after titration. Periodic reassessment and adjustment necessary.

ADVERSE REACTIONS
CNS: *somnolence, tremors, dizziness,* headache, insomnia, *nervousness, myoclonus, fatigue, EEG changes, seizures,* extrapyramidal reactions, asthenia, aggressiveness.
CV: postural hypotension, palpitations, tachycardia.
EENT: otitis media (in children), *abnormal vision,* laryngitis, pharyngitis, rhinitis.
GI: *dry mouth, constipation, nausea, dyspepsia, increased appetite,* diar-

---

rhea, *anorexia,* abdominal pain, eructation, *nausea.*
GU: *urinary hesitancy,* urinary tract infection, dysmenorrhea, *ejaculation failure,* impotence.
Hematologic: anemia, bone marrow suppression.
Skin: *diaphoresis,* rash, pruritus, photosensitivity, dry skin.
Other: myalgia, weight gain, *altered libido.*

INTERACTIONS
Barbiturates: decreased TCA blood levels. Monitor for decreased antidepressant effect.
Cimetidine, methylphenidate: increased TCA blood levels. Monitor for enhanced antidepressant effect.
Clonidine, epinephrine, norepinephrine: increased hypertensive effect. Use with caution.
CNS depressants, ethanol: enhanced CNS depression. Avoid concomitant use.
MAO inhibitors: may cause hyperpyretic crisis, seizures, coma, or death. Don't use together.

CONTRAINDICATIONS
Contraindicated in patients with hypersensitivity to drug or other tricyclic antidepressants, who have taken MAO inhibitors within the previous 14 days, and in patients during acute recovery period after MI.

NURSING CONSIDERATIONS
• Use cautiously in patients with history of seizure disorders or with brain damage of varying etiology; in patients receiving other seizure threshold-lowering drugs; in patients at risk for suicide; in patients with history of urine retention or angle-closure glaucoma, increased intraocular pressure, CV disease, impaired hepatic or renal function, or hyperthyroidism; in patients with tumors of the adrenal medulla; in patients receiving thyroid medication or electroconvulsive ther-

apy; and in those undergoing elective surgery.
• Know that total daily dose may be taken at bedtime after titration. During titration, dosage may be divided.
• Do not withdraw drug abruptly.
• Because hypertensive episodes have occurred during surgery in patients receiving TCAs, know that drug should be gradually discontinued several days before surgery.
• Be aware that adverse anticholinergic effects can occur rapidly.
• Relieve dry mouth with sugarless candy or gum. Saliva substitutes may be necessary.
• Monitor for urine retention and constipation. Increase fluids, and suggest stool softener or high-fiber diet as needed.
• Warn patients to avoid hazardous activities requiring alertness and good psychomotor coordination, especially during titration. Daytime sedation and dizziness may occur.
• Tell patients to avoid alcohol while taking this drug.
• Warn patient not to withdraw drug suddenly.
• To prevent photosensitivity reactions, advise patients to use sunblock, wear protective clothing, and avoid prolonged exposure to strong sunlight.

---

desipramine hydrochloride
Norpramin**, Pertofran‡, Pertofrane

Pregnancy Risk Category: NR

HOW SUPPLIED
Tablets: 10 mg, 25 mg, 50 mg, 75 mg, 100 mg, 150 mg
Capsules: 25 mg, 50 mg

ACTION
Unknown but a tricyclic antidepressant (TCA) that increases the amount of norepinephrine, serotonin, or both in the CNS by blocking their reuptake by the presynaptic neurons.

ONSET, PEAK, DURATION
Onset unknown but thought to occur in 2 to 4 weeks or longer. Serum levels peak within 4 to 6 hours. Duration unknown.

INDICATIONS & DOSAGE
Depression –
Adults: 100 to 200 mg P.O. daily in divided doses, increased to maximum of 300 mg daily. Or entire dosage can be given at h.s.
Elderly patients and adolescents: 25 to 100 mg P.O. daily in divided doses, increased gradually to maximum of 150 mg daily if needed.

ADVERSE REACTIONS
CNS: *drowsiness, dizziness,* excitation, tremors, weakness, confusion, headache, nervousness, EEG changes, *seizures,* extrapyramidal reactions.
CV: orthostatic hypotension, *tachycardia, ECG changes,* hypertension (especially during surgery).
EENT: *blurred vision,* tinnitus, mydriasis.
GI: *dry mouth, constipation,* nausea, vomiting, anorexia, paralytic ileus.
GU: *urine retention.*
Skin: rash, urticaria, photosensitivity.
Other: *diaphoresis,* hypersensitivity reaction.
After abrupt withdrawal of long-term therapy: nausea, headache, malaise (does not indicate addiction).

INTERACTIONS
Barbiturates, CNS depressants, ethanol: enhanced CNS depression. Avoid concomitant use.
Cimetidine, methylphenidate: may increase desipramine serum levels. Monitor for adverse reactions.
Clonidine, epinephrine, norepinephrine: increased hypertensive effect. Use with caution.
MAO inhibitors: may cause severe excitation, hyperpyrexia, or seizures,

usually with high dosage. Use with caution.

CONTRAINDICATIONS
Contraindicated in patients with hypersensitivity to drug, who have taken MAO inhibitors within the previous 14 days, and in patients during acute recovery phase of MI.

NURSING CONSIDERATIONS
• Use with extreme caution in patients with CV disease, history of urine retention, or glaucoma, thyroid disease, or those taking thyroid medication, and in patients with history of seizure disorder.
• Do not withdraw drug abruptly.
• Because hypertensive episodes have occurred during surgery in patients receiving TCAs, know that drug should be gradually discontinued several days before surgery.
• If signs of psychosis occur or increase, expect the doctor to reduce dosage. Record mood changes. Monitor patients for suicidal tendencies, and allow them only a minimum supply of the drug.
• Know that because desipramine produces less anticholinergic effects than other TCAs, it is often prescribed for cardiac patients.
• Be aware that adverse anticholinergic effects can occur rapidly.
• Relieve dry mouth with sugarless hard candy or gum. Saliva substitutes may be necessary.
• Check for urine retention and constipation. Increase fluids, and suggest stool softener or high-fiber diet, as needed.
• Advise patients to take full dose at bedtime.
• Warn patients to avoid hazardous activities that require alertness and good psychomotor coordination until CNS effects of the drug are known. Drowsiness and dizziness usually subside after a few weeks.
• Tell patients to avoid alcohol while

taking this drug because it may antagonize effects of desipramine.

• Warn patient not to stop drug therapy suddenly.

• Advise patients to consult their doctors before taking any other prescription or OTC medications.

• To prevent photosensitivity reactions, advise patients to use sunblock, wear protective clothing, and avoid prolonged exposure to strong sunlight.

doxepin hydrochloride
Adapin, Deptran‡, Novo-Doxepin†, Sinequan, Triadapin†

Pregnancy Risk Category: NR

HOW SUPPLIED
Capsules: 10 mg, 25 mg, 50 mg, 75 mg, 100 mg, 150 mg
Oral concentrate: 10 mg/ml

ACTION
Unknown but a tricyclic antidepressant (TCA) that increases the amount of norepinephrine, serotonin, or both in the CNS by blocking their reuptake by the presynaptic neurons.

ONSET, PEAK, DURATION
Onset unknown but thought to take 2 to 4 weeks or longer. Serum levels peak within 2 hours. Duration unknown.

INDICATIONS & DOSAGE
Depression and/or anxiety –
Adults: initially, 25 to 75 mg P.O. daily in divided doses, to maximum of 300 mg daily. Alternatively, entire maintenance dosage may be given once daily with a maximum dose of 150 mg P.O.

ADVERSE REACTIONS
CNS: *drowsiness, dizziness,* excitation, tremors, weakness, confusion, headache, nervousness, EEG changes, *seizures,* extrapyramidal reactions.

CV: *orthostatic hypotension, tachycardia, ECG changes,* hypertension.
EENT: *blurred vision,* tinnitus, mydriasis.
GI: *dry mouth, glossitis, constipation,* nausea, vomiting, anorexia, paralytic ileus.
GU: *urine retention.*
Skin: rash, urticaria, photosensitivity.
Other: *diaphoresis,* hypersensitivity reaction.
After abrupt withdrawal of long-term therapy: nausea, headache, malaise (does not indicate addiction).

INTERACTIONS
Barbiturates, CNS depressants, ethanol: enhanced CNS depression. Avoid concomitant use.
Cimetidine, methylphenidate: may increase doxepin serum levels. Monitor for increased adverse reactions.
Clonidine, epinephrine, norepinephrine: increased hypertensive effect. Use with caution.
MAO inhibitors: may cause severe excitation, hyperpyrexia, or seizures, usually with high dosage. Avoid concomitant use.

CONTRAINDICATIONS
Contraindicated in patients with hypersensitivity to drugs, glaucoma, or tendency to urinary retention.

NURSING CONSIDERATIONS
• Be aware that dosage should be reduced in elderly or debilitated patients, adolescents, and those receiving other medications (especially anticholinergics).
• Do not withdraw drug abruptly.
• Because hypertensive episodes have occurred during surgery in patients receiving TCAs, be aware that drug should be gradually discontinued several days before surgery.
• If signs of psychosis occur or increase, expect doctor to reduce dosage. Record mood changes. Monitor

---

*Liquid form contains alcohol.
**May contain tartrazine.

Common reactions are in italics; *life-threatening,* in bold italics.

patients for suicidal tendencies, and allow them only a minimum supply of the drug.

• Doxepin has strong anticholinergic effects; it is one of the most sedating TCAs. Also be aware that adverse anticholinergic effects can occur rapidly.

• Relieve dry mouth with sugarless hard candy or gum. Saliva substitutes may be necessary.

• Check for urine retention and constipation. Increase fluids, and suggest stool softener or high-fiber diet, as needed.

• Tell patient to dilute oral concentrate with 120 ml of water, milk, or juice (orange, grapefruit, tomato, prune, or pineapple). Incompatible with carbonated beverages.

• Advise patients to take full dose at bedtime but warn them of possible morning orthostatic hypotension.

• Warn patients to avoid hazardous activities that require alertness and good psychomotor coordination until CNS effects of the drug are known. Drowsiness and dizziness usually subside after a few weeks.

• Tell patients to avoid alcohol while taking this drug.

• Warn patient not to stop drug therapy suddenly.

• Advise patients to consult their doctors before taking any other prescription or OTC medications.

• To prevent photosensitivity reactions, advise patients to use sunblock, wear protective clothing, and avoid prolonged exposure to strong sunlight.

---

fluoxetine hydrochloride
Prozac, Prozac-20‡

Pregnancy Risk Category: B

HOW SUPPLIED
Pulvules: 10 mg, 20 mg
Oral solution: 20 mg/5 ml

ACTION
Unknown but presumed to be linked to its inhibition of CNS neuronal uptake of serotonin.

ONSET, PEAK, DURATION
Onset occurs in 1 to 4 weeks. Serum levels peak in 6 to 8 hours. Duration unknown.

INDICATIONS & DOSAGE
Depression, obsessive-compulsive disorder –
Adults: initially, 20 mg P.O. in the morning; dosage increased according to patient response. May be given b.i.d. in the morning and at noon. Maximum dosage is 80 mg/day.

ADVERSE REACTIONS
CNS: *nervousness, anxiety, insomnia, headache, drowsiness, tremor, dizziness, asthenia,* abnormal dreams.
CV: palpitations, flushing, bradycardia, ***arrhythmias.***
EENT: nasal congestion, pharyngitis, cough, sinusitis, visual disturbances, tinnitus.
GI: *nausea, diarrhea, dry mouth, anorexia, dyspepsia,* constipation, abdominal pain, vomiting, taste change, flatulence, increased appetite.
GU: sexual dysfunction, urine retention.
Respiratory: upper respiratory infection, respiratory distress.
Skin: *rash, pruritus, urticaria.*
Other: flulike syndrome, muscle pain, *weight loss,* edema, lymphadenopathy, diaphoresis.

INTERACTIONS
Flecainide, carbamazepine, vinblastine: increased serum levels of these drugs. Monitor serum levels and the patient for adverse effects.
Insulin, oral antidiabetic agents: altered blood glucose levels and possible altered requirements for antidiabetic medication. Adjust dosage as ordered.

Lithium, tricyclic antidepressants: risk of increased adverse CNS effects. Avoid concomitant use.

Phenytoin: increased plasma phenytoin levels and risk of toxicity. Monitor serum phenytoin levels and adjust dosage as ordered.

Tryptophan: increased toxic reaction exhibited by agitation, GI distress, and restlessness. Do not use together.

Warfarin, other highly protein-bound agents: may increase plasma levels of fluoxetine or other highly protein-bound drugs. Monitor closely.

CONTRAINDICATIONS
Contraindicated in patients hypersensitive to the drug and in patients taking MAO inhibitors within 14 days of starting therapy.

NURSING CONSIDERATIONS
• Use cautiously in patients at high risk for suicide and in patients with history of hepatic, renal, or CV disease; diabetes mellitus; or history of seizures.

• Because elderly or debilitated patients and patients with renal or hepatic dysfunction may require lower dosages or less frequent dosing.

• Use antihistamines or topical corticosteroids as ordered to treat rashes or pruritus.

• Tell patients to avoid taking drug in the afternoon because fluoxetine commonly causes nervousness and insomnia.

• May cause dizziness or drowsiness in some patients. Warn patients to avoid driving or other hazardous activities that require alertness and good psychomotor coordination until CNS effects of the drug are known.

• Advise patients to consult their doctors before taking any other prescription or OTC medications.

• Warn patients to avoid food high in tryptophan, including meats, poultry, fish, liver, kidney, eggs, nuts, peanut butter, broad beans, and wheat germ.

imipramine hydrochloride
Apo-Imipramine†, Imiprin‡, Impril†, Janimine**, Melipramine‡, Norfranil, Novopramine†, Tipramine, Tofranil**

imipramine pamoate
Tofranil-PM**

Pregnancy Risk Category: NR

HOW SUPPLIED
imipramine hydrochloride
Tablets: 10 mg, 25 mg, 50 mg
Injection: 12.5 mg/ml
imipramine pamoate
Capsules: 75 mg, 100 mg, 125 mg, 150 mg

ACTION
Unknown but a tricyclic antidepressant (TCA) that increases the amount of norepinephrine, serotonin, or both in the CNS by blocking their reuptake by the presynaptic neurons.

ONSET, PEAK, DURATION
Onset unknown but thought to take 2 to 4 weeks or longer. Peak plasma concentrations occur within 1 to 2 hours after oral administration and 30 minutes after I.M. administration. Duration unknown.

INDICATIONS & DOSAGE
Depression –
Adults: 75 to 100 mg P.O. or I.M. daily in divided doses, increased in 25- to 50-mg increments up to maximum dosage of 300 mg daily. Or, entire dosage may be given h.s. (using pamoate salt).
Childhood enuresis –
Children 6 years and over:
25 mg P.O. 1 hour before bedtime. If no response within 1 week, increased to 50 mg if child is under 12 years; increased to 75 mg for children 12 years and over. In either case, maximum dosage is 2.5 mg/kg/day.

---

*Liquid form contains alcohol.   *Common* reactions are in italics; *life-threatening,* in bold italics.
**May contain tartrazine.

ADVERSE REACTIONS

CNS: *drowsiness, dizziness,* excitation, tremors, weakness, confusion, headache, nervousness, EEG changes, *seizures,* extrapyramidal reactions.
CV: *orthostatic hypotension, tachycardia, ECG changes,* hypertension.
EENT: *blurred vision,* tinnitus, mydriasis.
GI: *dry mouth, constipation,* nausea, vomiting, anorexia, paralytic ileus.
GU: *urine retention.*
Skin: rash, urticaria, photosensitivity.
Other: *diaphoresis,* hypersensitivity reaction.
After abrupt withdrawal of long-term therapy: nausea, headache, malaise (does not indicate addiction).

INTERACTIONS

Barbiturates, CNS depressants, ethanol: enhanced CNS depression. Avoid concomitant use.
Cimetidine, methylphenidate: may increase imipramine serum levels. Monitor for adverse reactions.
Clonidine, epinephrine, norepinephrine: increased hypertensive effect. Use with caution.
MAO inhibitors: may cause hyperpyretic crisis, severe seizures, and fatalities. Avoid concomitant use.

CONTRAINDICATIONS

Contraindicated during acute recovery phase of MI, in patients with hypersensitivity to drug, and in those receiving MAO inhibitors.

NURSING CONSIDERATIONS

• Use with extreme caution in patients at risk for suicide; in patients with history of urine retention or angle-closure glaucoma, increased intraocular pressure, CV disease, impaired hepatic function; or hyperthyroidism, history of seizure disorder, impaired renal function; and in patients receiving thyroid medications. Injectable form contains sulfites, which may cause allergic reactions in hypersensitive individuals.
• Be aware that reduced dosage in elderly or debilitated persons, adolescents, and patients with aggravated psychotic symptoms is necessary.
• Do not withdraw drug abruptly.
• Because of hypertensive episodes during surgery in patients receiving TCAs, be aware that drug should be gradually discontinued several days before surgery.
• If signs of psychosis occur or increase, expect doctor to reduce dosage. Record mood changes. Monitor patients for suicidal tendencies, and allow them only a minimum supply of the drug.
• To prevent relapse in children receiving the drug for enuresis, be aware that drug should be withdrawn gradually.
• Check for urine retention and constipation. Increase fluids, and suggest stool softener or a high-fiber diet, as needed.
• Relieve dry mouth with sugarless hard candy or gum. Saliva substitutes may be necessary.
• Advise patients to take full dose at bedtime but warn them of possible morning orthostatic hypotension.
• If the child is an "early night" bedwetter, tell parents it may be more effective to divide dosage and administer the first dose earlier in the day if approved by doctor.
• Tell patients to avoid alcohol while taking this drug.
• Warn patients to avoid hazardous activities that require alertness and good psychomotor coordination until CNS effects of the drug are known. Drowsiness and dizziness usually subside after a few weeks.
• Warn patient not to stop drug suddenly.
• Advise patients to consult their doctors before taking any other prescription or OTC medications.
• To prevent photosensitivity reac-

tions, advise patient to use sunblock, wear protective clothing, and avoid prolonged exposure to strong sunlight.

---

isocarboxazid
Marplan

Pregnancy Risk Category: NR

HOW SUPPLIED
Tablets: 10 mg

ACTION
Unknown. An MAO inhibitor that probably promotes accumulation of neurotransmitters by inhibiting their metabolism.

ONSET, PEAK, DURATION
Onset in 7 to 10 days although up to 4 to 8 weeks may be needed to achieve full therapeutic effect. Peak levels occur within 3 to 5 days. Effects persist for up to 10 days after therapy is stopped.

INDICATIONS & DOSAGE
Depression –
Adults: 30 mg P.O. daily as a single dose or in divided doses. Reduced to 10 to 20 mg daily when condition improves.

ADVERSE REACTIONS
CNS: *dizziness,* vertigo, weakness, headache, hyperactivity, hyperreflexia, tremors, muscle twitching, mania, *insomnia,* confusion, memory impairment, fatigue.
CV: *orthostatic hypotension, **arrhythmias,*** paradoxical hypertension.
EENT: blurred vision.
GI: dry mouth, *anorexia,* nausea, diarrhea, constipation.
Skin: rash.
Other: peripheral edema, diaphoresis, weight changes, altered libido.
After abrupt withdrawal from drug therapy: restlessness, anxiety, hallucinations, headache, weakness.

INTERACTIONS
Amphetamines, antihistamines, ephedrine, levodopa, meperidine, metaraminol, methylphenidate, phenylephrine, phenylpropanolamine, sympathomimetics: enhanced pressor effects of these drugs. Avoid concomitant use.
Barbiturates, dextromethorphan, ethanol, methotrimeprazine, narcotics, other sedatives, tricyclic antidepressants: unpredictable interactions. Use these agents with caution and in reduced dosages.
Insulin, oral antidiabetic agents: increased risk of hypoglycemia. Use with caution in reduced dosages.
Foods high in tyramine, tryptophan: risk of hypertensive crisis. Avoid concomitant use.

CONTRAINDICATIONS
• Contraindicated in elderly or debilitated patients; in patients with hypersensitivity to the drug, severe hepatic or renal impairment, CHF, pheochromocytoma, hypertension, or CV or cerebrovascular disease; in patients with severe or frequent headaches; and in patients who are currently receiving or have received fluoxetine therapy within 5 weeks.
• Also contraindicated with foods containing tryptophan or tyramine; during therapy with other MAO inhibitors (including phenelzine, tranylcypromine) or within 10 days of such therapy; and within 10 days of elective surgery requiring general anesthetic, cocaine, or local anesthetic containing sympathomimetic vasoconstrictors.

NURSING CONSIDERATIONS
• Use cautiously in patients at risk for suicide; and in patients with Parkinson's disease, impaired renal function, hyperthyroidism, diabetes, or seizure disorders.
• Obtain baseline blood pressure, heart rate, CBC, and liver function

---

*Liquid form contains alcohol.   *Common* reactions are in italics; ***life-threatening,*** in bold italics.
**May contain tartrazine.

test results before beginning therapy as ordered, and continue to monitor throughout treatment.
• Be aware that dosage is usually reduced to maintenance level as soon as possible.
• Do not withdraw drug abruptly.
• Know that in most patients, MAO inhibitors should be discontinued 14 days before elective surgery to avoid drug interactions that may occur during anesthetic procedure.
• If the patient develops symptoms of overdose (palpitations, frequent headaches, or severe orthostatic hypotension), withhold dose and notify the doctor.
• Have phentolamine available to counteract severe hypertension.
• Monitor patients closely for suicidal tendencies, and allow them only a minimum supply of the drug.
• Continue precautions 10 days after discontinuation of the drug because it has long-lasting effects.
• Warn patients to avoid foods high in tryptophan (broad beans) or tyramine (aged cheese, Chianti wine, beer, avocados, chicken livers, chocolate, bananas, soy sauce, meat tenderizers, salami, bologna) and large amounts of caffeine.
• Tell patients to avoid alcohol while taking this drug.
• Advise patients to consult doctor before taking any other prescription or OTC medications. Severe adverse effects can occur if MAO inhibitors are taken with OTC cold, hay-fever, or diet preparations.
• Because MAO inhibitors may suppress chest pain in patients with angina, warn such patients to perform moderate activities and to avoid overexertion.
• To prevent dizziness from orthostatic hypotension, tell patient to get out of bed slowly, sitting up first for 1 minute. Supervise walking.
• Warn patient not to stop drug suddenly.

• Tell patient to weigh himself biweekly. Teach patients how to check for edema and urine retention.

---

maprotiline hydrochloride
Ludiomil

Pregnancy Risk Category: B

HOW SUPPLIED
Tablets: 25 mg, 50 mg, 75 mg

ACTION
Unknown. A tetracyclic antidepressant similar to tricyclic derivatives. Probably increases the amount of norepinephrine, serotonin, or both in the CNS by blocking their reuptake by the presynaptic neurons.

ONSET, PEAK, DURATION
Onset usually occurs in 2 to 3 weeks although sometimes it occurs within 7 days. Serum levels peak in 12 hours. Duration unknown.

INDICATIONS & DOSAGE
Depression –
Adults: initially, 75 mg P.O. daily for patients with mild to moderate depression, increased to 150 mg daily, if needed. Maximum dosage is 225 mg daily.

ADVERSE REACTIONS
CNS: *drowsiness, dizziness,* excitation, *seizures,* tremor, weakness, confusion, headache, nervousness, extrapyramidal reactions.
CV: *orthostatic hypotension, tachycardia, ECG changes.*
EENT: *blurred vision,* tinnitus, mydriasis.
GI: dry mouth, *constipation,* nausea, vomiting, anorexia, paralytic ileus.
GU: *urine retention.*
Skin: rash, urticaria, photosensitivity.
Other: *diaphoresis,* hypersensitivity reaction.
After abrupt withdrawal of long-

term therapy: nausea, headache, malaise (does not indicate addiction).

INTERACTIONS
Barbiturates: decreased maprotiline blood levels. Monitor for decreased antidepressant effect.
Cimetidine, methylphenidate: may increase maprotiline serum levels. Monitor for adverse reactions.
Clonidine, epinephrine, norepinephrine: increased hypertensive effect. Use with caution.
CNS depressants, ethanol: enhanced CNS depression. Avoid concomitant use.
MAO inhibitors: may cause severe excitation, hyperpyrexia, or seizures, usually with high dosage. Use with caution.

CONTRAINDICATIONS
Contraindicated during acute recovery phase of MI and in patients with hypersensitivity to drug, seizure disorders, or within 14 days of MAO inhibitor therapy.

NURSING CONSIDERATIONS
• Use with extreme caution in patients with history of MI or CV disease. Use cautiously in patients with suicidal tendency, increased intraocular pressure, or history of urine retention or angle-closure glaucoma.
• Know that dosage needs to be reduced in elderly or debilitated patients and adolescents.
• Do not withdraw drug abruptly.
• Because maprotiline shares toxic potentials with tricyclic antidepressants and may cause hypertensive episodes during surgery, know that dosage should be gradually discontinued several days before surgery.
• If signs of psychosis occur or increase, expect doctor to reduce dosage. Record mood changes. Monitor patients for suicidal tendencies, and allow them only a minimum supply of the drug.

• Relieve dry mouth with sugarless hard candy or gum. Saliva substitutes may be necessary.
• Check for urine retention and constipation. Increase fluids, and suggest stool softener or high-fiber diet, as needed.
• Warn patients to avoid activities that require alertness and good psychomotor coordination until CNS effects of the drug are known. Drowsiness and dizziness usually subside after a few weeks.
• Advise patients to take full dose at bedtime, but warn them of possible morning orthostatic hypotension.
• Tell patients to avoid alcohol while taking this drug.
• Warn patient not to withdraw drug suddenly.
• Advise patients to consult their doctors before taking any other prescription or OTC medications.
• To prevent photosensitivity reactions, advise patients to use sunblock, wear protective clothing, and avoid prolonged exposure to strong sunlight.

nefazodone hydrochloride
Serzone

Pregnancy Risk Category: C

HOW SUPPLIED
Tablets: 100 mg, 150 mg, 200 mg, 250 mg

ACTION
Not precisely defined. Nefazodone inhibits neuronal uptake of serotonin (5-HT-2) and norepinephrine; it also occupies serotonin and alpha$_1$-adrenergic receptors in the CNS.

ONSET, PEAK, DURATION
Onset and duration unknown. Serum levels peak in about 1 hour.

INDICATIONS & DOSAGE
Depression –
Adults: initially, 200 mg/day P.O. in

two divided doses. Dosage increased in increments of 100 to 200 mg/day at intervals of no less than 1 week, p.r.n. Usual dosage range is 300 to 600 mg/day.

ADVERSE REACTIONS
CNS: headache, *somnolence, dizziness, asthenia,* insomnia, *light-headedness, confusion,* memory impairment, paresthesia, vasodilation, abnormal dreams, decreased concentration, ataxia, incoordination, taste perversion, psychomotor retardation, tremor, hypertonia.
CV: postural hypotension, hypotension, peripheral edema.
EENT: *blurred vision, abnormal vision,* tinnitus, visual field defect.
GI: *dry mouth, nausea, constipation,* dyspepsia, diarrhea, increased appetite, vomiting.
GU: urinary frequency, urinary tract infection, urine retention.
Respiratory: pharyngitis, cough.
Skin: pruritus, rash.
Other: infection, flu syndrome, chills, fever, neck rididity, vaginitis, breast pain, thirst, arthralgia.

INTERACTIONS
Alprazolam, triazolam: coadministration with nefazodone potentiates the effects of these drugs. Do not administer concurrently. However, if necessary, dosage of alprazolam and triazolam may need to be reduced greatly.
Astemizole, terfenadine: may cause decreased metabolism, leading to increased levels of these antihistamines and cardiotoxicity. Avoid concomitant use.
CNS active drugs: may alter CNS activity. Use together cautiously.
Digoxin: may increase digoxin level. Use together cautiously and monitor digoxin levels.
MAO inhibitors: may cause severe excitation, hyperpyrexia, seizures, delirium, or coma. Avoid concomitant use.
Other highly bound plasma protein

drugs: may increase incidence and severity of adverse reactions. Monitor patient closely.

CONTRAINDICATIONS
Contraindicated in patients with hypersensitivity to the drug or to other phenylpiperazine antidepressants. Also contraindicated within 14 days of MAO inhibitor therapy and in coadministration with terfenadine or astemizole.

NURSING CONSIDERATIONS
• Use cautiously in patients with CV or cerebrovascular disease that could be exacerbated by hypotension (such as history of MI, angina, or CVA) and conditions that would predispose patients to hypotension (such as dehydration, hypovolemia, and treatment with antihypertensives). Also use cautiously in patients with a history of mania.
• Know that at least 1 week should be allowed after stopping nefazodone before patient is started on an MAO inhibitor and that at least 14 days should be allowed before a patient is started on nefazodone after MAO inhibitor therapy has been discontinued.
• Record mood changes. Monitor patients for suicidal tendencies, and allow them only a minimum supply of the drug.
• Warn patient not to engage in hazardous activity until drug's CNS effects are known.
• Instruct male patients who experience prolonged or inappropriate erections to stop drug immediately and notify doctor.
• Instruct female patients to notify doctor if they become pregnant or intend to become pregnant during therapy.
• Instruct patient not to take alcoholic beverages while taking this drug.
• Tell patient who develops a rash, hives, or a related allergic reaction to notify doctor.

• Inform patient that several weeks of therapy may be required to obtain the full antidepressant effect. Once improvement is seen, advise patient not to discontinue drug until directed by doctor.

nortriptyline hydrochloride
Allegron‡, Aventyl*, Nortab‡, Pamelor*

Pregnancy Risk Category: NR

HOW SUPPLIED
Tablets: 10 mg‡, 25 mg‡
Capsules: 10 mg, 25 mg, 50 mg, 75 mg
Oral solution: 10 mg/5 ml (4% alcohol)

ACTION
Unknown but a tricyclic antidepressant (TCA) that increases the amount of norepinephrine, serotonin, or both in the CNS by blocking their reuptake by the presynaptic neurons.

ONSET, PEAK, DURATION
Onset unknown but thought to take at least 2 to 4 weeks or longer. Peak plasma concentrations occur within 7 to 8.5 hours. Duration unknown.

INDICATIONS & DOSAGE
Depression –
Adults: 25 mg P.O. t.i.d. or q.i.d., gradually increased to maximum of 150 mg daily. Or, entire dosage may be given h.s.

ADVERSE REACTIONS
CNS: *drowsiness, dizziness,* excitation, *seizures,* tremor, weakness, confusion, headache, nervousness, EEG changes, extrapyramidal reactions.
CV: *tachycardia, ECG changes,* hypertension.
EENT: *blurred vision,* tinnitus, mydriasis.
GI: dry mouth, *constipation,* nausea, vomiting, anorexia, paralytic ileus.
GU: *urine retention.*
Skin: rash, urticaria, photosensitivity.
Other: *diaphoresis,* hypersensitivity reaction.
After abrupt withdrawal of long-term therapy: nausea, headache, malaise (does not indicate addiction).

INTERACTIONS
Barbiturates, CNS depressants, ethanol: enhanced CNS depression. Avoid concomitant use.
Cimetidine, methylphenidate: may increase nortriptyline serum levels. Monitor for adverse reactions.
Clonidine, epinephrine, norepinephrine: increased hypertensive effect. Use with caution.
MAO inhibitors: may cause severe excitation, hyperpyrexia, or seizures, usually with high dosage. Use with caution.

CONTRAINDICATIONS
Contraindicated during acute recovery phase of MI, and in patients with hypersensitivity to drug or MAO therapy within past 14 days.

NURSING CONSIDERATIONS
• Use with extreme caution in patients with glaucoma, suicidal tendency, history of urine retention or seizures, CV disease, or hyperthyroidism and in those receiving thyroid medication.
• Know that dosage should be reduced in elderly or debilitated patients and adolescents.
• Do not withdraw drug abruptly.
• Because hypertensive episodes have occurred during surgery in patients receiving TCAs, know that dosage should be gradually discontinued several days before surgery.
• If signs of psychosis occur or increase, expect doctor to reduce dosage. Record mood changes. Monitor patients for suicidal tendencies, and

---

*Liquid form contains alcohol.   *Common* reactions are in italics; *life-threatening,* in bold italics.
**May contain tartrazine.

allow them only a minimum supply of the drug.
• Be aware that adverse anticholinergic effects can occur rapidly. Has anticholinergic effects similar to other TCAs.
• Relieve dry mouth with sugarless hard candy or gum. Saliva substitutes may be necessary.
• Check for urine retention and constipation. Increase fluids, and suggest stool softener or high-fiber diet, as needed.
• Whenever possible, advise patients to take full dose at bedtime to reduce the risk of orthostatic hypotension.
• Warn patients to avoid activities that require alertness and good psychomotor coordination until CNS effects of the drug are known. Drowsiness and dizziness usually subside after a few weeks.
• Tell patients to avoid alcohol while taking this drug.
• Warn patient not to stop drug suddenly.
• Advise patients to consult their doctors before taking any other prescription or OTC medications.
• To prevent photosensitivity reactions, advise patients to use sunblock, wear protective clothing, and avoid prolonged exposure to strong sunlight.

paroxetine hydrochloride
Paxil

Pregnancy Risk Category: B

HOW SUPPLIED
Tablets: 20 mg, 30 mg

ACTION
Unknown but presumed to be linked to its inhibition of CNS neuronal uptake of serotonin.

ONSET, PEAK, DURATION
Onset usually occurs within 1 to 4 weeks. Serum levels peak in 2 to 8 hours. Duration unknown.

INDICATIONS & DOSAGE
Depression –
Adults: initially, 20 mg P.O. daily, preferably in the morning as indicated. If patient does not respond after full antidepressant effect has occurred, dosage increased in 10-mg/day increments at weekly intervals, to a maximum of 50 mg daily.
Elderly or debilitated patients; patients with severe hepatic or renal disease: initially, 10 mg P.O. daily, preferably in the morning as indicated. If patient does not respond after full antidepressant effect has occurred, dosage increased in 10-mg/day increments at weekly intervals, to a maximum of 40 mg daily.

ADVERSE REACTIONS
CNS: blurred vision, *somnolence, dizziness, insomnia, tremor, nervousness,* anxiety, paresthesia, confusion.
CV: palpitations, vasodilation, postural hypotension.
EENT: lump or tightness in throat, dysgeusia.
GI: *dry mouth, nausea, constipation, diarrhea, decreased appetite* or increased appetite, flatulence, vomiting, dyspepsia, increased appetite.
GU: ejaculatory disturbances, male genital disorders including anorgasmy, erectile difficulties, delayed ejaculation or orgasm, impotence, and sexual dysfunction), urinary frequency, other urinary disorder, female genital disorder (including anorgasmy, difficulty with orgasm).
Skin: rash.
Other: *asthenia, diaphoresis,* hyponatremia, myopathy, myalgia, myasthenia, decreased libido, yawn, taste perversion.

INTERACTIONS
Cimetidine: decreased hepatic metabolism of paroxetine, leading to risk of toxicity. Dosage adjustments may be necessary.

Digoxin: may decrease digoxin levels. Monitor closely.

MAO inhibitors: may increase risk of serious, sometimes fatal, adverse reactions. Avoid concomitant use.

Phenobarbital, phenytoin: may alter pharmacokinetics of both drugs. Dosage adjustments may be necessary.

Procyclidine: may increase procyclidine levels. Monitor for excessive anticholinergic effects.

Tryptophan: may increase incidence of adverse reactions, such as diaphoresis, headache, nausea, and dizziness. Avoid concomitant use.

Warfarin: increased risk of bleeding. Use concomitantly with caution.

CONTRAINDICATIONS
Contraindicated in patients taking MAO inhibitors.

NURSING CONSIDERATIONS
• Use cautiously in patients with a history of seizure disorders or mania and in those with severe, concomitant systemic illness.
• Use cautiously in patients at risk for volume depletion, and monitor appropriately.
• Don't administer paroxetine with, or within 14 days of discontinuing, MAO inhibitor therapy. Allow at least 2 weeks after discontinuing paroxetine before starting treatment with an MAO inhibitor as ordered.
• If signs of psychosis occur or increase, expect doctor to reduce dosage. Record mood changes. Monitor patients for suicidal tendencies, and allow them only a minimum supply of the drug.
• Warn patients to avoid activities that require alertness and good psychomotor coordination until CNS effects of the drug are known.

phenelzine sulfate
Nardil

Pregnancy Risk Category: C

HOW SUPPLIED
Tablets: 15 mg

ACTION
Unknown. An MAO inhibitor that probably promotes accumulation of neurotransmitters by inhibiting their metabolism.

ONSET, PEAK, DURATION
Onset occurs in 7 to 10 days although up to 4 to 8 weeks may be needed to achieve full therapeutic effect. Peak levels occur in 2 to 4 hours. Effects persist for up to 10 days after therapy is stopped.

INDICATIONS & DOSAGE
Depression –
Adults: 15 mg P.O. daily t.i.d., increased rapidly to 60 mg daily. Maximum dosage is 90 mg daily. Then dosage can usually be reduced to 15 mg daily.

ADVERSE REACTIONS
CNS: *dizziness,* vertigo, headache, hyperactivity, hyperreflexia, tremors, muscle twitching, mania, jitters, *insomnia,* confusion, memory impairment, drowsiness, weakness, fatigue.
CV: paradoxical hypertension, palpitations, *orthostatic hypotension,* **arrhythmias.**
GI: dry mouth, *anorexia,* nausea, constipation.
Other: peripheral edema, diaphoresis, weight changes.

INTERACTIONS
Amphetamines, antihistamines, ephedrine, levodopa, meperidine, metaraminol, methylphenidate, phenylephrine, phenylpropanolamine, sympathomimetics: enhanced pressor effects. Avoid concomitant use.

---

*Liquid form contains alcohol.   *Common* reactions are in italics; *life-threatening,* in bold italics.
**May contain tartrazine.

Barbiturates, dextromethorphan, ethanol, methotrimeprazine, narcotics, other sedatives, tricyclic antidepressants: unpredictable interaction. Use these agents with caution and in reduced dosage.
Insulin, oral antidiabetic agents: increased risk of hypoglycemia. Use with caution and in reduced dosages.
Foods high in tryptophan, tyramine: may precipitate hypertensive crisis. Avoid concomitant use.

CONTRAINDICATIONS
● Contraindicated in patients with hypersensitivity to drug, CHF, pheochromocytoma, hypertension, liver disease, and CV disease.
● Also contraindicated during therapy with other MAO inhibitors (isocarboxazid, tranylcypromine) or within 10 days of such therapy or within 10 days of elective surgery requiring general anesthesia, cocaine, or local anesthesia containing sympathomimetic vasoconstrictors.

NURSING CONSIDERATIONS
● Use cautiously with antihypertensive agents containing thiazide diuretics, with spinal anesthetics, and in patients at risk for suicide, diabetes, or seizure disorders.
● Obtain baseline blood pressure, heart rate, CBC, and liver function test results before therapy, and continue to monitor throughout treatment.
● Be aware dosage usually is reduced to maintenance level as soon as possible.
● In most patients, discontinue MAO inhibitors 14 days before elective surgery as ordered to avoid drug interactions that may occur during the anesthetic procedure.
● Monitor patients closely for suicidal tendencies, and allow them only a minimum supply of the drug.
● If patients develop symptoms of overdose (severe hypotension, palpi-

tations, or frequent headaches), withhold dose and notify the doctor.
● Have phentolamine available to combat severe hypertension.
● Continue precautions 10 days after stopping drug because it has long-lasting effects.
● Warn patients to avoid foods high in tryptophan (broad beans) or tyramine (aged cheese, Chianti wine, beer, avocados, chicken livers, chocolate, bananas, soy sauce, meat tenderizers, salami, bologna) and large amounts of caffeine.
● Tell patients to avoid alcohol while taking drug.
● Advise patients to consult doctor before taking any other prescription or OTC medications. Severe adverse effects can occur if MAO inhibitors are taken with OTC cold, hay-fever, or diet preparations.
● Warn patients about the probability of orthostatic hypotension. Supervise walking. Tell patients to get out of bed slowly, sitting up first for 1 minute.
● Because MAO inhibitors may suppress chest pain in patients with angina, warn such patients to perform moderate activities and to avoid overexertion.

---

protriptyline hydrochloride
Triptil†, Vivactil

Pregnancy Risk Category: NR

HOW SUPPLIED
Tablets: 5 mg, 10 mg

ACTION
Unknown but a tricyclic antidepressant (TCA) that increases the amount of norepinephrine, serotonin, or both in the CNS by blocking their reuptake by the presynaptic neurons.

ONSET, PEAK, DURATION
Onset unknown although therapeutic effect thought to take 2 to 4 weeks or

---

longer. Serum levels peak in 24 to 30 hours. Duration unknown.

INDICATIONS & DOSAGE
Depression—
Adults: 15 to 40 mg P.O. daily in divided doses, increasing gradually to maximum of 60 mg daily.

ADVERSE REACTIONS
CNS: excitation, *seizures,* tremor, weakness, confusion, headache, nervousness, EEG changes, extrapyramidal reactions.
CV: *tachycardia, ECG changes,* orthostatic hypotension, hypertension.
EENT: *blurred vision,* tinnitus, mydriasis.
GI: *dry mouth, constipation,* nausea, vomiting, anorexia, paralytic ileus.
GU: *urine retention.*
Skin: rash, urticaria, photosensitivity.
Other: *diaphoresis,* hypersensitivity reaction.
After abrupt withdrawal of long-term therapy: nausea, headache, malaise (does not indicate addiction).

INTERACTIONS
Barbiturates: decreased TCA blood levels. Monitor for decreased antidepressant effect.
Cimetidine, methylphenidate: may increase protriptyline serum levels. Monitor for adverse reactions.
Clonidine, epinephrine, norepinephrine: increased hypertensive effect. Use with caution.
CNS depressants, ethanol: enhanced CNS depression. Avoid concomitant use.
MAO inhibitors: may cause severe excitation, hyperpyrexia, seizures, or death, usually with high dosage. Use with caution.

CONTRAINDICATIONS
Contraindicated during acute recovery phase of MI, in patients with hypersensitivity to the drug, and within 14 days of MAO inhibitor therapy.

NURSING CONSIDERATIONS
• Use cautiously in elderly patients; in patients with history of seizures, suicidal tendencies, history of urine retention, increased intraocular pressure, CV disorders, hyperthyroidism, and in those receiving thyroid medications.
• Know that dosage should be reduced in elderly or debilitated patients and adolescents.
• Do not withdraw drug abruptly.
• Because hypertensive episodes have occurred during surgery in patients receiving TCAs, know that drug should be gradually discontinued several days before surgery.
• If signs of psychosis occur or increase, expect doctor to reduce dosage. Record mood changes. Monitor patients for suicidal tendencies, and allow them only a minimum supply of the drug. To prevent insomnia, avoid late-day dosing.
• Know that protriptyline has strong anticholinergic effects.
• Relieve dry mouth with sugarless hard candy or gum. Saliva substitutes may be necessary.
• Check for urine retention and constipation. Increase fluids, and suggest stool softener or high-fiber diet, as needed.
• Tell patients to avoid alcohol while taking this drug.
• Warn patient not to withdraw drug suddenly.
• Advise patients to consult doctor before taking any other prescription or OTC medications.
• To prevent photosensitivity reactions, advise patients to use sunblock, wear protective clothing, and avoid prolonged exposure to strong sunlight.

---

*Liquid form contains alcohol.
**May contain tartrazine.

Common reactions are in italics; *life-threatening,* in bold italics.

sertraline hydrochloride
Zoloft

Pregnancy Risk Category: B

HOW SUPPLIED
Tablets: 50 mg, 100 mg

ACTION
Unknown but presumed to be linked to its inhibition of neuronal uptake of serotonin in the CNS.

ONSET, PEAK, DURATION
Onset occurs in 2 to 4 weeks. Serum levels peak 4½ to 8½ hours after dose. Duration unknown.

INDICATIONS & DOSAGE
Depression –
Adults: 50 mg P.O. daily. Dosage adjusted as tolerated and needed; clinical trials involved dosage of 50 to 200 mg daily. Dosage adjustments should be made at intervals of no less than 1 week.

ADVERSE REACTIONS
CNS: *headache, tremor, dizziness, insomnia, somnolence,* syncope, paresthesia, hypoesthesia, hyperesthesia, twitching, hypertonia, confusion, ataxia, abnormal coordination or gait, vertigo, hyperkinesia, hypokinesia, mania.
CV: palpitations, chest pain, postural hypotension, hypertension, hypotension, edema, peripheral ischemia, tachycardia.
EENT: nystagmus.
GI: *dry mouth, nausea, diarrhea, loose stools, dyspepsia,* vomiting, flatulence, anorexia, abdominal pain, increased appetite, dysphagia.
GU: male sexual dysfunction.
Skin: rash, acne, alopecia, pruritus, erythematous or maculopapular rash, cold or clammy skin, dry skin.
Other: *diaphoresis,* flushing, myalgia.

INTERACTIONS
Diazepam, tolbutamide: decreased clearance of these drugs. Clinical significance unknown; however, monitor patients for increased drug effects.
MAO inhibitors: may cause serious sometimes fatal reactions including myoclonus rigidity, mental status changes, hyperthermia, autonomic nervous system instability, rapid fluctuations of vital signs, delirium, coma, and death. Avoid concomitant use.
Warfarin, other highly protein-bound drugs: may increase plasma levels of sertraline or other highly bound drug. Small (8%) increases in PT have been seen with concomitant use of warfarin. Monitor closely.

CONTRAINDICATIONS
None known.

NURSING CONSIDERATIONS
● Use cautiously in patients at risk for suicide, and in those with seizure disorder, major affective disorder, or diseases or conditions that affect metabolism or hemodynamic responses.
● Administer sertraline once daily, either in the morning or evening. May be given with or without food.
● Know that sertraline should not be administered with, or within 14 days of discontinuing, MAO inhibitor therapy. Allow 14 days after discontinuing sertraline before starting treatment with an MAO inhibitor as ordered.
● Record mood changes. Monitor patients for suicidal tendencies, and allow them only a minimum supply of the drug.
● Know that drug may change several laboratory values — increases in serum cholesterol and triglyceride levels, decreases in uric acid concentrations, and elevations in AST and ALT (usually within the first 9 weeks of therapy). AST and ALT values return to normal after discontinuing

---

drug; clinical significance is unknown.

• Advise patients to use caution when performing hazardous tasks that require alertness and to avoid alcohol while taking this drug. Drugs that influence the CNS may impair judgment.

• Caution patients to check with doctor or pharmacist before taking any OTC medications.

---

tranylcypromine sulfate
Parnate

Pregnancy Risk Category: NR

HOW SUPPLIED
Tablets: 10 mg

ACTION
Unknown. An MAO inhibitor that probably promotes accumulation of neurotransmitters by inhibiting MAO.

ONSET, PEAK, DURATION
Onset in 48 hours to 3 weeks may be needed to achieve full therapeutic effect. Peak levels occur in 1 to 3.5 hours. Effects persist for up to 10 days after therapy is stopped.

INDICATIONS & DOSAGE
Depression –
Adults: 10 mg P.O. t.i.d. Increased by 10 mg P.O. daily at 1- to 3-week intervals to maximum of 60 mg daily, if necessary, after 2 weeks of initial therapy.

ADVERSE REACTIONS
CNS: *dizziness,* vertigo, headache, overstimulation, numbness, paresthesia, tremors, jitters, confusion, memory impairment.
CV: *orthostatic hypotension, tachycardia,* paradoxical hypertension, palpitations.
EENT: blurred vision, tinnitus.
GI: dry mouth, *anorexia,* nausea, diarrhea, constipation, abdominal pain.
GU: impotence, SIADH, urinary retention, retarded ejaculation.
Skin: rash.
Other: edema, hepatitis, muscle spasm, myoclonic jerks, hematologic disorders, chills.

INTERACTIONS
Amphetamines, antihistamines, ephedrine, levodopa, meperidine, metaraminol, methylphenidate, phenylephrine, phenylpropanolamine, sympathomimetics: enhanced pressor effects of these drugs. Avoid concomitant use.
Barbiturates, dextromethorphan, ethanol, methotrimeprazine, narcotics, other sedatives, tricyclic antidepressants: enhanced adverse CNS effects. Use with caution and in reduced dosage.
Buspirone: may elevate blood pressure. Monitor closely.
Insulin, oral antidiabetic agents: increased risk of hypoglycemia. Use with caution and in reduced dosages.
Foods high in tryptophan, tyramine: may cause hypertensive crisis. Avoid concomitant use.

CONTRAINDICATIONS
• Contraindicated in patients receiving MAO inhibitors or dibenzazepine derivatives; sympathomimetics (including amphetamines); some CNS depressants (including narcotics and alcohol); selective serotonin reuptake inhibitors; antihypertensive, diuretic, antihistaminic, sedative or anesthetic drugs; bupropion hydrochloride, buspirone hydrocholoride, dextromethorphan, meperidine; cheese or other foods with a high tyramine or tryptophan content; or excessive quantities of caffeine.
• Also contraindicated in patients with a confirmed or suspected cerebrovascular defect, CV disease, hypertension, or history of headache

---

and in those undergoing elective surgery.

NURSING CONSIDERATIONS
• Use cautiously with antiparkinsonian drugs or spinal anesthetics; in patients with renal disease, diabetes, seizure disorder, Parkinson's disease, or hyperthyroidism; and in patients at risk for suicide.
• Obtain baseline blood pressure, heart rate, CBC, and liver function test results before beginning therapy, and continue to monitor throughout treatment.
• Know that dosage usually is reduced to maintenance level as soon as possible.
• Do not withdraw drug abruptly.
• In most patients, discontinue MAO inhibitors 14 days before elective surgery as ordered to avoid drug interactions that may occur during the anesthetic procedure.
• Monitor patients for suicidal tendencies, and allow them only a minimum supply of the drug.
• If patients develop symptoms of overdose (palpitations, severe hypotension, or frequent headaches), withhold dose and notify the doctor.
• Have phentolamine available to combat severe hypertension.
• Continue precautions for 10 days after stopping drug because it has long-lasting effects.
• Warn patients to avoid foods high in tyramine or tryptophan and large amounts of caffeine. Tranylcypromine is the MAO inhibitor most often reported to cause hypertensive crisis with ingestion of foods high in tyramine, including aged cheese, Chianti wine, beer, avocados, chicken livers, chocolate, bananas, soy sauce, meat tenderizers, salami, and bologna.
• Tell patients to avoid alcohol while taking this drug.
• To prevent dizziness resulting from orthostatic hypotension, tell patients to get out of bed slowly, sitting up for 1 minute first.
• Because MAO inhibitors may suppress anginal pain, warn such patients to moderate activities to avoid overexertion.
• Advise patients to consult their doctors before taking any other prescription or OTC medications. Severe adverse effects can occur if MAO inhibitors are taken with OTC cold, hay fever, or diet preparations.
• Warn patient not to stop drug suddenly.

trazodone hydrochloride
Desyrel, Trazon, Trialodine
Pregnancy Risk Category: C

HOW SUPPLIED
Tablets: 50 mg, 100 mg, 150 mg, 300 mg

ACTION
Unknown although it inhibits serotonin uptake in the brain. Not a tricyclic derivative.

ONSET, PEAK, DURATION
Onset occurs in 2 to 4 weeks or longer. Plasma levels peak after 1 hour if taken on an empty stomach, 2 hours if taken with food. Duration unknown.

INDICATIONS & DOSAGE
Depression –
Adults: initial dosage, 150 mg P.O. daily in divided doses; increased by 50 mg daily q 3 to 4 days as needed. Average dosage ranges from 150 mg to 400 mg daily. Maximum daily dosage is 600 mg.

ADVERSE REACTIONS
CNS: *drowsiness, dizziness,* nervousness, fatigue, confusion, tremors, weakness, hostility, anger, nightmares, vivid dreams.

CV: orthostatic hypotension, tachycardia, bradycardia.
EENT: blurred vision, tinnitus.
GI: dry mouth, dysgeusia, constipation, nausea, vomiting, anorexia.
GU: urine retention, priapism possibly leading to impotence, hematuria.
Hematologic: anemia.
Skin: rash, urticaria.
Other: diaphoresis.

INTERACTIONS
Antihypertensives: increased hypotensive effect of trazodone. Antihypertensive dosage may have to be decreased.
Clonidine, CNS depressants, ethanol: enhanced CNS depression.
Digoxin, phenytoin: may increase serum levels of these drugs. Monitor for toxicity.
MAO inhibitors: no clinical experience. Use together with extreme caution.

CONTRAINDICATIONS
Contraindicated during initial recovery phase of MI or in patients with hypersensitivity to drug.

NURSING CONSIDERATIONS
• Use cautiously in patients with cardiac disease and in patients at risk for suicide.
• Administer after meals or a light snack for optimal absorption and to decrease incidence of dizziness.
• Record mood changes. Monitor patients for suicidal tendencies, and allow them only minimum supply of the drug.
• Inform male patient that priapism is a potential problem in men taking trazodone; it may require surgical intervention.
• Warn patients to avoid activities that require alertness and good psychomotor coordination until CNS effects of the drug are known. Drowsiness and dizziness usually subside after the first few weeks.

• Teach patients' families how to recognize signs of suicidal tendency or suicidal ideation.

---

trimipramine maleate
Apo-Trimip†, Novo-Tripramine†, Rhotrimine†, Surmontil

Pregnancy Risk Category: C

HOW SUPPLIED
Tablets: 25 mg‡
Capsules: 25 mg, 50 mg, 100 mg

ACTION
Unknown but a tricyclic antidepressant (TCA) that increases the amount of norepinephrine, serotonin, or both in the CNS by blocking their reuptake by the presynaptic neurons.

ONSET, PEAK, DURATION
Onset unknown although thought to occur in 2 to 4 weeks or longer. Plasma concentrations peak in 2 hours. Duration unknown.

INDICATIONS & DOSAGE
Depression –
Adults: 75 to 100 mg P.O. daily in divided doses, increased to 200 to 300 mg daily. Dosages over 300 mg daily not recommended in hospitalized patients; over 200 mg in outpatient.

ADVERSE REACTIONS
CNS: *drowsiness, dizziness,* excitation, tremors, weakness, confusion, headache, nervousness, EEG changes, *seizures,* extrapyramidal reactions.
CV: *orthostatic hypotension, tachycardia, ECG changes,* hypertension.
EENT: *blurred vision,* tinnitus, mydriasis.
GI: *dry mouth, constipation,* nausea, vomiting, anorexia, paralytic ileus.
GU: *urine retention.*
Skin: rash, urticaria, photosensitivity.
Other: *diaphoresis,* hypersensitivity reaction.

---

*Liquid form contains alcohol.
May contain tartrazine.*   *Common* reactions are in italics; ***life-threatening,* in bold italics.

After abrupt withdrawal of long-term therapy: nausea, headache, malaise (does not indicate addiction).

INTERACTIONS
Barbiturates: decreased TCA blood levels. Monitor for decreased antidepressant effect.
Cimetidine, methylphenidate: may increase trimipramine serum levels. Monitor for increased adverse reactions.
Clonidine, epinephrine, norepinephrine: increased hypertensive effect. Use with caution.
CNS depressants, ethanol: enhanced CNS depression. Avoid concomitant use.
MAO inhibitors: may cause severe excitation, hyperpyrexia, or seizures, usually with high dosage. Use with caution.

CONTRAINDICATIONS
Contraindicated during acute recovery phase of MI and in patients with hypersensitivity to drug or receiving MAO inhibitor therapy within 14 days.

NURSING CONSIDERATIONS
• Use with extreme caution in patients with CV disease, history of urine retention or angle-closure glaucoma, increased intraocular pressure, hyperthyroidism, impaired hepatic function, or history of seizures and in those receiving thyroid medications, guanethidine, or similiar agents.
• Know that dosage should be reduced in elderly or debilitated persons and adolescents.
• Do not withdraw drug abruptly.
• Because hypertensive episodes have occurred during surgery in patients receiving TCAs, be aware that dosage should be gradually discontinued several days before surgery.
• If signs of psychosis occur or increase, expect doctor to reduce dosage. Record mood changes. Monitor

patients for suicidal tendencies, and allow them only a minimum supply of the drug.
• Relieve dry mouth with sugarless hard candy or gum. Saliva substitutes may be necessary.
• Check for urine retention and constipation. Increase fluids, and suggest stool softener or high-fiber diet, as needed.
• To avoid daytime sedation, tell patients to take full dose at bedtime. Warn them about possible morning orthostatic hypotension.
• Warn patients to avoid hazardous activities that require alertness and good psychomotor coordination until CNS effects of the drug are known. Drowsiness and dizziness usually subside after a few weeks.
• Tell patients to avoid alcohol while taking this drug.
• Warn patient not to stop drug suddenly.
• Advise patients to consult doctor before taking any other prescription or OTC medications.
• To prevent photosensitivity reactions, advise patients to use sunblock, wear protective clothing, and avoid prolonged exposure to strong sunlight.

---

venlafaxine hydrochloride
Effexor

Pregnancy Risk Category: C

HOW SUPPLIED
Tablets: 25 mg, 37.5 mg, 50 mg, 75 mg, 100 mg

ACTION
Blocks reuptake of norepinephrine and serotonin into neurons in the CNS.

ONSET, PEAK, DURATION
Onset unknown but thought to take several weeks. Peak and duration unknown.

INDICATIONS & DOSAGE
Depression –
Adults: initially, 75 mg P.O. daily, in two or three divided doses with food. Dosage increased as tolerated and needed in increments of 75 mg/day at intervals of no less than 4 days. For moderately depressed outpatients, usual maximum dosage is 225 mg/day; in certain severely depressed patients, dosage may be as high as 375 mg/day.

ADVERSE REACTIONS
CNS: *headache, somnolence, dizziness, nervousness, insomnia,* anxiety.
CV: hypertension.
EENT: blurred vision.
GI: *nausea, constipation,* vomiting, *dry mouth.*
GU: abnormal ejaculation, impotence.
Other: tremor, diaphoresis, asthenia, weight loss.

INTERACTIONS
MAO inhibitors: may precipitate a syndrome similar to neuroleptic malignant syndrome (myoclonus, hyperthermia, seizures, and death). Do not start venlafaxine within 14 days of discontinuing therapy with an MAO inhibitor, and don't start MAO inhibitor therapy within 7 days of stopping venlafaxine.

CONTRAINDICATIONS
Contraindicated in patients hypersensitive to the drug. Also contraindicated for use within 14 days of an MAO inhibitor.

NURSING CONSIDERATIONS
• Use cautiously in patients with renal impairment, diseases or conditions that could affect hemodynamic responses or metabolism, and in those with history of mania or seizures.
• Know that total daily dosage should be reduced by 50% in patients with hepatic impairment. In patients with moderate renal impairment (glomerular filtration rate of 10 to 70 ml/minute), total daily dosage should be reduced by 25%. In patients undergoing hemodialysis, know that dose should be withheld until dialysis session is completed and daily dosage reduced by 50%.
• Carefully monitor blood pressure. Venlafaxine therapy is associated with sustained, dose-dependent increases in blood pressure. Greatest increases (averaging about 7 mm Hg above baseline) occur in patients taking 375 mg daily.
• Patients who have received drug for 6 weeks or more should gradually discontinue drug by tapering dosage over a 2-week period as instructed by doctor.

---

*Liquid form contains alcohol.   *Common* reactions are in italics; *life-threatening,* in bold italics.
**May contain tartrazine.

32

Antianxiety agents

ß **alprazolam** XANAX
buspirone hydrochloride
chlordiazepoxide
chlordiazepoxide hydrochloride
clorazepate dipotassium
ß **diazepam** Valium
doxepin hydrochloride
   (See Chapter 31, ANTIDEPRESSANTS.)
hydroxyzine embonate
hydroxyzine hydrochloride
hydroxyzine pamoate
ß **lorazepam** Ativan
meprobamate Equanil
midazolam hydrochloride
oxazepam
prazepam

COMBINATION PRODUCTS
EQUAGESIC: meprobamate 200 mg
and aspirin 325 mg.
LIBRAX: chlordiazepoxide hydrochloride 5 mg and clidinium bromide 2.5
mg.
LIMBITROL DS: chlordiazepoxide
10 mg and amitriptyline hydrochloride 25 mg.

---

alprazolam
Apo-Alpraz†, Novo-Alprazol†, Nu-
Alpraz†, Xanax
Controlled Substance Schedule IV
Pregnancy Risk Category: D

HOW SUPPLIED
Tablets: 0.25 mg, 0.5 mg, 1 mg, 2 mg
Oral solution: 0.5 mg/5 ml, 1 mg/ml
(concentrate)

ACTION
Unknown. A benzodiazepine that
probably potentiates the effects of
gamma-aminobutyric acid, an inhibitory neurotransmitter, and depresses
the CNS at the limbic and subcortical
levels of the brain.

ONSET, PEAK, DURATION
Onset and duration unknown. Serum
levels peak within 1 to 2 hours.

INDICATIONS & DOSAGE
Anxiety –
Adults: usual initial dose, 0.25 to 0.5
mg P.O. t.i.d. Maximum dosage is 4
mg daily in divided doses.
**Elderly or debilitated patients or
advanced liver disease:** usual initial
dose, 0.25 mg P.O. b.i.d. or t.i.d.
Maximum dosage is 4 mg daily in divided doses.
Panic disorders –
Adults: 0.5 mg P.O. t.i.d., increased
at intervals of 3 to 4 days in increments of no more than 1 mg. Maximum dosage is 10 mg daily in divided
doses.

ADVERSE REACTIONS
CNS: *drowsiness, light-headedness,*
headache, confusion, hostility, anterograde amnesia, restlessness, psychosis.
CV: transient hypotension, tachycardia.
EENT: visual disturbances.
GI: dry mouth, nausea, vomiting,
constipation, discomfort.
GU: incontinence, urine retention,
menstrual irregularities.

INTERACTIONS
Cimetidine: increased sedation. Monitor carefully.
Digoxin: may increase serum levels of
digoxin, increasing toxicity. Monitor
closely.
Ethanol, other CNS depressants: increased CNS depression. Avoid concomitant use.
Smoking: increased clearance of benzodiazepines. Monitor for lack of effect.

Tricyclic antidepressants: increased plasma levels of tricyclic antidepressants. Monitor for toxicity.

CONTRAINDICATIONS

Contraindicated in patients with hypersensitivity to drug or other benzodiazepines or acute angle-closure glaucoma.

NURSING CONSIDERATIONS

• Use cautiously in patients with hepatic, renal, or pulmonary disease.
• Also know that drug should not be prescribed for everyday stress or for long-term use (more than 4 months).
• Know that drug should not be withdrawn abruptly after long-term use; withdrawal symptoms may occur. Abuse or addiction is possible.
• Monitor liver, renal, and hematopoietic function studies periodically in patients receiving repeated or prolonged therapy as ordered.
• Warn patients to avoid hazardous activities that require alertness and good psychomotor coordination until CNS effects of the drug are known.
• Tell patients to avoid alcohol while taking this drug.

---

buspirone hydrochloride
BuSpar

Pregnancy Risk Category: B

HOW SUPPLIED
Tablets: 5 mg, 10 mg

ACTION
Unknown. May inhibit neuronal firing and reduce serotonin turnover in cortical, amygdaloid, and septohippocampal tissue.

ONSET, PEAK, DURATION
Onset unknown but for therapeutic effect, possibly 1 to 2 weeks; optimal results, possibly 3 to 4 weeks. Serum levels peak within 40 to 90 minutes. Duration unknown.

INDICATIONS & DOSAGE
Anxiety disorders; short-term relief of anxiety –
Adults: initially, 5 mg P.O. t.i.d. Dosage increased at 3-day intervals in 5 mg increments. Usual maintenance dosage is 20 to 30 mg daily in divided doses. Do not exceed 60 mg daily.

ADVERSE REACTIONS
CNS: *dizziness, drowsiness,* nervousness, excitement, insomnia, headache.
GI: dry mouth, nausea, diarrhea.
Other: fatigue.

INTERACTIONS
Ethanol, other CNS depressants: increased CNS depression. Avoid concomitant use.
MAO inhibitors: may elevate blood pressure. Avoid concomitant use.

CONTRAINDICATIONS
Contraindicated in patients hypersensitive to the drug or use within 14 days of an MAO inhibitor.

NURSING CONSIDERATIONS
• Use cautiously in patients with hepatic or renal failure.
• Monitor patient closely for adverse CNS reactions. Buspirone is less sedating than other antianxiety agents and does not produce any serious functional impairment. However, CNS effects in individual patients may be unpredictable.
• Be aware that drug has shown no potential for abuse and has not been classified as a controlled substance. However, it is not recommended for relief of everyday stress.
• Before initiating buspirone therapy in patients already being treated with benzodiazepines, warn them against stopping the benzodiazepine abruptly; withdrawal reaction may occur.
• Tell patients to take drug with food.
• Warn patients to avoid hazardous activities that require alertness and

---

*Liquid form contains alcohol.
May contain tartrazine. *Common* reactions are in italics; **life-threatening, in bold italics.

good psychomotor coordination until CNS effects of the drug are known.

---

chlordiazepoxide
Libritabs

chlordiazepoxide hydrochloride
Apo-Chlordiazepoxide†, Librium, Lipoxide, Novopoxide†, Solium†
Controlled Substance Schedule IV

Pregnancy Risk Category: NR

HOW SUPPLIED
chlordiazepoxide
Tablets: 5 mg, 10 mg, 25 mg
chlordiazepoxide hydrochloride
Capsules: 5 mg, 10 mg, 25 mg
Powder for injection: 100 mg/ampule

ACTION
Unknown. Thought to depress the CNS at the limbic and subcortical levels of the brain.

ONSET, PEAK, DURATION
Onset and duration unknown. Plasma levels peak in 30 minutes to 4 hours.

INDICATIONS & DOSAGE
Mild to moderate anxiety –
Adults: 5 to 10 mg P.O. t.i.d. or q.i.d.
Children over 6 years: 5 mg P.O. b.i.d. to q.i.d. Maximum dosage is 10 mg P.O. b.i.d. or t.i.d.
Severe anxiety –
Adults: 20 to 25 mg P.O. t.i.d. or q.i.d.
Withdrawal symptoms of acute alcoholism –
Adults: 50 to 100 mg P.O., I.M., or I.V. Repeated in 2 to 4 hours as needed. Maximum dosage is 300 mg daily.
Preoperative apprehension and anxiety –
Adults: 5 to 10 mg P.O. t.i.d. or q.i.d. on day preceding surgery; or 50 to 100 mg I.M. 1 hour before surgery.

Note: Parenteral form not recommended in children under 12 years.

ADVERSE REACTIONS
CNS: *drowsiness, lethargy, hangover,* fainting, restlessness, psychosis, *suicidal tendencies.*
CV: *thrombophlebitis,* transient hypotension.
EENT: visual disturbances.
GI: nausea, vomiting, abdominal discomfort.
GU: incontinence, urine retention, menstrual irregularities.
Skin: *swelling, pain at injection site.*

INTERACTIONS
Cimetidine: increased sedation. Monitor carefully.
Digoxin: increased serum digoxin levels and risk of toxicity. Monitor closely.
Ethanol, other CNS depressants: increased CNS depression. Avoid concomitant use.
Smoking: increased clearance of benzodiazepines. Monitor for lack of effect.

CONTRAINDICATIONS
Contraindicated in patients hypersensitive to the drug.

NURSING CONSIDERATIONS
● Use cautiously in patients with mental depression, porphyria, or hepatic or renal disease.
● Know that drug should be avoided during pregnancy, especially during first trimester.
● Know that dosage should be reduced in elderly or debilitated patients.
● Also know that drug should not be prescribed regularly for everyday stress.
● Injectable form (as hydrochloride) comes in two types of ampules – as diluent and as powdered drug. Read directions carefully.

---

†Available in Canada only.   ‡Available in Australia only.   ◇Available OTC.

• Do not mix injectable form with any other parenteral drug.

• Warn patients to avoid hazardous activities that require alertness and good psychomotor coordination until CNS effects of the drug are known.

• Tell patients to avoid alcohol while taking this drug.

• Keep powder away from light and refrigerate; mix just before use and discard remainder.

• For I.M. use, add 2 ml of diluent to powder and agitate gently until clear. Use immediately. I.M. form may be erratically absorbed.

• Recommended for I.M. use only, but may be given intravenously.

• **I.V. use:** Use 5 ml of 0.9% sodium chloride solution or sterile water for injection as diluent; do not give packaged diluent intravenously. Administer over 1 minute.

• When giving drug intravenously, be sure equipment and personnel needed for emergency airway management are available. Monitor respirations every 5 to 15 minutes and before each repeated I.V. dose.

• Monitor liver, renal, and hematopoietic function studies periodically in patients receiving repeated or prolonged therapy as ordered.

• Possibility of abuse and addiction exists. Drug should be withdrawn abruptly after long-term administration; withdrawal symptoms may occur.

• May cause false-positive reaction in the Gravindex pregnancy test. May also interfere with certain tests for urine 17-ketosteroids.

clorazepate dipotassium
Apo-Clorazepate†, Gen-XENE, Novoclopate†, Tranxene, Tranxene-SD, Tranxene-T-Tab
Controlled Substance Schedule IV

Pregnancy Risk Category: NR

HOW SUPPLIED
Tablets: 3.75 mg, 7.5 mg, 11.25 mg, 15 mg, 22.5 mg
Capsules: 3.75 mg, 7.5 mg, 15 mg

ACTION
Unknown. A benzodiazepine that probably facilitates the action of the inhibitory neurotransmitter gamma-aminobutyric acid. Depresses the CNS at the limbic and subcortical levels of the brain and suppresses the spread of seizure activity produced by epileptogenic foci in the cortex, thalamus, and limbic structures.

ONSET, PEAK, DURATION
Onset and duration unknown. Plasma levels peak within ½ to 2 hours.

INDICATIONS & DOSAGE
Acute alcohol withdrawal–
Adults: day 1 – 30 mg P.O. initially, followed by 30 to 60 mg P.O. in divided doses; day 2 – 45 to 90 mg P.O. in divided doses; day 3 – 22.5 to 45 mg P.O. in divided doses; day 4 – 15 to 30 mg P.O. in divided doses; then gradually reduce dosage to 7.5 to 15 mg daily.
Anxiety–
Adults: 15 to 60 mg P.O. daily.
Adjunct in partial seizure disorder–
Adults and children over 12 years: Maximum recommended initial dosage is 7.5 mg P.O. t.i.d. Dosage increases should be no greater than 7.5 mg/week. Maximum dosage should not exceed 90 mg daily.
Children 9 and 12 years: Maximum recommended initial dosage is 7.5 mg P.O. b.i.d. Dosage increases should be no greater than 7.5 mg/week. Maximum dosage should not exceed 60 mg daily.

ADVERSE REACTIONS
CNS: *drowsiness, lethargy, hangover,* fainting, restlessness, psychosis.
CV: transient hypotension.
EENT: visual disturbances.

---

*Liquid form contains alcohol.
**May contain tartrazine.
Common reactions are in italics; **life-threatening,** in bold italics.

GI: nausea, vomiting, abdominal discomfort, dry mouth
GU: urine retention, incontinence.

INTERACTIONS
Cimetidine: increased sedation. Monitor carefully.
Digoxin: may increase serum levels of digoxin, increasing toxicity. Monitor closely.
Ethanol, other CNS depressants: increased CNS depression. Avoid concomitant use.
Smoking: increased clearance of benzodiazepines. Monitor for lack of effect.

CONTRAINDICATIONS
Contraindicated in patients with hypersensitivity to the drug and acute angle-closure glaucoma.

NURSING CONSIDERATIONS
• Know that drug should be avoided during pregnancy, especially first trimester.
• Use cautiously in patients with suicidal tendencies, renal or hepatic impairment, or history of drug abuse.
• Know that dosage should be reduced in elderly or debilitated patients.
• Monitor liver, renal, and hematopoietic function studies periodically in patients receiving repeated or prolonged therapy as ordered.
• Possibility of abuse and addiction exists. Do not withdraw drug abruptly after prolonged use; withdrawal symptoms may occur.
• Warn patients to avoid activities that require alertness and good psychomotor coordination until CNS effects of the drug are known.
• Tell patients to avoid alcohol while taking this drug.
• Tell patient sugarless chewing gum or hard candy can relieve dry mouth.

diazepam
Apo-Diazepam†, Atenex‡, Diazemuls†‡, Diazepam Intensol, Ducene‡, Novodipam†, PMS Diazepam†, T-Quil, Valium, Valrelease, Vazepam, Vivol†, Zetran
Controlled Substance Schedule IV

Pregnancy Risk Category: NR

HOW SUPPLIED
Tablets: 2 mg, 5 mg, 10 mg
Capsules (extended-release): 15 mg
Oral solution: 5 mg/5 ml, 5 mg/ml
Injection: 5 mg/ml
Sterile emulsion for injection: 5 mg/ml†

ACTION
Unknown. A benzodiazepine that probably depresses the CNS at the limbic and subcortical levels of the brain. Suppresses spread of seizure activity produced by epileptogenic foci in the cortex, thalamus, and limbic structures.

ONSET, PEAK, DURATION
Onset occurs 30 minutes after oral dose, 1 to 5 minutes after I.V. injection. Plasma levels peak 30 minutes to 2 hours after oral dose, immediately after I.V. injection; peak levels after administration of injectable emulsion occur 15 minutes after I.V. injection, 2 hours after I.M. injection. Effects persist 3 to 8 hours after oral dose, 15 minutes to 1 hour after I.V. injection.

INDICATIONS & DOSAGE
Anxiety –
Adults: depending on severity 2 to 10 mg P.O. 2 to 4 times daily or 15 to 30 mg extended release capsules P.O. once daily. Alternatively, 2 to 10 mg I.M. or I.V. q 3 to 4 hours, if needed.
Children 6 months and older: 1 to 2.5 mg P.O. 3 to 4 times daily, increased gradually as needed and tolerated.

---

†Available in Canada only.   ‡Available in Australia only.   ◊Available OTC.

Acute alcohol withdrawal –
Adults: 10 mg P.O. 3 or 4 times first 24 hours, reduced to 5 mg P.O. 3 or 4 times daily as needed. Alternatively, initially, 10 mg I.M. or I.V., then 5 to 10 mg I.M. or I.V. in 3 to 4 hours, if necessary.
Before endoscopic procedures –
Adults: I.V. dose titrated to desired sedative response (up to 20 mg). Alternatively, 5 to 10 mg I.M. 30 minutes before procedure.
Muscle spasm –
Adults: 2 to 10 mg P.O. 2 to 4 times daily or 15 to 30 mg extended release capsules once daily. Alternatively, 5 to 10 mg I.M. or I.V. initially, then 5 to 10 mg I.M. or I.V. in 3 to 4 hours as needed. For tetatnus, larger doses may be required.
Children over 30 days to 5 years: 1 to 2 mg I.M. or I.V. slowly repeated q 3 to 4 hours p.r.n.
Children 5 years or older: 5 to 10 mg I.M. or I.V. q 3 to 4 hours p.r.n.
Preoperative sedation –
Adults: 10 mg I.M. (preferred) or I.V. before surgery
Cardioversion –
Adults: 5 to 15 mg I.V. within 5 to 10 minutes prior to procedure
Adjunct in seizure disorders –
Adults: 2 to 10 mg P.O. 2 to 4 times daily.
Children 6 months and older: 1 to 2.5 mg P.O. 3 or 4 times daily initially; increased as tolerated and needed.
Status epilepticus and severe recurrent seizures –
Adults: 5 to 10 mg I.V. (preferred) or I.M. initially. Repeated q 10 to 15 minutes p.r.n. up to a maximum dose of 30 mg. Repeated in 2 to 4 hours if necessary.
Children over 30 days to 5 years: 0.2 to 0.5 mg I.V. slowly q 2 to 5 minutes up to a maximum of 5 mg. Repated in 2 to 4 hours if necessary.
Children 5 years and older: 1 mg I.V. q 2 to 5 minutes up to maximum

of 10 mg. Repeated in 2 to 4 hours if necessary.

ADVERSE REACTIONS
CNS: *drowsiness, lethargy, hangover, ataxia,* fainting, depression, restlessness, anterograde amnesia, psychosis, slurred speech, tremor.
CV: transient hypotension, bradycardia, ***cardiovascular collapse.***
EENT: diplopia, blurred vision, nystagmus.
GI: nausea, vomiting, abdominal discomfort.
GU: incontinence, urine retention.
Respiratory: respiratory depression.
Skin: rash, urticaria, desquamation.
Other: physical or psychological dependence, ***acute withdrawal syndrome*** after sudden discontinuation in physically dependent persons, *pain, phlebitis at injection site.*

INTERACTIONS
Cimetidine: increased sedation. Monitor carefully.
Digoxin: may increase serum levels of digoxin, increasing toxicity. Monitor closely.
Ethanol, other CNS depressants: increased CNS depression. Avoid concomitant use.
Phenobarbital: increased effects of both drugs. Use together cautiously.
Smoking: increased clearance of benzodiazepines. Monitor for lack of effect.

CONTRAINDICATIONS
Contraindicated in patients with hypersensitivity or angle-closure glaucoma; in patients experiencing shock, coma, or acute alcohol intoxication (parenteral form); and in children under 6 months (oral form).

NURSING CONSIDERATIONS
• Know that drug should be avoided during pregnancy, especially first trimester.
• Use cautiously in patients with liver

or renal impairment, depression, or chronic open-angle glaucoma; and in elderly and debilitated patients.

• Be aware dosage should be reduced in elderly or debilitated patients because they may be more susceptible to the adverse CNS effects of the drug.

• When oral concentrate solution is used, dilute the dose just before administering. Use water, juice, or carbonated beverages, or mix with semisolid food such as applesauce or pudding.

• I.V. route is the most reliable parenteral route; I.M. administration is not recommended because absorption is variable and injection is painful.

• **I.V. use:** Give at rate not exceeding 5 mg/minute. When injecting, administer directly into the vein. If this is impossible, inject slowly through the infusion tubing as near to the vein insertion site as possible. Watch daily for phlebitis at injection site.

• Avoid extravasation. Do not inject into small veins.

• Do not mix injectable form with other drugs because diazepam is incompatible with most drugs.

• Monitor respirations every 5 to 15 minutes and before each repeated I.V. dose. Have emergency resuscitation equipment and oxygen at bedside.

• Do not store parenteral solution in plastic syringes.

• Parenteral emulsion – a stabilized oil-in-water emulsion – should appear milky white and uniform. Avoid mixing with any other drugs or solutions, and avoid infusion sets or containers made from polyvinyl chloride. If dilution is necessary, drug may be mixed with I.V. fat emulsion. Use the admixture within 6 hours.

• Monitor periodic liver, renal, and hematopoietic function studies in patients receiving repeated or prolonged therapy as ordered.

• Possibility of abuse and addiction exists. Do not withdraw drug abruptly

after long-term use; withdrawal symptoms may occur.

• Warn patients to avoid activities that require alertness and good psychomotor coordination until CNS effects of the drug are known.

• Tell patients to avoid alcohol while taking this drug.

hydroxyzine embonate‡
Atarax

hydroxyzine hydrochloride
Anxanil, Apo-Hydroxyzine†, Atarax*, Atozine, Durrax, E-Vista, Hydroxacen, Hyzine-50, Multipax†, Novohydroxyzin†, Quiess, Vistacon-50, Vistaject-25, Vistaject-50, Vistaquel, Vistaril, Vistazine-50

hydroxyzine pamoate
Hy-Pam, Vamate, Vistaril

Pregnancy Risk Category: NR

HOW SUPPLIED
hydroxyzine embonate‡
Capsules: 25 mg, 50 mg
hydroxyzine hydrochloride
Tablets: 10 mg, 25 mg, 50 mg, 100 mg
Capsules: 10 mg†‡, 25 mg†‡, 50 mg†‡
Syrup: 10 mg/5 ml
Injection: 25 mg/ml, 50 mg/ml
hydroxyzine pamoate
Capsules: 25 mg, 50 mg, 100 mg
Oral suspension: 25 mg/5 ml

ACTION
Unknown. A piperazine antihistamine that may be due to a suppression of activity in certain key regions of the subcortical area of the CNS.

ONSET, PEAK, DURATION
Onset occurs in 15 to 30 mnutes with oral administration, almost immediately with I.V. administration. Serum levels peak about 2 hours after oral dose, immediately after I.V. administration. Effects persist 4 to 6 hours.

INDICATIONS & DOSAGE

Anxiety –
Adults: 50 to 100 mg P.O. q.i.d.
Children under 6 years: 50 mg P.O. daily in divided doses.
Children 6 years and over: 50 to 100 mg P.O. daily in divided doses.
Preoperative and postoperative adjunctive therapy –
Adults: 25 to 100 mg I.M. q 4 to 6 hours.
Children: 1.1 mg/kg I.M. q 4 to 6 hours.
Pruritus due to allergies –
Adults: 25 mg P.O. t.i.d. or q.i.d.
Children under 6 years: 50 mg P.O. daily in divided doses.
Children 6 years and over: 50 to 100 mg P.O. daily in divided doses.
Psychiatric and emotional emergencies, including acute alcoholism –
Adults: 50 to 100 mg I.M. q 4 to 6 hours p.r.n.
Nausea and vomiting (excluding nausea and vomiting of pregnancy) –
Adults: 25 to 100 mg I.M.
Children: 1.1 mg/kg I.M.
Prepartum and postpartum adjunctive therapy –
Adults: 25 to 100 mg I.M.

ADVERSE REACTIONS

CNS: *drowsiness,* involuntary motor activity.
GI: *dry mouth.*
Other: marked discomfort at I.M. injection site.

INTERACTIONS

Ethanol, other CNS depressants: increased CNS depression. Avoid concomitant use.

CONTRAINDICATIONS

Contraindicated in patients hypersensitive to the drug and during early pregnancy.

NURSING CONSIDERATIONS

- Know that dosage should be reduced in elderly or debilitated patients.
- Parenteral form (hydroxyzine hydrochloride) for I.M. use only; never administer intravenously. Z-track injection method is preferred.
- Aspirate I.M. injection carefully to prevent inadvertent intravascular injection. Inject deeply into a large muscle mass.
- If the patient is taking other CNS drugs, observe for excessive sedation.
- Be aware that drug may cause false elevations of urine 17-hydroxycorticosteroids, depending on test method used.
- Warn patients to avoid hazardous activities that require alertness and good psychomotor coordination until CNS effects of the drug are known.
- Tell patients to avoid alcohol while taking this drug.
- To relieve dry mouth, suggest sugarless hard candy or gum.

lorazepam

Alzapam, Apo-Lorazepam†,
Ativan, Lorazepam Intensol, Novo-
Lorazem†, Nu-Loraz†
Controlled Substance Schedule IV

Pregnancy Risk Category: NR

HOW SUPPLIED

Tablets: 0.5 mg, 1 mg, 2 mg
Tablets (sublingual): 0.5 mg†, 1 mg†, 2 mg†
Oral solution (concentrated): 2 mg/ml
Injection: 2 mg/ml, 4 mg/ml

ACTION

Unknown. Probably stimulates gamma-aminobutyric (GABA) receptors in the ascending reticular activating system.

ONSET, PEAK, DURATION

Onset occurs within 1 to 5 minutes after I.V. administration, 15 to 30 min-

---

*Liquid form contains alcohol.
**May contain tartrazine.

Common reactions are in italics; *life-threatening,* in bold italics.

ANTIANXIETY AGENTS **433**

utes after I.M. injection, 1 to 6 hours after oral administration. Plasma levels peak within 1 to 1½ hours. Effects persist for 12 to 24 hours.

INDICATIONS & DOSAGE
Anxiety –
Adults: 2 to 6 mg P.O. daily in divided doses. Maximum dosage is 10 mg daily.
Insomnia due to anxiety –
Adults: 2 to 4 mg P.O. h.s.
Premedication before operative procedure –
Adults: 0.05 mg/kg I.M. 2 hours before procedure. Total dosage should not exceed 4 mg. Alternatively, 2 mg total or 0.044 mg/kg whichever is smaller. Larger doses up to 0.05 mg/kg I.V. up to a total of 4 mg may be required.

ADVERSE REACTIONS
CNS: *drowsiness, lethargy, hangover,* fainting, anterograde amnesia, restlessness, psychosis.
CV: transient hypotension.
EENT: visual disturbances.
GI: dry mouth, abdominal discomfort.
GU: incontinence, urine retention.
Other: *acute withdrawal syndrome* following sudden discontinuation in physically dependent persons.

INTERACTIONS
Digoxin: may increase serum levels of digoxin, increasing toxicity. Monitor closely.
Ethanol, other CNS depressants: increased CNS depression. Avoid concomitant use.
Smoking: increased clearance of benzodiazepines. Monitor for lack of effect.

CONTRAINDICATIONS
Contraindicated in patients with acute angle-closure glaucoma or hypersensitivity to drug, other benzodiaze-

pines or its vehicle (used in parenteral dosage form).

NURSING CONSIDERATIONS
• Know that drug should be avoided during pregnancy, especially first trimester.
• Use cautiously in patients with pulmonary, renal, or hepatic impairment. Also use cautiously in elderly, acutely ill or debilitated patients.
• Know that dosage should be reduced in elderly or debilitated patients. Preoperative I.V. dose not to exceed 2 mg in patients over 50.
• For I.M. administration, inject deeply into a muscle mass. Don't dilute.
• **I.V. use:** Give slowly, at rate not exceeding 2 mg/minute. Dilute with an equal volume of sterile water for injection, 0.9% sodium chloride injection, or dextrose 5% injection.
• Monitor respirations every 5 to 15 minutes and before each repeated I.V. dose. Have emergency resuscitation equipment and oxygen available.
• Refrigerate parenteral form to prolong shelf life.
• Monitor liver, renal, and hematopoietic function studies periodically in patients receiving repeated or prolonged therapy as ordered.
• Possibility of abuse and addiction exists. Do not withdraw drug abruptly after long-term use; withdrawal symptoms may occur.
• Warn patients to avoid hazardous activities that require alertness or good psychomotor coordination until CNS effects of the drug are known.
• Tell patients to avoid alcohol while taking this drug.
• As a premedication before surgery, lorazepam provides substantial preoperative amnesia. Patient teaching requires extra care to ensure adequate recall. Provide written materials or inform a family member, if possible.

meprobamate

Apo-Meprobamate†, Equanil**,
Meprospan-200, Meprospan-400,
Miltown-200, Miltown-400, Miltown-
600, Probate, Trancot
Controlled Substance Schedule IV

Pregnancy Risk Category: NR

HOW SUPPLIED
Tablets: 200 mg, 400 mg, 600 mg
Capsules (sustained-release): 200 mg,
400 mg

ACTION
Unknown. It appears to act at multiple
sites in the central nervous system.

ONSET, PEAK, DURATION
Unknown.

INDICATIONS & DOSAGE
Anxiety –
Adults: 1.2 to 1.6 g P.O. daily in
three or four equally divided doses.
Maximum dosage is 2.4 g daily. Alternatively, 400 to 800 mg sustained-
release capsule P.O. b.i.d.
Children 6 to 12 years: 200 to 600
mg P.O. b.i.d. or t.i.d. Or, 200 mg
sustained-release capsule P.O. b.i.d.
Not recommended for children under
6 years.

ADVERSE REACTIONS
CNS: *drowsiness,* ataxia, dizziness,
slurred speech, headache, vertigo,
seizures.
CV: palpitation, tachycardia, hypotension.
GI: anorexia, nausea, vomiting, diarrhea, stomatitis.
Hematologic: *aplastic anemia,*
thrombocytopenia, leukopenia, eosinophilia.
Skin: pruritus, urticaria, erythematous maculopapular rash.
**After abrupt withdrawal of long-
term therapy:** severe generalized
tonic-clonic seizures.

INTERACTIONS
Ethanol, other CNS depressants: increased CNS depression. Avoid concomitant use.

CONTRAINDICATIONS
Contraindicated in patients hypersensitive to meprobamate or related compounds (such as carisoprodol, mebu-
tamate, tybamate, and carbromal) and
in patients with porphyria.

NURSING CONSIDERATIONS
● Know that drug should be avoided
during pregnancy, especially first
trimester.
● Use cautiously in patients with impaired hepatic or renal function, seizure disorders, or suicidal tendencies.
● Be aware that dosage should be reduced in elderly or debilitated patients.
● Give drug with meals to reduce GI
distress.
● Possibility of abuse and addiction
exists with long-term use. Withdraw
drug gradually over 2 weeks to avoid
withdrawal symptoms.
● Know that drug may interfere with
certain laboratory tests for urinary
17-ketogenic steroids and 17-hy-
droxycorticosteroids.
● Periodically monitor CBC and renal
and liver function tests in patients receiving high doses as ordered.
● Warn patients to avoid hazardous
activities that require alertness and
good psychomotor coordination until
CNS effects of the drug are known.
● Tell patients to avoid alcohol while
taking this drug.
● Tell patients to report any unusual
bruising or bleeding, fever, or sore
throat. These symptoms may indicate
serious hematologic toxicity.

---

*Liquid form contains alcohol. *Common* reactions are in italics; **life-threatening,** in bold italics.
**May contain tartrazine.

midazolam hydrochloride
Hypnovel‡, Versed
Controlled Substance Schedule IV

Pregnancy Risk Category: D

HOW SUPPLIED
Injection: 1 mg/ml, 5 mg/ml

ACTION
Unknown. Thought to depress CNS at the limbic and subcortical levels of the brain by potentiating the effects of gamma-aminobutyric acid (GABA).

ONSET, PEAK, DURATION
Onset occurs 1½ to 5 minutes after I.V. injection, within 15 minutes of I.M. injection. Peak effect occurs rapidly after I.V. administration, within 15 to 60 minutes after I.M. injection. Effects typically persist about 2 hours, but may last up to 6 hours.

INDICATIONS & DOSAGE
Preoperative sedation (to induce sleepiness or drowsiness and relieve apprehension) –
Adults: 0.07 mg to 0.08 mg/kg I.M. approximately 1 hour before surgery.
Conscious sedation before short diagnostic or endoscopic procedures –
Adults: initially, small dose not to exceed 2.5 mg I.V. administered slowly; repeated in 2 minutes if needed in small increments of initial dose over at least a 2-minute period to achieve desired effect. A total dose of up to 5 g may be used (3.5 mg for elderly or debilitated patients and patients with decreased pulmonary reserve).
Induction of general anesthesia –
Adults: 0.3 to 0.35 mg/kg I.V. over 20 to 30 seconds if patient has not received any preanesthesia medication or 0.2 to 0.25 mg/kg I.V. over 20 to 30 seconds if patient has received preanesthesia medication. Additional increments of 25% of the initial dose may be needed to complete induction.

ADVERSE REACTIONS
CNS: headache, oversedation, involuntary movements, combativeness, amnesia.
CV: variations in blood pressure and pulse rate.
GI: *nausea,* vomiting, *hiccups.*
Respiratory: *decreased respiratory rate,* apnea.
Skin: *pain and tenderness at injection site.*

INTERACTIONS
Ethanol or other CNS depressants: may increase the risk of apnea. Avoid concomitant use. Prepare to adjust dosage of midazolam if used with opiates or other CNS depressants.

CONTRAINDICATIONS
Contraindicated in patients with hypersensitivity to drug, acute angle-closure glaucoma, shock, coma, or acute alcohol intoxication.

NURSING CONSIDERATIONS
• Use cautiously in patients with uncompensated acute illness and in elderly or debilitated patients.
• Before administering, have oxygen and resuscitation equipment available in case of severe respiratory depression. Excessive dosage or rapid infusion has been associated with respiratory arrest, particularly in elderly or debilitated patients.
• May be mixed in the same syringe with morphine sulfate, meperidine, atropine sulfate, or scopolamine.
• When injecting I.M., give deep into a large muscle mass.
• **I.V. use:** Administer slowly over at least 2 minutes, and wait at least 2 minutes when titrating doses to effect.
• When administering I.V., take care to avoid extravasation.
• Monitor blood pressure, heart rate and rhythm, respirations, airway integrity, and arterial oxygen saturation during procedure, especially in patients premedicated with narcotics.

• Midazolam's beneficial amnestic effect diminishes a patient's recall of perioperative events. However, this effect requires extra caution when teaching patients. Written information, family member instruction, and follow-up contact may be required to ensure that the patient has adequate information.

oxazepam
Alepam‡, Apo-Oxazepam†, Murelax‡, Novoxapam†, Ox-Pam†, Serax**, Serepax‡, Zapex†
Controlled Substance Schedule IV

Pregnancy Risk Category: NR

HOW SUPPLIED
Tablets: 10 mg, 15 mg, 30 mg
Capsules: 10 mg, 15 mg, 30 mg

ACTION
Unknown. Believed to stimulate GABA receptors in the ascending reticular activating system.

ONSET, PEAK, DURATION
Onset and duration unknown. Serum levels peak in about 3 hours.

INDICATIONS & DOSAGE
Alcohol withdrawal –
Adults: 15 to 30 mg P.O. t.i.d. or q.i.d.
Severe anxiety –
Adults: 15 to 30 mg P.O. t.i.d. or q.i.d.
Mild to moderate anxiety –
Adults: 10 to 15 mg P.O. t.i.d. or q.i.d.

ADVERSE REACTIONS
CNS: *drowsiness, lethargy, hangover,* fainting.
CV: transient hypotension.
GI: nausea, vomiting, abdominal discomfort.
Hematologic: *leukopenia* (rare).
Hepatic: *hepatic dysfunction.*

INTERACTIONS
Digoxin: may increase serum levels of digoxin, increasing toxicity. Monitor closely.
Ethanol, cimetidine, other CNS depressants: increased CNS depression. Avoid concomitant use.
Smoking: increased clearance of benzodiazepines. Monitor for lack of effect.

CONTRAINDICATIONS
Contraindicated in patients hypersensitive to the drug.

NURSING CONSIDERATIONS
• Know that drug should be avoided during pregnancy, especially first trimester.
• Use cautiously in elderly patients and in patients with a history of drug abuse or in whom a drop in blood pressure might lead to cardiac problems.
• Know that dosage should be reduced in elderly or debilitated patients.
• Monitor liver, renal, and hematopoietic function studies periodically in patients receiving repeated or prolonged therapy as ordered.
• Possibility of abuse and addiction exists. Do not stop drug abruptly; withdrawal symptoms may occur.
• Warn patients to avoid hazardous activities that require alertness or good psychomotor coordination until CNS effects of the drug are known.
• Tell patients to avoid alcohol while taking this drug.

prazepam
Centrax
Controlled Substance Schedule IV

Pregnancy Risk Category: NR

HOW SUPPLIED
Tablets: 5 mg, 10 mg
Capsules: 5 mg, 10 mg, 20 mg

---

*Liquid form contains alcohol.
**May contain tartrazine.
Common reactions are in italics; *life-threatening,* in bold italics.

ACTION
Unknown. Believed to potentiate the effects of gamma-aminobutyric acid, an inhibitory neurotransmitter. Depresses the CNS at the limbic and sub-cortical levels of the brain.

ONSET, PEAK, DURATION
Unknown.

INDICATIONS & DOSAGE
Anxiety –
Adults: 20 to 60 mg P.O. daily in divided doses, or 20 to 40 mg h.s.

ADVERSE REACTIONS
CNS: *drowsiness, lethargy, hangover,* dizziness, ataxia, fainting.
CV: transient hypotension.
GI: dry mouth, nausea, vomiting, abdominal discomfort.
Skin: rash.

INTERACTIONS
Cimetidine: increased sedation. Monitor carefully.
Digoxin: may increase serum levels of digoxin, increasing toxicity. Monitor closely.
Ethanol, other CNS depressants: increased CNS depression. Avoid concomitant use.
Smoking: increased clearance of benzodiazepines. Monitor for lack of effect.

CONTRAINDICATIONS
Contraindicated in patients with hypersensitivity to drug or acute angle-closure glaucoma.

NURSING CONSIDERATIONS
● Know that drug should be avoided during pregnancy, especially first trimester.
● Use cautiously in elderly patients or patients with renal or hepatic impairment.
● Know that dosage should be reduced in elderly or debilitated patients.

● Monitor liver, renal, and hemato-poietic function studies periodically in patients receiving repeated or prolonged therapy as ordered.
● Possibility of abuse and addiction exists. Do not stop drug abruptly; withdrawal symptoms may occur.
● Warn patients to avoid activities that require alertness or good psychomotor coordination until CNS effects of the drug are known.
● Tell patients to avoid alcohol while taking this drug.

33

Antipsychotics

chlorpromazine hydrochloride
chlorprothixene
clozapine
fluphenazine decanoate
fluphenazine enanthate
fluphenazine hydrochloride
haloperidol
haloperidol decanoate
haloperidol lactate
loxapine hydrochloride
loxapine succinate
mesoridazine besylate
molindone hydrochloride
perphenazine
pimozide
prochlorperazine
   (See Chapter 51, ANTIEMETICS.)
promazine hydrochloride
risperidone
thioridazine hydrochloride
thiothixene
thiothixene hydrochloride
trifluoperazine hydrochloride

COMBINATION PRODUCTS

ETRAFON 2-10: perphenazine 2 mg and amitriptyline hydrochloride 10 mg.
ETRAFON-A: perphenazine 2 mg and amitriptyline hydrochloride 25 mg.
ETRAFON-FORTE: perphenazine 4 mg and amitriptyline hydrochloride 25 mg.
TRIAVIL 2-10, TRIAVIL 4-10, TRIA-VIL 2-25 are identical to Etrafon products above. Triavil also is available as TRIAVIL 4-25 (perphenazine 4 mg and amitriptyline hydrochloride 25 mg) and TRIAVIL 4-50 (perphenazine 4 mg and amitriptyline hydrochloride 50 mg).

chlorpromazine hydrochloride

Chlorpromanyl-5†, Chlorpromanyl-20†, Chlorpromanyl-40†, Largactil†‡, Novo-Chlorpromazine†, Ormazine, Thorazine, Thor-Prom

Pregnancy Risk Category: NR

HOW SUPPLIED

Tablets: 10 mg, 25 mg, 50 mg, 100 mg, 200 mg
Capsules (controlled-release): 30 mg, 75 mg, 150 mg, 200 mg, 300 mg
Oral concentrate: 30 mg/ml, 100 mg/ml
Syrup: 10 mg/5ml
Injection: 25 mg/ml
Suppositories: 25 mg, 100 mg

ACTION

Unknown. An aliphatic phenothiazine that probably blocks postsynaptic dopamine receptors in the brain and inhibits the medullary chemoreceptor trigger zone.

ONSET, PEAK, DURATION

Onset for full antipsychotic effects, 6 weeks or longer. Onset for other effects highly variable as well as for peak and duration.

INDICATIONS & DOSAGE

Psychosis –
Adults: initially, 25 to 75 mg P.O. daily in two to four divided doses. Dosage increased by 20 to 50 mg twice weekly until symptoms are controlled. Up to 800 mg daily may be required in some patients. Or, 25 to 50 mg I.M. q 1 to 4 hours p.r.n. Should be switched to oral therapy as soon as possible.
Children 6 months and older: 0.55

---

*Liquid form contains alcohol.
**May contain tartrazine.

Common reactions are in italics; ***life-threatening,*** in bold italics.

mg/kg P.O. or I.M. q 4 to 6 hours; or 1.1 mg/kg P.R. q 6 to 8 hours. Maximum I.M. dose in children under 5 years or weighing less than 22.7 kg is 40 mg. Maximum I.M. dose in children 5 to 12 years or weighing 22.7 to 45.5 kg is 75 mg.

Nausea and vomiting –
Adults: 10 to 25 mg P.O. q 4 to 6 hours, p.r.n.; or 50 to 100 mg P.R. q 6 to 8 hours, p.r.n. or 25 mg I.M. (if no hypotension occurs), 25 to 50 mg I.M. q 3 to 4 hours p.r.n. until vomiting stops.

Children 6 months and older: 0.55 mg/kg P.O. or I.M. q 4 to 6 hours; or 1.1 mg/kg P.R. q 6 to 8 hours. Maximum I.M. dose in children under 5 years or weighing less than 22.7 kg is 40 mg. Maximum I.M. dose in children 5 to 12 years or weighing 22.7 to 45.5 kg is 75 mg.

Intractable hiccups, acute intermittent porphyria –
Adults: 25 to 50 mg P.O. t.i.d. or q.i.d. If symptoms persist for 2 to 3 days, 25 to 50 mg I.M. If symptoms still persist 25 to 50 mg diluted in 500 to 1000 ml of saline and infused slowly.

Tetanus –
Adults: 25 to 50 mg I.V. or I.M. t.i.d. or q.i.d.
Children 6 months or older: 0.55 mg/kg I.M. or I.V. q 6 to 8 hours. Maximum parenteral dosage in children weighing less than 22.7 kg. is 40 mg daily; for children weighing 22.7 to 45.5 kg is 75 mg, except in severe cases.

Surgery –
Adults: preoperatively, 25 to 50 mg P.O. 2 to 3 hours before surgery or 12.5 to 25 mg I.M. 1 to 2 hours before surgery; during surgery, 12.5 mg I.M. repeated in 30 minutes if needed or fractional 2 mg doses I.V. at 2 minute intervals up to a maximum dose of 25 mg; post-operatively, 10 to 25 mg P.O. q 4 to 6 hours or 12.5 mg to 25

mg I .M. repeated in 1 hour if needed.
Children 6 months and older: preoperatively, 0.55 mg/kg P.O. 2 to 3 hours before surgery or I.M. 1 to 2 hours before surgery; during surgery, 0.275 mg/kg I.M. repeated in 30 minutes if needed or fractional 1 mg doses I.V. at 2 minute intervals up to a total of 0.275 mg/kg, may repeat fractional I.V. regimen in 30 minutes if needed; postoperatively, 0.55 mg/kg P.O. or I.M. q 4 to 6 hours (oral dose) or 1 hour (I.M. dose) if needed and hypotension does not occur.

ADVERSE REACTIONS
CNS: *extrapyramidal reactions* (moderate incidence), *sedation* (high incidence), *tardive dyskinesia,* pseudoparkinsonism, dizziness.
CV: *orthostatic hypotension,* tachycardia, ECG changes.
EENT: ocular changes, blurred vision.
GI: *dry mouth, constipation.*
GU: *urine retention,* menstrual irregularities, gynecomastia, inhibited ejaculation.
Hematologic: transient leukopenia, *agranulocytosis,* hyperprolactinemia.
Hepatic: cholestatic jaundice, abnormal liver function test results.
Skin: *mild photosensitivity,* allergic reactions, *I. M. injection site pain,* sterile abscess.
Other: *neuroleptic malignant syndrome.*
After abrupt withdrawal of long-term therapy: gastritis, nausea, vomiting, dizziness, tremors.

INTERACTIONS
Antacids: inhibited absorption of oral phenothiazines. Separate antacid and phenothiazine doses by at least 2 hours.
Anticholinergics (including antidepressants and antiparkinsonian agents): increased anticholinergic ac-

tivity, aggravated parkinsonian symptoms. Use with caution.
Barbiturates, lithium: may decrease phenothiazine effect. Observe patient.
Centrally acting antihypertensives: decreased antihypertensive effect.
Ethanol, other CNS depressants: increased CNS depression. Avoid concomitant use.
Propranolol: increased levels of both propranolol and chlorpromazine.
Warfarin: decreased effect of oral anticoagulants. Monitor PT.

CONTRAINDICATIONS
Contraindicated in patients with hypersensitivity or in patients experiencing CNS depression, bone marrow suppression, subcortical damage, and coma.

NURSING CONSIDERATIONS
• Use cautiously in elderly or debilitated patients and in patients with hepatic or renal disease; severe CV disease (may cause sudden drop in blood pressure); exposure to extreme heat or cold (including antipyretic therapy), to organophosphate insecticides; respiratory disorders; hypocalcemia; seizure disorders (may lower seizure threshold); severe reactions to insulin or electroconvulsive therapy; glaucoma; or prostatic hyperplasia.
• Use cautiously in acutely ill or dehydrated children.
• Obtain baseline measures of blood pressure before starting therapy and monitor regularly. Watch for orthostatic hypotension, especially with parenteral administration. Monitor blood pressure before and after I.M. administration. Keep patient supine for 1 hour afterward and advise him to get up slowly.
• **I.V. use:** For direct injection, drug may be diluted with 0.9% sodium chloride injection and administered into a large vein or through the tubing of a free-flowing I.V. solution. Do not

exceed 1 mg/minute for adults or 0.5 mg/minute for children. Drug also may be given as an intermittent I.V. infusion; dilute with 50 or 100 ml of a compatible solution and infuse over 30 minutes. Chlorpromazine is compatible with most common I.V. solutions, including D_5W, Ringer's injection, lactated Ringer's injection, and 0.9% sodium chloride injection.
• Slight yellowing of injection or concentrate is common; does not affect potency. Discard markedly discolored solutions.
• Give deep I.M. only in upper outer quadrant of buttocks. Massage slowly afterward to prevent sterile abscess. Injection stings.
• Wear gloves when preparing solutions, and prevent any contact with skin and clothing. Oral liquid and parenteral forms can cause contact dermatitis.
• Protect liquid concentrate from light. Dilute with fruit juice, milk, or semisolid food just before administration.
• Monitor patient for tardive dyskinesia. Be aware that tardive dyskinesia may occur after prolonged use. It may not appear until months or years later and may disappear spontaneously or persist for life despite discontinuation of drug.
• Watch for symptoms of neuroleptic malignant syndrome. It is rare, but frequently fatal. It is not necessarily related to length of drug use or type of neuroleptic, but over 60% of affected patients are men.
• Monitor therapy with weekly bilirubin tests during first month; periodic blood tests (CBC and liver function); and ophthalmic tests (long-term use) as ordered.
• Do not withdraw drug abruptly unless required by severe adverse reactions.
• Withhold dose and notify doctor if patient develops jaundice, symptoms of blood dyscrasia (fever, sore throat,

---

*Liquid form contains alcohol. *Common* reactions are in italics; *life-threatening,* in bold italics.
**May contain tartrazine.

infection, cellulitis, weakness), persistent extrapyramidal reactions (longer than a few hours), or any such reaction in pregnancy or in children.
• Know that acute dystonic reactions may be treated with diphenhydramine.
• Warn patients to avoid activities that require alertness or good psychomotor coordination until CNS effects of the drug are known. Drowsiness and dizziness usually subside after first few weeks.
• Tell patients to avoid alcohol while taking this drug.
• Have patients report urine retention or constipation.
• Tell patients to use sunblock and to wear protective clothing to avoid photosensitivity reactions. Chlorpromazine causes higher incidence of photosensitivity than any other drug in its class.
• Tell patient to relieve dry mouth with sugarless gum or hard candy.

---

chlorprothixene
Taractan**, Tarasan†

Pregnancy Risk Category: NR

HOW SUPPLIED
Tablets: 10 mg, 25 mg, 50 mg, 100 mg
Oral concentrate: 100 mg/5 ml (fruit)
Injection: 12.5 mg/ml

ACTION
Unknown. A thioxanthene that probably blocks postsynaptic dopamine receptors in the brain.

ONSET, PEAK, DURATION
Onset unknown but may take several weeks. Peak unknown. Effects pesist for up to 12 hours after I.M. administration, unknown for oral form.

INDICATIONS & DOSAGE
Psychotic disorders –
Adults and adolescents: initially, 25

to 50 mg P.O. or I.M. t.i.d. or q. Increased gradually to maximum of 600 mg daily.
Children 6 to 12 years: 10 to 25 mg P.O. t.i.d. or q.i.d.

ADVERSE REACTIONS
CNS: extrapyramidal reactions (low incidence), tardive dyskinesia, *sedation,* pseudoparkinsonism, EEG changes, dizziness.
CV: *orthostatic hypotension,* tachycardia, ECG changes.
EENT: ocular changes, *blurred vision.*
GI: *dry mouth, constipation.*
GU: *urine retention,* dark urine, menstrual irregularities, gynecomastia, inhibited ejaculation.
Hematologic: transient leukopenia, *agranulocytosis,* hyperprolactinemia.
Hepatic: cholestatic jaundice, abnormal liver function test results.
Skin: *mild photosensitivity,* allergic reactions, I.M. injection site pain, sterile abscess.
Other: weight gain; increased appetite; rarely, *neuroleptic malignant syndrome.*
After abrupt withdrawal of long-term therapy: gastritis, nausea, vomiting, dizziness, tremors, feeling of warmth or cold, diaphoresis, tachycardia, headache, insomnia.

INTERACTIONS
Anticholinergics: potentiated central anticholinergic effects. Use together cautiously.
Centrally acting antihypertensives: decreased antihypertensive effect. Monitor blood pressure.
Ethanol: increased CNS depression. Avoid concomitant use.
Other CNS depressants: increased CNS depression. Use together cautiously.

CONTRAINDICATIONS
Contraindicated in patients with hypersensitivity, blood dyscrasia, CNS

---

depression, bone marrow suppression, or circulatory collapse.

NURSING CONSIDERATIONS

• Use cautiously in elderly or debilitated patients and in patients with hepatic disease, CV disease (may cause sudden drop in blood pressure), seizure disorders (may lower seizure threshold), glaucoma, or prostatic hyperplasia.

• Also use cautiously in patients with peptic ulcer, respiratory disorders, urine retention, or Parkinson's disease.

• Obtain baseline measures of blood pressure before starting therapy and monitor regularly. Watch for orthostatic hypotension, especially with parenteral administration, because adrenergic blockage is high. Keep patients in a supine position for 1 hour afterward and advise them to change positions slowly.

• Give deep I.M. only in upper outer quadrant of buttocks or midlateral thigh. Massage slowly afterward to prevent sterile abscess. Injection stings.

• Protect medication from light. Slight yellowing of injection or concentrate is common; does not affect potency. Discard markedly discolored solutions.

• Dilute liquid concentrate with fruit juice, milk, or semisolid food just before administration.

• Oral liquid form can cause contact dermatitis. Wear gloves when preparing, and prevent any contact with skin and clothing.

• Monitor patient for tardive dyskinesia. Tardive dyskinesia may occur after prolonged use. It may not appear until months or years later and may disappear spontaneously or persist for life despite discontinuation of drug.

• Watch for symptoms related to neuroleptic malignant syndrome. It is rare, but frequently fatal. It is not necessarily related to length of drug use or type of neuroleptic, but over 60% of affected patients are men.

• Monitor therapy with weekly bilirubin tests during first month; periodic blood tests (CBC and liver function) before and during therapy; and ophthalmic tests (long-term therapy) as ordered.

• Do not withdraw drug abruptly unless required by severe adverse reactions.

• Withhold dose and notify doctor if patient develops symptoms of blood dyscrasia (fever, sore throat, infection, cellulitis, weakness), jaundice, or persistent extrapyramidal reactions (longer than a few hours), especially in children.

• Acute dystonic reactions may be treated with diphenhydramine.

• Warn patients to avoid activities that require alertness or good psychomotor coordination until CNS effects of the drug are known. Drowsiness and dizziness usually subside after first few weeks.

• Tell patients to avoid alcohol while taking this drug.

• Tell patient to relieve dry mouth with sugarless gum or hard candy.

• Have patients report urine retention or constipation.

• Tell patients to use sunblock and to wear protective clothing to avoid photosensitivity reactions.

clozapine
Clozaril

Pregnancy Risk Category: B

HOW SUPPLIED
Tablets: 25 mg, 100 mg

ACTION
Unknown. Binds to dopaminergic receptors (both D-1 and D-2) within the limbic system of the CNS and may interfere with adrenergic, cholinergic, histaminergic, and serotoninergic receptors.

---

*Liquid form contains alcohol.
May contain tartrazine.   *Common* reactions are in italics; ***life-threatening,* in bold italics.

fluphenazine enanthate
Depot injection: 25 mg/ml
fluphenazine hydrochloride
Tablets: 1 mg, 2.5 mg, 5 mg, 10 mg
Oral concentrate: 5 mg/ml (contains 1% alcohol)
Elixir: 2.5 mg/5 ml (with 14% alcohol)
I.M. injection: 2.5 mg/ml

ACTION
Unknown. A piperazine phenothiazine that probably blocks postsynaptic dopamine receptors in the brain.

ONSET, PEAK, DURATION
Following administration of fluphenazine hydrochloride, onset occurs within 1 hour although full therapeutic effect may take up to several weeks. Serum levels peak within 1.5 to 2 hours following I.M. administration; 0.5 hours after oral administration. Effects persist for 6 to 8 hours. Following I.M. administration of fluphenazine decanoate or enanthate, the onset of action occurs within 24 to 72 hours and duration of action is 1 to 6 weeks.

INDICATIONS & DOSAGE
Psychotic disorders –
Adults: initially, 1.25 to 10 mg hydrochloride P.O. daily in divided doses q 6 to 8 hours; may increase cautiously to 20 mg. Higher doses (50 to 100 mg) have been given. Maintenance dosage is 1 to 5 mg P.O. daily. I.M. doses are one-third to one-half of oral doses. Use lower dosages for elderly patients (1 to 2.5 mg daily). Alternatively, 12.5 to 25 mg of long-acting esters (decanoate or enanthate) I.M. or S.C. q 1 to 6 weeks; maintenance dosage is 25 to 100 mg, p.r.n.

ADVERSE REACTIONS
CNS: *extrapyramidal reactions* (high incidence), *tardive dyskinesia,* sedation (low incidence), pseudoparkinsonism, EEG changes, dizziness.
CV: *orthostatic hypotension,* tachycardia, ECG changes.
EENT: ocular changes, *blurred vision.*
GI: *dry mouth, constipation.*
GU: *urine retention,* dark urine, menstrual irregularities, gynecomastia, inhibited ejaculation.
Hematologic: transient leukopenia, *agranulocytosis,* hyperprolactinemia.
Hepatic: cholestatic jaundice, abnormal liver function test results.
Skin: *mild photosensitivity,* allergic reactions.
Other: weight gain; increased appetite; rarely, *neuroleptic malignant syndrome.*
After abrupt withdrawal of long-term therapy: gastritis, nausea, vomiting, dizziness, tremors, feeling of warmth or cold, diaphoresis, tachycardia, headache, insomnia.

INTERACTIONS
Antacids: inhibited absorption of oral phenothiazines. Separate antacid and phenothiazine doses by at least 2 hours.
Anticholinergics: increased anticholinergic effects. Avoid concomitant use.
Barbiturates, lithium: may decrease phenothiazine effect. Observe patient.
Centrally acting antihypertensives: decreased antihypertensive effect. Monitor blood pressure.
Ethanol, other CNS depressants: increased CNS depression. Avoid concomitant use.

CONTRAINDICATIONS
Contraindicated in patients with hypersensitivity or in patients experiencing coma, CNS depression, bone marrow suppression or other blood dyscrasia, subcortical damage, or liver damage.

NURSING CONSIDERATIONS

• Use cautiously in elderly or debilitated patients and in those with pheochromocytoma; severe CV disease (may cause sudden drop in blood pressure); peptic ulcer; exposure to extreme heat or cold (including antipyretic therapy) or phosphorus insecticides; respiratory disorder; hypocalcemia; seizure disorder (may lower seizure threshold); severe reactions to insulin or electroconvulsive therapy; mitral insufficiency; glaucoma; or prostatic hyperplasia. Use parenteral form cautiously in asthmatic patients and patients allergic to sulfites.

• Prolixin Concentrate and Permitil Concentrate are 10 times more concentrated than Prolixin elixir (5 mg/ml vs. 0.5 mg/ml). Check dosage order carefully.

• Dilute liquid concentrate with water, fruit juice, milk, or semisolid food just before administration.

• For long-acting forms (decanoate and enanthate), which are oil preparations, use a dry needle of at least 21G. Allow 24 to 96 hours for onset of action. Note and report adverse reactions in patients taking these drug forms.

• Oral liquid and parenteral forms can cause contact dermatitis. Wear gloves when preparing solutions, and prevent contact with skin and clothing.

• Protect medication from light. Slight yellowing of injection or concentrate is common; does not affect potency. Discard markedly discolored solutions.

• Monitor patient for tardive dyskinesia. Tardive dyskinesia may occur after prolonged use. It may not appear until months or years later and may disappear spontaneously or persist for life despite discontinuation of drug.

• Watch patient for neuroleptic malignant syndrome. It is rare, but frequently fatal. It is not necessarily related to length of drug use or type of

neuroleptic, but over 60% of affected patients are men.

• Monitor therapy with weekly bilirubin tests during first month; periodic blood tests (CBC and liver function); and periodic renal function and ophthalmic tests (long-term use) as ordered.

• Withhold dose and notify doctor if patient develops symptoms of blood dyscrasia (fever, sore throat, infection, cellulitis, weakness), persistent extrapyramidal reactions (longer than a few hours) especially in pregnant patients or in children.

• Acute dystonic reactions may be treated with diphenhydramine.

• Warn patients to avoid activities that require alertness and good psychomotor coordination until CNS effects of the drug are known. Drowsiness and dizziness usually subside after first few weeks.

• Tell patients to avoid alcohol while taking this drug.

• Tell patient to relieve dry mouth with sugarless gum or hard candy.

• Have patient report urine retention or constipation.

• Tell patients to use sunblock and to wear protective clothing to avoid photosensitivity reactions.

• Do not withdraw drug abruptly unless severe adverse reactions occur.

• Tell patients that drug may discolor urine.

---

haloperidol

Apo-Haloperidol†, Haldol**, Halperon, Novo-Peridol†, Peridol†, Serenace‡

haloperidol decanoate

Haldol Decanoate, Haldol LA†

haloperidol lactate

Haldol

Pregnancy Risk Category: C

HOW SUPPLIED
haloperidol
Tablets: 0.5 mg, 1 mg, 2 mg, 5 mg, 10 mg, 20 mg
haloperidol decanoate
Injection: 50 mg/ml, 100 mg/ml
haloperidol lactate
Oral concentrate: 2 mg/ml
Injection: 5 mg/ml

ACTION
Unknown. A butyrophenone that probably blocks postsynaptic dopamine receptors in the brain.

ONSET, PEAK, DURATION
Onset unknown. Serum levels peak in 3 to 6 hours with oral dose, 10 to 20 minutes with I.M. injection (lactate), or 3 to 9 days with long-acting I.M. injection (decanoate). Duration unknown.

INDICATIONS & DOSAGE
Psychotic disorders —
Adults and children 12 and older: dosage varies for each patient. Initial range, 0.5 to 5 mg P.O. b.i.d. or t.i.d.; or 2 to 5 mg I.M. q 4 to 8 hours although q 1 hour administration may be needed until control obtained. Maximum dosage is 100 mg P.O. daily.
Children ages 3 to 12: 0.05 mg/kg to 0.15 mg/kg P.O. daily. Severely disturbed children may require higher doses.
Chronic psychotic patients who require prolonged therapy –
Adults: 50 to 100 mg I.M. haloperidol decanoate q 4 weeks.
Non-psychotic behavior disorders –
Children ages 3 to 12 : 0.05 mg/kg P.O. daily. Maximum daily dosage is 6 mg.
Tourette syndrome –
Adults: 0.5 to 5 mg P.O. b.i.d. or t.i.d. or p.r.n.
Children 3 to 12: 0.075 mg/kg P.O. daily.

ADVERSE REACTIONS
CNS: *severe extrapyramidal reactions* (high incidence), *tardive dyskinesia,* sedation (low incidence).
CV: cardiovascular effects (low incidence with therapeutic dosages).
EENT: *blurred vision.*
GU: urine retention, menstrual irregularities, gynecomastia.
Hematologic: transient leukopenia and leukocytosis.
Skin: rash.
Other: rarely, *neuroleptic malignant syndrome.*

INTERACTIONS
Ethanol, other CNS depressants: increased CNS depression. Avoid concomitant use.
Lithium: lethargy and confusion with high doses. Monitor the patient.
Methyldopa: may cause symptoms of dementia or psychosis. Monitor the patient.

CONTRAINDICATIONS
Contraindicated in patients with hypersensitivity or in patients experiencing parkinsonism, coma, or CNS depression.

NURSING CONSIDERATIONS
• Use cautiously in elderly and debilitated patients; in patients with history of seizures or EEG abnormalities, severe CV disorders, allergies, glaucoma, or urine retention; and in conjunction with anticonvulsant, anticoagulant, antiparkinsonian, or lithium medications.
• Know that elderly patients usually require lower initial doses and a more gradual dosage titration.
• Do not administer the decanoate form intravenously.
• When changing from tablets to decanoate injection, know that patient should be given 10 to 15 times the oral dose once a month (maximum 100 mg).
• Protect medication from light. Slight yellowing of injection or con-

centrate is common; does not affect potency. Discard markedly discolored solutions.
• Do not withdraw drug abruptly unless required by severe adverse reactions.
• Monitor patient for tardive dyskinesia. It may occur after prolonged use. It may not appear until months or years later and may disappear spontaneously or persist for life despite discontinuation of drug.
• Watch patient for neuroleptic malignant syndrome. It is rare, but frequently fatal. It is not necessarily related to length of drug use or type of neuroleptic, but over 60% of affected patients are men.
• Know that acute dystonic reactions may be treated with diphenhydramine.
• Least sedating of the antipsychotic agents. However, warn patients to avoid activities that require alertness and good psychomotor coordination until CNS effects of the drug are known. Drowsiness and dizziness usually subside after a few weeks.
• Tell the patient to avoid alcohol while taking this drug.
• Tell patient to relieve dry mouth with sugarless gum or hard candy.

loxapine hydrochloride
Loxapac†, Loxitane C, Loxitane IM

loxapine succinate
Loxapac†, Loxitane

Pregnancy Risk Category: NR

HOW SUPPLIED
loxapine hydrochloride
Oral concentrate: 25 mg/ml
Injection: 50 mg/ml
loxapine succinate
Capsules: 5 mg, 10 mg, 25 mg, 50 mg
Tablets: 5 mg†, 10 mg†, 25 mg†, 50 mg†

ACTION
Unknown. A dibenzoxazepine that probably blocks postsynaptic dopamine receptors in the brain.

ONSET, PEAK, DURATION
Onset of action occurs in 30 minutes. Serum levels peak in 1.5 to 3 hours. Effects persist up to 12 hours.

INDICATIONS & DOSAGE
Psychotic disorders –
Adults: 10 mg P.O. b.i.d. to q.i.d., rapidly increasing to 60 to 100 mg P.O. daily for most patients; dosage varies from patient to patient. If patient unable to take oral dose, 12.5 to 50 mg I.M. q 4 to 6 hours or longer, both dose and interval depending on patient response.

ADVERSE REACTIONS
CNS: *extrapyramidal reactions* (moderate incidence), *sedation* (moderate incidence), *tardive dyskinesia,* pseudoparkinsonism, EEG changes, dizziness.
CV: *orthostatic hypotension,* tachycardia, ECG changes.
EENT: *blurred vision.*
GI: *dry mouth, constipation.*
GU: *urine retention,* dark urine, menstrual irregularities, gynecomastia.
Hematologic: transient leukopenia.
Skin: *mild photosensitivity,* allergic reactions.
Other: weight gain; increased appetite; rarely, ***neuroleptic malignant syndrome.***

INTERACTIONS
Ethanol, other CNS depressants: increased CNS depression. Avoid concomitant use.

CONTRAINDICATIONS
Contraindicated in patients with hypersensitivity to dibenzoxazepines and in patients experiencing coma, severe CNS depression, or drug-induced depressed states.

---

*Liquid form contains alcohol.
May contain tartrazine.*   *Common* reactions are in italics; ***life-threatening,* in bold italics.

NURSING CONSIDERATIONS

- Use with extreme caution in patients with seizure disorder, CV disorder, glaucoma, and history of urine retention.
- Obtain baseline measures of blood pressure before starting therapy and monitor regularly.
- Dilute liquid concentrate with orange or grapefruit juice just before giving.
- Monitor patient for tardive dyskinesia. It may occur after prolonged use. It may not appear until months or years later and may disappear spontaneously or persist for life despite discontinuation of drug.
- Monitor patient for neuroleptic malignant syndrome. It is rare, but frequently fatal. It is not necessarily related to length of drug use or type of neuroleptic, but over 60% of affected patients are men.
- Know that acute dystonic reactions may be treated with diphenhydramine.
- Warn patients to avoid activities that require alertness and good psychomotor coordination until CNS effects of the drug are known. Drowsiness and dizziness usually subside after first few weeks.
- Tell patients to avoid alcohol while taking this drug.
- Advise patients to get up slowly to avoid orthostatic hypotension.
- Tell patient to relieve dry mouth with sugarless gum or hard candy.
- Tell patient periodic eye examinations are recommended.

---

mesoridazine besylate
Serentil* **, Serentil Concentrate

Pregnancy Risk Category: NR

HOW SUPPLIED
Tablets: 10 mg, 25 mg, 50 mg, 100 mg
Oral concentrate: 25 mg/ml (0.6% alcohol)

Injection: 25 mg/ml

ACTION
Unknown. A piperidine phenothiazine and the major sulfoxide metabolite of thioridazine that probably blocks postsynaptic dopamine receptors in the brain.

ONSET, PEAK, DURATION
Onset of antipsychotic effect is gradual (up to several weeks) and variable between patients. Peak and duration not clearly defined.

INDICATIONS & DOSAGE
Alcoholism –
Adults and children over 12 years: 25 mg P.O. b.i.d. up to maximum of 200 mg daily.
Behavioral problems associated with chronic organic mental syndrome –
Adults and children over 12 years: 25 mg P.O. t.i.d. up to maximum of 300 mg daily.
Psychoneurotic manifestations (anxiety) –
Adults and children over 12 years: 10 mg P.O. t.i.d. up to maximum of 150 mg daily.
Schizophrenia –
Adults and children over 12 years: initially, 50 mg P.O. t.i.d. or 25 mg I.M. repeated in 30 to 60 minutes, p.r.n. Maximum dosage is 400 mg daily.

ADVERSE REACTIONS
CNS: extrapyramidal reactions (low incidence), *tardive dyskinesia, sedation* (high incidence), EEG changes, dizziness.
CV: *orthostatic hypotension,* tachycardia, ECG changes.
EENT: *ocular changes, blurred vision,* retinitis pigmentosa.
GI: *dry mouth, constipation.*
GU: *urine retention,* dark urine, menstrual irregularities, gynecomastia, inhibited ejaculation.

Hematologic: transient leukopenia, *agranulocytosis,* hyperprolactinemia.
Hepatic: cholestatic jaundice, abnormal liver function test results.
Skin: *mild photosensitivity,* allergic reactions, pain at I.M. injection site, sterile abscess.
Other: weight gain; increased appetite; rarely, *neuroleptic malignant syndrome.*
After abrupt withdrawal of long-term therapy: gastritis, nausea, vomiting, dizziness, tremors, feeling of warmth or cold, diaphoresis, tachycardia, headache, insomnia.

INTERACTIONS
Antacids: inhibited absorption of oral phenothiazines. Separate antacid and phenothiazine doses by at least 2 hours.
Anticholinergics: may increase anticholinergic effects. Use together cautiously.
Barbiturates: may decrease phenothiazine effect. Observe patient.
Ethanol: increased CNS depression. Avoid concomitant use.
Other CNS depressants: increased CNS depression. Use together cautiously.

CONTRAINDICATIONS
Contraindicated in patients with hypersensitivity to the drug or experiencing severe CNS depression or comatose states.

NURSING CONSIDERATIONS
• Obtain baseline measures of blood pressure before starting therapy and monitor regularly. Watch for orthostatic hypotension, especially with parenteral administration.
• Oral liquid and parenteral forms may cause contact dermatitis. Wear gloves when preparing solutions, and prevent contact with skin and clothing.
• Give deep I.M. only in upper outer quadrant of buttocks. Massage slowly

afterward to prevent sterile abscess. Injection may sting.
• Protect medication from light. Slight yellowing of injection or concentrate is common; does not affect potency. Discard markedly discolored solutions.
• Monitor patient for tardive dyskinesia. It may occur after prolonged use. It may not appear until months or years later and may disappear spontaneously or persist for life despite discontinuation of drug.
• Assess patient for neuroleptic malignant syndrome. It is rare, but frequently fatal. It is not necessarily related to length of drug use or type of neuroleptic, but over 60% of affected patients are men.
• Withhold dose and notify the doctor if patient develops jaundice, symptoms of blood dyscrasia (fever, sore throat, infection, cellulitis, weakness), persistent extrapyramidal reactions (longer than a few hours), especially in pregnant patients or in children.
• Monitor therapy with weekly bilirubin tests during first month; periodic blood tests (CBC and liver function); and ophthalmic tests (long-term use) as ordered.
• Know that acute dystonic reactions may be treated with diphenhydramine.
• Do not withdraw drug abruptly unless required by severe adverse reactions.
• Warn patients to avoid activities that require alertness and good psychomotor coordination until CNS effects of the drug are known. Drowsiness and dizziness usually subside after a few weeks.
• Advise patients to change position slowly.
• Tell patients to avoid alcohol while taking this drug.
• Have patients report urine retention or constipation.

---

*Liquid form contains alcohol.   *Common* reactions are in italics; *life-threatening,* in bold italics.
**May contain tartrazine.

• Tell patients that drug may discolor urine.

• Instruct patient to relieve dry mouth with sugarless gum or hard candy.

• Tell patients to use sunblock and to wear protective clothing to avoid photosensitivity reactions.

---

molindone hydrochloride
Moban

Pregnancy Risk Category: NR

HOW SUPPLIED
Tablets: 5 mg, 10 mg, 25 mg, 50 mg, 100 mg
Oral solution: 20 mg/ml

ACTION
Unknown. A dihydroindolone that probably blocks postsynaptic dopamine receptors in the brain.

ONSET, PEAK, DURATION
Onset unknown but thought to take several weeks. Serum levels peak in 1.5 hours. Effects persist for 24 to 36 hours.

INDICATIONS & DOSAGE
Psychotic disorders –
Adults: initially, 50 to 75 mg P.O. daily, then increased to 100 to 225 mg/day in 3 or 4 days. Maintenance dosage as follows: mild severity — 5 to 15 mg P.O. t.i.d. to q.i.d.; moderate severity — 10 to 25 mg P.O. t.i.d. or q.i.d.; or severe severity — 225 mg/day P.O.

ADVERSE REACTIONS
CNS: *extrapyramidal reactions* (moderate incidence), *tardive dyskinesia, sedation* (moderate incidence), pseudoparkinsonism, EEG changes, dizziness.
CV: *orthostatic hypotension,* tachycardia, ECG changes.
EENT: *blurred vision.*
GI: *dry mouth, constipation.*
GU: *urine retention,* dark urine, menstrual irregularities, gynecomastia, inhibited ejaculation.
Hematologic: transient leukopenia, hyperprolactinemia.
Hepatic: cholestatic jaundice, abnormal liver function test results.
Skin: *mild photosensitivity,* allergic reactions.
Other: rarely, *neuroleptic malignant syndrome.*

INTERACTIONS
Ethanol, other CNS depressants: increased CNS depression. Avoid concomitant use.

CONTRAINDICATIONS
Contraindicated in patients with hypersensitivity to drug or experiencing coma or severe CNS depression.

NURSING CONSIDERATIONS
• Use cautiously when increased physical activity would be harmful because this agent increases activity and in patients subject to seizures (may lower seizure threshold).

• Know that drug may be administered in a single daily dose.

• Monitor patient for tardive dyskinesia. It may occur after prolonged use. It may not appear until months or years later and may disappear spontaneously or persist for life despite discontinuation of drug.

• Assess patient for neuroleptic malignant syndrome. It is rare, but frequently fatal. It is not necessarily related to length of drug use or type of neuroleptic, but over 60% of affected patients are men.

• Know that acute dystonic reactions may be treated with diphenhydramine.

• Warn patients to avoid activities that require alertness or good psychomotor coordination until CNS effects of the drug are known. Drowsiness and dizziness usually subside after first few weeks.

---

†Available in Canada only.   ‡Available in Australia only.   ◇Available OTC.

• Tell patients to avoid alcohol while taking this drug.
• Tell patient to relieve dry mouth with sugarless gum or hard candy.

perphenazine
Apo-Perphenazine†, PMS-Perphenazine†, Trilafon, Trilafon Concentrate

Pregnancy Risk Category: NR

HOW SUPPLIED
Tablets: 2 mg, 4 mg, 8 mg, 16 mg
Oral concentrate: 16 mg/5ml
Syrup: 2 mg/5 ml†
Injection: 5 mg/ml

ACTION
Unknown. Probably blocks postsynaptic dopamine receptors in the brain and inhibits the medullary chemoreceptor trigger zone.

ONSET, PEAK, DURATION
Onset of antipsychotic effect is gradual (up to several weeks) and variable between patients. Peak and duration not clearly defined.

INDICATIONS & DOSAGE
Psychosis in non-hospitalized patients –
Adults: initially, 4 to 8 mg P.O. t.i.d., reduced as soon as possible to minimum effective dosage.
Children over 12: lowest adult dose.
Psychosis in hospitalized patients –
Adults: initially, 8 to 16 mg P.O. b.i.d., t.i.d., or q.i.d., increased to 64 mg daily as needed. Alternatively, 5 to 10 mg I.M. q 6 hours p.r.n. Maximum dosage is 30 mg.
Children over 12: lowest limit of adult dosage.
Severe nausea and vomiting –
Adults: 8 to 16 mg P.O. daily in divided doses up to maximum of 24 mg. Alternatively, 5 to 10 mg I.M. p.r.n.

ADVERSE REACTIONS
CNS: *extrapyramidal reactions* (high incidence), *tardive dyskinesia,* sedation (low incidence), pseudoparkinsonism, EEG changes, dizziness.
CV: *orthostatic hypotension,* tachycardia, ECG changes.
EENT: ocular changes, *blurred vision.*
GI: *dry mouth, constipation.*
GU: *urine retention,* dark urine, menstrual irregularities, gynecomastia, inhibited ejaculation.
Hematologic: transient leukopenia, hyperprolactinemia, *agranulocytosis.*
Hepatic: cholestatic jaundice, abnormal liver function test results.
Skin: *mild photosensitivity,* allergic reactions, pain at I.M. injection site, sterile abscess.
Other: weight gain; increased appetite; rarely, *neuroleptic malignant syndrome.*
After abrupt withdrawal of long-term therapy: gastritis, nausea, vomiting, dizziness, tremors, feeling of warmth or cold, diaphoresis, tachycardia, headache, insomnia.

INTERACTIONS
Antacids: inhibited absorption of oral phenothiazines. Separate antacid and phenothiazine doses by at least 2 hours.
Barbiturates: may decrease phenothiazine effect. Observe patient.
Ethanol, other CNS depressants: increased CNS depression. Avoid concomitant use.

CONTRAINDICATIONS
Contraindicated in patients with hypersensitivity to the drug; in patients experiencing coma; in those with CNS depression, blood dyscrasia, bone marrow depression, liver damage, or subcortical damage; and in those receiving large doses of CNS depressants.

---

*Liquid form contains alcohol.   *Common* reactions are in italics; *life-threatening,* in bold italics.
**May contain tartrazine.

NURSING CONSIDERATIONS

• Use cautiously with other CNS depressants or anticholinergics, and in elderly or debilitated patients.

• Also use cautiously in patients with alcohol withdrawal, psychic depression, suicidal tendency, severe adverse reactions to other phenothiazines, impaired renal function, and respiratory disorders.

• Obtain baseline measures of blood pressure before starting therapy and monitor regularly. Watch for orthostatic hypotension, especially with parenteral administration. Keep patient supine for 1 hour afterward; advise him to change positions slowly.

• Prevent contact dermatitis by keeping drug away from skin and clothes. Wear gloves when preparing liquid forms.

• Dilute liquid concentrate with fruit juice, milk, carbonated beverage, or semisolid food just before giving. Exceptions: Oral concentrate causes turbidity or precipitation in colas, black coffee, grape or apple juice, or tea. Do not mix with these liquids.

• Protect drug from light. Slight yellowing of injection or concentrate is common; does not affect potency. Discard markedly discolored solutions.

• Give deep I.M. only in upper outer quadrant of buttocks. Massage slowly afterward to prevent sterile abscess. Injection may sting.

• Monitor patient for tardive dyskinesia. It may occur after prolonged use. It may not appear until months or years later and may disappear spontaneously or persist for life despite discontinuation of drug.

• Assess patient for neuroleptic malignant syndrome. It is rare, but frequently fatal. It is not necessarily related to length of drug use or type of neuroleptic, but over 60% of affected patients are men.

• Know that acute dystonic reactions may be treated with diphenhydramine.

• Monitor therapy with weekly bilirubin tests during first month; periodic blood tests (CBC and liver function); and ophthalmic tests (long-term use) as ordered.

• Do not withdraw drug abruptly unless required by severe adverse reactions.

• Withhold dose and notify doctor if patient develops jaundice, symptoms of blood dyscrasia (fever, sore throat, infection, cellulitis, weakness), or persistent extrapyramidal reactions (longer than a few hours).

• Warn patients to avoid activities that require alertness or good psychomotor coordination until CNS effects of the drug are known. Drowsiness and dizziness usually subside after a few weeks.

• Tell patients to avoid alcohol while taking this drug.

• Advise patients to report urine retention or constipation.

• Tell patients to use sunblock and to wear protective clothing to avoid photosensitivity reactions.

• Tell patient to relieve dry mouth with sugarless gum or hard candy.

---

pimozide
Orap

Pregnancy Risk Category: C

HOW SUPPLIED
Tablets: 2 mg, 4mg†, 10 mg†

ACTION
Unknown. Although thought to block dopamine non selectively at both the pre- and post-synaptic receptors on neurons in the CNS.

ONSET, PEAK, DURATION
Onset and duration unknown. Serum levels peak within 4 to 12 hours.

INDICATIONS & DOSAGE
Suppression of motor and phonic tics in patients with Tourette syndrome refractory to first line therapy—
Adults and children over 12 years: initially, 1 to 2 mg P.O. daily in divided doses. Then increased every other day as needed. Maximum dosage is 10 mg daily.

ADVERSE REACTIONS
CNS: *parkinsonian-like symptoms,* other extrapyramidal symptoms (dystonia, akathisia, hyperreflexia, opisthotonos, oculogyric crisis), *tardive dyskinesia, sedation.*
CV: *ECG changes (prolonged QT interval),* hypotension.
EENT: visual disturbances.
GI: *dry mouth, constipation.*
GU: impotence.
Other: rarely, ***neuroleptic malignant syndrome;*** muscle rigidity.

INTERACTIONS
Ethanol, other CNS depressants: increased CNS depression. Avoid concomitant use.
Phenothiazines, tricyclic antidepressants, antiarrhythmics: increased incidence of ECG abnormalities. Monitor patient closely.

CONTRAINDICATIONS
Contraindicated in patients with hypersensitivity to drug, in the treatment of simple tics or tics other than those associated with Tourette syndrome, concurrent drug therapy known to cause motor and phonic tics, congenital long QT syndrome or history of arrhythmias, patients with severe toxic CNS depression, and patients experiencing coma.

NURSING CONSIDERATIONS
• Use cautiously in patients with hepatic or renal dysfunction, glaucoma, prostatic hyperplasia, seizure disorder, or EEG abnormalities.
• Perform an ECG before treatment begins and periodically thereafter as ordered. Monitor for prolonged QT interval.
• Monitor patient for tardive dyskinesia. It may occur after prolonged use. It may not appear until months or years later and may disappear spontaneously or persist for life despite discontinuation of drug.
• Assess patient for neuroleptic malignant syndrome. It is rare, but frequently fatal. It is not necessarily related to length of drug use or type of neuroleptic, but over 60% of affected patients are men.
• Know that acute dystonic reactions may be treated with diphenhydramine.
• Know that concurrent administration of other drugs that prolong the QT interval, such as antiarrhythmics should be avoided.
• Monitor patients who also are taking anticonvulsants for increased seizure activity. Pimozide may lower the seizure threshold.
• Warn patients not to stop taking drug abruptly and not to exceed prescribed dosage.
• Tell patients to avoid alcohol while taking this drug.
• Tell patients to use sugarless hard candy, gum, and liquids to relieve dry mouth.

promazine hydrochloride
Primazine, Prozine-50, Sparine**

Pregnancy Risk Category: NR

HOW SUPPLIED
Tablets: 25 mg, 50 mg, 100 mg
Injection: 25 mg/ml, 50 mg/ml

ACTION
Unknown. An aliphatic phenothiazine that probably blocks postsynaptic dopamine receptors in the brain.

---

*Liquid form contains alcohol.   *Common* reactions are in italics; ***life-threatening,*** in bold italics.
**May contain tartrazine.

ONSET, PEAK, DURATION
Onset of antipsychotic effect is gradual (up to several weeks) and variable between patients. Peak and duration unknown.

INDICATIONS & DOSAGE
Psychosis –
Adults: 10 to 200 mg P.O. or I.M. q 4 to 6 hours, up to 1 g daily as needed. For acutely agitated patients, initial dose is 50 to 150 mg I.M. or I.V.; repeat within 30 minutes if necessary up to a total of 300 mg.
Children over 12 years: 10 to 25 mg P.O. or I.M. q 4 to 6 hours.

ADVERSE REACTIONS
CNS: *extrapyramidal reactions* (moderate incidence), *tardive dyskinesia, sedation* (high incidence), pseudoparkinsonism, EEG changes, dizziness.
CV: *orthostatic hypotension,* tachycardia, ECG changes.
EENT: ocular changes, blurred vision.
GI: *dry mouth, constipation.*
GU: *urine retention,* dark urine, menstrual irregularities, gynecomastia, inhibited ejaculation.
Hematologic: transient leukopenia, *agranulocytosis,* hyperprolactinemia.
Hepatic: cholestatic jaundice, abnormal liver function test results.
Skin: *mild photosensitivity,* allergic reactions, pain at I.M. injection site, sterile abscess.
Other: weight gain; increased appetite; rarely, *neuroleptic malignant syndrome.*
After abrupt withdrawal of long-term therapy: gastritis, nausea, vomiting, dizziness, tremors, feeling of warmth or cold, diaphoresis, tachycardia, headache, insomnia.

INTERACTIONS
Antacids: inhibited absorption of oral phenothiazines. Use together cautiously. Separate antacid and phenothiazine doses by at least 2 hours.
Anticholinergics (including antidepressants and antiparkinsonian agents): increased anticholinergic activity, aggravated parkinsonian symptoms. Use together cautiously.
Barbiturates, lithium: may decrease phenothiazine effect. Observe patient.
Centrally acting antihypertensives: decreased antihypertensive effect. Monitor blood pressure.
Ethanol: increased CNS depression. Avoid concomitant use.
Other CNS depressants: increased CNS depression. Use together cautiously.

CONTRAINDICATIONS
Contraindicated in patients with hypersensitivity to the drug or in patients experiencing coma or CNS depression, bone marrow suppression, or subcortical damage.

NURSING CONSIDERATIONS
• Use cautiously in elderly or debilitated patients and in patients with hepatic or renal disease, severe CV disease (may cause sudden drop in blood pressure); exposure to extreme heat or cold (including antipyretic therapy) or to organophosphate insecticides; respiratory disorder; hypocalcemia; seizure disorder (may lower seizure threshold); severe reactions to insulin or electroconvulsive therapy; glaucoma; or prostatic hyperplasia.
• Monitor blood pressure with patient lying and standing before starting therapy, and routinely throughout course of treatment.
• Prevent contact dermatitis by keeping drug away from skin and clothes. Wear gloves when preparing liquid forms.
• Dilute liquid concentrate with fruit juice, milk, semisolid food, or chocolate-flavored drinks just before giving. For best taste, use at least 10 ml diluent per 25 mg drug.
• Protect drug from light. Slight yel-

lowing of injection or concentrate is common; does not affect potency. Discard markedly discolored solutions.

• Give deeply I.M. only in upper outer quadrant of buttocks. Massage slowly afterward to prevent sterile abscess. Injection may sting.

• Watch for orthostatic hypotension, especially with parenteral administration. Keep the patient supine for 1 hour afterward and advise patient to change positions slowly.

• Monitor patient for tardive dyskinesia. It may occur after prolonged use. It may not appear until months or years later and may disappear spontaneously or persist for life despite discontinuation of drug.

• Assess patient for neuroleptic malignant syndrome. It is rare, but frequently fatal. It is not necessarily related to length of drug use or type of neuroleptic, but over 60% of affected patients are men.

• Monitor therapy with weekly bilirubin tests during first month; periodic blood tests (CBC and liver function); and ophthalmic tests (long-term use) as ordered.

• Do not withdraw drug abruptly unless required by severe adverse reactions.

• Withhold dose and notify doctor if patient develops jaundice, symptoms of blood dyscrasia (fever, sore throat, infection, cellulitis, weakness), persistent extrapyramidal reactions (longer than a few hours), especially in pregnant patients or in children.

• Know that acute dystonic reactions may be treated with diphenhydramine.

• Warn patients to avoid activities that require alertness or good psychomotor coordination until CNS effects of the drug are known. Drowsiness and dizziness usually subside after a few weeks.

• Tell patients to avoid alcohol while taking this drug.

• Have patients report urine retention or constipation.

• Tell patients to use sunblock and to wear protective clothing to avoid photosensitivity reactions.

• Tell patient to relieve dry mouth with sugarless gum or hard candy.

risperidone
Risperdal

Pregnancy Risk Category: C

HOW SUPPLIED
Tablets: 1 mg, 2 mg, 3 mg, 4 mg

ACTION
Blocks dopamine and serotonin receptors; also blocks alpha$_1$, alpha$_2$, and histamine$_1$ receptors in the CNS.

ONSET, PEAK, DURATION
Onset and duration unknown. Plasma levels peak in about 1 hour.

INDICATIONS & DOSAGE
Psychosis –
Adults: initially, 1 mg P.O. b.i.d. Increased in increments of 1 mg b.i.d. on the second and third day of treatment to a target dose of 3 mg b.i.d. At least 1 week must pass before dosage is adjusted further.
Elderly or debilitated patients, hypotensive patients, or patients with severe renal or hepatic impairment: initially, 0.5 mg P.O. b.i.d. Increased in increments of 0.5 mg b.i.d. on the second and third day of treatment to a target dosage of 1.5 mg P.O. b.i.d. At least 1 week must pass before dosage increased further.

ADVERSE REACTIONS
CNS: *somnolence, extrapyramidal symptoms, headache, insomnia, agitation, anxiety,* tardive dyskinesia, aggressiveness.
CV: tachycardia, chest pain, orthostatic hypotension, prolonged QT interval.

---

*Liquid form contains alcohol.
**May contain tartrazine.
Common reactions are in italics; **life-threatening,** in bold italics.

EENT: rhinitis, coughing, upper respiratory infection, sinusitis, pharyngitis, abnormal vision.
GI: *constipation, nausea, vomiting, dyspepsia.*
Skin: rash, dry skin, photosensitivity.
Other: arthralgia; back pain; fever; rarely, ***neuroleptic malignant syndrome.***

INTERACTIONS
Carbamazepine: increased clearance of risperidone, leading to decreased effectiveness. Monitor closely.
Clozapine: decreased clearance of risperidone, increasing toxicity. Monitor closely.
Ethanol, CNS depressants: additive CNS depression. Avoid concomitant use.
Levodopa: antagonized effects. Don't use together.

CONTRAINDICATIONS
Contraindicated in patients hypersensitive to the drug. Also contraindicated in breast-feeding patients.

NURSING CONSIDERATIONS
• Use cautiously in patients with prolonged QT interval, cardiovascular disease, cerebrovascular disease, dehydration, hypovolemia, history of seizures, exposure to extreme heat, or conditions that could affect metabolism or hemodynamic responses.
• Obtain baseline measures of blood pressure before starting therapy and monitor regularly. Watch for orthostatic hypotension, especially during initial dosage titration. Warn patient to rise slowly, avoid hot showers, and use extra caution during the first few days of therapy to avoid fainting.
• Monitor patient for tardive dyskinesia. It may occur after prolonged use. It may not appear until months or years later and may disappear spontaneously or persist for life despite discontinuation of drug.
• Assess patient for neuroleptic ma-

lignant syndrome. It is rare, but frequently fatal. It is not necessarily related to length of drug use or type of neuroleptic, but over 60% of affected patients are men.
• Warn patients to avoid activities that require alertness or good psychomotor coordination until CNS effects of the drug are known. Drowsiness and dizziness usually subside after a few days.
• Tell patients to avoid alcohol while taking this drug.
• Advise patients to use caution in hot weather to prevent heatstroke because the drug may interfere with thermoregulation.
• Tell patients to use sunblock and to wear protective clothing to avoid photosensitivity reactions.
• Tell patients to notify their doctors if they are or plan to become pregnant during therapy.

---

thioridazine hydrochloride
Aldazine‡, Apo-Thioridazine†, Mellaril*, Mellaril Concentrate, Novoridazine†, PMS Thioridazine†

Pregnancy Risk Category: NR

HOW SUPPLIED
Tablets: 10 mg, 15 mg, 25 mg, 50 mg, 100 mg, 150 mg, 200 mg
Oral suspension: 25 mg/5 ml, 100 mg/5 ml
Oral concentrate: 30 mg/ml, 100 mg/ml (3% to 4.2% alcohol)

ACTION
Unknown. A piperidine phenothiazine that probably blocks postsynaptic dopamine receptors in the brain.

ONSET, PEAK, DURATION
Onset of antipsychotic effect is gradual (up to several weeks) and variable between patients. Peak and duration unknown.

INDICATIONS & DOSAGE
Psychosis—
Adults: initially, 50 to 100 mg P.O. t.i.d., with gradual increments up to 800 mg daily in divided doses, if needed. Dosage varies.
Short term treatment of moderate to marked depression with variable degrees of anxiety, treatment of multiple symptoms, such as agitation, anxiety, depressed mood, tension, sleep disturbances, and fears in geriatric patients—
Adults: Initially 25 mg P.O. daily. Maximum daily dosage is 200 mg.
Children age 2 to 12 years: 0.5 to 3 mg/kg P.O. daily in divided doses.

ADVERSE REACTIONS
CNS: extrapyramidal reactions (low incidence), *tardive dyskinesia, sedation* (high incidence), EEG changes, dizziness.
CV: *orthostatic hypotension,* tachycardia, ECG changes.
EENT: *ocular changes, blurred vision,* retinitis pigmentosa.
GI: *dry mouth, constipation.*
GU: *urine retention,* dark urine, menstrual irregularities, gynecomastia, inhibited ejaculation.
Hematologic: transient leukopenia, *agranulocytosis,* hyperprolactinemia.
Hepatic: cholestatic jaundice.
Skin: *mild photosensitivity,* allergic reactions.
Other: weight gain; increased appetite; rarely, *neuroleptic malignant syndrome.*
After abrupt withdrawal of long-term therapy: gastritis, nausea, vomiting, dizziness, tremors, feeling of warmth or cold, diaphoresis, tachycardia, headache, insomnia.

INTERACTIONS
Antacids: inhibited absorption of oral phenothiazines. Separate antacid and phenothiazine doses by at least 2 hours.
Barbiturates, lithium: may decrease phenothiazine effect. Observe patient.
Centrally acting antihypertensives: decreased antihypertensive effect. Monitor blood pressure.
Ethanol: increased CNS depression. Avoid concomitant use.
Other CNS depressants: increased CNS depression. Use together cautiously.

CONTRAINDICATIONS
Contraindicated in patients with hypersensitivity to the drug or in patients experiencing coma or CNS depression, or severe hypertensive or hypotensive cardiac disease.

NURSING CONSIDERATIONS
● Use cautiously in elderly or debilitated patients and in patients with hepatic disease; CV disease; exposure to extreme heat or cold (including antipyretic therapy) or to organophosphate insecticides; respiratory disorder; hypocalcemia; seizure disorder; or severe reactions to insulin or electroconvulsive therapy.
● Remember that different liquid formulations have different concentrations. Check dosage carefully.
● Prevent contact dermatitis by keeping drug away from skin and clothes. Wear gloves when preparing liquid forms.
● Dilute liquid concentrate with water or fruit juice just before giving.
● Be sure to shake suspension well before using.
● Monitor patient for tardive dyskinesia. It may occur after prolonged use. It may not appear until months or years later and may disappear spontaneously or persist for life despite discontinuation of drug.
● Assess patient for neuroleptic malignant syndrome. It is rare, but frequently fatal. It is not necessarily related to length of drug use or type of neuroleptic, but over 60% of affected patients are men.

---

*Liquid form contains alcohol.
**May contain tartrazine.

Common reactions are in italics; *life-threatening,* in bold italics.

- Monitor therapy with weekly bilirubin tests during first month; periodic blood tests (CBC and liver function); and ophthalmic tests (long-term therapy) as ordered.
- Do not withdraw abruptly unless required by severe adverse reactions.
- Withhold dose and notify the doctor if patient develops jaundice, symptoms of blood dyscrasia (fever, sore throat, infection, cellulitis, weakness), or persistent extrapyramidal reactions (longer than a few hours), especially in pregnant patients or in children.
- Know that acute dystonic reactions may be treated with diphenhydramine.
- Warn patients to avoid activities that require alertness or good psychomotor coordination until CNS effects of the drug are known. Drowsiness and dizziness usually subside after a few weeks.
- Tell patient to watch for orthostatic hypotension, especially with parenteral administration. Advise patient to change positions slowly.
- Tell patients to avoid alcohol while taking this drug.
- Have patients report urine retention or constipation.
- Tell patients that drug may discolor the urine.
- Tell patients to watch for and notify doctor of blurred vision.
- Advise patient to relieve dry mouth with sugarless gum or hard candy.
- Tell patients to use sunblock and to wear protective clothing to avoid photosensitivity reactions.

---

thiothixene
Navane

thiothixene hydrochloride
Navane*

Pregnancy Risk Category: NR

HOW SUPPLIED
thiothixene
Capsules: 1 mg, 2 mg, 5 mg, 10 mg, 20 mg
thiothixene hydrochloride
Oral concentrate: 5 mg/ml (7% alcohol)
Injection: 2 mg/ml, 5 mg/ml

ACTION
Unknown. A thioxanthene that probably blocks postsynaptic dopamine receptors in the brain.

ONSET, PEAK, DURATION
Onset of antipsychotic effect is gradual (up to several weeks). Peak and duration unknown.

INDICATIONS & DOSAGE
Mild to moderate psychosis –
Adults: initially, 2 mg P.O. t.i.d. Increased gradually to 15 mg daily as needed.
Severe psychosis –
Adults: initially, 5 mg P.O. b.i.d. Increased gradually to 15 to 30 mg daily as needed. Maximum recommended dosage is 60 mg daily. Alternatively, 4 mg I.M. b.i.d. or q.i.d. Maximum dosage is 30 mg I.M. daily. An oral form should supplant the injectable form as soon as possible.

ADVERSE REACTIONS
CNS: *extrapyramidal reactions* (high incidence), *tardive dyskinesia,* sedation (low incidence), pseudoparkinsonism, EEG changes, dizziness.
CV: *orthostatic hypotension,* tachycardia, ECG changes.
EENT: ocular changes, *blurred vision.*
GI: *dry mouth, constipation.*
GU: *urine retention,* dark urine, menstrual irregularities, gynecomastia, inhibited ejaculation.
Hematologic: transient leukopenia, *agranulocytosis,* hyperprolactinemia.
Hepatic: cholestatic jaundice.
Skin: *mild photosensitivity,* allergic

reactions, pain at I.M. injection site, sterile abscess.

Other: weight gain; increased appetite; rarely, ***neuroleptic malignant syndrome***.

After abrupt withdrawal of long-term therapy: gastritis, nausea, vomiting, dizziness, tremors, feeling of warmth or cold, diaphoresis, tachycardia, headache, insomnia.

INTERACTIONS

Ethanol, other CNS depressants: increased CNS depression. Avoid concomitant use.

CONTRAINDICATIONS

Contraindicated in patients with hypersensitivity to the drug or in patients experiencing circulatory collapse, coma, CNS depression, or blood dyscrasia.

NURSING CONSIDERATIONS

• Use with extreme caution in patients with history of seizure disorder or in a state of alcohol withdrawal.

• Use cautiously in elderly or debilitated patients; and in patients with CV disease (may cause sudden drop in blood pressure), exposure to extreme heat, glaucoma, and prostatic hyperplasia.

• Prevent contact dermatitis by keeping drug off skin and clothes. Wear gloves when preparing liquid forms.

• Dilute liquid concentrate with fruit juice, milk, or semisolid food just before administering.

• Slight yellowing of injection or concentrate is common; does not affect potency. Discard markedly discolored solutions.

• Give I.M. only in upper outer quadrant of buttocks or midlateral thigh. Massage slowly afterward to prevent sterile abscess. Injection may sting.

• Monitor patient for tardive dyskinesia. It may occur after prolonged use; may not appear until months or years later and may disappear sponta-

neously or persist for life, despite discontinuation of drug.

• Assess patient for neuroleptic malignant syndrome. It is rare, but frequently fatal. Not necessarily related to length of drug use or type of neuroleptic, but over 60% of affected patients are men.

• Do not withdraw abruptly unless required by severe adverse reactions.

• Withhold dose and notify doctor if patient develops jaundice, symptoms of blood dyscrasia (fever, sore throat, infection, cellulitis, weakness), persistent extrapyramidal reactions (longer than a few hours), especially in pregnant patients.

• Monitor therapy with weekly bilirubin tests during first month; periodic blood tests (CBC and liver function); and ophthalmic tests (long-term use) as ordered.

• Know that acute dystonic reactions may be treated with diphenhydramine.

• Watch for orthostatic hypotension, especially with parenteral administration. Keep the patient in supine position for 1 hour afterward and advise him to change positions slowly.

• Warn patients to avoid activities that require alertness or good psychomotor coordination until CNS effects of the drug are known. Drowsiness and dizziness usually subside after a few weeks.

• Tell patients to avoid alcohol while taking this drug.

• Have patient report urine retention or constipation.

• Tell patient to relieve dry mouth with sugarless gum or hard candy.

• Tell patients to use sunblock and to wear protective clothing to avoid photosensitivity reactions.

---

*Liquid form contains alcohol.
**May contain tartrazine.

Common reactions are in italics; ***life-threatening,*** in bold italics.

trifluoperazine hydrochloride

Apo-Trifluoperazine†, Calmazine‡,
Novo-Flurazine†, PMS
Trifluoperazine†, Solazine†,
Stelazine, Stelazine Concentrate,
Terfluzine†, Terfluzine
Concentrate†

Pregnancy Risk Category: NR

HOW SUPPLIED
Tablets (regular and film-coated):
1 mg, 2 mg, 5 mg, 10 mg
Oral concentrate: 10 mg/ml
Injection: 2 mg/ml

ACTION
Unknown. A piperazine phenothiazine that probably blocks postsynaptic dopamine receptors in the brain.

ONSET, PEAK, DURATION
Onset of antipsychotic effect is gradual (up to several weeks) and variable between patients. Peak and duration unknown.

INDICATIONS & DOSAGE
Anxiety states –
Adults: 1 to 2 mg P.O. b.i.d. Maximum dosage is 6 mg/day and drug should not be used longer than 12 weeks for this indication.
Schizophrenia and other psychotic disorders –
Adults: 2 to 5 mg P.O. b.i.d., gradually increased until therapeutic response. Or 1 to 2 mg deep I.M. q 4 to 6 hours, p.r.n. More than 6 mg I.M. in 24 hours is rarely required.
Children 6 to 12 years (hospitalized or under close supervision): 1 mg P.O. daily or b.i.d.; may increase gradually to 15 mg daily if needed.

ADVERSE REACTIONS
CNS: *extrapyramidal reactions* (high incidence), *tardive dyskinesia,* pseudoparkinsonism, dizziness, drowsiness, insomnia.

CV: *orthostatic hypotension,* tachycardia, ECG changes.
EENT: ocular changes, *blurred vision.*
GI: *dry mouth, constipation.*
GU: *urine retention,* dark urine.
Hematologic: transient leukopenia, *agranulocytosis,* hyperprolactinemia.
Hepatic: cholestatic jaundice.
Skin: *photosensitivity,* allergic reactions, pain at I.M. injection site, sterile abscess, rash, skin reactions.
Other: weight gain; rarely, *neuroleptic malignant syndrome* (fever, tachycardia, tachypnea, profuse diaphoresis), menstrual irregularities, gynecomastia, inhibited lactation.

After abrupt withdrawal of long-term therapy: gastritis, nausea, vomiting, dizziness, tremors, feeling of warmth or cold, diaphoresis, tachycardia, headache, insomnia, anorexia, muscle rigidity, altered mental status and evidence of autonomic instability.

INTERACTIONS
Antacids: inhibited absorption of oral phenothiazines. Separate antacid and phenothiazine doses by at least 2 hours.
Barbiturates, lithium: may decrease phenothiazine effect. Monitor the patient.
Centrally acting antihypertensives: decreased antihypertensive effect. Monitor blood pressure.
Ethanol: increased CNS depression. Avoid concomitant use.
Other CNS depressants: increased CNS depression. Use together cautiously.
Propranolol: increased levels of both propranolol and trifluoperazine. Monitor closely.
Warfarin: decreased effect of oral anticoagulants. Monitor P.T.

CONTRAINDICATIONS
Contraindicated in patients with hypersensitivity to phenothiazines or in

---

†Available in Canada only.　　　　‡Available in Australia only.　　　　◇Available OTC.

patients experiencing coma, CNS depression, bone marrow suppression, or liver damage.

NURSING CONSIDERATIONS
• Use cautiously in elderly or debilitated patients and in patients with CV disease (may cause drop in blood pressure), exposure to extreme heat, seizure disorder, glaucoma, or prostatic hyperplasia.
• Although there is little likelihood of contact dermatitis, persons with known sensitivity to phenothiazine drugs should avoid direct contact. Wear gloves when preparing liquid forms.
• Dilute liquid concentrate with 60 ml of tomato or fruit juice, carbonated beverages, coffee, tea, milk, water, or semisolid food just before giving.
• Protect drug from light. Slight yellowing of injection or concentrate is common; does not affect potency. Discard markedly discolored solutions.
• Give deeply I.M. only in upper outer quadrant of buttocks. Massage slowly afterward to prevent sterile abscess. Injection may sting.
• Watch for orthostatic hypotension, especially with parenteral administration. Keep the patient supine for 1 hour afterward, and advise him to change positions slowly.
• Monitor patient for tardive dyskinesia. It may occur after prolonged use. It may not appear until months or years later, and may disappear spontaneously or persist for life despite discontinuation of drug.
• Assess patient for neuroleptic malignant syndrome. It is rare, but frequently fatal. It is not necessarily related to length of drug use or type of neuroleptic, but over 60% of affected patients are men.
• Do not withdraw drug abruptly unless severe adverse reactions occur.
• Withhold dose and notify doctor if patient develops jaundice, symptoms of blood dyscrasia (fever, sore throat, infection, cellulitis, weakness), persistent extrapyramidal reactions (longer than a few hours), especially in pregnant patients or in children.
• Monitor therapy with weekly bilirubin tests during first month; periodic blood tests (CBC and liver function); and ophthalmic tests (long-term use) as ordered.
• Know that acute dystonic reactions may be treated with diphenhydramine.
• Warn patients to avoid activities that require alertness or good psychomotor coordination until CNS effects of the drug are known. Drowsiness and dizziness usually subside after a few weeks.
• Tell patients to avoid alcohol while taking this drug.
• Have patients report urine retention or constipation.
• Tell patients to use sunblock and to wear protective clothing to avoid photosensitivity reactions.
• Tell patient to relieve dry mouth with sugarless gum or hard candy.

---

*Liquid form contains alcohol.   *Common* reactions are in italics; ***life-threatening***, in bold italics.
**May contain tartrazine.

amphetamine sulfate
benzphetamine hydrochloride
caffeine
dextroamphetamine sulfate
diethylpropion hydrochloride
doxapram hydrochloride
fenfluramine hydrochloride
mazindol
methamphetamine hydrochloride
methylphenidate hydrochloride
pemoline
phendimetrazine tartrate
phentermine hydrochloride

COMBINATION PRODUCTS
None.

---

amphetamine sulfate
Controlled Substance Schedule II

Pregnancy Risk Category: C

HOW SUPPLIED
Tablets: 5 mg, 10 mg

ACTION
Unknown. Probably promotes nerve impulse transmission by releasing stored norepinephrine from nerve terminals in the brain. Main sites of activity appear to be the cerebral cortex and the reticular activating system.

ONSET, PEAK, DURATION
Unknown.

INDICATIONS & DOSAGE
Attention deficit disorder with hyperactivity –
Children 3 to 5 years: 2.5 mg P.O. daily, with 2.5-mg increments weekly, p.r.n.
Children 6 years and older: 5 mg P.O. daily, with 5-mg increments weekly, p.r.n. Give first dose on awakening; additional doses (1 or 2) at intervals of 4 to 6 hours.
Narcolepsy –
Adults: 5 to 60 mg P.O. daily in divided doses.
Short-term adjunct in exogenous obesity –
Adults: 5 to 30 mg P.O. daily in divided doses 30 to 60 minutes before meals.

ADVERSE REACTIONS
CNS: *restlessness,* tremor, *hyperactivity, talkativeness, insomnia,* irritability, dizziness, headache, chills, dysphoria.
CV: *tachycardia, palpitations,* hypertension, hypotension.
GI: dry mouth, metallic taste, nausea, vomiting, cramps, diarrhea, constipation, anorexia, weight loss.
GU: impotence.
Skin: urticaria.
Other: altered libido.

INTERACTIONS
Ammonium chloride, ascorbic acid: decreased serum levels and increased renal excretion of amphetamine. Monitor for decreased amphetamine effect.
Antacids, sodium bicarbonate, acetazolamide: increased renal reabsorption. Monitor for enhanced effect.
Antihypertensives: reversal of antihypertensive action. Monitor blood pressure.
Caffeine: may increase amphetamine and related amine effects. Avoid concomitant use.
Haloperidol, phenothiazines, tricyclic antidepressants: increased CNS effect. Avoid concomitant use.
Insulin, oral antidiabetic agents: may decrease antidiabetic agent requirements. Monitor blood glucose level.

---

†Available in Canada only.   ‡Available in Australia only.   ◇Available OTC.

MAO inhibitors: severe hypertension; possible hypertensive crisis. Don't use together or within 14 days after an MAO inhibitor has been discontinued.

CONTRAINDICATIONS
Contraindicated in patients with hypersensitivity or idiosyncrasy to the sympathomimetic amines, symptomatic CV disease, hyperthyroidism, moderate to severe hypertension, glaucoma, advanced arteriosclerosis, or history of drug abuse; within 14 days of MAO inhibitor therapy; and in agitated patients.

NURSING CONSIDERATIONS
● Use cautiously in elderly, debilitated, or hyperexcitable patients; or those with psychopathic personalities or history of suicidal or homicidal tendencies.
● Know that drug is not recommended for first-line treatment of obesity or for treatment of obesity in children under 12 years. Use as an anorexigenic agent is prohibited in some states.
● Be aware that drug should not be used to combat fatigue.
● Make sure obese patient is on a weight-reduction program. Give drug 30 to 60 minutes before meals. Monitor dietary intake and count calories, if necessary.
● If tolerance to anorexigenic effect develops, know that drug should be discontinued. Notify doctor.
● To avoid sleep interference, tell patient to take drug at least 6 hours before bedtime.
● Warn the patient to avoid activities that require alertness or good psychomotor coordination until CNS effects of the drug are known.
● Tell the patient to avoid drinks containing caffeine, which increase the effects of amphetamines and related amines.

● Tell the patient to report signs of excessive stimulation.
● Inform patient fatigue may result as drug effects wear off. The patient will need more rest.

benzphetamine hydrochloride
Didrex**
Controlled Substance Schedule III
Pregnancy Risk Category: X

HOW SUPPLIED
Tablets: 25 mg, 50 mg

ACTION
Unknown. Probably promotes nerve impulse transmission by releasing stored norepinephrine from nerve terminals in the brain. Main sites of activity appear to be the cerebral cortex and the reticular activating system.

ONSET, PEAK, DURATION
Onset and peak unknown. Effects persist for about 4 hours.

INDICATIONS & DOSAGE
Short-term adjunct in exogenous obesity —
Adults: 25 to 50 mg P.O. daily, b.i.d. or t.i.d. Increased as needed in dosage or interval.

ADVERSE REACTIONS
CNS: *restlessness,* tremor, *hyperactivity, talkativeness, insomnia,* irritability, dizziness, headache, chills, dysphoria.
CV: *tachycardia, palpitations,* hypertension, hypotension.
GI: dry mouth, metallic taste, nausea, vomiting, cramps, diarrhea, constipation, anorexia, weight loss.
GU: impotence.
Skin: urticaria.
Other: altered libido.

---

*Liquid form contains alcohol.   *Common* reactions are in italics; *life-threatening,* in bold italics.
**May contain tartrazine.

INTERACTIONS

Ammonium chloride, ascorbic acid: decreased serum levels and increased renal excretion of benzphetamine.
Antacids, sodium bicarbonate, acetazolamide: increased renal reabsorption. Monitor for enhanced effects.
Caffeine: may increase amphetamine and related amine effects. Avoid concomitant use.
Insulin, oral antidiabetic agents: may decrease antidiabetic agent requirement. Monitor blood glucose levels.
MAO inhibitors: severe hypertension; possible hypertensive crisis. Don't use together or within 14 days after MAO inhibitor has been discontinued.
Phenothiazines, haloperidol, tricyclic antidepressants: increased CNS effects. Avoid concomitant use.

CONTRAINDICATIONS

Contraindicated in patients with hypersensitivity or idiosyncrasy to sympathomimetic amines; within 14 days of MAO inhibitor therapy; in those with symptomatic CV disease, hyperthyroidism, moderate to severe hypertension, glaucoma, advanced arteriosclerosis, or history of drug abuse; and in agitated patients.

NURSING CONSIDERATIONS

• Use cautiously in patients with diabetes mellitus and mild hypertension.
• Use in conjunction with a weight-reduction program. Monitor dietary intake and count calories, if necessary. Give 30 to 60 minutes before meals.
• Give a single daily dose in mid-morning or mid-afternoon according to patient's eating habits.
• If tolerance to anorexigenic effect develops, know that drug should be discontinued. Notify doctor.
• To avoid sleep interference, tell patient to take drug at least 6 hours before bedtime.
• Warn the patient to avoid activities that require alertness or good psychomotor coordination until CNS effects of the drug are known.
• Tell patients to avoid drinks containing caffeine, which increase the effects of amphetamines and related amines.
• Tell the patient to report signs of excessive stimulation.
• Inform the patient fatigue may result as drug effects wear off. The patient will need more rest.

caffeine

Caffedrine Caplets◊, Dexitac◊, No Doz◊, Quick Pep◊, Vivarin◊

Pregnancy Risk Category: C

HOW SUPPLIED

Tablets: 100 mg◊, 150 mg◊, 200 mg◊
Capsules (timed-release): 200 mg◊, 250 mg◊
Injection: caffeine (125 mg/ml) with sodium benzoate (125 mg/ml)

ACTION

Inhibits phosphodiesterase, the enzyme that degrades cAMP.

ONSET, PEAK, DURATION

Onset and duration unknown. Serum levels peak within 50 to 75 minutes after oral administration.

INDICATIONS & DOSAGE

CNS stimulant –
Adults: 100 to 200 mg anhydrous caffeine P.O. p.r.n.

ADVERSE REACTIONS

CNS: *stimulation, insomnia,* restlessness, nervousness, mild delirium, headache, excitement, agitation, muscle tremors, twitches.
CV: *tachycardia, palpitations.*
GI: nausea, vomiting.
GU: *diuresis.*
Skin: hyperesthesia.
Other: dehydration, fever, hypergly-

cemia, abrupt withdrawal symptoms (headache, irritability).

INTERACTIONS
Beta-adrenergic agonists, cimetidine, fluoroquinolones, oral contraceptives, phenylpropanolamine, theophylline: excessive CNS stimulation. Avoid concomitant use.

CONTRAINDICATIONS
Contraindicated in patients with hypersensitivity to the drug.

NURSING CONSIDERATIONS
• Use cautiously in patients with history of peptic ulcer, symptomatic arrhythmias, or palpitations, and during the first several days to weeks after an acute MI.
• Know that caffeine does not reverse alcohol intoxication or CNS depressant effects of alcohol. Overvigorous therapy with caffeine may aggravate depression in an already depressed patient.
• Be aware single dose should not exceed 1 g.
• Restrict caffeine-containing beverages in patients who experience palpitations. Caffeine content: cola beverages, 17 to 55 mg/180 ml; tea, 40 to 100 mg/180 ml; instant coffee, 60 to 180 mg/180 ml; brewed coffee, 100 to 150 mg/180 ml; decaffeinated coffee, 1 to 6 mg/180 ml.
• Be alert for signs of overdose: GI pain, mild delirium, insomnia, diuresis, dehydration, and fever. Treat with short-acting barbiturates, gastric emesis, or lavage as ordered.
• Monitor patient for tolerance or psychological dependence.
• Be aware that sudden discontinuation of caffeine may cause headache and irritability.

dextroamphetamine sulfate
Dexedrine* **, Dexedrine Spansule, Oxydess II, Robese, Spancap #1
Controlled Substance Schedule II
Pregnancy Risk Category: C

HOW SUPPLIED
Tablets: 5 mg, 10 mg
Capsules (sustained-release): 5 mg, 10 mg, 15 mg

ACTION
Unknown. Probably promotes nerve impulse transmission by releasing stored norepinephrine from nerve terminals in the brain. Main sites of activity appear to be the cerebral cortex and the reticular activating system. In children with hyperkinesis, amphetamines have a paradoxical calming effect.

ONSET, PEAK, DURATION
Unknown.

INDICATIONS & DOSAGE
Narcolepsy –
Adults: 5 to 60 mg P.O. daily in divided doses.
Children 6 to 12 years: 5 mg P.O. daily, with 5-mg increments weekly, p.r.n.
Children 12 years and older: 10 mg P.O. daily, with 10-mg increments weekly, p.r.n. Give first dose on awakening; additional doses (1 or 2) at intervals of 4 to 6 hours.
Short-term adjunct in exogenous obesity –
Adults and children 12 years and older: 5 to 30 mg P.O. daily 30 to 60 minutes before meals in divided doses of 5 to 10 mg. Alternatively, one 10- or 15-mg sustained-release capsule daily as a single dose in the morning.
Attention deficit disorder with hyperactivity –
Children 3 to 5 years: 2.5 mg P.O.

---

daily, with 2.5-mg increments weekly, p.r.n.

Children 6 years and older: 5 mg P.O. once daily or b.i.d., with 5-mg increments weekly, p.r.n. Only in rare cases will it be necessary to exceed a total of 40 mg/day.

ADVERSE REACTIONS

CNS: *restlessness,* tremor, *insomnia,* dizziness, headache, chills, overstimulation, dysphoria.

CV: *tachycardia, palpitations,* hypertension.

GI: dry mouth, unpleasant taste, diarrhea, constipation, anorexia, weight loss and other GI disturbances.

GU: impotence.

Skin: urticaria.

Other: altered libido.

INTERACTIONS

Acidifying agents, ammonium chloride, ascorbic acid: decreased blood levels and increased renal clearance of dextroamphetamine. Monitor for decreased amphetamine effects.

Adrenergic blockers: adrenergic blockers inhibited by amphetamines. Avoid concomitant use.

Alkalizing agents, antacids, sodium bicarbonate, acetazolamide: increased renal reabsorption. Monitor for enhanced amphetamine effects.

Antihistamines: Amphetamines may counteract the sedative effects of antihistamines.

Caffeine: may increase amphetamine and related amine effects.

Chlorpromazine: Inhibits the central stimulant effects of amphetamines. Can be used to treat amphetamine poisoning.

Insulin, oral antidiabetic agents: may decrease antidiabetic agent requirements. Monitor blood glucose levels.

Lithium carbonate: may inhibit antiobesity and stimulating effects of amphetamines.

MAO inhibitors: severe hypertension; possible hypertensive crisis. Don't use together or within 14 days after MAO inhibitor has been discontinued.

Meperidine: amphetamines potentiate analgesic effect. Use together cautiously.

Methenamine therapy: increased urinary excretion of amphetamines and efficacy reduced. Monitor effects.

Norepinephrine: Amphetamines enhance the adrenergic effect of norepinephrine.

Phenobarbital, phenytoin: amphetamines may delay absorption. Monitor closely.

Phenothiazines, haloperidol, tricyclic antidepressants: increased CNS effects. Avoid concomitant use.

Propoxyphene: in cases of propoxyphene overdose, amphetamine CNS stimulation is potentiated and fatal convulsions can occur.

Veratrum alkaloids: amphetamines inhibit the hypotensive effect of veratrum alkaloids. Monitor blood pressure closely.

CONTRAINDICATIONS

Contraindicated in patients with hypersensitivity or idiosyncrasy to the sympathomimetic amines; within 14 days of MAO inhibitor therapy; and in those with hyperthyroidism, moderate to severe hypertension, symptomatic CV disease, glaucoma, advanced arteriosclerosis, and history of drug abuse.

NURSING CONSIDERATIONS

• Use cautiously in patients with motor and phonic tics, Tourette syndrome, and in agitated states.

• Be aware drug not recommended for first-line treatment of obesity. Use as an anorexigenic agent is prohibited in some states.

• Be aware drug is not to be used to prevent fatigue.

• Make sure the obese patient is on a weight-reduction program. Give 30 to 60 minutes before meals.

• Give at least 6 hours before bedtime to avoid sleep interference.
• If tolerance to anorexigenic effect develops, know that drug should be discontinued. Notify doctor.
• Warn patients to avoid activities that require alertness or good psychomotor coordination until CNS effects of the drug are known.
• Tell the patient to avoid drinks containing caffeine, which increase the effects of amphetamines and related amines.
• Tell patient fatigue may result as drug effects wear off. Patients will need more rest.
• Have patients report signs of excessive stimulation.

diethylpropion hydrochloride
M-Orexic, Nobesine†, Nobesine-75†, Propion†, Tenuate, Tenuate Dospan, Tepanil, Tepanil Ten-Tab

Controlled Substance Schedule IV

Pregnancy Risk Category: B

HOW SUPPLIED
Tablets: 25 mg
Tablets (extended-release): 75 mg
Capsules (extended-release): 75 mg†

ACTION
Unknown. Probably promotes nerve impulse transmission by releasing stored norepinephrine from nerve terminals in the brain. Main sites of activity appear to be the cerebral cortex and the reticular activating system.

ONSET, PEAK, DURATION
Onset and peak unknown. Effects of regular-release tablets persist for 4 hours; effects of extended-release tablets and and capsules, 12 hours.

INDICATIONS & DOSAGE
Short-term adjunct in exogenous obesity –
Adults: 25 mg P.O. before meals

t.i.d.; or 75 mg extended-release tablet or capsule P.O. in midmorning.

ADVERSE REACTIONS
CNS: headache, *nervousness,* dizziness.
CV: *tachycardia, palpitations,* elevated blood pressure, ***pulmonary hypertension.***
EENT: blurred vision.
GI: dry mouth, nausea, abdominal cramps, diarrhea, constipation.
GU: impotence.
Hematologic: decreased blood glucose levels.
Skin: urticaria.
Other: altered libido, changes in menstruation.

INTERACTIONS
Caffeine: may increase amphetamine and related amine effects. Avoid concomitant use.
Guanethidine: decrease antihypertensive effect. Monitor blood pressure.
Insulin, oral antidiabetic agents: may decrease antidiabetic agent requirements. Monitor blood glucose levels.
MAO inhibitors: hypertension; possible hypertensive crisis. Don't use together or within 14 days after MAO inhibitor has been discontinued.

CONTRAINDICATIONS
Contraindicated in patients with hypersensitivity or idiosyncrasy to sympathomimetic amines; within 14 days of MAO inhibitor therapy; in those with hyperthyroidism, severe hypertension, advanced arteriosclerosis, glaucoma, or history of drug abuse; and in agitated patients.

NURSING CONSIDERATIONS
• Use cautiously in patients with mild to moderate hypertension, symptomatic CV disease (including arrhythmias), or seizure disorder.
• Give drug at least 6 hours before bedtime to avoid sleep interference although it rarely causes insomnia.

---

*Liquid form contains alcohol.   *Common* reactions are in italics; *life-threatening,* in bold italics.
**May contain tartrazine.

- Be sure the patient also is on a weight-reduction program.
- Monitor patient for habituation or psychic dependence.
- Monitor blood sugars. May alter insulin requirements.
- If tolerance to anorexigenic effect develops, notify doctor as drug will need to be discontinued.
- Tell the patient to avoid drinks containing caffeine, which increase the effects of diethylpropion and related amines.
- Tell the patient to report signs of excessive stimulation.
- Tell patient fatigue may result as drug effects wear off. The patient will need more rest.

---

doxapram hydrochloride
Dopram

Pregnancy Risk Category: B

HOW SUPPLIED
Injection: 20 mg/ml (benzyl alcohol 0.9%)

ACTION
Not clearly defined. Acts either directly on the central respiratory centers in the medulla or indirectly on the chemoreceptors.

ONSET, PEAK, DURATION
Onset occurs in 20 to 40 seconds. Levels peak in 1 to 2 minutes. Effects persist for 5 to 12 minutes.

INDICATIONS & DOSAGE
Postanesthesia respiratory stimulation, drug-induced CNS depression, chronic pulmonary disease associated with acute hypercapnia –
Adults: 0.5 to 1 mg/kg of body weight (up to 2 mg/kg in CNS depression) by I.V. injection or infusion. Repeated q 5 minutes if needed. Maximum dosage is 4 mg/kg.
COPD –
Adults: 1 to 2 mg/minute by I.V. infu-

sion. Maximum dosage is 3 mg/minute for a maximum duration of 2 hours.

ADVERSE REACTIONS
CNS: *seizures, headache,* dizziness, apprehension, disorientation, pupillary dilation, bilateral Babinski's signs, paresthesia.
CV: *chest pain and tightness, variations in heart rate, hypertension,* lowered T waves.
EENT: sneezing, *laryngospasm.*
GI: nausea, vomiting, diarrhea.
GU: urine retention, bladder stimulation with incontinence.
Respiratory: cough, *bronchospasm.*
Skin: pruritus.
Other: hiccups, rebound hypoventilation, fever, muscle spasms, diaphoresis, flushing.

INTERACTIONS
MAO inhibitors, sympathomimetics: potentiate adverse cardiovascular effects. Use together cautiously.

CONTRAINDICATIONS
Contraindicated in patients with seizure disorders; head injury; CV disorders; frank uncompensated heart failure; severe hypertension; CVA; respiratory failure or incompetence secondary to neuromuscular disorders, muscle paresis, flail chest, obstructed airway, pulmonary embolism, pneumothorax, restrictive respiratory disease, acute bronchial asthma, or extreme dyspnea; or hypoxia not associated with hypercapnia.

NURSING CONSIDERATIONS
- Use cautiously in patients with bronchial asthma, severe tachycardia or arrhythmias, cerebral edema or increased CSF pressure, hyperthyroidism, pheochromocytoma, or metabolic disorders.
- Establish adequate airway before administering drug. Prevent patients

---

from aspirating vomitus by placing them on their side.
• **I.V. use:** Administer slowly; rapid infusion may cause hemolysis. Doxapram is physically incompatible with strongly alkaline drugs such as thiopental sodium, aminophylline, or sodium bicarbonate.
• Avoid extravasation, which may lead to thrombophlebitis and local skin irritation.
• Monitor blood pressure, heart rate, deep tendon reflexes, and arterial blood gases before giving drug and every 30 minutes afterward.
• Be alert for signs of overdosage: hypertension, tachycardia, arrhythmias, skeletal muscle hyperactivity, and dyspnea. Discontinue drug and notify doctor if patients show signs of increased arterial carbon dioxide or oxygen tension, or if mechanical ventilation is started.
• Be aware that drug is used only in surgical or emergency department situations.

fenfluramine hydrochloride
Ponderal†, Ponderal Pacaps†, Ponderax‡, Ponderax Pacaps‡, Pondimin, Pondimin Extentabs
Controlled Substance Schedule IV

Pregnancy Risk Category: C

HOW SUPPLIED
Tablets: 20 mg
Capsules (sustained-release): 60 mg†‡

ACTION
Unknown. Stimulates ventromedian nucleus of the hypothalamus. Also may affect serotonin metabolism.

ONSET, PEAK, DURATION
Onset occurs in 1 to 2 hours. Peak unknown. Effects persist for 4 to 6 hours.

INDICATIONS & DOSAGE
Short-term adjunct in exogenous obesity –
Adults: initially, 20 mg P.O. t.i.d. before meals. Maximum dosage is 40 mg t.i.d. Dosage adjusted according to patient response.

ADVERSE REACTIONS
CNS: *drowsiness,* dizziness, incoordination, headache, euphoria or depression, anxiety, *insomnia,* weakness, fatigue, agitation.
CV: *palpitations,* hypotension, hypertension, chest pain.
EENT: eye irritation, blurred vision.
GI: dry mouth, *diarrhea,* nausea, vomiting, abdominal pain, constipation.
GU: dysuria, increased urinary frequency, impotence.
Skin: rash, urticaria, burning sensation.
Other: diaphoresis, chills, fever, increased libido.

INTERACTIONS
Centrally acting antihypertensives: decreased antihypertensive effect. Monitor blood pressure.
Ethanol, CNS depressants: enhanced CNS depression. Don't use together.
Insulin, oral antidiabetic agents: may decrease antidiabetic agent requirements. Monitor blood glucose levels.
MAO inhibitors: severe hypertension; possible hypertensive crisis. Don't use together or within 14 days after an MAO inhibitor has been discontinued.

CONTRAINDICATIONS
Contraindicated in patients with psychotic disorders, severe hypertension, glaucoma, hypersensitivity to sympathomimetic amines, symptomatic CV disease (including arrhythmias), alcoholism, or history of drug abuse.

---

*Liquid form contains alcohol.
**May contain tartrazine.

Common reactions are in italics; **life-threatening,** in bold italics.

NURSING CONSIDERATIONS

• Use cautiously in patients with mild to moderate hypertension and history of mental depression.

• Make sure patient is on a weight-reduction program.

• Monitor patient for tolerance or physical or psychological dependence.

• Have patients report signs of excessive sedation, depression, or excessive stimulation. Monitor blood pressure.

• Tell patient to avoid alcohol while taking this drug.

• Tell patient not to discontinue abruptly; may precipitate an acute depressive reaction.

---

mazindol
Mazanor, Sanorex
Controlled Substance Schedule IV

Pregnancy Risk Category: NR

HOW SUPPLIED
Tablets: 1 mg, 2 mg

ACTION
Unknown. Probably inhibits neuronal uptake of norepinephrine and dopamine.

ONSET, PEAK, DURATION
Onset occurs in 30 to 60 minutes. Peak unknown. Effects persist 10 to 15 hours.

INDICATIONS & DOSAGE
Short-term adjunct in exogenous obesity –

Adults: 1 mg P.O. t.i.d. 1 hour before meals, or 2 mg P.O. daily 1 hour before lunch in a single dose. Lowest effective dosage should be used.

ADVERSE REACTIONS
CNS: *nervousness,* restlessness, dizziness, *insomnia,* dysphoria, headache, depression, drowsiness, weakness, tremor.
CV: *palpitations, tachycardia.*

GI: dry mouth, dysgeusia, nausea, constipation, diarrhea.
GU: urinary hestitancy, impotence.
Hematologic: decreased blood glucose levels.
Skin: rash, clamminess, pallor.
Other: shivering, diaphoresis, altered libido.

INTERACTIONS
Caffeine: may increase amphetamine and related amine effects. Avoid concomitant use.
Centrally acting antihypertensives: decreased antihypertensive effect. Monitor blood pressure.
Insulin, oral antidiabetic agents: may decrease antidiabetic agent requirements. Monitor blood glucose levels.
MAO inhibitors: severe hypertension; possible hypertensive crisis. Don't use together or within 14 days after an MAO inhibitor has been discontinued.

CONTRAINDICATIONS
Contraindicated in patients with symptomatic glaucoma, hypersensitivity or idiosyncrasy to drug, severe hypertension, CV disease (including arrhythmias) or history of drug abuse; within 14 days of MAO inhibitor therapy; and in agitated patients.

NURSING CONSIDERATIONS
• Use cautiously in patients with mild to moderate hypertension.

• Give at least 6 hours before bedtime to avoid sleep interference.

• Make sure the patient also is on a weight-reduction program.

• Monitor patient for tolerance or physical or psychological dependence may develop.

• Warn the patient to avoid activities that require alertness or good psychomotor coordination until CNS effects of the drug are known.

• Tell the patient to avoid drinks containing caffeine, which increase the

---

effects of amphetamines and related amines.
• Tell the patient to report signs of excessive stimulation.
• Inform patient fatigue may result as drug effects wear off. The patient will need more rest.

---

methamphetamine hydrochloride
Desoxyn, Desoxyn Gradumet
Controlled Substance Schedule II
Pregnancy Risk Category: C

HOW SUPPLIED
Tablets: 5 mg, 10 mg
Tablets (long-acting): 5 mg, 10 mg, 15 mg**

ACTION
Unknown. Probably promotes nerve impulse transmission by releasing stored norepinephrine from nerve terminals in the brain. Main sites of activity appear to be the cerebral cortex and the reticular activating system. In children with hyperkinesis, methamphetamine has a paradoxical calming effect.

ONSET, PEAK, DURATION
Onset and peak unknown. Effects persist up to 24 hours.

INDICATIONS & DOSAGE
Attention deficit disorder with hyperactivity –
Children 6 years and older: 2.5 to 5 mg P.O. once daily or b.i.d., with 5-mg increments weekly, p.r.n. Usual effective dosage is 20 to 25 mg daily.
Short-term adjunct in exogenous obesity –
Adults: 2.5 to 5 mg P.O. b.i.d. to t.i.d., 30 minutes before meals; or 10- to 15-mg long-acting tablet daily before breakfast.

ADVERSE REACTIONS
CNS: *nervousness, insomnia,* irritability, *talkativeness,* dizziness, headache, hyperexcitability, tremor.
CV: hypertension, hypotension, *tachycardia, palpitations,* arrhythmias.
EENT: blurred vision, mydriasis.
GI: dry mouth, metallic taste, nausea, vomiting, abdominal cramps, diarrhea, constipation, anorexia.
GU: impotence.
Skin: urticaria.
Other: altered libido.

INTERACTIONS
Ammonium chloride, ascorbic acid: decreased serum levels and increased renal excretion of methamphetamine. Monitor for decreased methamphetamine effects.
Antacids, sodium bicarbonate, acetazolamide: increased renal reabsorption. Monitor for enhanced effects.
Caffeine: may increase amphetamine and related amine effects. Avoid concomitant use.
Insulin, oral antidiabetic agents: may decrease antidiabetic agent requirements. Monitor blood glucose levels.
MAO inhibitors: severe hypertension; possible hypertensive crisis. Don't use together or within 14 days after MAO inhibitor has been discontinued.
Phenothiazines, haloperidol, tricyclic antidepressants: increased CNS effects. Avoid concomitant use.

CONTRAINDICATIONS
Contraindicated in patients with moderate to severe hypertension, hyperthyroidism, symptomatic CV disease, advanced arteriosclerosis, glaucoma, hypersensitivity or idiosyncrasy to sympathomimetic amines, history of drug abuse; within 14 days of MAO inhibitor therapy; and in agitated patients.

---

*Liquid form contains alcohol.
**May contain tartrazine.

Common reactions are in italics; **life-threatening,** in bold italics.

NURSING CONSIDERATIONS
- Use cautiously in patients who are elderly, debilitated, asthenic, psychopathic, or who have a history of suicidal or homicidal tendencies.
- Be aware that drug is not recommended for first-line treatment of obesity. Use as an anorexigenic agent is prohibited in some states.
- Give at least 6 hours before bedtime to avoid sleep interference.
- When used for obesity, be sure patient is on a weight-reduction program.
- If tolerance to anorexigenic effect develops, notify doctor as drug will need to be discontinued.
- Warn the patient of high potential for abuse. Advise him drug should not be used to prevent fatigue.
- Tell patient to never crush sustained-release tablets.
- Warn the patient to avoid activities that require alertness or good psychomotor coordination until CNS effects of the drug are known.
- Monitor blood sugar levels. May alter insulin needs in patients with diabetes.
- Tell the patient to avoid drinks containing caffeine, which increase the effects of amphetamines and related amines.
- Have the patient report signs of excessive stimulation.

---

methylphenidate hydrochloride
PMS-Methylphenidate‡, Ritalin, Ritalin-SR

Controlled Substance Schedule II

Pregnancy Risk Category: NR

HOW SUPPLIED
Tablets: 5 mg, 10 mg, 20 mg
Tablets (sustained-release): 20 mg

ACTION
Unknown. Probably promotes nerve impulse transmission by releasing stored norepinephrine from nerve terminals in the brain. Main site of activity appears to be the cerebral cortex and the reticular activating system. In children with hyperkinesis, methylphenidate has a paradoxical calming effect.

ONSET, PEAK, DURATION
Onset and duration unknown. Peak levels occur about 2 hours after regular-release tablets, 4 or 5 hours after sustained-release tablets.

INDICATIONS & DOSAGE
Attention deficit disorder with hyperactivity (ADDH) –
Children 6 years and older: initial dose, 5 to 10 mg P.O. daily before breakfast and lunch, with 5- to 10-mg increments weekly p.r.n., up to 60 mg daily.
Narcolepsy –
Adults: 10 mg P.O. b.i.d. or t.i.d. 30 to 45 minutes before meals. Dosage varies with patient needs.

ADVERSE REACTIONS
CNS: *nervousness, insomnia,* Tourette syndrome, dizziness, headache, akathisia, dyskinesia, *seizures.*
CV: *palpitations,* angina, *tachycardia,* changes in blood pressure and pulse rate.
EENT: dry throat.
GI: nausea, abdominal pain, anorexia, weight loss.
Hematologic: thrombocytopenia, thrombocytopenic purpura.
Skin: rash, urticaria, *exfoliative dermatitis, erythema multiforme.*
Other: delayed growth.

INTERACTIONS
Caffeine: may increase amphetamine and related amine effects. Avoid concomitant use.
Centrally acting antihypertensives: decreased antihypertensive effect. Monitor blood pressure.
MAO inhibitors: severe hypertension;

---

possible hypertensive crisis. Don't use together or within 14 days after an MAO inhibitor has been discontinued. *Tricyclic antidepressants:* increased plasma levels of these drugs. Avoid concomitant use.

CONTRAINDICATIONS
Contraindicated in patients with hypersensitivity to drug, glaucoma, motor tics, family history of or diagnosis of Tourette syndrome, or history of marked anxiety, tension, or agitation.

NURSING CONSIDERATIONS
• Use cautiously in patients with history of drug abuse, hypertension, history of seizures, or EEG abnormalities.
• Know that it is the drug of choice for ADDH. Usually discontinued after puberty.
• Know that drug should not be used to prevent fatigue.
• Give at least 6 hours before bedtime to prevent insomnia. Administer after meals to reduce appetite-suppressant effects.
• May precipitate Tourette syndrome in children. Monitor especially at start of therapy.
• Observe for signs of excessive stimulation. Monitor blood pressure.
• Monitor results of periodic CBC, differential, and platelet counts with long-term use.
• Monitor height and weight in children on prolonged therapy. May delay growth spurt, but children will attain normal height when drug is discontinued.
• Monitor patient for tolerance or psychological dependence.
• Warn the patient against chewing sustained-release tablets.
• Warn the patient to avoid activities that require alertness or good psychomotor coordination until CNS effects of the drug are known.
• Tell the patient to avoid drinks containing caffeine, which increase the effects of amphetamines and related amines.
• May decrease seizure threshold in patients with seizure disorders. Advise patients to notify doctor if seizure occurs.
• Inform patient fatigue may result as drug effects wear off. The patient will need more rest.

pemoline
Cylert, Cylert Chewable
Controlled Substance Schedule IV
Pregnancy Risk Category: B

HOW SUPPLIED
Tablets: 18.75 mg, 37.5 mg, 75 mg
Tablets (chewable): 37.5 mg

ACTION
Unknown. Probably promotes nerve impulse transmission by releasing stored norepinephrine from nerve terminals in the brain. Main sites of activity appear to be the cerebral cortex and the reticular activating system.

ONSET, PEAK, DURATION
Onset and duration unknown. Serum levels peak 2 to 4 hours after dose.

INDICATIONS & DOSAGE
Attention deficit disorder with hyperactivity –
Children 6 years and older: initially, 37.5 mg P.O. in the morning. Daily dosage raised by 18.75 mg weekly as needed. Effective dosage range is 56.25 to 75 mg daily; maximum dosage is 112.5 mg daily.

ADVERSE REACTIONS
CNS: *insomnia,* malaise, dyskinetic movements, irritability, fatigue, mild depression, dizziness, headache, drowsiness, hallucinations, nervousness (with large doses), *seizures, Tourette syndrome,* psychosis.
CV: *tachycardia* (with large doses).

---

*Liquid form contains alcohol.
**May contain tartrazine.

Common reactions are in italics; *life-threatening,* in bold italics.

GI: anorexia, abdominal pain, nausea, diarrhea.
Hepatic: elevated liver enzymes.
Skin: rash.

INTERACTIONS
Insulin, oral antidiabetic agents: may decrease antidiabetic agent requirements. Monitor blood glucose levels.

CONTRAINDICATIONS
Contraindicated in patients with hepatic dysfunction and hypersensitivity or idiosyncrasy to the drug.

NURSING CONSIDERATIONS
• Use cautiously in patients with impaired renal function.
• Be aware drug is structurally dissimilar to amphetamines or methylphenidate. However, may produce similar adverse reactions, including lowered seizure threshold. Has greater potential for abuse and dependence than previously thought.
• To avoid sleep interference, give at least 6 hours before bedtime.
• May precipitate Tourette syndrome in children. Monitor especially at start of therapy.
• Closely monitor patients on long-term therapy for possible blood or hepatic function abnormalities and for growth suppression.

phendimetrazine tartrate
Adipost, Anorex SR, Appecon, Bontril PDM, Bontril Slow-Release, Dyrexan OD, Malibar A, Melfiat-105 Unicelles, Metra, Neocurb, Obalan, Obe-Del, Obezine, Panrexin M, Panrexin MTP, Parzine, Phenazine, Phendiet, Phendiet-105, Phendimet, Phentra, Prelu-2, PT-105, Rexigen, Rexigen Forte, Tega-Nil, Trimcaps, Trimstat, Wehless, Weightrol, Wescoid, X-Trozine, X-Trozine LA
Controlled Substance Schedule IV

Pregnancy Risk Category: NR

HOW SUPPLIED
Tablets: 35 mg
Capsules: 35 mg
Capsules (sustained-release): 105 mg

ACTION
Unknown. Probably promotes nerve impulse transmission by releasing stored norepinephrine from nerve terminals in the brain. Main sites of activity appear to be the cerebral cortex and the reticular activating system.

ONSET, PEAK, DURATION
Onset and peak unknown. Effects persist about 4 hours.

INDICATIONS & DOSAGE
Short-term adjunct in exogenous obesity –
Adults: 35 mg P.O. b.i.d. or t.i.d., 1 hour before meals. Maximum dosage is 70 mg t.i.d. or 1 (105 mg) sustained-release capsule P.O. once daily in the morning. Lowest effective dosage should be used and adjusted to individual response.

ADVERSE REACTIONS
CNS: *nervousness,* dizziness, *insomnia,* tremor, headache.
CV: *tachycardia, palpitations,* elevated blood pressure.
EENT: blurred vision.

GI: dry mouth, nausea, abdominal cramps, diarrhea, constipation.
GU: dysuria.

INTERACTIONS
Ammonium chloride, ascorbic acid: decreased serum levels and increased renal excretion of phendimetrazine. Monitor for decreased phendimetrazine effects.
Antacids, sodium bicarbonate, acetazolamide: increased renal reabsorption. Monitor for enhanced effects.
Caffeine: may increase CNS stimulation. Avoid concomitant use.
MAO inhibitors: severe hypertension; possible hypertensive crisis. Don't use together or within 14 days after MAO inhibitor has been discontinued.
Phenothiazines, haloperidol, tricyclic antidepressants: increased CNS effect. Avoid concomitant use.

CONTRAINDICATIONS
• Contraindicated in patients with hypersensitivity or idiosyncrasy to sympathomimetic amines, advanced arteriosclerosis, hyperthyroidism, moderate to severe hypertension, symptomatic CV disease, or glaucoma.
• Also contraindicated in patients in agitated states or those who are highly nervous, have a history of drug abuse, or have received MAO inhibitors in the last 14 days.

NURSING CONSIDERATIONS
• Use cautiously in patients with mild hypertension.
• Give at least 6 hours before bedtime to avoid sleep interference.
• Make sure the patient also is on a weight-reduction program.
• Monitor patient for habituation and tolerance.
• Warn the patient to avoid activities that require alertness or good psychomotor coordination until CNS effects of the drug are known.
• Tell the patient to avoid drinks containing caffeine, which increase the effects of amphetamines and related amines.
• Tell the patient to report signs of excessive stimulation.
• Inform patient fatigue may result as drug effects wear off. The patient will need more rest.

---

phentermine hydrochloride
Adipex-P, Duromine‡, Fastin, Obe-Mar, Obe-Nix, Obephen, Oby-Trim, Panshape-M, Phentercot, Phentride, Phentride Caplets, Phentrol, Phentrol-2, Phentrol-4, Phentrol-5, T-Diet, Teramine, Wilpowr, Zantryl
Controlled Substance Schedule IV

Pregnancy Risk Category: NR

HOW SUPPLIED
Tablets: 8 mg, 30 mg, 37.5 mg
Capsules: 15 mg, 18.75 mg, 30 mg, 37.5 mg
Capsules (resin complex, sustained-release): 15 mg, 30 mg

ACTION
Unknown. Probably promotes nerve impulse transmission by releasing stored norepinephrine from nerve terminals in the brain. Main sites of activity appear to be the cerebral cortex and the reticular activating system.

ONSET, PEAK, DURATION
Onset and peak unknown. Effects persist 12 to 14 hours.

INDICATIONS & DOSAGE
Short-term adjunct in exogenous obesity –
Adults: 8 mg P.O. t.i.d. half hour before meals; or 15 to 30 mg (resin complex) daily 2 hours after breakfast.

ADVERSE REACTIONS
CNS: overstimulation, headache, euphoria, dysphoria, dizziness, *insomnia.*

---

*Liquid form contains alcohol.
**May contain tartrazine.

Common reactions are in italics; ***life-threatening,*** in bold italics.

CV: *palpitations, tachycardia,* increased blood pressure.
GI: dry mouth, dysgeusia, constipation, diarrhea, and other GI disturbances.
GU: impotence.
Skin: urticaria.
Other: altered libido.

INTERACTIONS
Ammonium chloride, ascorbic acid: decreased plasma levels and increased renal excretion of phentermine. Monitor for decreased phentermine effects.
Antacids, sodium bicarbonate, acetazolamide: increased renal reabsorption. Monitor for enhanced effects.
Caffeine: may increase CNS stimulation.
Insulin, oral antidiabetic agents: may alter antidiabetic agent requirements. Monitor blood glucose levels.
MAO inhibitors: severe hypertension; possible hypertensive crisis. Don't use together or within 14 days after MAO inhibitor has been discontinued.
Phenothiazines, haloperidol, tricyclic antidepressants: increased CNS effects. Avoid concomitant use.

CONTRAINDICATIONS
Contraindicated in patients with hyperthyroidism, moderate to severe hypertension, advanced arteriosclerosis, symptomatic CV disease, glaucoma, or hypersensitivity or idiosyncrasy to sympathomimetic amines; within 14 days of MAO inhibitor therapy; and in agitated patients.

NURSING CONSIDERATIONS
● Use cautiously in patients with mild hypertension.
● Use in conjunction with a weight-reduction program.
● Give at least 6 hours before bedtime to avoid sleep interference.
● Monitor patient for tolerance or dependence.
● Tell the patient to avoid drinks con-

taining caffeine, which increase the effects of amphetamines and related amines.
● Tell the patient to report signs of excessive stimulation.
● Tell patient fatigue may result as drug effects wear off. The patient will need more rest.

amantadine hydrochloride
(See Chapter 17, ANTIVIRALS.)
benztropine mesylate
biperiden hydrochloride
biperiden lactate
bromocriptine mesylate
carbidopa-levodopa
levodopa
pergolide mesylate
procyclidine hydrochloride
selegiline hydrochloride
trihexyphenidyl hydrochloride

COMBINATION PRODUCTS
MADOPAR‡: levodopa 200 mg and benserazide 50 mg.
MADOPAR HBS‡: levodopa 100 mg and benserazide 25 mg.
MADOPAR Q‡: levodopa 50 mg and benserazide 12.5 mg.
SINEMET 10-100: carbidopa 10 mg and levodopa 100 mg.
SINEMET 25-100: carbidopa 25 mg and levodopa 100 mg.
SINEMET 25-250: carbidopa 25 mg and levodopa 250 mg.
SINEMET CR: carbidopa 50 mg and levodopa 200 mg, in extended-release tablets.

benztropine mesylate
Apo-Benztropine†, Bensylate†, Cogentin, PMS Benztropine†

Pregnancy Risk Category: NR

HOW SUPPLIED
Tablets: 0.5 mg, 1 mg, 2 mg
Injection: 1 mg/ml in 2-ml ampules

ACTION
Unknown. Thought to block central cholinergic receptors, helping to balance cholinergic activity in the basal ganglia.

ONSET, PEAK, DURATION
Onset occurs within 15 minutes of parenteral use, or within 1 to 2 hours of oral use. Peak unknown. Effects persist 24 hours.

INDICATIONS & DOSAGE
Drug-induced extrapyramidal disorders (except tardive dyskinesia)
Adults: 1 to 4 mg P.O. or I.M. once or twice daily.
Acute dystonic reaction –
Adults: 1 to 2 mg I.V. or I.M. followed by 1 to 2 mg P.O. b.i.d. to prevent recurrence.
Parkinsonism –
Adults: 0.5 to 6 mg P.O. daily. Initial dose is 0.5 mg to 1 mg. Then increased by 0.5 mg q 5 to 6 days. Dosage adjusted to meet individual requirements.

ADVERSE REACTIONS
CNS: disorientation, restlessness, irritability, incoherence, hallucinations, headache, sedation, depression, muscular weakness.
CV: palpitations, tachycardia, paradoxical bradycardia, flushing.
EENT: dilated pupils, blurred vision, photophobia, difficulty swallowing.
GI: dry mouth, *constipation,* nausea, vomiting, epigastric distress.
GU: urinary hesitancy, urine retention.
   Some adverse reactions may result from atropine-like toxicity and are dose-related.

INTERACTIONS
Amantadine, phenothiazines, tricyclic antidepressants: additive anticholinergic adverse reactions, such as confusion and hallucinations. Reduce dosage before administering.

---

*Liquid form contains alcohol.
**May contain tartrazine.

Common reactions are in italics; *life-threatening,* in bold italics.

CONTRAINDICATIONS
Contraindicated in patients with hypersensitivity to drug or its components and acute angle-closure glaucoma. Also contraindicated in children under age 3.

NURSING CONSIDERATIONS
• Use cautiously in patients exposed to hot weather or in patients with mental disorders; and in children age 3 and older.
• To help prevent GI distress, administer after meals.
• **I.V. use:** Rarely used because of small difference in onset as compared to I.M. route.
• Monitor vital signs carefully. Watch closely for adverse reactions, especially in elderly or debilitated patients. Call the doctor promptly.
• Be aware that drug produces atropine-like adverse reactions and may aggravate tardive dyskinesia.
• Watch for intermittent constipation, abdominal distention, and abdominal pain; may indicate onset of paralytic ileus.
• Never discontinue this drug abruptly. Dosage must be reduced gradually.
• Warn patient to avoid activities that require alertness until CNS effects of the drug are known. If the patient is to receive a single daily dose, tell him to take it at bedtime.
• Advise patient to report signs of urinary hesitancy or urine retention.
• Tell patient to relieve dry mouth with cool drinks, ice chips, sugarless gum or hard candy.
• Advise patient to limit activities during hot weather because drug-induced anhydrosis may result in hyperthermia.

biperiden hydrochloride
Akineton

biperiden lactate
Akineton Lactate
Pregnancy Risk Category: C

HOW SUPPLIED
biperiden hydrochloride
Tablets: 2 mg
biperiden lactate
Injection: 5 mg/ml in 1-ml ampules

ACTION
Unknown. Blocks central cholinergic receptors, helping to balance cholinergic activity in the basal ganglia.

ONSET, PEAK, DURATION
Onset occurs within 30 minutes of parenteral use, within 1 hour of oral use. Peak unknown. Effects persist 1 to 8 hours after I.V. use, 6 to 12 hours after oral use.

INDICATIONS & DOSAGE
Drug-induced extrapyramidal disorders –
Adults: 2 mg P.O. once daily b.i.d. or t.i.d., depending on severity. Usual dosage is 2 mg daily, or 2 mg I.M. or I.V. q half hour, not to exceed four doses or 8 mg total daily.
Parkinsonism –
Adults: 2 mg P.O. t.i.d. or q.i.d. Some patients may require as much as 16 mg per day.

ADVERSE REACTIONS
CNS: disorientation, euphoria, restlessness, irritability, incoherence, dizziness, increased tremor.
CV: transient postural hypotension (with parenteral use).
EENT: blurred vision.
GI: dry mouth, *constipation,* nausea, vomiting, epigastric distress.
GU: urinary hesitancy, urine retention.
Skin: rash, urticaria.
  Adverse reactions are dose-related and may resemble atropine toxicity.

---

†Available in Canada only.   ‡Available in Australia only.   ◊ Available OTC.

INTERACTIONS
Amantadine, phenothiazines, tricyclic antidepressants: excessive CNS anticholinergic effects. Avoid concomitant use.
Antacids: decreased biperiden absorption. Administer antacids at least 1 hour after biperiden.

CONTRAINDICATIONS
Contraindicated in patients with hypersensitivity to the drug, angle-closure glaucoma, bowel obstruction, or megacolon.

NURSING CONSIDERATIONS
• Use cautiously in patients with prostatic hyperplasia, arrhythmias, manifest glaucoma, and seizure disorder.
• To decrease adverse GI effects, give oral doses with or after meals.
• **I.V. use:** Administer very slowly.
• When giving parenterally, keep patient in supine position. Parenteral administration may cause transient postural hypotension and coordination disturbances.
• Monitor vital signs carefully. Watch closely for adverse reactions, especially in elderly or debilitated patients. Call the doctor promptly.
• Monitor patient for tolerance. If it develops, notify doctor because dosage will need to be increased.
• Know that in severe parkinsonism, tremors may increase as spasticity is relieved.
• Warn the patient to avoid activities that require alertness until CNS effects of the drug are known.
• Because of possible dizziness, help patient when he gets out of bed.
• Advise the patient to report signs of urinary hesitancy or urine retention.
• Advise patient to relieve dry mouth with cool drinks, ice chips, sugarless gum, or hard candy.

bromocriptine mesylate
Parlodel

Pregnancy Risk Category: NR

HOW SUPPLIED
Tablets: 2.5 mg
Capsules: 5 mg

ACTION
Inhibits secretion of prolactin and acts as a dopamine-receptor agonist by activating postsynaptic dopamine receptors.

ONSET, PEAK, DURATION
Antiparkinsonian effects occur in 30 to 90 minutes; effects on serum prolactin, within 2 hours. Antiparkinsonian effects peak in 1 to 3 hours. Peak effects on serum prolactin occur within 8 hours. Antiparkinsonian effects persist for 12 to 18 hours; effects on serum prolactin, about 24 hours.

INDICATIONS & DOSAGE
Amenorrhea and galactorrhea associated with hyperprolactinemia; female infertility –
Adults: 1.25 to 2.5 mg P.O. daily. Increased by 2.5 mg daily at 3- to 7-day intervals until desired effect is achieved. Therapeutic dosage ranges from 2.5 to 5 mg/day. Safety and efficacy of doses greater than 100 mg daily have not been established.
Prevention of postpartum lactation –
Adults: 2.5 mg P.O. b.i.d. with meals for 14 days. Treatment may be extended for up to 21 days, if necessary.
Parkinson's disease –
Adults: 1.25 mg P.O. b.i.d. with meals. Dosage increased q 14 to 28 days, up to 100 mg daily as needed.
Acromegaly –
Adults: 1.25 to 2.5 mg P.O. with h.s. snack for 3 days. An additional 1.25 to 2.5 mg may be added q 3 to 7 days until patient receives therapeutic benefit. Maximal dosage is 100 mg/day.

ADVERSE REACTIONS

CNS: confusion, hallucinations, uncontrolled body movements, *dizziness, headache,* fatigue, mania, delusions, nervousness, insomnia, depression, *seizures.*
CV: *hypotension,* orthostatic hypotension, hypertension, CVA, syncope.
EENT: nasal congestion, tinnitus, blurred vision.
GI: *nausea,* vomiting, *abdominal cramps,* constipation, diarrhea.
GU: urine retention, urinary frequency.
Respiratory: *pulmonary infiltration and pleural effusion.*
Skin: coolness and pallor of fingers and toes.

INTERACTIONS

Antihypertensives: increased hypotensive effects. Adjust dosage of the antihypertensive.
Haloperidol, loxapine, methyldopa, metoclopramide, MAO inhibitors, phenothiazines, reserpine: interferes with bromocriptine's effects. Bromocriptine dosage may need to be increased.
Levodopa: additive effects. Adjust dosage of levodopa.
Oral contraceptives, estrogens, progestins: interfere with effects of bromocriptine. Concurrent use not recommended.

CONTRAINDICATIONS

Contraindicated in patients with hypersensitivity to ergot derivatives, uncontrolled hypertension, or toxemia of pregnancy.

NURSING CONSIDERATIONS

• Use cautiously in patients with impaired renal or hepatic function and history of MI with residual arrhythmias.
• Be aware patients with impaired renal function may require dosage adjustments.
• Know that for Parkinson's disease,

bromocriptine usually is given in addition to either levodopa or carbidopa-levodopa.
• Give drug with meals.
• Monitor patient for adverse reactions. Incidence of adverse reactions is high (about 68%), particularly at beginning of therapy; however, most are mild to moderate, with nausea being the most common. Minimize adverse reactions by gradually titrating doses to effective levels as ordered. Adverse reactions are more frequent when drug is used for Parkinson's disease.
• Monitor blood pressure closely in patients who receive bromocriptine for suppression of postpartum lactation. In such patients, transient hypotension is common; however, hypertension, seizures, and CVA have also been reported.
• Know that baseline and periodic evaluations of cardiac, hepatic, renal, and hematopoietic function are recommended during prolonged therapy.
• May lead to early postpartum conception. Test for pregnancy every 4 weeks or whenever period is missed after menses resumes.
• Advise patients to use contraceptive methods other than oral contraceptives or subdermal implants during treatment.
• Orthostatic hypotension is common. Advise patients to avoid dizziness and fainting by rising slowly to an upright position and avoiding sudden position changes.
• Advise patients that it may take 6 to 8 weeks or longer for menses to resume and galactorrhea to be suppressed.
• Inform postpartum patient that when therapy is discontinued, patients may experience mild to moderate rebound breast secretion, congestion, or engorgement.

carbidopa-levodopa
Sinemet, Sinemet CR

Pregnancy Risk Category: NR

HOW SUPPLIED
Tablets: carbidopa 10 mg with levodopa 100 mg (Sinemet 10-100), carbidopa 25 mg with levodopa 100 mg (Sinemet 25-100), carbidopa 25 mg with levodopa 250 mg (Sinemet 25-250)
Tablets (extended-release): carbidopa 50 mg with levodopa 200 mg (Sinemet CR)

ACTION
Unknown for levodopa. Thought to be decarboxylated to dopamine, countering the depletion of striatal dopamine in extrapyramidal centers. Carbidopa inhibits the peripheral decarboxylation of levodopa without affecting levodopa's metabolism within the CNS. Therefore, more levodopa is available to be decarboxylated to dopamine in the brain.

ONSET, PEAK, DURATION
Onset and duration unknown. Peak serum levels occur in about 40 minutes for regular-release tablets, or 2½ hours for extended-release tablets.

INDICATIONS & DOSAGE
Idiopathic Parkinson's disease, postencephalitic parkinsonism, and symptomatic parkinsonism resulting from carbon monoxide or manganese intoxication –
Adults: 1 tablet of 25 mg carbidopa/100 mg levodopa P.O. daily t.i.d. followed by an increase of 1 tablet every day or every other day as necessary to a maximum daily dosage of 8 tablets. 25 mg carbidopa/250 mg levodopa or 10 mg carbidopa/100 mg levodopa tablets are substituted as required to obtain maximum response. Optimum daily dosage must be determined by careful titration for each patient.

Patients treated with conventional tablets may receive extended-release tablets; dosage is calculated on current levodopa intake. Initially, extended-release tablets given equal to 10% more levodopa per day; increased as needed and tolerated to 30% more levodopa per day. Administered in divided doses at intervals of 4 to 8 hours.

ADVERSE REACTIONS
CNS: *choreiform, dystonic, dyskinetic movements; involuntary grimacing, head movements, myoclonic body jerks, ataxia,* tremors, muscle twitching; bradykinetic episodes; psychiatric disturbances, memory loss, nervousness, anxiety, disturbing dreams, euphoria, malaise, fatigue; severe depression, suicidal tendencies, dementia, delirium, hallucinations (may necessitate reduction or withdrawal of drug).
CV: *orthostatic hypotension,* **cardiac irregularities,** flushing, hypertension, phlebitis.
EENT: blepharospasm, blurred vision, diplopia, mydriasis or miosis, widening of palpebral fissures, activation of latent Horner's syndrome, oculogyric crises, nasal discharge, excessive salivation.
GI: *dry mouth,* bitter taste, *nausea, vomiting, anorexia,* weight loss may occur at start of therapy; constipation; flatulence; diarrhea; *epigastric pain; bleeding* (rare).
GU: urinary frequency, urine retention, urinary incontinence, darkened urine, excessive and inappropriate sexual behavior, priapism.
Hematologic: *hemolytic anemia.*
Hepatic: hepatotoxicity.
Other: dark perspiration, hyperventilation, hiccups.

INTERACTIONS
Antihypertensives: additive hypotensive effects. Use together cautiously.

---

*Liquid form contains alcohol.
**May contain tartrazine.

Common reactions are in italics; *life-threatening*, in bold italics.

MAO inhibitors: risk of severe hypertension. Avoid concomitant use.

Papaverine, phenytoin: antagonism of antiparkinsonian actions. Don't use together.

Phenothiazines and other antipsychotics: may antagonize antiparkinsonian actions. Use together cautiously.

CONTRAINDICATIONS

Contraindicated in patients with hypersensitivity to drug, acute angle-closure glaucoma, melanoma, or undiagnosed skin lesions, and within 14 days of MAO inhibitor therapy.

NURSING CONSIDERATIONS

• Use cautiously in patients with severe CV, renal, hepatic, endocrine, or pulmonary disorders; history of peptic ulcer; psychiatric illness; MI with residual arrhythmias; bronchial asthma; emphysema; and well-controlled, chronic open-angle glaucoma.

• Know that if the patient is being treated with levodopa, the drug should be discontinued at least 8 hours before starting carbidopa-levodopa.

• Know that carbidopa-levodopa typically decreases amount of levodopa needed by 75%, reducing the incidence of adverse reactions.

• Be aware that therapeutic and adverse reactions occur more rapidly with carbidopa-levodopa than with levodopa alone. Observe and monitor vital signs, especially while adjusting dosage. Report significant changes.

• Carefully monitor patients receiving antihypertensives.

• Muscle twitching and blepharospasm (twitching of eyelids) may be early signs of drug overdose; report immediately.

• Know that patients receiving long-term therapy should be tested regularly for diabetes and acromegaly and should have periodic tests of liver, renal, and hematopoietic function as ordered.

• Depending on reagent and test method used, expect possible false-positive increases in levels of uric acid, urine ketones, urine catecholamines, and urine vanillylmandelic acid.

• False-positive tests for urine glucose can occur if reagents using copper sulfate are used; false-negative results can occur with tests that use glucose enzymatic methods. An accurate measure can be obtained if the paper strip is only partially immersed in the urine sample. Urine will migrate up the strip, as with an ascending chromatographic system. Read only the top of the strip.

• Assess the patient for signs and symptoms of GI intolerance. To minimize GI upset, tell patient to take the drug with food.

• Warn the patient and his family not to increase dosage without doctor's orders.

• Warn the patient of possible dizziness and orthostatic hypotension, especially at start of therapy. Tell the patient to change position slowly and dangle legs before getting out of bed. Elastic stockings may control this adverse reaction in some patients.

• Instruct the patient to report adverse reactions and therapeutic effects.

• Inform patient pyridoxine (vitamin B_6) does not reverse the beneficial effects of carbidopa-levodopa. Multivitamins can be taken without losing control of symptoms.

---

levodopa
Dopar, Larodopa
Pregnancy Risk Category: NR

HOW SUPPLIED
Tablets: 100 mg, 250 mg, 500 mg
Capsules: 100 mg, 250 mg, 500 mg

ACTION
Unknown. Thought to be decarboxylated to dopamine, countering the depletion of striatal dopamine in extrapyramidal centers, which is thought to produce parkinsonism.

ONSET, PEAK, DURATION
Onset for maximal effects, 3 weeks to 6 months.Plasma levels peak in 1 to 3 hours. Effects persist for about 5 hours although it varies.

INDICATIONS & DOSAGE
Idiopathic parkinsonism, postencephalitic parkinsonism, and symptomatic parkinsonism after carbon monoxide or manganese intoxication or in association with cerebral arteriosclerosis —
Adults and children over 12 years: initially, 0.5 to 1 g P.O. daily, divided in 2 or more doses with food; increased by no more than 0.75 g daily q 3 to 7 days, until usual maximum daily dosage of 8 g is reached. Dosage carefully adjusted to patient requirements, tolerance, and response. Higher dosage requires close supervision.

ADVERSE REACTIONS
CNS: *aggressive behavior; choreiform, dystonic, and dyskinetic movements; involuntary grimacing, head movements, myoclonic body jerks, ataxia, tremors, muscle twitching; bradykinetic episodes; psychiatric disturbances; memory loss, mood changes, nervousness, anxiety, disturbing dreams, euphoria, malaise, fatigue; severe depression, suicidal tendencies, dementia, delirium, hallucinations* (may necessitate reduction or withdrawal of drug).
CV: *orthostatic hypotension,* cardiac irregularities, flushing, hypertension, phlebitis.
EENT: blepharospasm, blurred vision, diplopia, mydriasis or miosis, widening of palpebral fissures, activation of latent Horner's syndrome, oculogyric crises, nasal discharge, excessive salivation.
GI: dry mouth, bitter taste, *nausea, vomiting, anorexia,* weight loss (may occur at start of therapy), constipation, flatulence, diarrhea, epigastric pain.
GU: urinary frequency, urine retention, incontinence, darkened urine, excessive and inappropriate sexual behavior, priapism.
Hematologic: *hemolytic anemia,* leukopenia.
Hepatic: hepatotoxicity.
Other: dark perspiration, hyperventilation, hiccups.

INTERACTIONS
Antacids: increased absorption of levodopa. Administer antacids 1 hour after levodopa.
Cocaine, sympathomimetic agents, inhalational halogen anesthetics: increased risk of arrhythmias. Monitor the patient closely.
MAO inhibitors, furazolidone, procarbazine: risk of severe hypertension. Avoid concomitant use.
Metoclopramide: accelerated gastric emptying of levodopa. Give metoclopramide 1 hour after levodopa.
Papaverine, phenothiazines and other antipsychotics, phenytoin, rauwolfia alkaloids: decreased levodopa effect.
Pyridoxine: reversal of antiparkinsonian effects. Check vitamin preparations and nutritional supplements for pyridoxine (vitamin B$_6$) content. Don't give together.
Foods high in protein: decreased absorption of levodopa. Don't give levodopa with high-protein foods.

CONTRAINDICATIONS
Contraindicated in concurrent therapy with MAO inhibitors within 14 days, and in patients with hypersensitivity to the drug, acute angle-closure glaucoma, melanoma, or undiagnosed skin lesions.

---

*Liquid form contains alcohol.
**May contain tartrazine.

Common reactions are in italics; *life-threatening,* in bold italics.

NURSING CONSIDERATIONS
• Use cautiously in patients with severe CV, renal, liver, and pulmonary disorders; peptic ulcer; psychiatric illness; MI with residual arrhythmias; bronchial asthma; emphysema; and endocrine disease.

• Patients who must undergo surgery should continue levodopa as long as oral intake is permitted, generally 6 to 24 hours before surgery. Drug should be resumed as soon as patient is able to take oral medication.

• Assess the patient for signs and symptoms of GI intolerance. To minimize GI upset, tell the patient to take the drug with food. However, taking the drug with high-protein meals can impair absorption and reduce effectiveness.

• Protect from heat, light, and moisture. If preparation darkens, it has lost potency and should be discarded.

• Carbidopa-levodopa typically decreases amount of levodopa needed by 75%, reducing the incidence of adverse reactions.

• Observe and monitor vital signs, especially while adjusting dosage. Report significant changes.

• Muscle twitching and blepharospasm (twitching of eyelids) may be early signs of drug overdose; report immediately.

• Be aware Coombs' test occasionally becomes positive during extended use. Expect uric acid elevations with colorimetric method but not with urate oxidase.

• Know that alkaline phosphatase, AST, ALT, lactate dehydrogenase, bilirubin, BUN, and protein-bound iodine show transient elevations in patients receiving levodopa; WBC count, hemoglobin, and hematocrit show occasional reductions.

• Depending on reagent and test method used, expect possible false-positive increases in levels of uric acid, urine ketones, urine catecholamines, and urine vanillylmandelic acid, depending on reagent and test method used.

• False-positive tests for urine glucose can occur if reagents using copper sulfate are used; false-negative results can occur with tests that use glucose enzymatic methods. An accurate measure can be obtained if the paper strip is only partially immersed in the urine sample. Urine will migrate up the strip, as with an ascending chromatographic system. Read only the top of the strip.

• Know that patients receiving long-term therapy should be tested regularly for diabetes and acromegaly; periodically monitor renal, liver, and hematopoietic function as ordered.

• Know that a doctor-supervised period of drug discontinuance (called a drug holiday) may reestablish the effectiveness of a lower dosage regimen.

• For patients who have difficulty swallowing pills, tell patients or family to crush tablets and mix with applesauce or baby food fruits.

• Warn the patient and family not to increase dosage without the doctor's orders. Daily dosage should not exceed 8 g.

• Warn the patient of possible dizziness and orthostatic hypotension, especially at start of therapy. Tell the patient to change position slowly and dangle legs before getting out of bed. Elastic stockings may control this adverse reaction in some patients.

• Advise the patient and his family that multivitamin preparations, fortified cereals, and certain OTC medications may contain pyridoxine (vitamin B_6), which can block the effects of levodopa by enhancing its peripheral metabolism.

pergolide mesylate
Permax

Pregnancy Risk Category: B

HOW SUPPLIED
Tablets: 0.05 mg, 0.25 mg, 1 mg

ACTION
A dopamine agonist that directly stimulates dopamine receptors in the nigrostriatal system.

ONSET, PEAK, DURATION
Unknown.

INDICATIONS & DOSAGE
Adjunctive treatment with carbidopa-levodopa in the management of the symptoms associated with Parkinson's disease –
Adults: initially, 0.05 mg P.O. daily for the first 2 days followed by increased dosage of 0.1 to 0.15 mg every third day over 12 days. Subsequent dosage increased by 0.25 mg every third day until optimum response is seen if needed. The drug usually is administered in divided doses t.i.d. Gradual reductions in carbidopa-levodopa dosage could be made during dosage titration.

ADVERSE REACTIONS
CNS: headache, asthenia, *dyskinesia, dizziness, hallucinations,* dystonia, confusion, *somnolence,* insomnia, anxiety, depression, tremor, abnormal dreams, personality disorder, psychosis, abnormal gait, akathisia, extrapyramidal syndrome, incoordination, akinesia, hypertonia, neuralgia, speech disorder, twitching.
CV: *orthostatic hypotension,* vasodilation, palpitations, hypotension, syncope, hypertension, ***arrhythmias, MI.***
EENT: *rhinitis,* epistaxis, abnormal vision, diplopia, eye disorder.
GI: dry mouth, dysgeusia, abdominal pain, *nausea, constipation,* diarrhea, dyspepsia, anorexia, vomiting.
GU: urinary frequency, urinary tract infection, hematuria.
Skin: rash, diaphoresis, paresthesia.
Other: flulike syndrome; chest, neck, and back pain; chills; infection; facial, peripheral, or generalized edema; weight gain; arthralgia; bursitis; myalgia.
Note: The above adverse reactions, although not always attributable to the drug, occurred in > 1% of the study population.

INTERACTIONS
Butyrophenones, metoclopramide, other dopamine antagonists, phenothiazines, thioxanthenes: may antagonize the effects of pergolide. Avoid concomitant use.

CONTRAINDICATIONS
Contraindicated in patients hypersensitive to the drug or to ergot alkaloids.

NURSING CONSIDERATIONS
• Use cautiously in patients prone to arrhythmias.
• Monitor blood pressure. Symptomatic orthostatic or sustained hypotension may occur in some patients, especially at the start of therapy.
• Inform patients of potential adverse reactions, especially hallucinations and confusion (27% incidence).
• Warn patients to avoid activities that could result in injury from orthostatic hypotension and syncope.

---

procyclidine hydrochloride
Kemadrin, PMS Procyclidine†, Procyclid†

Pregnancy Risk Category: NR

HOW SUPPLIED
Tablets: 5 mg

ACTION
Unknown. Blocks central cholinergic receptors, helping to balance cholinergic activity in the basal ganglia.

---

*Liquid form contains alcohol.   *Common* reactions are in italics; ***life-threatening,*** in bold italics.
**May contain tartrazine.

ONSET, PEAK, DURATION
Onset occurs within 1 hour. Peak effects occur in 1 to 3 hours. Effects persist about 4 hours.

INDICATIONS & DOSAGE
Parkinsonism, drug-induced extrapyramidal symptoms –
Adults: initially, 2.5 mg P.O. t.i.d. after meals. Increased as needed to 5 mg P.O. t.i.d. after meals and, occasionally, 5 mg P.O. h.s.

ADVERSE REACTIONS
CNS: light-headedness, giddiness.
EENT: blurred vision, mydriasis.
GI: *dry mouth, constipation,* nausea, vomiting, epigastric distress.
Skin: rash.
Other: muscle weakness.

INTERACTIONS
None significant.

CONTRAINDICATIONS
Contraindicated in patients with acute angle-closure glaucoma.

NURSING CONSIDERATIONS
• Use cautiously in patients with tachycardia, hypotension, urine retention, and prostatic hyperplasia.
• To minimize GI distress, give after meals.
• Watch closely for mental confusion, disorientation, agitation, hallucinations, and psychotic symptoms, especially in elderly patients. Call the doctor promptly if these occur.
• Be aware that in severe parkinsonism, tremors may increase as spasticity is relieved.
• Warn the patient to avoid activities that require alertness until CNS effects of the drug are known.
• Tell patient to relieve dry mouth with cool drinks, ice chips, sugarless gum or hard candy.

selegiline hydrochloride (L-deprenyl hydrochloride)
Eldepryl

Pregnancy Risk Category: C

HOW SUPPLIED
Tablets: 5 mg

ACTION
Unknown. Probably acts by selectively inhibiting MAO type B (found mostly in the brain). At higher-than-recommended doses, it is a nonselective inhibitor of MAO, including MAO type A (found in the GI tract). It also may directly increase dopaminergic activity by decreasing the reuptake of dopamine into nerve cells. Its active metabolites, amphetamine and methamphetamine, may contribute to this effect.

ONSET, PEAK, DURATION
Onset and duration unknown. Serum levels peak in 0.5 to 2 hours.

INDICATIONS & DOSAGE
Adjunctive treatment with carbidopa-levodopa in the management of the symptoms associated with Parkinson's disease –
Adults: 10 mg P.O. daily, taken as 5 mg at breakfast and 5 mg at lunch. After 2 or 3 days of therapy, gradual decrease of carbidopa-levodopa dosage is attempted.

ADVERSE REACTIONS
CNS: *dizziness,* increased tremor, chorea, loss of balance, restlessness, increased bradykinesia, facial grimacing, stiff neck, dyskinesia, involuntary movements, twitching, increased apraxia, behavioral changes, fatigue, headache.
CV: orthostatic hypotension, hypertension, hypotension, *arrhythmias,* palpitations, new or increased anginal pain, tachycardia, peripheral edema, syncope.

EENT: blepharospasm.
GI: dry mouth, dysgeusia, *nausea,* vomiting, constipation, weight loss, anorexia or poor appetite, dysphagia, diarrhea, heartburn.
GU: slow urination, transient nocturia, prostatic hyperplasia, urinary hesitancy, urinary frequency, urine retention, sexual dysfunction.
Skin: rash, hair loss.
Other: malaise, diaphoresis.

INTERACTIONS
Adrenergic agents: possible increased pressor response, particularly in patients who have taken an overdose of selegiline. Use together cautiously.
Foods high in tyramine: possible hypertensive crisis. Monitor blood pressure.

CONTRAINDICATIONS
Contraindicated in patients with hypersensitivity to the drug and in patients receiving meperidine.

NURSING CONSIDERATIONS
• Be aware that some patients experience increased adverse reactions associated with levodopa and require a 10% to 30% reduction of carbidopa-levodopa dosage.
• Warn patients to move cautiously at the start of therapy because they may experience dizziness.
• Advise patients not to take more than 10 mg daily because a greater amount will not improve efficacy and may increase adverse reactions.

trihexyphenidyl hydrochloride
Aparkane†, Apo-Trihex†, Artane*, Artane Sequels, Novohexidyl†, Trihexane, Trihexy-2, Trihexy-5

Pregnancy Risk Category: NR

HOW SUPPLIED
Tablets: 2 mg, 5 mg
Capsules (sustained-release): 5 mg

Elixir: 2 mg/5 ml

ACTION
Unknown. Blocks central cholinergic receptors, helping to balance cholinergic activity in the basal ganglia.

ONSET, PEAK, DURATION
Onset occurs within 1 hour. Peak unknown. Effects persist for 6 to 12 hours.

INDICATIONS & DOSAGE
All forms of Parkisonism, drug-induced parkinsonism, and adjunctive treatment to levodopa in the management of parkinsonism –
Adults: 1 mg P.O. first day, 2 mg second day; then increased by 2 mg q 3 to 5 days until total of 6 to 10 mg is given daily. Usually given t.i.d. with meals, sometimes given q.i.d. (last dose before bedtime) or switched to extended-release form b.i.d. Postencephalitic parkinsonism may require total daily dosage of 12 to 15 mg.

ADVERSE REACTIONS
CNS: nervousness, dizziness, headache, restlessness, hallucinations, euphoria, amnesia.
CV: tachycardia.
EENT: blurred vision, mydriasis, increased intraocular pressure.
GI: *dry mouth,* constipation, *nausea.*
GU: urinary hesitancy, urine retention.

INTERACTIONS
Amantadine: additive anticholinergic adverse reactions, such as confusion and hallucinations. Reduce dosage of trihexyphenidyl before administering.

CONTRAINDICATIONS
Contraindicated in patients hypersensitive to the drug.

NURSING CONSIDERATIONS
• Use cautiously in patients with glaucoma; cardiac, hepatic, or renal disorders; obstructive disease of the

---

*Liquid form contains alcohol.   *Common* reactions are in italics; *life-threatening,* in bold italics.
**May contain tartrazine.

GI and GU tracts; and prostatic hyperplasia.

• Be aware that dosage may need to be gradually increased in patients who develop a tolerance to the drug.

• Monitor patient closely. Adverse reactions are dose-related and usually transient.

• Know that gonioscopic evaluation and monitoring of intraocular pressure are needed, especially in patients over 40 years.

• Alert patient that drug may cause nausea if given before meals.

• Tell patient to avoid activities that require alertness until CNS effects of the drug are known.

• Advise the patient to report signs of urinary hesitancy or urine retention.

• Tell patient to relieve dry mouth with cool drinks, ice chips, sugarless gum or hard candy.

fluvoxamine maleate
lithium carbonate
lithium citrate
nicotine polacrilex
nicotine transdermal system
sumatriptan succinate
tacrine hydrochloride

COMBINATION PRODUCTS
None.

fluvoxamine maleate
Luvox

Pregnancy Risk Category: C

HOW SUPPLIED
Tablets: 50 mg, 100 mg

ACTION
Unknown. Selectively inhibits the neuronal uptake of serotonin, which is thought to improve obsessive-compulsive disorders.

ONSET, PEAK, DURATION
Onset and duration unknown. Serum levels peak in 3 to 8 hours.

INDICATIONS & DOSAGE
Obsessive-compulsive disorder –
Adults: initially, 50 mg P.O. daily at h.s. Increased in 50-mg increments every 4 to 7 days until maximum benefit achieved. Maximum daily dosage is 300 mg. Total daily doses of more than 100 mg should be given in two divided doses.

ADVERSE REACTIONS
CNS: *headache, asthenia, somnolence, insomnia, nervousness,* dizziness, tremors, anxiety, vasodilation, hypertonia, *agitation,* depression, CNS stimulation, taste perversion.
CV: palpitations.

EENT: amblyopia.
GI: *nausea,* diarrhea, constipation, dyspepsia, anorexia, *vomiting,* flatulence, tooth disorder, dysphagia, dry mouth.
GU: decreased libido, abnormal ejaculation, urinary frequency, impotence, anorgasmia, urine retention.
Respiratory: upper respiratory tract infection, dyspnea, yawning.
Skin: sweating.
Other: flulike syndrome, chills.

INTERACTIONS
Astemizole, terfenadine: may cause decreased metabolism, leading to increased levels of these antihistamines and cardiotoxicity. Avoid concomitant use.
Benzodiazepines, theophylline, warfarin: reduced clearance of these drugs by fluvoxamine. Use together cautiously (except for diazepam, which should not be administered together with fluvoxamine). Dosage adjustments may be necessary.
Carbamazepine, clozapine, methadone, metopranolol, propranolol, tricyclic antidepressants: elevated serum levels of these drugs caused by fluvoxamine. Use together cautiously. Monitor patient closely for adverse reactions. Dosage adjustments may be necessary.
Diltiazem: bradycardia may occur. Monitor heart rate.
Lithium, tryptophan: may enhance effects of fluvoxamine. Use together cautiously.
MAO inhibitors: may cause severe excitation, hyperpyrexia, myoclonus, delirium, and coma. Avoid concomitant use.

---

*Liquid form contains alcohol.   *Common* reactions are in italics; **life-threatening,** in bold italics.
**May contain tartrazine.

CONTRAINDICATIONS
Contraindicated in patients with hypersensitivity to the drug or to other phenylpiperazine antidepressants and within 14 days of MAO inhibitor therapy.

NURSING CONSIDERATIONS
• Use cautiously in patients with hepatic dysfunction, concomitant conditions that may affect hemodynamic responses or metabolism, or history of mania or seizures.
• Know that at least 14 days should be allowed after stopping fluvoxamine before patient is started on an MAO inhibitor and that at least 14 days should be allowed before a patient is started on fluvoxamine after MAO inhibitor therapy has been discontinued.
• Record mood changes. Monitor patients for suicidal tendencies, and allow them only a minimum supply of the drug.
• Warn patient not to engage in hazardous activity until drug's CNS effects are known.
• Advise patient to avoid alcoholic beverages while taking this drug.
• Alert patient that smoking may decrease effectiveness of the drug.
• Instruct female patients who become pregnant or intend to become pregnant during therapy to notify doctor.
• Tell patient who develops a rash, hives, or a related allergic reaction to notify doctor.
• Inform patient that several weeks of therapy may be required to obtain the full antidepressant effect. Once improvement is seen, advise patient not to discontinue the drug until directed by doctor.
• Advise patient to check with doctor before taking any OTC medication; drug interactions can occur.

lithium carbonate
Carbolith†, Duralith†, Eskalith, Eskalith CR, Lithane**, Lithicarb‡, Lithizine†, Lithobid, Lithonate, Lithotabs, Priadel‡

lithium citrate
Cibalith-S*

Pregnancy Risk Category: NR

HOW SUPPLIED
lithium carbonate
Tablets: 250 mg‡, 300 mg (300 mg = 8.12 mEq lithium)
Tablets (controlled-release): 300 mg, 400 mg‡, 450 mg
Capsules: 150 mg, 300 mg, 600 mg
lithium citrate
Syrup (sugarless): 8 mEq (of lithium) per 5 ml
   Note: 5 ml lithium citrate (liquid) contains 8 mEq lithium, equal to 300 mg lithium carbonate.

ACTION
Unknown. Probably alters chemical transmitters in the CNS, possibly by interfering with ionic pump mechanisms in brain cells, and may compete with or replace sodium ions.

ONSET, PEAK, DURATION
Onset of clinical effects usually within 1 to 3 weeks. Serum levels peak in 0.5 to 3 hours depending on dosage form used. Duration unknown.

INDICATIONS & DOSAGE
Prevention or control of mania –
Adults: 300 to 600 mg P.O. up to q.i.d., increasing on the basis of blood levels to achieve optimal dosage. Recommended therapeutic lithium blood levels: 1 to 1.5 mEq/L for acute mania; 0.6 to 1.2 mEq/L for maintenance therapy; and 2 mEq/L as maximum dosage.

ADVERSE REACTIONS

CNS: tremors, drowsiness, headache, confusion, restlessness, dizziness, psychomotor retardation, stupor, lethargy, *coma,* blackouts, epileptiform seizures, EEG changes, worsened organic mental syndrome, impaired speech, ataxia, muscle weakness, incoordination.

CV: *reversible ECG changes, arrhythmias,* hypotension, *peripheral vascular collapse,* (rare).

EENT: tinnitus, blurred vision.

GI: dry mouth, metallic taste, nausea, vomiting, anorexia, diarrhea, *thirst,* abdominal pain, flatulation, indigestion.

GU: *polyuria,* glycosuria, renal toxicity with long-term use, decreased creatinine clearance, albuminuria.

Hematologic: *leukocytosis with leukocyte count of 14,000 to 18,000/mm³* (reversible).

Skin: pruritus, rash, diminished or absent sensation, drying and thinning of hair, psoriasis, acne, alopecia.

Other: transient hyperglycemia, goiter, hypothyroidism (lowered T_3, T_4, and protein-bound iodine, but elevated ^{131}I [radioactive iodine] uptake), hyponatremia, ankle and wrist edema.

INTERACTIONS

Aminophylline, sodium bicarbonate, urine alkalinizers: increased lithium excretion. Avoid salt loads and monitor lithium levels.

Carbamazepine, indomethacin, methyldopa, piroxicam, probenecid: increased effect of lithium. Monitor for lithium toxicity.

Diuretics: increased reabsorption of lithium by kidneys, with possible toxic effect. Use with extreme caution, and monitor lithium and electrolyte levels (especially sodium).

Neuroleptics: may cause encephalopathy. Watch for signs and symptoms (lethargy, tremors, extrapyramidal symptoms), and stop drug if it occurs.

Neuromuscular blockers: may cause prolonged paralysis or weakness. Monitor patient closely.

Thyroid hormones: may induce hypothyroidism. Monitor thyroid function.

CONTRAINDICATIONS

Contraindicated if therapy cannot be closely monitored.

NURSING CONSIDERATIONS

• Know that drug should not be administered during pregnancy.

• Use with extreme caution in patients receiving neuroleptics, neuromuscular blockers, and diuretics; in elderly or debilitated patients; and in patients with thyroid disease, seizure disorder, renal or CV disease, severe debilitation or dehydration, and sodium depletion.

• Be aware determination of lithium blood concentration is crucial to the safe use of the drug. Drug should not be used in patients who can't have regular lithium blood level checks.

• Monitor baseline ECG, thyroid and renal studies, as well as electrolyte levels as ordered. Monitor lithium blood levels 8 to 12 hours after first dose, usually before morning dose, two or three times weekly first month, then weekly to monthly during maintenance therapy.

• Know that with blood levels of lithium below 1.5 mEq/L, adverse reactions usually remain mild.

• Check fluid intake and output, especially when surgery is scheduled.

• Weigh the patient daily; check for signs of edema or sudden weight gain.

• Adjust fluid and salt ingestion to compensate if excessive loss occurs as a result of protracted diaphoresis or diarrhea. Under normal conditions, patients should have fluid intake of 2,500 to 3,000 ml daily and a balanced diet with adequate salt intake.

• Check urine specific gravity and report level below 1.005, which may indicate diabetes insipidus.

---

*Liquid form contains alcohol.
**May contain tartrazine.

Common reactions are in italics; *life-threatening,* in bold italics.

• May alter glucose tolerance in diabetics. Monitor blood glucose closely.
• Perform outpatient follow-up of thyroid and renal functions every 6 to 12 months. Palpate thyroid to check for enlargement.
• Tell patient to take drug with plenty of water and after meals to minimize GI upset.
• Explain to patients that lithium has a narrow therapeutic margin of safety. A blood level that is even slightly high can be dangerous.
• Warn patients and their families to watch for signs of toxicity (diarrhea, vomiting, tremor, drowsiness, muscle weakness, ataxia) and to expect transient nausea, polyuria, thirst, and discomfort during first few days. Patients should withhold one dose and call the doctor if toxic symptoms appear, but not stop drug abruptly.
• Warn ambulatory patients to avoid hazardous activities that require alertness and good psychomotor coordination until CNS effects of the drug are known.
• Tell patients not to switch brands of lithium or to take other prescription or OTC drugs without their doctor's guidance.
• Inform patients that they should carry medical identification card.

---

nicotine polacrilex (nicotine-polacrilin resin complex)
Nicorette, Nicorette DS

Pregnancy Risk Category: C

HOW SUPPLIED
Chewing gum: 2 mg/square, 4 mg/square

ACTION
Provides nicotine, which stimulates nicotinic acetylcholine receptors in the CNS, neuromuscular junction, autonomic ganglia, and adrenal medulla.

ONSET, PEAK, DURATION
Onset and duration unknown. Serum levels peak within 15 to 30 minutes after the patient begins to chew the gum.

INDICATIONS & DOSAGE
Relief of nicotine withdrawal symptoms in patients undergoing smoking cessation –
Adults: initially, one 2-mg square; highly dependent patients should start treatment with 4-mg squares. Patients should chew one piece of gum slowly and intermittently for 30 minutes whenever the urge to smoke occurs. Most patients require 9 to 12 pieces of gum daily during the first month. For patients using 4-mg squares, maximum dosage is 20 pieces daily. For patients using 2-mg squares, maximum dosage is 30 pieces daily.

ADVERSE REACTIONS
CNS: dizziness, light-headedness.
CV: atrial fibrillation.
EENT: throat soreness, jaw muscle ache (from chewing).
GI: nausea, vomiting, indigestion.
Other: hiccups.

INTERACTIONS
Beta blockers, methylxanthines, propoxyphene, propranolol: decreased metabolism of these agents, increasing therapeutic effects. Dosage adjustments of these agents may be necessary.

CONTRAINDICATIONS
Contraindicated in nonsmokers; in patients with recent MI, life-threatening arrhythmias, severe or worsening angina pectoris, or active temporomandibular joint disease; and during pregnancy.

NURSING CONSIDERATIONS
• Use cautiously in patients with hyperthyroidism, pheochromocytoma, insulin-dependent diabetes, peptic ul-

---

cer disease, history of esophagitis, oral or pharyngeal inflammation, or dental conditions that might be exacerbated by chewing gum.

• Know that smokers most likely to benefit from nicotine gum are those with high "physical" nicotine dependence — those who smoke more than 15 cigarettes daily, prefer brands of cigarettes with high nicotine levels, usually inhale the smoke, smoke the first cigarette within 30 minutes of arising, find the first morning cigarette the hardest to give up, smoke most frequently during the morning, find it difficult to refrain from smoking in places where it's forbidden, or smoke even when ill and confined to bed during the day.

• Instruct patients to chew gum slowly and intermittently (chew several times, then place between cheek and gums) for about 30 minutes to promote slow and even buccal absorption of nicotine. Fast chewing tends to produce more adverse reactions.

• Be sure that patient reads and understands the patient instruction sheet included in the package.

• Emphasize the importance of withdrawing the gum gradually.

• Tell patient that successful abstainers will begin to gradually withdraw gum usage after 3 months. Use of the gum for longer than 6 months is not recommended. For gradual withdrawal, cut gum in halves or quarters and mix with other sugarless gum.

---

nicotine transdermal system
Habitrol, Nicoderm, Nicotrol, ProStep

Pregnancy Risk Category: D

HOW SUPPLIED
Transdermal system: designed to release nicotine at a fixed rate
Habitrol — 21 mg/day, 14 mg/day, 7 mg/day

Nicoderm — 21 mg/day, 14 mg/day, 7 mg/day
ProStep — 22 mg/day, 11 mg/day

ACTION
Provides nicotine, which stimulates nicotinic acetylcholine receptors in the CNS, neuromuscular junction, autonomic ganglia, and adrenal medulla.

ONSET, PEAK, DURATION
Users of Habitrol exhibit peak serum levels 5 to 6 hours after application; Nicoderm, 4 hours after application; Nicotrol, 3 to 6 hours; ProStep, 9 hours after application. Duration is variable.

INDICATIONS & DOSAGE
Relief of nicotine withdrawal symptoms in patients undergoing smoking cessation —
Adults: initially, 1 trandermal system, delivering the largest available dosage of nicotine in its dosage series, applied once daily in the morning to a nonhairy part of body and removed before retiring. After 4 to 12 weeks (dependent on the brand used) dosage tapered to next largest available dosage of nicotine in its dosage series followed in 2 to 4 weeks by lowest nicotine dosage system in series being used. Drug is then stopped in 2 to 4 weeks.

ADVERSE REACTIONS
CNS: somnolence, dizziness, *headache, insomnia.*
EENT: pharyngitis, sinusitis.
GI: abdominal pain, constipation, dyspepsia, nausea.
GU: dysmenorrhea.
Skin: *local or systemic erythema, pruritus, burning at application site,* cutaneous hypersensitivity, rash.
Other: back pain, myalgia, diaphoresis.

---

*Liquid form contains alcohol.   *Common* reactions are in italics; *life-threatening,* in bold italics.
**May contain tartrazine.

INTERACTIONS
Acetaminophen, caffeine, imipramine, oxazepam, pentazocine, propranolol, theophylline: may decrease induction of hepatic enzymes that help metabolize certain drugs. Dosage reductions may be necessary.
Adrenergic agonists, such as isoproterenol or phenylephrine: may decrease circulating catecholamines. Dosage increases may be necessary.
Adrenergic antagonists, such as prazosin or labetalol: may decrease circulating catecholamines. Dosage reductions may be necessary.
Insulin: may increase amount of subcutaneous insulin absorbed. Dosage reduction of insulin may be necessary.

CONTRAINDICATIONS
Contraindicated in patients with hypersensitivity to nicotine or any component of the transdermal system. Also contraindicated in nonsmokers; in patients with recent MI, life-threatening arrhythmias, and severe or worsening angina pectoris.

NURSING CONSIDERATIONS
• Use cautiously in patients with hyperthyroidism, pheochromocytoma, hypertension, insulin-dependent diabetes, or peptic ulcer disease.
• Health care workers' exposure to nicotine within transdermal systems probably is minimal; however, avoid unnecessary contact with the system. Wash hands with water alone because soap can enhance absorption.
• Use of the transdermal system for more than 3 months should be discouraged. Chronic nicotine consumption by any route can be dangerous and habit-forming.
• Patients should be warned not to smoke. If they continue to smoke while using the system, they may experience serious adverse effects because peak serum nicotine levels will be substantially higher than those achieved by smoking alone.

• Be sure that patient reads and understands the patient information that is dispensed with the drug.
• Advise patients to apply the patch promptly because the nicotine can evaporate from the transdermal system once it is removed from its protective packaging. Patch should not be altered in any way (folded or cut) before application. Do not store at temperatures above 86° F (30° C).
• Teach patients proper disposal of the transdermal system. After removal, fold the patch in half, bringing the adhesive sides together. If the system comes in a protective pouch, place the used patch in the pouch that contained the system. Careful disposal is necessary to prevent accidental poisoning of children or pets.
• Tell patients who experience persistent or severe local skin reactions or generalized rash to immediately discontinue use of the patch and contact the doctor.
• Inform patients that patients who cannot stop cigarette smoking during the initial 4 weeks of therapy probably will not benefit from the continued use of the drug. Patients who were unsuccessful may benefit from counseling to identify factors that led to treatment failure. Encourage patient to minimize or eliminate factors contributing to treatment failure and to try again, possibly after some interval before the next attempt.

sumatriptan succinate
Imitrex
Pregnancy Risk Category: C

HOW SUPPLIED
Tablets: 100 mg (base)†
Injection: 6 mg/0.5 ml (12 mg/ml) in 0.5-ml prefilled syringes and vials

ACTION
Unknown. Thought to selectively activate vascular serotonin (5-hydroxy-

tryptamine, 5-HT) receptors. Stimulation of the specific receptor subtype 5-HT_1, present on cranial arteries and the dura mater, causes vasoconstriction of cerebral vessels but has minimal effects on systemic vessels, tissue perfusion, and blood pressure.

ONSET, PEAK, DURATION
Onset occurs within 10 to 20 minutes after S.C. injection, or 30 minutes after oral administration. Serum levels peak about 12 minutes after S.C. injection, within 1½ hours after oral administration. Peak effect occurs within 1 to 2 hours after S.C. administration, within 2 to 4 hours after oral administration. Duration unknown.

INDICATIONS & DOSAGE
Acute migraine attacks (with or without aura) –
Adults: 6 mg S.C. Maximum recommended dosage is two 6-mg injections daily.
   Where available, give 100 mg P.O. If a beneficial response occurs, repeat dosage in 4 hours. Do not give more than 300 mg P.O. within 24 hours.

ADVERSE REACTIONS
CNS: *dizziness, vertigo,* drowsiness, headache, anxiety, malaise, fatigue, weakness, dysphagia.
CV: *atrial fibrillation, ventricular fibrillation, ventricular tachycardia, MI, ECG changes such as ischemic ST-segment elevation* (rare).
EENT: discomfort of throat, nasal cavity or sinus, mouth, jaw, or tongue; altered vision.
GI: abdominal discomfort.
Skin: local reactions, flushing.
Other: *tingling; warm or hot sensation; burning sensation; heaviness, pressure or tightness;* feeling of strangeness; tight feeling in head; cold sensation; pressure or tightness in chest; neck pain; myalgia; muscle cramps; diaphoresis.

INTERACTIONS
Ergot and ergot derivatives: prolonged vasospastic effects. Don't use these drugs and sumatriptan within 24 hours of sumatriptan dosage.

CONTRAINDICATIONS
Contraindicated in patients with hypersensitivity to the drug; in patients with uncontrolled hypertension or ischemic heart disease (such as angina pectoris, Prinzmetal's angina, history of MI, or documented silent ischemia); in patients with hemiplegic or basilar migraine; in patients taking ergotamine; and within 14 days of MAO therapy.

NURSING CONSIDERATIONS
• Use cautiously in patients who are pregnant or intend to become pregnant.
• Also use cautiously in patients who may have unrecognized coronary artery disease (CAD), such as postmenopausal women; male patients over age 40; or patients with risk factors such as hypertension, hypercholesterolemia, obesity, diabetes, smoking, or family history of CAD.
• When giving the drug to patients at risk for unrecognized CAD, consider administering the first dose in the doctor's office. Serious adverse cardiac effects can follow S.C. administration of this drug, but such events are rare.
• After S.C. injection, most patients experience relief within 1 to 2 hours.
• Redness or pain at the injection site should subside within 1 hour after the injection.
• Be sure patients understand that drug is intended only to treat a migraine attack, not to prevent or reduce the number of attacks.
• Tell patients who are pregnant or intend to become pregnant not to use this drug. Advise them to discuss with the doctor the risks and benefits of using the drug during pregnancy.

---

*Liquid form contains alcohol.
**May contain tartrazine.   *Common* reactions are in italics; *life-threatening,* in bold italics.

• Tell patients drug may be given at any time during a migraine attack, but should be given as soon as symptoms appear.

• Drug is available in a spring-loaded injector system that facilitates self-administration. Review detailed information with patient. Be sure the patient understands how to load the injector, administer the injection, and dispose of the used syringes.

• Tell patients who feel persistent or severe chest pain to call the doctor immediately. Patients who feel pain or tightness in the throat or experience wheezing, heart throbbing, rash, lumps, hives, or swollen eyelids, face, or lips should stop using the drug and call the doctor.

---

tacrine hydrochloride
Cognex

Pregnancy Risk Category: C

HOW SUPPLIED
Capsules: 10 mg, 20 mg, 30 mg, 40 mg

ACTION
Reversibly inhibits the enzyme cholinesterase in the CNS, allowing the buildup of acetylcholine and thereby temporarily improving cognitive function in patients with Alzheimer's disease.

ONSET, PEAK, DURATION
Onset and duration unknown. Serum levels peak in 0.5 to 3 hours.

INDICATIONS & DOSAGE
Mild to moderate dementia of the Alzheimer's type –
Adults: initially, 10 mg P.O. q.i.d. After 6 weeks and if the patient tolerates treatment and there are no transaminase elevations, dosage increased to 20 mg P.O. q.i.d. After 6 weeks, dosage titrated upward to 30 mg P.O. q.i.d. If still tolerated, dosage in-creased to 40 mg P.O. q.i.d. after another 6 weeks.

ADVERSE REACTIONS
CNS: anorexia, agitation, ataxia.
GI: nausea, vomiting, diarrhea, dyspepsia, loose stools, changes in stool color.
Skin: rash, jaundice.
Other: *elevations in transaminases* (especially ALT), myalgia.

INTERACTIONS
Anticholinergics: may decrease the effectiveness of anticholinergics. Monitor closely.
Cholinesterase inhibitors, cholinergics (such as bethanechol): additive effects. Monitor for toxicity.
Succinylcholine: enhanced neuromuscular blockade and prolonged duration of action. Monitor closely.
Theophylline: increased theophylline serum levels and prolonged theophylline half-life. Carefully monitor theophylline plasma levels, and adjust dosage as ordered.
Food: decreased absorption of tacrine if taken concomitantly. Take drug 1 hour before a meal.

CONTRAINDICATIONS
Contraindicated in patients hypersensitive to the drug or acridine derivatives. Also contraindicated in patients who have previously developed tacrine-related jaundice, which has been confirmed with an elevated total bilirubin level of more than 3 mg/dl.

NURSING CONSIDERATIONS
• Use cautiously in patients with sick sinus syndrome or bradycardia; in patients at risk for peptic ulceration (including patients taking NSAIDs or those with history of peptic ulcer); and in patients with history of hepatic disease. Also use cautiously in patients with renal disease, asthma, prostatic hyperplasia, or other urinary outflow impairment.

• Have the patient take the drug between meals whenever possible. If GI upset becomes a problem, the drug may be taken with meals, although doing so may reduce plasma levels by 30% to 40%.

• Know that if the drug is discontinued for 4 weeks or more, the full dosage titration and monitoring schedule must be restarted.

• Monitor serum ALT levels weekly during the first 18 weeks of therapy as ordered. If ALT is modestly elevated after the first 18 weeks of monitoring (twice the upper limit of normal range), continue weekly monitoring. If no problems are detected, frequency of serum determinations is decreased to once every 3 months. On each occasion that dosage is increased, resume weekly monitoring for at least 6 weeks as ordered.

• Patient and family members should understand that this drug does not alter the underlying degenerative disease, but can alleviate symptoms. Effect of therapy depends upon drug administration at regular intervals.

• Remind caregivers that dosage titration is an integral part of the safe use of this drug. Abrupt discontinuation or a large reduction in daily dosage (80 mg or more per day) may precipitate behavioral disturbances and a decline in cognitive function.

• Advise the patient and caregivers to immediately report any significant adverse effects or changes in status.

Cholinergics (parasympathomimetics)

ambenonium chloride
bethanechol chloride
edrophonium chloride
neostigmine bromide
neostigmine methylsulfate
physostigmine salicylate
pyridostigmine bromide

COMBINATION PRODUCTS
None.

---

ambenonium chloride
Mytelase

Pregnancy Risk Category: NR

HOW SUPPLIED
Tablets: 10 mg

ACTION
Inhibits the destruction of acetylcholine released from the parasympathetic and somatic efferent nerves. Acetylcholine accumulates, promoting increased stimulation of the receptor.

ONSET, PEAK, DURATION
Onset and peak unknown. Effects persist for 4 to 8 hours.

INDICATIONS & DOSAGE
Symptomatic treatment of myasthenia gravis in patients who cannot take neostigmine bromide or pyridostigmine bromide –
Adults: dosage individualized for each patient, but usually ranges from 5 to 25 mg P.O. t.i.d. or q.i.d. Starting dose usually is 5 mg P.O. t.i.d. or q.i.d. Increased and adjusted at 1- to 2-day intervals to avoid drug accumulation and overdosage. Usual dosage range is 5 to 25 mg P.O. t.i.d. or q.i.d., but some patients may require as much as 75 mg b.i.d. to q.i.d.

ADVERSE REACTIONS
CNS: headache, dizziness, muscle weakness, incoordination, *seizures,* mental confusion, tremor or nervousness, sweating.
CV: bradycardia, hypotension.
EENT: miosis, lacrimation.
GI: *nausea, vomiting, diarrhea, abdominal cramps,* increased salivation.
GU: urinary frequency, incontinence.
Respiratory: bronchospasm, *bronchoconstriction,* increased bronchial secretions, *respiratory paralysis*.
Other: muscle cramps, sweating.

INTERACTIONS
Aminoglycosides, anesthetics, atropine, corticosteroids, magnesium, procainamide, quinidine: prolonged or enhanced muscle weakness. Monitor closely.
Mecamylamine, other ganglionic blockers: increased toxicity. Avoid concomitant use.

CONTRAINDICATIONS
Contraindicated in patients with mechanical obstruction of intestine or urinary tract and in patients receiving ganglionic blocking agents.

NURSING CONSIDERATIONS
● Use with extreme caution in patients with bronchial asthma. Use cautiously in patients with seizure disorder, bradycardia, recent coronary occlusion, vagotonia, hyperthyroidism, arrhythmias, postoperative atelectasis, and pneumonia.
● Discontinue all other cholinergics as ordered before administering this drug.
● Know that large doses should be avoided in patients with decreased GI motility or megacolon.
● Administer each dose exactly as or-

---

dered, on time. Amount and frequency of dosing should vary with the patient's activity level. The doctor probably will order larger doses when the patient is fatigued, for example, in the afternoon and at mealtime.
• Give with milk or food to produce fewer adverse muscarinic reactions.
• Monitor vital signs frequently, especially respirations, and document. Always have atropine injection readily available and be prepared to give 0.5 to 1 mg S.C. or slow I.V. push as ordered. Provide respiratory support as needed.
• Watch the patient very closely for adverse reactions, particularly if total dosage is greater than 200 mg daily. When adverse reactions indicate drug toxicity, notify the doctor immediately.
• If muscle weakness is severe, know that the doctor must determine if it is caused by drug toxicity or exacerbation of myasthenia gravis. A test dose of edrophonium I.V. will aggravate drug-induced weakness, but will temporarily relieve weakness resulting from the disease.
• Monitor for weakness occurring 30 to 60 minutes after administering dose, a warning sign of drug toxicity. Notify the doctor immediately.
• Seek approval, when indicated, for hospitalized patients to have bedside supply of tablets. Patients with long-standing disease often insist on taking pills themselves.
• Record the patient's variations in muscle strength. Show the patient how to monitor himself.
• Be aware that patients may develop resistance to drug.
• When given for myasthenia gravis, explain that this drug will relieve symptoms of ptosis, double vision, difficulty in chewing and swallowing, and trunk and limb weakness. Stress the importance of taking this drug exactly as ordered.
• Explain to the patient and his family

that ambenonium chloride is a chronic drug. Teach them about the disease and the drug's effect on symptoms.
• Advise patient to wear medical identification bracelet indicating myasthenia gravis.

---

bethanechol chloride
Duvoid, Urabeth, Urecholine, Urocarb Liquid‡, Urocarb Tablets‡

Pregnancy Risk Category: C

HOW SUPPLIED
Tablets: 5 mg, 10 mg, 25 mg, 50 mg
Injection: 5 mg/ml

ACTION
Directly stimulates cholinergic receptors, mimicking the action of acetylcholine.

ONSET, PEAK, DURATION
Onset occurs within 5 to 15 minutes of S.C. dose, within 30 to 90 minutes of oral dose. Serum levels peak 15 to 30 minutes after S.C. administration, about 1 hour after oral dose. Effects persist for about 2 hours after S.C. administration, up to 6 hours after oral administration, depending on dose.

INDICATIONS & DOSAGE
Acute postoperative and postpartum nonobstructive (functional) urine retention, neurogenic atony of urinary bladder with urine retention –
Adults: 10 to 50 mg P.O. b.i.d. to q.i.d. Or, 2.5 to 5 mg S.C. Never give I.M. or I.V. When used for urine retention, some patients may require 50 to 100 mg P.O. per dose. Use such doses with extreme caution.
   Test dose is 2.5 mg S.C. repeated at 15- to 30-minute intervals to total of four doses to determine the minimal effective dose; then minimal effective dose used q 6 to 8 hours. All doses must be adjusted individually.

ADVERSE REACTIONS
CNS: headache, malaise.
CV: bradycardia, hypotension, reflex tachycardia.
EENT: lacrimation, miosis.
GI: *abdominal cramps, diarrhea,* excessive salivation, nausea, vomiting, belching, borborygmus, esophageal spasms.
GU: urinary urgency.
Respiratory: *bronchoconstriction,* increased bronchial secretions.
Skin: flushing, sweating.

INTERACTIONS
Atropine, anticholinergic agents, procainamide, quinidine: may reverse cholinergic effects. Observe for lack of drug effect.
Cholinergic agonists, anticholinesterase agents: may cause additive effects, or increase toxicity. Avoid concomitant use.
Ganglionic blockers: may cause hypotension. Avoid concomitant use.

CONTRAINDICATIONS
Contraindicated for I.M. or I.V. use and in patients with hypersensitivity to drug or any of its components; in patients with uncertain strength or integrity of bladder wall; when increased muscular activity of GI or urinary tract is harmful; in patients with mechanical obstructions of GI or urinary tract; in patients with hyperthyroidism, peptic ulceration, latent or active bronchial asthma, pronounced bradycardia or hypotension, vasomotor instability, cardiac or coronary artery disease, seizure disorder, Parkinson's disease, spastic GI disturbances, acute inflammatory lesions of the GI tract, peritonitis, or marked vagotonia.

NURSING CONSIDERATIONS
• Use cautiously in pregnant patients.
• Give on empty stomach; otherwise, may cause nausea and vomiting.
• *Never* give I.M. or I.V.; could cause circulatory collapse, hypotension, severe abdominal cramping, bloody diarrhea, shock, or cardiac arrest.
• Monitor vital signs frequently, especially respirations. Always have atropine injection readily available and be prepared to give 0.5 mg S.C. or slow I.V. push as ordered. Provide respiratory support if needed.
• Watch for toxicity, especially with S.C. administration. Edrophonium not effective against muscle relaxation caused by bethanechol.
• Watch closely for adverse reactions that may indicate drug toxicity.
• If used to treat urine retention, ensure that bedpan is available. Monitor fluid intake and output.
• Know that oral drug absorption is poor and variable, requiring larger oral doses. Oral and S.C. doses are *not* interchangeable.

edrophonium chloride
Enlon, Reversol, Tensilon
Pregnancy Risk Category: NR

HOW SUPPLIED
Injection: 10 mg/ml in 1-ml ampules or in 10-ml or 15-ml vials

ACTION
Inhibits the destruction of acetylcholine released from the parasympathetic and somatic efferent nerves. Acetylcholine accumulates, promoting increased stimulation of the receptor.

ONSET, PEAK, DURATION
Onset occurs within 30 to 60 seconds of I.V. administration, within 2 to 10 minutes of I.M. injection. Peak unknown. Effects persist for 5 to 10 minutes after I.V. administration, 5 to 30 minutes after I.M. injection. Duration of action is extremely short.

INDICATIONS & DOSAGE

As a curare antagonist (to reverse non-depolarizing neuromuscular blocking action) –

Adults: 10 mg I.V. given over 30 to 45 seconds. Dose may be repeated as necessary to 40 mg maximum dosage. Larger dosages may potentiate effect of curare.

Diagnostic aid in myasthenia gravis (Tensilon test) –

Adults: 1 to 2 mg I.V. over 15 to 30 seconds, then 8 mg if no response (increase in muscular strength) occurs. Alternatively, 10 mg I.M. If cholinergic reaction occurs, 2 mg I.M. 30 minutes later is given to rule out false-negative response.

Children over 34 kg: 2 mg I.V. If no response within 45 seconds, 1 mg q 45 seconds to maximum of 10 mg. Alternatively, 5 mg I.M.

Children up to 34 kg: 1 mg I.V. If no response within 45 seconds, 1 mg q 45 seconds to maximum of 5 mg. Alternatively, 2 mg I.M.

I.M. route may be used in children because of difficulty with I.V. route: for children under 34 kg, 2 mg I.M.; for children over 34 kg, 5 mg I.M. Expect same reactions as with I.V. test, but these appear after 2- to 10-minute delay.

Infants: 0.5 mg to 1 mg I.M. or S.C.

To differentiate myasthenic crisis from cholinergic crisis –

Adults: 1 mg I.V. If no response in 1 minute, dose repeated once. Increased muscular strength confirms myasthenic crisis; no increase or exaggerated weakness confirms cholinergic crisis.

ADVERSE REACTIONS

CNS: *seizures,* weakness, dysarthria, dysphagia, sweating.
CV: hypotension, bradycardia, AV block.
EENT: excessive lacrimation, diplopia, miosis, conjunctival hyperemia.

GI: nausea, vomiting, *diarrhea, abdominal cramps,* excessive salivation.
GU: urinary frequency, incontinence.
Respiratory: *paralysis, bronchospasm, laryngospasm,* increased bronchial secretions.
Other: muscle cramps, muscle fasciculation.

INTERACTIONS

Aminoglycosides, anesthetics: prolonged or enhanced muscle weakness. Monitor closely.
Corticosteroids, magnesium, procainamide, quinidine: may antagonize cholinergic effects. Observe for lack of drug effect.
Digitalis glycosides: may increase the heart's sensitivity to edrophonium. Use together cautiously.

CONTRAINDICATIONS

Contraindicated in patients with hypersensitivity to anticholinesterase agents and in those with mechanical obstruction of the intestine or urinary tract.

NURSING CONSIDERATIONS

• Use cautiously in patients with bronchial asthma or cardiac arrhythmias.
• Stop all other cholinergics before giving this drug, as ordered.
• **I.V. use:** For easier parenteral administration, use tuberculin syringe with an I.V. needle. When giving drug to differentiate myasthenic crisis from cholinergic crisis, observe patient's muscle strength closely.
• Monitor vital signs frequently, especially respirations. Always have atropine injection readily available and be prepared to give 0.5 to 1 mg S.C. or slow I.V. push as ordered. Provide respiratory support as needed.
• Watch closely for adverse reactions; may indicate toxicity.
• Keep in mind that the drug is effective against muscle relaxation induced

---

*Liquid form contains alcohol.
May contain tartrazine. *Common* reactions are in italics; **life-threatening, in bold italics.

by decamethonium bromide and succinylcholine chloride.

• Be aware that this cholinergic has the most rapid onset but shortest duration; therefore, it is not used to treat myasthenia gravis.

---

neostigmine bromide
Prostigmin

neostigmine methylsulfate
Prostigmin

Pregnancy Risk Category: C

HOW SUPPLIED
neostigmine bromide
Tablets: 15 mg
neostigmine methylsulfate
Injection: 0.25 mg/ml, 0.5 mg/ml, 1 mg/ml

ACTION
Inhibits the destruction of acetylcholine released from the parasympathetic and somatic efferent nerves. Acetylcholine accumulates, promoting increased stimulation of the receptor.

ONSET, PEAK, DURATION
Onset occurs 4 to 8 minutes after I.V. administration, 20 to 30 minutes after I.M. injection, or 45 to 75 minutes after oral administration. Peak levels occur within 1 to 2 hours, with considerable individual variations. Effects persist for 2 to 4 hours.

INDICATIONS & DOSAGE
Treatment of myasthenia gravis –
Adults: 15 to 30 mg P.O. t.i.d. (range is 15 to 375 mg daily); or 0.5 to 2 mg S.C., I.M., or I.V. q 1 to 3 hours.
Children: 7.5 to 15 mg P.O. t.i.d. or q.i.d.
Dosage must be highly individualized, depending on response and tolerance of adverse effects. Therapy may be required day and night.
Diagnosis of myasthenia gravis –

Adults: 0.022 mg/kg I.M. 30 minutes after 0.4 to 0.6 mg of atropine sulfate.
Children: 0.025 to 0.04 mg/kg. I.M. after 0.11 mg/kg atropine sulfate S.C.
Postoperative abdominal distention and bladder atony –
Adults: 0.5 to 1 mg I.M. or S.C. q 4 to 6 hours.
Antidote for nondepolarizing neuromuscular blocking agents –
Adults: 0.5 to 2.5 mg I.V. slowly. Repeat p.r.n. to a total of 5 mg. Before antidote dose, 0.6 to 1.2 mg atropine sulfate is given I.V.
Note: 1:1,000 solution of injectable solution contains 1 mg/ml; 1:2,000 solution contains 0.5 mg/ml.

ADVERSE REACTIONS
CNS: dizziness, headache, muscle weakness, mental confusion, jitters, sweating.
CV: bradycardia, hypotension.
EENT: blurred vision, lacrimation, miosis.
GI: *nausea, vomiting, diarrhea, abdominal cramps,* excessive salivation.
GU: urinary frequency.
Respiratory: *depression, bronchospasm, bronchoconstriction.*
Skin: rash (with bromide form).
Other: *muscle cramps,* muscle fasciculations.

INTERACTIONS
Atropine, anticholinergic agents, corticosteroids, magnesium sulfate, procainamide, aminoglycosides, quinidine: may reverse cholinergic effects. Observe for lack of drug effect.

CONTRAINDICATIONS
Contraindicated in patients with hypersensitivity to cholinergics or to bromide and in those with peritonitis or mechanical obstruction of the intestine or urinary tract.

NURSING CONSIDERATIONS
• Use cautiously in patients with bronchial asthma, bradycardia, sei-

---

zure disorders, recent coronary occlusion, vagotonia, hyperthyroidism, arrhythmias, and peptic ulcer.

• Stop all other cholinergics before giving this drug as ordered.

• In myasthenia gravis, schedule doses before periods of fatigue. For example, if the patient has dysphagia, schedule dose 30 minutes before each meal.

• **I.V. use:** Give at a slow, controlled rate not to exceed 1 mg/minute in adults and 0.5 mg/minute in children.

• Monitor vital signs frequently, especially respirations. Have atropine injection available and be prepared to give as ordered; provide respiratory support as needed.

• Monitor and document the patient's response after each dose. Optimum dosage is difficult to judge. Observe closely for improvement in strength, vision, and ptosis 45 to 60 minutes after each dose. Show the patient how to observe and record variations in muscle strength.

• Although drug is frequently used to reverse the effects of nondepolarizing neuromuscular blockers in patients who have undergone surgery, be aware that it may actually worsen the blockade produced by succinylcholine.

• If patient's muscle weakness is severe, keep in mind that the doctor determines if it is caused by drug-induced toxicity or exacerbation of myasthenia gravis. Test dose of edrophonium I.V. will aggravate drug-induced weakness, but will temporarily relieve weakness caused by disease.

• Be aware that I.M. neostigmine may be used instead of edrophonium to diagnose myasthenia gravis. May be preferable to edrophonium when limb weakness is the only symptom.

• When drug is used to prevent abdominal distention and GI distress, be aware that the doctor may order a rectal tube inserted to help passage of gas.

• Know that patients sometimes develop a resistance to neostigmine.

• If appropriate, obtain a doctor's order for a hospitalized patient to have bedside supply of tablets. Patients with long-standing disease often insist on self-administration.

• Tell the patient to take the drug with food or milk to reduce adverse GI reactions.

• When using for myasthenia gravis, explain that this drug will relieve ptosis, double vision, difficulty in chewing and swallowing, and trunk and limb weakness. Stress importance of taking drug exactly as ordered. Explain that drug may have to be taken for life.

• Advise patient to wear medical identification bracelet indicating myasthenia gravis.

physostigmine salicylate (eserine salicylate)
Antilirium

Pregnancy Risk Category: NR

HOW SUPPLIED
Injection: 1 mg/ml

ACTION
Inhibits the destruction of acetylcholine released from the parasympathetic and somatic efferent nerves. Acetylcholine accumulates, promoting increased stimulation of the receptor.

ONSET, PEAK, DURATION
Onset occurs within 3 to 5 minutes of injection. Peak levels occur within 5 minutes of I.V. injection, 20 to 30 minutes after I.M. injection. Effects persist for 30 to 60 minutes after parenteral use.

INDICATIONS & DOSAGE
To reverse the CNS toxicity associated with clinical or toxic dosages of drugs

capable of producing anticholinergic syndrome –
Adults: 0.5 to 2 mg I.M. or I.V. (1 mg/minute I.V.) repeated q 20 minutes as necessary if life-threatening signs recur (coma, seizures, arrhythmias). Additional doses of 1 to 4 mg I.M. or I.V. q 30 to 60 minutes may be given.
Children: Reserved for life-threatening situations only. 0.02 mg/kg I.M. or slow I.V. repeated q 5 to 10 minutes until response is obtained. Maximum dosage is 2 mg.

ADVERSE REACTIONS
CNS: *seizures,* hallucinations, muscle twitching, muscle weakness, ataxia, *restlessness, excitability, sweating.*
CV: irregular pulse, palpitations, bradycardia, hypotension.
EENT: miosis.
GI: nausea, vomiting, epigastric pain, *diarrhea, excessive salivation.*
GU: urinary urgency.
Respiratory: *bronchospasm,* bronchial constriction, dyspnea.

INTERACTIONS
Atropine, anticholinergic agents, procainamide, quinidine: may reverse cholinergic effects. Observe for lack of drug effect.
Ganglionic blockers: may decrease blood pressure. Avoid concomitant use.

CONTRAINDICATIONS
Contraindicated in patients with mechanical obstruction of the intestine or urogenital tract, asthma, gangrene, diabetes, CV disease, or vagotonia and in those receiving choline esters or depolarizing neuromuscular blocking agents.

NURSING CONSIDERATIONS
• Use cautiously in pregnant patients.
• **I.V. use:** Give I.V. at controlled rate; use direct injection at no more than 1 mg/minute.

• Use only clear solution. Darkening may indicate loss of potency.
• Monitor vital signs frequently, especially respirations. Position the patient to ease breathing. Have atropine injection available and be prepared to give 0.5 mg S.C. or slow I.V. push as ordered. Provide respiratory support as needed. Best administered in presence of a doctor.
• Watch closely for adverse reactions, particularly CNS disturbances. Put up side rails of the bed if the patient becomes restless or hallucinates. Adverse reactions may indicate drug toxicity.
• Know that effectiveness is often immediate and dramatic, but may be transient and may require repeated doses.

pyridostigmine bromide
Mestinon*, Mestinon†, Mestinon Timespan, Regonol
Pregnancy Risk Category: NR

HOW SUPPLIED
Tablets: 60 mg
Tablets (extended-release): 180 mg
Syrup: 60 mg/5 ml
Injection: 5 mg/ml in 2-ml ampules or 5-ml vials

ACTION
Inhibits the destruction of acetylcholine released from the parasympathetic and somatic efferent nerves. Acetylcholine accumulates, promoting increased stimulation of the receptor.

ONSET, PEAK, DURATION
Onset occurs within 2 to 5 minutes of I.V. injection, 15 minutes after I.M. injection, 20 to 45 minutes after oral ingestion of regular-release tablets or syrup, 30 to 60 minutes after ingestion of extended-release tablets. Levels peak within 1 to 2 hours of oral administration. Effects persist for 2 to

3 hours after parenteral use, 3 to 6 hours after regular-release tablets or syrup, 6 to 12 hours after extended-release tablets.

INDICATIONS & DOSAGE

Antidote for nondepolarizing neuromuscular blocking agents –
Adults: 10 to 20 mg I.V. preceded by atropine sulfate 0.6 to 1.2 mg I.V.
Myasthenia gravis –
Adults: 60 to 120 mg P.O. q 3 or 4 hours. Usual dosage is 600 mg daily but higher dosage may be needed (up to 1,500 mg daily). For I.M. or I.V. use, ⅓₀ of oral dosage is given. Dosage must be adjusted for each patient, depending on response and tolerance of adverse effects. Alternatively, 180 to 540 mg timed-release tablets (1 to 3 tablets) P.O. b.i.d., with at least 6 hours between doses.
Children: 7 mg/kg or 200 mg/m² daily in five or six divided doses.
Supportive treatment of neonates born to myasthenic mothers –
Neonates: 0.05 to 0.15 mg/kg I.M. q 4 to 6 hours. Dosage decreased daily until drug can be withdrawn.

ADVERSE REACTIONS

CNS: headache (with high doses), weakness, sweating, *seizures.*
CV: bradycardia, hypotension, thrombophlebitis.
EENT: miosis.
GI: abdominal cramps, nausea, vomiting, diarrhea, excessive salivation.
Respiratory: *bronchospasm, bronchoconstriction,* increased bronchial secretions.
Skin: rash.
Other: muscle cramps, muscle fasciculations.

INTERACTIONS

Aminoglycosides, anesthetics: may decrease response to pyridostigmine. Use together cautiously.
Atropine, anticholinergic agents, corticosteroids, magnesium, procain-amide, quinidine: may antagonize cholinergic effects. Observe for lack of drug effect.
Ganglionic blockers: increased risk of hypotension. Monitor closely.

CONTRAINDICATIONS

Contraindicated in patients with hypersensitivity to anticholinesterase agents and in those with mechanical obstruction of the intestine or urinary tract.

NURSING CONSIDERATIONS

• Use cautiously in patients with bronchial asthma, bradycardia, and arrhythmias.
• Stop all other cholinergics before giving this drug, as ordered.
• **I.V. use:** Administer I.V. injection no faster than 1 mg/minute. If I.V. administration is too rapid, bradycardia and seizures may result. Monitor vital signs frequently, especially respirations. Position patient to ease breathing. Have atropine injection readily available and be prepared to give as ordered; provide respiratory support as needed.
• Don't crush the timed-release (Timespan or Supraspan) tablets.
• When using sweet syrup for patients who have difficulty swallowing, give over ice chips if the patient can't tolerate flavor.
• Monitor and document patient's response after each dose. Optimum dosage is difficult to judge.
• If patient's muscle weakness is severe, keep in mind that the doctor determines if it is caused by drug-induced toxicity or exacerbation of myasthenia gravis. Test dose of edrophonium I.V. will aggravate drug-induced weakness, but will temporarily relieve weakness caused by disease.
• In the United States, be aware that Regonol contains benzyl ethanol preservative that may cause toxicity in neonates if administered in high doses. The Canadian formulation of

---

*Liquid form contains alcohol.
**May contain tartrazine.

Common reactions are in italics; *life-threatening,* in bold italics.

this drug does not contain benzyl ethanol.

• If appropriate, obtain a doctor's order for a hospitalized patient to have bedside supply of tablets. Patients with long-standing disease often insist on self-administration.

• When using for myasthenia gravis, stress importance of taking drug exactly as ordered, on time, in evenly spaced doses. If the doctor has ordered extended-release tablets, explain that patients must take tablets at the same time each day, at least 6 hours apart. Explain that patients may have to take drug for life.

• Advise patient to wear medical identification bracelet indicating myasthenia gravis.

atropine sulfate
  (See Chapter 21, ANTIARRHYTHMICS.)
belladonna leaf
clidinium bromide
dicyclomine hydrochloride
glycopyrrolate
hyoscyamine
hyoscyamine sulfate
mepenzolate bromide
propantheline bromide
scopolamine
scopolamine butylbromide
scopolamine hydrobromide

COMBINATION PRODUCTS
BARBIDONNA ELIXIR*: atropine sulfate 0.034 mg/5 ml, phenobarbital 21.6 mg/5 ml, hyoscyamine hydrobromide or sulfate 0.174 mg/5 ml, scopolamine hydrobromide 0.01 mg/5 ml, and ethanol 15%.
BARBIDONNA NO. 2 TABLETS: atropine sulfate 0.025 mg, scopolamine hydrobromide 0.0074 mg, hyoscyamine hydrobromide or sulfate 0.1286 mg, and phenobarbital 32 mg.
BARBIDONNA TABLETS: atropine sulfate 0.025 mg, scopolamine hydrobromide 0.0074 mg, hyoscyamine hydrobromide or sulfate 0.1286 mg, and phenobarbital 16 mg.
CHARDONNA-2: belladonna extract 15 mg and phenobarbital 15 mg.
DONNATAL ELIXIR*: atropine sulfate 0.0194 mg/5 ml, scopolamine hydrobromide 0.0065 mg/5 ml, ethanol 23%, hyoscyamine hydrobromide or sulfate 0.1037 mg/5 ml, and phenobarbital 16 mg/5 ml.
DONNATAL EXTENTABS: atropine sulfate 0.0582 mg, scopolamine hydrobromide 0.0195 mg, hyoscyamine sulfate 0.3111 mg, and phenobarbital 48.6 mg.
DONNATAL NO. 2 TABLETS: atropine sulfate 0.0194 mg, scopolamine hydrobromide 0.0065 mg, hyoscyamine hydrobromide or sulfate 0.1037 mg, and phenobarbital 32.4 mg.
DONNATAL TABLETS AND CAPSULES: atropine sulfate 0.0194 mg, scopolamine hydrobromide 0.0065 mg, hyoscyamine hydrobromide or sulfate 0.1037 mg, and phenobarbital 16 mg.
KINESED TABLETS: atropine sulfate 0.02 mg, scopolamine hydrobromide 0.007 mg, hyoscyamine hydrobromide or sulfate 0.1 mg, and phenobarbital 16 mg.
LIBRAX CAPSULES: clidinium bromide 2.5 mg and chlordiazepoxide hydrochloride 5 mg.

---

belladonna leaf
(used to prepare extract and tincture)
Belladonna Tincture USP*

Pregnancy Risk Category: NR

HOW SUPPLIED
Oral solution: 27 to 33 mg belladonna alkaloids/100 ml in 67% alcohol solution

ACTION
Blocks acetylcholine, which decreases GI motility and inhibits gastric acid secretion.

ONSET, PEAK, DURATION
Unknown.

INDICATIONS & DOSAGE
Adjunctive therapy for peptic ulceration, irritable bowel syndrome, functional GI disorders, and neurogenic bowel disturbances –
Adults: 0.6 to 1 ml P.O. t.i.d. or q.i.d.
Children: 0.1 ml/kg or 2.5 ml/m²

---

*Liquid form contains alcohol.
**May contain tartrazine.
Common reactions are in italics; *life-threatening,* in bold italics.

tincture P.O. t.i.d. or q.i.d. Total dosage should not exceed 3.5 ml/day.

ADVERSE REACTIONS
CNS: headache, insomnia, drowsiness, dizziness, *confusion or excitement in elderly patients,* nervousness, weakness.
CV: *palpitations,* tachycardia.
EENT: *blurred vision,* mydriasis, increased intraocular pressure, cycloplegia, photophobia.
GI: *dry mouth,* dysphagia, heartburn, loss of taste, *constipation,* nausea, vomiting.
GU: *urinary hesitancy, urine retention,* impotence.
Skin: urticaria, decreased sweating or possible anhidrosis, other dermal manifestations.
Other: fever, allergic reactions.
Note: Overdose may cause curare-like effects, such as respiratory paralysis.

INTERACTIONS
Amantadine, antihistamines, antiparkinsonian agents, disopyramide, glutethimide, meperidine, phenothiazines, procainamide, quinidine, tricyclic antidepressants: additive adverse effects. Avoid concomitant use.
Antacids: decreased absorption of oral anticholinergics. Separate administration times by 2 to 3 hours.
Ketoconazole: anticholinergics may interfere with ketoconazole absorption. Avoid concomitant use.
Methotrimeprazine: anticholinergics may enhance risk of extrapyramidal reactions. Avoid concomitant use.

CONTRAINDICATIONS
Contraindicated in patients with angle-closure glaucoma, obstructive uropathy, obstructive disease of the GI tract, severe ulcerative colitis, myasthenia gravis, hypersensitivity to anticholinergics, paralytic ileus, intestinal atony, unstable cardiovascular status in acute hemorrhage, or toxic megacolon.

NURSING CONSIDERATIONS
• Use cautiously in patients with autonomic neuropathy, hyperthyroidism, coronary artery disease, arrhythmias, CHF, hypertension, hiatal hernia associated with reflux esophagitis, GI infections, hepatic or renal disease, partial obstructive uropathy, and ulcerative colitis and in patients over 40 years because of increased incidence of glaucoma. Also use cautiously in patients in hot or humid environments. Drug-induced heatstroke can develop.
• Give 30 minutes to 1 hour before meals and h.s. Bedtime dose can be larger; give at least 2 hours after last meal of the day.
• Administer smaller doses to elderly patients.
• Monitor the patient's vital signs and urine output carefully.
• Instruct the patient to avoid driving and other hazardous activities if he is drowsy, dizzy, or has blurred vision; to drink plenty of fluids to help prevent constipation; and to report any skin rash or local eruption.
• Instruct the patient to use sugarless gum or hard candy to relieve dry mouth.

---

clidinium bromide
Quarzan
Pregnancy Risk Category: NR

HOW SUPPLIED
Capsules: 2.5 mg, 5 mg

ACTION
Blocks acetylcholine, which decreases GI motility and inhibits gastric acid secretion.

ONSET, PEAK, DURATION
Onset occurs within 1 hour of administration. Peak unknown. Effects persist up to 3 hours.

INDICATIONS & DOSAGE
Adjunctive therapy for peptic ulcerations —
Adults: 2.5 to 5 mg P.O. t.i.d. or q.i.d. before meals and h.s.
Elderly or debilitated patients: 2.5 mg P.O. t.i.d.

ADVERSE REACTIONS
CNS: headache, insomnia, drowsiness, dizziness, *confusion or excitement in elderly patients,* nervousness, weakness.
CV: *palpitations,* tachycardia.
EENT: *blurred vision,* mydriasis, increased intraocular pressure, cycloplegia, photophobia.
GI: *dry mouth,* dysphagia, heartburn, loss of taste, nausea, vomiting, *paralytic ileus, constipation.*
GU: *urinary hesitancy, urine retention,* impotence.
Skin: urticaria, decreased sweating or possible anhidrosis, other dermal manifestations.
Other: fever, allergic reactions.
   Note: Overdose may cause curare-like effects, such as respiratory paralysis.

INTERACTIONS
Amantadine, antihistamines, antiparkinsonian agents, disopyramide, glutethimide, meperidine, phenothiazines, procainamide, quinidine, tricyclic antidepressants: additive adverse effects. Avoid concomitant use.
Antacids: decreased absorption of oral anticholinergics. Separate administration times by 2 to 3 hours.
Ketoconazole: anticholinergics may interfere with ketoconazole absorption. Avoid concomitant use.
Methotrimeprazine: anticholinergics may enhance risk of extrapyramidal reactions. Avoid concomitant use.

CONTRAINDICATIONS
Contraindicated in patients with angle-closure glaucoma, obstructive uropathy, obstructive disease of the GI tract, severe ulcerative colitis, myasthenia gravis, hypersensitivity to anticholinergics, paralytic ileus, intestinal atony, unstable cardiovascular status in acute hemorrhage, or toxic megacolon.

NURSING CONSIDERATIONS
• Use cautiously in patients with autonomic neuropathy, hyperthyroidism, coronary artery disease, arrhythmias, CHF, hypertension, hiatal hernia associated with reflux esophagitis, GI infections, hepatic or renal disease, partial obstructive uropathy, and ulcerative colitis and in patients over 40 years because of increased incidence of glaucoma. Also use cautiously in patients in hot or humid environments. Drug-induced heatstroke may develop.
• Give 30 minutes to 1 hour before meals and h.s. Bedtime dose can be larger; give at least 2 hours after last meal of the day.
• Monitor the patient's vital signs and urine output carefully.
• Assess the patient for dysphagia, which may cause aspiration.
• Keep in mind that dosage should be individualized according to severity of symptoms and occurrence of adverse reactions.
• Be aware that no conclusive evidence exists that clidinium aids in healing, decreasing recurrence of, or preventing complications of peptic ulcerations.
• Instruct the patient to avoid driving and other hazardous activities if he is drowsy, dizzy, or has blurred vision; to drink plenty of fluids to help prevent constipation; and to report any rash or skin eruption.
• Instruct the patient to use sugarless gum or hard candy to relieve dry mouth.

dicyclomine hydrochloride

Antispas, A-Spas, Bentyl,
Bentylol†, Byclomine, Dibent,
Di-Spaz, Formulex†, Lomine†,
Merbentyl‡, Or-Tyl, Spasmoban†,
Spasmoject

Pregnancy Risk Category: B

HOW SUPPLIED
Tablets: 10 mg‡, 20 mg
Capsules: 10 mg, 20 mg
Syrup: 5 mg/5 ml‡, 10 mg/5 ml
Injection: 10 mg/ml

ACTION
Unknown. Appears to exert a nonspecific, nondirect spasmolytic action on smooth muscle. Also possesses local anesthetic properties that may be partly responsible for spasmolysis.

ONSET, PEAK, DURATION
Onset and duration unknown. Peak effects occur 1 to 1½ hours after administration.

INDICATIONS & DOSAGE
Irritable bowel syndrome and other functional GI disorders–
Adults: initially, 20 mg P.O. q.i.d., increased to 40 mg q.i.d.; or, 20 mg I.M. q 4 to 6 hours.
Children 2 years and older: 10 mg P.O. t.i.d. or q.i.d.
Children 6 months to 2 years: 5 to 10 mg P.O. t.i.d. to q.i.d.

ADVERSE REACTIONS
CNS: *headache; dizziness;* insomnia; drowsiness; nervousness, confusion, excitement (in elderly patients).
CV: *palpitations,* tachycardia.
EENT: blurred vision, increased intraocular pressure, mydriasis.
GI: nausea, vomiting, *constipation, dry mouth,* abdominal distention, heartburn, paralytic ileus.
GU: *urinary hesitancy, urine retention,* impotence.
Skin: urticaria, decreased sweating or possible anhidrosis, other dermal manifestations.
Other: fever; allergic reactions. Dicyclomine is a synthetic tertiary derivative that may have atropine-like adverse reactions.
Note: Overdose may cause curare-like effects, such as respiratory paralysis.

INTERACTIONS
Amantadine, antihistamines, antiparkinsonian agents, disopyramide, glutethimide, meperidine, phenothiazines, procainamide, quinidine, tricyclic antidepressants: additive adverse effects. Avoid concomitant use.
Antacids: decreased absorption of oral anticholinergics. Separate administration times by 2 to 3 hours.
Ketoconazole: anticholinergics may interfere with ketoconazole absorption. Avoid concomitant use.
Methotrimeprazine: anticholinergics may enhance risk of extrapyramidal reactions. Avoid concomitant use.

CONTRAINDICATIONS
Contraindicated in patients with obstructive uropathy, obstructive disease of the GI tract, reflux esophagitis, severe ulcerative colitis, myasthenia gravis, hypersensitivity to anticholinergics, unstable cardiovascular status in acute hemorrhage, or glaucoma. Also contraindicated in breast-feeding patients and in children under 6 months.

NURSING CONSIDERATIONS
• Use cautiously in patients with autonomic neuropathy, hyperthyroidism, coronary artery disease, arrhythmias, CHF, hypertension, hiatal hernia, hepatic or renal disease, prostatic hypertrophy, and ulcerative colitis.
• Give 30 minutes to 1 hour before meals and h.s.. Bedtime dose can be larger; give at least 2 hours after last meal of the day.
• Do not use S.C. or I.V.

- Be prepared to adjust dosage according to patient's needs and response, as ordered. Doses up to 40 mg P.O. q.i.d. have been used in adults, but safety and efficacy for more than 2 weeks has not been established.
- Monitor patient's vital signs and urine output carefully.
- Instruct the patient to avoid driving and other hazardous activities if he is drowsy, dizzy, or has blurred vision; to drink plenty of fluids to help prevent constipation; and to report any rash or skin eruption.
- Instruct the patient to use sugarless gum or hard candy to relieve dry mouth.

---

glycopyrrolate
Robinul, Robinul Forte

Pregnancy Risk Category: B

HOW SUPPLIED
Tablets: 1 mg, 2 mg
Injection: 0.2 mg/ml

ACTION
Inhibits cholinergic (muscarinic) actions of acetylcholine on autonomic effectors innervated by postganglionic cholinergic nerves.

ONSET, PEAK, DURATION
Onset occurs in 1 minute after I.V. administration, 15 to 30 minutes after S.C. or I.M. injection. Serum levels peak in 30 to 45 minutes after I.M. injection. Vagal blocking effects persist about 3 hours; effect on secretions, up to 7 hours.

INDICATIONS & DOSAGE
Blockade of adverse cholinergic effects caused by anticholinesterase agents used to reverse neuromuscular blockade –
Adults and children: 0.2 mg I.V. for each 1 mg neostigmine or 5 mg of pyridostigmine. May be given I.V.

without dilution or may be added to dextrose injection and given by infusion.
Preoperatively to diminish secretions and block cardiac vagal reflexes –
Adults: 0.0044 mg/kg of body weight I.M. 30 to 60 minutes before anesthesia.
Children 2 years and older: 0.0044 mg/kg I.M. 30 to 60 minutes before anesthesia.
Children under 2 years: 0.0088 mg/kg I.M. 30 minutes before anesthesia.
Adjunctive therapy in peptic ulcerations and other GI disorders –
Adults: 1 to 2 mg P.O. t.i.d. or 0.1 mg I.M. t.i.d. or q.i.d. Dosage must be individualized. Maximum P.O. dosage is 8 mg/day.

ADVERSE REACTIONS
CNS: disorientation, irritability, incoherence, weakness, nervousness, drowsiness, dizziness, headache, confusion or excitement (in elderly patients).
CV: palpitations, tachycardia, paradoxical bradycardia.
EENT: *dilated pupils, blurred vision,* photophobia, increased intraocular pressure, difficulty swallowing.
GI: *constipation, dry mouth,* nausea, vomiting, epigastric distress.
GU: *urinary hesitancy, urine retention,* impotence.
Respiratory: *bronchial plugging.*
Skin: urticaria, decreased sweating or anhidrosis, other dermal manifestations.
Other: burning at injection site, fever, loss of taste, abdominal distention.

INTERACTIONS
Amantadine, antihistamines, antiparkinsonian agents, disopyramide, glutethimide, meperidine, phenothiazines, procainamide, quinidine, tricyclic antidepressants: additive adverse effects. Avoid concomitant use.
Antacids: decreased absorption of

---

oral anticholinergics. Separate administration times by 2 to 3 hours.
Ketoconazole: anticholinergics may interfere with ketoconazole absorption. Avoid concomitant use.
Methotrimeprazine: anticholinergics may enhance risk of extrapyramidal reactions. Avoid concomitant use.

CONTRAINDICATIONS
Contraindicated in patients with hypersensitivity to drug and in those with glaucoma, obstructive uropathy, obstructive disease of the GI tract, myasthenia gravis, paralytic ileus, intestinal atony, unstable cardiovascular status in acute hemorrhage, severe ulcerative colitis, or toxic megacolon.

NURSING CONSIDERATIONS
• Use cautiously in patients with autonomic neuropathy, hyperthyroidism, coronary artery disease, arrhythmias, CHF, hypertension, hiatal hernia, hepatic or renal disease, and ulcerative colitis. Also use cautiously in patients in hot or humid environments. Drug-induced heatstroke is possible.
• Administer 30 minutes to 1 hour before meals.
• **I.V. use:** Administer by direct injection without dilution. Alternatively, inject into the tubing of a free-flowing I.V. solution.
• Don't mix with I.V. solution containing sodium bicarbonate or alkaline solutions with a pH > 6. Alkaline drugs, such as barbiturates (thiopental, methohexital, secobarbital, pentobarbital), chloramphenicol, dexamethasone, dimenhydrinate, diazepam, methylprednisolone, and pentazocine, are incompatible with glycopyrrolate.
• Check all dosages carefully; slight overdose can lead to toxicity.
• Monitor vital signs carefully. Watch closely for adverse reactions, especially in elderly or debilitated patients. Call the doctor promptly if they occur.
• Be aware that elderly patients typically receive smaller dosages.
• Warn patients to avoid activities that require alertness until drug's CNS effects are known.
• Advise patients to report signs of urinary hesitancy or urine retention.

hyoscyamine
Cystospaz

hyoscyamine sulfate
Anaspaz, Bellaspaz, Cystospaz, Cystospaz-M, Gastrosed, Levsin*, Levsinex Timecaps, Levsin S/L

Pregnancy Risk Category: C

HOW SUPPLIED
hyoscyamine
Tablets: 0.15 mg
hyoscyamine sulfate
Tablets: 0.125 mg, 0.13 mg, 0.15 mg
Capsules (extended-release): 0.375 mg
Elixir: 125 mcg/5 ml
Oral solution: 0.125 mg/ml
Injection: 0.5 mg/ml

ACTION
Competitively blocks acetylcholine, which decreases GI motility and inhibits gastric acid secretion.

ONSET, PEAK, DURATION
Onset occurs within 2 minutes after I.V. injection, 5 to 20 minutes after oral elixir, 20 to 30 minutes after oral tablets. Serum levels peak within 15 to 30 minutes after parenteral use, 30 to 60 minutes after oral use. Effects persist for 4 to 12 hours.

INDICATIONS & DOSAGE
GI tract disorders caused by spasm; adjunctive therapy for peptic ulcerations –
Adults and children 12 years or older: 0.125 to 0.25 mg P.O. or S.L.

t.i.d. or q.i.d. before meals and h.s.; 0.375 mg extended-release form P.O. q 8 to 12 hours; or 0.25 to 0.5 mg (1 or 2 ml) I.M., I.V., or S.C. b.i.d. to q.i.d. (Oral medication substituted when symptoms are controlled.) Maximum daily dosage is 1.5 mg.
Children 2 to 12 years: one-half of adult dose P.O., not to exceed 0.75 mg daily.
Children under 2 years: one-quarter of adult dose P.O., not to exceed 0.075 mg daily.

ADVERSE REACTIONS
CNS: headache, insomnia, drowsiness, dizziness, *confusion or excitement in elderly patients,* nervousness, weakness.
CV: *palpitations,* tachycardia.
EENT: *blurred vision,* mydriasis, increased intraocular pressure, cycloplegia, photophobia.
GI: *dry mouth,* dysphagia, *constipation,* heartburn, loss of taste, nausea, vomiting, *paralytic ileus.*
GU: *urinary hesitancy, urine retention,* impotence.
Skin: urticaria, decreased sweating or possible anhidrosis, other dermal manifestations.
Other: fever, allergic reactions.
Note: Overdose may cause curare-like effects, such as respiratory paralysis.

INTERACTIONS
Amantadine, antihistamines, antiparkinsonian agents, disopyramide, glutethimide, meperidine, phenothiazines, procainamide, quinidine, tricyclic antidepressants: additive adverse effects. Avoid concomitant use.
Antacids: decreased absorption of oral anticholinergics. Separate administration times by 2 to 3 hours.
Ketoconazole: anticholinergics may interfere with ketoconazole absorption. Avoid concomitant use.
Methotrimeprazine: anticholinergics may enhance risk of extrapyramidal reactions. Avoid concomitant use.

CONTRAINDICATIONS
Contraindicated in patients with glaucoma, obstructive uropathy, obstructive disease of the GI tract, severe ulcerative colitis, myasthenia gravis, hypersensitivity to anticholinergics, paralytic ileus, intestinal atony, unstable cardiovascular status in acute hemorrhage, or toxic megacolon.

NURSING CONSIDERATIONS
• Use cautiously in patients with autonomic neuropathy, hyperthyroidism, coronary artery disease, arrhythmias, CHF, hypertension, hiatal hernia associated with reflux esophagitis, hepatic or renal disease, and ulcerative colitis. Also use cautiously in patients in hot or humid environments. Drug-induced heatstroke can develop.
• Give 30 minutes to 1 hour before meals and h.s. Bedtime dose can be larger; give at least 2 hours after the last meal of the day.
• Monitor the patient's vital signs and urine output carefully.
• Be aware that injection contains sodium metabisulfite, which may cause allergic reaction in certain individuals.
• Instruct the patient to avoid driving and other hazardous activities if he is drowsy, dizzy, or has blurred vision; to drink plenty of fluids to help prevent constipation; and to report any rash or skin eruption.
• Instruct the patient to use sugarless gum or hard candy to relieve dry mouth.

---

mepenzolate bromide
Cantil**

Pregnancy Risk Category: NR

HOW SUPPLIED
Tablets: 25 mg

ACTION
Blocks acetylcholine, which decreases GI motility and inhibits gastric acid secretion.

ONSET, PEAK, DURATION
Unknown.

INDICATIONS & DOSAGE
Adjunctive therapy in treating peptic ulceration, irritable bowel syndrome, and neurogenic bowel disturbances –
Adults: 25 to 50 mg P.O. t.i.d. to q.i.d. with meals and h.s. Dosage adjusted to individual patient's needs.

ADVERSE REACTIONS
CNS: headache, insomnia, drowsiness, dizziness, *confusion or excitement in elderly patients,* nervousness, weakness.
CV: *palpitations,* tachycardia.
EENT: *blurred vision,* mydriasis, increased intraocular pressure, cycloplegia, photophobia.
GI: *dry mouth,* dysphagia, heartburn, loss of taste, nausea, *constipation,* vomiting, *paralytic ileus.*
GU: *urinary hesitancy, urine retention,* impotence.
Skin: urticaria, decreased sweating or possible anhidrosis, other dermal manifestations.
Other: fever, allergic reactions.
Note: Overdose may cause curare-like effects, such as respiratory paralysis.

INTERACTIONS
Amantadine, antihistamines, antiparkinsonian agents, disopyramide, glutethimide, meperidine, phenothiazines, procainamide, quinidine, tricyclic antidepressants: additive adverse effects. Avoid concomitant use.
Antacids: decreased absorption of oral anticholinergics. Separate administration times by 2 to 3 hours.
Ketoconazole: anticholinergics may interfere with ketoconazole absorption. Avoid concomitant use.

Methotrimeprazine: anticholinergics may enhance risk of extrapyramidal reactions. Avoid concomitant use.

CONTRAINDICATIONS
Contraindicated in patients with angle-closure glaucoma, obstructive uropathy, obstructive disease of the GI tract, severe ulcerative colitis, myasthenia gravis, hypersensitivity to anticholinergics, paralytic ileus, intestinal atony, unstable cardiovascular status in acute hemorrhage, or toxic megacolon. Contains tartrazine, which may precipitate an allergic reaction in certain individuals, especially those hypersensitive to aspirin.

NURSING CONSIDERATIONS
• Use cautiously in patients with autonomic neuropathy, hyperthyroidism, coronary artery disease, arrhythmias, CHF, hypertension, hiatal hernia associated with reflux esophagitis, hepatic or renal disease, and ulcerative colitis. Also use cautiously in patients in hot or humid environments. Drug-induced heatstroke can develop.
• Give with meals and h.s.
• Monitor the patient's vital signs and urine output carefully.
• Instruct the patient to avoid driving and other hazardous activities if he is drowsy, dizzy, or has blurred vision; to drink plenty of fluids to help prevent constipation; and to report any rash or skin eruption.
• Instruct the patient to use sugarless gum or hard candy to relieve dry mouth.

---

propantheline bromide
Panthelinę‡, Pro-Banthine, Propanthel†

Pregnancy Risk Category: C

HOW SUPPLIED
Tablets: 7.5 mg, 15 mg

ACTION
Blocks acetylcholine, which decreases GI motility and inhibits gastric acid secretion.

ONSET, PEAK, DURATION
Onset unknown. Serum levels may peak in 2 hours. Effects persist for 6 hours.

INDICATIONS & DOSAGE
Adjunctive treatment of peptic ulceration –
Adults: 15 mg P.O. t.i.d. before meals, and 30 mg h.s.
Elderly patients: 7.5 mg P.O. t.i.d. before meals.

ADVERSE REACTIONS
CNS: headache, insomnia, drowsiness, dizziness, *confusion or excitement in elderly patients,* nervousness, weakness.
CV: *palpitations,* tachycardia.
EENT: *blurred vision,* mydriasis, increased intraocular pressure, cycloplegia, photophobia.
GI: *dry mouth,* dysphagia, constipation, heartburn, loss of taste, nausea, vomiting, paralytic ileus.
GU: *urinary hesitancy, urine retention,* impotence.
Skin: urticaria, decreased sweating or possible anhidrosis, other dermal manifestations.
Other: fever, allergic reactions.
  Note: Overdose may cause curare-like effects, such as respiratory paralysis.

INTERACTIONS
Amantadine, antihistamines, antiparkinsonian agents, disopyramide, glutethimide, meperidine, phenothiazines, procainamide, quinidine, tricyclic antidepressants: additive adverse effects. Avoid concomitant use.
Antacids: decreased absorption of oral anticholinergics. Separate administration times by 2 to 3 hours.
Digoxin: increased serum digoxin levels. Monitor closely for digitalis toxicity.
Ketoconazole: anticholinergics may interfere with ketoconazole absorption. Avoid concomitant use.
Methotrimeprazine: anticholinergics may enhance risk of extrapyramidal reactions. Avoid concomitant use.

CONTRAINDICATIONS
Contraindicated in patients with angle-closure glaucoma, obstructive uropathy, obstructive disease of the GI tract, severe ulcerative colitis, myasthenia gravis, hypersensitivity to anticholinergics, paralytic ileus, intestinal atony, unstable cardiovascular status in acute hemorrhage, or toxic megacolon.

NURSING CONSIDERATIONS
● Use cautiously in patients with autonomic neuropathy, hyperthyroidism, coronary artery disease, arrhythmias, CHF, hypertension, hiatal hernia associated with reflux esophagitis, hepatic or renal disease, and ulcerative colitis. Also use cautiously in patients in hot or humid environments. Drug-induced heatstroke can develop.
● Give 30 minutes to 1 hour before meals and h.s. Bedtime doses can be larger; give at least 2 hours after last meal of the day.
● Monitor the patient's vital signs and urine output carefully.
● Instruct the patient to avoid driving and other hazardous activities if he is drowsy, dizzy, or has blurred vision; to drink plenty of fluids to help prevent constipation; and to report any rash or skin eruption.
● Instruct patient to use sugarless gum or hard candy to relieve dry mouth.

---

*Liquid form contains alcohol.   *Common* reactions are in italics; *life-threatening,* in bold italics.
**May contain tartrazine.

scopolamine (hyoscine)
Scop‡, Transderm-Scōp,
Transderm-V†

scopolamine butylbromide
(hyoscine butylbromide)
Buscospan†‡

scopolamine hydrobromide
(hyoscine hydrobromide)

Pregnancy Risk Category: C

HOW SUPPLIED
scopolamine
Transdermal patch: 1.5 mg
scopolamine butylbromide
Capsules: 0.25 mg
Suppositories: 10 mg†
Tablets: 10 mg†
scopolamine hydrobromide
Injection: 0.3, 0.4, 0.5, 0.6, and 1
mg/ml in 1-ml vials and ampules;
0.86 mg/ml in 0.5-ml ampules

ACTION
Inhibits muscarinic actions of acetylcholine on autonomic effectors innervated by postganglionic cholinergic
neurons. Also may affect neural pathways originating in the labyrinth (inner ear) to inhibit nausea and vomiting.

ONSET, PEAK, DURATION
Onset occurs within 30 minutes after
parenteral administration, 30 to 60
minutes after oral administration, unknown with transdermal patch. Peak
unknown. Effects persist about 4
hours after parenteral administration,
4 to 6 hours after oral administration,
and up to 72 hours after applying
transdermal patch.

INDICATIONS & DOSAGE
Spastic states –
Adults: 10 to 20 mg P.O. t.i.d. or
q.i.d. Dosage adjusted as needed. Or,
10 to 20 mg (butylbromide) S.C.,
I.M., or I.V. t.i.d. or q.i.d.

*Preoperatively to reduce secretions
and block cardiac vagal reflexes –*
Adults: 0.2 to 0.6 mg (hydrobromide) I.M. 30 to 60 minutes before
induction of anesthesia.
Children 8 to 12 years: 300 mcg (hydrobromide) I.M. 45 minutes before
induction of anesthesia.
Children 3 to 8 years: 200 mcg (hydrobromide) I.M. 45 minutes before
induction of anesthesia.
Children 7 months to 3 years: 150
mcg (hydrobromide) I.M. 45 minutes
before induction of anesthesia.
Infants 4 to 7 months: 100 mcg (hydrobromide) I.M. or I.V. 45 minutes
before induction of anesthesia.
*Prevention of nausea and vomiting as-
sociated with motion sickness –*
Adults: one Transderm-Scōp or
Transderm-V patch (a circular flat
unit) programmed to deliver 0.5 mg
scopolamine daily over 3 days (72
hours), applied to the skin behind the
ear several hours before the antiemetic is required. Or, 300 to 600
mcg (hydrobromide) S.C., I.M., or
I.V.
Children: 6 mcg/kg or 200 mcg/m² of
body surface (hydrobromide) S.C.,
I.M., or I.V.

ADVERSE REACTIONS
CNS: disorientation, restlessness, irritability, dizziness, drowsiness, headache, confusion.
CV: palpitations, tachycardia, paradoxical bradycardia.
EENT: dilated pupils, blurred vision,
photophobia, increased intraocular
pressure, difficulty swallowing.
GI: *constipation, dry mouth, nausea,
vomiting, epigastric distress.*
GU: urinary hesitancy, urine retention.
Respiratory: bronchial plugging, depressed respirations.
Skin: rash, flushing, dryness, contact
dermatitis (with transdermal patch).
Other: fever.
   Adverse reactions may be caused by

pending atropine-like toxicity and are dose-related. Individual tolerance varies greatly.

Many adverse reactions (such as dry mouth, constipation) are an expected extension of the drug's pharmacologic activity.

INTERACTIONS
Centrally acting anticholinergics (tricyclic antidepressants, antihistamines, phenothiazines): increased incidence of adverse CNS reactions.
Digoxin: increased digoxin levels.
Ethanol, CNS depressants: increased incidence of CNS depression.

CONTRAINDICATIONS
Contraindicated in patients with angle-closure glaucoma, obstructive uropathy, obstructive disease of the GI tract, asthma, chronic pulmonary disease, myasthenia gravis, paralytic ileus, intestinal atony, unstable cardiovascular status in acute hemorrhage, or toxic megacolon.

NURSING CONSIDERATIONS
• Use cautiously in patients with autonomic neuropathy, hyperthyroidism, coronary artery disease, arrhythmias, CHF, hypertension, hiatal hernia associated with reflux esophagitis, hepatic or renal disease, and ulcerative colitis and in children under 6 years. Also use cautiously in patients in hot or humid environments. Drug-induced heatstroke possible.
• **I.V. use:** Keep in mind that intermittent and continuous infusions are not recommended. For direct injection, dilute with sterile water and inject diluted drug at ordered rate through patent I.V. line.
• Protect I.V. solutions from freezing and light, and store at room temperature.
• Raise the bed's side rails as a precaution because some patients become temporarily excited or disoriented. Symptoms disappear when sedative effect is complete.
• Know that in therapeutic doses, scopolamine may produce amnesia, drowsiness, and euphoria; may need to reorient the patient.
• Be aware that tolerance may develop when given over a long time.
• Advise the patient to apply patch the night before a planned trip. Transdermal method releases a controlled therapeutic amount of scopolamine. Transderm-Scōp is effective if applied 2 to 3 hours before experiencing motion, but more effective if applied 12 hours before.
• Advise the patient to wash and dry hands thoroughly before and after applying the transdermal patch on dry skin behind the ear and before touching the eye, as pupil may dilate. After removing the system, discard it. Wash hands and application site thoroughly.
• Tell patient that, if patch becomes displaced, to remove and replace it with another patch on a fresh skin site behind the ear.
• Alert the patient to the possibility of withdrawal symptoms (nausea, vomiting, headache, dizziness) if the transdermal system is used longer than 72 hours.
• Warn the patient against driving and other activities that require alertness until drug's CNS effects are known.
• Have the patient ask the pharmacist for the brochure that comes with the transdermal product.
• Advise the patient to report signs of urinary hesitancy or urine retention.
• Instruct the patient to use sugarless gum or hard candy to help minimize dry mouth.

---

*Liquid form contains alcohol.   *Common* reactions are in italics; *life-threatening*, in bold italics.
**May contain tartrazine.

Adrenergics (sympathomimetics)

dobutamine hydrochloride
dopamine hydrochloride
mephentermine sulfate
metaraminol bitartrate
norepinephrine bitartrate
phenylephrine hydrochloride
pseudoephedrine hydrochloride
pseudoephedrine sulfate

COMBINATION PRODUCTS
ENTEX: phenylephrine hydrochloride
5 mg, phenylpropanolamine hydrochloride 45 mg, and guaifenesin 400
mg.
ENTEX LIQUID: phenylephrine hydrochloride 5 mg/5 ml, phenylpropanolamine hydrochloride 20 mg/5 ml, and
guaifenesin 100 mg/5 ml (alcohol 5%).
ENTEX PSE: pseudophedrine 120 mg
and guaifenesin 600 mg.
SEMPREX-D: acrivastine 8 mg and
pseudoephedrine hydrochloride 60
mg.

---

dobutamine hydrochloride
Dobutrex

Pregnancy Risk Category: NR

HOW SUPPLIED
Injection: 12.5 mg/ml in 20-ml vials
(parenteral)

ACTION
Directly stimulates beta₁ receptors of
the heart to increase myocardial contractility and stroke volume. At therapeutic dosages, decreases peripheral
vascular resistance (afterload), reduces ventricular filling pressure
(preload), and may facilitate AV node
conduction. Net result is increased
cardiac output.

ONSET, PEAK, DURATION
Onset occurs in 1 to 2 minutes, up to
10 minutes, if I.V. infusion rate is
slow. Peak effects usually occur
within 10 minutes of starting I.V. infusion. Effects persist for less than 5
minutes after infusion is stopped.

INDICATIONS & DOSAGE
*To increase cardiac output in the
short-term treatment of cardiac decompensation caused by depressed
contractility, such as during refractory heart failure, and as adjunct in
cardiac surgery –*
Adults: 2.5 to 10 mcg/kg/minute I.V.
infusion. Infusion rates up to 40 mcg/
kg/minute may be needed (rare).

ADVERSE REACTIONS
CNS: headache.
CV: *increased heart rate, hyperten-
sion, PVCs,* angina, nonspecific chest
pain.
GI: nausea, vomiting.
Respiratory: shortness of breath.
Other: mild leg cramps or tingling
sensation.

INTERACTIONS
Beta blockers: may antagonize dobutamine effects. Do not use together.
General anesthetics: greater incidence
of ventricular arrhythmias.

CONTRAINDICATIONS
Contraindicated in patients with hypersensitivity to the drug or any component of the formulation and in those
with idiopathic hypertrophic subaortic stenosis.

NURSING CONSIDERATIONS
• Use cautiously in patients with a
history of hypertension. Drug may

---

precipitate an exaggerated pressor response.
• Do not mix with sodium bicarbonate injection because the drug is incompatible with alkaline solutions. Infusions for up to 72 hours produce no more adverse effects than shorter infusions.
• Before initiating therapy with dobutamine, correct hypovolemia with plasma volume expanders, as ordered.
• Administer a digitalis glycoside before dobutamine as ordered. Because drug increases AV node conduction, patients with atrial fibrillation may develop a rapid ventricular rate.
• **I.V. use:** Administer using a central venous catheter or large peripheral vein. Titrate infusion according to the doctor's orders and the patient's condition. Use an infusion pump.
• Dilute concentrate for injection before administration. Compatible solutions include D_5W, 0.45% sodium chloride injection, 0.9% sodium chloride injection, and lactated Ringer's injection. The contents of one vial (250 mg) diluted with 1,000 ml of solution yields a concentration of 250 mcg/ml; diluted with 500 ml, a concentration of 500 mcg/ml; diluted with 250 ml, a concentration of 1,000 mcg/ml. Maximum concentration should not exceed 5 mg/ml.
• Avoid extravasation; may cause an inflammatory response. Change I.V. sites regularly to avoid phlebitis.
• Do not administer through the same I.V. line with other drugs. Drug is incompatible with heparin, hydrocortisone sodium succinate, cefazolin, cefamandole, neutral cephalothin, penicillin, and ethacrynate sodium.
• Keep in mind that I.V. solutions remain stable for 24 hours.
• Be aware that oxidation of drug may slightly discolor admixtures containing dobutamine. This does not indicate a significant loss of potency provided drug is used within 24 hours of reconstitution.

• Continuously monitor ECG, blood pressure, pulmonary capillary wedge pressure, cardiac condition, and urine output.
• Monitor serum electrolytes, as ordered. Drug may lower serum potassium levels.
• Be aware that drug is a unique agent that increases contractility of failing heart without inducing marked tachycardia, except at high doses.

---

dopamine hydrochloride
Dopastat, Intropin, Revimine†‡

Pregnancy Risk Category: C

HOW SUPPLIED
Injection: 40 mg/ml, 80 mg/ml, 160 mg/ml parenteral concentrate for injection for I.V. infusion; 0.8 mg/ml (200 or 400 mg) in dextrose 5%; 1.6 mg/ml (400 or 800 mg) in dextrose 5%, 3.2 mg/ml (800 mg) in dextrose 5% parenteral injection for I.V. infusion.

ACTION
Stimulates dopaminergic, beta-adrenergic, and alpha-adrenergic receptors of the sympathetic nervous system.

ONSET, PEAK, DURATION
Onset occurs within 5 minutes of starting I.V. infusion. Peak unknown. Effects subside within 10 minutes of discontinuing infusion.

INDICATIONS & DOSAGE
To treat shock and correct hemodynamic imbalances; to improve perfusion to vital organs; to increase cardiac output; to correct hypotension—
Adults: initially, 1 to 5 mcg/kg/minute by I.V. infusion. Dosage titrated to desired hemodynamic or renal response; infusion may be increased by 1 to 4 mcg/kg/minute at 10- to 30-minute intervals.

ADVERSE REACTIONS

CNS: headache.

CV: *arrhythmias,* ectopic beats, tachycardia, anginal pain, palpitations, *hypotension.* Less frequently, bradycardia, widening of QRS complex, conduction disturbances, vasoconstriction, hypertension.

GI: nausea, vomiting.

Other: necrosis and tissue sloughing with extravasation, piloerection, dyspnea.

INTERACTIONS

Alpha blockers, beta blockers: may antagonize dopamine's effects.

Ergot alkaloids: extreme elevations in blood pressure. Don't use together.

Inhalation anesthetics: increased risk of arrhythmias or hypertension. Monitor closely.

MAO inhibitors: may cause hypertensive crisis. Avoid if possible.

Phenytoin: may lower blood pressure of dopamine-stabilized patients. Monitor carefully.

CONTRAINDICATIONS

Contraindicated in patients with uncorrected tachyarrhythmias, pheochromocytoma, or ventricular fibrillation.

NURSING CONSIDERATIONS

• Use cautiously in patients with occlusive vascular disease, cold injuries, diabetic endarteritis, and arterial embolism; in pregnant patients; and in those taking MAO inhibitors.

• **I.V. use:** Use a central line or large vein, such as in the antecubital fossa, to minimize risk of extravasation. Watch infusion site carefully for signs of extravasation; if it occurs, stop infusion immediately and call doctor. Extravasation may require treatment by infiltration of the area with 5 to 10 mg phentolamine and 10 to 15 ml 0.9% sodium chloride solution. Don't mix with alkaline solutions. Use D_5W, 0.9% sodium chloride solution, or a combination of D_5W and 0.9% sodium chloride solution. Mix just before use.

• Use a continuous infusion pump to regulate flow rate.

• Do not mix other drugs in I.V. container with dopamine. Do not give alkaline drugs (for example, sodium bicarbonate or phenytoin sodium) through I.V. line containing dopamine.

• During infusion, frequently monitor ECG, blood pressure, cardiac output, central venous pressure, pulmonary capillary wedge pressure, pulse rate, urine output, and color and temperature of extremities.

• If a disproportionate rise in diastolic pressure (a marked decrease in pulse pressure) is observed in patients receiving dopamine, decrease infusion rate as ordered and observe carefully for further evidence of predominant vasoconstrictor activity, unless such an effect is desired.

• Observe patients closely for adverse effects. If they develop, the doctor will adjust or discontinue dosage.

• Check urine output often. If urine flow decreases without hypotension, notify doctor because dosage may need to be reduced.

• After drug is stopped, watch closely for sudden drop in blood pressure. Taper dosages slowly to evaluate stability of blood pressure, as ordered.

• Remember that drug is not a substitute for blood or fluid volume deficit. If deficit exists, replace fluid before administering vasopressors, as ordered.

• Be aware that acidosis decreases effectiveness of dopamine.

• Know that most patients are satisfactorily maintained on dosage less than 20 mcg/kg/minute.

• Keep in mind that patient response depends on dosage and pharmacologic effect. Dosages of 0.5 to 2 mcg/kg/minute predominantly stimulate dopamine receptors and produce vasodilation of the renal vasculature. Dosages of 2 to 10 mcg/kg/minute stimulate beta-adrenergic receptors for a positive inotropic effect. Higher dosages also stimulate alpha-adrenergic receptors, causing vasoconstriction and increased blood pressure.

• Discard after 24 hours (dopamine solutions deteriorate after 24 hours) or earlier if solution is discolored.

---

mephentermine sulfate
Wyamine

Pregnancy Risk Category: NR

HOW SUPPLIED
Injection: 15 mg/ml, 30 mg/ml

ACTION
Unknown. Appears to indirectly stimulate beta- and alpha-adrenergic receptors by releasing norepinephrine.

ONSET, PEAK, DURATION
Onset occurs immediately after I.V. administration, within 5 to 15 minutes after I.M. injection. Peak unknown. Effects persist for 15 to 30 minutes after I.V. administration, 1 to 4 hours after I.M. injection.

INDICATIONS & DOSAGE
Hypotension after spinal anesthesia –
Adults: 30 to 45 mg I.V. as a single injection, then 30 mg I.V. repeated p.r.n. for maintenance of blood pressure, continuous I.V. infusion of 0.1% solution of mephentermine in D_5W.
Children: 0.4 mg/kg I.M. or I.V.
Hypotension after spinal anesthesia during obstetric procedures –
Adults: initially, 15 mg I.V., then repeated p.r.n.
Prevention of hypotension during spinal anesthesia –
Adults: 30 to 45 mg I.M. 10 to 20 minutes before anesthesia.

ADVERSE REACTIONS
CNS: euphoria, nervousness, anxiety, tremor, incoherence, drowsiness, *seizures,* visual hallucinations (with large doses).
CV: *arrhythmias, marked elevation of blood pressure (with large doses),* AV block, tachycardia.

INTERACTIONS
Antihypertensives, guanethidine, nitrates phenothiazines, reserpine: decreased effects of these adrenergic blocking agents.
Beta-adrenergic blocking agents, rauwolfia alkaloids: mutual inhibition of therapeutic effects.
CNS stimulants, mazindol, methylphenidate, sympathomimetics: increased CNS stimulation.
Digitalis glycosides, levodopa, inhalation anesthetics: increased risk of arrhythmias.
Ergot alkaloids, oxytocin: enhanced vasoconstriction.
Inhalation anesthetics: increased risk of hypertension. Monitor closely.
MAO inhibitors: may precipitate hypertension, headache, and related symptoms. Don't use together.
Maprotiline, tricyclic antidepressants: decreased pressure of mephentermine.
Thyroid hormones: enhanced risk of coronary insufficiency.

CONTRAINDICATIONS
Contraindicated in patients with hypersensitivity to the drug and in those with hypotension resulting from hemorrhage, except in emergencies.

NURSING CONSIDERATIONS
• Use cautiously in patients with CV disease, hyperthyroidism, hypertension, and chronic illness.
• Remember that the drug is not a substitute for blood or fluid volume deficit. If deficit exists, replace fluid before administering vasopressors, as ordered.

---

*Liquid form contains alcohol.
**May contain tartrazine.

Common reactions are in italics; *life-threatening,* in bold italics.

• **I.V. use:** Administer at 1 to 5 mg/ minute. Can be given undiluted; I.V. drug is not irritating to tissue and extravasation is not dangerous. To prepare 0.1% I.V. solution, add 16.6 ml of mephentermine (30 mg/ml) to 500 ml of D_5W.

• Don't mix with I.V. hydralazine or epinephrine, which are physically incompatible with mephentermine.

• During infusion, frequently monitor ECG, blood pressure, cardiac output, central venous pressure, pulmonary capillary wedge pressure, pulse rate, urine output, and color and temperature of extremities. Titrate infusion rate according to findings and the doctor's guidelines. Use a continuous infusion pump to regulate flow rate.

• During infusion, check blood pressure every 2 minutes until stabilized; then check every 10 to 15 minutes.

• Know that the I.M. route may be used because drug is not irritating to tissue.

• Monitor blood pressure until stable, even after discontinuing drug.

• Observe patients closely for adverse effects. If they develop, the doctor will adjust or discontinue dosage.

• Keep in mind that hypercapnia, hypoxia, or acidosis may reduce effectiveness or increase adverse effects. Identify and correct before and during administration, as ordered.

• Be aware that the drug may increase uterine contractions during third trimester of pregnancy.

---

metaraminol bitartrate
Aramine

Pregnancy Risk Category: C

HOW SUPPLIED
Injection: 10 mg/ml

ACTION
Stimulates alpha- and beta₁-adrenergic receptors within the sympathetic nervous system.

ONSET, PEAK, DURATION
Onset occurs in 1 to 2 minutes after I.V. administration, 10 minutes after I.M. administration, 5 to 20 minutes after S.C administration. Peak unknown. Effects last 20 minutes after I.V. administration, up to 90 minutes after S.C. or I.M. administration.

INDICATIONS & DOSAGE
Prevention of hypotension associated with spinal anesthesia –
Adults: 2 to 10 mg I.M. or S.C.
Treatment of hypotension associated with spinal anesthesia –
Adults: 0.5 to 5 mg by direct I.V. injection, followed by I.V. infusion titrated to maintain blood pressure.
Children: 0.01 mg/kg as single I.V. injection; 1 mg/25 ml of D_5W as I.V. infusion. Rate adjusted to maintain blood pressure in normal range. Alternatively, 0.1 mg/kg I.M. as single dose, p.r.n. At least 10 minutes should elapse before dosage increased because maximum effect is not immediately apparent.

ADVERSE REACTIONS
CNS: apprehension, restlessness, dizziness, headache, tremor, weakness, *seizures* (with excessive use).
CV: hypertension; hypotension; precordial pain; palpitations; *arrhythmias,* including sinus or *ventricular tachycardia;* bradycardia; premature supraventricular contractions; AV dissociation.
GI: nausea, vomiting.
GU: decreased urine output.
Respiratory: respiratory distress.
Skin: flushing, pallor, sweating.
Other: abscess, hyperglycemia, necrosis, sloughing upon extravasation, *metabolic acidosis (in hypovolemia),* increased body temperature.

INTERACTIONS
Beta-adrenergic blockers: mutual inhibition of drug effects, with possible

---

†Available in Canada only.   ‡Available in Australia only.   ◇Available OTC.

hypertension, bradycardia, and heart block. Avoid concomitant use.
Cocaine, digitalis glycosides, doxapram, ergot alkaloids, general anesthetics, levodopa, maprotiline, other sympathomimetics, thyroid hormones, tricyclic antidepressants: increased risk of adverse cardiac effects. Monitor closely.
Furazolidone, MAO inhibitors, procarbazine: may cause severe hypertension (hypertensive crisis) and increase action of metaraminol. Avoid this combination.
Guanadrel, guanethidine: metaraminol may decrease the hypotensive effect of these drugs; guanadrel and guanethidine may enhance the pressor effect of metaraminol. Avoid concomitant use.

CONTRAINDICATIONS

Contraindicated in patients with hypersensitivity to the drug and in patients receiving anesthesia with cyclopropane and halogenated hydrocarbon anesthetics.

NURSING CONSIDERATIONS

• Use cautiously in patients with heart disease, hypertension, peripheral vascular disease, thyroid disease, diabetes, cirrhosis, history of malaria, or sulfite sensitivity and in patients receiving digitalis glycosides.
• Do not mix metaraminol with other drugs.
• **I.V. use:** To prepare an I.V. infusion, mix 15 to 100 mg in 500 ml of 0.9% sodium chloride solution or D_5W. Adjust rate to maintain blood pressure.
• During infusion, check blood pressure every 5 minutes until stabilized; then check every 15 minutes. Frequently monitor ECG, blood pressure, cardiac output, central venous pressure, pulmonary capillary wedge pressure, pulse rate, urine output, and color and temperature of extremities.

Titrate infusion rate according to findings and the doctor's guidelines.
• Use a central venous catheter or large vein, such as in the antecubital fossa, to minimize risk of extravasation. Use a continuous infusion pump to regulate infusion flow rate and a piggyback setup so I.V. line remains open if drug is stopped. Watch infusion site carefully for signs of extravasation. If it occurs, stop infusion immediately and call the doctor.
• To treat extravasation, infiltrate site promptly with 10 to 15 ml of 0.9% sodium chloride injection containing 5 to 10 mg phentolamine. Use a fine needle.
• Keep in mind that blood pressure should be raised to slightly less than the patient's normal level. Be careful to avoid excessive blood pressure response. Headache may be a symptom of hypertension. Rapidly induced hypertensive response can cause acute pulmonary edema, arrhythmias, and cardiac arrest.
• Allow at least 10 minutes between doses. Drug effects are not always immediately apparent.
• Observe patients closely for adverse effects. If they develop, notify the doctor, who will adjust or discontinue dosage.
• Keep emergency drugs on hand to reverse effects of metaraminol: atropine for reflex bradycardia; phentolamine to decrease vasopressor, effects; and propranolol for arrhythmias.
• Know that drug is not a substitute for blood or fluid volume deficit. If deficit exists, replace fluid before administering vasopressors, as ordered.
• Report persistent decreased urine output. Urine output may decrease initially, then increase as blood pressure returns to normal level.
• Closely monitor patients with diabetes; insulin dosage may need to be adjusted.
• When discontinuing drug, gradually

---

*Liquid form contains alcohol.   *Common* reactions are in italics; *life-threatening*, in bold italics.
**May contain tartrazine.

slow infusion rate, as ordered. Continue monitoring vital signs, watching for possible severe drop in blood pressure. Keep equipment nearby to resume drug, if necessary. Do not reinstate vasopressor therapy until the systolic blood pressure falls below 70 to 80 mm Hg, as ordered.

• Be aware that because of prolonged action, a cumulative effect is possible. With an excessive vasopressor response, elevated blood pressure may persist after drug is stopped.

• Keep solution in light-resistant container, away from heat.

---

norepinephrine bitartrate (levarterenol bitartrate, noradrenaline acid tartrate)
Levophed

Pregnancy Risk Category: C

HOW SUPPLIED
Injection: 1 mg/ml

ACTION
Stimulates alpha- and beta$_1$-adrenergic receptors within the sympathetic nervous system.

ONSET, PEAK, DURATION
Onset and peak immediately after I.V. infusion begins. Effects persist for 1 to 2 minutes after I.V. infusion ends.

INDICATIONS & DOSAGE
To restore blood pressure in acute hypotensive states –
Adults: initially, 8 to 12 mcg/minute I.V. infusion, then adjusted to maintain normal blood pressure. Average maintenance dosage is 2 to 4 mcg/minute.
Children: 2 mcg/m^2/minute I.V. infusion; dosage adjusted based on patient response.
Severe hypotension during cardiac arrest –
Children: initial I.V. infusion rate is 0.1 mcg/kg/minute. Rate adjusted according to patient response.

ADVERSE REACTIONS
CNS: *headache,* anxiety, weakness, dizziness, tremor, restlessness, insomnia.
CV: bradycardia, *severe hypertension,* marked increase in peripheral resistance, decreased cardiac output, *arrhythmias, ventricular tachycardia, fibrillation,* bigeminal rhythm, AV dissociation, precordial pain.
GU: decreased urine output.
Respiratory: respiratory difficulties.
Other: fever, metabolic acidosis, hyperglycemia, increased glycogenolysis, irritation with extravasation, swelling and enlargement of thyroid.

INTERACTIONS
Alpha-adrenergic blocking agents: may antagonize drug effects.
Antihistamines, ergot alkaloids, guanethidine, methyldopa: when given with sympathomimetics, may cause severe hypertension (hypertensive crisis). Don't give together.
Inhalation anesthetics: increased risk of arrhythmias. Monitor closely.
MAO inhibitors: increased risk of hypertensive crisis.

CONTRAINDICATIONS
Contraindicated in patients with mesenteric or peripheral vascular thrombosis, profound hypoxia, hypercapnia, or hypotension resulting from blood volume deficits and during cyclopropane and halothane anesthesia.

NURSING CONSIDERATIONS
• Use with extreme caution in patients receiving MAO inhibitors or triptyline or imipramine type antidepressants. Use cautiously in patients with sulfite sensitivity.
• **I.V. use:** Use a central venous catheter or a large vein, such as in the antecubital fossa, to minimize risk of extravasation. Administer in dextrose

---

5% in 0.9% sodium chloride injection; 0.9% sodium chloride injection alone is not recommended. Use continuous infusion pump to regulate infusion flow rate and a piggyback setup so I.V. line remains open if norepinephrine is stopped.
• During infusion, frequently monitor ECG, blood pressure, cardiac output, central venous pressure, pulmonary capillary wedge pressure, pulse rate, urine output, and color and temperature of extremities. Titrate infusion rate according to findings and the doctor's guidelines. In previously hypertensive patients, blood pressure should be raised no higher than 40 mm Hg below preexisting systolic pressure.
• Check site frequently for signs of extravasation. If it occurs, stop infusion immediately and call the doctor. He may counteract effect by infiltrating area with 5 to 10 mg phentolamine and 10 to 15 ml of 0.9% sodium chloride solution. Also check for blanching along course of infused vein; may progress to superficial sloughing.
• If prolonged I.V. therapy is necessary, change injection site frequently.
• Keep emergency drugs on hand to reverse effects of norepinephrine: atropine for reflex bradycardia; phentolamine for increased vasopressor effects; and propranolol for arrhythmias.
• Never leave patients unattended during infusion. Also, check blood pressure every 2 minutes until stabilized; then check every 5 minutes.
• Report decreased urine output to the doctor immediately.
• Know that drug is not a substitute for blood or fluid volume deficit. If deficit exists, replace fluid before administering vasopressors.
• When discontinuing drug, gradually slow infusion rate, as ordered. Continue monitoring vital signs, watching

for possible severe drop in blood pressure.
• Be aware that norepinephrine solutions deteriorate after 24 hours.
• Protect drug from light. Discard discolored solutions or solutions that contain a precipitate.

phenylephrine hydrochloride
Neo-Synephrine

Pregnancy Risk Category: C

HOW SUPPLIED
Injection: 10 mg/ml

ACTION
Predominantly stimulates alpha-adrenergic receptors in the sympathetic nervous system.

ONSET, PEAK, DURATION
Onset occurs immediately after I.V. administration, within 10 to 15 minutes after S.C. or I.M. injection. Peak unknown. Effects persist for 15 to 20 minutes after I.V. administration, ½ to 2 hours after I.M. injection, 50 minutes to 1 hour after S.C. injection.

INDICATIONS & DOSAGE
Hypotensive emergencies during spinal anesthesia –
Adults: initially, 0.1 to 0.2 mg I.V., then subsequent doses of 0.1 to 0.2 mg, p.r.n.
Maintenance of blood pressure during spinal or inhalation anesthesia –
Adults: 2 to 3 mg S.C. or I.M. 3 or 4 minutes before anesthesia.
Children: 0.044 mg to 0.088 mg/kg S.C. or I.M.
Prolongation of spinal anesthesia –
Adults: 2 to 5 mg added to anesthetic solution.
Vasoconstrictor for regional anesthesia –
Adults: 1 mg phenylephrine added to 20 ml local anesthetic.
Mild to moderate hypotension –

---

*Liquid form contains alcohol.
**May contain tartrazine.

Common reactions are in italics; ***life-threatening***, in bold italics.

Adults: 2 to 5 mg S.C. or I.M.; repeated in 1 to 2 hours as needed and tolerated. Initial dose should not exceed 5 mg. Alternatively, 0.1 to 0.5 mg slow I.V., not to be repeated more often than 10 to 15 minutes.
Children: 0.1 mg/kg I.M. or S.C.; repeated in 1 to 2 hours as needed and tolerated.
Severe hypotension and shock (including drug-induced) –
Adults: 10 mg in 250 to 500 ml of D₅W or 0.9% sodium chloride injection. I.V. infusion started at 100 to 180 mcg/minute, then decreased to a maintenance infusion of 40 to 60 mcg/minute when blood pressure stabilizes.
Paroxysmal supraventricular tachycardia –
Adults: initially, 0.5 mg rapid I.V.; subsequent doses should not exceed the preceding dose by more than 0.1 to 0.2 mg and should not exceed 1 mg.

ADVERSE REACTIONS
CNS: *headache, restlessness, lightheadedness, weakness, seizures.*
CV: palpitations, bradycardia, *arrhythmias,* hypertension, anginal pain, decreased cardiac output.
EENT: blurred vision.
GI: vomiting.
Skin: pilomotor response, feeling of coolness.
Other: tachyphylaxis (may occur with continued use), decreased organ perfusion (with prolonged use), tissue sloughing with extravasation.

INTERACTIONS
Alpha-adrenergic blockers, phenothiazines: decreased vasopressor response. Monitor closely.
Beta-adrenergic blockers: block cardiostimulatory effects. Monitor closely.
MAO inhibitors: may cause severe hypertension (hypertensive crisis). Don't use together.

Oxytocics, tricyclic antidepressants (TCAs): increased pressor response. Observe patient.

CONTRAINDICATIONS
Contraindicated in patients with hypersensitivity to the drug and in those with severe hypertension or ventricular tachycardia.

NURSING CONSIDERATIONS
• Use with extreme caution in patients with heart disease, hyperthyroidism, severe atherosclerosis, bradycardia, partial heart block, myocardial disease, or sulfite sensitivity and in elderly patients.
• **I.V. use:** For direct injection, dilute 10 mg (1 ml) with 9 ml sterile water for injection to provide a solution containing 1 mg/ml. I.V. infusions are usually prepared by adding 10 mg of drug to 500 ml of D₅W or 0.9% sodium chloride injection. The initial infusion rate is usually 100 to 180 mcg/minute; the maintenance infusion rate is usually 40 to 60 mcg/minute.
• With prolonged I.V. infusions, avoid abrupt withdrawal. During infusion, frequently monitor ECG, blood pressure, cardiac output, central venous pressure, pulmonary capillary wedge pressure, pulse rate, urine output, and color and temperature of extremities. Titrate infusion rate according to findings and the doctor's guidelines. Use a continuous infusion pump to regulate flow rate.
• Use a central venous catheter or a large vein, as in the antecubital fossa, to minimize risk of extravasation. Use a continuous infusion pump to regulate infusion flow rate.
• Monitor blood pressure frequently; avoid severe increase. Maintain blood pressure slightly below the patient's normal level, as ordered. In previously normotensive patients, maintain systolic blood pressure at 80 to 100 mm Hg; in previously hypertensive

patients, maintain systolic blood pressure at 30 to 40 mm Hg below usual level.

• To treat extravasation, infiltrate site promptly with 10 to 15 ml of 0.9% sodium chloride injection containing 5 to 10 mg phentolamine, as ordered. Use a fine needle.

• Remember that drug causes little or no CNS stimulation.

• Keep in mind that drug is incompatible with butacaine sulfate, alkalis, ferric salts, and oxidizing agents.

---

pseudoephedrine hydrochloride

Afrinol Repetabs◇, Allerid◇, Cenafed◇, Children's Sudafed Liquid◇, Congestac N.D. caplets†◇, Decofed◇, De Fed-60◇, Dorcol Children's Decongestant◇, Drixoral Non-Drowsy Formula◇, Efidac/24◇, Eltor 120†◇, Genaphed◇, Halofed◇, Halofed Adult Strength◇, Maxenal†◇, Myfedrine◇, NeoFed◇, Novafed◇, Ornex Cold†◇, PediaCare Infants' Oral Decongestant Drops◇, Pseudo◇, Pseudofrin†◇, Pseudogest◇, Robidrine◇, Sinufed◇, Sinustat◇, Sudafed◇, Sudafed 12 Hour◇, Sudafed-60◇, Sudrin◇, Sufedrin◇

pseudoephedrine sulfate

Afrinol Repetabs, Drixoral‡

Pregnancy Risk Category: C

HOW SUPPLIED

pseudoephedrine hydrochloride
Tablets: 30 mg◇, 60 mg◇
Tablets (extended-release): 120 mg◇, 240 mg◇
Capsules: 60 mg
Capsules (extended-release): 120 mg
Oral solution: 15 mg/5 ml◇, 30 mg/5 ml◇, 7.5 mg/0.8 ml◇
Syrup: 30 mg/5 ml
pseudoephedrine sulfate
Tablets (extended-release): 120 mg

(60 mg immediate-release, 60 mg delayed-release)◇

ACTION

Stimulates alpha-adrenergic receptors in the respiratory tract, producing vasoconstriction.

ONSET, PEAK, DURATION

Onset occurs in 15 to 30 minutes. Serum levels peak within 30 to 60 minutes. Effects persist for 3 to 4 hours after administration of tablets, oral solution, and syrup, 8 to 12 hours after administration of extended-release capsules and tablets.

INDICATIONS & DOSAGE

Nasal and eustachian tube decongestion –
Adults: 60 mg P.O. q 4 hours. Maximum dosage is 240 mg daily. Or, 120 mg extended-release tablet P.O. q 12 hours or 240 mg extended-release (Efidac/24) once daily.
Children ages 6 to 12: 30 mg P.O. regular-release form q 4 to 6 hours. Maximum dosage is 120 mg daily.
Children ages 2 to 6: 15 mg P.O. regular-release form q 4 to 6 hours. Maximum dosage is 60 mg/day.
Children over age 12: 120 mg P.O. q 12 hours, or 240 mg P.O. (Efidac/24) once daily.
Relief of nasal congestion –
Adults: 120 mg q 12 hours.

ADVERSE REACTIONS

CNS: *anxiety,* transient stimulation, tremor, dizziness, headache, insomnia, *nervousness.*
CV: arrhythmias, *palpitations,* tachycardia.
GI: anorexia, nausea, vomiting, dry mouth.
GU: difficulty urinating.
Respiratory: respiratory difficulty.
Skin: pallor.

INTERACTIONS
Antihypertensives: may attenuate hypotensive effect.
MAO inhibitors: may cause severe hypertension (hypertensive crisis).
Don't use together.

CONTRAINDICATIONS
Contraindicated in patients with severe hypertension or severe coronary artery disease, in patients receiving MAO inhibitors, and in breast-feeding patients. Extended-release preparations are contraindicated for children under age 12.

NURSING CONSIDERATIONS
• Use cautiously in patients with hypertension, cardiac disease, diabetes, glaucoma, hyperthyroidism, and prostatic hyperplasia.
• Do not crush or break extended-release forms.
• Be aware that elderly patients are more sensitive to the drug's effects.
• Warn against using OTC products containing other sympathomimetics.
• Tell the patient not to take drug within 2 hours of bedtime because it can cause insomnia.
• Tell the patient to relieve dry mouth with sugarless gum or hard candy.
• Tell the patient to stop drug if he becomes unusually restless and to notify the doctor promptly.

**dihydroergotamine mesylate
ergotamine tartrate
methysergide maleate
propranolol hydrochloride**
(See Chapter 22, ANTIANGINALS.)

COMBINATION PRODUCTS
BELLERGAL-S**, BEL-PHEN-ERGOT
S, PHENERBEL-S: ergotamine tartrate
0.6 mg, levorotatory belladonna alkaloids 0.2 mg, and phenobarbital 40
mg.
CAFERGOT, ERCAF, WIGRAINE: ergotamine tartrate 1 mg and caffeine
100 mg.
CAFERGOT SUPPOSITORIES: ergotamine tartrate 2 mg and caffeine 100
mg.
HYDERGINE: dihydroergocornine
mesylate 0.167 mg, dihydroergocris-
tine mesylate 0.167 mg, and dihy-
droergocryptine mesylate 0.167 mg.
WIGRAINE SUPPOSITORIES: ergotamine tartrate 2 mg and caffeine 100
mg.

---

dihydroergotamine mesylate
D.H.E. 45, Dihydergot‡,
Dihydroergotamine-Sandoz†

Pregnancy Risk Category: X

HOW SUPPLIED
Injection: 1 mg/ml

ACTION
Causes peripheral vasoconstriction
primarily by stimulating alpha-adrenergic receptors; may abort vascular
headaches by direct vasoconstriction
of dilated carotid artery bed with a
decline in amplitude of pulsations.

ONSET, PEAK, DURATION
Onset occurs within 5 minutes of I.V.
administration, within 15 to 30 minutes of I.M. injection. Serum levels
peak within 15 minutes of I.V. administration, 30 minutes after I.M. injection, 15 to 45 minutes after S.C. injection. Effects persist for about 8
hours after parenteral use.

INDICATIONS & DOSAGE
*To prevent or abort vascular or mi-
graine headache –*
Adults: 1 mg I.M. or I.V. Repeated
q 1 to 2 hours, p.r.n., up to total of
2 mg I.V. or 3 mg I.M. per attack.
Maximum weekly dosage is 6 mg.

ADVERSE REACTIONS
CNS: dizziness.
CV: numbness and tingling in fingers
and toes, transient tachycardia or bra-
dycardia, precordial distress and
pain, increased arterial pressure.
GI: *nausea, vomiting.*
Skin: itching.
Other: weakness in legs, muscle pain
in extremities, localized edema.

INTERACTIONS
Erythromycin, other macrolides: may
cause symptoms of ergot toxicity. Vasodilators (nitroprusside, nifedipine,
or prazosin) may be ordered to treat
such an attack. Monitor closely.
Propranolol and other beta blockers:
blocked natural pathway for vasodilation in patients receiving ergot alkaloids; may result in excessive vasoconstriction and cold extremities.
Watch closely if drugs are used together.

CONTRAINDICATIONS
Contraindicated in patients with hypersensitivity to the drug, during

---

*Liquid form contains alcohol. *Common* reactions are in italics; *life-threatening,* in bold italics.
**May contain tartrazine.

pregnancy or breast-feeding, and in patients with peripheral and occlusive vascular disease, coronary artery disease, uncontrolled hypertension, severe hepatic or renal dysfunction, and sepsis.

NURSING CONSIDERATIONS
• Know that the drug is most effective when used at first sign of migraine or soon after onset.
• **I.V. use:** Directly inject solution into the vein over 3 minutes. Continuous and intermittent infusion are not recommended.
• Avoid prolonged administration; don't exceed recommended dosage, as ordered. Adjust to most effective minimal dosage, as ordered, for best results.
• Be alert for ergotamine rebound, or an increase in frequency and duration of headache, which may occur when drug is stopped.
• Protect ampules from heat and light. Discard if solution is discolored.
• Instruct patients to lie down and relax in a quiet, low-light environment after administration of drug.
• Tell patients to report any feeling of coldness in extremities or of tingling in fingers and toes. Severe vasoconstriction may result in tissue damage. Keep extremities warm and administer vasodilators as ordered.
• Help patients evaluate underlying causes of stress, which may precipitate attacks.

---

ergotamine tartrate
Ergodryl Mono‡, Ergomar, Ergostat, Gynergen†

Pregnancy Risk Category: X

HOW SUPPLIED
Capsules: 1 mg‡
Tablets: 1 mg†
Tablets (sublingual): 2 mg

Aerosol inhaler: 360 mcg/metered spray†
Suppositories: 2 mg

ACTION
Stimulates alpha-adrenergic receptors, causing peripheral vasoconstriction. Also inhibits reuptake of norepinephrine, increasing vasoconstrictor activity.

ONSET, PEAK, DURATION
Onset and duration variable. Serum levels peak in ½ to 3 hours or longer after oral dose, unknown for other routes of administration.

INDICATIONS & DOSAGE
Vascular or migraine headache –
Adults: initially, 2 mg P.O. or S.L., then 1 to 2 mg P.O. q hour or S.L. q ½ hour, to maximum of 6 mg daily and 10 mg weekly. Alternatively, use of aerosol inhaler: 1 spray (360 mcg) initially, repeated q 5 minutes p.r.n. to a maximum of 6 sprays (2.16 mg) per 24 hours or 15 sprays (5.4 mg) per week.

Patient also may use rectal suppositories. Initially, 2 mg P.R. at onset of the attack, repeated in 1 hour p.r.n. Maximum dosage is 2 suppositories per attack or 5 suppositories per week.

ADVERSE REACTIONS
CV: numbness and tingling in fingers and toes, transient tachycardia or bradycardia, precordial distress and pain, increased arterial pressure, angina pectoris, peripheral vasoconstriction.
GI: nausea, vomiting, diarrhea, abdominal cramps, ischemic colitis.
Skin: itching.
Other: weakness in legs, muscle pain in extremities, localized edema, pruritus.

INTERACTIONS
Erythromycin, other macrolides: may cause symptoms of ergot toxicity. Vasodilators (nitroprusside, nifedipine, or prazosin) may be ordered to treat such an attack. Monitor closely.
Propranolol and other beta blockers: blocked natural pathway for vasodilation in patients receiving ergot alkaloids; may result in excessive vasoconstriction. Watch closely if drugs are used together.

CONTRAINDICATIONS
Contraindicated in patients with hypersensitivity to ergot alkaloids, during pregnancy, and in patients with peripheral and occlusive vascular diseases, coronary artery disease, hypertension, hepatic or renal dysfunction, severe pruritus, or sepsis.

NURSING CONSIDERATIONS
• Obtain an accurate dietary history from the patient to determine if a relationship exists between certain foods and onset of headache.
• Be aware that drug is most effective when used during prodromal stage of headache or as soon as possible after onset.
• Avoid prolonged administration; don't exceed recommended dosage.
• Provide a quiet, low-light environment to help patients relax.
• Be alert for ergotamine rebound, or an increase in frequency and duration of headache, which may occur if drug is suddenly discontinued.
• Tell patients not to eat, drink, or smoke while the tablet is dissolving. S.L. tablet is preferred during early stage of attack because of its rapid absorption.
• Warn patients not to increase dosage without first consulting the doctor.
• Advise patient to avoid prolonged exposure to cold weather whenever possible. Cold may increase many of the adverse reactions to the drug.

• Instruct patients on long-term therapy to check for and report feeling of coldness in extremities or of tingling in fingers and toes. Severe vasoconstriction may result in tissue damage. Keep extremities warm and administer vasodilators as ordered.
• Instruct patients how to use inhaler correctly.
• Help patient evaluate underlying causes of stress, which may precipitate attacks.

---

methysergide maleate
Deseril‡, Sansert**
Pregnancy Risk Category: X

HOW SUPPLIED
Tablets: 1 mg‡, 2 mg

ACTION
Unknown. Specifically blocks serotonin (a neurotransmitter) in the peripheral nervous system. In CNS, drug may act as a serotonin agonist.

ONSET, PEAK, DURATION
Onset occurs within 1 to 2 days after therapy initiated. Peak unknown. Effects persist for 1 to 2 days.

INDICATIONS & DOSAGE
Prevention of frequent, severe, uncontrollable, or disabling migraine or vascular headaches –
Adults: 4 to 8 mg P.O. daily with meals.

ADVERSE REACTIONS
CNS: insomnia, drowsiness, *euphoria, vertigo,* ataxia, *light-headedness,* hyperesthesia, weakness, hallucinations or feelings of disassociation, rapid speech, lethargy.
CV: ***fibrotic thickening of cardiac valves and aorta, inferior vena cava, and common iliac branches (retroperitoneal fibrosis);*** vasoconstriction, causing chest pain, abdominal pain, vascular insufficiency of lower limbs;

---

cold, numb, painful extremities with or without paresthesia and diminished or absent pulses; postural hypotension; tachycardia; peripheral edema; murmurs; bruits.

EENT: nasal congestion, visual disturbances.

GI: nausea, vomiting, diarrhea, constipation, epigastric pain.

Hematologic: neutropenia, eosinophilia.

Respiratory: *pulmonary fibrosis* (causing dyspnea, tightness and pain in chest, pleural friction rubs, and effusion).

Skin: hair loss, dermatitis, sweating, flushing, rash.

Other: arthralgia, myalgia.

INTERACTIONS
Beta blockers: may result in peripheral ischemia by cold extremities and possible gangrene. Monitor closely.

CONTRAINDICATIONS
Contraindicated in patients with severe hypertension or arteriosclerosis, peripheral vascular insufficiency, renal or hepatic disease, coronary artery disease (CAD), phlebitis or cellulitis of lower limbs, collagen diseases, fibrotic processes, or valvular heart disease; in debilitated patients; and during pregnancy.

NURSING CONSIDERATIONS
• Use cautiously in patients with peptic ulcerations or suspected CAD. ECG and cardiac status evaluation advisable before giving to patients over 40 years. Also use cautiously in patients sensitive to aspirin or tartrazine.

• Know that the drug is indicated only for patients who are unresponsive to other drugs and who can be kept under close medical supervision.

• Gradually introduce medication, as ordered, and administer with meals to prevent GI effects.

• Give drug for 3 weeks before evaluating effectiveness.

• Monitor laboratory studies of cardiac and renal function, blood count, and erythrocyte sedimentation rate before and during therapy.

• Because of its slow onset of action, do not use drug for treatment of migraine or vascular headache.

• Do not use to treat tension (muscle contraction) headaches.

• Be aware that drug may be withdrawn gradually every 6 months; then restarted after at least 3 weeks.

• Instruct patients to keep daily weight record and report unusually rapid weight gain. Teach patients to check for peripheral edema. Explain and suggest low-salt diet if necessary.

• Tell patients not to stop drug abruptly; may cause rebound headaches. Stop gradually over 2 to 3 weeks.

• Tell patients to promptly report any of the following symptoms the doctor: cold, numb, or painful hands and feet; leg cramps when walking; and pelvic, chest, or flank pain.

Skeletal muscle relaxants

baclofen
carisoprodol
chlorphenesin carbamate
chlorzoxazone
cyclobenzaprine hydrochloride
dantrolene sodium
methocarbamol
orphenadrine citrate

COMBINATION PRODUCTS
NORGESIC: orphenadrine citrate
25 mg, aspirin 385 mg, and caffeine
30 mg.
NORGESIC FORTE: orphenadrine citrate 50 mg, aspirin 770 mg, and caffeine 60 mg.
ROBAXISAL: methocarbamol 400 mg
and aspirin 325 mg.
SOMA COMPOUND: carisoprodol 200
mg and aspirin 325 mg.
SOMA COMPOUND WITH CODEINE:
carisoprodol 200 mg, aspirin 325 mg,
caffeine 32 mg, and codeine phosphate 16 mg.

baclofen
Clofen‡, Lioresal, Lioresal
Intrathecal

Pregnancy Risk Category: NR

HOW SUPPLIED
Tablets: 10 mg, 20 mg, 25 mg‡
Intrathecal injection: 500 mcg/ml,
2,000 mcg/ml

ACTION
Unknown. Appears to reduce transmission of impulses from the spinal
cord to skeletal muscle.

ONSET, PEAK, DURATION
Onset occurs hours to weeks after oral
administration, ½ to 1 hour after intrathecal administration. Serum levels
peak 2 to 3 hours after an oral dose;
peak effects occur about 4 hours after
intrathecal administration. Effects of
intrathecal injection persist for about
4 to 8 hours, unknown for oral administration.

INDICATIONS & DOSAGE
*Spasticity in multiple sclerosis, spinal
cord injury –*
Adults: initially, 5 mg P.O. t.i.d. for
3 days then 10 mg t.i.d. for 3 days, 15
mg t.i.d. for 3 days, 20 mg t.i.d. for 3
days. Increased according to response
up to maximum of 80 mg daily.
*Management of severe spasticity in patients who do not respond to or cannot
tolerate oral baclofen therapy –*
Adults: *Screening phase –* After a test
dose to check responsiveness, drug is
administered by an implantable infusion pump. The test dose is 1 ml of a
50-mcg/ml dilution administered into
the intrathecal space by barbotage
over 1 minute or more. Significantly
decreased severity or frequency of
muscle spasm or reduced muscle tone
should be evident within 4 to 8 hours.
If the response is inadequate, a second screening dose of 75 mcg/1.5 ml
is given 24 hours after the first. If response is still inadequate, a final test
dose of 100 mcg/2 ml is given 24
hours later. Patients unresponsive to
the 100-mcg dose shouldn't be considered candidates for the implantable
pump.
Maintenance therapy – initial dose titrated based on the screening dose
that elicited an adequate response.
This effective dose is doubled and administered over 24 hours. However, if
the screening dose efficacy was maintained for 12 hours or more, the dose
is not doubled. After the first 24
hours, the dose is increased slowly as
needed and tolerated by 10% to 30%

daily. During prolonged maintenance therapy, daily dose may be increased by 10% to 40% if needed; if the patient experiences adverse effects, dosage may be decreased by 10% to 20%. Maintenance dosages have ranged from 12 mcg to 1,500 mcg daily; however, experience with dosages over 1,000 mcg daily is limited. Most patients need 300 to 800 mcg daily.

ADVERSE REACTIONS
CNS: *drowsiness, dizziness,* headache, *weakness, fatigue,* confusion, insomnia, dysarthria, *seizures.*
CV: hypotension.
EENT: nasal congestion, blurred vision.
GI: *nausea,* constipation.
GU: urinary frequency.
Hepatic: increased AST and alkaline phosphatase levels.
Skin: rash, pruritus.
Other: ankle edema, excessive perspiration, hyperglycemia, weight gain.

INTERACTIONS
Ethanol, CNS depressants: increased CNS depression. Avoid concomitant use.

CONTRAINDICATIONS
Contraindicated in patients with hypersensitivity to the drug.

NURSING CONSIDERATIONS
• Use cautiously in patients with impaired renal function or seizure disorder or when spasticity is used to maintain motor function.
• Give oral form with meals or with milk to prevent GI distress.
• Know that orally administered drug should not be used to treat muscle spasm caused by rheumatic disorders, cerebral palsy, Parkinson's disease, or CVA because efficacy hasn't been established. Do not administer intrathecal injection by I.V., I.M., S.C., or epidural route.

• Watch for sensitivity reactions, such as fever, skin eruptions, and respiratory distress.
• Watch for increased incidence of seizures in patients with seizure disorder.
• Be aware that amount of relief determines if dosage (and drowsiness) can be reduced.
• Do not withdraw drug abruptly after long-term use unless required by severe adverse reactions; may precipitate hallucinations or rebound spasticity.
• Keep in mind that treatment for oral overdose is supportive only; emesis should not be induced or a respiratory stimulant used in obtunded patients.
• Know that experience with long-term intrathecal use suggests that about 10% of patients may develop tolerance to the drug. In some cases, this may be treated by hospitalizing the patient and slowly withdrawing the drug over a 2-week period.
• Tell patients to avoid activities that require alertness until drug's CNS effects are known. Drowsiness usually is transient.
• Tell patients to avoid alcohol while taking this drug.
• Advise the patient to follow the doctor's orders regarding rest and physical therapy.

carisoprodol
Rela, Sodol, Soma, Soprodol, Soridol

Pregnancy Risk Category: NR

HOW SUPPLIED
Tablets: 350 mg

ACTION
Unknown. Drug appears to modify central perception of pain without modifying pain reflexes. Blocks interneuronal activity in descending reticular activating system and in spinal cord.

ONSET, PEAK, DURATION
Onset occurs within 30 minutes.
Serum levels peak within 4 hours. Effects persist for 4 to 6 hours.

INDICATIONS & DOSAGE
As an adjunct in acute, painful musculoskeletal conditions—
Adults: 350 mg P.O. t.i.d. and h.s.

ADVERSE REACTIONS
CNS: *drowsiness, dizziness,* vertigo, ataxia, tremor, agitation, irritability, headache, depressive reactions, insomnia.
CV: orthostatic hypotension, tachycardia, facial flushing.
GI: nausea, vomiting, hiccups, increased bowel activity, epigastric distress.
Hematologic: eosinophilia.
Respiratory: asthmatic episodes.
Skin: rash, *erythema multiforme,* pruritus.
Other: fever, angioedema, *anaphylaxis.*

INTERACTIONS
Ethanol, CNS depressants: increased CNS depression. Avoid concomitant use.

CONTRAINDICATIONS
Contraindicated in patients with hypersensitivity to related compounds (for example, meprobamate or tybamate) or intermittent porphyria.

NURSING CONSIDERATIONS
• Use cautiously in patients with impaired hepatic or renal function.
• Watch for idiosyncratic reactions after first to fourth dose (weakness, ataxia, visual and speech difficulties, fever, skin eruptions, and mental changes) and for severe reactions, including bronchospasm, hypotension, and anaphylactic shock. Withhold dose and notify the doctor immediately of any unusual reactions.
• Record amount of relief to help the

doctor determine whether dosage can be reduced.
• Do not stop drug abruptly; mild withdrawal effects, such as insomnia, headache, nausea, and abdominal cramps, may result.
• Warn patients to avoid activities that require alertness until drug's CNS effects are known. Drowsiness is transient.
• Advise patients to avoid combining drug with alcohol or other CNS depressants.
• Advise patients to follow doctor's orders regarding rest and physical therapy.

chlorphenesin carbamate
Maolate**

Pregnancy Risk Category: NR

HOW SUPPLIED
Tablets: 400 mg

ACTION
Unknown. Probably modifies central perception of pain without modifying pain reflexes. Blocks interneuronal activity in descending reticular activating system and in spinal cord.

ONSET, PEAK, DURATION
Onset and duration unknown. Serum levels peak within 1 to 3 hours.

INDICATIONS & DOSAGE
As an adjunct to rest, physical therapy, and other measures for relief in short-term, acute, painful musculoskeletal conditions—
Adults: initial dose is 800 mg P.O. t.i.d. Maintenance dosage is 400 mg P.O. q.i.d. for maximum of 8 weeks.

ADVERSE REACTIONS
CNS: *drowsiness, dizziness,* confusion, headache, weakness. Dose-related adverse reactions include paradoxical stimulation, agitation, insomnia, nervousness, headache.

---

*Liquid form contains alcohol.   *Common* reactions are in italics; ***life-threatening,*** in bold italics.
**May contain tartrazine.

GI: *nausea, GI distress.*
Hematologic: thrombocytopenia, leukopenia, ***agranulocytosis.***
Other: *anaphylaxis.*

INTERACTIONS
Ethanol, CNS depressants: increased CNS depression. Avoid concomitant use.

CONTRAINDICATIONS
Contraindicated in patients with hypersensitivity to the drug.

NURSING CONSIDERATIONS
• Use cautiously in patients with hepatic disease or impaired renal function and in patients with hypersensitivity to aspirin because tablets contain tartrazine.
• Administer with meals or milk to prevent GI distress.
• Know that amount of relief determines if dosage (and drowsiness) can be reduced.
• Watch for sensitivity reactions, such as fever, skin eruptions, and respiratory distress. Withhold dose and notify doctor of unusual reactions.
• Monitor CBC and platelet studies in patients on long-term therapy. Watch for unusual bleeding and infections that may indicate blood dyscrasia.
• Be aware that safe use for periods over 8 weeks has not been established.
• Tell patients to avoid activities that require mental alertness, such as driving, until drug's adverse CNS effects are known.
• Advise patients to avoid combining drug with alcohol or other CNS depressants.

---

chlorzoxazone
Paraflex, Parafon Forte DSC, Strifon Forte DSC

Pregnancy Risk Category: NR

HOW SUPPLIED
Tablets: 250 mg
Caplets: 500 mg

ACTION
Unknown. Appears to modify central perception of pain without modifying pain reflexes. Blocks interneuronal activity in descending reticular activating system and in spinal cord.

ONSET, PEAK, DURATION
Onset occurs within 1 hour. Serum levels peak within 1 to 2 hours. Effects persist for 3 to 4 hours.

INDICATIONS & DOSAGE
As an adjunct in acute, painful musculoskeletal conditions –
Adults: 250 to 750 mg P.O. t.i.d. or q.i.d.
Children: 20 mg/kg P.O. or 600 mg/m² daily in divided doses t.i.d. or q.i.d.

ADVERSE REACTIONS
CNS: *drowsiness, dizziness, lightheadedness,* malaise, headache, overstimulation, tremor.
GI: anorexia, nausea, vomiting, heartburn, abdominal distress, constipation, diarrhea.
GU: urine discoloration (orange or purple-red).
Hematologic: anemia, agranulocytosis.
Hepatic: hepatic dysfunction.
Skin: urticaria, redness, itching, petechiae, bruising.

INTERACTIONS
Ethanol, CNS depressants: increased CNS depression. Avoid concomitant use.

CONTRAINDICATIONS
Contraindicated in patients with hypersensitivity to the drug or impaired hepatic function.

NURSING CONSIDERATIONS

• Use cautiously in patients with history of drug allergies.
• Give with meals or milk to prevent GI distress.
• Know that the amount of relief determines if dosage (and drowsiness) can be reduced.
• Watch for signs of hepatic dysfunction. If they occur, withhold dose and notify the doctor.
• Warn patients to avoid activities that require alertness until drug's CNS effects are known.
• Warn patients to avoid combining with alcohol or other CNS depressants.
• Tell patients that the drug may discolor urine orange or purple-red.
• Advise patients to follow the doctor's orders regarding physical activity.

---

cyclobenzaprine hydrochloride
Flexeril

Pregnancy Risk Category: B

HOW SUPPLIED
Tablets: 10 mg

ACTION
Unknown.

ONSET, PEAK, DURATION
Onset occurs within 1 hour. Serum levels peak in 3 to 8 hours. Effects persist for 12 to 24 hours.

INDICATIONS & DOSAGE
Short-term treatment of muscle spasm –
Adults: 10 mg P.O. t.i.d. for 7 days. Maximum dosage is 60 mg daily; maximum duration of treatment is 2 to 3 weeks.

ADVERSE REACTIONS
CNS: *drowsiness,* euphoria, weakness, headache, insomnia, nightmares, paresthesia, dizziness, depression, visual disturbances, **seizures.**
CV: tachycardia.
EENT: blurred vision, dry mouth.
GI: abdominal pain, dyspepsia, abnormal taste, constipation.
GU: urine retention.
Skin: rash, urticaria, pruritus.
Other: with high doses, watch for adverse reactions similiar to those of other TCAs.

INTERACTIONS
Anticholinergics: additive anticholinergic effects. Avoid concomitant use.
Ethanol, CNS depressants: may cause additive CNS depression. Avoid concomitant use.
MAO inhibitors: may exacerbate CNS depression or anticholinergic effects. Don't give within 14 days after discontinuing MAO inhibitors.

CONTRAINDICATIONS
Contraindicated in patients who have received MAO inhibitors within 14 days; during acute recovery phase of MI; and in patients with hyperthyroidism, hypersensitivity to the drug, heart block, arrhythmias, conduction disturbances, or CHF.

NURSING CONSIDERATIONS
• Use cautiously in patients with history of urine retention, acute angle-closure glaucoma, and increased intraocular pressure and in elderly or debilitated patients.
• Be alert for nausea, headache, and malaise, which may occur if drug is stopped abruptly after long-term use.
• Watch for symptoms of overdose, including possible cardiac toxicity. Notify the doctor immediately and have physostigmine available.
• Advise patients to report urinary hesitancy or urine retention. If constipation is a problem, increase fluid intake and suggest a stool softener.
• Warn patients to avoid activities

---

*Liquid form contains alcohol.   *Common* reactions are in italics; **life-threatening,** in bold italics.
**May contain tartrazine.

that require alertness until drug's CNS effects are known.
• Warn patients to avoid combining with alcohol or other CNS depressants.
• Tell patients that dry mouth may be relieved with sugarless candy or gum.

dantrolene sodium
Dantrium, Dantrium Intravenous
Pregnancy Risk Category: NR

HOW SUPPLIED
Capsules: 25 mg, 50 mg, 100 mg
Injection: 20 mg/vial

ACTION
Acts directly on skeletal muscle to interfere with intracellular calcium movement.

ONSET, PEAK, DURATION
Onset and duration unknown. Peak levels occur 5 hours after oral administration.

INDICATIONS & DOSAGE
Spasticity and sequelae secondary to severe chronic disorders (such as multiple sclerosis, cerebral palsy, spinal cord injury, CVA) –
Adults: 25 mg P.O. daily. Increased gradually in increments of 25 mg, up to 100 mg b.i.d. to q.i.d., to maximum of 400 mg daily.
Children: initially, 0.5 mg/kg P.O. b.i.d.; increased to t.i.d. then q.i.d. Dosage increased as needed by 0.5 mg/kg daily to 3 mg/kg b.i.d. to q.i.d. Maximum dosage is 100 mg q.i.d.
Management of malignant hyperthermia crisis –
Adults and children: 1 mg/kg I.V. initially; dose repeated as needed up to cumulative dosage of 10 mg/kg.
Prevention or attenuation of malignant hyperthermia crisis in susceptible patients who require surgery –
Adults: 4 to 8 mg/kg P.O. daily in three to four divided doses for 1 to 2 days before procedure. Final dose administered 3 to 4 hours before procedure.
Prevention of recurrence of malignant hyperthermia crisis –
Adults: 4 to 8 mg/kg/day P.O. in four divided doses for up to 3 days after hyperthermic crisis.

ADVERSE REACTIONS
CNS: *muscle weakness, drowsiness,* dizziness, light-headedness, malaise, headache, confusion, nervousness, insomnia, hallucinations, *seizures.*
CV: tachycardia, blood pressure changes.
EENT: excessive lacrimation, auditory or visual disturbances.
GI: anorexia, constipation, cramping, dysphagia, metallic taste, severe diarrhea, bleeding.
GU: urinary frequency, hematuria, incontinence, nocturia, dysuria, crystalluria, difficulty achieving erection.
Hepatic: hepatitis.
Respiratory: pleural effusion.
Skin: eczematous eruption, pruritus, urticaria, photosensitivity.
Other: abnormal hair growth, drooling, diaphoresis, myalgia, chills, fever.

INTERACTIONS
Ethanol, CNS depressants: increased CNS depression. Avoid concomitant use.
Intravenous verapamil: may result in cardiovascular collapse. Stop verapamil before administering I.V. dantrolene.

CONTRAINDICATIONS
Contraindicated in patients when spasticity is used to maintain motor function, in those with upper motor neuron disorders, for spasms in rheumatic disorders, in patients with active hepatic disease, and in breast-feeding patients.

NURSING CONSIDERATIONS
• Use cautiously in patients with severely impaired cardiac or pulmonary function or preexisting hepatic disease, in women, and in patients over 35 years.
• Obtain liver function tests at the beginning of therapy.
• For optimum drug effect, give daily dosage in four divided doses.
• Give with meals or milk to prevent GI distress.
• Prepare oral suspension for single dose by dissolving capsule contents in juice or other suitable liquid. For multiple doses, use acid vehicle, such as citric acid in USP syrup; refrigerate. Use within several days.
• **I.V. use:** Administer as soon as malignant hyperthermia reaction is recognized, as ordered. Reconstitute each vial by adding 60 ml of sterile water for injection and shaking vial until clear. Don't use a diluent that contains a bacteriostatic agent. Protect contents from light and use within 6 hours. Be careful to avoid extravasation.
• Watch for hepatitis (fever and jaundice), severe diarrhea, severe weakness, or sensitivity reactions (fever and skin eruptions). Withhold dose and notify the doctor.
• Know that amount of relief in patient determines if dosage (and drowsiness) can be reduced.
• Tell patients to use caution when eating to avoid choking. Some patients may experience difficulty swallowing during therapy.
• Warn patients to avoid driving and other hazardous activities until drug's CNS effects are known.
• Advise patients to avoid combining with alcohol and other CNS depressants.
• Tell patients to avoid photosensitivity reactions by using sunblock and wearing protective clothing, to report abdominal discomfort or GI problems immediately, and to follow the doctor's orders regarding rest and physical therapy.

---

methocarbamol
Delaxin, Marbaxin-750, Robaxin, Robomol-500, Robomol-750

Pregnancy Risk Category: NR

HOW SUPPLIED
Tablets: 500 mg, 750 mg
Injection: 100 mg/ml

ACTION
Unknown. Probably modifies central perception of pain without modifying pain reflexes.

ONSET, PEAK, DURATION
Onset is immediate after I.V. administration; within ½ hour after oral administration. Peak levels occur immediately after I.V. administration, or within 2 hours of an oral dose. Duration unknown.

INDICATIONS & DOSAGE
As an adjunct in acute, painful musculoskeletal conditions –
Adults: 1.5 g P.O. q.i.d. for 2 to 3 days, then 1 g P.O. q.i.d., or not more than 500 mg (5 ml) I.M. into each gluteal region. Repeated q 8 hours p.r.n. Or 1 to 3 g daily (10 to 30 ml) I.V. directly into vein at 3 ml/minute, or 10 ml may be added to no more than 250 ml of D₅W or 0.9% sodium chloride solution. Maximum dosage is 3 g daily.
Supportive therapy in tetanus management –
Adults: 1 to 2 g by direct I.V. or 1 to 3 g as infusion q 6 hours.
Children: 15 mg/kg I.V. q 6 hours.

ADVERSE REACTIONS
CNS: drowsiness, dizziness, lightheadedness, headache, syncope, mild muscular incoordination (with I.M. or I.V. use), *seizures* (with I.V. use only).

---

*Liquid form contains alcohol.
**May contain tartrazine.

Common reactions are in italics; *life-threatening*, in bold italics.

CV: hypotension, bradycardia (with I.M. or I.V. use).
GI: nausea, anorexia, GI upset, metallic taste.
GU: hematuria (with I.V. use only), discoloration of urine.
Hematologic: hemolysis, decreased hemoglobin (with I.V. use only).
Skin: urticaria, pruritus, rash.
Respiratory: thrombophlebitis.
Other: extravasation (with I.V. use only), fever, flushing, *anaphylactic reactions* (with I.M. or I.V. use).

INTERACTIONS
Ethanol, CNS depressants: increased CNS depression. Avoid concomitant use.

CONTRAINDICATIONS
Contraindicated in patients with hypersensitivity to the drug, impaired renal function (injectable form), or seizure disorder (injectable form).

NURSING CONSIDERATIONS
• Give tablets with meals or milk to prevent GI distress.
• Prepare liquid by crushing tablets into water or sodium chloride solution. Give through nasogastric tube.
• In tetanus management, be aware methocarbamol is used with tetanus antitoxin, penicillin; tracheotomy; and aggressive supportive care. Long course of I.V. methocarbamol therapy is required.
• **I.V. use:** Dilute 10 ml of drug in not more than 250 ml of solution. Use D_5W or 0.9% sodium chloride injection. Infuse slowly; maximum rate is 300 mg (3 ml)/minute.
• Know that drug irritates veins; may cause phlebitis, aggravate seizures, and cause fainting if injected rapidly. Make sure the patient remains in a supine position during infusion. Drug is an irritant; avoid extravasation.
• Give I.M. deeply, only into upper outer quadrant of buttocks, with maximum of 5 ml in each buttock.

• Do not give subcutaneously.
• Watch for orthostatic hypotension, especially with parenteral administration. Keep the patient in a supine position for 15 minutes afterward, and supervise ambulation. Advise the patient to get up slowly.
• Watch for sensitivity reactions, such as fever and skin eruptions.
• Have epinephrine, antihistamines, and corticosteroids available.
• Monitor CBC periodically during prolonged therapy.
• Know that drug may interfere with urine tests for 5-hydroxyindoleacetic acid and vanillylmandelic acid.
• Tell patients urine may turn green, black, or brown.
• Advise patients to follow the doctor's orders regarding physical activity.
• Warn patients to avoid activities that require alertness until drug's CNS effects are known.
• Advise patients to avoid combining with alcohol or other CNS depressants.

orphenadrine citrate
Banflex, Flexoject, Flexon, K-Flex, Marflex, Myolin, Neocyten, Noradex, Norflex, O-Flex, Orflagen, Orphenate

Pregnancy Risk Category: NR

HOW SUPPLIED
Tablets: 100 mg
Tablets (extended-release): 100 mg
Injection: 30 mg/ml

ACTION
Unknown. Appears to modify central perception of pain without modifying pain reflexes. Blocks interneuronal activity in descending reticular activating system and in spinal cord.

ONSET, PEAK, DURATION
Onset occurs immediately with I.V. use, within 5 minutes of I.M. injec-

tion, or within 1 hour of oral administration. Peak levels occur immediately after I.V. infusion, within 30 minutes of I.M. injection, within 2 hours of tablet ingestion, or within 6 to 8 hours of extended-release tablet ingestion. Duration unknown.

INDICATIONS & DOSAGE
Adjunctive treatment in painful, acute musculoskeletal conditions –
Adults: 100 mg P.O. b.i.d., or 60 mg I.V. or I.M. q 12 hours, p.r.n. For maintenance therapy, patient switched to oral therapy beginning 12 hours after last parenteral dose.

ADVERSE REACTIONS
CNS: disorientation, restlessness, irritability, weakness, *drowsiness,* headache, dizziness, hallucinations, insomnia.
CV: palpitations, tachycardia.
EENT: dilated pupils, blurred vision, difficulty swallowing, increased intraocular pressure.
GI: constipation, *dry mouth,* nausea, vomiting, paralytic ileus, epigastric distress.
GU: urinary hesitancy or urine retention.
Hematologic: *aplastic anemia.*
Other: *anaphylaxis.*

INTERACTIONS
Ethanol, CNS depressants, propoxyphene: increased CNS depression. Avoid concomitant use.

CONTRAINDICATIONS
Contraindicated in patients with hypersensitivity to the drug and in those with glaucoma; prostatic hyperplasia; pyloric, duodenal, or bladder-neck obstruction; myasthenia gravis; and peptic ulceration.

NURSING CONSIDERATIONS
• Use cautiously in elderly or debilitated patients or in those with tachycardia, cardiac disease, arrhythmias, or sulfite sensitivity.
• Check all dosages carefully; a slight overdose can lead to toxicity. Early signs are excessive dry mouth, dilated pupils, blurred vision, skin flushing, and fever.
• **I.V. use:** Inject drug over approximately 5 minutes while the patient is supine. Wait 5 to 10 minutes and then help the patient to sit up.
• When given I.V., assess for paradoxical initial bradycardia; usually disappears in 2 minutes.
• Monitor CBC, hepatic function, and urinalysis in patients receiving long-term therapy as ordered.
• Monitor vital signs carefully.
• Have patients report urinary hesitancy and urine retention. Have patients void before taking the drug.
• Advise patient to relieve dry mouth with cool drinks, sugarless gum or hard candy.
• Warn patients to avoid tasks that require alertness until drug's CNS effects are known.
• Advise patients to avoid combining with alcohol or other CNS depressants.

---

*Liquid form contains alcohol.   *Common* reactions are in italics; ***life-threatening,*** in bold italics.
**May contain tartrazine.

atracurium besylate
doxacurium chloride
gallamine triethiodide
metocurine iodide
mivacurium chloride
pancuronium bromide
pipecuronium bromide
rocuronium bromide
succinylcholine chloride
tubocurarine chloride
vecuronium bromide

COMBINATION PRODUCTS
None.

atracurium besylate
Tracrium

Pregnancy Risk Category: C

HOW SUPPLIED
Injection: 10 mg/ml

ACTION
A nondepolarizing neuromuscular blocking agent that prevents acetylcholine from binding to receptors on the muscle end plate, thus blocking depolarization and resulting in skeletal muscle paralysis.

ONSET, PEAK, DURATION
Onset occurs within 2 minutes. Peak effects occur in 3 to 5 minutes. Twenty-five percent of muscle twitch strength returns in 35 to 45 minutes; 95% recovery evident in 60 to 70 minutes.

INDICATIONS & DOSAGE
Adjunct to general anesthesia, to facilitate endotracheal intubation and to provide skeletal muscle relaxation during surgery or mechanical ventilation –
Dosage depends on anesthetic used, individual needs, and response. Dosages given here are representative and must be adjusted.
Adults and children over 2 years: 0.4 to 0.5 mg/kg by I.V. bolus. Maintenance dosage of 0.08 to 0.10 mg/kg within 20 to 45 minutes of initial dose should be administered during prolonged surgical procedures. Maintenance dosages may be administered q 12 to 25 minutes in patients receiving balanced anesthesia. For prolonged procedures, a constant infusion of 5 to 9 mcg/kg/minute may be used.
Children 1 month to 2 years: initial dose, 0.3 to 0.4 mg/kg. Frequent maintenance doses may be needed.

ADVERSE REACTIONS
CV: increased heart rate, bradycardia, hypotension.
Skin: *skin flushing,* erythema, pruritus, urticaria.
Respiratory: *prolonged dose-related apnea,* wheezing, increased bronchial secretions.

INTERACTIONS
Aminoglycoside antibiotics (including amikacin, gentamicin, kanamycin, neomycin, streptomycin); polymyxin antibiotics (polymyxin B sulfate, colistin); clindamycin; quinidine; general anesthetics (such as halothane, enflurane, and isoflurane): potentiated neuromuscular blockade, leading to increased skeletal muscle relaxation and prolongation of effect. Use cautiously during surgical and postoperative periods.
Lithium, magnesium salts, opioid analgesics: potentiated neuromuscular blockade, leading to increased skeletal muscle relaxation and possible respiratory paralysis. Reduce dose of atracurium.

CONTRAINDICATIONS
Contraindicated in patients with hypersensitivity to the drug.

NURSING CONSIDERATIONS
• Use cautiously in patients with CV disease; severe electrolyte disorders; bronchogenic carcinoma; hepatic, renal, or pulmonary impairment; neuromuscular diseases; and myasthenia gravis and in elderly or debilitated patients.
• Administer sedatives or general anesthetics before neuromuscular blockers, as ordered. Neuromuscular blockers don't obtund consciousness or alter the pain threshold.
• Make sure to explain all events and happenings to the patient because he can still hear.
• Administer analgesics, as ordered, for pain. Remember that patient can have pain but not be able to express it.
• Use this drug only under direct medical supervision by personnel skilled in the use of neuromuscular blockers and techniques for maintaining a patent airway. Don't use unless facilities and equipment for mechanical ventilation, oxygen therapy, and intubation and an antagonist are immediately available.
• **I.V. use:** Drug usually is administered by rapid I.V. bolus injection but may be given by intermittent infusion or continuous infusion. At concentrations of 0.2 mg/ml to 0.5 mg/ml, atracurium is compatible for 24 hours in D_5W, 0.9% sodium chloride injection, or dextrose 5% in 0.9% sodium chloride injection.
• Do not use lactated Ringer's solution. In lactated Ringer's injection, atracurium is stable for 8 hours at a concentration of 0.5 mg/ml. However, because of an increased rate of drug degradation in this solution, it is not recommended.
• Do not administer by I.M. injection.

• Do not mix with acidic or alkaline solutions (precipitate may form).
• Keep airway clear. Have emergency respiratory support equipment (endotracheal equipment, ventilator, oxygen, atropine, edrophonium, neostigmine, and epinephrine) immediately available.
• Once spontaneous recovery starts, be prepared to reverse atracurium-induced neuromuscular blockade with an anticholinesterase agent (such as neostigmine or edrophonium), as ordered. Usually administered together with an anticholinergic (such as atropine).
• Monitor respirations closely until the patient is fully recovered from neuromuscular blockade, as evidenced by tests of muscle strength (hand grip, head lift, and ability to cough).
• Be aware that a nerve stimulator and train-of-four monitoring are recommended to confirm antagonism of neuromuscular blockade and recovery of muscle strength. Before attempting pharmacologic reversal with neostigmine, some evidence of spontaneous recovery should be seen.
• Know that prior administration of succinylcholine doesn't prolong duration of action, but quickens onset and may deepen neuromuscular blockade.
• Keep in mind that atracurium has a longer duration of action than succinylcholine and a shorter duration of action than tubocurarine or pancuronium.

doxacurium chloride
Nuromax

Pregnancy Risk Category: C

HOW SUPPLIED
Injection: 1 mg/ml

ACTION
A nondepolarizing neuromuscular blocking agent that competes with

acetylcholine for receptor sites at the motor end plate; because this action may be antagonized by cholinesterase inhibitors, doxacurium is considered a competitive antagonist.

ONSET, PEAK, DURATION
Onset occurs within 5 minutes. Peak effects are dose-dependent and occur within 3 to 9 minutes. Effects persist 1 to 4 hours.

INDICATIONS & DOSAGE
To provide skeletal muscle relaxation during surgery as an adjunct to general anesthesia –
Dosage is highly individualized. Note that all times of onset and duration of neuromuscular blockade are averages and considerable individual variation is normal.
Adults: 0.05 mg/kg rapid I.V. produces adequate conditions for endotracheal intubation in 5 minutes in about 90% of patients when used as part of a thiopental-narcotic induction technique. Lower doses may require longer delay before intubation is possible. Neuromuscular blockade at this dose will last for an average of 100 minutes.
Children over 2 years: an initial dose of 0.03 mg/kg I.V. administered during halothane anesthesia produces effective blockade in 7 minutes with duration of 30 minutes. Under the same conditions, 0.05 mg/kg produces a blockade in 4 minutes with duration of 45 minutes.
Maintenance of neuromuscular blockade during long procedures –
Adults and children: after initial dose of 0.5 mg/kg I.V., maintenance doses of 0.005 to 0.01 mg/kg will prolong neuromuscular blockade for an average of 30 minutes. Children usually require more frequent administration of maintenance doses.

ADVERSE REACTIONS
Respiratory: dyspnea, respiratory depression, *respiratory insufficiency or apnea*.
Other: prolonged muscle weakness.

INTERACTIONS
Alkaline solutions (such as barbiturate solutions): physically incompatible; precipitate may form. Do not administer through same I.V. line.
Aminoglycosides (gentamicin, kanamycin, neomycin, and streptomycin), bacitracin, colistimethate, colistin, polymyxin B, tetracyclines: potentiated neuromuscular blockade leading to increased skeletal muscle relaxation and prolongation of effect. Use together cautiously.
Carbamazepine, phenytoin: may prolong the time to maximal block or shorten the duration of block with neuromuscular blocking agents.
Inhalation anesthetics, quinidine: may enhance the activity (or prolonged action) of nondepolarizing neuromuscular blocking agents.
Magnesium salts: may enhance neuromuscular blockade. Monitor for excessive weakness.

CONTRAINDICATIONS
Contraindicated in patients with hypersensitivity to the drug and in neonates. The drug contains benzyl ethanol, which has been associated with fatalities in newborns.

NURSING CONSIDERATIONS
● Use cautiously, possibly at reduced dosage, in debilitated patients; in patients with metastatic cancer, severe electrolyte disturbances, or neuromuscular diseases; and in those in whom potentiation or difficulty in reversal of neuromuscular blockade is anticipated. Patients with myasthenia gravis or myasthenic syndrome (Eaton-Lambert syndrome) are particularly sensitive to the effects of nondepolarizing relaxants. Shorter-acting

agents are recommended for use in such patients.

• Because of the lack of data supporting safety, be aware that this drug is not recommended for use in patients requiring prolonged mechanical ventilation in the intensive care unit, before or after administration of nondepolarizing neuromuscular blocking agents, or during cesarean section.

• To avoid distress to the patient, do not administer the drug until the patient's consciousness is obtunded by general anesthetic. Doxacurium has no effect on consciousness or pain threshold.

• **I.V. use:** Prepare drug for I.V. use with D_5W, 0.9% sodium chloride injection, dextrose 5% in 0.9% sodium chloride injection, lactated Ringer's injection, and dextrose 5% in lactated Ringer's injection.

• When diluted as directed, keep in mind that doxacurium is compatible with alfentanil, fentanyl, and sufentanil.

• Recommend that the product be administered immediately after reconstitution. Diluted solutions are stable for 24 hours at room temperature; however, because reconstitution dilutes the preservative, risk of contamination increases. Unused solutions should be discarded after 8 hours.

• Use drug only under direct medical supervision by personnel skilled in the use of neuromuscular blocking agents and techniques for maintaining a patent airway. Do not use unless facilities and equipment for mechanical ventilation, oxygen therapy, and intubation and an antagonist are within reach.

• Be aware that a nerve stimulator and train-of-four monitoring are recommended to document antagonism of neuromuscular blockade and recovery of muscle strength. Before attempting pharmacologic reversal with neostigmine, some evidence of spontaneous recovery should be evident.

• Because the drug has minimal vagolytic action, monitor for bradycardia, which may occur during anesthesia.

• Monitor respirations closely until the patient is fully recovered from neuromuscular blockade, as evidenced by tests of muscle strength (hand grip, head lift, and ability to cough).

• Know that higher initial doses may be required in patients with severe burns and in some patients with severe liver disease. Higher doses (0.8 mg/kg) will produce intubating conditions more rapidly (4 minutes), with neuromuscular blockade for 160 minutes or more. Consequently, these higher doses should be reserved for long procedures. Administration during steady-state anesthesia with enflurane, halothane, or isoflurane may allow 33% reduction of dose.

• Know that experimental evidence suggests that acid-base and electrolyte balance may influence the actions of nondepolarizing neuromuscular blockers. Alkalosis may counteract the paralysis and acidosis may enhance it.

• Be aware that the drug is not metabolized; it is excreted in urine and bile. Therefore, patients with renal or hepatic insufficiency may require dosage adjustment.

• Keep in mind that the dosage should be adjusted to ideal body weight in obese patients (patients 30% or more above their ideal weight) to avoid prolonged neuromuscular blockade.

gallamine triethiodide
Flaxedil

Pregnancy Risk Category: C

HOW SUPPLIED
Injection: 20 mg/ml

ACTION
A nondepolarizing neuromuscular blocking agent that prevents acetyl-

---

*Liquid form contains alcohol.
**May contain tartrazine.

Common reactions are in italics; *life-threatening,* in bold italics.

choline from binding to the receptors on the muscle end plate, thus blocking depolarization and resulting in skeletal muscle paralysis.

ONSET, PEAK, DURATION
Onset occurs in 1 to 2 minutes. Peak effects occur in 3 to 5 minutes. Effects persist for 15 to 30 minutes.

INDICATIONS & DOSAGE
Adjunct to anesthesia to induce skeletal muscle relaxation; to facilitate intubation, reduction of fractures and dislocations; to lessen muscle contractions in pharmacologically or electrically induced seizures; to assist with mechanical ventilation –
Dosage depends on anesthetic used, individual needs, and response. Dosages are representative and must be adjusted.
Adults and children over 1 month: initially, 1 mg/kg I.V. to maximum of 100 mg, regardless of patient's weight; then 0.5 mg to 1 mg/kg q 30 to 40 minutes.
Children under 1 month but over 5 kg (11 lb): initially, 0.25 to 0.75 mg/ kg I.V., then additional doses of 0.1 to 0.5 mg/kg q 30 to 40 minutes, as needed.

ADVERSE REACTIONS
CV: tachycardia.
Respiratory: *respiratory paralysis, dose-related prolonged apnea,* increased oropharyngeal secretions.
Other: residual muscle weakness, allergic or idiosyncratic hypersensitivity reactions.

INTERACTIONS
Aminoglycoside antibiotics (amikacin, gentamicin, kanamycin, neomycin, streptomycin); polymyxin antibiotics (polymyxin B sulfate, colistin); clindamycin; quinidine; general anesthetics (such as halothane, enflurane, isoflurane: potentiated neuromuscular blockade, leading to increased skeletal muscle relaxation and prolongation of effect. Monitor closely.
Narcotic analgesics, I.V. diazepam: potentiated neuromuscular blockade, leading to increased skeletal muscle relaxation and possible respiratory paralysis. Reduce dose of gallamine.

CONTRAINDICATIONS
Contraindicated in patients with hypersensitivity to iodides, impaired renal function, and myasthenia gravis; in patients in shock; and in those in whom tachycardia may be hazardous.

NURSING CONSIDERATIONS
• Use cautiously in elderly or debilitated patients, in patients sensitive to sulfites, and in patients undergoing cesarean section. Also use cautiously in patients with cardiac, hepatic, or pulmonary impairment; respiratory depression; myasthenic syndrome of lung cancer or bronchogenic carcinoma; dehydration; thyroid disorders; collagen diseases; porphyria; and electrolyte disturbances.
• Administer sedatives or general anesthetics before neuromuscular blockers, as ordered. Neuromuscular blockers do not obtund consciousness or alter pain threshold.
• Make sure to explain all events and happenings to the patient because he can still hear.
• Administer analgesics, as ordered, for pain.
• Use drug only under direct medical supervision by personnel skilled in the use of neuromuscular blockers and techniques for maintaining a patent airway. Do not use unless facilities and equipment for artificial respiration, mechanical ventilation, oxygen therapy, and intubation and an antagonist are within reach.
• Keep airway clear. Have emergency respiratory support equipment (endotracheal equipment, ventilator, oxygen, atropine, edrophonium, neostig-

mine, and epinephrine) immediately available.
• **I.V. use:** Give by direct I.V. injection over 30 to 90 seconds.
• Do not mix solution with meperidine or barbiturate solutions.
• Protect drug from light or excessive heat; use only fresh solutions.
• Know that a nerve stimulator and train-of-four monitoring are recommended to confirm antagonism of neuromuscular blockade and recovery of muscle strength. Before attempting pharmacologic reversal, some evidence of spontaneous recovery should exist.
• Take vital signs every 15 minutes, and monitor for developing tachycardia. Notify doctor immediately of significant changes.
• Monitor baseline electrolyte determinations (electrolyte imbalance can potentiate neuromuscular effects).
• Monitor respirations closely until patient is fully recovered from neuromuscular blockade, as evidenced by tests of muscle strength (hand grip, head lift, and ability to cough).

---

metocurine iodide
Metubine Iodide

Pregnancy Risk Category: C

HOW SUPPLIED
Injection: 2 mg/ml

ACTION
A nondepolarizing neuromuscular blocking agent that prevents acetylcholine from binding to receptors on the muscle end plate, thus blocking depolarization.

ONSET, PEAK, DURATION
Onset occurs in 1 to 4 minutes. Peak effects occur in 3 to 5 minutes. Effects persist for 35 to 60 minutes; may take more than 6 hours for more than 50% of muscle twitch strength to return.

INDICATIONS & DOSAGE
Adjunct to anesthesia to induce skeletal muscle relaxation; to facilitate intubation, reduction of fractures and dislocations –
Adults: 0.2 to 0.4 mg/kg for endotracheal intubation; supplemented with 0.5 to 1 mg for additional surgical relaxation.
Lessen muscle contractions in pharmacologically or electrically induced seizures –
Adults: 1.75 to 5.5 mg I.V.

ADVERSE REACTIONS
CV: hypotension secondary to histamine release, ganglionic blockade with rapid dose or overdose.
GI: reduced motility and tone.
Respiratory: *dose-related prolonged apnea, bronchospasm.*
Other: residual muscle weakness, increased oropharyngeal secretions, allergic or idiosyncratic hypersensitivity reactions.

INTERACTIONS
Alkaline solutions, such as barbiturates, meperidine, or morphine: instability when combined in same syringe. Do not administer in same syringe.
Aminoglycoside antibiotics (including amikacin, gentamicin, kanamycin, neomycin, streptomycin); polymyxin antibiotics (polymyxin B sulfate, colistin); clindamycin; quinidine; general anesthetics (such as halothane, enflurane, isoflurane), furosemide, thiazide diuretics, and beta-adrenergic blocking agents: potentiated neuromuscular blockade, leading to increased skeletal muscle relaxation and possible respiratory paralysis. Use cautiously during surgical and postoperative periods.
Opioid analgesics: potentiated neuromuscular blockade, leading to increased skeletal muscle relaxation and possible respiratory paralysis. Use

---

with extreme caution, and reduce dose of metocurine iodide.

CONTRAINDICATIONS

Contraindicated in patients with hypersensitivity to iodides or in whom histamine release is a hazard (asthmatic or atopic patients).

NURSING CONSIDERATIONS

• Use cautiously in elderly or debilitated patients. Also use cautiously in patients with cardiac, renal, hepatic, or pulmonary impairment; respiratory depression; myasthenia gravis; myasthenic syndrome of lung cancer or bronchogenic cancer; dehydration; thyroid disorders; collagen diseases; porphyria; electrolyte disturbances; hyperthermia; hypotension; or shock. Also use large doses cautiously in patients undergoing cesarean section.

• Know that metocurine should only be used by personnel skilled in airway management.

• Administer sedatives or general anesthetics before neuromuscular blockers, as ordered. Neuromuscular blockers do not obtund consciousness or alter pain threshold.

• Make sure to explain all events and happenings to the patient because he can still hear.

• Administer analgesics, as ordered, for pain.

• Keep airway clear. Have emergency respiratory support equipment (endotracheal equipment, ventilator, oxygen, atropine, edrophonium, epinephrine, and neostigmine) immediately available.

• **I.V. use:** Give by direct I.V. injection over 30 to 90 seconds. Dosage depends on anesthetic used, individual needs, and response. Dosages given are representative and must be adjusted. Administer as sustained injection over 30 to 60 seconds. Adults given cyclopropane, 2 to 4 mg I.V. (2.68 mg average); given ether, 1.5 to 3 mg I.V. (2.1 mg average); given ni-

trous oxide, 4 to 7 mg I.V. (4.79 mg average) with supplemental injections of 0.5 to 1 mg in 25 to 90 minutes, repeated p.r.n.

• Do not administer I.M.

• Store solution away from heat and sunlight. Do not mix with barbiturates (precipitate will form). Use fresh solutions only.

• Know that a nerve stimulator and train-of-four monitoring are recommended to document antagonism of neuromuscular blockade and recovery of muscle strength. Before attempting pharmacologic reversal with neostigmine, some evidence of spontaneous recovery should be seen.

• Monitor baseline electrolyte determinations (electrolyte imbalance, especially potassium, calcium, and magnesium as ordered, can potentiate neuromuscular effects) and vital signs, especially respiration.

• Monitor respirations closely until patient is fully recovered from neuromuscular blockade, as evidenced by tests of muscle strength (hand grip, head lift, and ability to cough).

• Measure fluid intake and output; renal dysfunction prolongs duration of action because drug is mainly unchanged before excretion.

• Be aware that dose of 1 mg is the therapeutic equivalent of 3 mg tubocurarine chloride.

---

mivacurium chloride
Mivacron

Pregnancy Risk Category: C

HOW SUPPLIED

Injection: 2 mg/ml in 5-ml and 10-ml vials

Infusion: 0.5 mg/ml in 50 ml of D_5W

ACTION

A nondepolarizing neuromuscular blocking agent that competes with acetylcholine for receptor sites at the motor end plate. Because this action may be antagonized by cholinesterase inhibitors, mivacurium is considered a competitive antagonist. The drug is a mixture of three stereoisomers, each possessing neuromuscular blocking activity.

ONSET, PEAK, DURATION
Onset occurs within 1 to 2 minutes. Peak effects occur in 2 to 5 minutes. 95% muscle twitch strength recovery within 20 to 35 minutes.

INDICATIONS & DOSAGE
As an adjunct to general anesthesia, to facilitate endotracheal intubation, and to relax skeletal muscles during surgery or mechanical ventilation —
Adults: dosage is highly individualized. Usually, 0.15 mg/kg I.V. push over 5 to 15 seconds provides adequate muscle relaxation within 2½ minutes for endotracheal intubation. Supplemental doses of 0.1 mg/kg I.V. q 15 minutes usually sufficient to maintain muscle relaxation.

Alternatively, maintain neuromuscular blockade with a continuous infusion of 4 mcg/kg/minute begun simultaneously with the initial dose, or 9 to 10 mcg/kg/minute started after evidence of spontaneous recovery caused by the initial dose. When used with isoflurane or enflurane anesthesia, dosage usually is reduced about 25%.
Children 2 to 12 years: 0.20 mg/kg I.V. push administered over 5 to 15 seconds. Neuromuscular blockade is usually evident in less than 2 minutes. Maintenance doses are generally required more frequently in children.

Alternatively, neuromuscular blockade maintained with a continuous I.V. infusion titrated to effect. Most children respond to 5 to 31 mcg/kg/minute (average 14 mcg/kg/minute).

ADVERSE REACTIONS
CNS: dizziness.
CV: *flushing,* hypotension, tachycardia, bradycardia, arrhythmias.
Respiratory: ***bronchospasm,*** wheezing, ***respiratory insufficiency or apnea.***
Skin: rash, urticaria, erythema.
Other: prolonged muscle weakness, phlebitis, muscle spasms.

INTERACTIONS
Alkaline solutions (such as barbiturate solutions): physically incompatible; precipitate may form. Do not administer through the same I.V. line.
Aminoglycosides (gentamicin, kanamycin, neomycin, and streptomycin), bacitracin, colistin, colistimethate, polymyxin B sulfate, tetracyclines: potentiated neuromuscular blockade, leading to increased skeletal muscle relaxation and prolongation of effect. Use together cautiously.
Carbamazepine, phenytoin: may prolong the time to maximal blockade or shorten the duration of blockade with neuromuscular blockers.
Inhalation anesthetics (especially isoflurane or enflurane), quinidine: may enhance the activity (or prolonged action) of nondepolarizing neuromuscular blockers. Monitor for excessive weakness.
Magnesium salts: may enhance neuromuscular blockade. Monitor for excessive weakness.

CONTRAINDICATIONS
Contraindicated in patients with hypersensitivity to the drug.

NURSING CONSIDERATIONS
● Use cautiously in patients with significant CV disease and in patients who may be adversely affected by release of histamine (such as asthmatic patients). To avoid hypotension, initial dose of the drug should be lower or drug should be given over longer periods of time (60 seconds).

---

*Liquid form contains alcohol.
**May contain tartrazine.

Common reactions are in italics; *life-threatening,* in bold italics.

• Also use cautiously, possibly at reduced dosage, in debilitated patients; in patients with metastatic cancer, severe electrolyte disturbances, or neuromuscular diseases; and in those in whom potentiation or difficulty in reversal of neuromuscular blockade is anticipated. Patients with myasthenia gravis or myasthenic syndrome (Eaton-Lambert syndrome) are particularly sensitive to effects of nondepolarizing relaxants. Test doses of 0.015 to 0.020 mg/kg may be used to assess the patient's sensitivity to the drug.

• Use very cautiously, if at all, in patients who are homozygous for the atypical plasma pseudocholinesterase gene. Drug is metabolized to inactive compounds by plasma pseudocholinesterase.

• Use only under direct medical supervision by personnel skilled in the use of neuromuscular blockers and techniques for maintaining a patent airway. Do not use unless facilities and equipment for artificial respiration, mechanical ventilation, oxygen therapy, and intubation and an antagonist are within reach.

• To avoid patient distress, do not administer until the patient's consciousness is obtunded by the general anesthetic because drug has no effect on consciousness or pain threshold.

• Administer a test dose to assess the patient's sensitivity to the drug. Patients with severe burns are known to develop resistance to nondepolarizing neuromuscular blockers; however, they also may have reduced plasma pseudocholinesterase activity.

• **I.V. use:** Prepare drug for I.V. use with D_5W, 0.9% sodium chloride injection, dextrose 5% in 0.9% sodium chloride injection, lactated Ringer's injection, and dextrose 5% in lactated Ringer's injection. Diluted solutions are stable for 24 hours at room temperature.

• Remember that when diluted as directed, mivacurium is compatible with alfentanil, fentanil, sufentanil, droperidol, and midazolam.

• For drug available as premixed infusion in D_5W, remove the protective outer wrap, then check container for minor leaks by squeezing the bag before administering. Do not add any other drugs to the container, and do not use the container in series connections.

• Be aware that a nerve stimulator and train-of-four monitoring are recommended to document antagonism of neuromuscular blockade and recovery of muscle strength. Before attempting pharmacologic reversal with neostigmine or edrophonium, some signs of spontaneous recovery should be evident.

• Monitor respirations closely until patient is fully recovered from neuromuscular blockade, as evidenced by tests of muscle strength (hand grip, head lift, and ability to cough).

• Know that experimental evidence suggests that acid-base and electrolyte balances may influence the actions of nondepolarizing neuromuscular blockers. Alkalosis may counteract the paralysis; acidosis may enhance it.

• Keep in mind that dosage should be adjusted to ideal body weight in obese patients (patients 30% or more above their ideal weight) to avoid prolonged neuromuscular blockade.

• Know that the duration of the drug effect is increased about 150% in patients with end-stage renal disease and 300% in patients with hepatic dysfunction.

• Be aware that like other neuromuscular blockers, dosage requirements for children are higher on a mg/kg basis than those for adults. Onset and recovery of neuromuscular blockade occur more rapidly in children.

---

†Available in Canada only.　　‡Available in Australia only.　　◊Available OTC.

pancuronium bromide
Pavulon

Pregnancy Risk Category: C

HOW SUPPLIED
Injection: 1 mg/ml, 2 mg/ml

ACTION
A nondepolarizing neuromuscular blocking agent that prevents acetylcholine from binding to receptors on the muscle end plate, thus blocking depolarization.

ONSET, PEAK, DURATION
Onset occurs in 30 to 45 seconds. Peak effects occur in 3 to 4½ minutes. Effects persist for 35 to 45 minutes; 90% of muscle twitch strength returns within 1 hour.

INDICATIONS & DOSAGE
Adjunct to anesthesia to induce skeletal muscle relaxation; to facilitate intubation; to lessen muscle contractions in pharmacologically or electrically induced seizures; to assist with mechanical ventilation –
Dosage depends on anesthetic used, individual needs, and response. Dosages are representative and must be adjusted.
Adults and children 1 month and over: initially, 0.04 to 0.1 mg/kg I.V.; then 0.01 mg/kg q 30 to 60 minutes.
Neonates up to 1 month: individualized.

ADVERSE REACTIONS
CV: tachycardia, increased blood pressure.
Respiratory: *prolonged dose-related apnea,* wheezing.
Skin: transient rashes.
Other: burning sensation, excessive sweating and salivation, residual muscle weakness, allergic or idiosyncratic hypersensitivity reactions.

INTERACTIONS
Aminoglycoside antibiotics (including amikacin, gentamicin, kanamycin, neomycin, streptomycin); polymyxin antibiotics (polymyxin B sulfate, colistin); clindamycin; quinidine; general anesthetics (such as halothane, enflurane, isoflurane): potentiated neuromuscular blockade, leading to increased skeletal muscle relaxation and prolongation of effect. Use cautiously during surgical and postoperative periods.
Lithium, opioid analgesics: potentiated neuromuscular blockade, leading to increased skeletal muscle relaxation and possible respiratory paralysis. Use with extreme caution, and reduce dose of pancuronium.
Succinylcholine: increased intensity and duration of neuromuscular blockade. Allow effects of succinylcholine to subside before administering pancuronium.

CONTRAINDICATIONS
Contraindicated in patients with hypersensitivity to bromides or preexisting tachycardia and in patients for whom even a minor increase in heart rate is undesirable.

NURSING CONSIDERATIONS
• Use cautiously in elderly or debilitated patients; in patients with renal, hepatic, or pulmonary impairment; and in those with respiratory depression, myasthenia gravis, myasthenic syndrome of lung cancer or bronchogenic carcinoma, dehydration, thyroid disorders, collagen diseases, porphyria, electrolyte disturbances, hyperthermia, and toxemic states. Also use large doses cautiously in patients undergoing cesarean section.
• Administer sedatives or general anesthetics before neuromuscular blockers, as ordered. Neuromuscular blockers do not obtund consciousness or alter the pain threshold.
• Make sure to explain all events and

---

*Liquid form contains alcohol.   *Common* reactions are in italics; ***life-threatening,*** in bold italics.
**May contain tartrazine.

happenings to the patient because he can still hear.

• Administer analgesics, as ordered, for pain.

• Have emergency respiratory support equipment (endotracheal equipment, ventilator, oxygen, atropine, edrophonium, epinephrine, and neostigmine) immediately available.

• **I.V. use:** Do not mix with alkaline solutions, such as barbiturate solutions, because precipitate will form; use only fresh solutions.

• Allow succinylcholine effects to subside before giving pancuronium, as ordered.

• Store in refrigerator. Do not store in plastic containers or syringes, although plastic syringes may be used for administration.

• Monitor baseline electrolyte determinations (electrolyte imbalance can potentiate neuromuscular effects) and vital signs, especially respirations and heart rate.

• Measure fluid intake and output; renal dysfunction may prolong duration of action because 25% of the drug is unchanged before excretion.

• Keep in mind that a nerve stimulator and train-of-four monitoring are recommended to confirm antagonism of neuromuscular blockade and recovery of muscle strength. Before attempting pharmacologic reversal with neostigmine, some evidence of spontaneous recovery should be seen.

• Monitor respirations closely until patient is fully recovered from neuromuscular blockade, as evidenced by tests of muscle strength (hand grip, head lift, and ability to cough).

• Once spontaneous recovery starts, be aware that pancuronium-induced neuromuscular blockade may be reversed with an anticholinesterase agent (such as neostigmine or edrophonium). Usually administered with an anticholinergic (such as atropine).

• Be aware that drug does not cause histamine release or hypotension, but may raise heart rate and blood pressure.

• Know that pancuronium should be used only by personnel skilled in airway management.

---

pipecuronium bromide
Arduan

Pregnancy Risk Category: C

HOW SUPPLIED
Powder for injection: 10 mg/vial

ACTION
A nondepolarizing neuromuscular blocking agent that competes with acetylcholine for receptor sites at the motor end plate. Because this action may be antagonized by cholinesterase inhibitors, pipecuronium is considered a competitive antagonist.

ONSET, PEAK, DURATION
Onset occurs in 1 to 2 minutes. Peak effects occur within 5 minutes. 25% to 50% of muscle twitch strength returns within 24 minutes.

INDICATIONS & DOSAGE
To provide skeletal muscle relaxation during surgery as adjunct to general anesthesia –
Dosage is highly individualized. The following doses may serve as a guide for use in nonobese patients with normal renal function.
Adults and children: initially, 70 to 85 mcg/kg I.V. provides conditions considered ideal for endotracheal intubation and maintains paralysis for 1 to 2 hours. If succinylcholine is used for endotracheal intubation, initial dose of 50 mcg/kg I.V. provides good relaxation for 45 minutes or more. Maintenance dose of 10 to 15 mcg/kg provides relaxation for about 50 minutes.

---

†Available in Canada only.   ‡Available in Australia only.   ◇Available OTC.

ADVERSE REACTIONS
CV: hypotension, bradycardia, hypertension, myocardial ischemia, *CVA,* thrombosis, atrial fibrillation, *ventricular extrasystole.*
GU: anuria.
Respiratory: dyspnea, respiratory depression, *respiratory insufficiency or apnea.*
Other: prolonged muscle weakness, increased creatinine levels.

INTERACTIONS
Aminoglycosides (gentamicin, kanamycin, neomycin, and streptomycin), bacitracin, colistimethate, colistin, polymyxin B sulfate, tetracyclines: potentiated neuromuscular blockade, leading to increased skeletal muscle relaxation and prolongation of effect. Use together cautiously.
Inhalation anesthetics, quinidine: enhanced activity (or prolonged action) of nondepolarizing neuromuscular blocking agents.
Magnesium salts: may enhance neuromuscular blockade. Monitor for excessive weakness.

CONTRAINDICATIONS
Contraindicated in patients with hypersensitivity to the drug.

NURSING CONSIDERATIONS
• Use cautiously and with dosage adjustments in patients with renal failure because the drug is excreted by the kidneys. No information is available regarding use of the drug in patients with hepatic disease.
• Use drug under direct medical supervision by personnel skilled in use of neuromuscular blockers and techniques for maintaining a patent airway. Do not use drug unless facilities and equipment for artificial respiration, mechanical ventilation, oxygen therapy, and intubation and an antagonist are within reach.
• Because of its prolonged duration of action, keep in mind that pipecuronium is recommended only for procedures that take 90 minutes or longer.
• Administer pipecuronium after succinylcholine when the latter is used to facilitate intubation. However, no evidence exists to support safe use of pipecuronium before succinylcholine to decrease adverse effects of the latter drug.
• Give patients sedatives or general anesthetics before neuromuscular blockers are administered, as ordered. Neuromuscular blockers do not obtund consciousness or alter pain threshold.
• **I.V. use:** Reconstitute with 10 ml solution before use to yield a solution of 1 mg/ml. Large volumes of diluent or addition of the drug to a hanging I.V. solution is not recommended.
• After reconstitution with sterile water for injection or other compatible I.V. solutions (such as 0.9% sodium chloride injection, D_5W, lactated Ringer's injection, dextrose 5% in 0.9% sodium chloride), know that the drug is stable for 24 hours if refrigerated.
• After reconstitution with any solution other than bacteriostatic water for injection, discard unused drug.
• After reconstitution with bacteriostatic water for injection, know that the drug is stable for 5 days at room temperature or in the refrigerator. Note that bacteriostatic water contains benzyl alcohol and is not intended for use in neonates.
• Store the powder at room temperature or in the refrigerator (36° to 86° F [2° to 30° C]).
• Monitor respirations closely until patient is fully recovered from neuromuscular blockade, as evidenced by tests of muscle strength (hand grip, head lift, and ability to cough).
• Because the drug has minimal vagolytic action, monitor for bradycardia during anesthesia, which may be common.
• Know that a nerve stimulator and

---

train-of-four monitoring are recommended to document antagonism of neuromuscular blockade and recovery of muscle strength. Before attempting pharmacologic reversal with neostigmine, some evidence of spontaneous recovery should be evident.

• Because of the lack of data supporting safety, know that this drug is not recommended for use in patients requiring prolonged mechanical ventilation in the intensive care unit, before or after administration of other nondepolarizing neuromuscular blockers, or during cesarean section.

• Be aware that patients with myasthenia gravis or myasthenic syndrome (Eaton-Lambert syndrome) are particularly sensitive to the effects of nondepolarizing relaxants. Shorter-acting agents are recommended for use in such patients.

• Keep in mind that the drug is not recommended for use in neonates and infants younger than 3 months. Limited evidence suggests that infants and children (ages 1 to 14) under balanced anesthesia or halothane anesthesia may be less sensitive than adults.

• Know that dosage should be adjusted to ideal body weight in obese patients (30% or more over their ideal weight) to avoid prolonged neuromuscular blockade.

• Be aware that experimental evidence suggests that acid-base and electrolyte balances may influence the actions of nondepolarizing neuromuscular blocking agents. Alkalosis may counteract the paralysis and acidosis may enhance it.

---

rocuronium bromide
Zemuron

Pregnancy Risk Category: B

HOW SUPPLIED
Injection: 10 mg/ml

ACTION
A nondepolarizing neuromuscular blocking agent that prevents acetylcholine from binding to receptors on the muscle end plate, thus blocking depolarization.

ONSET, PEAK, DURATION
Onset occurs within 1 minute. Peak effects occur within 2 minutes in most patients. Duration is dose-dependent; 25% recovery of muscle twitch strength occurs within 22 to 67 minutes.

INDICATIONS & DOSAGE
Adjunct to general anesthesia, to facilitate endotracheal intubation and to provide skeletal muscle relaxation during surgery or mechanical ventilation –
Dosage depends on anesthetic used, individual needs, and response. Dosages are representative and must be adjusted.
Adults and children: initially, 0.6 mg/kg I.V. bolus. In most patients, tracheal intubation may be performed within 2 minutes; muscle paralysis should last about 22 minutes. A maintenance dosage of 0.1 mg/kg should provide an additional 12 minutes of muscle relaxation; 0.15 mg/kg will add 17 minutes; or 0.2 mg/kg will add 24 minutes to the duration of effect.

ADVERSE REACTIONS
CV: tachycardia, abnormal ECG, arrhythmias (rare).
GI: nausea, vomiting.
Respiratory: asthma.
Local: rash, edema.
Other: hiccups.

INTERACTIONS
Aminoglycoside antibiotics (including amikacin, gentamicin, kanamycin, neomycin, streptomycin); polymyxin antibiotics (polymyxin B sulfate, colistin); anticonvulsants; clindamycin; quinidine; general anesthetics (such

---

as halothane, enflurane, isoflurane); opiate analgesics: potentiated neuromuscular blockade, leading to increased skeletal muscle relaxation and potentiation of effect. Use cautiously during surgical and postoperative periods.

CONTRAINDICATIONS
Contraindicated in patients with hypersensitivity to bromides.

NURSING CONSIDERATIONS
• Use cautiously in patients with altered circulation time caused by CV disease, old age, and edematous states; hepatic disease; severe obesity; bronchogenic carcinoma; electrolyte disturbances; and neuromuscular disease.
• Administer sedatives or general anesthetics before neuromuscular blockers, as ordered. Neuromuscular blockers do not obtund consciousness or alter the pain threshold.
• Make sure to explain all events and happenings to the patient because he can still hear.
• Administer analgesics, as ordered, for pain.
• Keep airway clear. Have emergency respiratory support equipment (endotracheal equipment, ventilator, oxygen, atropine, edrophonium, epinephrine, and neostigmine) immediately available.
• **I.V. use:** Administer by rapid I.V. injection. Alternatively, give by continuous I.V. infusion. Infusion rates are highly individualized but have ranged from 0.004 to 0.16 mg/kg/minute. Compatible solutions include D_5W, 0.9% sodium chloride injection, dextrose 5% in 0.9% sodium chloride injection, sterile water for injection, and lactated Ringer's injection.
• Store reconstituted solution in refrigerator. Discard after 24 hours.
• Know that a nerve stimulator and train-of-four monitoring are recommended to confirm antagonism of

neuromuscular blockade and recovery of muscle strength. Before attempting pharmacologic reversal with neostigmine, some evidence of spontaneous recovery should be evident.
• Keep in mind that prior administration of succinylcholine may enhance neuromuscular blocking effect and duration of action.
• Monitor patients with liver disease because they may require higher doses of the drug to achieve adequate muscle relaxation. However, such patients exhibit prolonged effects from the drug.
• Know that rocuronium should be used only by personnel skilled in airway management.
• Be aware that unlike many other nondepolarizing neuromuscular blockers, rocuronium has no effect on the CV system. Also, the drug causes no histamine release and therefore no histamine-related hypersensitivity reactions, such as bronchospasm, hypotension, or tachycardia.
• Monitor respirations closely until patient is fully recovered from neuromuscular blockade, as evidenced by tests of muscle strength (hand grip, head lift, and ability to cough).
• Know that rocuronium is well tolerated in patients with renal failure.
• Be alert that rocuronium provides conditions for intubation within 3 minutes. Effect lasts 25 to 40 minutes.
• Because of lack of clinical experience with the drug, be aware that the drug it is not recommended for use during rapid sequence induction for cesarean section.

succinylcholine chloride (suxamethonium chloride)
Anectine, Anectine Flo-Pack, Quelicin, Scoline‡, Sucostrin
Pregnancy Risk Category: C

HOW SUPPLIED
Injection: 20 mg/ml, 50 mg/ml, 100 mg/ml; 100 mg/vial, 500 mg/vial, 1 g/vial

ACTION
A depolarizing neuromuscular blocking agent that prolongs depolarization of the muscle end plate.

ONSET, PEAK, DURATION
Onset occurs in 30 seconds to 1 minute after I.V. use; 2 to 3 minutes after I.M. use. Peak effects occur in 1 to 2 minutes after I.V. use. Effects persist 4 to 10 minutes after I.V. use, 10 to 30 minutes after I.M. use.

INDICATIONS & DOSAGE
Adjunct to anesthesia to induce skeletal muscle relaxation; to facilitate intubation and assist with mechanical ventilation or orthopedic manipulations (drug of choice); to lessen muscle contractions in pharmacologically or electrically induced seizures –
Dosage depends on anesthetic used, individual needs, and response. Dosages are representative and must be adjusted.
Adults: 25 to 75 mg I.V., then 2.5 mg/minute, p.r.n., or 2.5 mg/kg I.M. up to maximum of 150 mg I.M. in deltoid muscle.
Children: 1 to 2 mg/kg I.M. or I.V. Maximum I.M. dosage is 150 mg. (Children may be less sensitive to succinylcholine than adults.)

ADVERSE REACTIONS
CV: bradycardia, tachycardia, hypertension, hypotension, *arrhythmias.*
EENT: increased intraocular pressure.
Respiratory: *prolonged respiratory depression, apnea.*
Other: malignant hyperthermia, muscle fasciculation, *postoperative muscle pain,* myoglobinemia, excessive salivation, allergic or idiosyncratic hypersensitivity reactions.

INTERACTIONS
Aminoglycoside antibiotics (including amikacin, gentamicin, kanamycin, neomycin, streptomycin); polymyxin antibiotics (polymyxin B sulfate, colistin); cholinesterase inhibitors (such as neostigmine, pyridostigmine, edrophonium, physostigmine, or echothiophate); general anesthetics (such as halothane, enflurane, isoflurane): potentiated neuromuscular blockade, leading to increased skeletal muscle relaxation and potentiation of effect. Use cautiously during surgical and postoperative periods.
Cyclophosphamide, lithium, MAO inhibitors: prolonged apnea. Use with caution.
Digitalis glycosides: may cause arrhythmias. Use together cautiously.
Methotrimeprazine, opioid analgesics: potentiated neuromuscular blockade, leading to increased skeletal muscle relaxation and possible respiratory paralysis. Use with extreme caution.
Parenteral magnesium sulfate: potentiated neuromuscular blockade, increased skeletal muscle relaxation, and possible respiratory paralysis. Use with caution, preferably with reduced doses.

CONTRAINDICATIONS
Contraindicated in patients with hypersensitivity to the drug and in patients with abnormally low plasma pseudocholinesterase, angle-closure glaucoma, malignant hyperthermia, or penetrating eye injuries.

NURSING CONSIDERATIONS
• Use cautiously in elderly or debilitated patients; in patients receiving quinidine or digitalis glycoside therapy; in patients with hepatic, renal, or pulmonary impairment; in those with respiratory depression, severe burns or trauma, electrolyte imbalances, hyperkalemia, paraplegia, spinal neuraxis injury, CVA, degenerative or

dystrophic neuromuscular disease, myasthenia gravis, myasthenic syndrome of lung cancer or bronchogenic carcinoma, dehydration, thyroid disorders, collagen diseases, porphyria, fractures, muscle spasms, eye surgery, and pheochromocytoma. Also use large doses cautiously in patients undergoing cesarean section.

• Administer sedatives or general anesthetics before neuromuscular blockers, as ordered. Neuromuscular blockers do not obtund consciousness or alter the pain threshold.

• Make sure to explain all events and happenings to the patient because he can still hear.

• Administer analgesics, as ordered, for pain.

• Keep airway clear. Have emergency respiratory support equipment (endotracheal equipment, ventilator, oxygen, atropine, and epinephrine) immediately available.

• **I.V. use:** Give test dose (10 mg I.M. or I.V.) after patient has been anesthetized. Normal response (no respiratory depression or transient depression for up to 5 minutes) indicates drug may be given. Do not give if patient develops respiratory paralysis sufficient to permit endotracheal intubation. (Recovery within 30 to 60 minutes.)

• **I.M. use:** give deep I.M., preferably high into deltoid muscle.

• Reassure patients that postoperative stiffness is normal and will soon subside.

• Store injectable form in refrigerator. Store powder form at room temperature in tightly closed container. Use immediately after reconstitution. Do not mix with alkaline solutions (thiopental sodium, sodium bicarbonate, or barbiturates).

• Monitor baseline electrolyte determinations and vital signs (check respiration every 5 to 10 minutes during infusion).

• Monitor respirations closely until patient is fully recovered from neuromuscular blockade, as evidenced by tests of muscle strength (hand grip, head lift, and ability to cough).

• Don't use reversing agents. Unlike nondepolarizing agents, neostigmine or edrophonium may worsen neuromuscular blockade.

• Know that repeated or continuous infusions of succinylcholine are not advised; may cause reduced response or prolonged muscle relaxation and apnea.

• Be aware that succinylcholine should be used only by personnel skilled in airway management.

• Know that succinylcholine is the drug of choice for short procedures (less than 3 minutes) and for orthopedic manipulations; use caution in fractures or dislocations.

tubocurarine chloride
Tubarine†

Pregnancy Risk Category: C

HOW SUPPLIED
Injection: 3 mg (20 units)/ml; 10 mg/ml‡

ACTION
A nondepolarizing neuromuscular blocking agent that prevents acetylcholine from binding to receptors on the muscle end plate, thus blocking depolarization.

ONSET, PEAK, DURATION
Onset occurs within 1 minute. Peak effects occur in 2 to 5 minutes. Effects persist for 20 to 40 minutes; 50% recovery of muscle twitch strength within 50 minutes, 90% recovery within 75 to 90 minutes.

INDICATIONS & DOSAGE
Adjunct to anesthesia to induce skeletal muscle relaxation; to facilitate intubation, orthopedic manipulations – Dosage depends on anesthetic used,

---

*Liquid form contains alcohol.
**May contain tartrazine.

Common reactions are in italics; ***life-threatening,*** in bold italics.

individual needs, and response. Dosages listed are representative and must be adjusted.

Adults: 1 unit/kg or 0.15 mg/kg I.V. slowly over 60 to 90 seconds. Average dose is initially, 40 to 60 units I.V. May give 20 to 30 units in 3 to 5 minutes. For longer procedures, give 20 units, p.r.n.

Children: 1 unit/kg or 0.15 mg/kg.
To assist with mechanical ventilation –
Adults and children: initially, 0.0165 mg/kg I.V. (average 1 mg or 7 units), then adjust subsequent doses to patient response.
To lessen muscle contractions in pharmacologically or electrically induced seizures –
Adults and children: 1 unit/kg or 0.15 mg/kg over 60 to 90 seconds. Initial dose is 20 units (3 mg) less than calculated dose.
Diagnosis of myasthenia gravis –
Adults: 4 to 33 mcg/kg as a single I.V. dose.

ADVERSE REACTIONS
CV: hypotension, circulatory depression.
Respiratory: *respiratory depression or apnea, bronchospasm.*
Other: profound and prolonged muscle relaxation, hypersensitivity reactions, idiosyncrasy, residual muscle weakness, increased salivation.

INTERACTIONS
Aminoglycoside antibiotics (including amikacin, gentamicin, kanamycin, neomycin, streptomycin); polymyxin antibiotics (polymyxin B sulfate, colistin); general anesthetics (such as halothane, enflurane, isoflurane): potentiated neuromuscular blockade, leading to increased skeletal muscle relaxation and potentiation of effect. Use cautiously during surgical and postoperative periods.
Amphotericin B, ethacrynic acid, furosemide, methotrimeprazine, opioid analgesics, propranolol, thiazide diuretics: potentiated neuromuscular blockade, leading to increased skeletal muscle relaxation and possible respiratory paralysis. Use with extreme caution during surgical and postoperative periods.
Quinidine: prolonged neuromuscular blockade. Use together with caution. Monitor closely.

CONTRAINDICATIONS
Contraindicated in patients with hypersensitivity to the drug and in patients for whom histamine release is a hazard (asthmatic patients).

NURSING CONSIDERATIONS
• Use cautiously in elderly or debilitated patients and in those with hepatic or pulmonary impairment, hypothermia, respiratory depression, myasthenia gravis, myasthenic syndrome of lung cancer or bronchogenic carcinoma, dehydration, thyroid disorders, collagen diseases, porphyria, electrolyte disturbances, fractures, and muscle spasms. Also use large doses cautiously in patients undergoing cesarean section.
• Keep airway clear. Have emergency respiratory support equipment (endotracheal equipment, ventilator, oxygen, atropine, edrophonium, epinephrine, and neostigmine) immediately available.
• Allow succinylcholine effects to subside before giving tubocurarine.
• Administer sedatives or general anesthetics before neuromuscular blockers, as ordered. Neuromuscular blockers do not obtund consciousness or alter the pain threshold.
• Make sure to explain all events and happenings to the patient because he still can hear.
• Administer analgesics, as ordered, for pain.
• Monitor baseline electrolyte determinations (electrolyte imbalance can potentiate neuromuscular blocking effects).

• **I.V. use:** Give I.V. over 60 to 90 seconds.
• Do not mix with barbiturates (precipitate will form). Use only fresh solutions and discard if discolored.
• Check vital signs every 15 minutes. Notify the doctor at once of changes.
• Measure fluid intake and output; renal dysfunction prolongs duration of action because much of drug is unchanged before excretion.
• Know that a nerve stimulator and train-of-four monitoring are recommended to confirm antagonism of neuromuscular blockade and recovery of muscle strength. Before attempting pharmacologic reversal with neostigmine, some evidence of spontaneous recovery should be evident.
• Monitor respirations closely until patient is fully recovered from neuromuscular blockade, as evidenced by tests of muscle strength (hand grip, head lift, and ability to cough).
• Know that only personnel skilled in airway management should administer tubocurarine.

vecuronium bromide
Norcuron

Pregnancy Risk Category: C

HOW SUPPLIED
Injection: 10 mg/vial

ACTION
A nondepolarizing neuromuscular blocking agent that prevents acetylcholine from binding to receptors on the muscle end plate, thus blocking depolarization.

ONSET, PEAK, DURATION
Onset occurs within 1 minute. Peak effects occur in 3 to 5 minutes. Effects persist for 25 to 30 minutes; 25% recovery of muscle twitch strength within 24 to 40 minutes, 95% recovery in 45 to 65 minutes.

INDICATIONS & DOSAGE
Adjunct to general anesthesia, to facilitate endotracheal intubation and to provide skeletal muscle relaxation during surgery or mechanical ventilation – Dosage depends on anesthetic used, individual needs, and response. Dosages are representative and must be adjusted.
Adults and children over age 9: initially, 0.08 to 0.10 mg/kg I.V. bolus. Maintenance doses of 0.010 to 0.015 mg/kg within 25 to 40 minutes of initial dose should be administered during prolonged surgical procedures. Maintenance doses may be given q 12 to 15 minutes in patients receiving balanced anesthesia.
Children under age 9: may require a slightly higher initial dose and also may require supplementation slightly more often than adults. Alternatively, drug may be given by continuous I.V. infusion of 1 mcg/kg/minute initially, then 0.8 to 1.2 mcg/kg/minute.

ADVERSE REACTIONS
CV: transient increases in heart rate.
Respiratory: *prolonged dose-related apnea.*
Other: redness, itching, induration.

INTERACTIONS
Aminoglycoside antibiotics (including amikacin, gentamicin, kanamycin, neomycin, streptomycin); polymyxin antibiotics (polymyxin B sulfate, colistin); clindamycin; quinidine; general anesthetics (such as halothane, enflurane, isoflurane): potentiated neuromuscular blockade, leading to increased skeletal muscle relaxation and potentiation of effect. Use cautiously during surgical and postoperative periods.
Opioid analgesics: potentiated neuromuscular blockade, leading to increased skeletal muscle relaxation and possible respiratory paralysis. Use with extreme caution, and reduce dose of vecuronium.

---

*Liquid form contains alcohol.   *Common* reactions are in italics; **life-threatening,** in bold italics.
**May contain tartrazine.

CONTRAINDICATIONS

Contraindicated in patients with hypersensitivity to bromides.

NURSING CONSIDERATIONS

• Use cautiously in elderly patients; in patients with altered circulation caused by CV disease and edematous states; and in those with hepatic disease, severe obesity, bronchogenic carcinoma, electrolyte disturbances, and neuromuscular disease.
• Keep airway clear. Have emergency respiratory support equipment (endotracheal equipment, ventilator, oxygen, atropine, edrophonium, epinephrine, and neostigmine) immediately available.
• Administer sedatives or general anesthetics before neuromuscular blockers, as ordered. Neuromuscular blockers do not obtund consciousness or alter the pain threshold.
• Make sure to explain all events and happenings to the patient because he can still hear.
• Administer analgesics, as ordered, for pain.
• **I.V. use:** Administer by rapid I.V. injection. Alternatively, 10 to 20 mg may be added to 100 ml of a compatible solution and given by I.V. infusion. Compatible solutions include D_5W, 0.9% sodium chloride injection, dextrose 5% in 0.9% sodium chloride injection, and lactated Ringer's injection.
• Do not mix with alkaline solutions.
• Store reconstituted solution in refrigerator. Discard after 24 hours.
• Know that a nerve stimulator and train-of-four monitoring are recommended to confirm antagonism of neuromuscular blockade and recovery of muscle strength. Before attempting pharmacologic reversal with neostigmine, some evidence of spontaneous recovery should be seen.
• Monitor respirations closely until patient is fully recovered from neuromuscular blockade as evidenced by

tests of muscle strength (hand grip, head lift, and ability to cough).
• Keep in mind that prior administration of succinylcholine may enhance the neuromuscular blocking effect and duration of action.
• Know that vecuronium is well tolerated in patients with renal failure.
• Know that the drug should be used only by personnel skilled in airway management.
• Be aware that unlike other nondepolarizing neuromuscular blockers, vecuronium has no effect on the CV system. Also, the drug causes no histamine release and therefore no histamine-related hypersensitivity reactions, such as bronchospasm, hypotension, or tachycardia.

Antihistamines

astemizole
azatadine maleate
brompheniramine maleate
chlorpheniramine maleate
clemastine fumarate
cyproheptadine hydrochloride
dexchlorpheniramine maleate
diphenhydramine hydrochloride
loratadine
methdilazine hydrochloride
promethazine hydrochloride
promethazine theoclate
terfenadine
trimeprazine tartrate
tripelennamine citrate
tripelennamine hydrochloride
triprolidine hydrochloride

COMBINATION PRODUCTS

ALLEREST MAXIMUM STRENGTH TABLETS◇: pseudoephedrine hydrochloride 30 mg and chlorpheniramine maleate 2 mg.

CHLOR-TRIMETON ALLERGY DECONGESTANT◇: chlorpheniramine maleate 4 mg and pseudoephedrine sulfate 60 mg.

CHLOR-TRIMETON DECONGESTANT REPETABS◇: chlorpheniramine maleate 8 mg and pseudoephedrine sulfate 120 mg.

CLARITIN-D: loratadine 5 mg and pseudoephedrine sulfate 120 mg.

CONDRIN-LA: phenylpropanolamine hydrochloride 75 mg and chlorpheniramine maleate 12 mg.

CONTAC CAPSULES◇: phenylpropanolamine 75 mg and chlorpheniramine maleate 8 mg.

CONTAC 12-HOUR CAPLETS◇: phenylpropanolamine 75 mg and chlorpheniramine maleate 8 mg.

CORICIDIN D TABLETS◇: chlorpheniramine maleate 2 mg, acetaminophen 325 mg, and phenylpropranolamine hydrochloride 12.5 mg.

DECONAMINE: pseudoephedrine hydrochloride 60 mg and chlorpheniramine maleate 4 mg.

DIMETAPP EXTENTABS: brompheniramine maleate 12 mg and phenylpropanolamine hydrochloride 75 mg.

DRIZE: phenylpropanolamine hydrochloride 75 mg and chlorpheniramine maleate 12 mg.

FEDAHIST: pseudoephedrine hydrochloride 60 mg and chlorpheniramine maleate 4 mg.

NALDECON: phenylephrine hydrochloride 10 mg, phenylpropanolamine hydrochloride 40 mg, phenyltoloxamine citrate 15 mg, and chlorpheniramine maleate 5 mg.

NOLAMINE: chlorpheniramine maleate 4 mg, phenindamine tartrate 24 mg, and phenylpropanolamine hydrochloride 50 mg.

NOVAFED A: pseudoephedrine hydrochloride 120 mg and chlorpheniramine maleate 8 mg.

NOVAHISTINE ELIXIR◇*: phenylephrine 5 mg, chlorpheniramine maleate 2 mg, and alcohol 5% per 5 ml.

ORNADE SPANSULES: phenylpropanolamine hydrochloride 75 mg and chlorpheniramine maleate 12 mg.

P-V TUSSIN SYRUP*: chlorpheniramine maleate 2 mg/5 ml, phenindamine tartrate 5 mg/5 ml, phenylephrine hydrochloride 5 mg/ 5 ml, and pyrilamine maleate 6 mg/5 ml.

SELDANE-D: terfenadine 60 mg and pseudoephedrine hydrochloride 120 mg.

SUDAFED PLUS◇: pseudoephedrine hydrochloride 60 mg and chlorpheniramine maleate 4 mg.

TAVIST-D◇: clemastine fumarate 1.34 mg and phenylpropanolamine 75 mg.

TRIAMINIC-12: phenylpropanolamine hydrochloride 75 mg and chlorpheniramine maleate 12 mg.

*Liquid form contains alcohol.   *Common* reactions are in italics; *life-threatening,* in bold italics.
**May contain tartrazine.

TRINALIN REPETABS: azatadine maleate 1 mg and pseudoephedrine sulfate 120 mg.

---

astemizole
Hismanal

Pregnancy Risk Category: C

HOW SUPPLIED
Tablets: 10 mg
Oral suspension: 2 mg/ml*‡

ACTION
Blocks effects of histamine at H_1 receptors. Astemizole is a nonsedating antihistamine; its chemical structure prevents entry into the CNS.

ONSET, PEAK, DURATION
Onset occurs within 24 hours. Serum levels peak within 1 hour. Duration unknown.

INDICATIONS AND DOSAGE
Relief of symptoms associated with chronic idiopathic urticaria and seasonal allergic rhinitis –
Adults and children over 12 years: 10 mg P.O. daily.

ADVERSE REACTIONS
CNS: headache, nervousness, dizziness, drowsiness.
CV: arrhythmias (with high plasma levels).
EENT: dry mouth, pharyngitis, conjunctivitis.
GI: nausea, diarrhea, abdominal pain, increased appetite.
Other: arthralgia, weight gain, cholestatic jaundice.

INTERACTIONS
Itraconazole, ketoconazole, macrolide antibiotics (such as erythromycin): risk of serious adverse cardiac reactions. Don't use together.

CONTRAINDICATIONS
Contraindicated in patients with hypersensitivity to astemizole and in patients taking the antifungal agents itraconazole or ketoconazole or macrolide antibiotics, including erythromycin.

NURSING CONSIDERATIONS
• Use cautiously in patients with hepatic or renal disease.
• Also use cautiously in patients with lower respiratory tract diseases (including asthma); drying effects can increase the risk of bronchial mucus plug formation.
• Ensure that patients know to take astemizole only once a day. If symptoms persist or worsen, warn patients not to increase dosage without consulting doctor. High doses may increase risk of arrhythmias.
• Instruct patient to take drug on an empty stomach at least 2 hours after a meal and to avoid eating for at least 1 hour after dosing.
• Warn patients to stop drug 4 days before allergy skin tests to preserve accuracy of tests.

---

azatadine maleate
Optimine, Zadine‡

Pregnancy Risk Category: B

HOW SUPPLIED
Tablets: 1 mg
Syrup: 0.5 mg/5 ml‡

ACTION
Competes with histamine for H_1-receptor sites on effector cells. Prevents, but does not reverse, histamine-mediated responses.

ONSET, PEAK, DURATION
Onset occurs within 15 to 60 minutes. Plasma levels peak within 4 hours. Effects persist for 12 hours.

---

†Available in Canada only.   ‡Available in Australia only.   ◊ Available OTC.

INDICATIONS & DOSAGE
Rhinitis, allergy symptoms, chronic urticaria –
Adults and children 12 years and older: 1 to 2 mg P.O. b.i.d. Maximum dosage is 4 mg daily.

ADVERSE REACTIONS
CNS: (especially in elderly patients) *drowsiness, dizziness,* vertigo, disturbed coordination.
CV: hypotension, palpitations.
GI: anorexia, nausea, vomiting, *dry mouth and throat,* epigastric distress.
GU: urine retention.
Hematologic: thrombocytopenia.
Respiratory: thick bronchial secretions.
Skin: urticaria, rash.

INTERACTIONS
CNS depressants: increased sedation. Use together cautiously.
MAO inhibitors: increased anticholinergic effects. Don't use together.

CONTRAINDICATIONS
Contraindicated in patients with acute asthmatic attacks and in breast-feeding patients.

NURSING CONSIDERATIONS
• Use cautiously in elderly patients and in patients with increased intraocular pressure, hyperthyroidism, CV or renal disease, hypertension, bronchial asthma, urine retention, prostatic hyperplasia, bladder-neck obstruction, and stenosing peptic ulcerations.
• Monitor blood counts during long-term therapy, as ordered; watch for signs of blood dyscrasias.
• Instruct patient to reduce GI distress by giving drug with food or milk.
• Tell patients to stop drug 4 days before allergy skin tests to preserve accuracy of tests.
• Warn patients to avoid alcohol and

activities that require alertness until drug's CNS effects are known.
• Inform patient that coffee or tea may reduce drowsiness. Sugarless gum, sugarless sour hard candy, or ice chips may relieve dry mouth.
• Tell patient to notify doctor if tolerance develops because a different antihistamine may need to be prescribed.

---

brompheniramine maleate
Bromphen*◇, Chlorphed◇, Codimal-A, Conjec-B◇, Cophene-B, Dehist, Diamine T.D., Dimetane*◇, Dimetane Extentabs◇, Histaject Modified, Nasahist B, ND-Stat Revised, Oraminic II, Veltane

Pregnancy Risk Category: C

HOW SUPPLIED
Tablets: 4 mg◇
Tablets (extended-release): 8 mg◇, 12 mg◇
Elixir: 2 mg/5 ml*◇
Injection: 10 mg/ml

ACTION
Competes with histamine for H_1-receptor sites on effector cells. Prevents, but does not reverse, histamine-mediated responses.

ONSET, PEAK, DURATION
Onset occurs in 15 to 60 minutes. Peak levels occur within 2 to 5 hours. Peak effects occur in 3 to 9 hours. Effects persist for 4 to 8 hours for regular release preparations, longer for extended-release preparations.

INDICATIONS & DOSAGE
Rhinitis, allergy symptoms –
Adults: 4 to 8 mg P.O. t.i.d. or q.i.d.; or 8 to 12 mg extended-release P.O. b.i.d. or t.i.d.; or 5 to 20 mg q 6 to 12 hours I.M., I.V., or S.C. Maximum dosage is 40 mg daily.
Children 6 years and over: 2 to 4 mg

---

*Liquid form contains alcohol. *Common* reactions are in italics; **life-threatening,** in bold italics.
**May contain tartrazine.

P.O. t.i.d. or q.i.d.; or 8 to 12 mg extended-release P.O. q 12 hours; or 0.5 mg/kg I.M., I.V., or S.C. daily in divided doses t.i.d. or q.i.d.
Children under 6 years: 0.5 mg/kg P.O., I.M., I.V., or S.C. daily in divided doses t.i.d. or q.i.d.

Note: Children under 12 years should use only as directed by a doctor.

ADVERSE REACTIONS
CNS: (especially in elderly patients) dizziness, tremors, irritability, insomnia, *drowsiness, stimulation.*
CV: hypotension, palpitations.
GI: anorexia, nausea, vomiting, *dry mouth and throat.*
GU: urine retention.
Hematologic: thrombocytopenia, *agranulocytosis.*
Skin: urticaria, rash.
Other: (after parenteral administration) local stinging, diaphoresis, syncope.

INTERACTIONS
CNS depressants: increased sedation. Use together cautiously.
MAO inhibitors: increased anticholinergic effects. Don't use together.

CONTRAINDICATIONS
Contraindicated in patients with hypersensitivity to any of the drug's ingredients; in those with acute asthmatic attacks, severe hypertension or coronary artery disease, angle-closure glaucoma, urine retention, and peptic ulcer; and within 14 days of MAO inhibitor therapy.

NURSING CONSIDERATIONS
• Use cautiously in elderly patients and in those with increased intraocular pressure, diabetes, ischemic heart disease, hyperthyroidism, hypertension, bronchial asthma, and prostatic hyperplasia.
• **I.V. use:** Injectable form containing 10 mg/ml can be given diluted or undiluted very slowly intravenously. Do not give the 100 mg/ml injection intravenously.
• Monitor blood count during long-term therapy, as ordered; observe for signs of blood dyscrasias.
• Instruct patient to reduce GI distress by giving drug with food or milk.
• Warn patients to avoid alcohol and activities that require alertness until drug's CNS effects are known.
• Tell patient that coffee or tea may reduce drowsiness. Causes less drowsiness than some other antihistamines.
• Inform patient that sugarless gum, sugarless sour hard candy, or ice chips may relieve dry mouth.
• Tell patient to notify doctor if tolerance develops because a different antihistamine may need to be prescribed.
• Instruct patients to stop drug 4 days before allergy skin tests to preserve accuracy of tests.

chlorpheniramine maleate
Aller-Chlor*◇, Allergex‡, Chlo-Amine◇, Chlor-100◇, Chlorate◇, Chlor-Niramine◇, Chlor-Pro, Chlor-Pro 10, Chlorspan-12, Chlortab-4, Chlortab-8, Chlor-Trimeton*◇, Chlor-Trimeton Allergy 12 Hour◇, Chlor-Tripolon†◇, Genallerate◇, Novopheniram‡◇, Pfeiffer's Allergy◇, Phenetron*, Piriton‡, Pyranistan◇, Telachlor, Teldrin◇, Trymegen◇
Pregnancy Risk Category: B

HOW SUPPLIED
Tablets: 4 mg◇
Tablets (chewable): 2 mg◇
Tablets (timed-release): 8 mg◇, 12 mg◇
Capsules (timed-release): 6 mg◇, 8 mg◇, 12 mg◇
Syrup: 2 mg/5 ml*◇
Injection: 10 mg/ml, 100 mg/ml

ACTION
Competes with histamine for H_1-receptor sites on effector cells. Prevents, but does not reverse, histamine-mediated responses.

ONSET, PEAK, DURATION
Onset occurs in 15 to 60 minutes. Peak concentrations occur 2 to 6 hours after oral dose, immediately after I.V. injection, unknown after I.M. administration. Effects persist up to 24 hours.

INDICATIONS & DOSAGE
Rhinitis, allergy symptoms –
Adults: 4 mg P.O. q 4 to 6 hours, not to exceed 24 mg/day; or 8 to 12 mg timed-release P.O. every 8 to 12 hours; or 5 to 40 mg I.M., I.V., or S.C. as a single dose.
Children 6 to 12 years: 2 mg P.O. q 4 to 6 hours, not to exceed 12 mg/day. Alternatively, may give 8 mg timed-release P.O. h.s.
Children 2 to 6 years: 1 mg P.O. q 4 to 6 hours.

ADVERSE REACTIONS
CNS: *stimulation,* sedation, *drowsiness* (especially in elderly patients), excitability (in children).
CV: hypotension, palpitations.
GI: epigastric distress, *dry mouth.*
GU: urine retention.
Respiratory: thick bronchial secretions.
Skin: rash, urticaria.
Other: (after parenteral administration) local stinging, burning sensation, pallor, weak pulse, transient hypotension.

INTERACTIONS
CNS depressants: increased sedation. Use together cautiously.
MAO inhibitors: increased anticholinergic effects. Don't use together.

CONTRAINDICATIONS
● Contraindicated in patients with acute asthmatic attacks.
● Antihistamines are not recommended for breast-feeding patients because small amounts of drug are excreted in breast milk.

NURSING CONSIDERATIONS
● Use cautiously in elderly patients and in those with increased intraocular pressure, hyperthyroidism, CV or renal disease, hypertension, bronchial asthma, urine retention, prostatic hyperplasia, bladder-neck obstruction, and stenosing peptic ulcerations.
● **I.V. use:** Drug is available in 10 mg/ml ampules for I.V. use; do not give the 100 mg/ml strength intravenously. Chlorpheniramine is compatible with most I.V. solutions. Check with pharmacist before mixing with any I.V. solutions to verify specific compatibilities. Give injection over 1 minute.
● If symptoms occur during or after parenteral dose, discontinue drug. Notify the doctor.
● Warn patients to avoid alcohol and other CNS depressants and driving or other activities that require alertness until drug's CNS effects are known.
● Tell patient that coffee or tea may reduce drowsiness. Sugarless gum, sugarless sour hard candy, or ice chips may relieve dry mouth.
● Advise patients to stop drug 4 days before allergy skin tests to preserve accuracy of tests.
● Tell patient to notify doctor if tolerance develops because a different antihistamine may need to be prescribed.
● Tell parents that drug, including extended-release products, should not be used in children under 12 years unless directed by doctor.

---

*Liquid form contains alcohol.   *Common* reactions are in italics; *life-threatening,* in bold italics.
**May contain tartrazine.

clemastine fumarate
Tavist, Tavist-1◊

Pregnancy Risk Category: B

HOW SUPPLIED
Tablets: 1.34 mg◊, 2.68 mg
Syrup: 0.67 mg per 5 ml

ACTION
Competes with histamine for H_1-receptor sites on effector cells. Prevents, but does not reverse, histamine-mediated responses.

ONSET, PEAK, DURATION
Onset occurs in 15 to 60 minutes. Peak levels occur in 2 to 4 hours; peak effects occur in 5 to 7 hours. Effects persist for 12 hours.

INDICATIONS & DOSAGE
Rhinitis, allergy symptoms –
Adults and children 12 years and over: 1.34 mg P.O. q 12 hours, or 2.68 mg P.O. once daily to t.i.d. as needed.
Children 6 to 12 years: 0.67 to 1.34 mg P.O. b.i.d.

ADVERSE REACTIONS
CNS: (especially in elderly patients) *sedation, drowsiness.*
CV: hypotension, palpitations, tachycardia.
GI: epigastric distress, anorexia, nausea, vomiting, constipation, *dry mouth.*
GU: urine retention.
Hematologic: hemolytic anemia, thrombocytopenia, *agranulocytosis.*
Respiratory: thick bronchial secretions.
Skin: rash, urticaria.

INTERACTIONS
CNS depressants: increased sedation. Use together cautiously.
MAO inhibitors: increased anticholinergic effects. Don't use together.

CONTRAINDICATIONS
Contraindicated in patients with hypersensitivity to drug or other antihistamines of similar chemical structure, in those with acute asthmatic attacks, and in neonates or premature infants and breast-feeding patients.

NURSING CONSIDERATIONS
• Use cautiously in elderly patients and in those with angle-closure glaucoma, increased intraocular pressure, hyperthyroidism, CV disease, hypertension, bronchial asthma, prostatic hyperplasia, bladder-neck obstruction, pyloruduodenal obstruction, and stenosing peptic ulcerations.
• Know that children under 12 years should use only as directed by a doctor.
• Monitor blood counts during long-term therapy, as ordered; observe for signs of blood dyscrasias.
• Warn patients to avoid alcohol and driving or other activities that require alertness until drug's CNS effects are known.
• Tell patient that coffee or tea may reduce drowsiness. Sugarless gum, sugarless sour hard candy, or ice chips may relieve dry mouth.
• Advise patients to stop drug 4 days before allergy skin tests to preserve accuracy of tests.
• Tell patient to notify doctor if tolerance develops because a different antihistamine may need to be prescribed.

cyproheptadine hydrochloride
Periactin

Pregnancy Risk Category: B

HOW SUPPLIED
Tablets: 4 mg
Syrup: 2 mg/5 ml

---

†Available in Canada only.   ‡Available in Australia only.   ◊ Available OTC.

ACTION
Competes with histamine for H_1-receptor sites on effector cells. Prevents, but does not reverse, histamine-mediated responses.

ONSET, PEAK, DURATION
Onset occurs in 15 to 60 minutes. Serum levels peak in 6 to 9 hours. Effects persist for 8 hours.

INDICATIONS & DOSAGE
Allergy symptoms, pruritus –
Adults: 4 to 20 mg P.O. daily in divided doses. Maximum dosage is 0.5 mg/kg daily.
Children 7 to 14 years: 4 mg P.O. b.i.d. or t.i.d. Maximum dosage is 16 mg daily.
Children 2 to 6 years: 2 mg P.O. b.i.d. or t.i.d. Maximum dosage is 12 mg daily.

ADVERSE REACTIONS
CNS: (especially in elderly patients) *drowsiness,* dizziness, headache, fatigue.
GI: nausea, vomiting, epigastric distress, *dry mouth.*
GU: urine retention.
Skin: rash.
Other: weight gain.

INTERACTIONS
CNS depressants: increased sedation. Use together cautiously.
MAO inhibitors: increased anticholinergic effects. Don't use together.

CONTRAINDICATIONS
Contraindicated in patients with hypersensitivity to drug or other drugs of similar chemical structure; in those with acute asthmatic attacks, angle-closure glaucoma, stenosing peptic ulcer, symptomatic prostatic hypertrophy, bladder-neck obstruction, and pyloroduodenal obstruction; in concurrent therapy with MAO inhibitors; in neonates or premature infants; in elderly or debilitated patients, and in breast-feeding patients.

NURSING CONSIDERATIONS
• Use cautiously in patients with increased intraocular pressure, hyperthyroidism, CV disease, hypertension, or bronchial asthma.
• Know that children under 14 years should use only as directed by a doctor.
• Reduce GI distress by giving drug with food or milk.
• Warn patients to avoid alcohol and driving or other activities that require alertness until drug's CNS effects are known.
• Tell patient that coffee or tea may reduce drowsiness. Sugarless gum, sugarless sour hard candy, or ice chips may relieve dry mouth.
• Advise patients to stop drug 4 days before allergy skin tests to preserve accuracy of tests.
• Instruct patient to notify doctor if tolerance develops because a different antihistamine may need to be prescribed.

dexchlorpheniramine maleate
Dexchlor, Poladex T.D., Polaramine*, Polaramine Repetabs
Pregnancy Risk Category: B

HOW SUPPLIED
Tablets: 2 mg
Tablets (timed-release): 4 mg, 6 mg
Syrup: 2 mg/5 ml*

ACTION
Competes with histamine for H_1-receptor sites on effector cells. Prevents, but does not reverse, histamine-mediated responses.

ONSET, PEAK, DURATION
Onset occurs in 15 to 60 minutes. Peak unknown. Effects persist for 4 to 8 hours.

---

*Liquid form contains alcohol.   *Common* reactions are in italics; *life-threatening,* in bold italics.
**May contain tartrazine.

INDICATIONS & DOSAGE

Rhinitis, allergy symptoms, contact dermatitis, pruritus –

Adults and children over 12 years: 2 mg P.O. q 4 to 6 hours, not to exceed 12 mg/day; or 4 to 6 mg timed-release P.O. b.i.d. or t.i.d.

Children 6 to 12 years: 1 mg P.O. q 4 to 6 hours, not to exceed 6 mg/day; or 4 mg timed-release tablet P.O. h.s.

Children 2 to 6 years: 0.5 mg P.O. q 4 to 6 hours, not to exceed 3 mg/ day.

ADVERSE REACTIONS

CNS: (especially in elderly patients) *drowsiness,* dizziness, *stimulation.*
GI: nausea, *dry mouth.*
GU: polyuria, dysuria, urine retention.

INTERACTIONS

CNS depressants: increased sedation. Use together cautiously.
MAO inhibitors: increased anticholinergic effects. Don't use together.

CONTRAINDICATIONS

● Contraindicated in patients with acute asthmatic attacks.
● Antihistamines are not recommended for use by breast-feeding patients because small amounts of drug are excreted in breast milk.

NURSING CONSIDERATIONS

● Use cautiously in elderly patients and in patients with increased intraocular pressure, hyperthyroidism, CV or renal disease, hypertension, bronchial asthma, urine retention, prostatic hyperplasia, bladder-neck obstruction, and stenosing peptic ulcer.
● Know that children under 6 years should use only as directed by a doctor. Timed-release tablets should not be used for children younger than 6 years.
● Warn patients to avoid alcohol and driving or other activities that require alertness until drug's CNS effects are known.
● Tell patient that coffee or tea may reduce drowsiness. Sugarless gum, sugarless sour hard candy, or ice chips may relieve dry mouth.
● Advise patients to stop drug 4 days before allergy skin tests to preserve accuracy of tests.
● Tell patient to notify doctor if tolerance develops because a different antihistamine may need to be prescribed.

diphenhydramine hydrochloride

Allerdryl†◇, AllerMax Caplets◇, Aller-med◇, Banophen◇, Banophen Caplets◇, Beldin◇, Belix◇, Bena-D 10, Bena-D 50, Benadryl◇, Benadryl 25◇, Benadryl Kapseals◇, Benahist 10, Benahist 50, Ben-Allergin-50, Benoject-10, Benoject-50, Benylin Cough◇, Bydramine Cough◇, Compoz◇, Diphenacen-50, Diphenadryl◇, Diphen Cough◇, Diphenhist◇, Diphenhist Captabs◇, Dormarex 2◇, Fynex◇, Genahist◇, Gen-D-phen◇, Hydramine◇, Hydramine Cough◇, Hydramyn◇, Hydril◇, Hyrexin-50, Insomnal†◇, Nervine Nighttime Sleep-Aid◇, Nidryl◇, Noradryl◇, Nordryl◇, Nordryl Cough◇, Nytol Maximum Strength◇, Nytol with DPH◇, Phendry◇, Phendry Children's Allergy Medicine◇, Sleep-Eze 3◇, Sominex Formula 2◇, Tusstat◇, Twilite Caplets◇, Uni-Bent Cough◇, Wehdryl-10, Wehdryl-50

Pregnancy Risk Category: B

HOW SUPPLIED

Tablets: 25 mg◇, 50 mg◇
Capsules: 25 mg◇, 50 mg◇
Elixir: 12.5 mg/5 ml (14% alcohol)*◇
Syrup: 12.5 mg/5 ml◇, 13.3 mg/5 ml (5% alcohol)◇
Injection: 10 mg/ml, 50 mg/ml

ACTION

Competes with histamine for H_1-receptor sites on effector cells. Prevents, but does not reverse, histamine-mediated responses, particularly histamine's effects on the smooth muscle of the bronchial tubes, GI tract, uterus, and blood vessels. Structurally related to local anesthetics, diphenhydramine provides local anesthesia by preventing initiation and transmission of nerve impulses. Also suppresses cough reflex by a direct effect in the medulla of the brain.

ONSET, PEAK, DURATION

Onset occurs within 15 minutes of oral administration, immediately after I.V. administration, unknown after I.M. administration. Serum levels peak and drug effects occur 1 to 4 hours after administration. Effects persist for 6 to 8 hours.

INDICATIONS & DOSAGE

Rhinitis, allergy symptoms, motion sickness, Parkinson's disease –
Adults and children 12 years and over: 25 to 50 mg P.O. t.i.d. or q.i.d.; or 10 to 50 mg deep I.M. or I.V. Maximum I.M. or I.V. dosage is 400 mg daily.
Children under 12 years: 5 mg/kg daily P.O., deep I.M., or I.V. in divided doses q.i.d. Maximum dosage is 300 mg daily.
Sedation –
Adults: 25 to 50 mg P.O., or deep I.M., p.r.n.
Nighttime sleep aid –
Adults: 50 mg P.O. h.s.
Nonproductive cough –
Adults: 25 mg P.O. q 4 to 6 hours (not to exceed 150 mg daily).
Children 6 to 12 years: 12.5 mg P.O. q 4 to 6 hours (not to exceed 75 mg daily).
Children 2 to 6 years: 6.25 mg P.O. q 4 to 6 hours (not to exceed 25 mg daily).

ADVERSE REACTIONS

CNS: (especially in elderly patients) *drowsiness,* confusion, insomnia, headache, vertigo.
CV: palpitations.
EENT: diplopia.
GI: *nausea,* vomiting, diarrhea, *dry mouth,* constipation.
GU: dysuria, urine retention.
Respiratory: nasal congestion.
Skin: urticaria, photosensitivity.

INTERACTIONS

CNS depressants: increased sedation. Use together cautiously.
MAO inhibitors: increased anticholinergic effects. Don't use together.

CONTRAINDICATIONS

Contraindicated in patients with hypersensitivity to the drug, during acute asthmatic attacks, and in newborns or premature neonates and breast-feeding women.

NURSING CONSIDERATIONS

• Use with extreme caution in patients with angle-closure glaucoma, prostatic hyperplasia, pyloroduodenal and bladder-neck obstruction, asthma or COPD, increased intraocular pressure, hyperthyroidism, CV disease, hypertension, and stenosing peptic ulcer.
• Know that children under 12 years should use only as directed by a doctor.
• Reduce GI distress by giving drug with food or milk.
• Alternate injection sites to prevent irritation. Administer I.M. injection deeply into large muscle.
• Instruct patients to take 30 minutes before travel to prevent motion sickness.
• Warn patients to avoid alcohol and driving or other hazardous activities that require alertness until drug's CNS effects are known.
• Tell patient that coffee or tea may reduce drowsiness. Sugarless gum,

---

*Liquid form contains alcohol.
**May contain tartrazine.

Common reactions are in italics; *life-threatening,* in bold italics.

sugarless sour hard candy, or ice chips may relieve dry mouth.
- Advise patients to stop drug 4 days before allergy skin tests to preserve accuracy of tests.
- Tell patient to notify doctor if tolerance develops because a different antihistamine may need to be prescribed.
- Warn patients of possible photosensitivity. Advise use of a sunblock.

loratadine
Claratyne‡, Claritin

Pregnancy Risk Category: B

HOW SUPPLIED
Tablets: 10 mg

ACTION
Blocks effects of histamine at H$_1$-receptor sites. Loratadine is a nonsedating antihistamine; its chemical structure prevents entry into the CNS.

ONSET, PEAK, DURATION
Onset occurs in 1 hour. Peak effects occur in 4 to 6 hours. Effects persist for at least 24 hours.

INDICATIONS & DOSAGE
Symptomatic treatment of seasonal allergic rhinitis –
Adults and children 12 years and over: 10 mg P.O. daily. Dosage for patients with hepatic failure is 10 mg P.O. every other day.

ADVERSE REACTIONS
CNS: headache, somnolence, fatigue.
GI: dry mouth.

INTERACTIONS
Erythromycin: increased loratadine plasma concentrations. Monitor patient closely.

CONTRAINDICATIONS
Contraindicated in patients with hypersensitivity to the drug.

NURSING CONSIDERATIONS
- Use cautiously in patients with liver impairment.
- Instruct patients to take drug at least 2 hours after a meal and to avoid eating for at least 1 hour after taking drug.
- Ensure that patients know to take drug only once daily. If symptoms persist or worsen, patients should contact the doctor.
- Advise patients to stop taking drug 4 days before allergy skin tests to preserve accuracy of tests.

methdilazine hydrochloride
Dilosyn †‡ Tacaryl*

Pregnancy Risk Category: B

HOW SUPPLIED
Tablets: 8 mg
Tablets (chewable): 3.6 mg methdilazine (equal to 4 mg methdilazine hydrochloride)
Syrup: 4 mg/5 ml*

ACTION
Competes with histamine for H$_1$-receptor sites on effector cells. Prevents, but does not reverse, histamine-mediated responses. A phenothiazine derivative.

OSET, PEAK, DURATION
Onset occurs in 15 to 60 minutes. Peak unknown. Effects persist for 6 to 12 hours.

INDICATIONS & DOSAGE
Allergic rhinitis, pruritus –
Adults: 8 mg P.O. b.i.d. to q.i.d. or 7.2 mg chewable tablets P.O. b.i.d. to q.i.d.
Children over 3 years: 4 mg P.O. b.i.d. to q.i.d. or 3.6 mg chewable tablets P.O. b.i.d. to q.i.d.

ADVERSE REACTIONS
CNS: (especially in elderly patients) *drowsiness,* dizziness, headache.

GI: nausea, *dry mouth and throat.*
GU: urine retention.
Hepatic: cholestatic jaundice.
Skin: rash.

INTERACTIONS
CNS depressants: increased sedation. Use together cautiously.
Epinephrine: methdilazine may block or reverse the effects of epinephrine. Other pressor agents should be used.
MAO inhibitors: increased anticholinergic effects. Don't use together.
Phenothiazines: increased effects. Don't use together.

CONTRAINDICATIONS
Contraindicated in patients experiencing acute asthmatic attacks; in patients with hypersensitivity to the drug; and in newborn or premature neonates and breast-feeding women.

NURSING CONSIDERATIONS
• Use with extreme caution in patients with angle-closure glaucoma, prostatic hyperplasia, pyloroduodenal and bladder-neck obstruction, stenosing peptic ulcer, asthma or COPD, increased intraocular pressure, hyperthyroidism, CV disease, and hypertension.
• Reduce GI distress by giving drug with food or milk.
• Available as chewable tablet for children. Instruct child to chew completely and swallow promptly; may cause local anesthetic effect in mouth, which increases the risk of choking.
• Warn patients to avoid alcohol and driving or other activities that require alertness until drug's CNS effects are known.
• Tell patient that coffee or tea may reduce drowsiness. Sugarless gum, sugarless sour hard candy, or ice chips may relieve dry mouth.
• Advise patients to stop drug 4 days before allergy skin tests to preserve accuracy of tests.

• Tell patient to notify doctor if tolerance develops because a different antihistamine may need to be prescribed.

promethazine hydrochloride
Anergan 25, Anergan 50, Histanil†, Pentazine, Phenameth, Phenazine 25, Phenazine 50, Phencen-50, Phenergan*, Phenergan-Fortis*, Phenergan-Plain*, Phenoject-50, PMS-Promethazine†, Pro-50, Prometh-25, Prometh-50, Promethegan, Prorex-25, Prorex-50, Prothazine†*, Prothazine Plain, V-Gan-25, V-Gan-50

promethazine theoclate
Avomine‡

Pregnancy Risk Category: NR

HOW SUPPLIED
promethazine hydrochloride
Tablets: 12.5 mg, 25 mg, 50 mg
Syrup: 5 mg/5 ml‡*, 6.25 mg/5 ml*, 10 mg/5 ml*, 25 mg/5 ml*
Injection: 25 mg/ml, 50 mg/ml
Suppositories: 12.5 mg, 25 mg, 50 mg
promethazine theoclate
Tablets: 25 mg‡

ACTION
Competes with histamine for H_1-receptor sites on effector cells. Prevents, but does not reverse, histamine-mediated responses. A phenothiazine derivative.

ONSET, PEAK, DURATION
Onset occurs in 15 to 60 minutes after oral administration, 20 minutes after I.M. injection and P.R. administration, 3 to 5 minutes after I.V. administration. Peak unknown. Effects persist up to 12 hours.

---

*Liquid form contains alcohol.   *Common* reactions are in italics; ***life-threatening,*** in bold italics.
**May contain tartrazine.

INDICATIONS & DOSAGE

Motion sickness –
Adults: 25 mg P.O. b.i.d.
Children: 12.5 to 25 mg P.O., I.M., or P.R. b.i.d.
Nausea –
Adults: 12.5 to 25 mg P.O., I.M., or P.R. q 4 to 6 hours, p.r.n.
Children: 12.5 to 25 mg I.M. or P.R. q 4 to 6 hours, p.r.n.
Rhinitis, allergy symptoms –
Adults: 12.5 mg P.O. q.i.d.; or 25 mg P.O. h.s.
Children: 6.25 to 12.5 mg P.O. t.i.d. or 25 mg P.O. or P.R. h.s.
Sedation –
Adults: 25 to 50 mg P.O. or I.M. h.s. or p.r.n.
Children: 12.5 to 25 mg P.O., I.M., or P.R. h.s.
Routine preoperative or postoperative sedation or adjunct to analgesics –
Adults: 25 to 50 mg I.M., I.V., or P.O.
Children: 12.5 to 25 mg I.M., I.V., or P.O.

ADVERSE REACTIONS

CNS: (especially in elderly patients) *sedation,* confusion, restlessness, tremors, *drowsiness.*
CV: hypotension.
EENT: transient myopia, nasal congestion.
GI: anorexia, nausea, vomiting, constipation, *dry mouth.*
GU: urine retention.
Hematologic: leukopenia, ***agranulocytosis.***
Other: photosensitivity.

INTERACTIONS

Anticholinergics, phenothiazines, tricyclic antidepressants: increased effects. Don't give together.
CNS depressants, ethanol: increased sedation. Use together cautiously.
Epinephrine: promethazine may block or reverse the effects of epinephrine. Other pressor agents should be used.

MAO inhibitors: increased extrapyramidal effects. Don't use together.
Levodopa: promethazine may decrease levodopa's antiparkinsonian action. Avoid concomitant use.
Lithium: promethazine may reduce GI absorption or enhance renal elimination of lithium. Avoid concomitant use.

CONTRAINDICATIONS

Contraindicated in patients with hypersensitivity to the drug; in those with intestinal obstruction, prostatic hyperplasia, bladder-neck obstruction, seizure disorders, coma, CNS depression, and stenosing peptic ulcerations; and in newborns and premature neonates, and breast-feeding women; and in acutely ill or dehydrated children.

NURSING CONSIDERATIONS

• Use cautiously in patients with pulmonary, hepatic, CV disease, or asthma.
• Know that pronounced sedative effect limits use in many ambulatory patients.
• Know that promethazine is used as an adjunct to analgesics (usually to increase sedation) and that it has no analgesic activity.
• Reduce GI distress by giving drug with food or milk.
• **I.V. use:** Don't give in a concentration greater than 25 mg/ml or at a rate exceeding 25 mg/minute. Shield I.V. infusion from direct light.
• Inject deep I.M. into large muscle mass. Don't administer via S.C. route. Rotate injection sites.
• Be aware that drug may be safely mixed with meperidine (Demerol) in the same syringe.
• In patients scheduled for a myelogram, discontinue drug 48 hours before procedure and do not resume drug until 24 hours after procedure, as ordered, because of the risk of seizures.

• Know that drug may cause false-positive immunologic urine pregnancy test (Gravindex). Also may interfere with blood typing of ABO group.

• When treating motion sickness, tell patient to take first dose 30 to 60 minutes before travel. On succeeding days of travel, patient should take dose upon rising and with evening meal.

• Warn patients to avoid alcohol and driving or other activities that require alertness until drug's CNS effects are known.

• Tell patient that coffee or tea may reduce drowsiness. Sugarless gum, sugarless sour hard candy, or ice chips may relieve dry mouth.

• Warn patients about possible photosensitivity and precautions to avoid it.

• Advise patient to stop drug 4 days before allergy skin tests to preserve accuracy of tests.

---

terfenadine
Seldane, Seldane Caplets†, Teldane‡

Pregnancy Risk Category: C

HOW SUPPLIED
Tablets: 60 mg, 120 mg†
Oral suspension†: 6 mg/ml

ACTION
Competes with histamine for H_1-receptor sites on effector cells. Prevents, but does not reverse, histamine-mediated responses.

ONSET, PEAK, DURATION
Onset occurs in 1 to 2 hours. Serum levels peak in 2 hours. Time to peak effect occurs in 3 to 4 hours. Effects persist for over 12 hours.

INDICATIONS & DOSAGE
Rhinitis, allergy symptoms –
Adults and children 12 years and over: 60 mg P.O. b.i.d. or 120 mg once daily.

ADVERSE REACTIONS
CNS: fatigue, dizziness, *headache,* sedation.
CV: *arrhythmias* (with high blood levels).
EENT: dry throat, nasal congestion.
GI: abdominal distress, nausea, dry mouth.
Other: alopecia, cholestatic jaundice, rash, urticaria.

INTERACTIONS
Cimetidine, ciprofloxacin, itraconazole, ketoconazole, macrolide antibiotics (erythromycin, troleandomycin): decreased hepatic metabolism of terfenadine, leading to increased serum levels and risk of serious arrhythmias. Avoid concomitant use.

CONTRAINDICATIONS
Contraindicated in patients with hypersensitivity to terfenadine; in those taking the antifungal agents itraconazole or ketoconazole or macrolide antibiotics, including erythromycin; and in patients with significant hepatic impairment.

NURSING CONSIDERATIONS
• Use cautiously in patients with cardiac disease.

• Be aware that terfenadine does not cause the degree of drowsiness and sedation associated with other antihistamines because it does not cross the blood-brain barrier; its anticholinergic and antiserotonin effects are mild.

• Instruct patients not to exceed prescribed dosage. If overdose occurs, monitor patient for arrhythmias.

• Instruct patient to keep well hydrated. Drug may cause a mild anticholinergic drying effect in patients with lower airway disease, such as asthma.

---

*Liquid form contains alcohol.   *Common* reactions are in italics; *life-threatening,* in bold italics.
**May contain tartrazine.

trimeprazine tartrate
Panectyl†, Temaril*, Vallergan‡
Pregnancy Risk Category: NR

HOW SUPPLIED
Tablets: 2.5 mg, 10 mg‡
Spansule capsules (sustained-release): 5 mg
Syrup: 2.5 mg/5 ml*, 7.5 mg/5 ml*‡, 30 mg/5 ml*‡

ACTION
Competes with histamine for H_1-receptor sites on effector cells. Prevents, but does not reverse, histamine-mediated responses. A phenothiazine derivative.

ONSET, PEAK, DURATION
Onset occurs in 15 to 60 minutes. Peak unknown. Effects persist for 3 to 6 hours.

INDICATIONS & DOSAGE
Pruritus –
Adults: 2.5 mg P.O. q.i.d.; or 5 mg timed-release P.O. b.i.d.
Children 3 years and over: 2.5 mg P.O. h.s. or t.i.d., p.r.n.
Children 6 months to 3 years: 1.25 mg P.O. h.s. or t.i.d., p.r.n.

ADVERSE REACTIONS
CNS: (especially in elderly patients) drowsiness, dizziness, confusion, headache, restlessness, tremors, irritability, insomnia; (in children) paradoxical excitation.
CV: hypotension, palpitations, tachycardia.
GI: anorexia, nausea, vomiting, *dry mouth and throat.*
GU: urinary frequency, urine retention.
Hematologic: *agranulocytosis,* leukopenia.
Skin: urticaria, rash, *photosensitivity.*

INTERACTIONS
Anticholinergics, MAO inhibitors, phenothiazines, tricyclic antidepressants: increased anticholinergic effect. Don't use together.
CNS depressants, ethanol: increased sedation. Use together cautiously.
Levodopa: trimeprazine may block levodopa's antiparkinsonian effects. Don't use together.
Lithium: trimeprazine may decrease GI absorption and enhance renal excretion of lithium. Don't use together.

CONTRAINDICATIONS
Contraindicated in patients with hypersensitivity to the drug or other phenothiazines; in those with acute asthmatic attacks, coma, CNS depression, and bone marrow depression; in neonates or premature infants; and in acutely ill or dehydrated children; and in breast-feeding patients.

NURSING CONSIDERATIONS
• Use with extreme caution in patients with angle-closure glaucoma, prostatic hypertrophy, stenosing peptic ulcer, pyloroduodenal or bladder-neck obstruction and in patients receiving MAO inhibitors.
• Know that children under 12 years should use only as directed by a doctor.
• Reduce GI distress by giving drug with food or milk.
• In patients scheduled for a myelogram, discontinue drug 48 hours before procedure, as ordered; do not continue drug until 24 hours after the procedure because of the risk of seizures.
• Monitor blood counts during long-term therapy, as ordered.
• Warn patients to avoid alcohol and driving or other activities that require alertness until drug's CNS effects are known.
• Tell patient that coffee or tea may reduce drowsiness. Sugarless gum,

---

sugarless sour hard candy, or ice chips may relieve dry mouth.
• Warn patients about risk of photosensitivity. Recommend use of a sunblock. If photosensitivity occurs, tell the patient to discontinue drug and call the doctor.
• Advise patients to stop drug 4 days before allergy skin tests to preserve accuracy of tests.

---

tripelennamine citrate
PBZ*

tripelennamine hydrochloride
PBZ, PBZ-SR, Pelamine, Pyribenzamine

Pregnancy Risk Category: NR

HOW SUPPLIED
tripelennamine citrate
Elixir: 37.5 mg/5 ml (equivalent to 25 mg/5 ml tripelennamine hydrochloride)*
tripelennamine hydrochloride
Tablets: 25 mg, 50 mg
Tablets (extended-release): 100 mg

ACTION
Competes with histamine for H_1-receptor sites on effector cells. Prevents, but does not reverse, histamine-mediated responses.

ONSET, PEAK, DURATION
Onset occurs in 15 to 60 minutes. Peak unknown. Effects persist for 4 to 6 hours.

INDICATIONS & DOSAGE
Rhinitis, allergy symptoms –
Adults: 25 to 50 mg P.O. q 4 to 6 hours; or 100 mg extended-release P.O. b.i.d. or t.i.d. Maximum dosage is 600 mg daily.
Children: 5 mg/kg P.O. daily in four to six divided doses. Maximum dosage is 300 mg daily.

ADVERSE REACTIONS
CNS: (especially in elderly patients) *drowsiness,* dizziness, confusion, restlessness, tremor, irritability, insomnia.
CV: palpitations.
GI: anorexia, diarrhea or constipation, *nausea, vomiting, dry mouth.*
GU: urinary frequency, urine retention.
Skin: urticaria, rash.
Other: thick bronchial secretions.

INTERACTIONS
CNS depressants: increased sedation. Use together cautiously.
MAO inhibitors: increased anticholinergic effects. Don't use together.

CONTRAINDICATIONS
Contraindicated in patients with hypersensitivity to the drug or any related compounds; in those with angle-closure glaucoma, stenosing peptic ulcer, symptomatic prostatic hypertrophy, pyloroduodenal or bladder-neck obstruction, and lower respiratory tract symptoms including asthma; and in premature infants, neonates, or breast-feeding patients.

NURSING CONSIDERATIONS
• Use cautiously in elderly patients and in patients with increased intra-ocular pressure, hyperthyroidism, CV disease, hypertension, or history of bronchial asthma.
• Know that extended-release preparations should not be used in children.
• Reduce GI distress by giving drug with food or milk.
• Warn patients to avoid alcohol and driving or other activities that require alertness until drug's CNS effects are known.
• Tell patient that coffee or tea may reduce drowsiness. Sugarless gum or sour hard candy, or ice chips may relieve dry mouth.
• Advise patients to stop drug 4 days

---

*Liquid form contains alcohol.   *Common* reactions are in italics; ***life-threatening,*** in bold italics.
**May contain tartrazine.

before allergy skin tests to preserve accuracy of tests.
• Tell patient to notify doctor if tolerance developes because a different antihistamine may need to be prescribed.

triprolidine hydrochloride
Alleract◇, Myidyl

Pregnancy Risk Category: C

HOW SUPPLIED
Tablets: 2.5 mg◇
Syrup*: 1.25 mg/5 ml◇

ACTION
Competes with histamine for H_1-receptor sites on effector cells. Prevents, but does not reverse, histamine-mediated responses.

ONSET, PEAK, DURATION
Onset occurs in 15 to 60 minutes. Peak levels occur in about 2 hours. Peak effects occur in 2 to 3 hours. Effects persist for 4 to 8 hours.

INDICATIONS & DOSAGE
Colds and allergy symptoms –
Adults and children 12 years and over: 2.5 mg P.O. q 4 to 6 hours. Maximum dosage is 10 mg/day.
Children 6 to 12 years: 1.25 mg P.O. q 4 to 6 hours. Maximum dosage is 5 mg/day.
Children 4 to 6 years: 0.938 mg P.O. q 4 to 6 hours. Maximum dosage is 3.744 mg/day.
Children 2 to 4 years: 0.625 mg P.O. q 4 to 6 hours. Maximum dosage is 2.5 mg/day.
Children 4 months to 2 years: 0.313 mg P.O. q 4 to 6 hours. Maximum dosage is 1.252 mg/day.

ADVERSE REACTIONS
CNS: (especially in elderly patients) *drowsiness,* dizziness, confusion, restlessness, insomnia, *stimulation.*

GI: anorexia, diarrhea or constipation, nausea, vomiting, *dry mouth.*
GU: urinary frequency, urine retention.
Skin: urticaria, rash.

INTERACTIONS
CNS depressants: increased sedation.
MAO inhibitors: increased anticholinergic effects. Don't use together.

CONTRAINDICATIONS
Contraindicated in patients with hypersensitivity to the drug, in those with acute asthma attacks, and in neonates, premature infants, and breast-feeding patients.

NURSING CONSIDERATIONS
• Use with extreme caution in patients with increased intraocular pressure, angle-closure glaucoma, hyperthyroidism, CV disease, hypertension, bronchial asthma, prostatic hyperplasia, bladder-neck obstruction, and stenosing peptic ulcerations.
• Know that children under 12 years should use only as directed by a doctor.
• Reduce GI distress by giving drug with food or milk.
• Warn patients to avoid alcohol and driving or other activities that require alertness until drug's CNS effects are known.
• Tell patient that coffee or tea may reduce drowsiness. Sugarless gum, sugarless sour hard candy, or ice chips may relieve dry mouth.
• Advise patients to stop drug 4 days before allergy skin tests to preserve accuracy of tests.

---

†Available in Canada only.   ‡Available in Australia only.   ◇Available OTC.

albuterol
albulterol sulfate
aminophylline
atropine sulfate
(See Chapter 21, ANTIARRHYTHMICS.)
bitolterol mesylate
dyphylline
ephedrine sulfate
epinephrine
epinephrine bitartrate
epinephrine hydrochloride
ethylnorepinephrine
  hydrochloride
ipratropium bromide
isoetharine hydrochloride
isoetharine mesylate
isoproterenol
isoproterenol hydrochloride
isoproterenol sulfate
metaproterenol sulfate
oxtriphylline
pirbuterol
salmeterol xinafoate
terbutaline sulfate
theophylline
theophylline sodium glycinate

COMBINATION PRODUCTS
Inhalants
DUO-MEDIHALER: isoproterenol hydrochloride 0.16 mg and phenylephrine bitartrate 0.24 mg per dose.
Oral bronchodilators
BRONCHIAL CAPSULES: 150 mg theophylline and 90 mg guaifenesin.
DILOR-G TABLETS: 200 mg dyphylline and 200 mg guaifenesin.
DYFLEX-G TABLETS: 200 mg dyphylline and 200 mg guaifenesin.
DYLINE-GG TABLETS: 200 mg dyphylline and 200 mg guaifenesin.
GLYCERYL-T CAPSULES: 150 mg theophylline and 90 mg guaifenesin.
MARAX*: theophylline 130 mg, ephedrine sulfate 25 mg, and hydroxyzine hydrochloride 10 mg.

NEOTHYLLINE-GG TABLETS: 200 mg dyphylline and 200 mg guaifenesin.
QUIBRON CAPSULES: 150 mg theophylline and 90 mg guaifenesin.
SYNOPHYLATE GG SYRUP*: 33.3 mg/5 ml guaifenesin and 100 mg/ml theophylline sodium glycinate.
THALFED◇: theophylline 120 mg, ephedrine hydrochloride 25 mg, and phenobarbital 8 mg.
Decongestants
ACTIFED◇: pseudoephedrine hydrochloride 60 mg and triprolidine hydrochloride 2.5 mg.
CONGESPIRIN◇: phenylephrine hydrochloride 1.25 mg and acetaminophen 81 mg.
DRISTAN◇: phenylephrine hydrochloride 5 mg, chlorpheniramine maleate 2 mg, and acetaminophen 325 mg.
NALDECON: phenylpropanolamine hydrochloride 40 mg, phenylephrine hydrochloride 10 mg, chlorpheniramine maleate 5 mg, and phenyltoloxamine citrate 15 mg.
ORNEX◇: phenylpropanolamine hydrochloride 18 mg and acetaminophen 325 mg.
SEMPREX-D: acrivastine 8 mg and pseudoephedrine hydrochloride 60 mg.

---

*Liquid form contains alcohol.   *Common* reactions are in italics; ***life-threatening,*** in bold italics.
**May contain tartrazine.

albuterol (salbutamol)
Asmol‡, Proventil, Respolin‡, Ventolin

albuterol sulfate (salbutamol sulphate)
Proventil, Proventil Repetabs, Respolin Autohaler Inhalation Device‡, Respolin Inhaler‡, Respolin Respirator Solution‡, Ventolin, Ventolin Obstetric Injection‡, Ventolin Rotacaps, Volmax

Pregnancy Risk Category: C

HOW SUPPLIED
albuterol
Aerosol inhaler: 90 mcg/metered spray, 100 mcg/metered spray‡
albuterol sulfate
Capsules for inhalation: 200 mcg
Tablets: 2 mg, 4 mg
Tablets (extended-release): 4 mg, 8 mg
Syrup: 2 mg/5 ml
Solution for inhalation: 0.083%, 0.5%
Injection: 1 mg/ml‡

ACTION
Relaxes bronchial and uterine smooth muscle by acting on beta$_2$-adrenergic receptors.

ONSET, PEAK, DURATION
Onset occurs within 5 to 15 minutes after inhalation, within 15 to 30 minutes after oral administration. Peak effect occurs 1 to 1½ hours after inhalation, 2 to 3 hours after oral administration. Effects persist for 3 to 6 hours after inhalation, up to 6 hours for syrup, up to 8 hours for tablets, about 12 hours for extended-release preparations.

INDICATIONS & DOSAGE
To prevent or treat bronchospasm in patients with reversible obstructive airway disease –

Adults and children 12 years and older: dosage and frequency vary with dosage form.
Aerosol inhalation – 1 to 2 inhalations q 4 to 6 hours. More frequent administration or a greater number of inhalations is not recommended.
Solution for inhalation – 2.5 mg t.i.d. or q.i.d. by nebulizer. To prepare solution, use 0.5 ml of the 0.5% solution diluted with 2.5 ml of 0.9% sodium chloride. Alternatively, use 3 ml of the 0.083% solution.
Capsules for inhalation – 200 mcg inhaled every 4 to 6 hours using a Rotahaler inhalation device. Some patients may need 400 mcg q 4 to 6 hours.
Oral tablets – 2 to 4 mg P.O. t.i.d. or q.i.d. Maximum dosage is 8 mg q.i.d.
Extended-release tablets – 4 to 8 mg P.O. q 12 hours. Maximum dosage is 16 mg b.i.d.
Children 6 to 13 years: 2 mg (1 teaspoonful) P.O. t.i.d. or q.i.d.
Children 2 to 5 years: 0.1 mg/kg P.O. t.i.d., not to exceed 2 mg (1 teaspoonful) t.i.d.
Adults over 65 years: 2 mg P.O. t.i.d. or q.i.d.
To prevent exercise-induced asthma –
Adults: 2 inhalations 15 minutes before exercise.
Prevention of premature labor‡ –
Adults: initially, 10 mcg/minute by continuous I.V. infusion (via an infusion pump). Dosage should be increased in 10-minute intervals until the desired response is achieved.

ADVERSE REACTIONS
CNS: *tremor, nervousness,* dizziness, insomnia, headache.
CV: tachycardia, palpitations, hypertension.
EENT: drying and irritation of nose and throat (with inhaled form).
GI: heartburn, nausea, vomiting.
Respiratory: *bronchospasm.*
Other: muscle cramps, hypokalemia (with high doses).

---

†Available in Canada only.   ‡Available in Australia only.   ◇Available OTC.

INTERACTIONS

CNS stimulants: increased CNS stimulation. Avoid concomitant use.
Levodopa: risk of arrhythmias. Monitor closely.
MAO inhibitors, tricyclic antidepressants: increased adverse CV effects.
Propranolol and other beta blockers: mutual antagonism. Monitor patient carefully.

CONTRAINDICATIONS

Contraindicated in patients with hypersensitivity to the drug or any component of the formulation.

NURSING CONSIDERATIONS

• Use cautiously in patients with CV disorders, including coronary insufficiency and hypertension; in patients with hyperthyroidism or diabetes mellitus; and in those who are unusually responsive to adrenergics.
• Use extended-release tablets cautiously in patients with preexisting GI narrowing.
• Know that pleasant-tasting syrup may be taken by children as young as 2 years. Contains no alcohol or sugar.
• Know that aerosol form may be prescribed for use 15 minutes before exercise to prevent exercise-induced bronchospasm.
• Know that patients may use tablets and aerosol concomitantly. Monitor closely for toxicity.
• **I.V. use:** where available, I.V. form may be used to prepare infusion using NaCl injection, glucose injection, or NaCl and glucose injection. Do not administer drug without dilution. Do not mix with any other medication. Discard unused diluted solution after 24 hours.
• When used to prevent premature labor, monitor maternal heart rate closely. It should not exceed 140 beats/minute.
• After uterine contractions have ceased, drip rate of drug should be maintained for 1 hour, then gradually

tapered at 50% increments in six hourly intervals. Do not continue infusions for more than 48 hours. If therapy needs to continue over 48 hours, doctor may prescribe 4 to 8 mg P.O. q.i.d.
• Warn patients about possibility of paradoxical bronchospasm. If this occurs, discontinue drug immediately.
• Teach patients to perform oral inhalation correctly. Give the following instructions for using metered-dose inhaler:
  — Clear nasal passages and throat.
  — Breathe out, expelling as much air from lungs as possible.
  — Place mouthpiece well into mouth as dose from inhaler is released, and inhale deeply.
  — Hold breath for several seconds, remove mouthpiece, and exhale slowly.
• If more than one inhalation is ordered, advise patient to wait at least 2 minutes before repeating procedure.
• Tell patients who also are using a steroid inhaler to use the bronchodilator first, then wait about 5 minutes before using the steroid. This allows bronchodilator to open air passages for maximum effectiveness.

aminophylline (theophylline and ethylenediamine)

Aminophyllin, Cardophyllin‡, Corophyllin†, Phyllocontin, Phyllocontin-350, Somophyllin, Somophyllin-DF

Pregnancy Risk Category: C

HOW SUPPLIED

Tablets: 100 mg, 200 mg
Tablets (extended-release): 225 mg, 350 mg†
Oral liquid: 105 mg/5 ml
Injection: 250 mg/10 ml, 500 mg/20 ml, 500 mg/2 ml, 100 mg/100 ml in 0.45% sodium chloride, 200 mg/100 ml in 0.45% sodium chloride

---

*Liquid form contains alcohol.
**May contain tartrazine.
Common reactions are in italics; **life-threatening,** in bold italics.

Rectal suppositories: 250 mg, 500 mg

ACTION
Inhibits phosphodiesterase, the enzyme that degrades cAMP. Results in relaxation of smooth muscle of the bronchial airways and pulmonary blood vessels.

ONSET, PEAK, DURATION
Onset occurs in 15 minutes after I.V. injection, 15 to 60 minutes after oral solution or tablets. Peak serum levels occur immediately after I.V. infusion; within 1 hour of oral solution; 2 hours after oral, uncoated tablets; 4 to 7 hours after extended-release capsules or tablets. Effects persist for variable lengths of time depending on patient's age, concurrent illnesses, and smoking status.

INDICATIONS & DOSAGE
Symptomatic relief of bronchospasm —
Patients not currently receiving theophylline products who require rapid relief of symptoms: loading dose is 6 mg/kg (equivalent to 4.7 mg/kg anhydrous theophylline) I.V. (less than or equal to 25 mg/minute), then maintenance infusion.
Adults (nonsmokers): 0.7 mg/kg/hour I.V. for 12 hours; then 0.5 mg/kg/hour.
Otherwise healthy adult smokers: 1 mg/kg/hour I.V. for 12 hours; then 0.8 mg/kg/hour.
Older patients and adults with cor pulmonale: 0.6 mg/kg/hour I.V. for 12 hours; then 0.3 mg/kg/hour.
Adults with CHF or liver disease: 0.5 mg/kg/hour I.V. for 12 hours; then 0.1 to 0.2 mg/kg/hour.
Children 9 to 16 years: 1 mg/kg/hour I.V. for 12 hours; then 0.8 mg/kg/hour.
Children 6 months to 9 years: 1.2 mg/kg/hour for 12 hours; then 1 mg/kg/hour.
Patients currently receiving theophylline products: aminophylline infusions of 0.63 mg/kg (0.5 mg/kg anhydrous theophylline) will increase plasma levels of theophylline by 1 mcg/ml. Some clinicians recommend a dose of 3.1 mg/kg (2.5 mg/kg anhydrous theophylline) if no obvious signs of theophylline toxicity are present.
Chronic bronchial asthma —
Highly individualized.
Adults: 600 to 1,600 mg P.O. daily in divided doses t.i.d. or q.i.d.
Children: 12 mg/kg P.O. daily in divided doses t.i.d. or q.i.d.
Note: Rectal dosage is the same as that recommended for oral dosage.

ADVERSE REACTIONS
CNS: *nervousness, restlessness, dizziness,* headache, *insomnia,* light-headedness, *seizures,* muscle twitching.
CV: *palpitations, sinus tachycardia,* extrasystoles, flushing, marked hypotension, increased respiratory rate.
GI: *nausea, vomiting, anorexia,* bitter aftertaste, dyspepsia, heavy feeling in stomach, diarrhea.
Skin: urticaria.
Other: irritation (with rectal suppositories).

INTERACTIONS
Adenosine: decreased antiarrhythmic effectiveness. Higher doses of adenosine may be necessary.
Alkali-sensitive drugs: reduced activity. Do not add to I.V. fluids containing aminophylline.
Barbiturates, carbamazepine, nicotine, phenytoin, rifampin: enhanced metabolism and decreased theophylline blood levels. Monitor for decreased aminophylline effect.
Beta-adrenergic blockers: antagonism. Propranolol and nadolol, especially, may cause bronchospasm in sensitive patients. Use together cautiously.
Cimetidine, influenza virus vaccine, macrolide antibiotics (such as erythromycin), oral contraceptives, quino-

lone antibiotics (such as ciprofloxacin): decreased hepatic clearance of theophylline; elevated theophylline levels. Monitor for signs of toxicity.
Ephedrine and other sympathomimetics: theophylline may exhibit synergistic toxicity with these agents, predisposing patients to development of cardiac arrhythmias.
Lithium: theophylline may increase secretion of lithium.

CONTRAINDICATIONS
Contraindicated in patients with hypersensitivity to xanthine compounds (caffeine, theobromine) and ethylenediamine and in patients with active peptic ulcer disease and seizure disorders (unless adequate anticonvulsant therapy is given).

NURSING CONSIDERATIONS
• Use cautiously in neonates and infants under age 1, young children, and elderly patients; also use cautiously in patients with CHF or other cardiac or circulatory impairment, COPD, cor pulmonale, renal or hepatic disease, hyperthyroidism, diabetes mellitus, peptic ulcer, severe hypoxemia, and hypertension.
• Relieve GI symptoms by giving oral drug with full glass of water at meals, although food in stomach delays absorption. No evidence exists that antacids reduce adverse GI reactions. Know that enteric-coated tablets also may delay and impair absorption.
• Before giving loading dose, ensure that patient has not had recent theophylline therapy.
• **I.V. use:** I.V. drug administration can cause burning; dilute with compatible I.V. solution and inject at a rate no faster than 25 mg/minute. Drug is compatible with most I.V. solutions except invert sugar, fructose, and fat emulsions.
• Suppositories are slowly and erratically absorbed. Administer rectal suppository if patients cannot take drug

orally, as ordered. Schedule after evacuation, if possible; may be retained better if given before meal. Advise patients to remain recumbent 15 to 20 minutes after insertion.
• Monitor vital signs; measure and record fluid intake and output. Expected clinical effects include improvement in quality of pulse and respiration.
• Aminophylline is a soluble salt of theophylline. Know that dosage is adjusted by monitoring response, tolerance, pulmonary function, and serum theophylline levels. Monitor serum theophylline levels as ordered. Theophylline concentrations should range from 10 to 20 mcg/ml; toxicity has been reported with levels above 20 mcg/ml.
• Be aware that patients who experience urticaria may still tolerate other theophylline preparations. Urticaria may be caused by the ethylenediamine salt.
• Supply instructions for home care and dosage schedule. Some patients may require an around-the-clock dosage schedule.
• Warn elderly patients that dizziness, a common adverse reaction at start of therapy, may occur.
• Warn patients to check with the doctor or pharmacist before combining aminophylline with other drugs. OTC remedies may contain ephedrine in combination with theophylline salts; excessive CNS stimulation may result.
• Advise patients to avoid switching brand without first checking with the doctor.

---

bitolterol mesylate
Tornalate

Pregnancy Risk Category: C

HOW SUPPLIED
Aerosol inhaler: 370 mcg/metered spray

---

*Liquid form contains alcohol.   *Common* reactions are in italics; *life-threatening*, in bold italics.
**May contain tartrazine.

ACTION
Relaxes bronchial smooth muscle by acting on beta$_2$-adrenergic receptors.

ONSET, PEAK, DURATION
Onset occurs in 3 to 4 minutes. Peak effects occur within ½ to 1 hour. Effects persist for 5 to 8 hours, may be only 2½ to 5 hours in steroid-dependent patients.

INDICATIONS & DOSAGE
To prevent or treat bronchial asthma and bronchospasm—
Adults and children over 12 years: to treat bronchospasm, two inhalations with an interval of at least 1 to 3 minutes, followed by a third inhalation, if needed. To prevent bronchospasm, the usual dosage is two inhalations q 8 hours. In either case, dosage should never exceed three inhalations q 6 hours or two inhalations q 4 hours.

ADVERSE REACTIONS
CNS: *tremor,* nervousness, headache, dizziness, light-headedness.
CV: palpitations, chest discomfort, tachycardia.
EENT: throat irritation, cough.
GI: nausea.
Other: dyspnea, *hypersensitivity.*

INTERACTIONS
None significant.

CONTRAINDICATIONS
Contraindicated in patients with hypersensitivity to the drug.

NURSING CONSIDERATIONS
• Use cautiously in patients with ischemic heart disease or hypertension, hyperthyroidism, diabetes mellitus, arrhythmias, seizure disorders, and history of unusual responsiveness to beta-adrenergic agonists.
• Monitor blood pressure regularly.
• Advise patients not to exceed recommended dosages. Too frequent use may cause tachycardia.

• Remind patients that beneficial effects last for up to 8 hours, longer than most other similar bronchodilators.
• Teach patients to perform oral inhalation correctly. Give the following instructions for using a metered-dose inhaler:
   — Clear nasal passages and throat.
   — Breathe out, expelling as much air from lungs as possible.
   — Place mouthpiece well into mouth as dose from inhaler is released, and inhale deeply and slowly for about 10 seconds.
   — Hold breath for several seconds, remove mouthpiece, and exhale slowly.
• If more than one inhalation is ordered, tell the patient to wait at least 2 minutes before repeating procedure.
• Tell patients who also are using a steroid inhaler to use bronchodilator first, then wait about 5 minutes before using steroid. This allows the bronchodilator to open air passages for maximum effectiveness.
• Tell patient that manufacturer recommends rinsing plastic mouthpiece daily with warm tap water, then drying it to ensure proper delivery of drug.

dyphylline
Dilor*, Dilor-400, Dyflex, Dyflex-400, Lufyllin*, Lufyllin-400, Neothylline, Protophylline†, Thylline

Pregnancy Risk Category: C

HOW SUPPLIED
Tablets: 200 mg, 400 mg
Elixir: 100 mg/15 ml, 160 mg/15 ml*
Injection: 250 mg/ml

ACTION
Unknown. Probably inhibits phosphodiesterase, the enzyme that degrades cAMP. Results in relaxation of

smooth muscle of the bronchial airways and pulmonary blood vessels.

ONSET, PEAK, DURATION
Onset occurs in 15 minutes to 1 hour. Peak levels occur within 1 hour. Effects persist for 4 to 6 hours.

INDICATIONS & DOSAGE
Relief of acute and chronic bronchial asthma and reversible bronchospasm associated with chronic bronchitis and emphysema –
Adults: up to 15 mg/kg P.O. q 6 hours. I.M. route is rarely used, but patients may receive 250 to 500 mg I.M. injected slowly at 6-hour intervals.

ADVERSE REACTIONS
CNS: *restlessness, dizziness,* headache, *insomnia,* light-headedness, *seizures,* muscle twitching.
CV: *palpitations, sinus tachycardia,* extrasystoles, flushing, marked hypotension, increased respiratory rate.
GI: *nausea, vomiting, anorexia,* bitter aftertaste, dyspepsia, heavy feeling in stomach.
Skin: urticaria.

INTERACTIONS
Probenecid: increased serum dyphylline levels. Monitor for adverse effects.

CONTRAINDICATIONS
Contraindicated in patients with hypersensitivity to the drug or related xanthine compounds.

NURSING CONSIDERATIONS
• Use cautiously in patients with severe cardiac disease, hypertension, hyperthyroidism, acute myocardial injury, or peptic ulcer.
• Know that dosage should be decreased in patients with renal insufficiency.
• Relieve gastric irritation by giving oral drug after meals; no evidence ex-

ists that antacids reduce this adverse reaction. May produce less gastric discomfort than theophylline.
• Do not administer intravenously.
• Discard injectable dyphylline if precipitate is present. Protect from light.
• Monitor vital signs; measure and record fluid intake and output. Expected clinical effects include improvement in quality of pulse and respirations.
• Be aware that because dyphylline is a theophylline analog, unlike other derivatives (such as aminophylline), it is not converted to theophylline in the bloodstream. No routine plasma assays exist for determining effective blood levels.
• Supply instructions for home care and dosage schedule.
• Warn elderly patients that dizziness, a common adverse reaction at start of therapy, may occur.
• Warn patients to check with the doctor or pharmacist before taking any other drugs. OTC remedies may contain ephedrine in combination with theophylline salts; excessive CNS stimulation may result.

ephedrine sulfate
Ephed II
Pregnancy Risk Category: C

HOW SUPPLIED
Tablets: 30 mg‡
Capsules: 25 mg, 50 mg
Injection: 25 mg/ml, 50 mg/ml

ACTION
Stimulates alpha- and beta-adrenergic receptors; a direct- and indirect-acting sympathomimetic.

ONSET, PEAK, DURATION
Onset occurs within 5 minutes of I.V. use, 10 to 20 minutes of I.M. use, 15 to 60 minutes after oral use. Peak unknown. Effects persist for 30 minutes

---

*Liquid form contains alcohol.
**May contain tartrazine.

Common reactions are in italics; *life-threatening*, in bold italics.

to 1 hour after I.M. or S.C. use, 3 to 5 hours after oral use.

INDICATIONS & DOSAGE
To correct hypotension –
Adults: 25 to 50 mg I.M. or S.C., or 10 to 25 mg I.V. p.r.n. to maximum of 150 mg/24 hours.
Children: 3 mg/kg or 100 mg/m² S.C. or I.V. daily, in four to six divided doses.
Bronchodilation or nasal decongestion –
Adults and children over age 12: 12.5 to 50 mg P.O. b.i.d., t.i.d., or q.i.d. Maximum dosage is 400 mg daily in six to eight divided doses.
Children over age 2: 2 to 3 mg/kg P.O. daily in four to six divided doses.

ADVERSE REACTIONS
CNS: *insomnia, nervousness,* dizziness, headache, muscle weakness, diaphoresis, euphoria, confusion, delirium.
CV: *palpitations,* tachycardia, hypertension.
EENT: dryness of nose and throat.
GI: nausea, vomiting, anorexia.
GU: urine retention, painful urination due to visceral sphincter spasm.

INTERACTIONS
Acetazolamide: increased serum ephedrine levels. Monitor for toxicity.
Alpha-adrenergic blocking agents: unopposed beta-adrenergic effects, resulting in hypotension.
Antihypertensives: decreased effects.
Beta-adrenergic blocking agents: unopposed alpha-adrenergic effects, resulting in hypertension.
Digitalis glycosides, general anesthetics (halogenated hydrocarbons): increased risk of ventricular arrhythmias.
Ergot alkaloids: enhanced vasoconstrictor activity.
Guanadrel, guanethidine: enhanced pressor effects of ephedrine.

Levodopa: enhanced risk of ventricular arrhythmias.
MAO inhibitors and tricyclic antidepressants: when given with sympathomimetics, may cause severe hypertension (hypertensive crisis).
Methyldopa, reserpine: may inhibit effects of ephedrine. Use together cautiously.

CONTRAINDICATIONS
Contraindicated in patients with hypersensitivity to ephedrine and other sympathomimetic drugs; in those with porphyria, severe coronary artery disease, arrhythmias, angle-closure glaucoma, psychoneurosis, angina pectoris, substantial organic heart disease, and CV disease; and in those taking MAO inhibitors.

NURSING CONSIDERATIONS
• Use with extreme caution in elderly men and in those with hypertension, hyperthyroidism, nervous or excitable states, diabetes, and prostatic hyperplasia.
• Know that hypoxia, hypercapnia, and acidosis, which may reduce effectiveness or increase the incidence of adverse reactions, must be identified and corrected before or during ephedrine administration.
• This drug is not a substitute for blood or fluid volume replenishment. Know that volume deficit must be corrected before administering vasopressors.
• **I.V. use:** Give 10 to 25 mg by I.V. injection slowly; repeat in 5 to 10 minutes if necessary. Compatible with most common I.V. solutions.
• To prevent insomnia, avoid giving within 2 hours before bedtime.
• Effectiveness decreases after 2 to 3 weeks, as tolerance develops. Doctor may need to increase dosage. Drug is not addictive.
• Warn patients not to take OTC drugs that contain ephedrine without informing the doctor.

---

†Available in Canada only.   ‡Available in Australia only.   ◊ Available OTC.

epinephrine (adrenaline)
Adrenalin◇, Bronkaid Mist◇, Bronkaid Mistometer†, Primatene Mist◇

epinephrine bitartrate
AsthmaHaler◇, Broniten Mist◇, Bronkaid Mist Suspension◇, Medihaler-Epi◇, Primatene Mist Suspension◇

epinephrine hydrochloride
Adrenalin Chloride◇, Epi-Pen, Epi-Pen Jr., Sus-Phrine

Pregnancy Risk Category: C

HOW SUPPLIED
Aerosol inhaler: 160 mcg◇, 200 mcg◇, 220 mcg◇, 250 mcg/metered spray◇
Nebulizer inhaler: 1% (1:100)†◇, 1.25%†◇, 2.25%†◇
Injection: 0.01 mg/ml (1:100,000), 0.1 mg/ml (1:10,000), 0.5 mg/ml (1:2,000), 1 mg/ml (1:1,000) parenteral; 5 mg/ml (1:200) parenteral suspension

ACTION
Stimulates alpha- and beta-adrenergic receptors within the sympathetic nervous system.

ONSET, PEAK, DURATION
Onset occurs immediately after I.V. injection, 3 to 5 minutes after inhalation, 6 to 15 minutes after S.C. injection, variable after I.M. use. Peak effects occur within 5 minutes of I.V. administration, within 30 minutes of S.C. injection. Effects persist for 1 to 3 hours after inhalation, less than 1 to about 4 hours after parenteral use.

INDICATIONS & DOSAGE
Bronchospasm, hypersensitivity reactions, anaphylaxis –
Adults: 0.1 to 0.5 ml of 1:1,000 S.C. or I.M. Repeated q 10 to 15 minutes, p.r.n. Or 0.1 to 0.25 ml of 1:1,000

(1 to 2.5 ml of a commercially available 1:10,000 injection or of a 1:10,000 dilution prepared by diluting 1 ml of a commercially available 1:1,000 injection with 10 ml of water for injection or 0.9% sodium chloride injection) I.V. slowly over 5 to 10 minutes.
Children: 0.01 ml (10 mcg) of 1:1,000/kg S.C.; repeated q 20 minutes to 4 hours, p.r.n. Or, 0.005 ml/kg of 1:200 (Sus-Phrine) S.C.; repeated q 8 to 12 hours, p.r.n.
Hemostasis –
Adults: 1:50,000 to 1:1,000, applied topically.
Acute asthmatic attacks –
Adults and children 4 years and over: 160 to 250 mcg (metered aerosol) which is equivalent to 1 inhalation, repeated once if necessary after at least 1 minute; subsequent doses should not be administered for at least 3 hours. Alternatively, 1% (1:100) solution of epinephrine or 2.25% solution of racepinephrine administered via a hand-bulb nebulizer as 1 to 3 deep inhalations, repeated q 3 hours as needed.
To prolong local anesthetic effect –
Adults and children: 0.1 to 0.2 mg (base) added to anesthetic spinal fluid mixture; 0.1 to 0.2 mg (base) in a 1:200,000 to 1:20,000 solution.
To restore cardiac rhythm in cardiac arrest –
Adults: 0.5 to 1 mg I.V. or into endotracheal tube. May be given intracardiac if no I.V. route or intratracheal route available. Some clinicians advocate higher dose (up to 5 mg), especially in patients who don't respond to usual I.V dose. Following initial I.V. administration, may be infused I.V. at a rate of 1 to 4 mcg/minute.
Children: 10 mcg/kg I.V. or 5 to 10 mcg (0.05 to 0.1 ml of 1:10,000)/kg intracardiac.
Note: 1 mg = 1 ml of 1:1,000 or 10 ml of 1:10,000.

ADVERSE REACTIONS

CNS: *nervousness,* tremor, euphoria, anxiety, coldness of extremities, vertigo, *headache,* diaphoresis, disorientation, agitation. In patients with Parkinson's disease, the drug increases rigidity and tremor.

CV: *palpitations;* widened pulse pressure; *hypertension; tachycardia; ventricular fibrillation; CVA;* anginal pain; ECG changes, including a decreased T-wave amplitude.

Other: pulmonary edema, dyspnea, pallor, hyperglycemia, glycosuria.

INTERACTIONS

Alpha-adrenergic blocking agents: hypotension due to unopposed beta-adrenergic effects.

Antihistamines, thyroid hormones, tricyclic antidepressants: when given with sympathomimetics, may cause severe adverse cardiac effects. Avoid giving together.

Beta blockers, such as propranolol: vasoconstriction and reflex bradycardia. Monitor patient carefully.

Digitalis glycosides, general anesthetics (halogenated hydrocarbons): increased risk of ventricular arrhythmias.

Doxapram, mazindol, methylphenidate: enhanced CNS stimulation or pressor effects.

Ergot alkaloids: enhanced vasoconstrictor activity.

Guanadrel, guanethidine: enhanced pressor effects of epinephrine.

Levodopa: enhanced risk of cardiac arrhythmias.

MAO inhibitors: increased risk of hypertensive crisis.

CONTRAINDICATIONS

• Contraindicated in patients with angle-closure glaucoma, shock (other than anaphylactic shock), organic brain damage, cardiac dilation, arrhythmias, coronary insufficiency, or cerebral arteriosclerosis. Also contraindicated in patients during general anesthesia with halogenated hydrocarbons or cyclopropane and in patients in labor (may delay second stage).

• Some commercial products contain sulfites: contraindicated in patients with sulfite allergies except when epinephrine is being used for treatment of serious allergic reactions or other emergency situations.

• In conjunction with local anesthetics, epinephrine is contraindicated for use in fingers, toes, ears, nose, or genitalia.

NURSING CONSIDERATIONS

• Use with extreme caution in patients with long-standing bronchial asthma and emphysema who have developed degenerative heart disease. Also use cautiously in elderly patients and in those with hyperthyroidism, CV disease, hypertension, psychoneurosis, and diabetes.

• Be aware that epinephrine is the drug of choice in emergency treatment of acute anaphylactic reactions.

• Discard epinephrine solutions after 24 hours or if solution is discolored or contains precipitate. Keep solution in light-resistant container, and don't remove before use.

• **I.V. use:** Don't mix with alkaline solutions. Use D_5W, 0.9% sodium chloride injection, lactated Ringer's injection, or combinations of dextrose in sodium chloride. Mix just before use.

• When administering I.V., monitor blood pressure, heart rate, and ECG when therapy is initiated and frequently thereafter.

• Avoid I.M. administration of parenteral suspension into buttocks. Gas gangrene may occur because epinephrine reduces oxygen tension of the tissues, encouraging the growth of contaminating organisms.

• Massage site after I.M. injection to counteract possible vasoconstriction. Repeated local injection can cause

necrosis resulting from vasoconstriction at injection site.
• Observe patients closely for adverse reactions. Notify doctor if adverse reactions develop; he may adjust dosage or discontinue drug.
• Know that if a sharp blood pressure rise occurs, rapid-acting vasodilators, such as nitrites or alpha-adrenergic blockers, can be given to counteract the marked pressor effect of large doses of epinephrine.
• Know that epinephrine is rapidly destroyed by oxidizing agents, such as iodine, chromates, nitrates, nitrites, oxygen, and salts of easily reducible metals (such as iron).
• Teach patients to perform oral inhalation correctly. Give the following instructions for using a metered-dose inhaler:
  — Clear nasal passages and throat.
  — Breathe out, expelling as much air from lungs as possible.
  — Place mouthpiece well into mouth as dose from inhaler is released, and inhale deeply.
  — Hold breath for several seconds, remove mouthpiece, and exhale slowly.
• If more than one inhalation is ordered, tell patients to wait at least 2 minutes before repeating procedure.
• Tell patients who also are using a steroid inhaler to use the bronchodilator first, then wait about 5 minutes before using steroid. This allows the bronchodilator to open air passages for maximum effectiveness.
• If patient has acute hypersensitivity reactions, such as to bee stings, it may be necessary to instruct him to self-inject epinephrine at home.

ethylnorepinephrine hydrochloride
Bronkephrine

Pregnancy Risk Category: C

HOW SUPPLIED
Injection: 2 mg/ml

ACTION
Relaxes bronchial smooth muscle by acting on beta-adrenergic receptors.

ONSET, PEAK, DURATION
Onset occurs in 6 to 12 minutes. Peak unknown. Effects persist for 1 to 2 hours.

INDICATIONS & DOSAGE
Bronchospasm caused by asthma –
Adults: 0.5 to 1 ml (1 to 2 mg) S.C. or I.M.
Children: 0.1 to 0.5 ml (0.2 to 1 mg) S.C. or I.M.

ADVERSE REACTIONS
CNS: *headache,* dizziness.
CV: changes in blood pressure, *elevation in pulse rate,* palpitations.
GI: nausea.

INTERACTIONS
Antihypertensives, nitrates: decreased effects of these agents.
Beta blockers: mutual inhibition of clinical effects.
CNS stimulants, xanthine derivatives: enhanced CNS stimulation.
Digitalis glycosides, levodopa, halogenated inhalation anesthetics, cyclopropane: increased risk of arrhythmias. Monitor closely.
Rauwolfia alkaloids, sympathomimetics: enhanced effects.
Thyroid hormones: increased risk of coronary insufficiency.

CONTRAINDICATIONS
Contraindicated in patients with hypersensitivity to the drug; in patients with tachyarrhythmias, tachycardia caused by digitalis toxicity, angle-closure glaucoma, or shock; and in those receiving general anesthesia with cyclopropane or halogenated inhalation anesthetics.

---

*Liquid form contains alcohol.   *Common* reactions are in italics; ***life-threatening***, in bold italics.
**May contain tartrazine.

NURSING CONSIDERATIONS
• Use cautiously in patients with CV disease or history of CVA.
• Know that drug is safer than epinephrine for use in hypertensive or severely ill patients in whom significant pressor effects are undesirable.
• Be aware that drug is valuable for use in children because of low incidence of adverse reactions; may be useful in diabetic asthmatic patients because of low glycogenolytic activity.
• Choose anatomic injection site carefully to avoid inadvertent intraneural or intravascular injection.

ipratropium bromide
Atrovent

Pregnancy Risk Category: B

HOW SUPPLIED
Inhaler: each metered dose supplies 18 mcg
Solution (for nebulizer): 0.025% (250 mcg/ml)‡
Nasal spray: each metered dose supplies 20 mcg

ACTION
Inhibits vagally mediated reflexes by antagonizing acetylcholine. An anticholinergic.

ONSET, PEAK, DURATION
Onset occurs in 5 to 15 minutes. Peak effects occur in 1 to 2 hours. Effects persist usually 3 to 4 hours; up to 6 hours in some patients.

INDICATIONS & DOSAGE
Bronchospasm associated with COPD –
Adults: 1 to 2 inhalations q.i.d. Additional inhalations may be needed. However, total inhalations should not exceed 12 in 24 hours. Alternatively, use inhalation solution where available. Give 250 to 500 mcg dissolved

in 0.9% sodium chloride and administer by nebulizer every 4 to 6 hours.
Children ages 5 to 12: give 125 to 250 mcg nebulizer solution dissolved in 0.9% sodium chloride and administer by nebulizer every 4 to 6 hours.
Seasonal allergic rhinitis‡ –
Adults: 2 sprays in each nostril b.i.d. Increase to t.i.d. or q.i.d. if needed. Maximum dosage is 8 sprays in each nostril daily.

ADVERSE REACTIONS
CNS: nervousness, dizziness, headache.
CV: palpitations.
EENT: cough, blurred vision.
GI: nausea, GI distress, dry mouth.
Skin: rash.

INTERACTIONS
Anticholinergics: increased anticholinergic effects. Avoid concomitant use.
Cromolyn sodium: will form a precipitate if mixed in the same nebulizer. Don't use together.

CONTRAINDICATIONS
Contraindicated in patients with hypersensitivity to the drug or to atropine or any of its derivatives and in those with a history of hypersensitivity to soyalecithin or related food products such as soybeans and peanuts.

NURSING CONSIDERATIONS
• Use cautiously in patients with angle-closure glaucoma, prostatic hyperplasia, and bladder-neck obstruction.
• Warn patients that ipratropium bromide is not effective for treating acute episodes of bronchospasm where rapid response is required.
• Teach patients to perform oral inhalation correctly. Give the following instructions for using a metered-dose inhaler:
  — Clear nasal passages and throat.

— Breathe out, expelling as much air from lungs as possible.

— Place mouthpiece well into mouth as dose from inhaler is released, and inhale deeply.

— Hold breath for several seconds, remove mouthpiece, and exhale slowly.

• Tell patients to avoid accidentally spraying into eyes. Temporary blurring of vision may result.

• If more than one inhalation is ordered, tell patients to wait at least 2 minutes before repeating procedure.

• Tell patients who also are using a steroid inhaler to use ipratropium first, then wait about 5 minutes before using the steroid. This allows the bronchodilator to open air passages for maximum effectiveness.

• Tell patients if a dose is missed to take as soon as remembered, unless it's almost time for the next dose. In that case, skip the missed dose. Do not double-dose.

• Advise the patient to use sugarless hard candy or gum, or a saliva substitute to relieve dry mouth.

isoetharine hydrochloride
Arm-a-Med Isoetharine, Bronkosol, Dey-Dose Isoetharine, Dey-Dose Isoetharine S/F, Dey-Lute Isoetharine S/F, Dispos-a-Med Isoetharine

isoetharine mesylate
Bronkometer

Pregnancy Risk Category: NR

HOW SUPPLIED
Aerosol inhaler: 340 mcg/metered spray
Nebulizer inhaler: 0.062%, 0.08%, 0.1%, 0.125%, 0.167%, 0.17%, 0.2%, 0.25%, 0.5%, 1% solution

ACTION
Relaxes bronchial smooth muscle by acting on beta$_2$-adrenergic receptors.

ONSET, PEAK, DURATION
Onset occurs in 1 to 6 minutes. Peak effects occur within 15 to 60 minutes. Effects persist 1 to 4 hours.

INDICATIONS & DOSAGE
Bronchial asthma and reversible bronchospasm that may occur with bronchitis and emphysema —
Adults: *hydrochloride form* — administered by hand nebulizer, oxygen aerosolization, or IPPB; use chart below.

Method	Dose	Dilutions
Hand nebulizer	3 to 7 inhalations	undiluted
Oxygen aerosolization	0.5 ml	1:3 with saline
IPPB	0.5 ml	1:3 with saline

mesylate form — 1 to 2 inhalations. Occasionally, more may be required.

ADVERSE REACTIONS
CNS: *tremor, headache,* dizziness, excitement.
CV: *palpitations,* increased heart rate, alterations in blood pressure.
GI: nausea, vomiting.

INTERACTIONS
Cyclopropane, digitalis glycosides, halogenated inhalation anesthetics, levodopa: increased risk of arrhythmias. Monitor closely.
Epinephrine and other sympathomimetic agents: may cause excessive tachycardia. Should not be used together with isoetharine.
Propranolol and other beta blockers: blocked bronchodilating effect of isoetharine. Monitor patient carefully if used together.

CONTRAINDICATIONS
Contraindicated in patients with hypersensitivity to the drug.

---

*Liquid form contains alcohol.
**May contain tartrazine.

Common reactions are in italics; ***life-threatening,*** in bold italics.

NURSING CONSIDERATIONS

• Use cautiously in patients with hyperthyroidism, hypertension, or coronary disease and in those with hypersensitivity to sympathomimetics.
• Although isoetharine has minimal effects on the heart, know that it should be used cautiously in patients receiving general anesthetics that sensitize the myocardium to sympathomimetic drugs.
• Monitor for severe paradoxical bronchoconstriction after excessive use. If bronchoconstriction occurs, discontinue immediately and notify doctor.
• Teach patients to perform oral inhalation correctly. Give the following instructions for using a metered-dose inhaler:
  — Clear nasal passages and throat.
  — Breathe out, expelling as much air from lungs as possible.
  — Place mouthpiece well into mouth as dose from inhaler is released, and inhale deeply.
  — Hold breath for several seconds, remove mouthpiece, and exhale slowly.
• If more than one inhalation is ordered, tell patients to wait at least 2 minutes before repeating procedure.
• Tell patients who also are using a steroid inhaler to use the bronchodilator first, then wait about 5 minutes before using the steroid. This allows the bronchodilator to open air passages for maximum effectiveness.
• Because of oxidation of drug when diluted with water, pink sputum mimicking hemoptysis may occur after inhaling isoetharine solution. Tell patients not to be concerned.
• Warn patient that excessive use can lead to decreased effectiveness.

isoproterenol (isoprenaline)

Aerolone, Dey-Dose Isoproterenol, Dispos-a-Med Isoproterenol, Isuprel, Vapo-Iso

isoproterenol hydrochloride

Isuprel, Isuprel Glossets, Isuprel Mistometer, Norisodrine Aerotrol

isoproterenol sulfate

Medihaler-Iso

Pregnancy Risk Category: C

HOW SUPPLIED

isoproterenol
Nebulizer inhaler: 0.25%, 0.5%, 1%
isoproterenol hydrochloride
Tablets (sublingual): 10 mg, 15 mg
Aerosol inhaler: 120 mcg or 131 mcg/metered spray
Injection: 20 mcg/ml, 200 mcg/ml
isoproterenol sulfate
Aerosol inhaler: 80 mcg/metered spray

ACTION

Relaxes bronchial smooth muscle by acting on beta$_2$-adrenergic receptors. As a cardiac stimulant, acts on beta$_1$-adrenergic receptors in the heart.

ONSET, PEAK, DURATION

Onset occurs immediately after I.V. use, 2 to 5 minutes after inhalation, 15 to 30 minutes after S.L. use. Peak unknown. Effects persist for ½ to 2 hours after inhalation, less than 1 hour after I.V. use, 1 to 2 hours after S.L. use.

INDICATIONS & DOSAGE

Bronchial asthma and reversible bronchospasm—
Adults: 10 to 15 mg hydrochloride S.L. q 6 to 8 hours. Daily S.L. dosage should not exceed 60 mg.
Children: 5 to 10 mg hydrochloride S.L. q 6 to 8 hours. Daily S.L. dosage should not exceed 30 mg.
Bronchospasm—
Adults and children: acute dyspneic episodes: 1 inhalation of sulfate form initially. Repeated if needed after 2 to 5 minutes.
  Maintenance dosage is 1 to 2 inha-

lations q.i.d. to six times daily. Repeated once more 10 minutes after second dose. No more than three doses should be administered for each attack.

Bronchospasm in COPD –
Administered via IPPB or for nebulization by compressed air or oxygen.
Adults: 2 ml of 0.125% or 2.5 ml of 0.1% solution (prepared by diluting 0.5 ml of 0.5% solution to 2 or 2.5 ml or by diluting 0.25 ml of 1% solution to 2 or 2.5 ml with water or 0.45% or 0.9% sodium chloride solution) up to five times daily.
Children: 2 ml of a 0.0625% solution or 2.5 ml of 0.05% solution (prepared by diluting 0.25 ml of 0.5% solution to 2 or 2.5 ml with water or 0.45%) or 0.9% sodium chloride solution) up to five times daily.

Heart block and ventricular arrhythmias –
Adults: (hydrochloride) initially, 0.02 to 0.06 mg I.V. Subsequent doses 0.01 to 0.2 mg I.V. or 5 mcg/minute I.V.; or 0.2 mg I.M. initially, then 0.02 to 1 mg, p.r.n.
Children: (hydrochloride) half of initial adult dose may be given.

Shock –
Adults and children: (hydrochloride) 0.5 to 5 mcg/minute by continuous I.V. infusion. Usual concentration is 1 mg (5 ml) in 500 ml D₅W. Rate adjusted according to heart rate, central venous pressure (CVP), blood pressure, and urine flow.

ADVERSE REACTIONS
CNS: *headache,* mild tremor, weakness, dizziness, nervousness, insomnia.
CV: *palpitations, tachycardia, anginal pain; blood pressure may rise and then fall.*
GI: nausea, vomiting.
Respiratory: bronchial edema and inflammation.
Other: diaphoresis, flushing of face, hyperglycemia.

INTERACTIONS
Epinephrine and other sympathomimetics: increased risk of arrhythmias.
Propranolol and other beta blockers: blocked bronchodilating effect of isoproterenol. Monitor patient carefully if used together.

CONTRAINDICATIONS
Contraindicated in patients with tachycardia caused by digitalis intoxication, in patients with preexisting arrhythmias (other than those that may respond to treatment with isoproterenol), and in those with angina pectoris.

NURSING CONSIDERATIONS
• Use cautiously in elderly patients and in patients with renal or CV disease, coronary insufficiency, diabetes, hyperthyroidism, or history of sensitivity to sympathomimetic amines.
• Know that drug is not a substitute for blood or fluid volume deficit. Volume deficit should be corrected before administering vasopressors.
• Do not use injection or inhalation solution if it is discolored or contains precipitate.
• **I.V. use:** Give by direct injection or I.V. infusion. For infusion, drug may be diluted with most common I.V. solutions. However, do not use with sodium bicarbonate injection; drug decomposes rapidly in alkaline solutions.
• If heart rate exceeds 110 beats/minute with I.V. infusion, notify the doctor. Doses sufficient to increase the heart rate to more than 130 beats/minute may induce ventricular arrhythmias.
• When administering I.V. isoproterenol to treat shock, closely monitor blood pressure, CVP, ECG, arterial blood gas measurements, and urine output. Carefully adjust infusion rate according to these measurements, as

*Liquid form contains alcohol.   *Common* reactions are in italics; **life-threatening**, in bold italics.
**May contain tartrazine.

ordered. Use a continuous infusion pump to regulate flow rate.
• If drug is administered via inhalation with oxygen, be sure oxygen concentration will not suppress respiratory drive.
• Follow same instructions for metered powder nebulizer, although deep inhalation is not necessary.
• Be aware that drug may aggravate ventilation-perfusion abnormalities; even while ease of breathing is improved, arterial oxygen tension may fall paradoxically.
• Be aware that isoproterenol may cause a slight rise in systolic blood pressure and a slight to marked drop in diastolic blood pressure.
• Monitor patient for adverse reactions.
• Teach patients to perform oral inhalation correctly. Give the following instructions for using a metered-dose inhaler:
   — Clear nasal passages and throat.
   — Breathe out, expelling as much air from lungs as possible.
   — Place mouthpiece well into mouth as dose from inhaler is released, and inhale deeply.
   — Hold breath for several seconds, remove mouthpiece, and exhale slowly.
• If more than one inhalation is ordered, tell patients to wait at least 2 minutes before repeating procedure.
• Tell patients who also are using a steroid inhaler to use the bronchodilator first, then wait about 5 minutes before using the steroid. This allows the bronchodilator to open air passages for maximum effectiveness.
• Warn patients using oral inhalant that drug may turn sputum and saliva pink.
• Teach patients to take S.L. tablet properly. Instruct patients to hold tablet under tongue, and not to swallow saliva until tablet dissolves and is absorbed. Instruct patients to rinse

mouth with water between doses to help prevent oropharyngeal dryness.
• Caution patients that prolonged use of S.L. tablets can cause tooth decay.
• Tell patient not to use drug at bedtime if possible; it interrupts sleep patterns.
• Tell patients to discontinue drug immediately and notify doctor if drug causes precordial distress or anginal pain or if an increase in chest tightness or dyspnea occurs.
• Patients may develop a tolerance to this drug; warn against overuse.

metaproterenol sulfate
Alupent, Arm-A-Med
Metaproterenol, Dey-Dose
Metaproterenol, Dey-Lute
Metaproterenol, Metaprel

Pregnancy Risk Category: C

HOW SUPPLIED
Tablets: 10 mg, 20 mg
Syrup: 10 mg/5 ml
Aerosol inhaler: 0.65 mg/metered spray
Nebulizer inhaler: 0.4%, 0.6%, 5% solution

ACTION
Relaxes bronchial smooth muscle by acting on beta$_2$-adrenergic receptors.

ONSET, PEAK, DURATION
Onset occurs in 1 minute with oral inhalation, in 5 to 30 minutes with aerosol nebulization, and in 15 minutes with oral administration. Peak effects occur within 1 hour. Effects persist for 1½ hours after inhalation, 1 to 4 hours after oral use.

INDICATIONS & DOSAGE
Acute episodes of bronchial asthma —
Adults and children: 2 to 3 inhalations. Do not repeat inhalations more often than q 3 to 4 hours. Do not exceed 12 inhalations daily.

Bronchial asthma and reversible bronchospasm –
Adults: 20 mg P.O. q 6 to 8 hours.
Children over 9 years or over 27 kg: 20 mg P.O. q 6 to 8 hours (0.4 mg to 0.9 mg/kg/dose t.i.d.).
Children 6 to 9 years or less than 27 kg: 10 mg P.O. q 6 to 8 hours (0.4 mg to 0.9 mg/kg/dose t.i.d.).

Alternatively, via IPPB or nebulizer:
Adults and children 12 years and over: 0.2 to 0.3 ml of 5% solution diluted in approximately 2.5 ml of 0.45% or 0.9% sodium chloride or 2.5 ml of a commercially available 0.4% or 0.6% solution q 4 hours p.r.n.
Children 6 to 12 years: 0.1 to 0.2 ml of a 5% solution diluted in 0.9% sodium chloride to final volume of 3 ml q 4 hours p.r.n.

ADVERSE REACTIONS

CNS: nervousness, weakness, drowsiness, tremor.
CV: tachycardia, hypertension, palpitations; *cardiac arrest (with excessive use)*.
GI: vomiting, nausea, bad taste in mouth.
Respiratory: paradoxical bronchiolar constriction with excessive use.

INTERACTIONS

Levodopa: risk of arrhythmias. Avoid concomitant use.
Propranolol and other beta blockers: blocked bronchodilating effect of metaproterenol. Monitor patient carefully if used together.

CONTRAINDICATIONS

Contraindicated in patients with hypersensitivity to the drug or any of its ingredients and in use during anesthesia with cyclopropane or halogenated hydrocarbon general anesthetics and in those with tachycardia and arrhythmias associated with tachycardia, peripheral or mesenteric vascular thrombosis, profound hypoxia or hypercapnia.

NURSING CONSIDERATIONS

● Use cautiously in patients with hypertension, hyperthyroidism, heart disease, diabetes, or cirrhosis and in those who are receiving digitalis glycosides.
● Know that metaproterenol reportedly produces less cardiac stimulation than other sympathomimetics, especially isoproterenol.
● Be aware that patients may use tablets and aerosol concomitantly. Monitor closely for toxicity.
● Know that inhalant solution can be administered by IPPB with drug diluted in 0.9% sodium chloride solution or via a hand nebulizer at full strength.
● Teach patients to perform oral inhalation correctly. Give the following instructions for using a metered-dose inhaler:
  — Clear nasal passages and throat.
  — Breathe out, expelling as much air from lungs as possible.
  — Place mouthpiece well into mouth as dose from inhaler is released, and inhale deeply.
  — Hold breath for several seconds, remove mouthpiece, and exhale slowly. Allow two minutes between inhalations.
● Store drug in light-resistant container.
● Tell patient that metaproterenol inhalations should precede steroid inhalations (when prescribed) by 10 to 15 minutes to maximize therapy.
● Tell patients who also are using a steroid inhaler to use the bronchodilator first, then wait about 5 minutes before using the steroid. This allows bronchodilator to open air passages for maximum effectiveness.
● If more than one inhalation is ordered, tell patients to wait at least 2 minutes before repeating procedure.
● Warn patients to discontinue imme-

---

*Liquid form contains alcohol.
**May contain tartrazine.   *Common* reactions are in italics; *life-threatening,* in bold italics.

diately if paradoxical bronchospasm occurs and to notify doctor.
• Warn patients to notify doctor if no response is derived from dosage or to request dosage adjustments.

oxtriphylline (choline salt of theophyllinate)
Choledyl*

Pregnancy Risk Category: C

HOW SUPPLIED
Tablets: 100 mg, 200 mg
Tablets (extended-release): 400 mg, 600 mg
Tablets (delayed-release): 100 mg, 200 mg
Elixir:* 100 mg/5 ml
Syrup: 50 mg/5 ml

ACTION
Inhibits phosphodiesterase, the enzyme that degrades cAMP. Results in relaxation of smooth muscle of the bronchial airways and pulmonary blood vessels. Oxtriphylline is equivalent to 64% anhydrous theophylline.

ONSET, PEAK, DURATION
Onset and duration unknown. Peak effects occur within 1 hour after oral solution, within 2 hours of oral tablets.

INDICATIONS & DOSAGE
Acute bronchial asthma and reversible bronchospasm associated with chronic bronchitis and emphysema –
Adults (nonsmokers): 4.7 mg/kg P.O. q 8 hours.
Adults (smokers) and children 9 to 16 years: 4.7 mg/kg q 6 hours.
Children 1 to 9 years: 6.2 mg/kg P.O. q 6 hours.
    If total daily maintenance dosage is established at approximately 800 to 1,200 mg, 1 sustained-action tablet q 12 hours may be substituted.

ADVERSE REACTIONS
CNS: *restlessness, dizziness,* headache, *insomnia,* light-headedness, *seizures,* muscle twitching.
CV: *palpitations, sinus tachycardia,* extrasystoles, flushing, marked hypotension.
GI: *nausea, vomiting, anorexia,* bitter aftertaste, dyspepsia, heavy feeling in stomach.
Respiratory: increased respiratory rate.
Skin: urticaria.

INTERACTIONS
Adenosine: decreased antiarrhythmic effectiveness. Higher doses of adenosine may be necessary.
Allopurinol (high-dose): increased serum theophylline levels. Monitor for toxicity.
Barbiturates, carbamazepine, nicotine, phenytoin, rifampin: enhanced metabolism and decreased theophylline blood levels. Monitor for decreased effect.
Beta-adrenergic blockers: antagonism. Propranolol and nadolol, especially, may cause bronchospasm in sensitive patients. Use together cautiously.
Cimetidine, influenza virus vaccine, macrolide antibiotics (such as erythromycin), oral contraceptives, quinolone antibiotics (such as ciprofloxacin): decreased hepatic clearance of theophylline; elevated theophylline levels. Monitor for signs of toxicity.
Lithium: increased renal excretion of lithium. Monitor for decreased effect.

CONTRAINDICATIONS
Contraindicated in patients with hypersensitivity to xanthines (caffeine, theobromine) and in patients with preexisting arrhythmias, especially tachyarrhythmias.

NURSING CONSIDERATIONS
• Use cautiously in young children, in elderly patients, and in those with

peptic ulceration, COPD, cardiac failure, cor pulmonale, renal or hepatic impairment, glaucoma, severe hypoxemia, hypertension, compromised cardiac or circulatory function, angina, acute MI, sulfite sensitivity, hyperthyroidism, and diabetes mellitus.
• Do not combine with products containing ephedrine; excessive CNS stimulation (nervousness, tremor, akathisia) may result.
• Administer drug after meals and at bedtime.
• Know that oxtriphylline is a soluble salt of theophylline. Dosage is adjusted by monitoring response, tolerance, pulmonary function, and serum theophylline levels. Ensure that theophylline concentrations range from 10 to 20 mcg/ml; toxicity has been reported with levels above 20 mcg/ml.
• Monitor therapy carefully. Individuals metabolize theophyllines at different rates. Dosage adjustments are necessary in elderly patients; in those with CHF, cor pulmonale, and hepatic disease; and in smokers.
• Store at 15° to 30° C (59° to 86° F). Protect elixir from light and tablets from moisture.
• Tell patients to report GI distress, palpitations, irritability, restlessness, nervousness, or insomnia; may indicate excessive CNS stimulation.
• Tell patient that tablets should not be chewed, crushed, or dissolved.

pirbuterol
Maxair

Pregnancy Risk Category: C

HOW SUPPLIED
Inhaler: 0.2 mg/metered dose

ACTION
Relaxes bronchial smooth muscle by acting on beta$_2$-adrenergic receptors.

ONSET, PEAK, DURATION
Onset occurs within 5 minutes. Peak effects occur in 30 to 60 minutes. Effects persist for 5 hours.

INDICATIONS AND DOSAGE
Prevention and reversal of bronchospasm, asthma –
Adults and children 12 years and over: 1 or 2 inhalations (0.2 to 0.4 mg) repeated q 4 to 6 hours. Not to exceed 12 inhalations daily.

ADVERSE REACTIONS
CNS: tremor, nervousness, dizziness, insomnia, headache.
CV: tachycardia, palpitations, increased blood pressure.
EENT: dryness or irritation of throat.

INTERACTIONS
MAO inhibitors, tricyclic antidepressants: may potentiate action of beta-adrenergic agonist on vascular system. Use together cautiously.
Propranolol and other beta-adrenergic blocking agents: decreased bronchodilating effects.

CONTRAINDICATIONS
Contraindicated in patients with hypersensitivity to pirbuterol.

NURSING CONSIDERATIONS
• Use cautiously in patients with CV disorders, hyperthyroidism, diabetes, and seizure disorders or in those who are unusually responsive to sympathomimetic amines.
• Teach patients to perform oral inhalation correctly. Give the following instructions for using a metered-dose inhaler:
   – Clear nasal passages and throat.
   – Breathe out, expelling as much air from lungs as possible.
   – Place mouthpiece well into mouth as dose from inhaler is released, and inhale deeply.
   – Hold breath for several seconds,

---

*Liquid form contains alcohol.   *Common* reactions are in italics; *life-threatening*, in bold italics.
**May contain tartrazine.

remove mouthpiece, and exhale slowly.

• If more than one inhalation is ordered, tell patients to wait at least 2 minutes before repeating procedure.

• Tell patients who also are using a steroid inhaler to use the bronchodilator first, then wait about 5 minutes before using the steroid. This allows the bronchodilator to open air passages for maximum effectiveness.

• Tell patients who experience increased bronchospasm after using drug to call the doctor.

• Advise patients to seek medical attention if a previously effective dosage does not control symptoms; this may signify worsening of the disease.

salmeterol xinafoate
Serevent

Pregnancy Risk Category: C

HOW SUPPLIED
Inhalation aerosol: 21 mcg per metered spray

ACTION
Not clearly defined. Selectively activates beta$_2$-adrenergic receptors, which results in bronchodilation. Also blocks the release of allergic mediators from mast cells lining the respiratory tract.

ONSET, PEAK, DURATION
Onset occurs in 10 to 20 minutes. Peak effects occur after about 3 hours; plasma levels peak within 45 minutes, but drug acts locally in the lung and its action is not dependent on plasma levels. Effects persist about 12 hours.

INDICATIONS & DOSAGE
Long-term maintenance treatment of asthma; prevention of bronchospasm in patients with nocturnal asthma or reversible obstructive airway disease who require regular treatment with short-acting beta agonists –
Adults and children over 12 years: two inhalations twice daily, one in the morning and one in the evening.

Not for use to treat acute symptoms.
Prevention of exercise-induced bronchospasm –
Adults and children 12 years and over: 2 inhalations at least 30 to 60 minutes before exercise.

ADVERSE REACTIONS
CNS: headache, sinus headache, tremor.
CV: tachycardia, palpitations.
EENT: upper respiratory infection, nasopharyngitis, nasal cavity or sinus disorder.
GI: stomachache.
Respiratory: cough, lower respiratory infection, *bronchospasm.*
Other: hypersensitivity reactions (such as rash, urticaria).

INTERACTIONS
Beta-adrenergic agonists, theophylline or other methylxanthines: possible adverse cardiac effects with excessive use. Monitor closely.
MAO inhibitors: risk of severe adverse cardiovascular effects. Avoid use within 14 days of MAO therapy.
Tricyclic antidepressants: risk of moderate to severe adverse cardiovascular effects. Use with extreme caution.

CONTRAINDICATIONS
Contraindicated in patients with hypersensitivity to the drug or any component of the formulation.

NURSING CONSIDERATIONS
• Use cautiously in patients with coronary insufficiency, arrhythmias, hypertension, other CV disorders, thyrotoxicosis, or seizure disorders and in patients who are unusually responsive to sympathomimetics.
• Remind patients to take drug at ap-

---

proximately 12-hour intervals for optimum effect and to take the drug even when feeling better.

• If the patient is taking the drug to prevent exercise-induced bronchospasm, tell him he should take it 30 to 60 minutes before exercise.

• Tell patient that although this drug is a beta agonist, do not use to treat acute bronchospasm. Patients must be provided with a short-acting beta agonist (such as albuterol) to treat such exacerbations.

• Tell patients to contact the doctor if the short-acting agonist no longer provides sufficient relief or if more than four inhalations are needed per day. This may be a sign that the asthma symptoms are worsening. Tell patient not to increase the dosage of salmeterol.

• If patients are taking an inhaled corticosteroid, they should continue to use it on a regular basis. Warn patients not to take any other medications without the doctor's consent.

terbutaline sulfate
Brethaire, Brethine, Bricanyl

Pregnancy Risk Category: B

HOW SUPPLIED
Tablets: 2.5 mg, 5 mg
Aerosol inhaler: 200 mcg/metered spray
Injection: 1 mg/ml

ACTION
Relaxes bronchial smooth muscle by acting on beta$_2$-adrenergic receptors. Also relaxes uterine muscle.

ONSET, PEAK, DURATION
Onset occurs within 15 minutes of S.C. injection, 5 to 30 minutes after inhalation, 1 to 2 hours after oral use. Peak effects occur within 30 minutes to 1 hour of S.C. injection, 1 to 2 hours after inhalation, or 2 to 3 hours after oral use. Effects persist about

1½ to 4 hours after S.C. injection, 3 to 6 hours after inhalation, or 4 to 8 hours after oral use.

INDICATIONS & DOSAGE
Bronchospasm in patients with reversible obstructive airway disease –
Adults and children over 11 years: 2 inhalations separated by a 60-second interval, repeated q 4 to 6 hours. Also may be administered 5 mg for adults and 2.5 mg for children over 11 years P.O. or 0.25 mg S.C. q 8 hours.

ADVERSE REACTIONS
CNS: *nervousness, tremor, headache,* drowsiness, sweating.
CV: palpitations, increased heart rate.
EENT: dryness and irritation of nose and throat (with inhaled form).
GI: vomiting, nausea.
Respiratory: *paradoxical bronchospasm with prolonged usage.*
Other: hypokalemia (with high doses).

INTERACTIONS
CNS stimulants: increased CNS stimulation. Avoid concomitant use.
Cyclopropane, digitalis glycosides, halogenated inhalation anesthetics, levodopa: increased risk of arrhythmias. Monitor closely, and avoid concomitant use with levodopa.
MAO inhibitors: when given with sympathomimetics, may cause severe hypertension (hypertensive crisis). Don't use together.
Propranolol and other beta blockers: blocked bronchodilating effects of terbutaline.

CONTRAINDICATIONS
Contraindicated in patients with hypersensitivity to the drug or sympathomimetic amines.

---

*Liquid form contains alcohol.
**May contain tartrazine.
Common reactions are in italics; *life-threatening*, in bold italics.

NURSING CONSIDERATIONS

• Use cautiously in patient with CV disorders, hyperthyroidism, diabetes, or seizure disorders.

• Give S.C. injections in lateral deltoid area.

• Protect injection from light. Do not use if discolored.

• Know that patients may use tablets and aerosol concomitantly. Monitor closely for toxicity.

• Ensure that patients and family members understand why drug is necessary.

• Teach patients to perform oral inhalation correctly. Give the following instructions for using a metered-dose inhaler:

    — Clear nasal passages and throat.

    — Breathe out, expelling as much air from lungs as possible.

    — Place mouthpiece well into mouth as dose from inhaler is released, and inhale deeply.

    — Hold breath for several seconds, remove mouthpiece, and exhale slowly.

• If more than one inhalation is ordered, tell patients to wait at least 2 minutes before repeating procedure.

• Tell patients who also are using a steroid inhaler to use bronchodilator first, then wait about 5 minutes before using steroid. This allows bronchodilator to open air passages for maximum effectiveness.

• Warn patients to discontinue the drug immediately and notify doctor if paradoxical bronchospasm occurs.

• Warn patient that tolerance may develop with prolonged use.

theophylline

Immediate-release liquids: Accurbron*, Aquaphyllin, Asmalix*, Bronkodyl*, Elixicon, Elixomin*, Elixophyllin*, Lanophyllin*, Lixolin, Slo-Phyllin, Theolair Liquid, Theon*
Immediate-release tablets and capsules: Bronkodyl, Elixophyllin, Nuelin‡, Slo-Phyllin, Somophyllin-T
Timed-release tablets: Constant-T, Duraphyl, Quibron-T/SR, Respbid, Sustaire, Theo-Dur, Theolair-SR, Theo-Time, Uniphyl
Timed-release capsules: Aerolate, Elixophyllin SR, Nuelin-SR‡, Slobid Gyrocaps, Slo-Phyllin, Somophyllin-CRT, Theo-24, Theobid Duracaps, Theobid Jr. Duracaps, Theochron, Theo-Dur Sprinkle, Theospan-SR, Theovent Long-Acting

theophylline sodium glycinate

Acet-Am†

Pregnancy Risk Category: C

HOW SUPPLIED
theophylline
Tablets: 100 mg, 125 mg, 200 mg, 250 mg, 300 mg
Tablets (chewable): 100 mg
Tablets (extended-release): 100 mg, 200 mg, 250 mg, 300 mg, 400 mg, 450 mg, 500 mg
Capsules: 100 mg, 200 mg
Capsules (extended-release): 50 mg, 60 mg, 65 mg, 75 mg, 100 mg, 125 mg, 130 mg, 200 mg, 250 mg, 260 mg, 300 mg
Elixir: 27 mg/5 ml, 50 mg/5 ml*
Oral solution: 27 mg/5 ml, 50 mg/5 ml
Syrup: 27 mg/5 ml, 50 mg/5 ml
Dextrose 5% injection: 200 mg in 50 ml or 100 ml; 400 mg in 100 ml, 250 ml, 500 ml, or 1,000 ml; 800 mg in 500 ml or 1,000 ml

---

†Available in Canada only.   ‡Available in Australia only.   ◇Available OTC.

theophylline sodium glycinate
Elixir: 110 mg/5 ml (equivalent to 55 mg anhydrous theophylline/5 ml)

ACTION
Inhibits phosphodiesterase, the enzyme that degrades cAMP. Results in relaxation of smooth muscle of the bronchial airways and pulmonary blood vessels.

ONSET, PEAK, DURATION
Onset occurs within 15 minutes of I.V. use, 15 minutes to 1 hour after oral use. Peak effects occur 15 to 30 minutes after I.V. use; 1 to 2 hours after oral use, except for enteric-coated tablets (peak in about 5 hours) and extended-release capsules and tablets (peak in 4 to 7 hours). Duration unknown.

INDICATIONS & DOSAGE
Oral theophylline for acute bronchospasm in patients not currently receiving theophylline –
Adults: (nonsmoker) 6 mg/kg P.O. followed by 2 to 3 mg/kg q 6 hours for 2 doses. Maintenance dosage is 3 mg/kg q 8 hours.
Otherwise healthy adult smokers: 6 mg/kg P.O. followed by 3 mg/kg q 6 hours for 3 doses. Maintenance dosage is 3 mg/kg q 6 hours.
Children 9 to 16 years: 6 mg/kg P.O. followed by 3 mg/kg q 6 hours for 3 doses. Maintenance dosage is 3 mg/kg q 6 hours.
Children 6 months to 9 years: 6 mg/kg P.O. followed by 4 mg/kg q 6 hours for 3 doses. Maintenance dosage is 4 mg/kg q 6 hours.
   Extended-release preparations should not be used for the treatment of acute bronchospasm.
Parenteral theophylline for patients not currently receiving theophylline –
Loading dose: 4.7 mg/kg I.V. slowly; then maintenance infusion.
Adults (nonsmokers): 0.55 mg/kg/

hour I.V. for 12 hours, then 0.39 mg/kg/hour.
Otherwise healthy adult smokers: 0.79 mg/kg/hour I.V. for 12 hours; then 0.63 mg/kg/hour.
Older adults with cor pulmonale: 0.47 mg/kg/hour I.V. for 12 hours; then 0.24 mg/kg/hour.
Adults with CHF or liver disease: 0.39 mg/kg/hour I.V. for 12 hours; then 0.08 to 0.16 mg/kg/hour.
Children 9 to 16 years: 0.79 mg/kg/hour I.V. for 12 hours; then 0.63 mg/kg/hour.
Children 6 months to 9 years: 0.95 mg/kg/hour I.V. for 12 hours; then 0.79 mg/kg/hour.
Oral and parenteral theophylline for acute bronchospasm in patients currently receiving theophylline –
Adults and children: each 0.5 mg/kg I.V. or P.O. (loading dose) will increase plasma levels by 1 mcg/ml. Ideally, dose is based on current theophylline level. In emergency situations, some clinicians recommend a 2.5 mg/kg P.O. dose of rapidly absorbed form if no obvious signs of theophylline toxicity are present.
Chronic bronchospasm –
Adults and children: 16 mg/kg or 400 mg P.O. daily (whichever is less) given in 3 or 4 divided doses at 6- to 8-hour intervals. Alternatively, 12 mg/kg or 400 mg P.O. daily (whichever is less) using an extended-release preparation given in 2 or 3 divided doses at 8- or 12-hour intervals. Dosage increased as tolerated at 2- to 3-day intervals to maximum dosage as follows:
Adults and children 16 years and over: 13 mg/kg or 900 mg P.O. daily (whichever is less).
Children 12 to 16 years: 18 mg/kg P.O. daily.
Children 9 to 12 years: 20 mg/kg P.O. daily.
Children to 9 years: 24 mg/kg P.O. daily.

---

*Liquid form contains alcohol.
**May contain tartrazine.

Common reactions are in italics; *life-threatening,* in bold italics.

ADVERSE REACTIONS

CNS: *restlessness, dizziness,* headache, *insomnia,* light-headedness, *seizures,* muscle twitching.
CV: *palpitations, sinus tachycardia,* extrasystoles, flushing, marked hypotension.
GI: *nausea, vomiting, anorexia,* bitter aftertaste, dyspepsia, heavy feeling in stomach, diarrhea.
Respiratory: increased respiratory rate.
Skin: urticaria.

INTERACTIONS

Adenosine: decreased antiarrhythmic effectiveness. Higher doses of adenosine may be necessary.
Barbiturates, carbamazepine, nicotine, phenytoin, rifampin: enhanced metabolism and decreased theophylline blood levels. Monitor for decreased effect.
Beta-adrenergic blockers: antagonism. Propranolol and nadolol, especially, may cause bronchospasm in sensitive patients. Use together cautiously.
Cimetidine, influenza virus vaccine, macrolide antibiotics (such as erythromycin), oral contraceptives, quinolone antibiotics (such as ciprofloxacin), caffeine: decreased hepatic clearance of theophylline; elevated theophylline levels. Monitor for signs of toxicity.
  Patients taking Theo-24 should take it on an empty stomach because food accelerates the drug's absorption.

CONTRAINDICATIONS

Contraindicated in patients with hypersensitivity to xanthine compounds (caffeine, theobromine) and in those with active peptic ulcer and seizure disorders.

NURSING CONSIDERATIONS

• Use cautiously in young children, infants under 1 year, and neonates; in elderly patients; and in those with COPD, cardiac failure, cor pulmonale, renal or hepatic disease, peptic ulceration, hyperthyroidism, diabetes mellitus, glaucoma, severe hypoxemia, hypertension, compromised cardiac or circulatory function, angina, acute MI, or sulfite sensitivity.
• Be careful not to confuse sustained-release dosage forms with standard-release dosage forms.
• **I.V. use:** Use commercially available infusion solution, or mix drug in D_5W. Use infusion pump for continuous infusion.
• Know that drug dosage may need to be increased in cigarette smokers and in habitual marijuana smokers because smoking causes the drug to be metabolized faster.
• Be aware that daily dosage may need to be decreased in patients with CHF or hepatic disease or in elderly patients because metabolism and excretion may be decreased. Monitor carefully, using blood levels, observation, examination, and patient interview. Give drug around-the-clock, using sustained-release product at bedtime.
• Monitor vital signs; measure and record fluid intake and output. Expected clinical effects include improvement in quality of pulse and respirations.
• Warn patient not to dissolve, crush, or chew slow-release products. Small children unable to swallow these can ingest (without chewing) the contents of bead-filled capsules sprinkled over soft food.
• Know that individuals metabolize xanthines at different rates; dosage determined by monitoring response, tolerance, pulmonary function, and serum theophylline levels. Serum theophylline concentrations should range from 10 to 20 mcg/ml; toxicity has been reported with levels above 20 mcg/ml.
• Supply instructions for home care and dosage schedule.

● Tell patient to relieve GI symptoms by taking oral drug with full glass of water after meals, although food in stomach delays absorption.

● Warn patients to take the drug regularly, as directed. Patients tend to want to take extra "breathing pills."

● Warn elderly patients that dizziness, a common adverse reaction at start of therapy, may occur.

● Warn patients to check with the doctor or pharmacist about *any* other drugs used. OTC remedies may contain ephedrine in combination with theophylline salts; excessive CNS stimulation may result.

---

benzonatate
codeine phosphate
(See Chapter 28, NARCOTIC AND OPIOID
ANALGESICS.)
codeine sulfate
(See Chapter 28, NARCOTIC AND OPIOID
ANALGESICS.)
dextromethorphan
hydrobromide
diphenhydramine hydrochloride
(See Chapter 43, ANTIHISTAMINES.)
guaifenesin
hydromorphone hydrochloride
(See Chapter 28, NARCOTIC AND OPIOID
ANALGESICS.)

COMBINATION PRODUCTS
Preparations are available in the following combinations:
• expectorants with decongestants or
antihistamines, or both
• antitussives with decongestants or
antihistamines, or both
• expectorants and antitussives
• expectorants and antitussives with
decongestants or antihistamines, or
both.

benzonatate
Tessalon

Pregnancy Risk Category: C

HOW SUPPLIED
Capsules: 100 mg

ACTION
Suppresses the cough reflex by direct
action on the cough center in the medulla. Also has local anesthetic action.

ONSET, PEAK, DURATION
Onset ocucrs in 15 to 20 minutes.
Peak unknown. Effects persist up to 8
hours.

INDICATIONS & DOSAGE
Symptomatic relief of cough –
Adults and children over 10 years:
100 mg P.O. t.i.d.; up to 600 mg daily
may be needed.

ADVERSE REACTIONS
CNS: dizziness, drowsiness, head-
ache, restlessness, *seizures.*
EENT: nasal congestion, burning
sensation in eyes.
GI: nausea, constipation.
Skin: rash.
Other: chills.

INTERACTIONS
None significant.

CONTRAINDICATIONS
Contraindicated in patients hypersensitive to the drug.

NURSING CONSIDERATIONS
• Use cautiously in patients hypersensitive to paramino-benzoic acid anesthetics (procaine, tetracaine) because
cross-sensitivity reactions may occur.
• Don't use benzonatate when cough
is a valuable diagnostic sign or is beneficial (as after thoracic surgery).
• Monitor cough type and frequency.
• Use with percussion and chest vibration.
• Maintain fluid intake to help liquefy sputum.
• Warn patients not to chew capsules
or dissolve in mouth. Produces either
local anesthesia that may result in aspiration or CNS stimulation that may
cause restlessness, tremor, and seizures.

---

†Available in Canada only. ‡Available in Australia only. ◇Available OTC.

dextromethorphan hydrobromide

Balminil D.M.◊, Benylin DM◊, Broncho-Grippol-DM†, Children's Hold◊, DM Syrup◊, Hold◊, Koffex†, Mediquell◊, Neo-DM†, Ornex-DM 15◊, Ornex-DM 30◊, Pertussin Cough Suppressant◊, Pertussin CS◊, Pertussin ES◊, Robidex†, Robitussin Pediatric◊, Sedatuss†, St. Joseph Cough Suppression for Children◊, Sucrets Cough Control Formula◊, Trocal◊, Vicks Formula 44 Pediatric Formula◊. More commonly available in combination products, such as Anti-Tuss DM Expectorant◊, Baytussin DM◊, Benylin Expectorant Cough Formula◊, Cheracol D Cough◊, Codistan No. 1◊, Efficol Cough Whip◊, Extra Action Cough◊, 2/G-DM Cough◊, Glycotuss dM◊, Guiamid D.M. Liquid◊, Guiatuss-DM◊, Halotussin-DM Expectorant◊, Kolephrin GG/DM◊, Mytussin DM◊, Naldecon Senior DX◊, Pertussin All-Night CS◊, Rhinosyn-DMX Expectorant◊, Robitussin-DM◊, Silexin Cough◊, Tolu-Sed DM◊, Tuss-DM◊, Unproco◊, Vicks Children's Cough Syrup◊

Pregnancy Risk Category: C

HOW SUPPLIED
Liquid (extended-release): 30 mg/5 ml◊
Lozenges: 5 mg◊, 7.5 mg◊
Solution: 3.5 mg/5 ml, 5 mg/5 ml*◊, 7.5 mg/5 ml*◊, 10 mg/5 ml*◊, 15 mg/5 ml*◊

ACTION
An antitussive that suppresses the cough reflex by direct action on the cough center in the medulla.

ONSET, PEAK, DURATION
Onset occurs within 30 minutes. Peak unknown. Effects persist 3 to 6 hours with conventional dosage forms; up to 12 hours with extended-release forms.

INDICATIONS & DOSAGE
Nonproductive cough –
Adults and children 12 years and over: 10 to 20 mg P.O. q 4 hours, or 30 mg q 6 to 8 hours. Or, 60 mg controlled-release liquid b.i.d. Maximum dosage is 120 mg daily.
Children 6 to 12 years: 5 to 10 mg P.O. q 4 hours, or 15 mg q 6 to 8 hours. Or, 30 mg controlled-release liquid b.i.d. Maximum dosage is 60 mg daily.
Children 2 to 6 years: 2.5 to 5 mg P.O. q 4 hours, or 7.5 mg q 6 to 8 hours. Or, 15 mg controlled-release liquid b.i.d. Maximum dosage is 30 mg daily.
  Dosages for children under 2 years must be individualized.

ADVERSE REACTIONS
CNS: drowsiness, dizziness.
GI: nausea, vomiting, stomach pain.

INTERACTIONS
MAO inhibitors: risk of hypotension, coma, hyperpyrexia, and death. Avoid concomitant use.

CONTRAINDICATIONS
Contraindicated in patients currently taking MAO inhibitors or within 2 weeks of discontinuing MAO inhibitors.

NURSING CONSIDERATIONS
● Use with caution in atopic children, sedated or debilitated patients, and in patients confined to the supine position. Also, use cautiously in patients with aspirin sensitivity.
● Don't use dextromethorphan when cough is a valuable diagnostic sign or is beneficial (as after thoracic surgery).

---

*Liquid form contains alcohol.
**May contain tartrazine.

Common reactions are in italics; ***life-threatening,*** in bold italics.

- Know that dextromethorphan 15 to 30 mg is equivalent to 8 to 15 mg codeine as an antitussive.
- Be aware that drug produces no analgesia or addiction and little or no CNS depression.
- Use drug with chest percussion and vibration.
- Monitor cough type and frequency.

guaifenesin
(glyceryl guaiacolate)
Anti-Tuss*◊, Balminil Expectorant†, Baytussin◊, Breonesin◊, Cremacoat 2◊, Gee-Gee◊, GG-CEN*◊, Glyate*◊, Glycotuss◊, Glytuss◊, Guiatuss*◊, Halotussin, Humibid L.A.◊, Hytuss◊, Hytuss-2X◊, Naldecon Senior EX◊, Neo-Spec†, Nortussin◊, Resyl†◊, Robafen◊, Robitussin*◊, S-T Expectorant◊

Pregnancy Risk Category: C

HOW SUPPLIED
Tablets: 100 mg◊, 200 mg◊
Capsules: 200 mg◊
Capsules (extended-release): 300 mg
Solution: 100 mg/5 ml*◊, 200 mg/5 ml*◊

ACTION
Increases production of respiratory tract fluids to help liquefy and reduce the viscosity of tenacious secretions.

ONSET, PEAK, DURATION
Unknown.

INDICATIONS & DOSAGE
Expectorant –
Adults and children 12 years of age and over: 200 to 400 mg P.O. q 4 hours, or 600 to 1,200 mg extended-release capsules q 12 hours. Maximum dosage is 2,400 mg daily.
Children 2 to 6 years: 50 to 100 mg P.O. q 4 hours. Maximum dosage is 600 mg daily.
Children 6 to 12 years: 100 to 200 mg P.O. q 4 hours. Maximum dosage is 1,200 mg daily.

ADVERSE REACTIONS
CNS: drowsiness.
GI: stomach pain, diarrhea, vomiting, and nausea occur with large doses.

INTERACTIONS
Heparin: increased risk of bleeding. Use together cautiously.

CONTRAINDICATIONS
Contraindicated in patients hypersensitive to the drug.

NURSING CONSIDERATIONS
- Be aware that drug is used to liquefy thick, tenacious sputum. Evidence that guaifenesin is effective as expectorant but no evidence to support role an antitussive.
- Know that drug may interfere with certain laboratory tests for 5-hydroxyindoleacetic acid and vanillylmandelic acid.
- Monitor cough type and frequency.
- Ensure that patients understand that persistent cough may indicate a serious condition and that they should contact a doctor if cough lasts longer than 1 week, recurs frequently, or is associated with high fever, rash, or severe headache.
- Advise patients to take each dose with a glass of water; increasing fluid intake may prove beneficial.
- Encourage deep-breathing exercises.

acetylcysteine
alpha, proteinase inhibitor
   (human)
beclomethasone dipropionate
beractant
colfosceril palmitate
cromolyn sodium
dexamethasone sodium
   phosphate inhalation
dornase alfa
flunisolide
nedocromil sodium
triamcinolone acetonide

COMBINATION PRODUCTS
None.

---

acetylcysteine
Airbron†, Mucomyst,
Mucomyst-10, Mucosil-10,
Mucosil-20, Parvolex†‡

Pregnancy Risk Category: NR

HOW SUPPLIED
Solution: 10%, 20%
Injection: 200 mg/ml†‡

ACTION
A mucolytic that increases production of respiratory tract fluids to help liquefy and reduce the viscosity of tenacious secretions. Also restores liver stores of glutathione to treat acetaminophen toxicity.

ONSET, PEAK, DURATION
Unknown.

INDICATIONS & DOSAGE
Pneumonia, bronchitis, tuberculosis, cystic fibrosis, emphysema, atelectasis (adjunct), complications of thoracic surgery and CV surgery –
Adults and children: 1 to 2 ml 10% or 20% solution by direct instillation into trachea as often as every hour; or 3 to 5 ml 20% solution or 6 to 10 ml 10% solution by nebulization q 2 to 6 hours p.r.n. Alternatively, where available 300 mg/kg by I.V. infusion in divided doses.
Acetaminophen toxicity –
Adults and children: initially, 140 mg/kg P.O., followed by 70 mg/kg P.O. q 4 hours for 17 doses. Or, where available 300 mg/kg by I.V. infusion.

ADVERSE REACTIONS
EENT: *rhinorrhea, hemoptysis.*
GI: *stomatitis, nausea, vomiting.*
Respiratory: ***bronchospasm*** (especially in asthmatic patients).

INTERACTIONS
Activated charcoal: limits acetylcysteine's effectiveness. Avoid concomitant use in treating acetaminophen toxicity.

CONTRAINDICATIONS
Contraindicated in patients hypersensitive to the drug.

NURSING CONSIDERATIONS
• Use cautiously in elderly or debilitated patients with severe respiratory insufficiency.
• Use plastic, glass, stainless steel, or another nonreactive metal when administering by nebulization. Hand-bulb nebulizers are not recommended because output is too small and particle size too large.
• Know that drug may have a foul taste or smell that some patients find distressing.
• Physically or chemically incompatible with tetracyclines, erythromycin lactobionate, amphotericin B, and ampicillin sodium. If administered by aerosol inhalation, these drugs should

---

*Liquid form contains alcohol.
**May contain tartrazine.

Common reactions are in italics; ***life-threatening,*** in bold italics.

be nebulized separately. Iodized oil, trypsin, and hydrogen peroxide are physically incompatible with acetylcysteine; don't add to nebulizer.
• Monitor cough type and frequency. For maximum effect, instruct patient to clear his airway by coughing before aerosol administration.
• **I.V. use:** To prepare I.V. infusion, dilute calculated dose in D_5W. Dilute initial dose (150 mg/kg) in 200 ml of D_5W and infuse over 15 minutes. Dilute second dose of 50 mg/kg in 500 ml of D_5W and give over 4 hours. Dilute final dose of 100 mg/kg in 1,000 ml of D_5W and infuse over 16 hours.
• After opening, store in refrigerator; use within 96 hours.
• Acetylcysteine is administered to treat acetaminophen overdose within 24 hours after ingestion. Start treatment immediately as prescribed; do not wait for results of acetaminophen blood levels.
• When used orally to treat acetaminophen overdose, dilute oral doses with cola, fruit juice, or water before administering. Dilute the 20% solution to a concentration of 5% (add 3 ml of diluent to each ml of acetylcysteine). If patient vomits within 1 hour of receiving loading or maintenance dose, repeat dose.

alpha₁ proteinase inhibitor (human)
Prolastin

Pregnancy Risk Category: C

HOW SUPPLIED
Injection: 500 mg, 1,000 mg

ACTION
Replaces alpha₁-proteinase in patients with alpha₁-antitrypsin deficiency.

ONSET, PEAK, DURATION
Onset occurs within a few weeks. Serum levels peak immediately after I.V. infusion. Duration unknown.

INDICATIONS & DOSAGE
Chronic replacement therapy in patients with congenital alpha₁-antitrypsin deficiency and demonstrable panacinar emphysema –
Adults: 60 mg/kg I.V. once weekly. May give at a rate of 0.08 ml/kg/minute or greater.

ADVERSE REACTIONS
Hematologic: possible viral transmission.

INTERACTIONS
Cigarette smoke: blocks drug's effects. Patients should not smoke.

CONTRAINDICATIONS
Contraindicated in patients with selective immunoglobulin A (IgA) deficiency who have known antibodies against IgA.

NURSING CONSIDERATIONS
• Use cautiously in patients at risk for circulatory overload.
• **I.V. use:** Store powder for injection in the refrigerator (36° to 46° F [2° to 8° C]). Reconstitute using the supplied diluent (sterile water for injection). After reconstitution, administer within 3 hours. Inject directly into vein; intermittent or continuous infusion is not recommended.
• Be aware that many commercial assays for alpha₁-proteinase inhibitor measure immunoreactivity of the protein and not inhibitor activity. Monitoring serum level may not accurately reflect clinical response.
• Explain to patients that product has been treated to minimize the risk of transmission of hepatitis and AIDS.

beclomethasone dipropionate
Aldecin Inhaler‡, Beclodisk†, Becloforte Inhaler‡, Beclovent, Beclovent Rotacaps†, Vanceril

Pregnancy Risk Category: NR

HOW SUPPLIED
Oral inhalation aerosol: 42 mcg/metered spray, 50 mcg/metered spray‡

ACTION
Unknown. Probably decreases inflammation, mainly by stabilizing leukocyte lysosomal membranes.

ONSET, PEAK, DURATION
Onset occurs in 1 to 4 weeks. Peak and duration unknown.

INDICATIONS & DOSAGE
Steroid-dependent asthma –
Adults and children 12 years of age and over: 2 to 4 inhalations t.i.d. or q.i.d. Maximum dosage is 20 inhalations daily.
Children 6 to 12 years: 1 to 2 inhalations t.i.d. or q.i.d. Maximum dosage is 10 inhalations daily.

ADVERSE REACTIONS
EENT: hoarseness, fungal infections of throat, throat irritation.
GI: dry mouth, fungal infections of mouth.

INTERACTIONS
None significant.

CONTRAINDICATIONS
Contraindicated in patients hypersensitive to any component of the formulation (fluorocarbons, oleic acid) and in those with status asthmaticus.

NURSING CONSIDERATIONS
• Use with extreme caution, if at all, in a patient with tuberculosis, fungal or bacterial infections, ocular herpes simplex or systemic viral infections.

• Not for use in patients with asthma controlled by bronchodilators or other noncorticosteroids alone or for those with nonasthmatic bronchial diseases.
• Use with caution in patients receiving systemic corticosteroid therapy.
• Be aware a spacer device may help ensure delivery of the proper dose.
• Check mucous membranes frequently for signs of fungal infection.
• Keep in mind that during times of stress (trauma, surgery, or infection) systemic corticosteroids may be needed to prevent adrenal insufficiency in previously steroid-dependent patients.
• Know that periodic measurement of growth and development may be necessary during high-dose or prolonged therapy in children.
• Taper oral glucocorticoid therapy slowly as ordered. Acute adrenal insufficiency and death have occurred in asthmatics who changed abruptly from oral corticosteroids to beclomethasone.
• Inform patients that beclomethasone doesn't provide relief for acute asthma attacks.
• Tell patients requiring a bronchodilator to use it several minutes before beclomethasone.
• Instruct patients to carry a medical identification card indicating need for supplemental systemic glucocorticoids during stress.
• Advise patients to allow 1 minute to elapse before taking subsequent puffs of medication and to hold breath for a few seconds to enhance action of drug.
• Instruct patients to contact their doctor if response to therapy decreases or if symptoms don't improve within 3 weeks; dosage may need to be adjusted. Tell patients not to exceed recommended dosage on their own.
• Tell patients to keep inhaler clean and unobstructed. Wash with warm water and dry thoroughly.
• Tell patients to prevent oral fungal in-

---

*Liquid form contains alcohol.
May contain tartrazine. *Common* reactions are in italics; **life-threatening, in bold italics.

fections by gargling or rinsing mouth with water after each use, but not to swallow the water.

• Tell patients to report symptoms associated with corticosteroid withdrawal, including fatigue, weakness, arthralgia, orthostatic hypotension, and dyspnea.

• Tell patient to store medication between 36° and 86° F (2° and 30° C). Advise patients to ensure delivery of the proper dose by gently warming canister to room temperature before using. Some patients carry the canister in a pocket to keep it warm.

beractant (natural lung surfactant)
Survanta

HOW SUPPLIED
Suspension for intratracheal instillation: 25 mg/ml

ACTION
Lowers the surface tension on alveolar surfaces during respiration and stabilizes the alveoli against collapse. An extract of bovine lung containing neutral lipids, fatty acids, surfactant-associated proteins, and phospholipids that mimics naturally occurring surfactant; palmitic acid, tripalmitin, and colfosceril palmitate are added to standardize the solution's composition.

ONSET, PEAK, DURATION
Onset occurs in ½ to 2 hours. Peak unknown. Effects persist for 2 to 3 days.

INDICATIONS & DOSAGE
Prevention of respiratory distress syndrome (RDS), also known as hyaline membrane disease, in premature neonates weighing 1,250 g or less at birth or having symptoms consistent with surfactant deficiency –
Neonates: 4 ml/kg intratracheally;

administer each dose in four quarter-doses, with a hand-held ventilator bag between quarter-doses at a rate of 60 breaths/minute and sufficient oxygen to prevent cyanosis. Give drug as soon as possible, preferably within 15 minutes of birth. Repeat in 6 hours if respiratory distress continues. Give no more than four doses in 48 hours.
Rescue treatment of RDS in premature infants –
Neonates: 4 ml/kg intratracheally; before administering, increase ventilator rate to 60 breaths/minute with an inspiratory time of 0.5 second and a fraction of inspired oxygen (FIO_2) of 1. Administer each dose in four quarter-doses, with a hand-held ventilator bag between quarter-doses at a rate of 60 breaths/minute and sufficient oxygen to prevent cyanosis. Give dose as soon as RDS is confirmed by X-ray, preferably within 8 hours of birth. Repeat in 6 hours if respiratory distress continues. Give no more than four doses in 48 hours.

ADVERSE REACTIONS
CV: transient bradycardia, vasoconstriction, hypotension.
Hematologic: decreased oxygen saturation, hypocapnia, hypercapnia.
Other: endotracheal tube reflux or blockage, pallor, *apnea.*

INTERACTIONS
None significant.

CONTRAINDICATIONS
None reported.

NURSING CONSIDERATIONS
• Beractant should be administered only by personnel experienced in the care of clinically unstable premature neonates. Such personnel should have knowledge of neonatal intubation and airway management.
• Accurate determination of weight is essential to proper measurement of dosage.

---

†Available in Canada only. ‡Available in Australia only. ◊Available OTC.

• Continuously monitor the neonate before, during, and after beractant administration. The endotracheal tube may be suctioned before giving the drug; allow the neonate to stabilize before proceeding with administration.

• Refrigerate at 36° to 46° F (2° to 8° C). Warm before administration by allowing drug to stand at room temperature for at least 20 minutes or by holding in hand for at least 8 minutes. Do not use artificial warming methods. Unopened vials that have been warmed to room temperature may be returned to the refrigerator within 8 hours; however, warm and return drug to the refrigerator only once. Vials are for single use only—discard unused drug.

• Beractant does not require sonication or reconstitution before use. Inspect contents before giving; ensure that the color is off-white to light brown and the contents are uniform. If settling occurs, swirl vial gently; do not shake. Some foaming is normal.

• Use a large-bore needle (20G or larger) to draw up drug; do not use a filter. Administer the drug using a #5 French end-hole catheter. Premeasure and shorten the catheter before use. Fill the catheter with beractant and discard any excess drug so only the total dose to be given remains in the syringe. Insert catheter into the neonate's endotracheal tube; make sure the catheter tip protrudes just beyond the end of the tube above the neonate's carina. Do not instill drug into a mainstem bronchus.

• Homogeneous distribution of the drug is important. In clinical trials, each dose of the drug was given in four quarter-doses, with the patient positioned differently after each administration. Each quarter-dose was given over 2 to 3 seconds; the catheter was removed and the patient ventilated between quarter-doses. With the head and body inclined slightly downward, the first quarter-dose was given with the head turned to the right; the second quarter-dose, with the head turned to the left. Then the head and body were inclined slightly upward; the third quarter-dose was given with the head turned to the right; the fourth quarter-dose, with the head turned to the left.

• Immediately after administration, moist breath sounds and crackles can occur. *Do not* suction the neonate for 1 hour unless other signs of airway obstruction are evident.

• Continuous monitoring of ECG and transcutaneous oxygen saturation are essential; frequent arterial blood pressure monitoring and frequent arterial blood gas sampling are highly desirable.

• Transient bradycardia and oxygen desaturation are common after dosing.

• Know that beractant can rapidly affect oxygenation and lung compliance. Peak ventilator inspiratory pressures may need to be adjusted if chest expansion improves substantially after drug administration. Notify doctor and adjust immediately as directed because lung overdistention and fatal pulmonary air leakage may result.

• Know that audiovisual materials that describe dosage and administration procedures are available from the manufacturer.

colfosceril palmitate
Exosurf Neonatal

HOW SUPPLIED
Suspension for intratracheal instillation: 10 ml

ACTION
Replaces a major component of naturally occurring lung surfactant (dipalmitoylphosphatidylcholine), which is deficient in premature neonates. The mixture also contains cetyl ethanol

---

*Liquid form contains alcohol.
May contain tartrazine.   *Common* reactions are in italics; ***life-threatening*, in bold italics.

(which acts as a spreading agent between the air-fluid interface) and tyloxapol, a long chain ethanol polymer (which acts as a dispersant).

ONSET, PEAK, DURATION
Unknown.

INDICATIONS & DOSAGE
Prevention of respiratory distress syndrome (RDS) in neonates weighing less than 1,350 g at risk for developing RDS; prophylactic treatment of neonates weighing more than 1,350 g with evidence of pulmonary insufficiency –
Neonates: administer 5 ml/kg intratracheally as soon as possible after delivery. If neonate is maintained on a mechanical ventilator, repeat dosage 12 and 24 hours later.
Rescue treatment of neonates with RDS –
Neonates: administer 5 ml/kg intratracheally as soon as possible after diagnosis of RDS. If the neonate is still mechanically ventilated, administer a second dose of 5 ml/kg 12 hours later.

ADVERSE REACTIONS
Respiratory: *pulmonary hemorrhage.*

INTERACTIONS
None significant.

CONTRAINDICATIONS
None reported.

NURSING CONSIDERATIONS
• Colfosceril should be administered only by personnel experienced in the care of clinically unstable premature neonates. Such personnel should have knowledge of neonatal intubation and airway management.
• Accurate determination of weight is essential to proper measurement of dosage.
• Know that colfosceril can rapidly affect oxygenation and lung compliance. Peak ventilator inspiratory pressures may need to be adjusted if chest expansion improves substantially after drug administration. Notify doctor and adjust immediately as directed because lung overdistention and fatal pulmonary air leakage may result.
• Continuous monitoring of ECG and transcutaneous oxygen saturation are essential; frequent arterial blood pressure monitoring and frequent arterial blood gas sampling are highly desirable. Continuously monitor the neonate before, during, and after drug administration.
• Reconstitute drug immediately before use with the supplied preservative-free sterile water for injection. Do not use solutions that contain antibacterial preservatives. After reconstitution, drug is stable for up to 12 hours at 36° to 86° F (2° to 30° C). Fill a 10-ml syringe with the supplied 8 ml of diluent using an 18G or 19G needle. Then, pierce the top of the vial and allow the vacuum to draw in the sterile water. Do not use vials without a vacuum. Aspirate as much of the 8 ml as possible out of vial while maintaining vacuum. Quickly release the syringe plunger. Repeat this final step at least three or four times to ensure adequate mixing of the vial contents.
• When drawing up the dose, use liquid below the froth. Each 8-ml vial contains sufficient material to administer a 5 ml/kg dose to a neonate weighing up to 1,600 g.
• Note that the suspension should have a homogeneous, milky white appearance. Do not use vials that appear to contain large flakes. If the suspension appears to separate, the vial may be shaken gently or swirled to resuspend the material.
• Suction the neonate before administering drug. Do not suction for 2 hours after dosing unless it is necessary.
• Special endotracheal tube adapters are available with each kit of surfactant. Ensure that adapter used corre-

sponds to the inside diameter of the neonate's endotracheal tube. Insert the adapter into the tube with a twisting motion and connect to the ventilator circuit. To administer the drug (in half-doses, 2.5 ml), remove the cap from side port of the adapter and attach syringe; do not interrupt mechanical ventilation. After dosing, remember to reattach cap.

• Instill each half-dose slowly over 1 to 2 minutes (30 to 50 mechanical breaths) in small bursts timed with inspiration. Administer first half-dose with the neonate in the midline position; then turn the neonate's head and torso 45 degrees to the right for 30 seconds to assist distribution of drug. Return the neonate to the midline position for the second half-dose and again administer over 1 to 2 minutes. After the second half-dose, turn the neonate's head and torso 45 degrees to the left for 30 seconds.

• When administering, monitor the neonate's facial expressions, skin color, chest expansion, heart rate, and endotracheal tube patency and position. If the neonate becomes dusky or agitated, heart rate slows, drug backs up in the endotracheal tube, or oxygen saturation decreases by more than 15%, discontinue the drug and modify peak inspiratory pressure, ventilator rate, or fraction of inspired oxygen FIO_2 as ordered. Note that rapid improvements in lung function may require rapid reductions in peak inspiratory pressure, ventilator rate, or FIO_2.

• Reduce ventilator rate immediately if the transcutaneous or arterial carbon dioxide measurements are less than 30 mm Hg. Failure to reduce the rate may result in hypocapnia, which can reduce blood flow to the brain.

• If the neonate becomes pink and the transcutaneous oxygen saturation exceeds 95%, reduce FIO_2 in a stepwise fashion until the saturation is 90% to 95%. Do so immediately because hyperoxia (an excess of systemic oxygen) may result.

• Monitor neonates for pulmonary hemorrhage.

cromolyn sodium (sodium cromoglycate)

Gastrocrom, Intal, Intal Aerosol Spray, Intal Nebulizer Solution, Nalcrom, Nasalcrom, Opticrom, Rynacrom†

Pregnancy Risk Category: B

HOW SUPPLIED
Capsules (for oral solution): 100 mg
Aerosol: 800 mcg/metered spray
Nasal solution: 5.2 mg/metered spray (40 mg/ml)
Solution (for nebulization): 20 mg/2 ml
Ophthalmic solution: 4% (with benzalkonium chloride 0.01%, EDTA 0.01%, and phenylethyl ethanol 0.4%)

ACTION
Inhibits the degranulation of sensitized mast cells that occurs after a patient's exposure to specific antigens. Also inhibits release of histamine and slow-reacting substance of anaphylaxis.

ONSET, PEAK, DURATION
Unknown.

INDICATIONS & DOSAGE
Adjunct in severe perennial bronchial asthma —
Adults and children 5 years and over: 2 metered sprays using inhaler q.i.d. at regular intervals. Alternatively, 20 mg via nebulization 4 times daily at regular intervals.
Prevention and treatment of allergic rhinitis —
Adults and children over 5 years: 1 spray in each nostril t.i.d or q.i.d. Maximal administration is six times daily.

---

*Liquid form contains alcohol. *Common* reactions are in italics; *life-threatening,* in bold italics.
**May contain tartrazine.

Prevention of exercise-induced bronchospasm–

Adults and children 5 years or over: 2 metered sprays inhaled no more than 1 hour before anticipated exercise.

Allergic ocular disorders–

Adults and children 4 years and older: 1 to 2 drops in each eye four to six times daily at regular intervals.

Systemic mastocytosis–

Adults and children over 12 years: 200 mg P.O. q.i.d. before meals and h.s.

Children 2 to 12 years: 100 mg P.O. q.i.d. 30 minutes before meals or h.s.

ADVERSE REACTIONS
CNS: dizziness, headache.
EENT: *irritation of the throat and trachea,* nasal congestion, pharyngeal irritation.
GI: nausea, esophagitis.
GU: dysuria, urinary frequency.
Respiratory: *bronchospasm* after inhalation of dry powder; *cough,* wheezing, *eosinophilic pneumonia.*
Skin: rash, urticaria.
Other: joint swelling and pain, lacrimation, swollen parotid gland, *angioedema.*

INTERACTIONS
None significant.

CONTRAINDICATIONS
Contraindicated in patients experiencing acute asthma attacks and status asthmaticus and in patients with hypersensitivity to drug.

NURSING CONSIDERATIONS
• Administer with caution in children. Use of cromolyn oral inhalation solution is *not* recommended in children under 2 years; cromolyn powder or aerosol for oral inhalation, not recommended in children under 5 years; and cromolyn nasal solution, not recomended in children under 6 years.
• Use inhalation form cautiously in patients with coronary artery disease or a history of arrhythmias.
• Know that drug should be used only when acute episode of asthma has been controlled, airway is cleared, and the patient can inhale independently.
• Be aware that oral cromolyn sodium should be used in full-term neonates and infants *only* for a severe, incapacitating disease when benefits clearly outweigh the risks.
• Dissolve powder in capsules for oral dose in hot water and further dilute with cold water before ingestion. Do not mix with fruit juice, milk, or food.
• Discontinue if the patient develops eosinophilic pneumonia, indicated by eosinophilia and infiltrates on chest X-ray film.
• Watch for recurrence of asthmatic symptoms when dosage is decreased, especially when corticosteroids are also used.
• Know that safety and efficacy of cromlyn sodium ophthalmic solution in children under 4 years have not been established.
• Tell patients esophagitis may be relieved by antacids or a glass of milk.

---

dexamethasone sodium phosphate inhalation
Decadron Phosphate Respihaler

Pregnancy Risk Category: NR

HOW SUPPLIED
Inhalation aerosol: 100 mcg/metered spray

ACTION
Unknown. Probably decreases inflammation, mainly by stabilizing leukocyte lysosomal membranes.

ONSET, PEAK, DURATION
Onset occurs in 1 to 4 weeks. Peak and duration unknown.

INDICATIONS & DOSAGE
Steroid-dependent asthma —
Adults: initially, 3 inhalations t.i.d. or q.i.d. Decreased as needed and tolerated; most patients respond to 2 inhalations b.i.d. Maximum dosage is 12 inhalations daily.
Children: 2 inhalations t.i.d. or q.i.d. Decreased as needed and tolerated; most patients respond to 2 inhalations b.i.d. Maximum dosage is 8 inhalations daily.

ADVERSE REACTIONS
EENT: hoarseness, fungal infections of throat, throat irritation.
GI: dry mouth, fungal infections of mouth.

INTERACTIONS
None significant.

CONTRAINDICATIONS
Contraindicated in patients hypersensitive to any component of the formulation (fluorocarbons, ethanol) and in those with status asthmaticus, persistent positive sputum cultures for candida albicans, or systemic fungal infections.

NURSING CONSIDERATIONS
• Not for use in patients with asthma controlled by bronchodilators or other noncorticosteroids alone or for those with nonasthmatic bronchial diseases.
• Use cautiously in patients with ocular herpes simplex, nonspecific ulcerative colitis, diverticulitis, fresh intestinal anastomoses, peptic ulcer, renal insufficiency, hypertension, osteoporosis, and myasthenia gravis.
• Know that a spacer device may help ensure delivery of the proper dose of medication.
• Check mucous membranes frequently for signs of fungal infection.
• Monitor patient for adverse effects. With prolonged use of high doses, systemic effects are likely because up to 50% of a dose is absorbed.

• Conduct periodic measurements of growth and development during high-dose or prolonged therapy in children.
• Know that during times of stress (trauma, surgery, or infection), systemic corticosteroids may be needed to prevent adrenal insufficiency in previously steroid-dependent patients.
• Taper oral glucocorticoid therapy slowly as ordered. Acute adrenal insufficiency and death have occurred in asthmatics who changed abruptly from oral corticosteroids to inhaled steroids. Be sure patients report symptoms associated with corticosteroid withdrawal, including fatigue, weakness, arthralgia, orthostatic hypotension, and dyspnea.
• Inform patients that dexamethasone doesn't provide relief for acute asthma attacks.
• Instruct patient to store medication between 36° and 86° F (2° and 30° C). Tell patients that this medication needs to be at room temperature when used. If the canister is cold, the proper dose may not be delivered.
• Advise patients to ensure delivery of the proper dose by gently warming the canister to room temperature before using. Some patients carry the canister in a pocket to keep it warm.
• Advise patients requiring bronchodilator to use it several minutes before dexamethasone.
• Tell patients to allow 1 minute to elapse before taking subsequent puffs of medication and to hold breath for a few seconds to enhance action of drug.
• Instruct patients to contact their doctor if response to therapy decreases or if symptoms don't improve within 3 weeks of initiating therapy; the doctor may need to adjust the dosage. Tell patients not to exceed recommended dosage on their own.
• Advise patients to prevent oral fungal infections by gargling or rinsing mouth with water after each use, but not to swallow water.

---

*Liquid form contains alcohol.
**May contain tartrazine.

Common reactions are in italics; ***life-threatening***, in bold italics.

- Teach patients to keep inhaler clean and unobstructed. Wash with warm water and dry thoroughly.
- Instruct patients to carry a card indicating need for supplemental systemic glucocorticoids during stress.

dornase alfa
Pulmozyme

Pregnancy Risk Category: B

HOW SUPPLIED
Inhalation solution: 2.5 mg/ampule (1 mg/ml)

ACTION
Hydrolyzes DNA in sputum of cystic fibrosis patients, causing decreased visosity and elasticity of pulmonary secretions.

ONSET, PEAK, DURATION
Significant improvement in lung function occurs within 3 days to 1 week. Reduction in respiratory tract infections takes weeks to months. Peak increases in baseline measurement of amount of air exhaled in first second of expiration occur after about 9 days of therapy. Duration unknown.

INDICATIONS & DOSAGE
To improve pulmonary function and decrease the frequency of moderate to severe respiratory infections in patients with cystic fibrosis –
Adults and children 5 years and over: one ampule (2.5 mg) inhaled once daily. Treatment usually takes 10 to 15 minutes. Use drug only with an approved nebulizer.

ADVERSE REACTIONS
EENT: *pharyngitis,* voice alteration, laryngitis, conjunctivitis.
Skin: rash, urticaria.
Other: chest pain.

INTERACTIONS
None significant.

CONTRAINDICATIONS
Contraindicated in patients hypersensitive to the drug or Chinese hamster ovary cell-derived products.

NURSING CONSIDERATIONS
- Know that drug is used in conjunction with other standard therapies for cystic fibrosis.
- Be aware that safety and efficacy in children under 5 years or with forced vital capacity less than 40% of normal value have not been established.
- Administer only with the following nebulizers and compressors: the Hudson T Up-draft II disposable jet nebulizer and the Marquest Acorn II disposable jet nebulizer in conjunction with the Pulmo-Aide compressor or the PARI LC Jet⁺ reusable nebulizer in conjunction with the PARI PRO-NEB compressor.
- Discard cloudy or discolored solution.
- Do not mix with other drugs in the nebulizer. Doing so could lead to a physical or chemical reaction that may inactivate dornase alfa.
- Refrigerate drug in its protective foil pouch.
- Remind the patient to breathe only through his mouth when using the nebulizer. If this is difficult, suggest use of a nose clip.
- Tell the patient that if he begins coughing during treatment to turn off the nebulizer without spilling the drug. To resume treatment, the patient should turn on the nebulizer and continue breathing through the mouthpiece until the nebulizer cup is empty or mist is no longer produced.

flunisolide
AeroBid

Pregnancy Risk Category: C

HOW SUPPLIED
Oral inhalant: 250 mcg/metered spray (at least 100 metered inhalations/container)

ACTION
Unknown. Probably decreases inflammation, mainly by stabilizing leukocyte lysosomal membranes.

ONSET, PEAK, DURATION
Onset occurs after 1 to 4 weeks of therapy. Peak and duration unknown.

INDICATIONS & DOSAGE
Steroid-dependent asthma –
Adults and children 6 years and over: 2 inhalations (500 mcg) b.i.d. Maximum daily dose is 4 inhalations b.i.d.

ADVERSE REACTIONS
CNS: headache.
EENT: watery eyes, throat irritation, hoarseness, nasopharyngeal fungal infections.
GI: nausea, vomiting, dry mouth, diarrhea.
Other: upper respiratory tract infection, cold symptoms.

INTERACTIONS
None significant.

CONTRAINDICATIONS
Contraindicated in patients hypersensitive to the drug and in those with status asthmaticus or respiratory infections.

NURSING CONSIDERATIONS
• Not recommended for use in patients with asthma controlled by bronchodilators or other noncorticosteroids alone or for those with nonasthmatic bronchial diseases.
• Know that a spacer device may help to ensure proper dosage administration.
• Store medication between 36° and 86° F (2° and 30° C).

• Withdraw drug slowly as ordered in patients who have received long-term oral corticosteroid therapy.
• Be aware that after withdrawal of systemic corticosteroids, patient may still need supplementation of systemic steroids if patient show signs and symptoms of adrenal insufficiency when exposed to trauma, surgery, or infections.
• Warn patients that flunisolide doesn't relieve emergency asthma attacks.
• Advise patients to ensure delivery of the proper dose by gently warming the canister to room temperature before using. Some patients carry the canister in a pocket to keep it warm.
• Tell patient who also is using a bronchodilator to use it several minutes before flunisolide.
• Instruct patients to allow 1 minute to elapse before repeating inhalations and to hold breath for a few seconds to enhance drug action.
• Teach patients to keep inhaler clean and unobstructed. Wash with warm water and dry thoroughly after use.
• Teach patients to check mucous membranes frequently for signs of fungal infection.
• Patients can prevent oral fungal infections by gargling or rinsing mouth with water after each inhaler use. Caution patients not to swallow the water.
• Advise parents of children receiving long-term therapy that the child should have periodic growth measurements and be checked for evidence of hypothalamic-pituitary-adrenal axis suppression.

---

nedocromil sodium
Tilade

Pregnancy Risk Category: B

HOW SUPPLIED
Inhalation aerosol: 1.75 mg/activation

ACTION
Reduces inflammatory changes in the airway by blocking the release of inflammation mediators (such as leukotrienes, histamine, and prostaglandins) from mast cells, eosinophils, monocytes, neutrophils, macrophages, and other immune cells.

ONSET, PEAK, DURATION
Onset occurs within days to 4 weeks. Time to peak concentration in an asthmatic patient occurs in 5 to 90 minutes. Effects persist for 6 to 12 hours.

INDICATIONS & DOSAGE
Maintenance in mild-to-moderate reversible obstructive airway disease –
Adults and children 12 years of age and over: 2 inhalations q.i.d., preferably at regular intervals.

ADVERSE REACTIONS
CNS: headache.
GI: nausea, vomiting.
RESP: upper respiratory tract infection, rhinitis.
Other: *unpleasant taste.*

INTERACTIONS
None significant.

CONTRAINDICATIONS
Contraindicated in patients hypersensitive to the formulation or in patients experiencing an acute asthmatic attack or acute bronchospasm.

NURSING CONSIDERATIONS
• Warn the patient that nedocromil has no direct bronchodilating action and cannot replace bronchodilators during an acute asthmatic attack.
• Tell the patient that drug is an adjunct to the regular bronchodilator regimen and may reduce the need for corticosteroids or bronchodilators.
• Emphasize to the patient that regular use of the drug will help him feel better. Most patients report benefits after 1 week of use; some require

longer treatment before any improvement.
• Teach the patient how to use the inhaler. Instruct him to shake canister immediately before use and to invert it just before actuation.
• Advise the patient to clean inhaler at least twice a week and to remove canister before rinsing inhaler in hot running water. Allow inhaler to air dry overnight.

---

triamcinolone acetonide
Azmacort

Pregnancy Risk Category: C

HOW SUPPLIED
Inhalation aerosol: 100 mcg/metered spray

ACTION
Unknown. Probably decreases inflammation, mainly by stabilizing leukocyte lysosomal membranes.

ONSET, PEAK, DURATION
Onset occurs in 1 to 4 weeks. Peak and duration unknown.

INDICATIONS & DOSAGE
Steroid-dependent asthma –
Adults: 2 inhalations t.i.d. to q.i.d. Maximum dosage is 16 inhalations daily. In some patients, maintenance can be accomplished when total daily dosage is given b.i.d.
Children 6 to 12 years: 1 to 2 inhalations t.i.d. to q.i.d. Maximum dosage is 12 inhalations daily.

ADVERSE REACTIONS
Most adverse reactions to corticosteroids are dose- or duration-dependent.
EENT: dry or irritated nose or throat, hoarseness.
Respiratory: cough.
Other: *oral candidiasis,* dry or irritated tongue or mouth.

INTERACTIONS
None significant.

CONTRAINDICATIONS
Contraindicated in patients hypersensitive to any component of the formulation and in those with status asthmaticus.

NURSING CONSIDERATIONS
• It is not known if drug is excreted in breast milk. Because of the risk of severe adverse effects, breast-feeding is not recommended.
• Use with extreme caution, if at all, in patients with tuberculosis of the respiratory tract; untreated fungal, bacterial, or systemic viral infections; or ocular herpes simplex.
• Use cautiously in patients receiving systemic corticosteroids.
• Know that patients who have recently been transferred to oral inhaled steroids from systemic administration of steroids may need to be placed back on systemic steroids during periods of stress or severe asthma attacks.
• Taper oral therapy slowly as ordered.
• Store medication between 36° and 86° F (2° and 30° C).
• Inform patients that inhaled corticosteroids don't provide relief for emergency asthma attacks.
• Advise patients to ensure delivery of the proper dose of medication by gently warming the canister to room temperature before using. Some patients carry the canister in a pocket to keep it warm.
• Patients requiring a bronchodilator should use it several minutes before triamcinolone. Tell patients to allow 1 minute to elapse before repeat inhalations and to hold breath for a few seconds to enhance drug action.
• Teach patients to check mucous membranes frequently for signs of fungal infection.
• Tell patients to prevent oral fungal infections by gargling or rinsing mouth with water after each use of the inhaler, but not to swallow the water.
• Tell patients to keep inhaler clean and unobstructed. Wash with warm water and dry thoroughly after use.
• Instruct patients to contact their doctor if response to therapy decreases; the doctor may need to adjust the dosage. Tell patients not to exceed recommended dosage on their own.
• Instruct patients to carry a card indicating their need for supplemental systemic glucocorticoids during stress.

---

*Liquid form contains alcohol.   *Common* reactions are in italics; *life-threatening*, in bold italics.
**May contain tartrazine.

47

Antacids, adsorbents, and antiflatulents

aluminum carbonate
aluminum hydroxide
aluminum phosphate
calcium carbonate
dihydroxyaluminum sodium
  carbonate
magaldrate
magnesium oxide
magnesium hydroxide
  (See Chapter 50, LAXATIVES.)
simethicone
sodium bicarbonate
  (See Chapter 64, ACIDIFIER AND
  ALKALINIZERS.)

COMBINATION PRODUCTS

ALKA-SELTZER WITH ASPIRIN,◊: sodium bicarbonate 1,916 mg, aspirin 325 mg, and citric acid 1,000 mg.
ALKA-SELTZER WITHOUT ASPIRIN◊: sodium bicarbonate 958 mg, citric acid 832 mg, and potassium bicarbonate 312 mg.
ALUDROX SUSPENSION◊: aluminum hydroxide 307 mg and magnesium hydroxide 103 mg.
CAMALOX TABLETS◊: aluminum hydroxide 225 mg, magnesium hydroxide 200 mg, and calcium carbonate 250 mg.
DI-GEL LIQUID◊: aluminum hydroxide 200 mg, magnesium hydroxide 200 mg, and simethicone 20 mg.
FLATULEX: simethicone 80 mg and activated charcoal 250 mg.
GAVISCON◊: aluminum hydroxide 31.7 mg and magnesium carbonate 137 mg.
GELUSIL◊: aluminum hydroxide 200 mg, magnesium hydroxide 200 mg, and simethicone 25 mg.
GELUSIL-II◊: aluminum hydroxide 400 mg, magnesium hydroxide 400 mg, and simethicone 30 mg.
MAALOX ◊: aluminum hydroxide 225 mg and magnesium hydroxide 200 mg.
MAALOX EXTRA STRENGTH TABLETS◊: aluminum hydroxide 400 mg and magnesium hydroxide 400 mg.
MAALOX PLUS TABLETS◊: aluminum hydroxide 200 mg, magnesium hydroxide 200 mg, and simethicone 25 mg.
MAALOX TC TABLETS◊: aluminum hydroxide 600 mg and magnesium hydroxide 300 mg.
MAGNATRIL◊: aluminum hydroxide 260 mg, magnesium hydroxide 130 mg, and magnesium trisilicate 455 mg.
MYLANTA TABLETS◊: aluminum hydroxide 200 mg, magnesium hydroxide 200 mg, and simethicone 20 mg.
MYLANTA-II TABLETS◊: aluminum hydroxide 400 mg, magnesium hydroxide 400 mg, and simethicone 40 mg.
RIOPAN PLUS CHEWABLE TABLETS◊: magaldrate 540 mg and simethicone 20 mg.
RIOPAN PLUS SUSPENSION◊: magaldrate 540 mg and simethicone 20 mg/5 ml.
TITRALAC PLUS SUSPENSION◊: calcium carbonate 500 mg and simethicone 20 mg.
TITRALAC TABLETS◊: calcium carbonate 420 mg and glycine 150 mg.
UNIVOL†◊: aluminum hydroxide and magnesium carbonate co-dried gel 300 mg and magnesium hydroxide 100 mg.
WINGEL◊: aluminum hydroxide 180 mg and magnesium hydroxide 160 mg.

---

†Available in Canada only.   ‡Available in Australia only.   ◊Available OTC.

aluminum carbonate
Basaljel◇

Pregnancy Risk Category: B

HOW SUPPLIED
Tablets or capsules: equivalent to aluminum hydroxide 500 mg◇
Oral suspension: equivalent to aluminum hydroxide 400 mg/5 ml◇

ACTION
An antacid that reduces total acid load in the GI tract, elevates gastric pH to reduce pepsin activity, strengthens the gastric mucosal barrier, and increases esophageal sphincter tone.

ONSET, PEAK, DURATION
Onset occurs in 20 minutes. Peak unknown. Effects persist for about 20 to 60 minutes in a fasting period and up to 3 hours if taken 1 hour after a meal.

INDICATIONS & DOSAGE
Antacid –
Adults: 5 to 10 ml of suspension P.O. q 2 hours p.r.n.; or 1 to 2 tablets or capsules P.O. q 2 hours p.r.n. Maximum dosage is 24 capsules, tablets, or teaspoonfuls per 24 hours.
To prevent formation of urinary phosphate stones (in conjunction with low-phosphate diet) –
Adults: 15 to 30 ml of suspension in water or juice P.O. 1 hour after meals and h.s.; or 2 to 6 tablets or capsules 1 hour after meals and h.s.

ADVERSE REACTIONS
GI: anorexia, *constipation,* intestinal obstruction.
Other: hypophosphatemia.

INTERACTIONS
Allopurinol, antibiotics (including quinolones and tetracyclines), corticosteroids, diflunisal, digoxin, ethambutol, histamine H$_2$ antagonists, iron, isoniazid, penicillamine, phenothiazines, thyroid hormones: decreased pharmacologic effect because of possible impaired absorption. Separate administration times.
Enteric-coated drugs: may release prematurely in stomach. Separate doses by at least 1 hour.

CONTRAINDICATIONS
None known.

NURSING CONSIDERATIONS
• Use cautiously in patients with chronic renal disease.
• Shake suspension well; give with small amount of water or fruit juice to facilitate passage.
• When administering through nasogastric tube, make sure tube is placed correctly and is patent; after instilling, flush tube with water to ensure passage to stomach and to clear tube.
• Monitor long-term, high-dose use in patients on restricted sodium intake. Each tablet, capsule, or 5 ml of suspension contains about 3 mg of sodium.
• Record amount and consistency of stools. Manage constipation with laxatives or stool softeners as ordered. Alternate with magnesium-containing antacids (if the patient does not have renal disease).
• Monitor serum phosphate levels.
• Watch for symptoms of hypophosphatemia with prolonged use (anorexia, malaise, muscle weakness); can also lead to resorption of calcium and bone demineralization.
• Because drug contains aluminum, keep in mind that it is used in patients with renal failure to help control hyperphosphatemia by binding with phosphate in the GI tract.
• Know that Basaljel liquid contains no sugar.
• Warn patients not to take aluminum carbonate indiscriminately or to switch antacids without their doctor's advice.

---

*Liquid form contains alcohol.
**May contain tartrazine. *Common* reactions are in italics; *life-threatening,* in bold italics.

aluminum hydroxide
ALternaGEL◊, Alu-Cap◊, Alu-Tab◊,
Amphojel◊, Basaljel◊, Dialume◊,
Nephrox◊

Pregnancy Risk Category: C

HOW SUPPLIED
Tablets: 300 mg◊, 500 mg◊, 600 mg◊
Capsules: 475 mg◊, 500 mg◊
Oral suspension: 320 mg/5 ml◊, 600 mg/5 ml◊

ACTION
An antacid that reduces total acid load in the GI tract, elevates gastric pH to reduce pepsin activity, strengthens the gastric mucosal barrier, and increases esophageal sphincter tone.

ONSET, PEAK, DURATION
Onset varies by dosage form; liquids are more rapid-acting than tablets or capsules. Peak unknown. Effects duration varies with gastric emptying time; 20 to 60 minutes in fasting patients, 3 hours when taken after meals.

INDICATIONS & DOSAGE
Antacid –
Adults: 500 to 600 mg P.O. (5 to 10 ml of most products) 1 hour after meals and h.s.; 300- or 600-mg tablet, chewed before swallowing, taken with milk or water five to six times daily after meals and h.s.

ADVERSE REACTIONS
GI: anorexia, *constipation,* intestinal obstruction.
Other: hypophosphatemia.

INTERACTIONS
Allopurinol, antibiotics (including quinolones and tetracyclines), corticosteroids, diflunisal, digoxin, ethambutol, H_2 antagonists, iron, isoniazid, penicillamine, phenothiazines, thyroid hormones: decreased pharmacologic effect because of possible im-
paired absorption. Separate administration times.
Enteric-coated drugs: may release prematurely in stomach. Separate doses by at least 1 hour.

CONTRAINDICATIONS
None known.

NURSING CONSIDERATIONS
• Use cautiously in patients with chronic renal disease.
• Shake suspension well; give with small amount of milk or water to facilitate passage.
• When administering through nasogastric tube, make sure tube is placed correctly and is patent; after instilling, flush tube with water to ensure passage to stomach and to clear tube.
• Monitor long-term, high-dose use in patient on restricted sodium intake. Each tablet, capsule, or 5 ml of suspension contains 2 to 3 mg of sodium.
• Record amount and consistency of stools. Manage constipation with laxatives or stool softeners as ordered; alternate with magnesium-containing antacids (if the patient does not have renal disease).
• Monitor serum phosphate levels.
• Watch for symptoms of hypophosphatemia with prolonged use (anorexia, malaise, and muscle weakness); can also lead to resorption of calcium and bone demineralization.
• Because drug contains aluminum, keep in mind that it is used in patients with renal failure to help control hyperphosphatemia by binding with phosphate in the GI tract.
• Advise patients not to take aluminum hydroxide indiscriminately or to switch antacids without their doctor's advice.

aluminum phosphate
Phosphaljel◊

Pregnancy Risk Category: NR

HOW SUPPLIED
Oral suspension: 233 mg/5 ml◇

ACTION
Provides supplemental phosphate.

ONSET, PEAK, DURATION
Onset occurs in about 20 minutes.
Peak unknown. Effects persist for 20
to 60 minutes in fasting patients, 3
hours when taken after meals.

INDICATIONS & DOSAGE
*To reduce fecal elimination of phos-
phorus –*
Adults: 15 to 30 ml undiluted P.O.
q 2 hours between meals and h.s.

ADVERSE REACTIONS
GI: *constipation,* intestinal obstruction.

INTERACTIONS
*Ciprofloxacin and other quinolones,
tetracyclines:* decreased antibiotic effect. Separate administration times.
Enteric-coated drugs: may release
prematurely in stomach. Separate
doses by at least 1 hour.

CONTRAINDICATIONS
None known.

NURSING CONSIDERATIONS
• Use cautiously in patients with
chronic renal disease.
• Shake suspension well; give alone
or with small amount of milk or
water.
• When administering through nasogastric tube, make sure tube is placed
correctly and is patent; after instilling, flush tube with water to ensure
passage to stomach and to clear tube.
• Record amount and consistency of
stools. Manage constipation with laxatives or stool softeners as ordered;
alternate with magnesium-containing
antacids (if the patient does not have
renal disease).
• Monitor patient closely, especially

with long-term use. Also monitor
long-term, high-dose use in patients
on restricted sodium intake.
• Know that the drug can reverse hypophosphatemia induced by aluminum hydroxide.
• Keep in mind that this drug is a very
weak antacid.
• Be aware that phosphaljel contains
no sugar.
• Advise patients not to take aluminum phosphate indiscriminately or to
switch antacids without their doctor's
advice.

---

calcium carbonate
Alka-Mints◇, Amitone◇, Calcilac◇,
Calcimax‡, Calglycine◇, Cal-Sup‡,
Chooz◇, Dicarbosil◇, Effercal-
600‡, Equilet◇, Genalac◇,
Mallamint◇, Rolaids Calcium
Rich◇, Titracid◇, Titralac◇,Titralac
Extra Strength◇, Titralac Plus◇,
Tums◇, Tums E-X◇, Tums Liquid
Extra Strength◇

Pregnancy Risk Category: NR

HOW SUPPLIED
Calcium carbonate contains 40% cal-
cium; 20 mEq calcium per gram.
Tablets (chewable): 350 mg◇, 420
mg◇, 500 mg◇, 750 mg, 850 mg,
1,000 mg, 1,250 mg‡
Tablets: 500 mg◇, 600 mg◇, 650
mg◇, 1,000 mg◇, 1,250 mg◇
Chewing gum: 500 mg/piece
Oral suspension: 1 g/5 ml◇, 250 mg/5
ml
Lozenges: 600 mg◇

ACTION
An antacid that reduces total acid load
in the GI tract, elevates gastric pH to
reduce pepsin activity, strengthens
the gastric mucosal barrier, and increases esophageal sphincter tone.

ONSET, PEAK, DURATION
Onset occurs within 20 minutes. Peak
unknown. Effects persist for 20 to 60

---

minutes in fasting patients, 3 hours when taken after meals.

INDICATIONS & DOSAGE
Antacid, calcium supplement –
Adults: 350 mg to 1.5 g P.O. or 2 pieces of chewing gum 1 hour after meals and h.s. p.r.n.

ADVERSE REACTIONS
GI: *constipation,* gastric distention, flatulence, rebound hyperacidity, *nausea.*

INTERACTIONS
Antibiotics (including quinolones and tetracyclines), hydantoins, iron, isoniazid, salicylates: decreased pharmacologic effect because of possible impaired absorption. Separate administration times.
Enteric-coated drugs: may release prematurely in stomach. Separate doses by at least 1 hour.
Milk and other foods high in vitamin D: possible milk-alkali syndrome (headache, confusion, distaste for food, nausea, vomiting, hypercalcemia, hypercalciuria, calcinosis, and hypophosphatemia). Avoid concomitant use.

CONTRAINDICATIONS
Contraindicated in patients with ventricular fibrillation or hypercalcemia.

NURSING CONSIDERATIONS
• Use cautiously, if at all, in patients with sarcoidosis, renal or cardiac disease, and in patients receiving cardiac glycosides.
• Record amount and consistency of stools. Manage constipation with laxatives or stool softeners as ordered.
• Monitor serum calcium levels, especially in patients with mild renal impairment.
• Watch for symptoms of hypercalcemia (nausea, vomiting, headache, mental confusion, and anorexia).
• Advise patients not to take calcium

carbonate indiscriminately or to switch antacids without their doctor's advice.

---

dihydroxyaluminum sodium carbonate
Rolaids◊

Pregnancy Risk Category: NR

HOW SUPPLIED
Tablets: 334 mg◊

ACTION
An antacid that reduces total acid load in the GI tract, elevates gastric pH to reduce pepsin activity, strengthens the gastric mucosal barrier, and increases esophageal sphincter tone.

ONSET, PEAK, DURATION
Onset occurs in 20 minutes. Peak unknown. Effects persist for 20 to 60 minutes in fasting patients, 3 hours when taken after meals.

INDICATIONS & DOSAGE
Antacid –
Adults: 1 to 2 tablets (334 to 668 mg) P.O., chewed well, p.r.n.

ADVERSE REACTIONS
GI: anorexia, *constipation,* intestinal obstruction.

INTERACTIONS
Allopurinol, antibiotics (including quinolones and tetracyclines), diflunisal, digoxin, iron, isoniazid, penicillamine, phenothiazines, quinidine: decreased pharmacologic effect because of possible impaired absorption. Separate administration times.
Enteric-coated drugs: may release prematurely in stomach. Separate doses by at least 1 hour.

CONTRAINDICATIONS
None known.

NURSING CONSIDERATIONS
• Use cautiously in patients with renal disease.
• Record amount and consistency of stools. Manage constipation with laxatives or stool softeners as ordered; alternate with magnesium-containing antacids (if the patient does not have renal disease).
• Monitor long-term, high-dose use in patients on restricted sodium intake. Has high sodium content (53 mg/tablet) and may increase sodium and water retention.
• Advise patient not to take dihydroxyaluminum sodium carbonate indiscriminately.

magaldrate (aluminum-magnesium complex)
Antiflux†, Lowsium◇, Riopan◇

Pregnancy Risk Category: NR

HOW SUPPLIED
Tablets: 480 mg◇
Tablets (chewable): 480 mg◇
Oral suspension: 540 mg/5 ml◇, 1,080 mg/5 ml◇

ACTION
An antacid that reduces total acid load in the GI tract, elevates gastric pH to reduce pepsin activity, strengthens the gastric mucosal barrier, and increases esophageal sphincter tone.

ONSET, PEAK, DURATION
Onset occurs within 20 minutes. Peak unknown. Effects persist for 20 to 60 minutes in fasting patients, 3 hours when taken after meals.

INDICATIONS & DOSAGE
Antacid –
Adults: 540 to 1,080 mg (5 to 10 ml) of suspension P.O. with water between meals and h.s.; or 480 to 960 mg tablets(1 to 2 tablets) P.O. with water between meals and h.s.; or 480 to 960 mg chewable tablets (1 to 2

tablets) P.O., chewed before swallowing, between meals and h.s.

ADVERSE REACTIONS
GI: mild constipation or diarrhea.

INTERACTIONS
Allopurinol, antibiotics (including quinolones and tetracyclines), diflunisal, digoxin, iron, isoniazid, penicillamine, phenothiazines, quinidine: decreased pharmacologic effect because of possible impaired absorption. Separate administration times.
Enteric-coated drugs: may release prematurely in stomach. Separate doses by at least 1 hour.

CONTRAINDICATIONS
Contraindicated in patients with severe renal disease.

NURSING CONSIDERATIONS
• Use cautiously in patients with mild kidney impairment.
• Shake suspension well; give with water to facilitate passage.
• When giving through nasogastric tube, make sure tube is placed properly and is patent. After instilling, flush tube with water to ensure passage to stomach and to clear tube.
• Record amount and consistency of stools.
• Monitor serum magnesium level in patients with mild kidney impairment. Symptomatic hypermagnesemia usually occurs only in severe renal failure.
• Keep in mind that drug is not typically used in patients with renal failure (although it contains aluminum) to help control hypophosphatemia because it contains magnesium, which may accumulate.
• Be aware that the drug has a very low sodium content and is good for patients on restricted sodium intake.
• Advise patients not to take magaldrate indiscriminately or to switch antacids without their doctor's advice.

magnesium oxide
Mag-Ox 400◇, Maox◇, Par-Mag◇, Uro-Mag◇

Pregnancy Risk Category: NR

HOW SUPPLIED
Tablets: 400 mg◇, 420 mg◇
Capsules: 140 mg◇
Oral suspension: 7.75%◇

ACTION
An antacid that reduces total acid load in the GI tract, elevates gastric pH to reduce pepsin activity, strengthens the gastric mucosal barrier, and increases esophageal sphincter tone.

ONSET, PEAK, DURATION
Onset occurs within 20 minutes. Peak unknown. Effects persist for 20 to 60 minutes in fasting patients, 3 hours when taken after meals.

INDICATIONS & DOSAGE
Antacid –
Adults: 140 mg P.O. with water or milk after meals and h.s.
Laxative –
Adults: 4 g P.O. with water or milk, usually h.s.
Oral replacement therapy in mild hypomagnesemia –
Adults: 400 to 840 mg P.O. daily. Monitor serum magnesium response.

ADVERSE REACTIONS
GI: *diarrhea,* nausea, abdominal pain.
Other: hypermagnesemia.

INTERACTIONS
Allopurinol, antibiotics (including quinolones and tetracyclines), diflunisal, digoxin, iron, isoniazid, penicillamine, phenothiazines, quinidine: decreased pharmacologic effect because of possible impaired absorption. Separate administration times.
Enteric-coated drugs: may release prematurely in stomach. Separate doses by at least 1 hour.

CONTRAINDICATIONS
Contraindicated in patients with severe renal disease.

NURSING CONSIDERATIONS
● Use cautiously in patients with mild renal impairment.
● When used as laxative, do not give other oral drugs 1 to 2 hours before or after treatment.
● Monitor serum magnesium levels. With prolonged use and some degree of renal impairment, watch for symptoms of hypermagnesemia (hypotension, nausea, vomiting, depressed reflexes, respiratory depression, and coma).
● If diarrhea occurs, be prepared to suggest alternative preparation.
● Advise patients not to take magnesium oxide indiscriminately or to switch antacids without their doctor's advice.

simethicone
Extra Strength Gas-X◇, Gas-Relief◇, Gas-X◇, Maximum Strength Gas-Relief◇, Maximum Strength Phazyme◇, Mylanta Gas◇, Mylanta Gas Maximum Strength◇, Mylanta Gas Regular Strength◇, Mylicon-80◇, Mylicon-125◇, Ovol†, Ovol-40†, Ovol-80†, Phazyme◇, Phazyme 55◇, Phazyme 95◇

Pregnancy Risk Category: NR

HOW SUPPLIED
Tablets: 40 mg◇, 50 mg◇, 60 mg◇, 80 mg◇, 95 mg◇, 125 mg◇
Capsules: 125 mg
Drops: 40 mg/0.6 ml◇

ACTION
By its defoaming action, disperses or prevents formation of mucus-surrounded gas pockets in the GI tract.

---

†Available in Canada only.   ‡Available in Australia only.   ◇Available OTC.

ONSET, PEAK, DURATION
Onset and peak is immediate. Duration unknown.

INDICATIONS & DOSAGE
Flatulence, functional gastric bloating—
Adults and children over 12 years:
40 to 125 mg after each meal and h.s.

ADVERSE REACTIONS
GI: expulsion of excessive liberated gas as belching, rectal flatus.

INTERACTIONS
None significant.

CONTRAINDICATIONS
Contraindicated in patients hypersensitive to the drug.

NURSING CONSIDERATIONS
• Tell patients to chew tablet before swallowing.
• Advise patients that medication does not prevent formation of gas.
• Encourage patients to change positions frequently and ambulate to aid in passing flatus.

chenodiol
monooctanoin
pancreatin
pancrelipase
ursodiol

COMBINATION PRODUCTS
DONNAZYME TABLETS: pancreatin 300 mg, pepsin 150 mg, bile salts 150 mg, hyoscyamine sulfate 0.0518 mg, atropine sulfate 0.0097 mg, scopolamine hydrobromide 0.0033 mg, and phenobarbital 8.1 mg.
ENTOZYME TABLETS: pancreatin 300 mg, pepsin 250 mg, and bile salts 150 mg.
PANCREASE CAPSULES: lipase 4,000 units, protease 25,000 units, and amylase 20,000 units in enteric-coated microspheres.

chenodiol
(chenodeoxycholic acid)
Chenix

Pregnancy Risk Category: X

HOW SUPPLIED
Tablets: 250 mg

ACTION
Unknown. Probably suppresses hepatic synthesis of both cholesterol and cholic acid. These actions contribute to biliary cholesterol desaturation and gradual dissolution of gallstones.

ONSET, PEAK, DURATION
Onset and duration unknown. Peak levels occur 50 minutes to 2 hours after a dose.

INDICATIONS & DOSAGE
Dissolution of radiolucent cholesterol stones (gallstones) when systemic disease or age precludes surgery –

Adults: 250 mg P.O. b.i.d. for the first 2 weeks, followed, as tolerated, by weekly increases of 250 mg/day, up to 13 to 16 mg/kg/day for up to 24 months.

ADVERSE REACTIONS
GI: *diarrhea,* cramps, heartburn, constipation, nausea, vomiting, anorexia, epigastric distress.
Hepatic: reversible elevated hepatic enzymes, possible liver toxicity.

INTERACTIONS
Aluminum-containing antacids, cholestyramine, clofibrate, colestipol, estrogens, oral contraceptives: decreased chenodiol effect. Monitor the patient carefully.

CONTRAINDICATIONS
Contraindicated in patients with known hepatocyte dysfunction, intrahepatic cholestasis, primary biliary cirrhosis, or sclerosing cholangitis, a gallbladder confirmed as nonvisualizing after two consecutive single doses of dye; radiopaque or radiolucent bile pigment stones; gallstone complications; or compelling reasons for gallbladder surgery, including unremitting acute cholecystitis, cholangitis, biliary obstruction, gallstone-induced pancreatitis, biliary fistula, and in pregnancy.

NURSING CONSIDERATIONS
• Be aware that treatment should be reserved for carefully selected patients.
• Monitor AST and ALT levels monthly for the first 3 months and every 3 months thereafter for duration of therapy as ordered.
• Monitor the patient for diarrhea which occurs in 30% to 40% of all pa-

tients. The doctor may reduce dosage until diarrhea subsides and may prescribe antidiarrheals. In some patients, however, persistent diarrhea will require discontinuation of chenodiol therapy.

• Monitor liver function test results periodically and oral cholecystogram or ultrasonogram every 6 to 9 months as ordered to observe for gallstone dissolution.

• Know that the drug is particularly effective in the dissolution of small, floatable gallstones.

• Keep in mind that the final dosage should not be less than 10 mg/kg/day; lower dosages are usually ineffective.

• Encourage compliance with the prescribed drug regimen and with scheduled follow-up appointments.

• Tell patients to immediately report worsening symptoms, such as sudden right upper quadrant pain, nausea, and vomiting.

---

monooctanoin
Moctanin

Pregnancy Risk Category: C

HOW SUPPLIED
Infusion: 120-ml bottles

ACTION
Dissolves gallstones by rendering them more soluble.

ONSET, PEAK, DURATION
Onset usually occurs within 72 hours. Peak and duration unknown.

INDICATIONS & DOSAGE
To solubilize cholesterol (radiolucent) gallstones that are retained in the biliary tract after cholecystectomy —
Adults: administered as a continuous infusion for 2 to 10 days (for elimination or size reduction of stones) through a catheter inserted directly into the common bile duct via a T

tube at a rate of 3 to 5 ml/hour and at a pressure of 10 cm H_2O.

ADVERSE REACTIONS
GI: *pain and discomfort, nausea, vomiting, diarrhea,* anorexia, indigestion.
Other: metabolic acidosis, fever.

INTERACTIONS
None significant.

CONTRAINDICATIONS
Contraindicated in patients with impaired hepatic function, biliary tract infection, or a history of recent duodenal ulceration or jejunitis; portosystemic shunting; acute pancreatitis, or any active life-threatening problems that would be complicated by perfusion into the biliary tract.

NURSING CONSIDERATIONS
• Be aware monooctanoin treatment should be initiated only by individuals experienced in infusion therapy.

• Because impaired liver function may lead to metabolic acidosis during monooctanoin administration, obtain routine liver function tests as ordered before perfusion therapy begins.

• Do not administer parenterally; for biliary tract infusion only.

• Dilute each vial with sterile water for injection. Diluting the drug will reduce solution viscosity and enhance bathing of the stone.

• Warm the solution to 60° to 80° F (16° to 27° C) before perfusion. Temperature of the solution should not fall below 65° F (18° C) during administration.

• Use a peristaltic infusion pump to regulate the infusion. Outpatients may use a battery-operated portable pump.

• Keep the pressure at 10 cm H_2O to help minimize GI and biliary tract irritation. Pressure must be kept below 15 cm H_2O.

• Reduce GI symptoms by slowing

---

*Liquid form contains alcohol.   *Common* reactions are in italics; ***life-threatening***, in bold italics.
**May contain tartrazine.

the infusion rate or discontinuing infusion during meals, as ordered.

pancreatin
Bioglan Panazyme‡, Creon, Creon 25, Dizymes Tablets◇, Donnazyme, Entozyme, Hi-Vegi-Lip Tablets◇, 4X Pancreatin 600 mg◇, 8X Pancreatin 900 mg◇, Pancrezyme 4X Tablets◇

Pregnancy Risk Category: C

HOW SUPPLIED
Bioglan Panazyme‡
Tablets: 468 mg pancreatin, 7,200 units lipase, 656 units protease, and 9,200 units amylase
Creon
Capsules (enteric-coated microspheres): 300 mg pancreatin, 8,000 units lipase, 13,000 units protease, and 30,000 units amylase
Creon 25
Capsules (enteric-coated microspheres): 300 mg pancreatin, 25,000 units lipase, 62,500 units protease, and 74,700 units amylase
Dizymes
Tablets (enteric-coated): 250 mg pancreatin, 6,750 units lipase, 41,250 units protease, and 43,750 units amylase◇
Donnazyme
Tablets: 500 mg pancreatin, 1,000 units lipase, 12,500 units protease, and 12,500 units amylase
8X Pancreatin 900 mg
Tablets (enteric-coated): 7,200 mg pancreatin, 22,500 units lipase, 180,000 units protease, and 180,000 units amylase◇
Entozyme
Tablets: 500 mg pancreatin, 600 units lipase, 7,500 units protease, and 7,500 units amylase
4X Pancreatin 600 mg
Tablets (enteric-coated): 2,400 mg pancreatin, 12,000 units lipase, 60,000 units protease, and 60,000 units amylase◇

Hi-Vegi-Lip
Tablets (enteric-coated): 2,400 mg pancreatin, 12,000 units lipase, 60,000 units protease, and 60,000 units amylase◇
Pancrezyme 4X
Tablets (enteric-coated): 2,400 mg pancreatin, 12,000 units lipase, 60,000 units protease, and 60,000 units amylase◇

ACTION
Replaces endogenous exocrine pancreatic enzymes and aids digestion of starches, fats, and proteins.

ONSET, PEAK, DURATION
Onset and peak unknown. Effects persist for 1 to 2 hours.

INDICATIONS & DOSAGE
Exocrine pancreatic secretion insufficiency; digestive aid in diseases associated with deficiency of pancreatic enzymes, such as cystic fibrosis –
Adults and children: dosage varies with condition being treated. Usual initial dosage is 8,000 to 24,000 units of lipase activity before or with each meal or snack. The total daily dose may also be given in divided doses at 1 to 2 hour intervals throughout the day.

ADVERSE REACTIONS
GI: nausea, diarrhea with high doses.
Other: hyperuricuria (with high doses).

INTERACTIONS
Antacids: may negate pancreatin's beneficial effect. Avoid concomitant use.

CONTRAINDICATIONS
Containdicated in patients with hypersensitivity to the drug, or to pork protein or enzymes, acute pancreatitis, and acute exacerbations of chronic pancreatitis.

NURSING CONSIDERATIONS

• Use with caution in pregnant or breast-feeding patients.

• Be aware that minimal USP standards dictate that each milligram of bovine or porcine pancreatin contain lipase 2 units, protease 25 units, and amylase 25 units.

• Monitor patient's dietary intake to ensure a proper balance of fat, protein, and starch intake to avoid indigestion. Dosage varies according to degree of maldigestion and malabsorption, amount of fat in diet, and enzyme activity of individual preparations.

• Keep in mind that a decreased number of bowel movements and improved stool consistency indicate effective therapy.

• Know that the drug is not effective in GI disorders unrelated to pancreatic enzyme deficiency.

• Be alert that enteric coating on some products may reduce availability of enzyme in upper portion of jejunum.

• Tell patient not to crush or chew enteric-coated dosage forms. However, capsules containing enteric-coated microspheres may be opened and the contents sprinkled on a small quantity of soft food or applesauce.

• Tell patient to store in airtight containers at room temperature.

---

pancrelipase

Cotazym Capsules, Cotazym-S Capsules, Creon 10 Capsules, Ilozyme Tablets, Ku-Zyme HP Capsules, Pancrease Capsules, Pancrease MT 4, Pancrease MT 10, Pancrease MT 16, Pancrelipase Capsules, Protilase Capsules, Ultrase MT 12, Ultrase MT 16, Ultrase MT 24, Viokase Powder, Viokase Tablets, Zymase Capsules

Pregnancy Risk Category: C

HOW SUPPLIED

Cotazym
Capsules: 8,000 units lipase, 30,000 units protease, 30,000 units amylase, and 25 mg calcium carbonate

Cotazym-S
Capsules (enteric-coated spheres): 5,000 units lipase, 20,000 units protease, and 20,000 units amylase

Creon
Capsules (enteric-coated microspheres): 10,000 units lipase, 13,000 units protease, and 30,000 units amylase

Ilozyme
Tablets: 11,000 units lipase, 30,000 units protease, and 30,000 units amylase

Ku-Zyme HP
Capsules: 8,000 units lipase, 30,000 units protease, and 30,000 units amylase

Pancrease
Capsules (enteric-coated microspheres): 4,000 units lipase, 25,000 units protease, and 20,000 units amylase

Pancrease MT 4
Capsules (enteric-coated microtablets): 4,000 units lipase, 12,000 units protease, and 30,000 units amylase

Pancrease MT 10
Capsules (enteric-coated microtablets): 10,000 units lipase, 30,000 units protease, and 30,000 units amylase

Pancrease MT 16
Capsules (enteric-coated microtablets): 16,000 units lipase, 48,000 units protease, and 48,000 units amylase

Pancrelipase
Capsules (enteric-coated pellets): 4,000 units lipase, 25,000 units protease, and 20,000 units amylase

Protilase
Capsules (enteric-coated spheres): 4,000 units lipase, 25,000 units protease, and 20,000 units amylase

Ultrase MT 12
Capsules (delayed-release): 12,000

---

*Liquid form contains alcohol.
May contain tartrazine.   *Common* reactions are in italics; ***life-threatening,* in bold italics.

units lipase, 39,000 units protease, and 39,000 units amylase

Ultrase MT 16
Capsules (delayed-release): 20,000 units lipase, 65,000 units protease, and 65,000 units amylase

Ultrase MT 24
Capsules (delayed-release): 24,000 units lipase, 78,000 units protease, and 78,000 units amylase

Viokase
Tablets: 8,000 units lipase, 30,000 units protease, and 30,000 units amylase
Powder: 16,800 units lipase, 70,000 units protease, and 70,000 units amylase per 0.7 g powder

Zymase
Capsules (enteric-coated spheres): 12,000 units lipase, 24,000 units protease, and 24,000 units amylase

ACTION
Replaces endogenous exocrine pancreatic enzymes and aids digestion of starches, fats, and proteins.

ONSET, PEAK, DURATION
Variable.

INDICATIONS & DOSAGE
Exocrine pancreatic secretion insufficiency, cystic fibrosis in adults and children, steatorrhea and other disorders of fat metabolism secondary to insufficient pancreatic enzymes –
Adults and children: dosage titrated to patient's response. Usual initial dosage is 4,000 to 33,000 units of lipase activity with each meal or snack.

ADVERSE REACTIONS
GI: *nausea,* cramping, diarrhea (high doses).

INTERACTIONS
Antacids: may destroy enteric coating and result in enhanced degradation of pancrelipase. Avoid concomitant use.

CONTRAINDICATIONS
Contraindicated in patients with severe hypersensitivity to pork, acute pancreatitis, or acute exacerbations of chronic pancreatic diseases.

NURSING CONSIDERATIONS
• Know that drug should be used only after confirmed diagnosis of exocrine pancreatic insufficiency. Not effective in GI disorders unrelated to enzyme deficiency.
• Know that lipase activity is greater than with other pancreatic enzymes.
• For infants, mix powder with applesauce and give with meals. Avoid contact with or inhalation of powder because it may be very irritating. Older children may take capsules with food.
• Monitor patient's stool. Know that adequate replacement decreases number of bowel movements and improves stool consistency.
• Be aware that minimal USP standards dictate that each mg of pancrelipase contain 24 units lipase, 100 units protease, and 100 units amylase.
• Be aware that dosage varies with degree of maldigestion and malabsorption, amount of fat in diet, and enzyme activity of individual preparations.
• Be aware that enteric coating on some products may reduce availability of enzyme in upper portion of jejunum.
• Advise patient not to crush or chew enteric-coated dosage forms.

---

ursodiol
Actigall

Pregnancy Risk Category: B

HOW SUPPLIED
Capsules: 300 mg

ACTION
Unknown. A naturally occurring bile acid that probably suppresses hepatic synthesis and secretion of cholesterol

as well as intestinal cholesterol absorption. After long-term administration, ursodiol can solubilize cholesterol from gallstones.

ONSET, PEAK, DURATION
Onset and duration unknown. Peak concentrations occur 1 to 3 hours after a dose.

INDICATIONS & DOSAGE
Dissolution of gallstones less than 20 mm in diameter in patients who are poor candidates for surgery or who refuse surgery –
Adults: 8 to 10 mg/kg P.O. daily in two or three divided doses.

ADVERSE REACTIONS
CNS: headache, fatigue, anxiety, depression, sleep disorders.
EENT: rhinitis.
GI: nausea, vomiting, dyspepsia, metallic taste, abdominal pain, biliary pain, cholecystitis, diarrhea, constipation, stomatitis, flatulence.
Respiratory: cough.
Skin: pruritus, rash, dry skin, urticaria, itching, hair thinning.
Other: arthralgia, myalgia, back pain.

INTERACTIONS
Aluminum-containing antacids, cholestyramine, colestipol: bind ursodiol and prevent its absorption.
Clofibrate, estrogens, oral contraceptives: increased hepatic cholesterol secretion; may counteract the effects of ursodiol.

CONTRAINDICATIONS
• Contraindicated in patients hypersensitive to ursodiol or other bile acids.
• Also contraindicated in patients with chronic hepatic disease, unremitting acute cholecystitis, cholangitis, biliary obstruction, gallstone-induced pancreatitis, or biliary fistula.

NURSING CONSIDERATIONS
• Be aware that ursodiol will not dissolve calcified cholesterol stones, radiolucent bile pigment stones, or radiopaque stones.
• Monitor liver function test results, including AST and ALT, at the beginning of therapy and after 1 month, 3 months, and then every 6 months during ursodiol therapy as ordered. Abnormal tests may indicate a worsening of the disease. A theoretical risk exists that a hepatotoxic metabolite of ursodiol may be formed in some patients.
• Know that therapy usually is long-term, with ultrasound images of the gallbladder taken at 6-month intervals. If partial stone dissolution does not occur within 12 months, eventual success is unlikely. Safety of use for longer than 24 months has not been established.
• Tell patients about alternative therapies, including "watchful waiting" (no intervention) and cholecystectomy since the relapse rate after bile acid therapy may be as high as 50% after 5 years.

---

*Liquid form contains alcohol.   *Common* reactions are in italics; *life-threatening*, in bold italics.
**May contain tartrazine.

49
Antidiarrheals

bismuth subgallate
bismuth subsalicylate
calcium polycarbophil
(See Chapter 50, LAXATIVES.)
**difenoxin hydrochloride and
atropine sulfate**
**diphenoxylate hydrochloride and
atropine sulfate**
kaolin and pectin mixtures
loperamide
octreotide acetate
opium tincture
opium tincture, camphorated

COMBINATION PRODUCTS
DONNAGEL-PG*: powdered opium
24 mg, kaolin 6 g, pectin 142.8 mg,
hyoscyamine sulfate 0.1037 mg, atropine sulfate 0.0194 mg, scopolamine
hydrobromide 0.0065 mg, and alcohol 5% in 30-ml suspension.
DONNAGEL SUSPENSION*: kaolin 6
g, pectin 142.8 mg, hyoscyamine sulfate 0.1037 mg, atropine sulfate
0.0194 mg, scopolamine hydrobromide 0.0065 mg, and alcohol 3.8% in
30-ml suspension.
PAREPECTOLIN*: opium 15 mg
(equivalent to paregoric 3.7 ml), kaolin 5.85 g, pectin 162 mg, and alcohol 0.69% in 30-ml suspension.

---

bismuth subgallate
Devrom◊

bismuth subsalicylate
Maximum Strength Pepto-Bismol
Liquid◊, Pepto-Bismol◊

Pregnancy Risk Category: NR

HOW SUPPLIED
bismuth subgallate
Tablets (chewable): 200 mg◊

bismuth subsalicylate
Tablets (chewable): 262.5 mg◊
Oral suspension: 262.5 mg/15 ml◊,
525 mg/15 ml◊

ACTION
Unknown. Has a mild water-binding
capacity; also may adsorb toxins and
provide protective coating for mucosa.

ONSET, PEAK, DURATION
Onset occurs within 1 hour. Peak and
duration unknown.

INDICATIONS & DOSAGE
Mild, nonspecific diarrhea –
Adults: 1 to 2 tablets (subgallate)
P.O. chewed or swallowed whole
t.i.d.; or 30 ml or 2 tablets (subsalicylate) P.O. q ½ to 1 hour, up to a maximum of eight doses and for no longer
than 2 days.
Children 3 to 6 years: 5 ml or ⅓ tablet P.O.
Children 6 to 9 years: 10 ml or ⅔
tablet P.O.
Children 9 to 12 years: 15 ml or 1
tablet P.O.

ADVERSE REACTIONS
GI: temporary darkening of tongue
and stools.
Other: salicylism (with high doses).

INTERACTIONS
Aspirin, other salicylates: risk of salicylate toxicity. Monitor closely.
*Oral anticoagulants, oral antidiabetic
agents:* theoretical risk of increased
effects of these agents after high
doses of bismuth subsalicylate. Monitor the patient closely.
Probenecid: theoretical risk of decreased uricosuric effects after high

doses of bismuth subsalicylate. Monitor the patient closely.
Tetracycline: decreased tetracycline absorption. Separate administration times by at least 2 hours.

CONTRAINDICATIONS
Contraindicated in patients hypersensitive to salicylates.

NURSING CONSIDERATIONS
• Use cautiously in patients already taking aspirin. Discontinue if tinnitus occurs.
• Avoid use before GI radiologic procedures because bismuth is radiopaque and may interfere with X-rays.
• Advise patients that bismuth subsalicylate contains a large amount of salicylate (each tablet provides 102 mg salicylate; the regular-strength liquid provides 130 mg/15 ml, and the extra-strength liquid yields 230 mg/15 ml).
• Instruct patients to chew tablets well or to shake liquid before measuring dose.
• Tell patients to call their doctor if diarrhea persists for more than 2 days or is accompanied by high fever.
• Tell patients to consult with the doctor before giving bismuth subsalicylate to children or teenagers during or after recovery from the flu or chicken pox.
• Inform patients that both the liquid and tablet forms of Pepto-Bismol are effective against traveler's diarrhea. Tablets may be more convenient to carry.

---

difenoxin hydrochloride and atropine sulfate
Lyspafen‡, Motofen
Controlled Substance Schedule IV

Pregnancy Risk Category: C

HOW SUPPLIED
Tablets: 0.5 mg (with atropine sulphate 0.025 mg)‡, 1 mg (with atropine sulfate 0.025 mg)

ACTION
Unknown. Probably exerts a direct effect on the intestinal wall to slow motility.

ONSET, PEAK, DURATION
Onset occurs within 30 minutes. Peak levels occur within 40 to 60 minutes. Duration unknown.

INDICATIONS AND DOSAGE
Adjunct in acute nonspecific diarrhea and acute exacerbations of chronic functional diarrhea –
Adults: initially, 2 mg P.O., then 1 mg P.O. after each loose bowel movement or 1 mg q 3 to 4 hours p.r.n. Do not exceed total dosage of 8 mg daily. Not recommended for use longer than 2 days.

ADVERSE REACTIONS
CNS: dizziness, light-headedness, drowsiness, headache, fatigue, nervousness, insomnia, confusion.
EENT: burning eyes, blurred vision.
GI: nausea, vomiting, dry mouth, epigastric distress, constipation.

INTERACTIONS
Barbiturates, CNS depressants, ethanol, narcotic agents, tranquilizers: enhanced CNS depression. Closely monitor patients.
MAO inhibitors: possible hypertensive crisis. Avoid concomitant use.

CONTRAINDICATIONS
• Contraindicated in patients hypersensitive to difenoxin or atropine, in children under 2 years, and in patients with diarrhea caused by pseudomembranous colitis associated with antibiotics.
• Also contraindicated in patients with jaundice and in those with diar-

---

*Liquid form contains alcohol. *Common* reactions are in italics; *life-threatening,* in bold italics.
**May contain tartrazine.

rhea from organisms that may penetrate the intestinal mucosa (including toxigenic *Escherichia coli, Salmonella,* or *Shigella*).

NURSING CONSIDERATIONS
• Use cautiously in patients with a history of drug abuse or in those currently receiving drugs with a high abuse potential. Difenoxin is the principal metabolite of diphenoxylate and is chemically related to meperidine.
• Know that atropine has been added to difenoxin to prevent abuse. The small dosage of atropine is unlikely to cause any significant clinical problems, but patients may experience dry mouth, tachycardia, urine retention, and flushing. Monitor for these effects.
• Monitor patients closely for fluid and electrolyte imbalance. Difenoxin-induced decreases in peristalsis may result in fluid retention in the colon, with subsequent dehydration and possibly delayed difenoxin intoxication.
• For overdose, observe patient for at least 48 hours. Respiratory depression may occur up to 30 hours after ingestion. Use gastric lavage, establishment of a patent airway, and mechanically assisted ventilation to treat overdose and naloxone to reverse respiratory depression. Know that because difenoxin has a longer duration of action than naloxone, repeated injections of naloxone are necessary.
• Advise patients to avoid hazardous activities that require mental alertness, such as driving or operating heavy machinery, until CNS effects of the drug are known.
• Advise patients to adhere to dosing schedule. Overdose with difenoxin may cause respiratory depression and coma. Encourage storing drug out of children's reach.

diphenoxylate hydrochloride and atropine sulfate
Diphenatol, Lofene, Logen, Lomenate, Lomotil*, Lonox, Lo-Trol, Nor-Mil
Controlled Substance Schedule V
Pregnancy Risk Category: C

HOW SUPPLIED
Tablets: 2.5 mg (with atropine sulfate 0.025 mg)
Liquid: 2.5 mg/5 ml (with atropine sulfate 0.025 mg/5 ml)*

ACTION
Unknown. Probably increases smooth muscle tone in the GI tract, inhibits motility and propulsion, and diminishes secretions.

ONSET, PEAK, DURATION
Onset occurs in 45 to 60 minutes after ingestion. Plasma levels peak about 3 hours after ingestion. Effects persist for 3 to 4 hours.

INDICATIONS & DOSAGE
Acute, nonspecific diarrhea–
Adults: initially, 5 mg P.O. q.i.d., then dosage adjusted as needed.
Children 2 to 12 years: 0.3 to 0.4 mg/kg liquid form P.O. daily in four divided doses. For maintenance, initial dosage reduced as needed up to 75%.

ADVERSE REACTIONS
CNS: *sedation, dizziness,* headache, drowsiness, lethargy, restlessness, depression, euphoria.
CV: tachycardia.
EENT: mydriasis.
GI: *dry mouth,* nausea, vomiting, abdominal discomfort or distention, *paralytic ileus,* anorexia, fluid retention in bowel (may mask depletion of extracellular fluid and electrolytes, especially in young children treated for acute gastroenteritis), possible

physical dependence with long-term use.
GU: urine retention.
Respiratory: respiratory depression.
Skin: pruritus, rash.
Other: *angioedema.*

INTERACTIONS
Barbiturates, CNS depressants, ethanol, narcotic agents, tranquilizers: enhanced CNS depression. Closely monitor patients.
MAO inhibitors: possible hypertensive crisis. Avoid concomitant use.

CONTRAINDICATIONS
Contraindicated in patients with hypersensitivity to diphenoxylate or atropine, acute diarrhea resulting from poison until toxic material is eliminated from GI tract, acute diarrhea caused by organisms that penetrate intestinal mucosa, or diarrhea resulting from antibiotic-induced pseudomembranous enterocolitis; also contraindicated in jaundiced patients and in children under 2 years.

NURSING CONSIDERATIONS
• Use cautiously in children 2 years and over; in patients with hepatic disease, narcotic dependence, or acute ulcerative colitis; and in pregnant patients. Stop therapy immediately if abdominal distention or other signs of toxic megacolon develop and notify doctor.
• Monitor fluid and electrolyte balance. Correct fluid and electrolyte disturbances before starting drug. Dehydration, especially in young children, may increase risk of delayed toxicity.
• Keep in mind that a dose of 2.5 mg is as effective as 5 ml camphorated opium tincture.
• Know that the drug is not indicated for treating antibiotic-induced diarrhea.
• Be aware that drug is unlikely to be

effective if no response occurs within 48 hours.
• Know that the risk of physical dependence increases with high dosage and long-term use. Atropine sulfate helps discourage abuse.
• Use naloxone as ordered to treat respiratory depression caused by overdose.
• Tell patients not to exceed recommended dosage.
• Warn patients not to use drug to treat acute diarrhea for longer than 2 days and to seek medical attention if diarrhea continues.
• Advise patients to avoid hazardous activities, such as driving, until CNS effects of the drug are known.

kaolin and pectin mixtures
Donnagel-MB*†, Kao-Con†, Kaopectate◊, Kaopectate Concentrated◊, Kao-tin◊, Kapectolin◊, K-P◊, K-Pek◊

Pregnancy Risk Category: NR

HOW SUPPLIED
Oral suspension: 5.2 mg kaolin and 260 mg pectin per 30 ml◊ (K-P◊); 5.85 g kaolin and 130 mg pectin per 30 ml◊ (Kaopectate◊, Kao-tin◊, Kapectolin◊, K-Pek◊); 5.91 g kaolin and 132 mg pectin per 30 ml◊ (Kaopectate◊), 6 g kaolin and 130 mg pectin per 30 ml◊ (Kaopectate†◊); 6 g kaolin and 143 mg pectin per 30 ml◊, with 3.8% ethanol (Donnagel-MB*†); 8.7 g kaolin and 195 mg pectin per 30 ml◊ (Kaopectate Concentrate◊); 8.8 g kaolin and 195 mg pectin per 30 ml◊ (Kao-Con†, Kaopectate Concentrated◊)

ACTION
Decreases the stool's fluid content, although *total* water loss seems to remain the same.

ONSET, PEAK, DURATION
Unknown.

INDICATIONS & DOSAGE

Mild, nonspecific diarrhea –
Adults: 60 to 120 ml regular strength suspension or 45 to 90 ml of the concentrated suspension P.O. after each bowel movement.
Children 3 to 6 years: 15 to 30 ml regular strength or 15 ml concentrated strength P.O. after each bowel movement.
Children 6 to 12 years: 30 to 60 ml regular strength or 30 ml concentrated strength P.O. after each bowel movement.
Children over 12 years: 60 ml regular strength or 45 ml concentrated strength P.O. after each bowel movement.

ADVERSE REACTIONS

GI: drug absorption of nutrients, other drugs, and enzymes; fecal impaction or ulceration in infants and elderly or debilitated patients after chronic use; constipation.

INTERACTIONS

Orally administered drugs: adsorption may occur. Separate administration times by at least 2 to 3 hours.

CONTRAINDICATIONS

None known.

NURSING CONSIDERATIONS

• Warn patient not to use drug to replace specific therapy for underlying cause.
• Advise patients not to use drug for more than 2 days.

loperamide

Imodium, Imodium A-D◇

Pregnancy Risk Category: B

HOW SUPPLIED

Tablets: 2 mg
Capsules: 2 mg◇
Oral liquid: 1 mg/5 ml◇

ACTION

Inhibits peristaltic activity, prolonging transit of intestinal contents.

ONSET, PEAK, DURATION

Onset unknown. Peak plasma levels occur about 2½ hours after oral liquid, 4 to 5 hours after capsules. Effects persist about 24 hours.

INDICATIONS & DOSAGE

Acute, nonspecific diarrhea –
Adults: initially, 4 mg P.O., then 2 mg after each unformed stool. Maximum dosage is 16 mg daily.
Children 2 to 6 years: 5 ml P.O. t.i.d. on first day. If diarrhea persists, contact doctor.
Children 6 to 8 years: 10 ml (2 mg) P.O. b.i.d. on first day. If diarrhea persists, contact doctor.
Children 8 to 12 years: 10 ml (2 mg) t.i.d. P.O. on first day. (Subsequent doses of 5 ml (1 mg)/10 kg of body weight may be administered after each unformed stool.) Maximum dosage is 6 mg daily.
Chronic diarrhea –
Adults: initially, 4 mg P.O., then 2 mg after each unformed stool until diarrhea subsides. Dosage adjusted to individual response.

ADVERSE REACTIONS

CNS: drowsiness, fatigue, dizziness.
GI: dry mouth; abdominal pain, distention, or discomfort; *constipation;* nausea; vomiting.
Skin: rash.

INTERACTIONS

None significant.

CONTRAINDICATIONS

Contraindicated in patients with hypersensitivity and when constipation must be avoided. Also contraindicated in children under 2 years.

NURSING CONSIDERATIONS
• Use cautiously in patients with hepatic disease.
• Be aware that the drug produces antidiarrheal action similar to diphenoxylate but without as many adverse CNS effects.
• Monitor children closely for CNS effects as they may be more sensitive to the CNS effects of the drug than adults.
• Advise patients not to exceed recommended dosage.
• In acute diarrhea, tell patient to discontinue drug and seek medical attention if no improvement occurs within 48 hours; in chronic diarrhea, notify doctor and discontinue drug if no improvement occurs after giving 16 mg daily for at least 10 days.
• Advise patient to stop drug immediately if abdominal distention or other symptoms develop in acute colitis and notify doctor.

octreotide acetate
Sandostatin

Pregnancy Risk Category: B

HOW SUPPLIED
Injection ampules: 0.05 mg, 0.1 mg, 0.5 mg
Injection-multidose vials: 0.2 mg/ml, 1 mg/ml

ACTION
Mimics the action of naturally occurring somatostatin.

ONSET, PEAK, DURATION
Onset occurs within 30 minutes. Peak levels occur within ½ hour. Effects persist up to 12 hours.

INDICATIONS & DOSAGE
Flushing and diarrhea associated with carcinoid tumors –
Adults: 0.1 to 0.6 mg daily S.C. in two to four divided doses for the first 2 weeks of therapy (usual daily dosage is 0.3 mg). Subsequent dosage based on individual response.
Watery diarrhea associated with vasoactive intestinal polypeptide secreting tumors (VIPomas) –
Adults: 0.2 to 0.3 mg daily S.C. in two to four divided doses for the first 2 weeks of therapy. Subsequent dosage based on individual response; typically, don't exceed 0.45 mg daily.
Acromegaly –
Adults: initially, 50 mcg S.C. t.i.d., then adjusted according to somatomedin C levels q 2 weeks.

ADVERSE REACTIONS
CNS: dizziness, light-headedness, fatigue.
GI: *nausea, diarrhea, abdominal pain or discomfort,* loose stools, vomiting, fat malabsorption, gallbladder abnormalities.
Skin: flushing, edema, wheal, erythema or pain at injection site.
Other: hyperglycemia, hypoglycemia, hypothyroidism, and pain, and/or burning at the S.C. injection site.

INTERACTIONS
Cyclosporine: may decrease plasma levels of cyclosporine.

CONTRAINDICATIONS
Contraindicated in patients hypersensitive to the drug or any of its components.

NURSING CONSIDERATIONS
• Monitor baseline thyroid function tests as ordered.
• Monitor somatomedin C levels q 2 weeks as ordered. Know that dosage adjustments are made on the basis of this level.
• Monitor laboratory tests periodically, such as thyroid function tests, urine 5-hydroxyindoleacetic acid, plasma serotonin, and plasma substance P (for carcinoid tumors), and plasma vasoactive intestinal peptide (for VIPomas).

---

*Liquid form contains alcohol.   *Common* reactions are in italics; *life-threatening*, in bold italics.
**May contain tartrazine.

• Monitor patients regularly for gallbladder disease, and tell them to report any signs of abdominal discomfort. May be associated with development of cholelithiasis by altering gallbladder motility or fat absorption.

• Monitor closely for symptoms of glucose imbalance. Mild, transient hypoglycemia or hyperglycemia may occur during octreotide therapy.

• Be alert that insulin-dependent diabetic patients and patients receiving oral antidiabetic agents or oral diazoxide may require dosage adjustments during therapy.

• Keep in mind that octreotide therapy may alter fluid and electrolyte balance and may require adjustment of other drugs used to control symptoms of the disease, such as beta blockers.

• Be aware that half-life may be altered in patients in end-stage renal failure who are receiving dialysis.

---

opium tincture*
Controlled Substance Schedule II

opium tincture, camphorated* (paregoric)
Controlled Substance Schedule III

Pregnancy Risk Category: NR

HOW SUPPLIED
opium tincture
Oral solution: equivalent to morphine 10 mg/ml*
opium tincture, camphorated
Oral solution: Each 5 ml contains morphine, 2 mg; anise oil, 0.2 ml; benzoic acid, 20 mg; camphor, 20 mg; glycerin, 0.2 ml; and ethanol to make 5 ml*

ACTION
Increases smooth muscle tone in the GI tract, inhibits motility and propulsion, and diminishes secretions.

ONSET, PEAK, DURATION
Unknown.

INDICATIONS & DOSAGE
Acute, nonspecific diarrhea –
Adults: 0.6 ml opium tincture (range 0.3 to 1 ml) P.O. q.i.d. Maximum dosage is 6 ml daily. Or, 5 to 10 ml camphorated opium tincture once daily, b.i.d., t.i.d., or q.i.d. until diarrhea subsides.
Children: 0.25 to 0.5 ml/kg camphorated opium tincture P.O. once daily, b.i.d., t.i.d., or q.i.d. until diarrhea subsides.

ADVERSE REACTIONS
CNS: dizziness, light-headedness.
GI: nausea, vomiting, physical dependence after long-term use.

INTERACTIONS
None significant.

CONTRAINDICATIONS
Contraindicated in patients with acute diarrhea resulting from poisoning until toxic material is removed from GI tract or in those with diarrhea caused by organisms that penetrate intestinal mucosa.

NURSING CONSIDERATIONS
• Use cautiously in patients with asthma, prostatic hyperplasia, hepatic disease, and history of opioid dependence.

• Mix with sufficient water to ensure passage to stomach.

• Know that a milky fluid forms when camphorated opium tincture is added to water.

• For overdose, use the narcotic antagonist naloxone, as ordered, to reverse respiratory depression.

• Keep in mind that opium content of opium tincture is 25 times greater than camphorated opium tincture. Camphorated opium tincture is more dilute, and teaspoonful doses are eas-

---

ier to measure than dropper quantities of opium tincture.
• Keep in mind that the drug is an effective and prompt-acting antidiarrheal, but unique because dosage can be adjusted precisely to patient's needs.
• Store in tightly capped, light-resistant container.
• Advise patients against using drug for more than 2 days; risk of physical dependence increases with long-term use.

50

Laxatives

bisacodyl
calcium polycarbophil
cascara sagrada
cascara sagrada aromatic fluidextract
cascara sagrada fluidextract
castor oil
docusate calcium
docusate potassium
docusate sodium
glycerin
lactulose
magnesium citrate
magnesium hydroxide
magnesium sulfate
methylcellulose
mineral oil
phenolphthalein, white
phenolphthalein, yellow
polyethylene glycol and electrolyte solution
psyllium
senna
sodium phosphates

COMBINATION PRODUCTS

AGORAL◊: mineral oil 28% and white phenolphthalein 1.3% in emulsion, with tragacanth, agar, egg albumin, acacia, and glycerin.
DIALOSE-PLUS◊: docusate sodium 100 mg and yellow phenophthalein 65 mg.
DOXIDAN◊: docusate calcium 60 mg and phenolphthalein 65 mg.
D-S-S PLUS◊: docusate sodium 100 mg and casanthranol 30 mg.
HALEY'S M-O◊: mineral oil (25%) and magnesium hydroxide.
KONDREMUL WITH CASCARA◊: heavy mineral oil 55%, cascara sagrada extract 660 mg/15 ml, and Irish moss as emulsifier.
KONDREMUL WITH PHENOLPHTHALEIN◊: heavy mineral oil 55%, white phenolphthalein 150 mg/15 ml, and Irish moss as emulsifier.
MODANE PLUS◊: docusate sodium 100 mg and white phenolphthalein 60 mg.
PERI-COLACE CAPSULES◊: docusate sodium 100 mg and casanthranol 30 mg.
PERI-COLACE SYRUP◊: docusate sodium 60 mg and casanthranol 30 mg/15 ml.
SENOKOT-S◊: docusate sodium 50 mg and standardized senna concentrate 187 mg.
UNILAX SOFTGEL◊: docusate sodium 230 mg and yellow phenolphthalein 130 mg.

bisacodyl

Bisac-Evac◊, Bisacolax†◊, Bisalax‡, Bisco-Lax**◊, Carter's Little Pills◊, Dacodyl◊, Deficol◊, Dulcolax◊, Durolax‡, Fleet Bisacodyl◊, Fleet Bisacodyl Prep◊, Fleet Laxative◊, Laxit†◊, Theralax◊

Pregnancy Risk Category: B

HOW SUPPLIED

Tablets (enteric-coated): 5 mg◊
Enema: 0.33 mg/dl◊, 10 mg/5 ml (microenema)‡
Powder for rectal solution (bisacodyl tannex): 1.5 mg bisacodyl and 2.5 g tannic acid
Suppositories: 5 mg◊, 10 mg◊

ACTION

Unknown. A stimulant laxative that increases peristalsis probably by direct effect on the smooth muscle of the intestine. Thought to either irritate the musculature or stimulate the colonic intramural plexus. Also promotes fluid accumulation in the colon and small intestine.

†Available in Canada only. ‡Available in Australia only. ◊Available OTC.

ONSET, PEAK, DURATION
Onset occurs 15 to 60 minutes after suppository, 6 to 12 hours after oral administration. Peak and duration variable among patients.

INDICATIONS & DOSAGE
Chronic constipation; preparation for delivery, surgery, or rectal or bowel examination –
Adults and children 12 years and over: 10 to 15 mg P.O. in evening or before breakfast. Up to 30 mg P.O. as needed and ordered, or 10 mg P.R. for evacuation before examination or surgery.
Children 6 to 12 years: 5 mg P.O. or P.R. h.s. or before breakfast.

ADVERSE REACTIONS
CNS: muscle weakness with excessive use.
GI: *nausea, vomiting, abdominal cramps,* diarrhea (with high doses), *burning sensation in rectum* (with suppositories), laxative dependence with long-term or excessive use.
Other: alkalosis, hypokalemia, tetany, protein-losing enteropathy in excessive use, fluid and electrolyte imbalance.

INTERACTIONS
Milk or antacids: gastric irritation or dyspepsia from prematue dissolution of enteric coating. Do not administer together.

CONTRAINDICATIONS
Contraindicated in patients with hypersensitivity, abdominal pain, nausea, vomiting, or other symptoms of appendicitis or acute surgical abdomen and in those with rectal bleeding, gastroenteritis, or intestinal obstruction.

NURSING CONSIDERATIONS
• Time administration of drug so as not to interfere with scheduled activities or sleep. Soft, formed stool usu-

ally produced 15 to 60 minutes after rectal administration.
• Before giving for constipation, determine if the patient has adequate fluid intake, exercise, and diet.
• Know that tablets and suppositories are used together to clean the colon before and after surgery and before barium enema.
• Insert suppository as high as possible into the rectum, and try to position the suppository against the rectal wall. Avoid embedding within fecal material because this may delay the onset of action.
• Use for short-term treatment as ordered. A stimulant laxative, this type of laxative is most abused. Discourage excessive use.
• Store tablets and suppositories at a temperature below 86° F (30° C).
• Advise the patient to swallow enteric-coated tablet whole to avoid GI irritation. Don't give within 1 hour of milk or antacid intake.
• Advise the patient to report adverse effects to the doctor.
• Teach the patient about dietary sources of bulk which include bran and other cereals, fresh fruit, and vegetables.

---

calcium polycarbophil
Equalactin◇, Fiberall◇, FiberCon◇, FiberLax◇, FiberNorm◇, Mitrolan◇

Pregnancy Risk Category: NR

HOW SUPPLIED
Tablets: 500 mg◇, 625 mg◇, 1,250 mg◇
Tablets (chewable): 500 mg◇

ACTION
A bulk-forming laxative that absorbs water and expands to increase bulk and moisture content of the stool. The increased bulk encourages peristalsis and bowel movement. As an antidiarrheal, absorbs free fecal water, thereby producing formed stools.

ONSET, PEAK, DURATION
Onset occurs in 12 to 24 hours. Peak effects may not occur for up to 3 days. Duration variable.

INDICATIONS & DOSAGE
Constipation –
Adults: 1 g P.O. q.i.d. as required. Maximum dosage is 6 g in 24-hour period.
Children 2 to 6 years: Use must be directed by doctor. 500 mg P.O. b.i.d. as required. Maximum dosage is 1.5 g in 24-hour period.
Children 6 to 12 years: 500 mg P.O. 1 to 3 times daily as required. Maximum dosage is 3 g in 24-hour period.
Diarrhea associated with irritable bowel syndrome, as well as acute non-specific diarrhea –
Adults: 1 g P.O. q.i.d. as required. Maximum dosage is 6 g in 24-hour period.
Children 2 to 6 years: Use must be directed by doctor. 500 mg P.O. b.i.d. as required. Maximum dosage is 1.5 g in 24-hour period.
Children 6 to 12 years: 500 mg P.O. t.i.d. as required. Maximum dosage is 3 g in 24-hour period.

ADVERSE REACTIONS
GI: abdominal fullness and increased flatus, intestinal obstruction.
Other: laxative dependence with long-term or excessive use.

INTERACTIONS
Tetracyclines: impaired absorption of tetracyclines. Avoid using together.

CONTRAINDICATIONS
Contraindicated in patients with signs of GI obstruction.

NURSING CONSIDERATIONS
• Before giving for constipation, determine if the patient has adequate fluid intake, exercise, and diet.
• Be aware that rectal bleeding or failure to respond to therapy may indicate need for surgery.
• Advise the patient to chew Equalactin or Mitrolan tablets thoroughly before swallowing and to drink a full glass of water with each dose. When used as an antidiarrheal, tell the patient not to drink a glass of water.
• Teach the patient about dietary sources of bulk which include bran and other cereals, fresh fruit, and vegetables.
• For severe diarrhea, advise the patient to repeat dose every half hour, but do not exceed maximum daily dosage.

---

cascara sagrada◊

cascara sagrada aromatic fluidextract*◊

cascara sagrada fluidextract*◊

Pregnancy Risk Category: C

HOW SUPPLIED
Tablets: 325 mg◊
Aromatic fluidextract: 1 g/ml*◊
Fluidextract: 1 g/ml*◊

ACTION
Unknown. A stimulant laxative that increases peristalsis probably by direct effect on the smooth muscle of the intestine. Thought to either irritate the musculature or stimulate the colonic intramural plexus. Also promotes fluid accumulation in the colon and small intestine.

ONSET, PEAK, DURATION
Onset occurs in 6 to 10 hours. Peak and duration variable.

INDICATIONS & DOSAGE
Acute constipation; preparation for bowel or rectal examination –
Adults and children 12 years and over: 0.3 to 1 g of cascara sagrada

P.O. once daily; 200 to 400 mg of cascara sagrada extract P.O. once daily; 0.5 to 1.5 ml of cascara sagrada fluid extract P.O. once daily, or 2 to 6 ml of aromatic cascara fluid extract P.O. once daily.

Children under 2 years: one-quarter adult dosage.

Children 2 to 12 years: one-half adult dosage.

ADVERSE REACTIONS
GI: *nausea;* vomiting; diarrhea; loss of normal bowel function with excessive use; *abdominal cramps,* especially in severe constipation; malabsorption of nutrients; "cathartic colon" (syndrome resembling ulcerative colitis radiologically and pathologically) in chronic misuse; discoloration of rectal mucosa after long-term use.
Other: hypokalemia, protein enteropathy, electrolyte imbalance (with excessive use), laxative dependence (with long-term or excessive use).

INTERACTIONS
None significant.

CONTRAINDICATIONS
Contraindicated in patients with abdominal pain, nausea, vomiting, or other symptoms of appendicitis or acute surgical abdomen; acute surgical delirium; fecal impaction; and intestinal obstruction or perforation.

NURSING CONSIDERATIONS
• Use cautiously when rectal bleeding is present.
• Before giving for constipation, determine if the patient has adequate fluid intake, exercise, and diet.
• Monitor serum electrolytes during prolonged use.
• Be aware that cascara sagrada aromatic fluidextract is less active and less bitter than nonaromatic fluidextract.
• Know that liquid preparations are more reliable than solid dosage forms.

• Warn patient that drug may turn alkaline urine red-pink and acidic urine yellow-brown.
• Teach the patient about dietary sources of bulk which include bran and other cereals, fresh fruit, and vegetables.

castor oil
Alphamul◇, Emulsoil◇, Fleet Flavored Castor Oil◇, Kellogg's Castor Oil◇, Minims Castor Oil‡, Neoloid◇, Purge◇

Pregnancy Risk Category: NR

HOW SUPPLIED
Oral liquid: 36.4% (Neoloid◇), 60% (Alphamul◇), 67% (Fleet◇), 95% (Emulsoil◇, Purge◇), 100% (Kellogg's◇, Minims◇).

ACTION
Unknown. A stimulant laxative that increases peristalsis probably by direct effect on the smooth muscle of the intestine. Thought to either irritate the musculature or stimulate the colonic intramural plexus. Also promotes fluid accumulation in the colon and small intestine.

ONSET, PEAK, DURATION
Onset occurs in 2 to 6 hours. Peak and duration variable.

INDICATIONS & DOSAGE
Preparation for rectal or bowel examination or for surgery –
Adults and children 12 years and older: 15 to 60 ml P.O.
Infants: up to 4 ml P.O. Increased dose produces no greater effect.
Children under 2 years: 1 to 5 ml P.O.
Children 2 to 12 years: 5 to 15 ml P.O.
 For all patients, administered as a single dose about 16 hours before surgery or procedure.

---

*Liquid form contains alcohol.   *Common* reactions are in italics; ***life-threatening,*** in bold italics.
**May contain tartrazine.

ADVERSE REACTIONS

GI: *nausea;* vomiting; diarrhea; loss of normal bowel function with excessive use; *abdominal cramps,* especially in severe constipation; malabsorption of nutrients; "cathartic colon" (syndrome resembling ulcerative colitis radiologically and pathologically) in chronic misuse; laxative dependence with long-term or excessive use. May cause constipation after catharsis.

GU: pelvic congestion in menstruating women.

Other: hypokalemia, protein-losing enteropathy, other electrolyte imbalances (with excessive use.)

INTERACTIONS
None significant.

CONTRAINDICATIONS
Contraindicated in patients with ulcerative bowel lesions; abdominal pain, nausea, vomiting, or other symptoms of appendicitis or acute surgical abdomen; and anal or rectal fissures, fecal impaction, or intestinal obstruction or perforation; and during menstruation or pregnancy.

NURSING CONSIDERATIONS
● Use cautiously in patients with rectal bleeding.
● Before giving for constipation, determine if the patient has adequate fluid intake, exercise, and diet.
● Give castor oil with juice or carbonated beverage to mask oily taste. Tell the patient to stir mixture and drink it promptly. Ice held in the mouth before taking drug will help prevent tasting it.
● Shake emulsion well before measuring dose. Emulsion is better tolerated but is more expensive. Store below 40° F (4.4° C). Don't freeze.
● Time drug administration so that it doesn't interfere with scheduled activities or sleep.
● Give on empty stomach for best results.
● Know that increased intestinal motility lessens absorption of concomitantly administered oral drugs. Separate administration times.
● Monitor serum electrolytes as ordered during prolonged use.
● Know that castor oil affects the small intestine. Regular use may cause excessive loss of water and salt.
● Keep in mind that drug is typically used before diagnostic testing or therapy requiring thorough evacuation of GI tract.
● Be aware that drug may be used as short-term treatment of acute constipation not responsive to milder laxatives. Not recommended for routine use.
● Be aware that failure to respond to drug may indicate acute condition requiring surgery.
● Tell the patient not to expect another bowel movement for 1 to 2 days after castor oil has emptied bowel.
● Teach the patient about dietary sources of bulk which include bran and other cereals, fresh fruit, and vegetables.

---

docusate calcium (dioctyl calcium sulfosuccinate)
Pro-Cal-Sof◇, Surfak◇

docusate potassium (dioctyl potassium sulfosuccinate)
Diocto-K◇, Kasof◇

docusate sodium (dioctyl sodium sulfosuccinate)
Afko-Lube◇, Colace◇, Coloxyl‡, Coloxyl Enema Concentrate‡, Dialose◇, Diocto◇, Dioeze◇, Diosuccin◇, Dio-Sul◇, Disonate◇, Di-Sosul◇, DOK-250◇, DOK Liquid◇, Doss◇, Doss 300◇, Doxinate◇, D-S-S◇, Duosol◇,

---

Genasoft◇, Laxinate 100◇,
Modane Soft◇, Molatoc◇, Pro-
Sof◇, Pro-Sof Liquid Concentrate◇,
Pro-Sof Liquid Plus◇, Regulax
SS◇, Regulex†◇, Regutol◇,
Stulex◇, Therevac Plus◇,
Therevac-SB◇

Pregnancy Risk Category: C

HOW SUPPLIED
docusate calcium
Capsules: 50 mg◇, 240 mg◇
docusate potassium
Capsules: 100 mg◇, 240 mg◇
docusate sodium
Tablets: 100 mg◇
Capsules: 50 mg◇, 60 mg◇, 100 mg◇,
240 mg◇, 250 mg◇
Oral liquid: 150 mg/15 ml◇
Oral solution: 50 mg/ml◇
Syrup: 50 mg/15 ml◇, 60 mg/15 ml◇
Enema concentrate: 18 g/100 ml
(must be diluted)‡

ACTION
A stool softener that reduces surface
tension of interfacing liquid contents
of the bowel. This detergent activity
promotes incorporation of additional
liquid into the stool, thus forming a
softer mass.

ONSET, PEAK, DURATION
Onset is variable; usually within 24 to
72 hours as is peak and duration.

INDICATIONS & DOSAGE
Stool softener –
**Adults and children older than 12
years:** 50 to 500 mg P.O. daily until
bowel movements are normal. Alternatively, give enema (where available). Dilute 1:24 with sterile water
before administration, and give 100 to
150 ml (retention enema), 300 to 500
ml (evacuation enema), or 0.5 to 1.5
liters (flushing enema).
Children under 3 years: 10 to 40 mg
docusate sodium P.O. daily.
Children 3 to 6 years: 20 to 60 mg
docusate sodium P.O. daily.

Children 6 to 12 years: 40 to 120 mg
docusate sodium P.O. daily.
  Higher dosages used for initial
therapy. Dosage adjusted to individual response. Usual dosage in children
and adults with minimal needs is 50
to 150 mg (calcium) P.O. daily.

ADVERSE REACTIONS
EENT: throat irritation.
GI: bitter taste, mild abdominal
cramping, diarrhea, laxative dependence (with long-term or excessive
use).

INTERACTIONS
Mineral oil: may increase mineral oil
absorption and cause toxicity and li-
poid pneumonia. Separate administration times.

CONTRAINDICATIONS
Contraindicated in patients hypersensitive to the drug and in those with intestinal obstruction, undiagnosed abdominal pain, vomiting or other signs
of appendicitis, fecal impaction, or
acute surgical abdomen.

NURSING CONSIDERATIONS
• Give liquid in milk, fruit juice, or
infant formula to mask bitter taste.
• Before giving for constipation, determine if the patient has adequate
fluid intake, exercise, and diet.
• Know that the drug is not for use in
treating existing constipation, but prevents constipation from developing.
• Be aware that the drug is laxative of
choice for patients who should not
strain during defecation, including
patients recovering from MI or rectal
surgery; for those with rectal or anal
disease that makes passage of firm
stool difficult; and for those with
postpartum constipation.
• Be aware that the drug acts within
24 to 48 hours to produce firm, semisolid stool.
• Know that the drug doesn't stimulate intestinal peristaltic movements.

---

*Liquid form contains alcohol.   *Common* reactions are in italics; ***life-threatening,*** in bold italics.
**May contain tartrazine.

• Store at 59° to 86° F (15° to 30° C), and protect liquid from light.
• Teach patient about dietary sources of bulk which include bran and other cereals, fresh fruit, and vegetables.
• Instruct patient to use only occasionally and don't use for more than 1 week without the doctor's knowledge.
• Tell patient to discontinue if severe cramping occurs and notify doctor.

glycerin
Fleet Babylax◊, Sani-Supp◊
Pregnancy Risk Category: NR

HOW SUPPLIED
Enema (pediatric): 4 ml/applicator◊
Suppositories: adult, children, and infant sizes◊

ACTION
A hyperosmolar laxative that draws water from the tissues into the feces and thus stimulates evacuation.

ONSET, PEAK, DURATION
Onset, peak and duration occur in 15 to 60 minutes.

INDICATIONS & DOSAGE
Constipation –
Adults and children 6 years and over: 2 to 3 g as a rectal suppository or 5 to 15 ml as an enema.
Children under 6 years: 1 to 1.7 g as a rectal suppository; or 2 to 5 ml as an enema.

ADVERSE REACTIONS
GI: *cramping pain,* rectal discomfort, hyperemia of rectal mucosa.

INTERACTIONS
None significant.

CONTRAINDICATIONS
Contraindicated in patients hypersensitive to the drug and in those with intestinal obstruction, undiagnosed abdominal pain, vomiting or other signs of appendicitis, fecal impaction, or acute surgical abdomen.

NURSING CONSIDERATIONS
• Know that drug is used mainly to reestablish proper toilet habits in laxative-dependent patients.
• Be aware that the drug must be retained for at least 15 minutes; usually acts within 1 hour. Entire suppository need not melt to be effective.

lactulose
Cephulac, Cholac, Chronulac, Constilac, Duphalac, Enulose, Generlac, Lactulax†, Portalac
Pregnancy Risk Category: B

HOW SUPPLIED
Syrup: 10 g/15 ml

ACTION
Produces an osmotic effect in the colon. Resulting distention promotes peristalsis. Also decreases blood ammonia, probably as a result of bacterial degradation, which decreases the pH of colon contents.

ONSET, PEAK, DURATION
Onset occurs in 24 to 48 hours. Peak and duration variable.

INDICATIONS & DOSAGE
Constipation –
Adults: 10 to 20 g (15 to 30 ml) P.O. daily.
To prevent and treat hepatic encephalopathy, including hepatic precoma and coma in patients with severe hepatic disease –
Adults: initially, 20 to 30 g (30 to 45 ml) P.O. t.i.d. or q.i.d., until two or three soft stools are produced daily. Usual dosage is 60 to 100 g daily in divided doses. Alternatively, 200 g (300 ml) diluted with 700 ml of water or saline solution and administered as a retention enema q 4 to 6 hours p.r.n.

ADVERSE REACTIONS
GI: abdominal cramps, belching, diarrhea, gaseous distention, flatulence.
Other: hypernatremia.

INTERACTIONS
Antacids, antibiotics, orally administered neomycin: decreased effectiveness of lactulose. Avoid concomitant use.

CONTRAINDICATIONS
Contraindicated in patients on a low-galactose diet.

NURSING CONSIDERATIONS
• Use cautiously in patients with diabetes mellitus.
• To minimize sweet taste, dilute with water or fruit juice or give with food.
• Prepare enema (not commercially available) by adding 200 g (300 ml) to 700 ml of water or 0.9% sodium chloride solution. The diluted solution is administered as a retention enema for 30 to 60 minutes. Use a rectal balloon catheter.
• If the enema is not retained for at least 30 minutes, be prepared to repeat dose.
• Monitor serum sodium level for possible hypernatremia, especially when giving in higher doses to treat hepatic encephalopathy.
• Be prepared to replace fluid loss.
• Store at room temperature, preferably below 86° F (30° C). Don't freeze.

magnesium citrate (citrate of magnesia)
Citroma◇, Citro-Mag†

magnesium hydroxide (milk of magnesia)
Milk of Magnesia◇, Philip's Milk of Magnesia◇

magnesium sulfate (epsom salts)◇
Pregnancy Risk Category: NR

HOW SUPPLIED
magnesium citrate
Oral solution: approximately 168 mEq magnesium/240 ml◇
magnesium hydroxide
Oral suspension: 7% to 8.5% (approximately 80 mEq magnesium/30 ml)◇
magnesium sulfate
Granules: approximately 40 mEq magnesium/5 g◇

ACTION
A saline laxative that produces an osmotic effect in the small intestine by drawing water into the intestinal lumen.

ONSET, PEAK, DURATION
Onset cocurs in ½ to 3 hours. Peak and duration variable.

INDICATIONS & DOSAGE
Constipation; to evacuate bowel before surgery –
Adults and children 12 years and older: 11 to 25 g magnesium citrate P.O. daily as a single dose or divided; 2.4 to 4.8 g (30 to 60 ml) magnesium hydroxide P.O. daily as a single dose or divided; 10 to 30 g magnesium sulfate P.O. daily as a single dose or divided.
Children 6 to 12 years: 5.5 to 12.5 g magnesium citrate P.O. daily as a single dose or divided; 1.2 to 2.4 g (15 to 30 ml) magnesium hydroxide P.O. daily as a single dose or divided; 5 to 10 g magnesium sulfate P.O. daily as a single dose or divided.
Children 2 to 6 years: 2.7 to 6.25 g magnesium citrate P.O. daily as a single dose or divided; 0.4 to 1.2 g (5 to 15 ml) magnesium hydroxide P.O. daily as a single dose or divided; 2.5 to 5 g magnesium sulfate P.O. daily as a single dose or divided.

Antacid –
Adults: 5 to 15 ml milk of magnesia
P.O. t.i.d. or q.i.d.

ADVERSE REACTIONS
GI: *abdominal cramping, nausea,
diarrhea,* laxative dependence with
long-term or excessive use.
Other: fluid and electrolyte disturbances with daily use.

INTERACTIONS
Orally administered drugs: impaired
absorption. Separate administration
times.

CONTRAINDICATIONS
Contraindicated in patients with abdominal pain, nausea, vomiting, or
other symptoms of appendicitis or
acute surgical abdomen and in those
with myocardial damage, heart block,
imminent delivery, fecal impaction,
rectal fissures, intestinal obstruction
or perforation, or renal disease.

NURSING CONSIDERATIONS
• Use cautiously in patients with rectal bleeding.
• Time drug administration so that it
doesn't interfere with scheduled activities or sleep. Drug produces watery stool in 3 to 6 hours.
• Before giving for constipation, determine if the patient has adequate
fluid intake, exercise, and diet.
• Chill magnesium citrate before use
to make it more palatable.
• Shake suspension well; give with
large amount of water when used as
laxative. When administering through
nasogastric tube, make sure tube is
placed properly and is patent. After
instilling, flush tube with water to ensure passage to stomach and maintain
tube patency.
• Monitor serum electrolytes as ordered during prolonged use. Magnesium may accumulate in patients with
renal insufficiency.

• Keep in mind that drug is for short-
term therapy.
• Know that magnesium sulfate is
more potent than other saline laxatives.
• Teach patient about dietary sources
of bulk which include bran and other
cereals, fresh fruit, and vegetables.
• Warn patients that frequent or prolonged use as a laxative may cause dependence.

methylcellulose
Citrucel◇, Cologel◇
Pregnancy Risk Category: NR

HOW SUPPLIED
Powder: 2 g/heaping tablespoon◇
Tablets: 500 mg◇

ACTION
A bulk-forming laxative that absorbs
water and expands to increase bulk
and moisture content of the stool. The
increased bulk encourages peristalsis
and bowel movement.

ONSET, PEAK, DURATION
Onset occurs in 12 to 24 hours. Peak
effects may not occur for up to 3 days.
Duration variable.

INDICATIONS & DOSAGE
Chronic constipation –
Adults: 1 to 3 heaping tablespoons in
8 oz (240 ml) cold water daily to t.i.d.
Usual dose up to 6 g daily (3 tablespoons).
Children 6 to 12 years: 1 to 1½ level
tablespoon in 4 oz (120 ml) cold water
daily to t.i.d. Usual dose up to 3 g
daily (1½ tablespoons).

ADVERSE REACTIONS
GI: *nausea,* vomiting, diarrhea (with
excessive use); esophageal, gastric,
small intestinal, or colonic strictures
when drug is chewed or taken in dry
form; *abdominal cramps,* especially
in severe constipation; laxative depen-

dence (with long-term or excessive use).

INTERACTIONS
None significant.

CONTRAINDICATIONS
Contraindicated in patients with abdominal pain, nausea, vomiting, or other symptoms of appendicitis or acute surgical abdomen and in those with intestinal obstruction or ulceration, disabling adhesions, or difficulty swallowing.

NURSING CONSIDERATIONS
Before giving for constipation, determine if the patient has adequate fluid intake, exercise, and diet.
• Be aware that the drug is especially useful in debilitated patients and in those with postpartum constipation, irritable bowel syndrome, diverticulitis, and colostomies. Also used to treat laxative abuse and to empty colon before barium enema examinations.
• Know that the drug is not absorbed systemically; nontoxic.
• Tell the patient to take drug with at least 8 oz of pleasant-tasting liquid to mask grittiness.
• Teach the patient about dietary sources of bulk which include bran and other cereals, fresh fruit, and vegetables.

mineral oil (liquid petrolatum)
Agoral Plain◇, Fleet Mineral Oil◇, Kondremul◇, Kondremul Plain◇, Lansoyl†, Liqui-Doss◇, Milkinol◇, Neo-Cultol◇, Petrogalar Plain◇, Zymenol◇

Pregnancy Risk Category: C

HOW SUPPLIED
Emulsion: 50%◇
Oral liquid: in pints, quarts, gallons◇
Enema: 120 ml◇, 133 ml◇

ACTION
A lubricant laxative that increases water retention in the stool by creating a barrier between colon wall and feces that prevents colonic reabsorption of fecal water.

ONSET, PEAK, DURATION
Onset occurs in 6 to 8 hours. Peak and duration variable.

INDICATIONS & DOSAGE
Constipation; preparation for bowel studies or surgery –
Adults and children 12 years and older: 5 to 45 ml P.O. h.s.; or 120 ml P.R. (as enema).
Children 6 to 12 years: 5 to 15 ml P.O. h.s.; or 30 to 60 ml P.R. (as enema).
Children 2 to 6 years: 30 to 60 ml P.R. (as enema).

ADVERSE REACTIONS
GI: *nausea;* vomiting; diarrhea (with excessive use); *abdominal cramps,* especially in severe constipation; decreased absorption of nutrients and fat-soluble vitamins, resulting in deficiency; slowed healing after hemorrhoidectomy.
Other: laxative dependence (with long-term or excessive use), pruritus, ***lipid pneumonia.***

INTERACTIONS
Docusate salts: may increase mineral oil absorption and cause lipid pneumonia. Separate administration times.
Fat-soluble vitamins (A, D, E, and K): possible decreased absorption after prolonged administration.

CONTRAINDICATIONS
Contraindicated in patients with abdominal pain, nausea, vomiting, or other symptoms of appendicitis or acute surgical abdomen and in those with fecal impaction or intestinal obstruction or perforation.

---

*Liquid form contains alcohol.   *Common* reactions are in italics; *life-threatening,* in bold italics.
**May contain tartrazine.

NURSING CONSIDERATIONS
• Use cautiously in young children; in elderly or debilitated patients because of susceptibility to lipid pneumonia through aspiration, absorption, and transport from intestinal mucosa; and in patients with rectal bleeding.
• Before giving for constipation, determine if the patient has adequate fluid intake, exercise, and diet.
• Give drug on an empty stomach because it delays passage of food from stomach; drug is more active on an empty stomach.
• Give with fruit juice or carbonated drink to disguise taste.
• Keep in mind that drug may be used when the patient needs to ease the strain of evacuation.
• Advise patient to take drug only at bedtime and not to take for more than 1 week.
• To avoid soiling clothing, advise the patient of possible rectal leakage from excessive dosages.
• Teach patient about dietary sources of bulk which include bran and other cereals, fresh fruit, and vegetables.

phenolphthalein, white
Alophen Pills◇, Feen-A-Mint◇, Medilax◇, Modane◇, Modane Mild◇, Phenolax Wafers**◇, Prulet◇

phenolphthalein, yellow
Espotabs◇, Evac-U-Gen◇, Evac-U-Lax◇, Ex-Lax◇, Ex-Lax Maximum Relief Formula◇, Ex-Lax Pills◇, Feen-A-Mint Gum◇, Lax-Pills◇

Pregnancy Risk Category: NR

HOW SUPPLIED
phenolphthalein white
Tablets: 60 mg◇, 65 mg ◇
Tablets (chewable): 60 mg◇, 64.8 mg◇
phenolphthalein yellow
Tablets (chewable): 80 mg◇, 90 mg◇, 97.2 mg◇
Chewing gum: 97.2 mg◇

ACTION
Unknown. A stimulant laxative that increases peristalsis probably by direct effect on the smooth muscle of the intestine. Thought either to irritate the musculature or stimulate the colonic intramural plexus. Also promotes fluid accumulation in the colon and small intestine.

ONSET, PEAK, DURATION
Onset occurs in 6 to 10 hours. Peak unknown. Effects persist 3 to 4 days.

INDICATIONS & DOSAGE
Constipation –
Adults and children 12 years and over: 30 to 270 mg P.O., preferably h.s.
Children 6 to 12 years: 30 to 60 mg P.O. h.s.
Children 2 to 6 years: 15 to 30 mg P.O. h.s.

ADVERSE REACTIONS
GI: diarrhea; *colic (with large doses):* factitious nausea; vomiting; loss of normal bowel function (with excessive use); *abdominal cramps,* especially in severe constipation; malabsorption of nutrients; "cathartic colon" (syndrome resembling ulcerative colitis radiologically and pathologically) with chronic misuse; reddish discoloration in alkaline feces or urine, laxative dependence (with long-term or excessive use).
Skin: dermatitis, pruritus, rash, pigmentation.
Other: hypersensitivity reactions.

INTERACTIONS
None significant.

CONTRAINDICATIONS
Contraindicated in patients with abdominal pain, nausea, vomiting, or other symptoms of appendicitis or acute surgical abdomen; in patients with fecal impaction or intestinal obstruction or perforation.

NURSING CONSIDERATIONS

• Use cautiously in patients with rectal bleeding.

• Before giving for constipation, determine if the patient has adequate fluid intake, exercise, and diet.

• Time drug administration so that it doesn't interfere with scheduled activities or sleep.

• Be aware that yellow phenolphthalein has been reported to be two to three times as potent as white phenolphthalein, but this has not been proved in clinical studies.

• Tell parents that children may mistake for candy. Keep out of reach.

• Warn the patient to avoid excessive sun exposure, not to use drug with any other product containing phenolphthalein, and to discontinue use if dermatoses occur. Phenolphthalein may cause drug-induced dermatoses.

• Warn the patient that the drug may discolor alkaline urine red-pink and acidic urine yellow-brown.

• Teach patient about dietary sources of bulk which include bran and other cereals, fresh fruit, and vegetables.

---

polyethylene glycol and electrolyte solution

Colovage, CoLyte, Glycoprep‡, GoLYTELY, NuLYTELY, OCL

Pregnancy Risk Category: C

HOW SUPPLIED

Powder for oral solution: polyethylene glycol (PEG) 3350 (6 g), anhydrous sodium sulfate (568 mg), sodium chloride (146 mg), potassium chloride (74.5 mg) per 100 ml (Colovage); PEG 3350 (120 g), sodium sulfate (3.36 g), sodium chloride (2.92 g), potassium chloride (1.49 g) per 2 liters (CoLyte); PEG 3350 (60 g), sodium chloride (1.46 g), potassium chloride (745 mg), sodium bicarbonate (1.68 g), sodium sulfate (5.68 g) per liter (Glycoprep‡); PEG 3350 (236 g), sodium sulfate (22.74 g), so-

dium bicarbonate (6.74g), sodium chloride (5.86 g), potassium chloride (2.97 g) per 4.8 liter (GoLYTELY); PEG 3350 (420 g), sodium bicarbonate (5.72 g), sodium chloride (11.2 g), potassium chloride (1.48 g) per 4 liters (NuLYTELY); PEG 3350 (6 g), sodium sulfate decahydrate (1.29 g), sodium chloride (146 mg), potassium chloride (75 mg), polysorbate-80 (30 mg) per 100 ml (OCL)

ACTION

PEG 3350, a nonabsorbable solution, acts as an osmotic agent. Sodium sulfate greatly reduces sodium absorption. The electrolyte concentration causes virtually no net absorption or secretion of ions.

ONSET, PEAK, DURATION

Onset occurs within 1 hour. Peak and duration variable.

INDICATIONS & DOSAGE

Bowel preparation before GI examination –

Adults: 240 ml P.O. q 10 minutes until 4 liters are consumed. Typically, administer 4 hours before examination, allowing 3 hours for drinking and 1 hour for bowel evacuation.

ADVERSE REACTIONS

GI: *nausea, bloating, cramps, vomiting.*

INTERACTIONS

Orally administered drugs: decreased absorption if administered within 1 hour of starting therapy. Administer at least 2 to 3 hours before starting therapy.

CONTRAINDICATIONS

Contraindicated in patients with GI obstruction or perforation, gastric retention, toxic colitis, or megacolon.

---

*Liquid form contains alcohol.   *Common* reactions are in italics; *life-threatening,* in bold italics.
**May contain tartrazine.

NURSING CONSIDERATIONS
• Use tap water to reconstitute powder. Shake vigorously to ensure that all powder is dissolved. Refigerate reconstituted solution but use within 48 hours.
• Do not add flavoring or additional ingredients to the solution or administer chilled solution. Hypothermia has been reported after ingestion of large amounts of chilled solution.
• Administer solution early in the morning if the patient is scheduled for a midmorning examination. Orally administered solution induces diarrhea (onset 30 to 60 minutes) that rapidly cleans the bowel, usually within 4 hours.
• When used as preparation for barium enema, administer solution the evening before the examination, to avoid interfering with barium coating of the colonic mucosa.
• Have the patient fast for 3 to 4 hours before taking the solution and thereafter ingest only clear fluids until the examination is complete.
• If administered to semiconscious patients or to patients with impaired gag reflex, take care to prevent aspiration.
• Be aware that no major shifts in fluid or electrolyte balance have been reported.

psyllium
Alramucil◊, Cillium◊, Fiberall◊, Fibrepur†◊, Hydrocil Instant◊, Karacil†◊, Konsyl◊, Metamucil◊, Metamucil Instant Mix◊, Metamucil Sugar-Free◊, Modane Bulk◊, Naturacil◊, Perdiem Plain◊, Prodiem Plain†◊, Pro-Lax◊, Reguloid◊, Serutan◊, Siblin◊, Syllact◊, Versabran◊, V-Lax◊

Pregnancy Risk Category: NR

HOW SUPPLIED
Chewable pieces: 1.7 g/piece◊
Effervescent powder: 3.4 g/packet◊, 3.7 g/packet◊
Granules: 2.5 g/tsp◊, 4.03 g/tsp◊
Powder: 3.3 g/tsp◊, 3.4 g/tsp◊, 3.5 g/tsp◊, 4.94 g/tsp◊
Wafers: 3.4 g/wafer◊

ACTION
A bulk-forming laxative that absorbs water and expands to increase bulk and moisture content of the stool, thus encouraging peristalsis and bowel movement.

ONSET, PEAK, DURATION
Onset occurs in 12 to 24 hours. Peak effects may not occur for 3 days. Duration variable.

INDICATIONS & DOSAGE
Constipation; bowel management –
Adults: 1 to 2 rounded teaspoonfuls P.O. in full glass of liquid once daily, b.i.d., or t.i.d., followed by second glass of liquid; or 1 packet dissolved in water once daily, b.i.d., or t.i.d.
Children over 6 years: 1 level teaspoonful P.O. in half a glass of liquid h.s.

ADVERSE REACTIONS
GI: nausea, vomiting, diarrhea (with excessive use); esophageal, gastric, small intestinal, or colonic strictures when drug is taken in dry form; abdominal cramps, especially in severe constipation.

INTERACTIONS
None significant.

CONTRAINDICATIONS
Contraindicated in patients with hypersensitivity to drug, abdominal pain, nausea, vomiting, or other symptoms of appendicitis and in those with intestinal obstruction or ulceration, disabling adhesions, or difficulty swallowing.

---

†Available in Canada only.   ‡Available in Australia only.   ◊Available OTC.

NURSING CONSIDERATIONS

● Before giving for constipation, determine if the patient has adequate fluid intake, exercise, and diet.

● Mix with at least 8 oz (240 ml) of cold, pleasant-tasting liquid, such as orange juice, to mask grittiness, and stir only a few seconds. Have the patient drink mixture immediately so it does not congeal. Follow with additional glass of liquid.

● For dosages in children under 6 years, consult the doctor.

● Know that drug may reduce appetite if taken before meals.

● Be aware that the drug is not absorbed systemically and is nontoxic. It is especially useful in debilitated patients and those with postpartum constipation, irritable bowel syndrome, and diverticular disease. Also useful to treat chronic laxative abuse and in combination with other laxatives to empty colon before barium enema examinations.

● Teach the patient how to properly mix medication. To enhance effect and prevent intestinal obstruction, tell the patient to take drug with plenty of water. Advise the patient that inhaling powder may cause allergic reactions.

● Tell the patient that laxative effect usually occurs in 12 to 24 hours, but may be delayed 3 days.

● Advise diabetic patients to check the label and use brand of psyllium that does not contain sugar.

● Teach the patient about dietary sources of bulk which include bran and other cereals, fresh fruit, and vegetables.

---

senna

Black-Draught◇, Fletcher's Castoria◇, Lax-Senna◇, Senexon◇, Senokot◇, Senolax◇, X-Prep Liquid*◇

Pregnancy Risk Category: C

HOW SUPPLIED

Tablets: 187 mg◇, 217 mg◇, 600 mg◇
Granules: 326 mg/tsp◇, 1.65 g/½ tsp◇
Suppositories: 652 mg◇
Syrup: 218 mg/5 ml◇

ACTION

Unknown. A stimulant laxative that increases peristalsis probably by direct effect on the smooth muscle of the intestine. Thought to either irritate the musculature or stimulate the colonic intramural plexus. Also promotes fluid accumulation in the colon and small intestine.

ONSET, PEAK, DURATION

Onset occurs in 6 to 10 hours. Peak and duration variable.

INDICATIONS & DOSAGE

Acute constipation; preparation for bowel or rectal examination –
Adults: dosage range for Senokot is 1 to 8 tablets P.O.; ½ to 4 teaspoonfuls of granules added to liquid P.O.; 1 to 2 suppositories P.R., h.s.; or 1 to 4 teaspoonfuls syrup P.O., h.s. Dosage for Black-Draught is 2 tablets or ¼ to ½ level teaspoonfuls of granules mixed with water.

X-Prep Liquid used solely as single dose for preradiographic bowel evacuation. Give 20 g powder dissolved in juice or 75 ml liquid P.O. between 2 p.m. and 4 p.m. on day before X-ray procedure. Use in divided doses, if needed, for elderly or debilitated patients.

Children over 27 kg: one-half adult dose of tablets, granules, or syrup (except Black-Draught tablets and granules – not recommended for children).
Children 1 month to 1 year: 1.25 to 2.5 ml Senokot syrup P.O. h.s.

ADVERSE REACTIONS

GI: *nausea;* vomiting; diarrhea; loss of normal bowel function with excessive use; *abdominal cramps,* espe-

---

*Liquid form contains alcohol.
**May contain tartrazine.

Common reactions are in italics; *life-threatening,* in bold italics.

cially in severe constipation; malabsorption of nutrients; "cathartic colon" (syndrome resembling ulcerative colitis radiologically) with chronic misuse; possible constipation after catharsis; yellow or yellow-green cast to feces; diarrhea in breast-feeding infants of mothers receiving senna; darkened pigmentation of rectal mucosa with long-term use (usually reversible within 4 to 12 months after stopping drug); laxative dependence with excessive use.
GU: red-pink discoloration in alkaline urine; yellow-brown color to acidic urine.
Other: protein-losing enteropathy, electrolyte imbalance (such as hypokalemia).

INTERACTIONS
None significant.

CONTRAINDICATIONS
Contraindicated in patients with ulcerative bowel lesions; with nausea, vomiting, abdominal pain, or other symptoms of appendicitis or acute surgical abdomen; fecal impaction; or intestinal obstruction or perforation.

NURSING CONSIDERATIONS
• Before giving for constipation, determine if the patient has adequate fluid intake, exercise, and diet.
• Limit diet to clear liquids after X-Prep Liquid is taken.
• Avoid exposing product to excessive heat or light.
• Know that drug is used for short-term treatment.
• Know that senna is one of the most effective laxatives for counteracting constipation caused by narcotic analgesics.
• Teach the patient about dietary sources of bulk which include bran and other cereals, fresh fruit, and vegetables.

sodium phosphates
Fleet Phospho-Soda◇

Pregnancy Risk Category: NR

HOW SUPPLIED
Liquid: 2.4 g/5 ml sodium phosphate and 900 mg sodium biphosphate/5 ml◇
Enema: 160 mg/ml sodium phosphate and 60 mg/ml sodium biphosphate◇

ACTION
A saline laxative that produces an osmotic effect in the small intestine by drawing water into the intestinal lumen.

ONSET, PEAK, DURATION
Onset occurs in ½ to 3 hours after oral use, 5 to 10 minutes after enema. Peak and duration variable after oral dose, complete upon evacuation following enema.

INDICATIONS & DOSAGE
Constipation –
Adults: 20 to 30 ml solution mixed with 120 ml cold water P.O.; or 60 to 135 ml P.R. (as enema).
Children: 5 to 15 ml solution mixed with 120 ml of cold water P.O.; or 67.5 ml P.R. (as enema).

ADVERSE REACTIONS
GI: *abdominal cramping.*
Other: fluid and electrolyte disturbances (hypernatremia, hyperphosphatemia) with daily use; laxative dependence with long-term or excessive use.

INTERACTIONS
None significant.

CONTRAINDICATIONS
Contraindicated in patients with abdominal pain, nausea, vomiting, or other symptoms of appendicitis or acute surgical abdomen; intestinal obstruction or perforation; edema; CHF;

megacolon; or impaired renal function and in patients on sodium-restricted diets.

NURSING CONSIDERATIONS
• Use cautiously in patients with large hemorrhoids or anal excoriations.
• Before giving for constipation, determine if the patient has adequate fluid intake, exercise, and diet.
• Be aware that up to 10% of sodium content of drug may be absorbed.
• Teach patient about dietary sources of bulk which include bran and other cereals, fresh fruit, and vegetables.

Common reactions are in italics; ***life-threatening,*** in bold italics.

51
Antiemetics

benzquinamide hydrochloride
buclizine hydrochloride
chlorpromazine hydrochloride
(See Chapter 33, ANTIPSYCHOTICS.)
cyclizine hydrochloride
cyclizine lactate
dimenhydrinate
diphenidol hydrochloride
dronabinol
granisetron hydrochloride
meclizine hydrochloride
metoclopramide hydrochloride
ondansetron hydrochloride
perphenazine
(See Chapter 33, ANTIPSYCHOTICS.)
prochlorperazine
prochlorperazine edisylate
prochlorperazine maleate
promethazine hydrochloride
(See Chapter 43, ANTIHISTAMINES.)
scopolamine
(See Chapter 38, ANTICHOLINERGICS.)
thiethylperazine maleate
trimethobenzamide
   hydrochloride

COMBINATION PRODUCTS
None.

---

benzquinamide
hydrochloride
Emete-Con

Pregnancy Risk Category: NR

HOW SUPPLIED
Injection: 50 mg/vial

ACTION
Unknown. Thought to act on the chemoreceptor trigger zone to inhibit nausea and vomiting.

ONSET, PEAK, DURATION
Onset occurs within 15 minutes.
Blood levels peak immediately after

I.V. injection or within 30 minutes after I.M. injection. Effects persist for 3 to 4 hours.

INDICATIONS & DOSAGE
Nausea and vomiting associated with anesthesia and surgery –
Adults: 50 mg I.M. (0.5 mg/kg to 1 mg/kg). Repeated in 1 hour and thereafter q 3 to 4 hours, p.r.n.; or 25 mg (0.2 mg/kg to 0.4 mg/kg) I.V. as a single dose, administered slowly (25 mg/minute).

ADVERSE REACTIONS
CNS: *drowsiness,* fatigue, insomnia, restlessness, headache, excitation, tremor, twitching, dizziness.
CV: sudden rise in blood pressure and transient arrhythmias (premature atrial and ventricular contractions, atrial fibrillation) after I.V. administration; hypertension; hypotension.
EENT: salivation, blurred vision.
GI: anorexia, nausea, dry mouth.
Skin: urticaria, rash.
Other: muscle weakness, flushing, hiccups, sweating, chills, fever.

INTERACTIONS
CNS depressants, ethanol: enhanced CNS depression. Avoid concomitant use.

CONTRAINDICATIONS
Contraindicated for I.V. use in patients with CV disease and within 15 minutes of administering preanesthetic or CV drugs. Also contraindicated in patients with hypersensitivity to the drug.

NURSING CONSIDERATIONS
• Be aware that use during pregnancy is not recommended.
• **I.V. use:** Reconstitute drug with 2.2

---

†Available in Canada only.   ‡Available in Australia only.   ◊ Available OTC.

ml of sterile water for injection or bacteriostatic water containing benzyl alcohol or propylparabens. Do not dilute further. Inject directly and slowly (25 mg/minute).
• Do not reconstitute with 0.9% sodium chloride injection.
• For I.M. use, give injections in large muscle mass. Use deltoid area only if well developed.
• Monitor blood pressure frequently.
• Like other antiemetics, be alert that drug may mask symptoms of ototoxicity, brain tumor, or intestinal obstruction.
• Store dry powder and reconstituted solution in a light-resistant container. Reconstituted solution is stable for 14 days at room temperature.

buclizine hydrochloride
Bucladin-S Softab**

Pregnancy Risk Category: NR

HOW SUPPLIED
Tablets (chewable): 50 mg

ACTION
Unknown. An antihistamine that may affect neural pathways originating in the labyrinth to inhibit nausea and vomiting, but exact mechanism of action is unknown.

ONSET, PEAK, DURATION
Onset and peak unknown. Effects persist for 4 to 6 hours.

INDICATIONS & DOSAGE
Prevention of motion sickness—
Adults: 50 mg P.O. at least ½ hour before beginning travel. If needed, repeat after 4 to 6 hours.
Vertigo—
Adults: 50 mg P.O., 1 to 3 times daily. Maintenance dosage is 50 mg b.i.d.

ADVERSE REACTIONS
CNS: *drowsiness,* headache, dizziness, jitters.
EENT: blurred vision.
GI: dry mouth.
GU: urine retention.

INTERACTIONS
CNS depressants, ethanol: additive CNS depression. Avoid concomitant use.

CONTRAINDICATIONS
Contraindicated in patients hypersensitive to the drug. Contains tartrazine, which may precipitate allergic reactions in certain individuals, including those allergic to aspirin.

NURSING CONSIDERATIONS
• Like other antiemetics, be alert that drug may mask symptoms of ototoxicity, intestinal obstruction, or brain tumor.
• Tell patients to place tablets in mouth and allow to dissolve without water, chew, or swallow them whole.
• Advise patients to avoid driving and other activities that require alertness until CNS effects of the drug are known.

cyclizine hydrochloride
Marezine◇

cyclizine lactate
Marezine, Marzine†

Pregnancy Risk Category: B

HOW SUPPLIED
cyclizine hydrochloride
Tablets: 50 mg◇
cyclizine lactate
Injection: 50 mg/ml†

ACTION
Unknown. An antihistamine that may affect neural pathways originating in the labyrinth to inhibit nausea and

---

*Liquid form contains alcohol.
**May contain tartrazine.

Common reactions are in italics; **life-threatening,** in bold italics.

vomiting, but the exact mechanism of action is unknown.

ONSET, PEAK, DURATION
Onset may occur in ½ to 1 hour. Peak unknown. Effects persist 4 to 6 hours.

INDICATIONS & DOSAGE
Prevention or treatment of motion sickness –
Adults and children 12 years and older: 50 mg P.O. (hydrochloride) ½ hour before travel, then q 4 to 6 hours, p.r.n., to maximum of 200 mg daily; or 50 mg I.M. (lactate) q 4 to 6 hours, p.r.n.
Children 6 to 12 years: 25 mg (hydrochloride) P.O. q 4 to 6 hours, p.r.n., to a maximum of 75 mg daily.

ADVERSE REACTIONS
CNS: *drowsiness,* dizziness, auditory and visual hallucinations.
CV: hypotension.
EENT: blurred vision.
GI: constipation, dry mouth.
GU: urine retention.

INTERACTIONS
CNS depressants, ethanol: additive CNS depression. Avoid concomitant use.

CONTRAINDICATIONS
Contraindicated in patients hypersensitive to the drug.

NURSING CONSIDERATIONS
• Use cautiously in patients with severe heart failure and after surgery.
• Like other antiemetics, be alert that drug may mask symptoms of ototoxicity, brain tumor, or intestinal obstruction.
• Store in cool place. When stored at room temperature, injection may turn slightly yellow; this change does not indicate loss of potency.
• Advise patients to avoid driving and other activities that require alertness

until CNS effects of the drug are known.

---

dimenhydrinate
Andrumin‡, Apo-Dimenhydrinate†, Calm X◊, Children's Dramamine◊, Dimetabs, Dinate, Dommanate, Dramamine◊*, Dramamine Chewable◊**, Dramamine Liquid◊*, Dramanate, Dramocen, Dramoject, Dymenate, Gravol†, Gravol L/A†, Hydrate, Marmine◊, Nauseatol†, Nico-Vert◊, Novo-Dimenate†, PMS-Dimenhydrinate†, Tega-Vert◊, Travamine†, Travs‡, Triptone Caplets◊, Vertab

Pregnancy Risk Category: B

HOW SUPPLIED
Tablets: 50 mg◊
Tablets (chewable): 50 mg◊
Capsules: 50 mg◊
Elixir: 15 mg/5 ml†
Syrup: 12.5 mg/4 ml*◊, 15.62 mg/5 ml
Injection: 50 mg/ml

ACTION
Unknown. An antihistamine that may affect neural pathways originating in the labyrinth to inhibit nausea and vomiting. Exact mechanism of action is unknown.

ONSET, PEAK, DURATION
Onset occurs immediately after I.V. administration, within 15 to 20 minutes of I.M. injection, within 20 to 30 minutes of oral administration. Peak unknown. Effects persist 3 to 6 hours.

INDICATIONS & DOSAGE
Prevention and treatment of motion sickness –
Adults and children 12 years and over: 50 to 100 mg P.O. q 4 to 6 hours; 50 mg I.M., p.r.n.; or 50 mg I.V. diluted in 10 ml sodium chloride injection, injected over 2 minutes. Maximum dosage is 400 mg daily.

Children 6 to 12 yeras: 25 to 50 mg P.O. q 6 to 8 hours, not to exceed 150 mg in 24 hours.
Children 2 to 6 years: 12.5 to 25 mg P.O. q 6 to 8 hours, not to exceed 75 mg in 24 hours.

ADVERSE REACTIONS
CNS: *drowsiness,* headache, incoordination, dizziness.
CV: palpitations, hypotension.
EENT: blurred vision, tinnitus, dry respiratory passages.
GI: dry mouth.

INTERACTIONS
CNS depressants, ethanol: additive CNS depression. Avoid concomitant use.

CONTRAINDICATIONS
None known.

NURSING CONSIDERATIONS
• Use cautiously in patients with seizures, acute angle-closure glaucoma, or enlarged prostate gland or in patients receiving ototoxic drugs.
• **I.V. use:** Before administration, dilute each ml of drug with 10 ml of sterile water for injection, D₅W, or 0.9% sodium chloride injection. Give by direct injection over not less than 2 minutes.
• Know that undiluted solution is irritating to veins and may cause sclerosis.
• Because incompatibilities are common, avoid mixing parenteral preparation with other drugs.
• Like other antiemetics, be alert that drug may mask symptoms of ototoxicity, brain tumor, or intestinal obstruction.
• Advise patients to avoid driving and other activities that require alertness until CNS effects of the drug are known.

diphenidol hydrochloride
Vontrol**

Pregnancy Risk Category: NR

HOW SUPPLIED
Tablets: 25 mg

ACTION
Unknown. Probably diminishes labrynthine function and vestibular stimulation and influences the chemoreceptor trigger zone to inhibit nausea and vomiting.

ONSET, PEAK, DURATION
Onset and duration unknown. Blood levels peak 1½ to 3 hours after a dose.

INDICATIONS & DOSAGE
Peripheral (labyrinthine) vertigo –
Adults: 25 to 50 mg P.O. q 4 hours, p.r.n.
Nausea and vomiting –
Adults: 25 to 50 mg P.O. q 4 hours, p.r.n.
Children over 23 kg: 0.88 mg/kg P.O. q 4 hours, not to exceed 5.5 mg/kg/24 hours. Usual dose is 25 mg.

ADVERSE REACTIONS
CNS: *drowsiness,* dizziness, sleep disturbances, *confusion,* auditory and visual hallucinations, disorientation.
CV: transient hypotension.
GI: dry mouth, nausea, indigestion, heartburn.
Skin: urticaria.

INTERACTIONS
None significant.

CONTRAINDICATIONS
Contraindicated in patients with anuria and hypersensitivity to drug.

NURSING CONSIDERATIONS
• Use cautiously in patients with glaucoma, pyloric stenosis, pylorospasm, obstructive lesions of GI or

---

*Liquid form contains alcohol.
**May contain tartrazine.*
Common reactions are in italics; ***life-threatening,*** in bold italics.

GU tract, prostatic hyperplasia, or organic cardiospasm (achalasia).
• Closely supervise patients. Patients usually are hospitalized when receiving drug. Monitor fluid intake and output; report any changes.
• Like other antiemetics, be alert that drug may mask symptoms of ototoxicity, brain tumor, intestinal obstruction, or other conditions.
• Stop drug if auditory or visual hallucinations, disorientation, or confusion occur and notify doctor.

---

dronabinol (delta-g-tetrahydrocannabinol)
Marinol
Controlled Substance Schedule II
Pregnancy Risk Category: C

HOW SUPPLIED
Capsules: 2.5 mg, 5 mg, 10 mg

ACTION
Unknown. A derivative of marijuana.

ONSET, PEAK, DURATION
Onset unknown. Serum levels peak in 2 to 4 hours. Effects persist for 4 to 6 hours.

INDICATIONS & DOSAGE
Nausea and vomiting associated with cancer chemotherapy –
Adults: 5 mg/m^2 P.O. 1 to 3 hours before administration of chemotherapy. Then same dose q 2 to 4 hours after chemotherapy for a total of four to six doses per day. If needed, dosage increased in increments of 2.5 mg/m^2 to a maximum of 15 mg/m^2 per dose.
Anorexia and weight loss in patients with AIDS –
Adults: 2.5 mg P.O. b.i.d. before lunch and dinner.

ADVERSE REACTIONS
CNS: *dizziness, drowsiness, euphoria, ataxia,* depersonalization, disorientation, hallucinations, head-
ache, irritability, memory lapse, muddled thinking, paranoia, perceptual difficulties, weakness, paresthesia.
CV: tachycardia, orthostatic hypotension.
GI: *dry mouth.*
Other: visual disturbances.

INTERACTIONS
CNS depressants, ethanol, psychotomimetic substances, sedatives: additive effects. Avoid concomitant use.

CONTRAINDICATIONS
Contraindicated in patients hypersensitive to sesame oil or cannabinoids.

NURSING CONSIDERATIONS
• Use cautiously in elderly, pregnant, or lactating patients and in those with heart disease, psychiatric illness, and history of drug abuse.
• Expect this drug to be prescribed only for patients who have not responded satisfactorily to other antiemetics.
• Know that dronabinol is the principal active substance present in *Cannabis sativa* (marijuana). This substance can produce both physical and psychological dependence and has a high potential for abuse.
• Keep in mind that CNS effects are intensified at higher drug dosages.
• Be aware that drug's effects may persist for days after treatment ends.
• To prevent panic and anxiety, tell the patient drug may induce unusual changes in mood or other adverse behavioral effects.
• Advise the patient against hazardous activities that require alertness until the CNS effects of the drug are known.
• Warn family members to ensure that the patient is supervised by a responsible person during and immediately after treatment.

---

†Available in Canada only.   ‡Available in Australia only.   ◇ Available OTC.

granisetron hydrochloride
Kytril

Pregnancy Risk Category: B

HOW SUPPLIED
Injection: 1 mg/ml
Tablets: 1 mg

ACTION
A selective antagonist of a specific type of serotonin receptor (5-HT$_3$) located in the CNS at the area postrema (chemoreceptor trigger zone) and in the peripheral nervous system on nerve terminals of the vagus nerve. Drug's blocking action may occur at both sites.

ONSET, PEAK, DURATION
Unknown.

INDICATIONS & DOSAGE
Prevention of nausea and vomiting associated with emetogenic cancer chemotherapy –

Adults and children 2 to 16 years: 10 mcg/kg I.V. infused over 5 minutes. Begin infusion within 30 minutes before administration of chemotherapy. Alternatively, 1 mg P.O. up to 1 hour before chemotherapy and dosage repeated 12 hours later.

ADVERSE REACTIONS
CNS: *headache, asthenia,* somnolence.
CV: hypertension.
GI: diarrhea, constipation.
Other: taste disorder, fever.

INTERACTIONS
None significant.

CONTRAINDICATIONS
Contraindicated in patients hypersensitive to the drug.

NURSING CONSIDERATIONS
● **I.V. use:** Dilute drug with 0.9% sodium chloride injection or D$_5$W to a volume of 20 to 50 ml. Infuse over 5 minutes beginning within 30 minutes before initiating chemotherapy, and only on the day(s) chemotherapy is given. Diluted solutions are stable for 24 hours at room temperature.
● Do not mix with other drugs; data regarding compatibility is limited.

meclizine hydrochloride (meclozine hydrochloride)
Ancolan‡, Antivert, Antivert/25◊, Antivert/50, Bonamine†, Bonine◊, Dizmiss◊, D-Vert 15, D-Vert 30, Meni-D, Ru-Vert M

Pregnancy Risk Category: B

HOW SUPPLIED
Tablets: 12.5 mg, 25 mg◊, 50 mg
Tablets (chewable): 25 mg◊
Capsules: 15 mg, 25 mg, 30 mg

ACTION
Unknown. An antihistamine that may affect neural pathways originating in the labyrinth to inhibit nausea and vomiting.

ONSET, PEAK, DURATION
Onset occurs in about 1 hour. Peak unknown. Effects persist 8 to 24 hours.

INDICATIONS & DOSAGE
Vertigo –
Adults: 25 to 100 mg P.O. daily in divided doses. Dosage varies with patient response.
Motion sickness –
Adults: 25 to 50 mg P.O. 1 hour before travel, repeated daily for duration of journey.

ADVERSE REACTIONS
CNS: *drowsiness,* fatigue.
EENT: blurred vision.
GI: dry mouth.

---

*Liquid form contains alcohol.   *Common* reactions are in italics; ***life-threatening,*** in bold italics.
**May contain tartrazine.

Identifying commonly prescribed tablets and capsules

One of the most critical responsibilities of any nurse is to ensure that the patient receives the right medication. This task becomes easier when the nurse can verify the appearance of drugs prescribed for the patient. The following section provides full-color photographs of some of the most commonly prescribed tablets and capsules in the United States (according to the latest annual survey from *American Druggist*, February 22, 1995). Shown here in actual size, the tablets and capsules are organized alphabetically for quick reference.

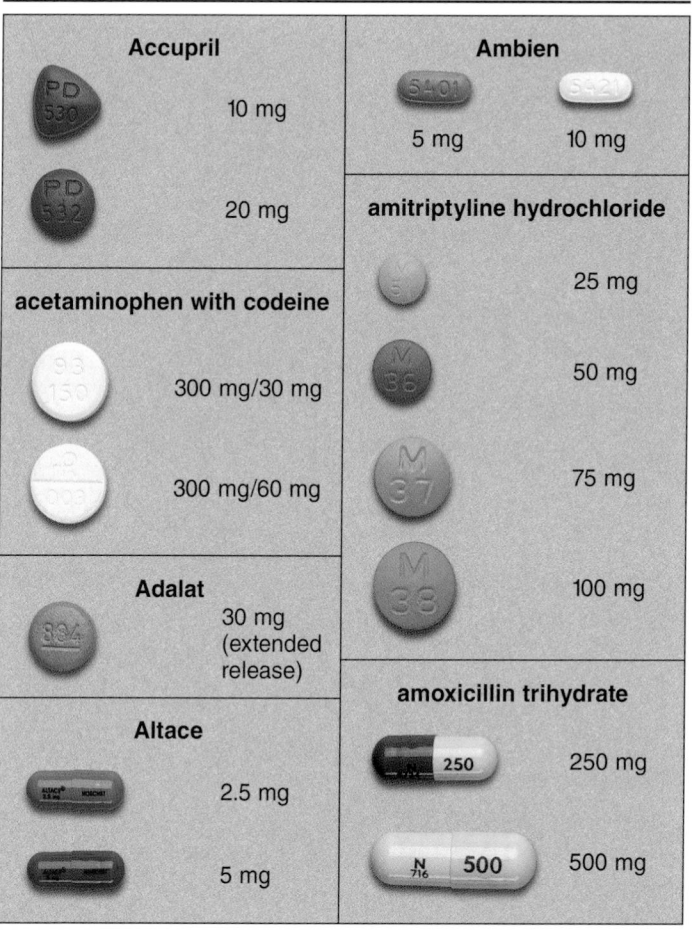

	Accupril	
		10 mg
		20 mg

acetaminophen with codeine

| | 300 mg/30 mg |
| | 300 mg/60 mg |

Adalat

30 mg (extended release)

Altace

| | 2.5 mg |
| | 5 mg |

Ambien

| 5 mg | 10 mg |

amitriptyline hydrochloride

	25 mg
	50 mg
	75 mg
	100 mg

amoxicillin trihydrate

| | 250 mg |
| | 500 mg |

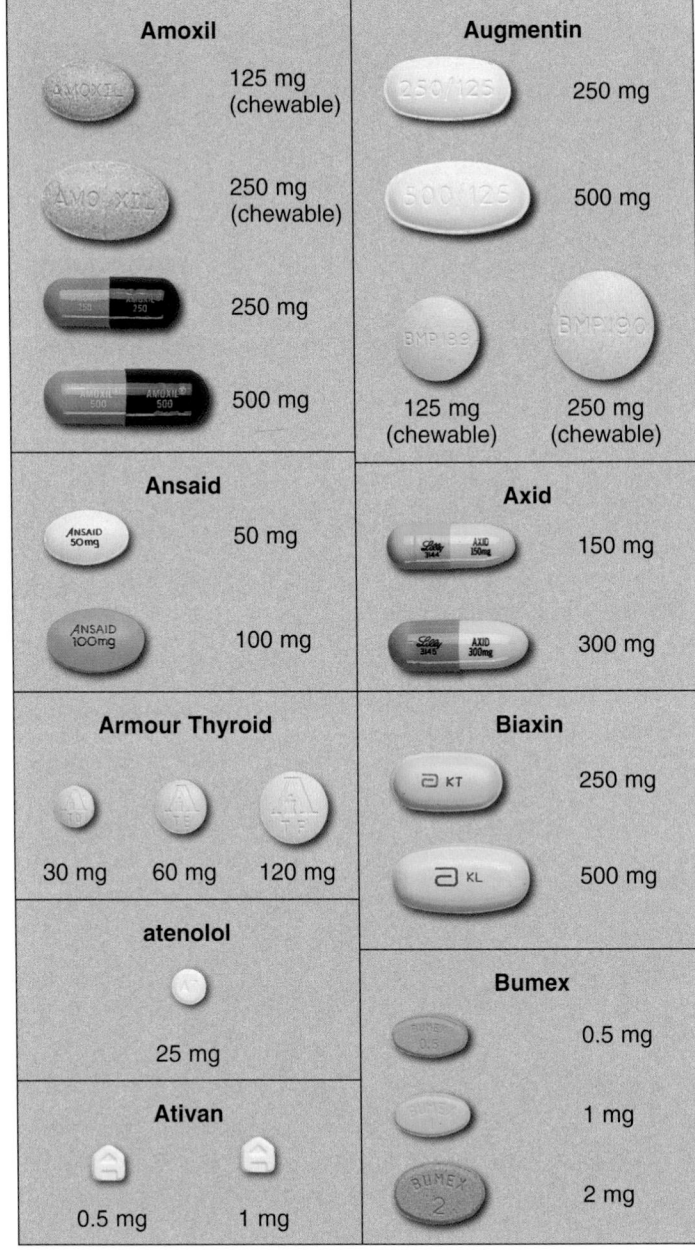

Amoxil

125 mg (chewable)

250 mg (chewable)

250 mg

500 mg

Augmentin

250 mg

500 mg

125 mg (chewable)

250 mg (chewable)

Ansaid

50 mg

100 mg

Axid

150 mg

300 mg

Armour Thyroid

30 mg 60 mg 120 mg

Biaxin

250 mg

500 mg

atenolol

25 mg

Bumex

0.5 mg

1 mg

2 mg

Ativan

0.5 mg 1 mg

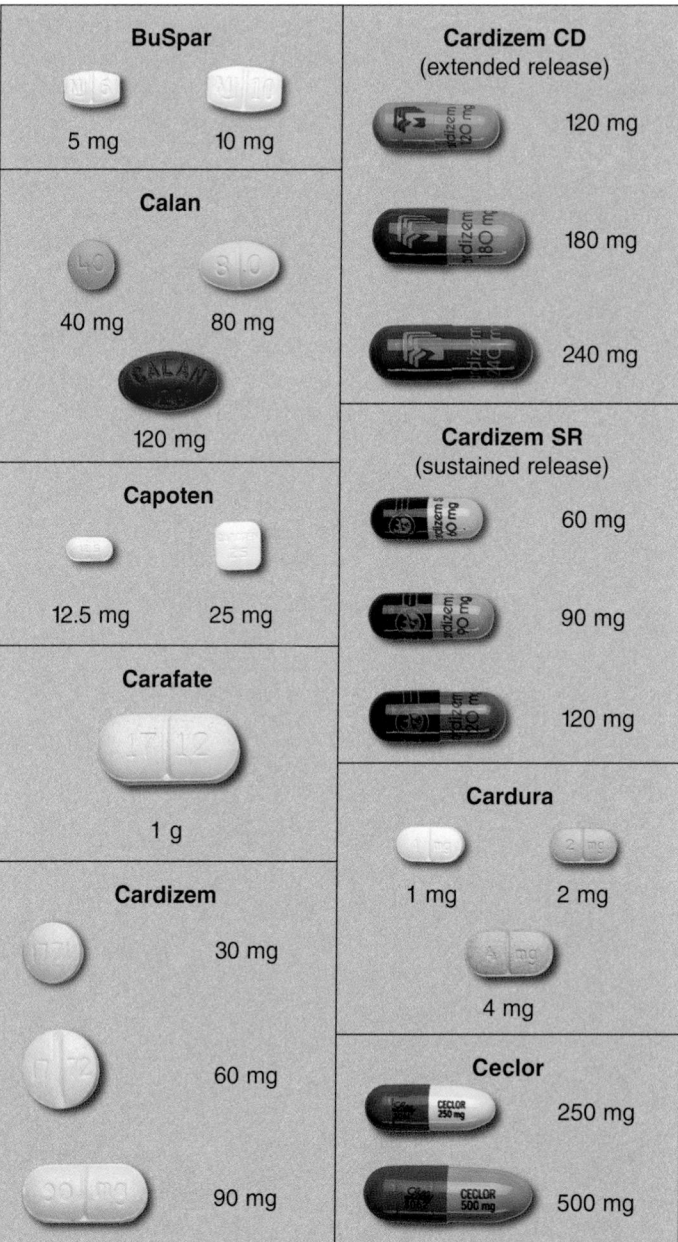

BuSpar

5 mg

10 mg

Calan

40 mg

80 mg

120 mg

Capoten

12.5 mg

25 mg

Carafate

1 g

Cardizem

30 mg

60 mg

90 mg

Cardizem CD
(extended release)

120 mg

180 mg

240 mg

Cardizem SR
(sustained release)

60 mg

90 mg

120 mg

Cardura

1 mg

2 mg

4 mg

Ceclor

250 mg

500 mg

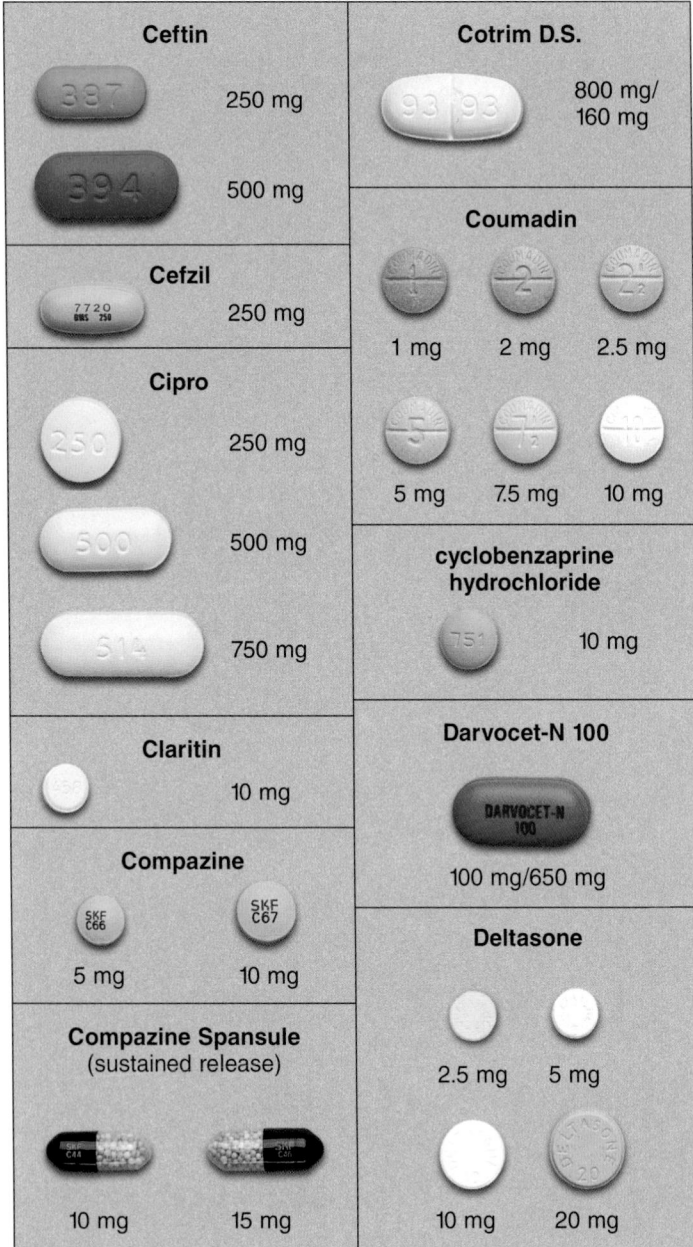

Ceftin
387 — 250 mg
394 — 500 mg

Cefzil
7720 BMS 250 — 250 mg

Cipro
250 — 250 mg
500 — 500 mg
514 — 750 mg

Claritin
10 mg

Compazine
SKF C66 — 5 mg
SKF C67 — 10 mg

Compazine Spansule
(sustained release)
10 mg
15 mg

Cotrim D.S.
93 93 — 800 mg/ 160 mg

Coumadin
1 — 1 mg
2 — 2 mg
2½ — 2.5 mg
5 — 5 mg
7½ — 7.5 mg
10 — 10 mg

cyclobenzaprine hydrochloride
751 — 10 mg

Darvocet-N 100
DARVOCET-N 100 — 100 mg/650 mg

Deltasone
2.5 mg
5 mg
10 mg
DELTASONE 20 — 20 mg

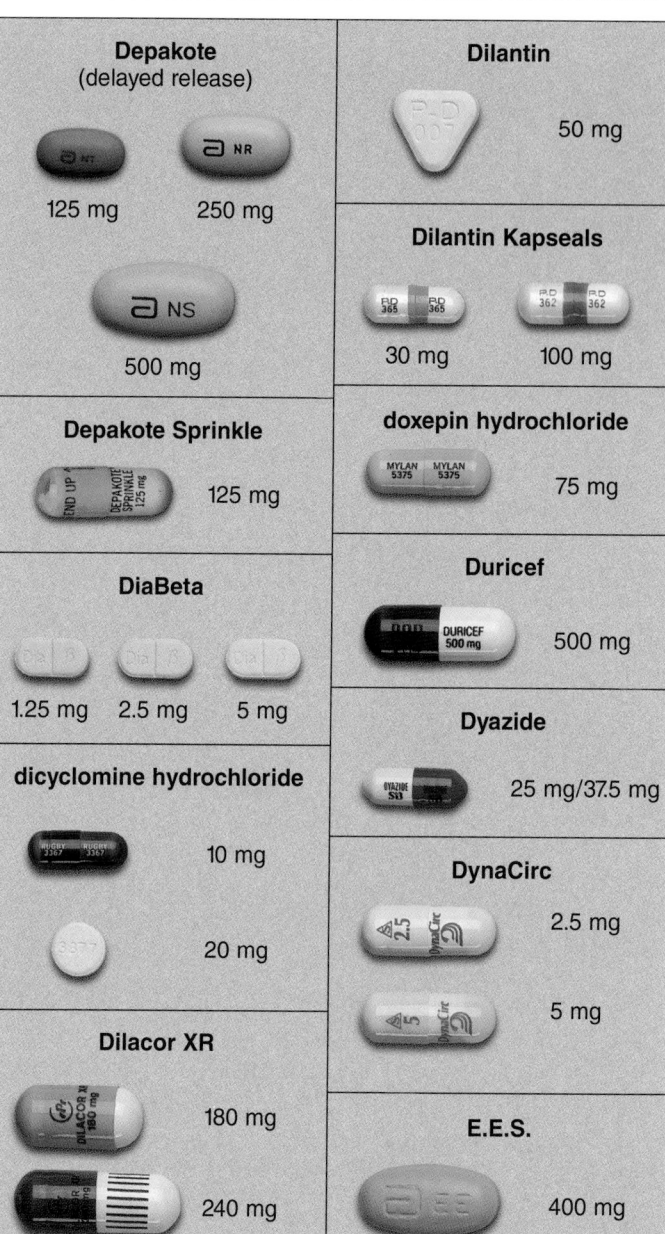

Depakote
(delayed release)

125 mg   250 mg

500 mg

Depakote Sprinkle

125 mg

DiaBeta

1.25 mg   2.5 mg   5 mg

dicyclomine hydrochloride

10 mg

20 mg

Dilacor XR

180 mg

240 mg

Dilantin

50 mg

Dilantin Kapseals

30 mg   100 mg

doxepin hydrochloride

75 mg

Duricef

500 mg

Dyazide

25 mg/37.5 mg

DynaCirc

2.5 mg

5 mg

E.E.S.

400 mg

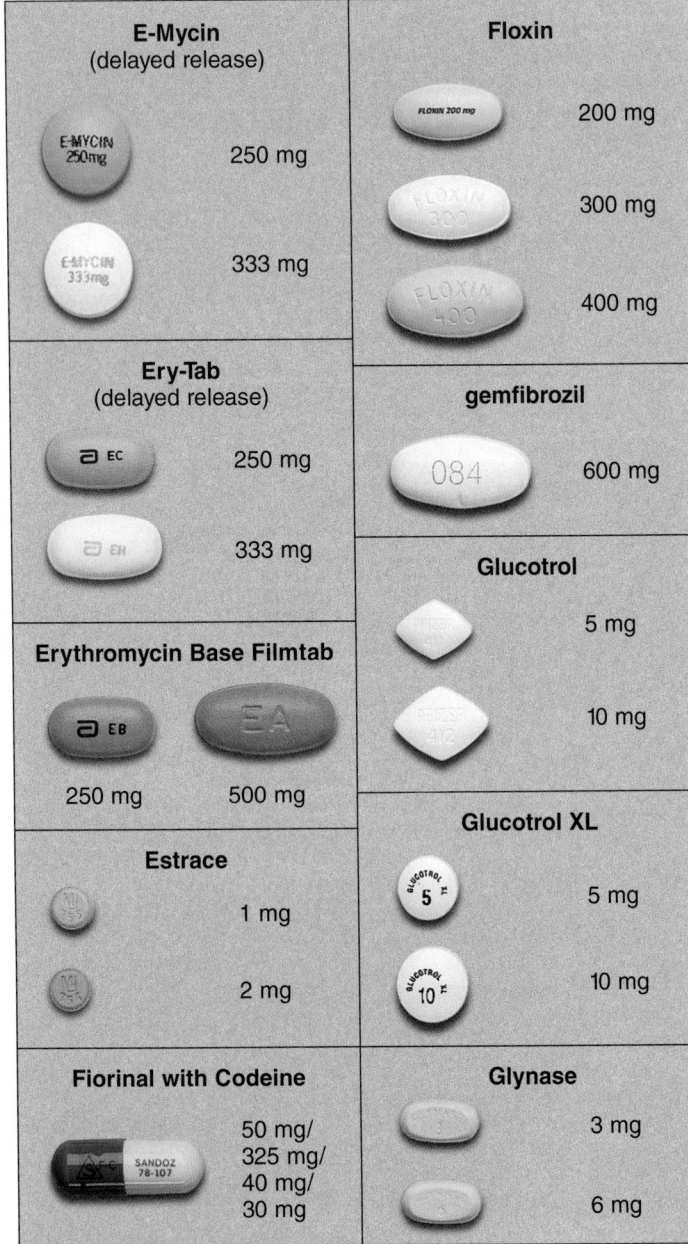

E-Mycin
(delayed release)

250 mg

333 mg

Ery-Tab
(delayed release)

250 mg

333 mg

Erythromycin Base Filmtab

250 mg   500 mg

Estrace

1 mg

2 mg

Fiorinal with Codeine

50 mg/
325 mg/
40 mg/
30 mg

Floxin

200 mg

300 mg

400 mg

gemfibrozil

600 mg

Glucotrol

5 mg

10 mg

Glucotrol XL

5 mg

10 mg

Glynase

3 mg

6 mg

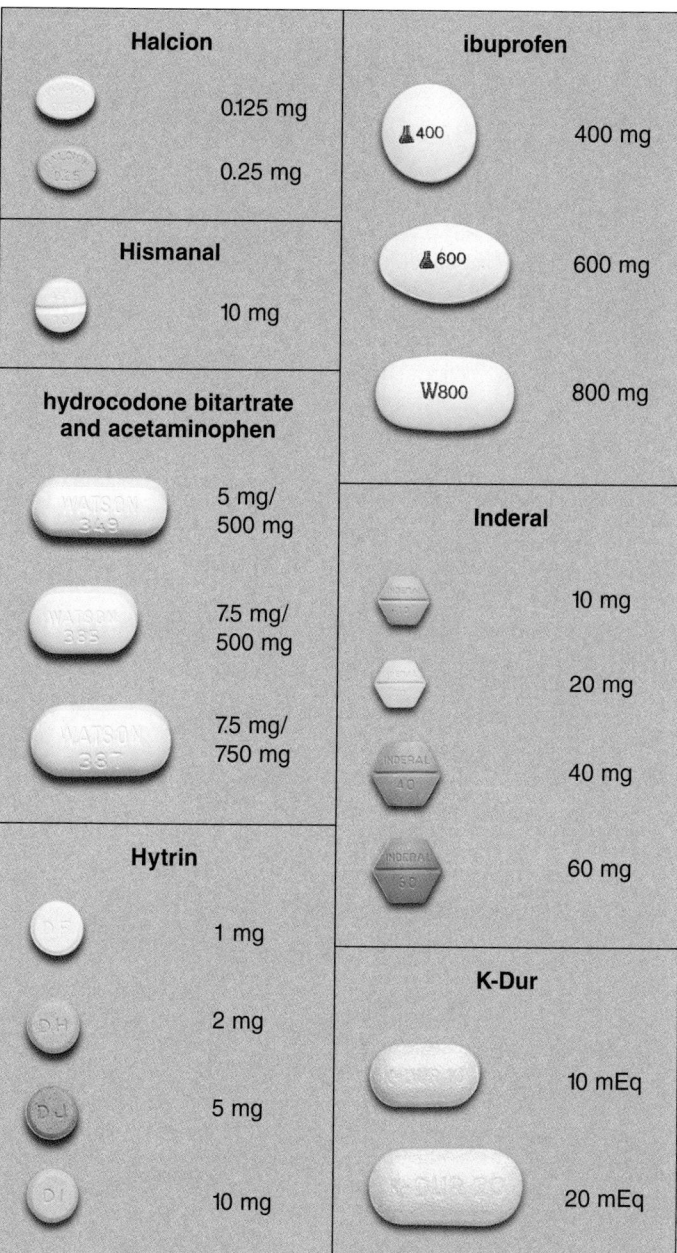

Halcion	
	0.125 mg
	0.25 mg

Hismanal	
	10 mg

hydrocodone bitartrate and acetaminophen

WATSON 349	5 mg/ 500 mg
WATSON 385	7.5 mg/ 500 mg
WATSON 387	7.5 mg/ 750 mg

Hytrin	
	1 mg
	2 mg
	5 mg
	10 mg

ibuprofen	
400	400 mg
600	600 mg
W800	800 mg

Inderal	
	10 mg
	20 mg
INDERAL 40	40 mg
INDERAL 60	60 mg

K-Dur	
	10 mEq
	20 mEq

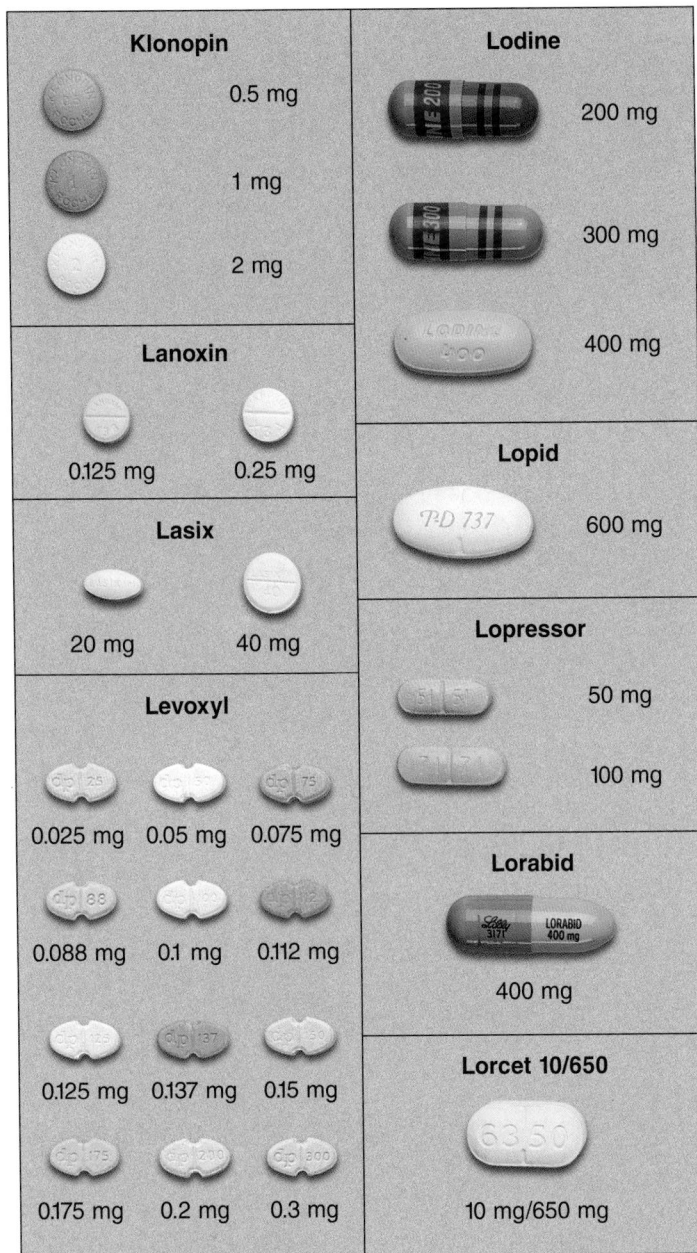

Klonopin

0.5 mg

1 mg

2 mg

Lanoxin

0.125 mg   0.25 mg

Lasix

20 mg   40 mg

Levoxyl

0.025 mg   0.05 mg   0.075 mg

0.088 mg   0.1 mg   0.112 mg

0.125 mg   0.137 mg   0.15 mg

0.175 mg   0.2 mg   0.3 mg

Lodine

200 mg

300 mg

400 mg

Lopid

600 mg

Lopressor

50 mg

100 mg

Lorabid

400 mg

Lorcet 10/650

10 mg/650 mg

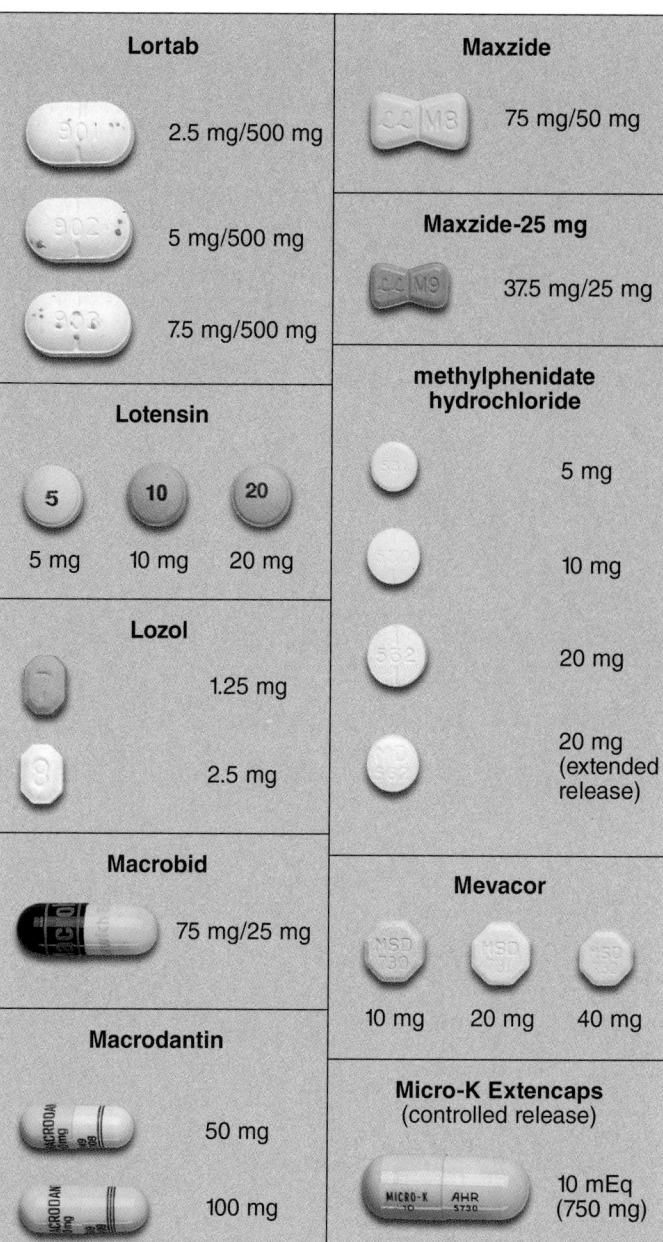

Lortab
2.5 mg/500 mg
5 mg/500 mg
7.5 mg/500 mg

Lotensin
5 mg   10 mg   20 mg

Lozol
1.25 mg
2.5 mg

Macrobid
75 mg/25 mg

Macrodantin
50 mg
100 mg

Maxzide
75 mg/50 mg

Maxzide-25 mg
37.5 mg/25 mg

methylphenidate hydrochloride
5 mg
10 mg
20 mg
20 mg (extended release)

Mevacor
10 mg   20 mg   40 mg

Micro-K Extencaps (controlled release)
10 mEq (750 mg)

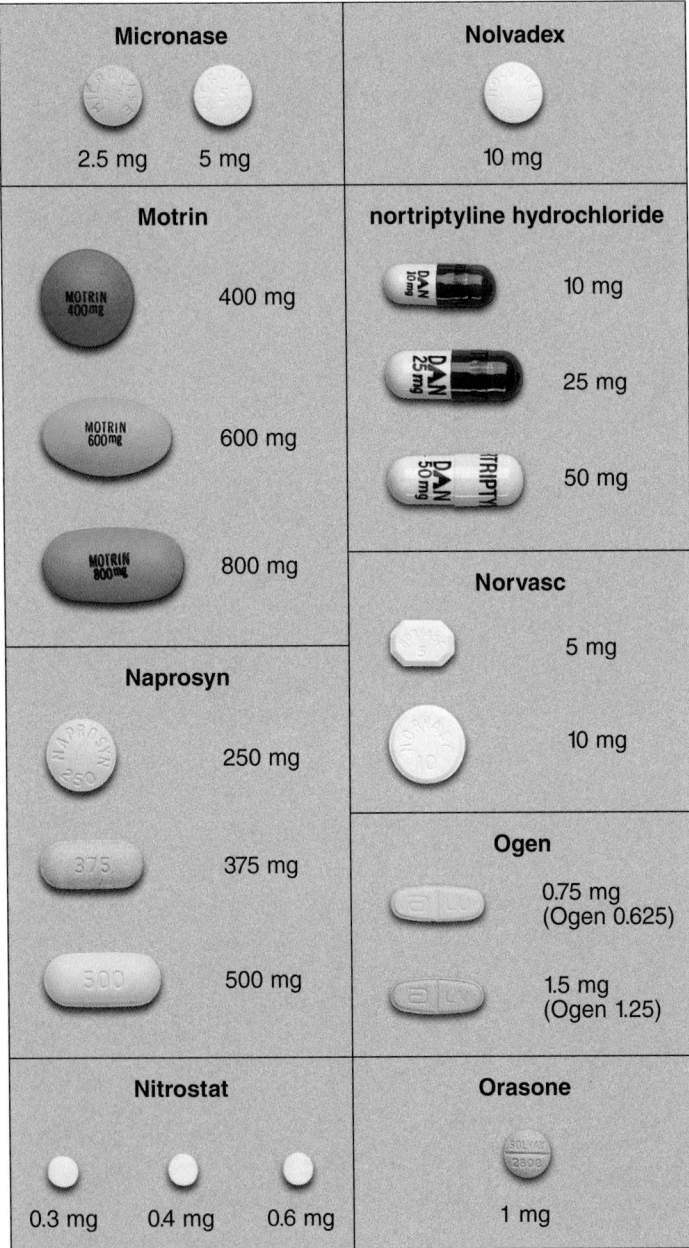

Micronase

2.5 mg   5 mg

Nolvadex

10 mg

Motrin

400 mg

600 mg

800 mg

nortriptyline hydrochloride

10 mg

25 mg

50 mg

Naprosyn

250 mg

375 mg

500 mg

Norvasc

5 mg

10 mg

Ogen

0.75 mg
(Ogen 0.625)

1.5 mg
(Ogen 1.25)

Nitrostat

0.3 mg   0.4 mg   0.6 mg

Orasone

1 mg

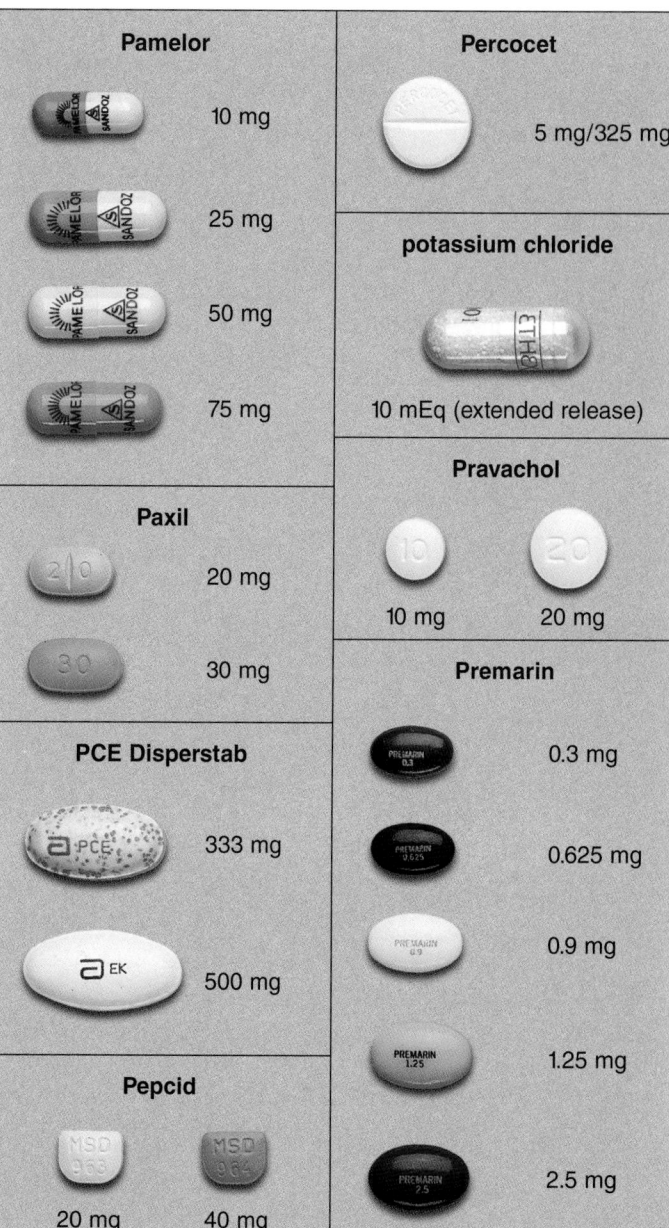

Pamelor

10 mg

25 mg

50 mg

75 mg

Paxil

20 mg

30 mg

PCE Disperstab

333 mg

500 mg

Pepcid

20 mg   40 mg

Percocet

5 mg/325 mg

potassium chloride

10 mEq (extended release)

Pravachol

10 mg   20 mg

Premarin

0.3 mg

0.625 mg

0.9 mg

1.25 mg

2.5 mg

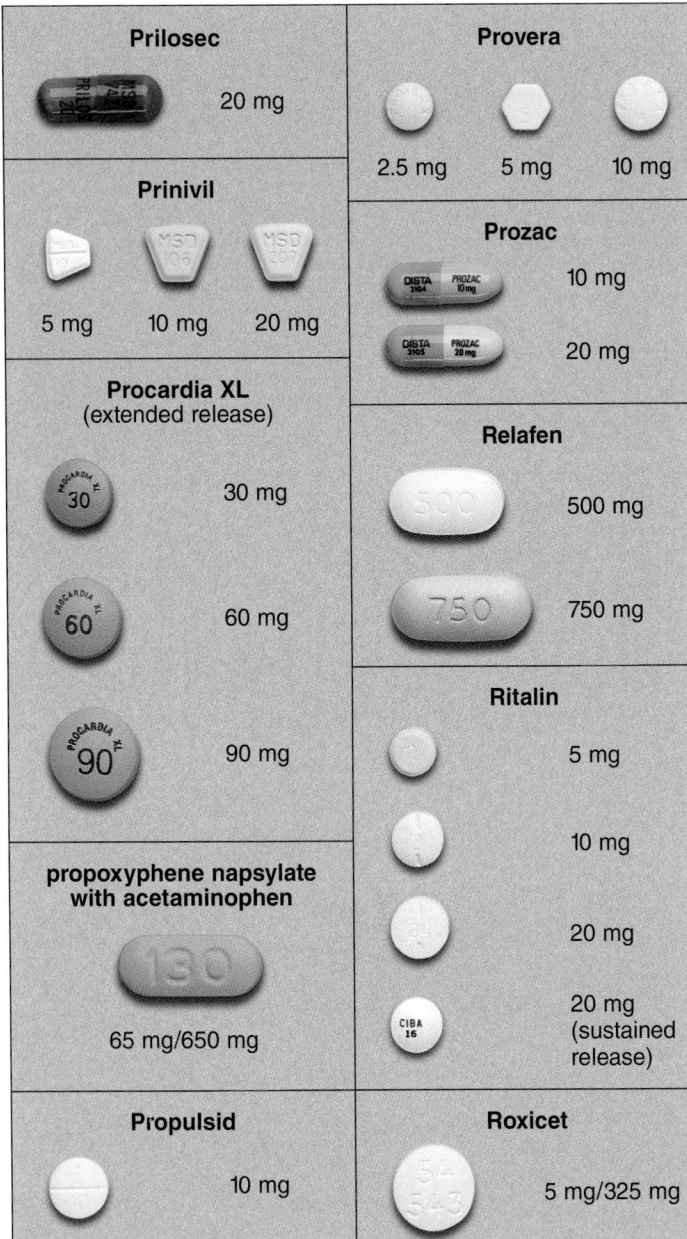

Prilosec

20 mg

Prinivil

5 mg 10 mg 20 mg

Procardia XL
(extended release)

30 mg

60 mg

90 mg

**propoxyphene napsylate
with acetaminophen**

65 mg/650 mg

Propulsid

10 mg

Provera

2.5 mg 5 mg 10 mg

Prozac

10 mg

20 mg

Relafen

500 mg

750 mg

Ritalin

5 mg

10 mg

20 mg

20 mg
(sustained
release)

Roxicet

5 mg/325 mg

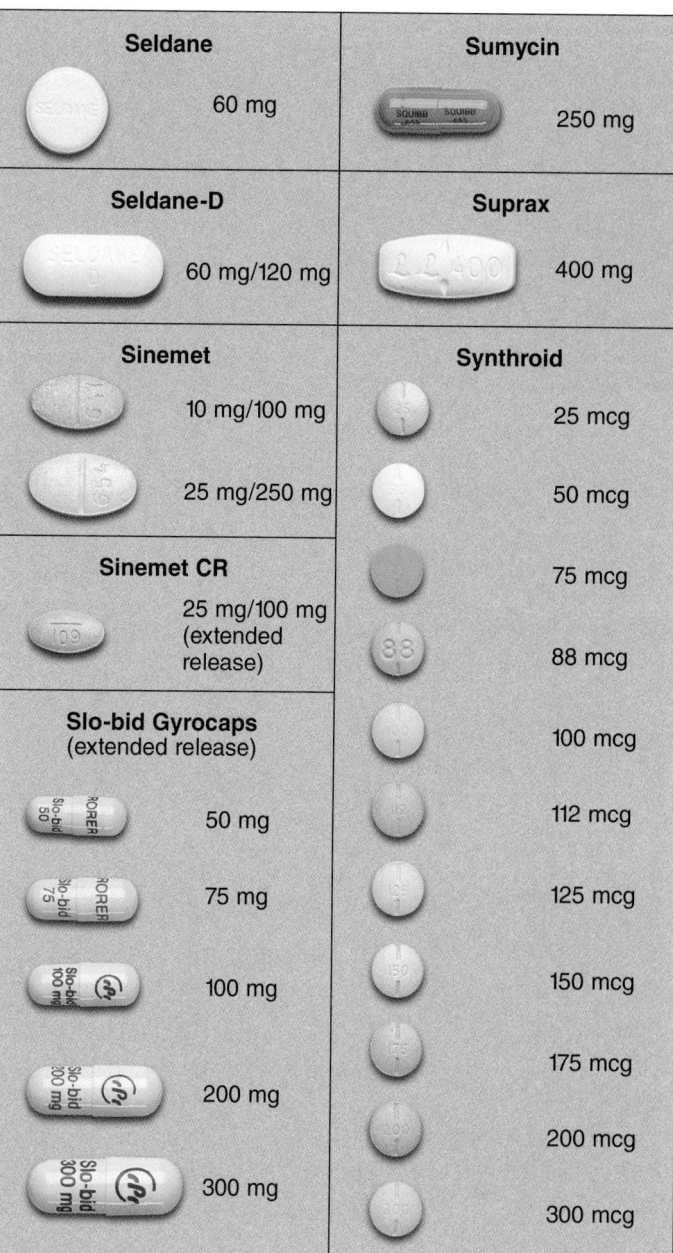

Seldane	
	60 mg

Sumycin	
	250 mg

Seldane-D	
	60 mg/120 mg

Suprax	
	400 mg

Sinemet	
	10 mg/100 mg
	25 mg/250 mg

Sinemet CR	
	25 mg/100 mg (extended release)

Slo-bid Gyrocaps (extended release)	
	50 mg
	75 mg
	100 mg
	200 mg
	300 mg

Synthroid	
	25 mcg
	50 mcg
	75 mcg
	88 mcg
	100 mcg
	112 mcg
	125 mcg
	150 mcg
	175 mcg
	200 mcg
	300 mcg

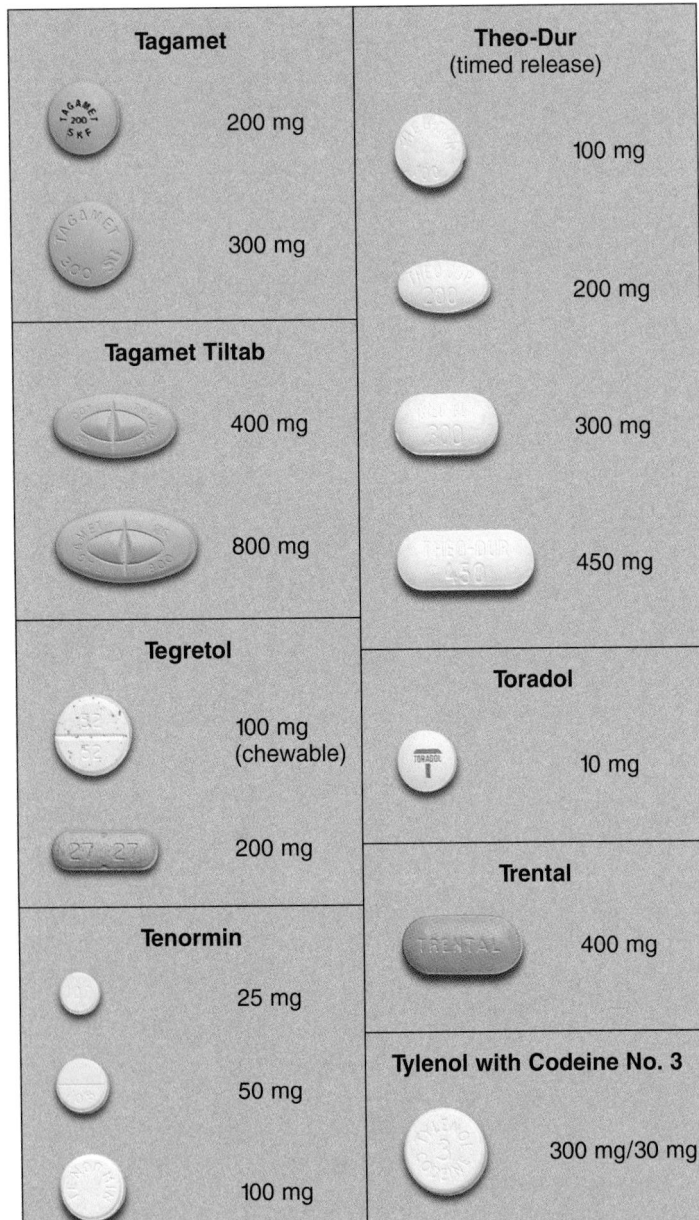

Tagamet

200 mg

300 mg

Tagamet Tiltab

400 mg

800 mg

Tegretol

100 mg (chewable)

200 mg

Tenormin

25 mg

50 mg

100 mg

Theo-Dur
(timed release)

100 mg

200 mg

300 mg

450 mg

Toradol

10 mg

Trental

400 mg

Tylenol with Codeine No. 3

300 mg/30 mg

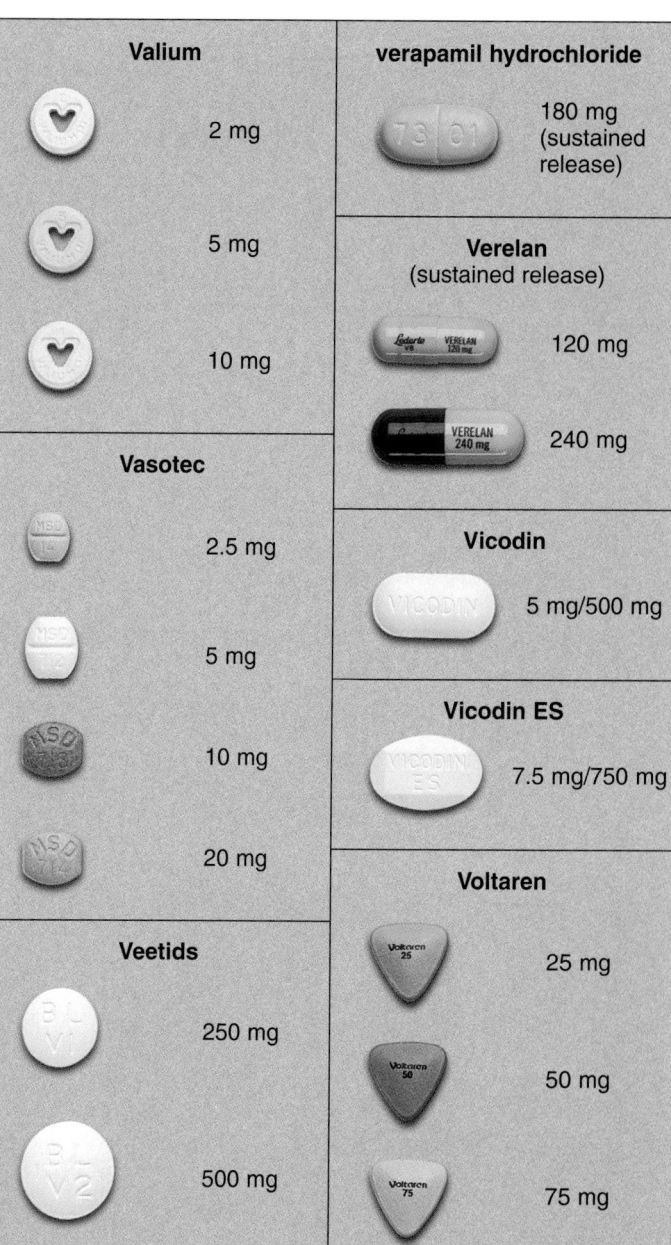

Valium	
	2 mg
	5 mg
	10 mg

Vasotec	
	2.5 mg
	5 mg
	10 mg
	20 mg

Veetids	
	250 mg
	500 mg

verapamil hydrochloride	
	180 mg (sustained release)

Verelan (sustained release)	
	120 mg
	240 mg

Vicodin	
	5 mg/500 mg

Vicodin ES	
	7.5 mg/750 mg

Voltaren	
	25 mg
	50 mg
	75 mg

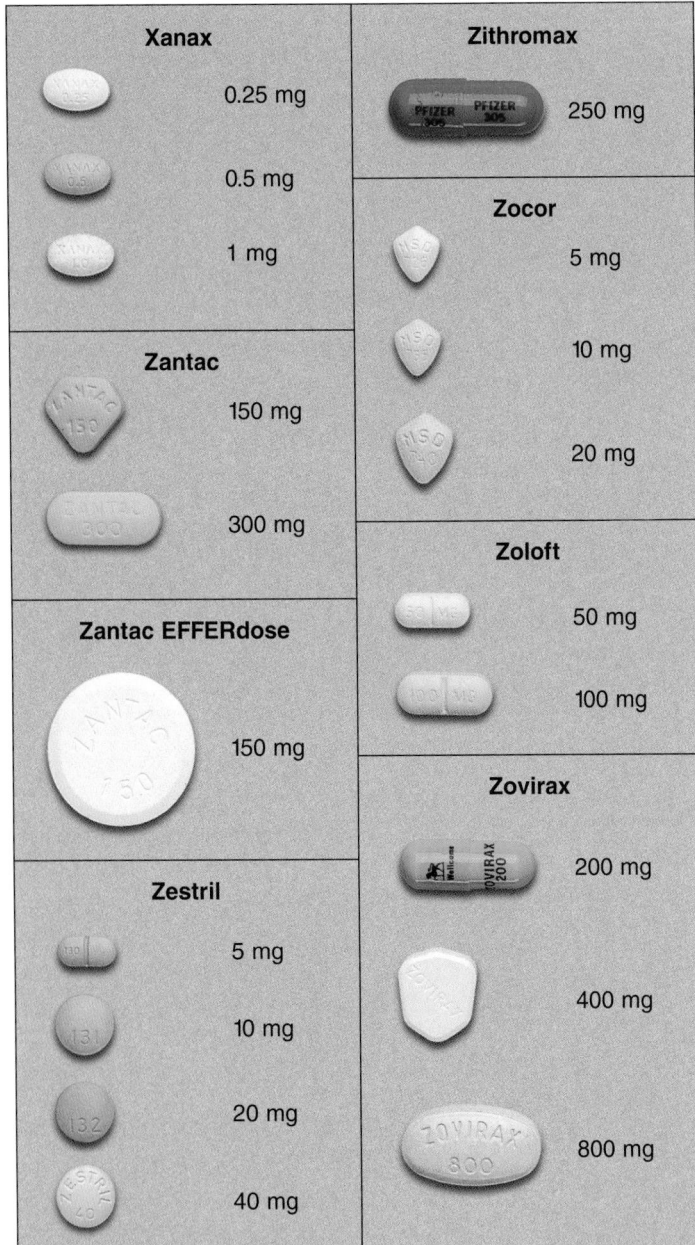

Xanax
0.25 mg
0.5 mg
1 mg

Zantac
150 mg
300 mg

Zantac EFFERdose
150 mg

Zestril
5 mg
10 mg
20 mg
40 mg

Zithromax
250 mg

Zocor
5 mg
10 mg
20 mg

Zoloft
50 mg
100 mg

Zovirax
200 mg
400 mg
800 mg

INTERACTIONS
CNS depressants: increased drowsiness.

CONTRAINDICATIONS
Contraindicated in patients hypersensitive to the drug.

NURSING CONSIDERATIONS
• Use cautiously in patients with asthma, glaucoma, or prostatic hyperplasia.
• Like other antiemetics, be alert that drug may mask symptoms of ototoxicity, brain tumor, or intestinal obstruction.
• Advise patients to avoid driving and other hazardous activities that require alertness until CNS effects of the drug are known.

---

metoclopramide hydrochloride
Apo-Metoclop†, Clopra, Emex†, Maxeran†, Maxolon, Maxolon High Dose‡, Octamide, Octamide PFS, Pramin‡, Reclomide, Reglan
Pregnancy Risk Category: B

HOW SUPPLIED
Tablets: 5 mg, 10 mg
Syrup: 5 mg/5 ml
Injection: 5 mg/ml

ACTION
Stimulates motility of the upper GI tract by increasing lower esophageal sphincter tone and blocks dopamine receptors at the chemoreceptor trigger zone.

ONSET, PEAK, DURATION
Onset occurs within 1 to 3 minutes of I.V. administration, 10 to 15 minutes after I.M. injection, 30 to 60 minutes after oral ingestion. Peak occurs in 1 to 2 hours after oral administration, unknown for parenteral administration. Effects persist for 1 to 2 hours.

INDICATIONS & DOSAGE
Prevention or reduction of nausea and vomiting induced by cisplatin and other chemotherapeutic agents –
Adults: 1 to 2 mg/kg I.V. 30 minutes before cancer chemotherapy then repeated q 2 hours for two doses, then q 3 hours for three doses.
Prevention or reduction of postoperative nausea and vomiting –
Adults: 10 to 20 mg I.M. near the end of the surgical procedure, repeated q 4 to 6 hours p.r.n.
To facilitate small-bowel intubation and to aid in radiologic examinations –
Adults and children over 14 years: 10 mg (2 ml) I.V. as a single dose over 1 to 2 minutes.
Children under 6 years: 0.1 mg/kg I.V.
Children 6 to 14 years: 2.5 to 5 mg I.V. (0.5 to 1 ml).
Delayed gastric emptying secondary to diabetic gastroparesis –
Adults: 10 mg P.O. for mild symptoms, slow I.V. for severe symptoms 30 minutes before meals and h.s. for 2 to 8 weeks, depending on response.
Gastroesophageal reflux disease –
Adults: 10 to 15 mg P.O. q.i.d., p.r.n., 30 minutes before meals and h.s.

ADVERSE REACTIONS
CNS: *restlessness, anxiety, drowsiness,* fatigue, *lassitude,* insomnia, headache, dizziness, extrapyramidal symptoms, tardive dyskinesia, dystonic reactions, sedation.
CV: transient hypertension.
GI: nausea, bowel disturbances.
Skin: rash.
Other: fever, prolactin secretion, loss of libido.

INTERACTIONS
Anticholinergics, opioid analgesics: antagonized GI motility effects of metoclopramide. Use together cautiously.

Butyrophenones, phenothiazines: increased risk of extrapyramidal effects. Monitor closely.
CNS depressants, ethanol: additive CNS depression. Avoid concomitant use.

CONTRAINDICATIONS
Contraindicated in patients in which stimulation of GI motility might be dangerous (for example, those with hemorrhage, obstruction, or perforation) and in those with hypersensitivity to drug, pheochromocytoma, or seizure disorder.

NURSING CONSIDERATIONS
• Use cautiously in patients with history of depression, Parkinson's disease, and hypertension.
• **I.V. use:** Give lower doses (10 mg or less) by direct injection over 1 to 2 minutes. Dilute doses larger than 10 mg in 50 ml of a compatible diluent and infuse over at least 15 minutes. Protection from light is unnecessary if the infusion mixture is administered within 24 hours.
• Know that the drug is compatible with D₅W, 0.9% sodium chloride injection, and dextrose 5% in sodium chloride 0.45%.
• Monitor blood pressure frequently in patients receiving I.V. form of the drug.
• Use diphenhydramine 25 mg I.V. as ordered to counteract the extrapyramidal adverse effects associated with high metoclopramide doses.
• Be aware that safety and effectiveness have not been established for therapy that continues longer than 12 weeks.
• Advise patients to avoid activities requiring alertness for 2 hours after taking each dose.

ondansetron hydrochloride
Zofran

Pregnancy Risk Category: B

HOW SUPPLIED
Tablets: 4 mg, 8 mg
Injection: 2 mg/ml, 4mg/ml

ACTION
A selective antagonist of a specific type of serotonin receptor (5-HT₃) located in the CNS at the area postrema (chemoreceptor trigger zone) and in the peripheral nervous system on nerve terminals of the vagus nerve. Drug's blocking action may occur at both sites.

ONSET, PEAK, DURATION
Unknown.

INDICATIONS & DOSAGE
Prevention of nausea and vomiting associated with emetogenic chemotherapy –
Adults and children 12 years and over: 8 mg P.O. 30 minutes before start of chemotherapy. Follow with 8 mg P.O. 4 and 8 hours after first dose. Then follow with 8 mg q 8 hours for 1 to 2 days. Alternatively, administer a single dose of 32 mg by I.V. infusion over 15 minutes beginning 30 minutes before chemotherapy; or three divided doses of 0.15 mg/kg I.V. (first dose given 30 minutes before chemotherapy; subsequent doses given 4 and 8 hours after first dose). Infuse drug over 15 minutes.
Children 4 to 12 years: 4 mg P.O. 30 minutes before start of chemotherapy. Follow with 4 mg P.O. 4 and 8 hours after first dose. Then follow with 4 mg q 8 hours for 1 to 2 days. Alternatively, three doses of 0.15 mg/kg I.V. Give first dose 30 minutes before chemotherapy; administer subsequent doses 4 and 8 hours after first dose. Infuse drug over 15 minutes.

---

*Liquid form contains alcohol.   *Common* reactions are in italics; ***life-threatening***, in bold italics.
**May contain tartrazine.

Prevention of postoperative nausea and vomiting –
Adults: 4 mg I.V. (undiluted) over 2 to 5 minutes.

ADVERSE REACTIONS
CNS: headache.
GI: *diarrhea, constipation.*
Hepatic: transient elevations in AST and ALT levels.
Respiratory: *bronchospasm (rare).*
Skin: rash.

INTERACTIONS
Drugs that alter hepatic drug metabolizing enzymes, such as phenobarbital or cimetidine: may alter pharmacokinetics of ondansetron. No dosage adjustment appears necessary.

CONTRAINDICATIONS
Contraindicated in patients hypersensitive to the drug.

NURSING CONSIDERATIONS
• Use cautiously in patients with liver failure.
• **I.V. use:** Dilute drug in 50 ml of D₅W injection or 0.9% sodium chloride injection before administration.
• Administer as I.V. infusion over 15 minutes.
• Know that drug is also stable for up to 48 hours after dilution in 5% dextrose in 0.9% sodium chloride injection, 5% dextrose in 0.45% sodium chloride injection, and 3% sodium chloride injection.

prochlorperazine
Compazine, PMS Prochlorperazine†, Prorazin†, Stemetil

prochlorperazine edisylate
Compa-Z, Compazine Syrup, Cotranzine, Ultrazine-10

prochlorperazine maleate
Anti-Naus‡, Chlorpazine, Compazine Spansule, PMS Prochlorperazine†, Prorazin†, Stemetil
Pregnancy Risk Category: NR

HOW SUPPLIED
prochlorperazine
Tablets: 5 mg, 10 mg
Injection: 5 mg/ml
Suppositories: 2.5 mg, 5 mg, 25 mg
prochlorperazine edisylate
Syrup: 1 mg/ml
prochlorperazine maleate
Tablets: 5 mg, 10 mg, 25 mg
Capsules (sustained-release): 10 mg, 15 mg, 30 mg

ACTION
Acts on the chemoreceptor trigger zone to inhibit nausea and vomiting; in larger doses, partially depresses the vomiting center.

ONSET, PEAK, DURATION
Onset 30 to 40 minutes after oral use, 60 minutes after rectal use, 10 to 20 minutes after I.M. use. Peak unknown. Effects persist 3 to 4 hours after regular-release preparations, 10 to 12 hours after sustained-release preparations, 3 to 4 hours after rectal or I.M. use.

INDICATIONS & DOSAGE
Preoperative nausea control –
Adults: 5 to 10 mg I.M. 1 to 2 hours before induction of anesthesia; repeat once in 30 minutes, if necessary. Or, 5 to 10 mg I.V. 15 to 30 minutes before induction of anesthesia; repeat once if necessary.
Severe nausea and vomiting –
Adults: 5 to 10 mg P.O., t.i.d. or q.i.d.; 15 mg sustained-release form P.O. on arising; 10 mg sustained-release form P.O. q 12 hours; 25 mg P.R., b.i.d.; or 5 to 10 mg I.M. repeated q 3 to 4 hours, p.r.n. Maximum I.M. dosage is 40 mg daily. Al-

ternatively, 2.5 to 10 mg I.V. at a rate not to exceed 5 mg/minute.

Children 9 to 13 kg: 2.5 mg P.O. or P.R. once daily or b.i.d. Maximum dosage is 7.5 mg daily. Or give 0.132 mg/kg by deep I.M. injection. Control usually is obtained with one dose.

Children 14 to 17 kg: 2.5 mg P.O. or P.R., b.i.d. or t.i.d. Maximum dosage is 10 mg daily. Or give 0.132 mg/kg by deep I.M. injection. Control usually is obtained with one dose.

Children 18 to 39 kg: 2.5 mg P.O. or P.R., t.i.d.; or 5 mg P.O. or P.R., b.i.d. Maximum dosage is 15 mg daily. Or, give 0.132 mg/kg by deep I.M. injection. Control usually is obtained with one dose.

To manage symptoms of psychotic disorders –

Adults: 5 to 10 mg P.O., t.i.d. or q.i.d.

Children 2 to 12 years: 2.5 mg P.O. or P.R., b.i.d. or t.i.d. Do not exceed 10 mg on day 1. Increase dosage gradually to recommended maximum (if necessary). In children 2 to 5 years, maximum daily dosage is 25 mg. In children 6 to 10 years, maximum daily dosage is 25 mg.

To manage symptoms of severe psychoses –

Adults: 10 to 20 mg I.M. repeated in 1 to 4 hours, if needed. Rarely, patients may receive 10 to 20 mg q 4 to 6 hours. Institute oral therapy after symptoms are controlled.

Children 2 to 12 years: 0.13 mg/kg I.M.

Non-psychotic anxiety –

Adults: 5 to 10 mg by deep I.M. injection q 3 to 4 hours, not to exceed 40 mg daily; or 5 to 10 mg P.O., t.i.d. or q.i.d. Alternatively, give 15 mg extended-release capsule once daily or 10 mg extended-release capsule q 12 hours.

ADVERSE REACTIONS

CNS: *extrapyramidal reactions,* sedation, pseudoparkinsonism, EEG changes, dizziness.

CV: *orthostatic hypotension,* tachycardia, ECG changes.

EENT: *ocular changes, blurred vision.*

GI: *dry mouth, constipation.*

GU: *urine retention,* dark urine, menstrual irregularities, inhibited ejaculation.

Hematologic: *transient leukopenia, agranulocytosis.*

Hepatic: *cholestatic jaundice.*

Skin: *mild photosensitivity,* allergic reactions, ***exfoliative dermatitis.***

Other: hyperprolactinemia, gynecomastia, weight gain, increased appetite.

INTERACTIONS

Antacids: inhibited absorption of oral phenothiazines. Separate antacid and phenothiazine doses by at least 2 hours.

Anticholinergics, including antidepressants and antiparkinsonian agents: increased anticholinergic activity and aggravated parkinsonian symptoms. Use together cautiously.

Barbiturates: may decrease phenothiazine effect. Monitor patient for decreased antiemetic effect.

CONTRAINDICATIONS

Contraindicated in patients hypersensitive to phenothiazines and in those with CNS depression including coma; during pediatric surgery; when using spinal or epidural anesthetic, adrenergic blockers, or ethanol; and in children under 2 years.

NURSING CONSIDERATIONS

• Use cautiously in patients with impaired CV function, glaucoma, seizure disorders; in those who have been exposed to extreme heat; and in children with acute illness.

• Dilute oral solution with tomato or

---

*Liquid form contains alcohol.
**May contain tartrazine.

Common reactions are in italics; ***life-threatening,*** in bold italics.

fruit juice, milk, coffee, carbonated beverage, tea, water or soup, or mix with pudding.
• **I.V. use:** 15 to 30 minutes before induction, add 20 mg of prochlorperazine per liter of D_5W and 0.9% sodium chloride solution. Infusion flow rate should not exceed 5 mg/minute. Maximum parenteral dosage is 40 mg daily. Infuse slowly, never as a bolus injection.
• For I.M. use, inject deeply into upper outer quadrant of gluteal region.
• Do not give subcutaneously or mix in syringe with another drug.
• To prevent contact dermatitis, avoid getting concentrate or injection solution on hands or clothing.
• Watch for orthostatic hypotension, especially when giving drug intravenously.
• Monitor CBC and liver function studies during prolonged therapy as ordered.
• Know that the drug is used only when vomiting can't be controlled by other measures or when only a few doses are required. If more than four doses are needed in 24 hours, notify the doctor.
• Know that the drug is not effective to treat motion sickness.
• Store in light-resistant container. Slight yellowing does not affect potency; discard extremely discolored solutions.
• Advise patients to wear protective clothing when exposed to sunlight.

---

thiethylperazine maleate
Norzine, Torecan**

Pregnancy Risk Category: X

HOW SUPPLIED
Tablets: 10 mg
Injection: 5 mg/ml
Suppositories: 10 mg

ACTION
Unknown. Probably acts on the chemoreceptor trigger zone to inhibit nausea and vomiting.

ONSET, PEAK, DURATION
Onset occurs in 30 minutes. Peak unknown. Effects persist 4 hours.

INDICATIONS & DOSAGE
Nausea and vomiting –
Adults: 10 mg P.O., I.M., or P.R. once daily, b.i.d. or t.i.d.

ADVERSE REACTIONS
CNS: *extrapyramidal reactions* (high incidence), sedation (low incidence), pseudoparkinsonism, EEG changes, dizziness, confusion (especially in elderly patients).
CV: *orthostatic hypotension,* tachycardia, ECG changes.
EENT: *ocular changes, blurred vision.*
GI: *dry mouth, constipation.*
GU: *urine retention,* dark urine, menstrual irregularities, inhibited ejaculation.
Hematologic: *transient leukopenia, agranulocytosis.*
Hepatic: *cholestatic jaundice.*
Skin: *mild photosensitivity,* allergic reactions.
Other: hyperprolactinemia, gynecomastia, weight gain, increased appetite.

INTERACTIONS
Antacids: inhibited absorption of oral phenothiazines. Separate antacid and phenothiazine doses by at least 2 hours.
Anticholinergics, including antidepressants and antiparkinsonian agents: increased anticholinergic activity and increased risk of parkinsonian-like symptoms. Use together cautiously.
Barbiturates: may decrease phenothiazine effect. Monitor patient for decreased antiemetic effect.

CONTRAINDICATIONS

Contraindicated in patients hypersensitive to phenothiazines, in those with severe CNS depression or hepatic disease, in patients experiencing coma, and in pregnancy.

NURSING CONSIDERATIONS

• Use cautiously in patients with aspirin hypersensitivity.
• Don't give intravenously. May cause severe hypotension.
• For nausea and vomiting associated with anesthesia and surgery, give deep I.M. injection shortly before or when terminating anesthesia.
• If drug gets on skin, wash off at once to prevent contact dermatitis.
• Know that the drug may effectively treat dizziness but not motion sickness.
• Use only when vomiting can't be controlled by other measures or when only a few doses are required.
• Store suppositories in tightly covered container and at temperatures below 77° F (25° C).
• Warn patients about hypotension and suggest they stay in bed for 1 hour after receiving drug.

---

trimethobenzamide hydrochloride

Arrestin, Benzacot, Bio-Gan, Stemetic, Tebamide, Tegamide, T-Gen, Ticon, Tigan, Triban, Tribenzagan

Pregnancy Risk Category: NR

HOW SUPPLIED

Capsules: 100 mg, 250 mg
Injection: 100 mg/ml
Suppositories: 100 mg, 200 mg

ACTION

Unknown. Probably acts on the chemoreceptor trigger zone to inhibit nausea and vomiting.

ONSET, PEAK, DURATION

Onset occurs 10 to 20 minutes after oral administration, 15 to 35 minutes after I.M. administration. Peak unknown. Effects persist 2 to 3 hours after I.M. administration, 3 to 4 hours after oral administration.

INDICATIONS & DOSAGE

Nausea and vomiting –
Adults: 250 mg P.O., t.i.d. or q.i.d.; or 200 mg I.M. or P.R., t.i.d. or q.i.d.
Prevention of postoperative nausea and vomiting –
Adults: 200 mg I.M. or P.R. as a single dose before or during surgery; if needed, repeat 3 hours after termination of anesthesia, p.r.n. Limit use to prolonged vomiting of known etiology.
Children under 13 kg: 100 mg P.R. t.i.d. or q.i.d.
Children 13 to 40 kg: 100 to 200 mg P.O. or P.R. t.i.d. or q.i.d.

ADVERSE REACTIONS

CNS: *drowsiness,* dizziness (in large doses).
CV: hypotension.
GI: diarrhea, exaggeration of preexisting nausea (in large doses).
Hepatic: *liver toxicity.*
Skin: hypersensitivity reaction.
Other: pain, stinging, burning, redness, swelling at I.M. injection site.

INTERACTIONS

CNS depressants, ethanol: additive CNS depression. Avoid concomitant use.

CONTRAINDICATIONS

Contraindicated in patients with hypersensitivity to drug. Suppositories are contraindicated in patients hypersensitive to benzocaine hydrochloride or similar local anesthetic.

NURSING CONSIDERATIONS

• Use cautiously in children.
• For I.M. administration, inject

---

deeply into upper outer quadrant of gluteal region to reduce pain and local irritation.

• Like other antiemetics, be alert that drug may mask signs of overdose of toxic agents or symptoms of intestinal obstruction, brain tumor, or other conditions.

• Withhold drug if skin hypersensitivity reaction occurs.

• Refrigerate suppositories.

• Advise patients of the possibility of drowsiness and dizziness, and caution against driving or other activities requiring alertness until CNS effects of the drug are known.

cimetidine
famotidine
lansoprazole
misoprostol
nizatidine
omeprazole
ranitidine hydrochloride
sucralfate

COMBINATION PRODUCTS
None.

cimetidine
Tagamet

Pregnancy Risk Category: B

HOW SUPPLIED
Tablets: 200 mg, 300 mg, 400 mg, 800 mg
Oral liquid: 300 mg/5 ml
Effervescent tablets: 800 mg‡
Injection: 100 mg/ml‡, 150 mg/ml; 300 mg in 50 ml 0.9% sodium chloride solution injection

ACTION
Competitively inhibits the action of histamine (H_2) at receptor sites of the parietal cells, decreasing gastric acid secretion.

ONSET, PEAK, DURATION
Onset unknown. Peak levels occur immediately after I.V. administration, unknown for I.M. administration, 45 to 90 minutes after oral dose. Effects persist for 4 to 5 hours after oral administration, unknown after parenteral administration. Therapeutic effects last 4 to 5 hours.

INDICATIONS & DOSAGE
Duodenal ulcer (short-term treatment) –
Adults and children 16 years and over: 800 mg P.O. h.s. Alternatively, 400 mg P.O. b.i.d. or 300 mg q.i.d. (with meals and h.s.). Treatment continued for 4 to 6 weeks unless endoscopy shows healing. For maintenance therapy, 400 mg h.s. For parenteral therapy, 300 mg diluted to 20 ml with 0.9% sodium chloride solution or other compatible I.V. solution I.V. push over 1 to 2 minutes q 6 hours; or 300 mg diluted in 50 ml D_5W or other compatible I.V. solution by I.V. infusion over 15 to 20 minutes q 6 hours; or 300 mg I.M. q 6 hours (no dilution necessary). Parenteral dosage increased by giving 300-mg doses more frequently to maximum daily dosage of 2,400 mg as needed. Alternatively, 900 mg/day (37.5 mg/hour) I.V. diluted in 100 to 1,000 ml of compatible solution by continuous I.V. infusion.
Active benign gastric ulceration –
Adults: 800 mg P.O. h.s., or 300 mg P.O. q.i.d., with meals and h.s., for up to 8 weeks.
Pathologic hypersecretory conditions (such as Zollinger-Ellison syndrome, systemic mastocytosis, and multiple endocrine adenomas) –
Adults and children 16 years and over: 300 mg P.O. q.i.d. with meals and h.s.; adjusted to individual needs. Maximum oral daily dosage is 2,400 mg.
For parenteral therapy, 300 mg diluted to 20 ml with 0.9% sodium chloride solution or other compatible I.V. solution by I.V. push over 1 to 2 minutes q 6 hours; or 300 mg diluted in 50 ml dextrose 5% solution or other compatible I.V. solution by I.V. infusion over 15 to 20 minutes q 6 hours. Parenteral dosage increased by giving 300-mg doses more frequently to

---

*Liquid form contains alcohol.
**May contain tartrazine.

Common reactions are in italics; *life-threatening*, in bold italics.

maximum daily dosage of 2,400 mg as needed.

Gastroesophageal reflux disease –
Adults: 800 mg P.O. b.i.d. or 400 mg q.i.d. before meals and h.s.

Prevention of upper GI bleeding in critically ill patients –
Adults: 50 mg/hour by continuous I.V. infusion for up to 7 days; 25 mg/hour to patients with creatinine clearance below 30 ml/minute/1.73 m².

ADVERSE REACTIONS
CNS: confusion, dizziness, headaches, peripheral neuropathy. **CV:** bradycardia.
GI: *mild and transient diarrhea.*
GU: transient elevations in serum creatinine levels.
Hematologic: *agranulocytosis, neutropenia, thrombocytopenia, aplastic anemia* (rare).
Hepatic: jaundice (rare).
Skin: acnelike rash, urticaria.
Other: hypersensitivity reactions, muscle pain, mild gynecomastia if used longer than 1 month.

INTERACTIONS
Antacids: interference with cimetidine absorption. Separate administration by at least 1 hour if possible.
Lidocaine, phenytoin, propranolol, some benzodiazepines, warfarin: inhibited hepatic microsomal enzyme metabolism of these drugs. Monitor serum levels of these drugs.

CONTRAINDICATIONS
Contraindicated in patients hypersensitive to the drug.

NURSING CONSIDERATIONS
• Use cautiously in elderly or debilitated patients because they may be more susceptible to cimetidine-induced confusion.
• Identify tablet strength when obtaining a drug history.
• **I.V. use:** Dilute I.V. solutions with 0.9% sodium chloride solution, D_5W

and dextrose 10% in water (and combinations of these), lactated Ringer's solution, or 5% sodium bicarbonate injection. Do not dilute with sterile water for injection.
• Don't infuse I.V. too rapidly; may cause bradycardia. When administering cimetidine I.V. in 100 ml of diluent solution, do not infuse so rapidly that circulatory overload is produced. Some authorities recommend infusing drug over at least 30 minutes, to minimize risk of adverse cardiac effects. Sometimes administered as continuous I.V. infusion. Use infusion pump if given in a total volume of 250 ml over 24 hours or less.
• Be aware that I.M. administration may be painful.
• Give tablets with meals to ensure a more consistent therapeutic effect.
• Schedule cimetidine dose at end of hemodialysis treatment. Hemodialysis reduces blood levels of cimetidine. Adjust dosage as ordered in patients with renal failure.
• Keep in mind that effectiveness in treatment of gastric ulcer not as great as in duodenal ulcer.
• Know that up to 10 g overdose has been reported without adverse reactions.
• Remind patients taking cimetidine once daily to take it at bedtime for best results.
• Urge patients to avoid cigarette smoking because it may increase gastric acid secretion and worsen disease.

famotidine
Pepcid, Pepcid AC◊, Pepcidine‡
Pregnancy Risk Category: B

HOW SUPPLIED
Tablets: 10 mg, 20 mg, 40 mg
Powder for oral suspension: 40 mg/5 ml after reconstitution
Injection: 10 mg/ml

ACTION
Competitively inhibits the action of histamine (H_2) at receptor sites of the parietal cells, decreasing gastric acid secretion.

ONSET, PEAK, DURATION
Onset occurs within 1 hour after oral or I.V. administration. Peak levels occur within 20 minutes of I.V. injection, 1 to 3 hours after oral administration. Effects persist up to 10 to 12 hours.

INDICATIONS & DOSAGE
Duodenal ulcer (short-term treatment) —
Adults: For acute therapy, 40 mg P.O. once daily h.s. or 20 mg P.O. b.i.d. For maintenance therapy, give 20 mg P.O. once daily h.s.
Benign gastric ulcer (short-term treatment) —
Adults: 40 mg P.O. daily h.s. for 8 weeks.
Pathologic hypersecretory conditions (such as Zollinger-Ellison syndrome) —
Adults: 20 mg P.O. q 6 hours up to 160 mg q 6 hours.
Hospitalized patients with intractable ulcerations or hypersecretory conditions or patients who cannot take oral medication —
Adults: 20 mg I.V. q 12 hours.
Gastroesophageal reflux disease (GERD) —
Adults: 20 mg P.O. b.i.d. for up to 6 weeks. For esophagitis caused by GERD, 20 to 40 mg b.i.d. for up to 12 weeks.
Prevention of heartburn —
Adults: 10 mg P.O. 1 hour before meals.

ADVERSE REACTIONS
CNS: *headache,* dizziness, hallucinations.
GI: diarrhea, constipation, nausea, flatulence.

GU: increased BUN and creatinine levels.
Hematologic: *thrombocytopenia* (rare).
Skin: acne, pruritus, rash.
Other: transient irritation at I.V. site.

INTERACTIONS
None significant.

CONTRAINDICATIONS
Contraindicated in patients hypersensitive to the drug.

NURSING CONSIDERATIONS
• **I.V. use:** To prepare I.V. injection, dilute 2 ml (20 mg) famotidine with compatible I.V. solution to a total volume of either 5 or 10 ml and inject over at least 2 minutes. Compatible solutions include sterile water for injection, 0.9% sodium chloride injection, D_5W or dextrose 10% in water injection, 5% sodium bicarbonate injection, and lactated Ringer's injection.
• Alternatively, give famotidine by intermittent I.V. infusion. Dilute 20 mg (2 ml) famotidine in 100 ml of compatible solution and infuse over 15 to 30 minutes. Solution is stable for 48 hours at room temperature after dilution.
• Store I.V. injection in refrigerator at 36° to 46° F (2° to 8° C).
• Store reconstituted suspension below 86° F (30° C). Discard after 30 days.
• Tell the patient to take famotidine with a snack if desired.
• Remind the patient that drug is most effective if taken at bedtime.
• Tell patients taking famotidine 20 mg b.i.d. to take at least one dose at bedtime.
• With doctor's knowledge, allow the patient to take antacids concomitantly, especially at the beginning of therapy when pain is severe.
• Urge the patient to avoid cigarette

---

*Liquid form contains alcohol.
**May contain tartrazine.

Common reactions are in italics; **life-threatening**, in bold italics.

smoking because it may increase gastric acid secretion and worsen disease.
• Advise the patient not to take drug for longer than 8 weeks unless the doctor specifically orders it.

lansoprazole
Prevacid

Pregnancy Risk Category: B

HOW SUPPLIED
Capsules (delayed release): 15 mg, 30 mg

ACTION
Inhibits the activity of the proton pump and binds to hydrogen/potassium adenosine triphosphatase, located at the secretory surface of the gastric parietal cells, to block the formation of gastric acid.

ONSET, PEAK, DURATION
Onset and duration unknown. Peak effects occur in 1.7 hours.

INDICATIONS & DOSAGE
Short-term treatment of active duodenal ulcer–
Adults: 15 mg P.O. daily before eating for 4 weeks.
Short-term treatment of erosive esophagitis–
Adults: 30 mg P.O. before eating for up to 8 weeks. If healing does not occur, an additional 8 weeks of therapy may be given.
Long-term treatment of pathological hypersecretory conditions, including Zollinger-Ellison syndrome–
Adults: initially, 60 mg P.O. once daily. Dosage increased as needed. Daily dosages of more than 120 mg should be administered in divided doses.

ADVERSE REACTIONS
CNS: headache, agitation, amnesia, anxiety, apathy, confusion, depression, dizziness or syncope, hallucina-

tions, hemiplegia, aggravated hostility, decreased libido, nervousness, paresthesia, thinking abnormality.
CV: chest pain, edema, angina, CVA, hypertension or hypotension, MI, palpitations, *shock,* vasodilation, cardiospasm.
EENT: amblyopia, deafness, eye pain, visual field deficits, otitis media, taste perversion, tinnitus.
GI: *diarrhea, nausea, abdominal pain,* halitosis, melena, anorexia, cholelithiasis, constipation, dry mouth, thirst, dyspepsia, dysphagia, eructation, esophageal stenosis, esophageal ulcer, esophagitis, fecal discoloration, flatulence, gastric nodules, fundic gland polyps, gastroenteritis, GI hemorrhage, hematemesis, increased appetite, increased salivation, rectal hemorrhage, stomatitis, tenesmus, ulcerative colitis.
GU: hematuria, impotence, renal calculi, albuminuria.
Hematologic: anemia, hemolysis.
Metabolic: diabetes mellitus, goiter, hyperglycemia, hypoglycemia, gout, weight gain or loss.
Musculoskeletal: arthritis or arthralgia, musculoskeletal pain, myalgia.
Respiratory: asthma, bronchitis, increased cough, dyspnea, epistaxis, hemoptysis, hiccups, pneumonia, upper respiratory tract inflammation.
Skin: acne, alopecia, pruritus, rash, urticaria.
Other: asthenia, candidiasis, fever, flulike syndrome, infection, malaise, abnormal menses, breast enlargement (gynecomastia), breast tenderness.

INTERACTIONS
Ampicillin esters, digoxin, iron salts, ketoconazole: lansoprazole may interfere with absorption. Monitor patient closely.
Sucralfate: delays lansoprazole absorption. Give lansoprazole at least 30 minutes prior to sucralfate.
Theophylline: may cause mild increase in theophylline clearance. Use

together cautiously. Dosage adjustment of theophylline may be necessary when lansoprazole is started or stopped.

CONTRAINDICATIONS
Contraindicated in patients hypersensitive to the drug.

NURSING CONSIDERATIONS
• Know that no dosage adjustment is necessary in patients with renal insufficiency or in elderly patients. For patients with severe liver disease, dosage adjustment may be necessary.
• Be aware that lansoprazole should not to be used as maintenance therapy for treatment of patients with duodenal ulcer or erosive esophagitis.
• Because it is not known if lansoprazole is excreted in breast milk, be aware that a decision to discontinue breast-feeding or the drug should be made when drug is prescribed for breast-feeding women.
• Instruct patient to take the drug before eating.
• Caution patient not to open, chew, or crush the capsules. The capsules should be swallowed whole.

---

misoprostol
Cytotec

Pregnancy Risk Category: X

HOW SUPPLIED
Tablets: 100 mcg, 200 mcg

ACTION
A synthetic prostaglandin E_1 analogue that replaces gastric prostaglandins depleted by NSAID therapy. Misoprostol also decreases basal and stimulated gastric acid secretion and may increase gastric mucus and bicarbonate production.

ONSET, PEAK, DURATION
Onset occurs in 30 minutes. Plasma levels peak within 10 to 15 minutes. Effects persist about 3 hours.

INDICATIONS & DOSAGE
Prevention of NSAID-induced gastric ulcer in elderly or debilitated patients at high risk for complications from gastric ulcer and in patients with a history of NSAID-induced ulcer —
Adults: 200 mcg P.O. q.i.d. with food. If dosage isn't tolerated, decreased to 100 mcg P.O. q.i.d.

ADVERSE REACTIONS
CNS: headache.
GI: *diarrhea, abdominal pain,* nausea, flatulence, dyspepsia, vomiting, constipation.
Other: hypermenorrhea, dysmenorrhea, spotting, cramps, menstrual disorders.

INTERACTIONS
Antacids: reduced plasma levels when administered concomitantly. Not considered significant.

CONTRAINDICATIONS
Contraindicated in pregnant or lactating patients.

NURSING CONSIDERATIONS
• Know that drug should not be routinely administered to women of childbearing age unless they are at high risk for developing ulcers or complications from NSAID-induced ulcers.
• Take special precautions to prevent use of drug during pregnancy. Make sure the patient is fully aware of the dangers of misoprostol to a fetus and that she receives both oral and written warnings regarding these dangers. Also ensure that the patient can comply with effective contraceptive means and that she has a negative serum pregnancy test within 2 weeks of initiating therapy.

---

*Liquid form contains alcohol.   *Common* reactions are in italics; *life-threatening*, in bold italics.
**May contain tartrazine.

• Instruct all patients not to share misoprostol. Remind them that when taken by a pregnant patient this drug may cause miscarriage, often with potentially life-threatening bleeding.
• Advise patient not to begin misoprostol therapy until the second or third day of the next normal menstrual period.

nizatidine
Axid, Tazac‡

Pregnancy Risk Category: C

HOW SUPPLIED
Capsules: 150 mg, 300 mg

ACTION
Competitively inhibits the action of histamine (H_2) at receptor sites of the parietal cells, decreasing gastric acid secretion.

ONSET, PEAK, DURATION
Onset occurs within 30 minutes. Peak levels occur in ½ to 3 hours. Effects persist up to 12 hours.

INDICATIONS & DOSAGE
Active duodenal ulcer –
Adults: 300 mg P.O. daily h.s. Alternatively, 150 mg P.O. b.i.d.
Maintenance therapy for duodenal ulcer –
Adults: 150 mg P.O. daily h.s.
Benign gastric ulcer –
Adults: 150 mg P.O. b.i.d. or 300 mg h.s. for 8 weeks.
Gastroesophageal reflux disease –
Adults: 150 mg P.O. b.i.d.
In patients with impaired renal function: If creatinine clearance is 20 to 50 ml/minute, 150 mg P.O. daily for treatment of active duodenal ulcer or 150 mg every other day for maintenance therapy; if creatinine clearance is below 20 ml/minute, 150 mg P.O. every other day for treatment or 150 mg every third day for maintenance.

ADVERSE REACTIONS
CNS: *somnolence.*
CV: arrhythmias.
Hematologic: *thrombocytopenia.*
Skin: *diaphoresis,* rash, urticaria, *exfoliative dermatitis.*
Other: liver damage, hyperuricemia, fever.

INTERACTIONS
Aspirin: possibly elevated serum salicylate levels (with high doses).
Tomato-based mixed-vegetable juices: may decrease potency of the drug when used concomitantly. Monitor diet.

CONTRAINDICATIONS
Contraindicated in patients hypersensitive to H_2-receptor antagonists.

NURSING CONSIDERATIONS
• Use cautiously and in reduced dosages in patients with impaired renal function.
• If necessary, open capsules and mix contents with apple juice. However, be aware that drug has been shown to lose some potency when combined with tomato-based mixed-vegetable juices. Check with pharmacist for compatibility.
• Know that nizatidine has not been associated with antiandrogenic activity and does not appear to affect hepatic drug-metabolizing enzyme systems.
• Be aware that false-positive test results for urobilinogen may occur.
• Urge patients to avoid cigarette smoking because it may increase gastric acid secretion and worsen disease.

omeprazole
Losec†‡, Prilosec

Pregnancy Risk Category: C

HOW SUPPLIED
Capsules (delayed-release): 20 mg

ACTION
Inhibits the activity of the acid (proton) pump, and binds to hydrogen/potassium adenosine triphosphatase, located at the secretory surface of the gastric parietal cells to block the formation of gastric acid.

ONSET, PEAK, DURATION
Onset occurs within 1 hour. Peak effects occur within 2 hours. Effects persist 3 days or more; may take 4 days for gastric acid production to return to normal.

INDICATIONS & DOSAGE
Erosive esophagitis; symptomatic, poorly responsive gastroesophageal reflux disease (GERD) –
Adults: 20 mg P.O. daily for 4 to 8 weeks. Patients with GERD should have failed initial therapy with an H₂ antagonist.
Pathologic hypersecretory conditions (such as Zollinger-Ellison syndrome) –
Adults: initially, 60 mg P.O. daily; dosage titrated according to patient response. If daily dosage exceeds 80 mg, administer in divided doses. Dosages up to 120 mg t.i.d. have been given. Continue therapy as long as clinically indicated.
Duodenal ulcer (short-term treatment) –
Adults: 20 mg P.O. daily for 4 to 8 weeks.

ADVERSE REACTIONS
CNS: headache, dizziness.
GI: *diarrhea, abdominal pain, nausea, vomiting, constipation, flatulence.*
Respiratory: cough.
Skin: rash.
Other: back pain.

INTERACTIONS
Ampicillin esters, iron derivatives, ketoconazole: may exhibit poor bioavailability in patients taking omeprazole

because optimal absorption of these drugs requires a low gastric pH.
Diazepam, phenytoin, warfarin: decreased hepatic clearance, possibly leading to increased serum levels. Monitor closely.

CONTRAINDICATIONS
Contraindicated in patients hypersensitive to the drug or any component of the formulation.

NURSING CONSIDERATIONS
• Know that dosage adjustments are not required for renal or hepatic impairment.
• Keep in mind that omeprazole increases its own bioavailability with repeated administration. Drug is labile in gastric acid; less drug is lost to hydrolysis because the drug increases gastric pH.
• Know that omeprazole should not be used for maintenance therapy. Most patients with duodenal ulcers heal within 4 weeks.
• Tell the patient to swallow capsules whole and not to open or crush.

---

ranitidine hydrochloride
Apo-Ranitidine†, Zantac*, Zantac-C†, Zantac EFFERdose

Pregnancy Risk Category: B

HOW SUPPLIED
Tablets: 150 mg, 300 mg
Dispersible tablets: 150 mg‡
Effervescent tablets: 150 mg
Effervescent granules: 150 mg
Syrup: 15 mg/ml*
Injection: 25 mg/ml
Infusion: 0.5 mg/ml in 100-ml containers

ACTION
Competitively inhibits the action of histamine (H₂) at receptor sites of the parietal cells, decreasing gastric acid secretion.

ONSET, PEAK, DURATION
Onset occurs within 1 hour. Peak effects occur in 1 to 3 hours. Effects persist up to 13 hours.

INDICATIONS & DOSAGE
Duodenal and gastric ulcer (short-term treatment); pathological hypersecretory conditions, such as Zollinger-Ellison syndrome –
Adults: 150 mg P.O. b.i.d. or 300 mg daily h.s. Alternatively, 50 mg I.V. or I.M. q 6 to 8 hours. Patients with Zollinger-Ellison syndrome may require dosages up to 6 g P.O. daily.
Maintenance therapy for duodenal ulcer –
Adults: 150 mg P.O. h.s.
Gastroesophageal reflux disease (GERD) –
Adults: 150 mg P.O. b.i.d.
Erosive esophagitis –
Adults: 150 mg P.O. q.i.d.

ADVERSE REACTIONS
CNS: headache, malaise, dizziness, confusion.
CV: bradycardia.
GI: nausea, constipation.
Hematologic: *neutropenia, thrombocytopenia.*
Hepatic: elevated liver enzymes, jaundice.
Skin: rash.
Other: burning and itching at injection site.

INTERACTIONS
Antacids: possible interference with ranitidine absorption. Stagger doses if possible.
Diazepam: decreased absorption of diazepam.
Glipizide: possible increased hypoglycemic effect. Adjust glipizide dosage as necessary.
Procainamide: possible decreased renal clearance of procainamide.
Warfarin: possible interference with warfarin clearance.

CONTRAINDICATIONS
Contraindicated in patients hypersensitive to the drug.

NURSING CONSIDERATIONS
• Use cautiously in patients with hepatic dysfunction. Adjust dosage in patients with impaired renal function as ordered.
• Avoid using aluminum-based needles or other equipment when mixing or administering drug. Drug is incompatible with aluminum.
• **I.V. use:** When administering by I.V. push, dilute to a total volume of 20 ml and inject over a period of 5 minutes. No dilution is necessary when administering I.M.
• To prepare I.V. injection, dilute 50 mg (2 ml) in 100 ml of compatible solution and infuse over 15 to 20 minutes. Compatible solutions include 0.9% sodium chloride injection, D_5W or $D_{10}W$ injection, 5% sodium bicarbonate injection, or lactated Ringer's injection.
• When administering by intermittent I.V. infusion, dilute 50 mg ranitidine in 100 ml of D_5W and infuse over 15 to 20 minutes. Alternatively, give by continuous I.V. infusion: 150 mg in 250 ml of compatible solution. Administer at 6.25 mg/hour using an infusion pump.
• When administering premixed I.V. infusion, give by slow I.V. drip (over 15 to 20 minutes). Do not add other drugs to the solution. If used with a primary I.V. fluid system, discontinue the primary solution during the infusion.
• Remind patients taking ranitidine once daily to take it at bedtime for best results.
• Instruct patient to take without regard to meals because absorption is not affected by food.
• Urge patients to avoid cigarette smoking because it may increase gastric acid secretion and worsen disease.

---

†Available in Canada only.   ‡Available in Australia only.   ◊Available OTC.

sucralfate
Carafate, SCF‡, Sulcrate†

Pregnancy Risk Category: B

HOW SUPPLIED
Tablets: 1 g

ACTION
Unknown. Probably adheres to and protects the ulcer's surface by forming a barrier.

ONSET, PEAK, DURATION
Onset and peak unknown. Effects persist for up to 6 hours.

INDICATIONS & DOSAGE
Short-term (up to 8 weeks) treatment of duodenal ulcer—
Adults: 1 g P.O. q.i.d. 1 hour before meals and h.s.
Maintenance therapy for duodenal ulcer—
Adults: 1 g P.O. b.i.d.

ADVERSE REACTIONS
CNS: dizziness, sleepiness.
GI: *constipation,* nausea, gastric discomfort, diarrhea, bezoar formation.

INTERACTIONS
Antacids: may decrease binding of drug to gastroduodenal mucosa, impairing effectiveness. Don't administer within 30 minutes of each other.
Cimetidine, ciprofloxacin, digoxin, norfloxacin, phenytoin, ranitidine, tetracycline, theophylline: decreased absorption. Separate administration times by at least 2 hours.

CONTRAINDICATIONS
None reported.

NURSING CONSIDERATIONS
● Use with caution in patients with chronic renal failure.
● Know that drug is minimally absorbed. Low incidence of adverse reactions.
● Monitor for severe, persistent constipation.
● Be aware that studies suggest that sucralfate is as effective as cimetidine in healing duodenal ulcer.
● Keep in mind that drug contains aluminum but isn't classified as an antacid.
● Tell patient for best results to take sucralfate on an empty stomach (1 hour before each meal and at bedtime).
● Tell patients to continue on prescribed regimen to ensure complete healing. Pain and ulcerative symptoms may subside within first few weeks of therapy.
● Urge patients to avoid cigarette smoking because it may increase gastric acid secretion and worsen disease.

---

*Liquid form contains alcohol.
**May contain tartrazine.

Common reactions are in italics; ***life-threatening,*** in bold italics.

53
Corticosteroids

betamethasone
betamethasone acetate and
  betamethasone sodium
  phosphate
betamethasone sodium
  phosphate
cortisone acetate
dexamethasone
dexamethasone acetate
dexamethasone sodium
  phosphate
fludrocortisone acetate
hydrocortisone
hydrocortisone acetate
hydrocortisone cypionate
hydrocortisone sodium
  phosphate
hydrocortisone sodium
  succinate
methylprednisolone
methylprednisolone acetate
methylprednisolone sodium
  succinate
prednisolone
prednisolone acetate
prednisolone sodium phosphate
prednisolone steaglate
prednisolone tebutate
prednisone
triamcinolone
triamcinolone acetonide
triamcinolone diacetate
triamcinolone hexacetonide

COMBINATION PRODUCTS
DECADRON PHOSPHATE WITH XY-LOCAINE: dexamethasone phosphate
4 mg and lidocaine hydrochloride 10
mg per ml.

---

betamethasone
Betnelan†, Betnesol†, Celestone*

---

betamethasone acetate and betamethasone sodium phosphate
Celestone Chronodose‡,
Celestone Soluspan

betamethasone sodium phosphate
Celestone Phosphate, Selestoject

Pregnancy Risk Category: NR

HOW SUPPLIED
betamethasone
Tablets: 600 mcg
Tablets (extended-release): 1 mg
Tablets (effervescent): 500 mcg†
Syrup: 600 mcg/5 ml
betamethasone acetate and betame-thasone sodium phosphate
Injection (suspension): betamethasone
acetate 3 mg and betamethasone so-dium phosphate (equivalent to 3-mg
base) per ml
betamethasone sodium phosphate
Tablets (effervescent): 500 mcg*
Injection: 4 mg (equivalent to 3-mg
base)/ml in 5-ml vials

ACTION
Not completely defined. Decreases
inflammation, mainly by stabilizing
leukocyte lysosomal membranes; sup-presses the immune response; stimu-lates bone marrow; and influences
protein, fat, and carbohydrate metab-olism.

ONSET, PEAK, DURATION
Onset prmpt. Peak unknown. Dura-tion variable but thought to persist for
3.25 days after oral administration, 7
to 14 days for parenteral administra-tion.

INDICATIONS & DOSAGE

Conditions with severe inflammation; conditions requiring immunosuppression –

Adults: 0.6 to 7.2 mg P.O. daily; or 0.5 to 9 mg I.M., I.V., or into joint or soft tissue daily; or 1.5 to 12 mg of sodium phosphate-acetate suspension into joint or soft tissue q 1 to 2 weeks, p.r.n.

ADVERSE REACTIONS

Most adverse reactions to corticosteroids are dose- or duration-dependent.

CNS: *euphoria, insomnia,* psychotic behavior, pseudotumor cerebri.
CV: *CHF,* hypertension, edema.
EENT: cataracts, glaucoma.
GI: *peptic ulceration,* GI irritation, increased appetite, pancreatitis.
Skin: delayed wound healing, acne, various skin eruptions.
Other: muscle weakness, osteoporosis, hirsutism, susceptibility to infections; hypokalemia, hyperglycemia, and carbohydrate intolerance; growth suppression in children; *acute adrenal insufficiency may follow increased stress (infection, surgery, or trauma) or abrupt withdrawal after long-term therapy.*
After abrupt withdrawal: rebound inflammation, fatigue, weakness, arthralgia, fever, dizziness, lethargy, depression, fainting, orthostatic hypotension, dyspnea, anorexia, hypoglycemia. *After prolonged use, sudden withdrawal may be fatal.*

INTERACTIONS

Aspirin, indomethacin, and other NSAIDs: increased risk of GI distress and bleeding. Give together cautiously.
Barbiturates, phenytoin, rifampin: decreased corticosteroid effect. Corticosteroid dosage may need to be increased.
Oral anticoagulants: altered dosage requirements. Monitor PT closely.

Potassium-depleting drugs, such as thiazide diuretics: enhanced potassium-wasting effects of betamethasone. Monitor serum potassium levels.
Skin-test antigens: decreased response. Defer skin testing until therapy is completed.
Toxoids and vaccines: decreased antibody response and increased risk of neurologic complications. Avoid concomitant use.

CONTRAINDICATIONS

Contraindicated in patients hypersensitive to the drug and in those with viral or bacterial infections (except in life-threatening situations) or systemic fungal infections.

NURSING CONSIDERATIONS

• Use with extreme caution in a patient with recent MI or peptic ulcer (used only in life-threatening situations).
• Use cautiously in patients with renal disease, hypertension, osteoporosis, diabetes mellitus, hypothyroidism, cirrhosis, diverticulitis, nonspecific ulcerative colitis, recent intestinal anastomoses, thromboembolic disorders, seizures, myasthenia gravis, CHF, tuberculosis, ocular herpes simplex, emotional instability, and psychotic tendencies. Because some formulations contain sulfite preservatives, also use cautiously in patients sensitive to sulfites.
• Know that drug should not be used for alternate-day therapy.
• Obtain baseline weight before starting therapy, and weigh patients daily; report any sudden weight gain to the doctor.
• For better results and less toxicity, give a once-daily dose in the morning.
• To reduce GI irritation, give with milk or food.
• To prevent muscle atrophy, give I.M. injection deeply. Rotate injection sites.

*Liquid form contains alcohol.   *Common* reactions are in italics; *life-threatening,* in bold italics.
**May contain tartrazine.

• **I.V. use:** Compatible with 0.9% sodium chloride, D₅W, lactated Ringer's injection, dextrose 5% in lactated Ringer's injection, and dextrose 5% in Ringer's injection.

• Be aware that drug should always be titrated to lowest effective dose.

• Monitor blood glucose and serum potassium levels regularly, as ordered. Diabetic patients may require adjustments in insulin dosage.

• Monitor for depression or mood changes, especially in patients receiving long-term therapy.

• Monitor for additional potassium depletion resulting from diuretics or amphotericin B therapy. Potassium supplements may be necessary for patients receiving long-term therapy.

• A calorie- or sodium-restricted diet with protein supplementation may be necessary for patients receiving long-term therapy.

• Know that elderly patients may be more susceptible to osteoporosis.

• Adrenal suppression may last up to 1 year after drug is stopped.

• Gradually reduce drug dosage after long-term therapy, as ordered.

• Observe for signs of infection, especially after steroid withdrawal.

• Tell patients not to stop drug abruptly or without the doctor's consent.

• Tell patients using the effervescent tablets to dissolve them in water immediately before ingestion.

• Teach patients about the drug's effects. Warn those on long-term therapy about cushingoid symptoms and to report sudden weight gain or swelling to the doctor.

• Make sure patients report symptoms associated with corticosteroid withdrawal, including fatigue, weakness, arthralgia, orthostatic hypotension, and dyspnea.

• Make sure patients understand to contact the doctor if symptoms are worsening or the medication is no longer effective. Tell patients not to

increase dosage without the doctor's consent.

• Advise elderly patient receiving long-term therapy to consider exercise or physical therapy. Also tell him to ask his doctor about vitamin D or calcium supplements.

• Advise patients receiving prolonged therapy to have periodic ophthalmic examinations.

• Tell patient to report slow healing.

• Instruct patients to carry a card indicating their need for supplemental glucocorticoids during stress.

---

cortisone acetate
Cortate‡, Cortone Acetate

Pregnancy Risk Category: NR

HOW SUPPLIED
Tablets: 5 mg, 10 mg, 25 mg
Injection (suspension): 25 mg/ml, 50 mg/ml

ACTION
Not completely defined. Decreases inflammation, mainly by stabilizing leukocyte lysosomal membranes; suppresses the immune response; stimulates bone marrow; and influences protein, fat, and carbohydrate metabolism.

ONSET, PEAK, DURATION
Highly variable.

INDICATIONS & DOSAGE
Adrenal insufficiency, allergy, inflammation —
Adults: 25 to 300 mg P.O. or 20 to 300 mg I.M. daily or on alternate days. Dosages are highly individualized, depending on severity of disease.

ADVERSE REACTIONS
Most adverse reactions to corticosteroids are dose- or duration-dependent.

CNS: *euphoria, insomnia,* psychotic behavior, pseudotumor cerebri.
CV: *CHF,* hypertension, edema.
EENT: cataracts, glaucoma.
GI: *peptic ulceration,* GI irritation, increased appetite, pancreatitis.
Skin: delayed wound healing, acne, various skin eruptions; atrophy at I.M. injection sites.
Other: muscle weakness, osteoporosis, hirsutism, susceptibility to infections; possible hypokalemia, hyperglycemia, and carbohydrate intolerance; growth suppression in children; *acute adrenal insufficiency may follow increased stress (infection, surgery, or trauma) or abrupt withdrawal after long-term therapy.*
After abrupt withdrawal: rebound inflammation, fatigue, weakness, arthralgia, fever, dizziness, lethargy, depression, fainting, orthostatic hypotension, dyspnea, anorexia, hypoglycemia. *After prolonged use, sudden withdrawal may be fatal.*

INTERACTIONS

Aspirin, indomethacin, and other NSAIDS: increased risk of GI distress and bleeding. Give together cautiously.
Barbiturates, phenytoin, rifampin: decreased corticosteroid effect. Increase corticosteroid dosage, as ordered.
Live attenuated virus vaccines, other toxoids and vaccines: decreased antibody response and increased risk of neurologic complications. Avoid concomitant use.
Oral anticoagulants: altered dosage requirements. Monitor PT closely.
Potassium-depleting drugs, such as thiazide diuretics: enhanced potassium-wasting effects of cortisone. Monitor serum potassium levels.
Skin-test antigens: decreased response. Defer skin testing until therapy is completed.

CONTRAINDICATIONS

Contraindicated in patients with hypersensitivity to drug or any of its ingredients or systemic fungal infections.

NURSING CONSIDERATIONS

• Use with extreme caution in a patient with recent MI.
• Use cautiously in patients with GI ulcer, renal disease, hypertension, osteoporosis, diabetes mellitus, hypothyroidism, cirrhosis, diverticulitis, nonspecific ulcerative colitis, recent intestinal anastomoses, thromboembolic disorders, seizures, myasthenia gravis, CHF, tuberculosis, ocular herpes simplex, emotional instability, and psychotic tendencies.
• To reduce GI irritation, give with milk or food.
• For better results and less toxicity, give a once-daily dose in the morning.
• I.M. route causes slow onset of action. Should not be used in acute conditions where a rapid effect is required. May be used on a twice-daily schedule matching diurnal variation. Rotate injection sites to prevent muscle atrophy.
• Mixing or diluting parenteral suspension may alter absorption rate and decrease the drug's effectiveness.
• Know that drug is not for I.V. use.
• Know that drug should always be titrated to lowest effective dose.
• Monitor serum electrolyte and blood glucose levels as ordered.
• Monitor patient for fluid and electrolyte imbalances. Patients may need low-sodium diet and potassium supplements.
• Monitor for additional potassium depletion resulting from diuretic or amphotericin B therapy.
• Know that elderly patients may be more susceptible to osteoporosis.
• Gradually reduce drug dosage after long-term therapy, as ordered.
• Observe for signs of infection, especially after steroid withdrawal.

---

*Liquid form contains alcohol.   *Common* reactions are in italics; *life-threatening,* in bold italics.
**May contain tartrazine.

• Tell patients not to discontinue drug abruptly or without the doctor's consent.
• Advise patient receiving long-term therapy to consider exercise or physical therapy. Also tell him to ask his doctor about vitamin D or calcium supplements.
• Tell patients to report slow healing.
• Warn patients on long-term therapy about cushingoid symptoms and to report sudden weight gain or swelling to the doctor.
• Instruct patients to carry a card indicating their need for supplemental glucocorticoids during stress.

dexamethasone
Decadron*, Deronil†, Dexamethasone Intensol*, Dexasone†, Dexone 0.5, Dexone 0.75, Dexone 1.5, Dexone 4, Hexadrol*, Mymethasone*

dexamethasone acetate
Dalalone D.P., Dalalone L.A., Decadron-LA, Decaject-L.A., Dexacen LA-8, Dexasone-LA, Dexone LA, Solurex-LA

dexamethasone sodium phosphate
Ak-Dex, Dalalone, Decadrol, Decadron Phosphate, Decaject, Dexacen-4, Dexone, Hexadrol Phosphate, Solurex

Pregnancy Risk Category: NR

HOW SUPPLIED
dexamethasone
Tablets: 0.25 mg, 0.5 mg, 0.75 mg, 1 mg, 1.5 mg, 2 mg, 4 mg, 6 mg
Oral solution: 0.5 mg/5 ml, 1 mg/ml
Elixir: 0.5 mg/5 ml*
dexamethasone acetate
Injection: 8 mg/ml, 16 mg/ml suspension
dexamethasone sodium phosphate
Injection: 4 mg/ml, 10 mg/ml, 20 mg/ml, 24 mg/ml

ACTION
Not clearly defined. Decreases inflammation, mainly by stabilizing leukocyte lysosomal membranes; suppresses the immune response; stimulates bone marrow; and influences protein, fat, and carbohydrate metabolism.

ONSET, PEAK, DURATION
Onset occurs within 1 hour after I.M. or I.V. administration; 1 to 2 hours after oral administration. Peak effects occur within 1 hour after I.M. or I.V. administration, within 1 to 2 hours after oral administration, or within 8 hours after use of the injectable suspension (acetate). Effects persist about 2½ days after oral use, 6 days after I.M. use (acetate), and up to 3 weeks after intralesional or intra-articular use (acetate or sodium phosphate).

INDICATIONS & DOSAGE
Cerebral edema–
Adults: initially, 10 mg (phosphate) I.V.; then 4 to 6 mg I.M. q 6 hours until symptoms subside (usually 2 to 4 days); then tapered over 5 to 7 days.
Inflammatory conditions, allergic reactions, neoplasias–
Adults: 0.75 to 9 mg/day P.O. or 0.5 to 9 mg/day (phosphate) I.M.; or 4 to 16 mg (acetate) I.M. into joint or soft tissue q 1 to 3 weeks; or 0.8 to 1.6 mg (acetate) into lesions q 1 to 3 weeks.
Shock–
Adults: 1 to 6 mg/kg (phosphate) I.V. as a single dose; or 40 mg I.V. q 2 to 6 hours, p.r.n.
Dexamethasone suppression test for Cushing's syndrome–
Adults: after determining baseline 24-hour urine levels of 17-hydroxycorticosteroids, 0.5 mg P.O. q 6 hours for 48 hours; 24-hour urine collection made for determination of 17-hydroxycorticosteroid excretion again during second 24 hours of dexamethasone administration.

ADVERSE REACTIONS

Most adverse reactions to corticosteroids are dose- or duration-dependent.

CNS: *euphoria, insomnia,* psychotic behavior, pseudotumor cerebri.

CV: *CHF,* hypertension, edema.

EENT: cataracts, glaucoma.

GI: *peptic ulceration,* GI irritation, increased appetite, pancreatitis.

Skin: delayed wound healing, acne, various skin eruptions; atrophy at I.M. injection sites.

Other: muscle weakness, osteoporosis, hirsutism, susceptibility to infections; hypokalemia, hyperglycemia, and carbohydrate intolerance; growth suppression in children; *acute adrenal insufficiency may follow increased stress (infection, surgery, or trauma) or abrupt withdrawal after long-term therapy.*

After abrupt withdrawal: rebound inflammation, fatigue, weakness, arthralgia, fever, dizziness, lethargy, depression, fainting, orthostatic hypotension, dyspnea, anorexia, hypoglycemia. *After prolonged use, sudden withdrawal may be fatal.*

INTERACTIONS

Aspirin, indomethacin, and other NSAIDs: increased risk of GI distress and bleeding. Give together cautiously.

Barbiturates, phenytoin, rifampin: decreased corticosteroid effect. Increase corticosteroid dosage, as ordered.

Oral anticoagulants: altered dosage requirements. Monitor PT closely.

Potassium-depleting drugs, such as thiazide diuretics: enhanced potassium-wasting effects of dexamethasone. Monitor serum potassium levels.

Skin-test antigens: decreased response. Defer skin testing until therapy is completed.

Toxoids and vaccines: decreased antibody response and increased risk of neurologic complications. Avoid concomitant use.

CONTRAINDICATIONS

Contraindicated in patients hypersensitive to any component of the drug and in those with systemic fungal infections.

NURSING CONSIDERATIONS

• Use with extreme caution in patient with recent MI.

• Use cautiously in patients with GI ulcer, renal disease, hypertension, osteoporosis, diabetes mellitus, hypothyroidism, cirrhosis, diverticulitis, nonspecific ulcerative colitis, recent intestinal anastomoses, thromboembolic disorders, seizures, myasthenia gravis, CHF, tuberculosis, ocular herpes simplex, emotional instability, and psychotic tendencies. Because some formulations contain sulfite preservatives, also use cautiously in patients sensitive to sulfites.

• For better results and less toxicity, give a once-daily dose in the morning.

• Give oral dose with food when possible.

• Give I.M. injection deeply into gluteal muscle. Rotate injection sites to prevent muscle atrophy. Avoid S.C. injection because atrophy and sterile abscesses may occur.

• **I.V. use:** When administering as direct injection, inject undiluted over at least 1 minute. When administering as an intermittent or continuous infusion, dilute solution according to the manufacturer's instructions and give over the prescribed duration. If used for continuous infusion, change solution every 24 hours.

• Always titrate to lowest effective dose as ordered.

• Monitor patients' weight, blood pressure, and serum electrolyte levels.

• Monitor for additional potassium depletion resulting from diuretic or amphotericin B therapy. Potassium supplements may be necessary.

• Watch for depression or psychotic episodes, especially in high-dose therapy.

---

*Liquid form contains alcohol.   Common reactions are in italics; **life-threatening,** in bold italics.
**May contain tartrazine.

• Diabetic patients may need increased insulin; monitor blood glucose levels.
• Know that drug may mask or exacerbate infections, including latent amebiasis.
• Know that elderly patients may be more susceptible to osteoporosis.
• Inspect patient's skin for petechiae.
• Gradually reduce drug dosage after long-term therapy as ordered.
• Tell patients not to discontinue drug abruptly or without the doctor's consent.
• Teach patients signs of early adrenal insufficiency: fatigue, muscular weakness, joint pain, fever, anorexia, nausea, dyspnea, dizziness, and fainting.
• Instruct patients to carry a card indicating their need for supplemental systemic glucocorticoids during stress, especially as dosage is decreased.
• Warn patients on long-term therapy about cushingoid symptoms and to report sudden weight gain or swelling to the doctor.
• Warn patients about easy bruising.
• Advise patients receiving long-term therapy to consider exercise or physical therapy. Give vitamin D or calcium supplements as ordered.
• Advise patients receiving long-term therapy to have periodic ophthalmic examinations.

fluldrocortisone acetate
Florinef

Pregnancy Risk Category: C

HOW SUPPLIED
Tablets: 0.1 mg

ACTION
Increases sodium reabsorption and potassium and hydrogen secretion at the nephrons' distal convoluted tubule.

ONSET, PEAK, DURATION
Onset and peak variable. Effects persist for 1 to 2 days.

INDICATIONS & DOSAGE
Adrenal insufficiency (partial replacement), adrenogenital syndrome –
Adults: 0.1 to 0.2 mg P.O. daily.

ADVERSE REACTIONS
CV: *sodium and water retention,* hypertension, cardiac hypertrophy, edema.
Other: hypokalemia.

INTERACTIONS
Potassium-depleting drugs, such as thiazide diuretics: enhanced potassium-wasting effects of fludrocortisone. Monitor serum potassium levels.

CONTRAINDICATIONS
Contraindicated in patients with hypersensitivity to drug or in patients with systemic fungal infections.

NURSING CONSIDERATIONS
• Use cautiously in patients with hypothyroidism, cirrhosis, ocular herpes simplex, emotional instability, and psychotic tendencies, nonspecific ulcerative colitis, diverticulitis, fresh intestinal anastomoses, active or latent peptic ulcer, renal insufficiency, hypertension, osteoporosis, and myasthenia gravis.
• Be aware that drug is used with cortisone or hydrocortisone in adrenal insufficiency.
• Monitor patient's blood pressure and serum electrolyte levels. If hypertension occurs, notify doctor and expect dosage to be decreased by 50%.
• Weigh patients daily; report sudden weight gain to the doctor.
• Watch for additional potassium depletion resulting from diuretic or amphotericin B therapy.
• Unless contraindicated, give low-sodium diet high in potassium and

---

protein. Be aware that potassium supplements may be needed.

• Tell patients to report worsening symptoms, such as hypotension, weakness, cramping, and palpitations, to the doctor.

• Warn patients that mild peripheral edema is common.

---

hydrocortisone
Cortef, Cortenema, Hydrocortone

hydrocortisone acetate
Cortifoam, Hydrocortone Acetate

hydrocortisone cypionate
Cortef

hydrocortisone sodium phosphate
Hydrocortone Phosphate

hydrocortisone sodium succinate
A-hydroCort, Solu-Cortef

Pregnancy Risk Category: NR

HOW SUPPLIED
hydrocortisone
Tablets: 5 mg, 10 mg, 20 mg
Enema: 100 mg/60 ml
hydrocortisone acetate
Injection: 25 mg/ml*, 50 mg/ml* suspension
Enema: 10% aerosol foam (provides 90 mg/application)
Suppositories: 25 mg
hydrocortisone cypionate
Oral suspension: 10 mg/5 ml
hydrocortisone sodium phosphate
Injection: 50 mg/ml solution
hydrocortisone sodium succinate
Injection: 100 mg/vial*, 250 mg/vial*, 500 mg/vial*, 1,000 mg/vial*

ACTION
Not clearly defined. Decreases inflammation, mainly by stabilizing leukocyte lysosomal membranes; suppresses the immune response; stimulates bone marrow; and influences protein, fat, and carbohydrate metabolism.

ONSET, PEAK, DURATION
Highly variable.

INDICATIONS & DOSAGE
Severe inflammation, adrenal insufficiency –
Adults: 5 to 30 mg P.O. b.i.d., t.i.d., or q.i.d. (as much as 80 mg q.i.d. may be given in acute situations); or initially, 100 to 250 mg succinate I.M. or I.V., and then 50 to 100 mg I.M., as indicated; or 15 to 240 mg phosphate I.M. or I.V. q 12 hours; or 5 to 75 mg acetate into joints or soft tissue. Dosage varies with size of joint. Local anesthetics often are injected with dose.
Shock –
Adults: initially, 50 mg/kg succinate I.V. repeated in 4 hours. Repeat dosage q 24 hours as needed. Alternatively, 100 to 500 mg to 2 g q 2 to 6 hours.
Children: 186 to 280 mcg/kg phosphate or succinate I.M. or I.V. t.i.d.
Adjunct for ulcerative colitis and proctitis –
Adults: 1 enema (100 mg) P.R. nightly for 21 days.

ADVERSE REACTIONS
Most adverse reactions to corticosteroids are dose- or duration-dependent.
CNS: *euphoria, insomnia,* psychotic behavior, pseudotumor cerebri.
CV: **CHF,** hypertension, edema.
EENT: cataracts, glaucoma.
GI: *peptic ulceration,* GI irritation, increased appetite, pancreatitis.
Skin: delayed wound healing, acne, various skin eruptions, easy bruising.
Other: muscle weakness, osteoporosis, hirsutism, susceptibility to infections; possible hypokalemia, hyperglycemia, and carbohydrate intolerance; growth suppression in chil-

---

*Liquid form contains alcohol.   *Common* reactions are in italics; **life-threatening,** in bold italics.
**May contain tartrazine.

dren; *acute adrenal insufficiency may occur with increased stress (infection, surgery, or trauma) or abrupt withdrawal after long-term therapy.* **After abrupt withdrawal:** rebound inflammation, fatigue, weakness, arthralgia, fever, dizziness, lethargy, depression, fainting, orthostatic hypotension, dyspnea, anorexia, hypoglycemia. *After prolonged use, sudden withdrawal may be fatal.*

INTERACTIONS

Aspirin, indomethacin, and other NSAIDs: increased risk of GI distress and bleeding. Give together cautiously.

Barbiturates, phenytoin, rifampin: decreased corticosteroid effect. Increase corticosteroid dosage, as ordered.

Live attenuated virus vaccines, other toxoids and vaccines: decreased antibody response and increased risk of neurologic complications. Avoid concomitant use.

Oral anticoagulants: altered dosage requirements. Monitor PT closely.

Potassium-depleting drugs, such as thiazide diuretics: enhanced potassium-wasting effects of hydrocortisone. Monitor serum potassium levels.

Skin-test antigens: decreased response. Defer skin testing until therapy is completed.

CONTRAINDICATIONS

Contraindicated in patients allergic to any component of the formulation, in those with systemic fungal infections, and in premature infants (succinate).

NURSING CONSIDERATIONS

• Use with extreme caution in patient with recent MI.

• Use cautiously in patients with GI ulcer, renal disease, hypertension, osteoporosis, diabetes mellitus, hypothyroidism, cirrhosis, diverticulitis, nonspecific ulcerative colitis, recent intestinal anastomoses, thromboembolic disorders, seizures, myasthenia gravis, CHF, tuberculosis, ocular herpes simplex, emotional instability, and psychotic tendencies.

• For better results and less toxicity, give a once-daily dose in the morning.

• Give oral dose with food when possible.

• **I.V. use:** Do not use the acetate or suspension form for I.V. use. When administering as direct injection, inject directly into vein or an I.V. line containing a free-flowing compatible solution over 30 seconds to several minutes. When administering as an intermittent or continuous infusion, dilute solution according to manufacturer's instructions and give over the prescribed duration. If used for continuous infusion, change solution every 24 hours.

• Hydrocortisone sodium phosphate may be added directly to D_5W or 0.9% sodium chloride for I.V. administration.

• Reconstitute hydrocortisone sodium succinate with bacteriostatic water or bacteriostatic sodium chloride solution before adding to I.V. solutions. When giving by direct I.V. injection, inject over at least 30 seconds. For infusion, dilute with D_5W, 0.9% sodium chloride, or dextrose 5% in 0.9% sodium chloride to a concentration of 1 mg/ml or less.

• Give I.M. injection deeply into gluteal muscle. Rotate injection sites to prevent muscle atrophy. Avoid S.C. injection because atrophy and sterile abscesses may occur.

• Do not confuse Solu-Cortef with Solu-Medrol (methylprednisolone sodium succinate).

• Know that injectable forms are not used for alternate-day therapy.

• Enema may produce same systemic effects as other forms of hydrocortisone. If enema therapy must exceed 21 days, discontinue gradually by reducing administration to every other night for 2 or 3 weeks, as ordered.

• Be aware high-dose therapy is usually not continued beyond 48 hours.
• Always titrate to lowest effective dose as ordered.
• Monitor patients' weight, blood pressure, and serum electrolyte levels.
• Unless contraindicated, give low-sodium diet high in potassium and protein. Administer potassium supplements as ordered. Watch for additional potassium depletion resulting from diuretic or amphotericin B therapy.
• Know that drug may mask or exacerbate infections, including latent amebiasis.
• Stress (fever, trauma, surgery, and emotional problems) may increase adrenal insufficiency. Increase dosage, as ordered.
• Watch for depression or psychotic episodes, especially during high-dose therapy.
• Inspect patients' skin for petechiae.
• Warn patients about easy bruising.
• Diabetic patients may need increased insulin; monitor blood glucose levels.
• Periodic measurement of growth and development may be necessary during high-dose or prolonged therapy in children.
• Know that elderly patients may be more susceptible to osteoporosis.
• Gradually reduce drug dosage after long-term therapy, as ordered.
• Teach patients signs of early adrenal insufficiency: fatigue, muscular weakness, joint pain, fever, anorexia, nausea, dyspnea, dizziness, and fainting.
• Instruct patients to carry a card identifying their need for supplemental systemic glucocorticoids during stress.
• Tell patients not to discontinue the drug abruptly or without the doctor's consent.
• Warn patients on long-term therapy about cushingoid symptoms and to report sudden weight gain or swelling to the doctor.

• Advise patient receiving long-term therapy to consider exercise or physical therapy. Also tell him to ask his doctor about vitamin D or calcium supplements.
• Advise patients receiving prolonged therapy to have periodic ophthalmic examinations.

methylprednisolone
Medrol**, Meprolone

methylprednisolone acetate
depMedalone-40, depMedalone-80, Depoject-40, Depoject-80, Depo-Medrol, Depopred-40, Depopred-80, Depo-Predate 40, Depo-Predate 80, Duralone-40, Duralone-80, Medralone-40, Medralone-80, Medrol Enpak

methylprednisolone sodium succinate
A-metha-Pred, Solu-Medrol

Pregnancy Risk Category: NR

HOW SUPPLIED
methylprednisolone
Tablets: 2 mg, 4 mg, 8 mg, 16 mg, 24 mg, 32 mg
methylprednisolone acetate
Injection (suspension): 20 mg/ml, 40 mg/ml, 80 mg/ml
Enema: 40 mg
methylprednisolone sodium succinate
Injection: 40 mg/vial, 125 mg/vial, 500 mg/vial, 1,000 mg/vial, 2,000 mg/vial

ACTION
Not clearly defined. Decreases inflammation, mainly by stabilizing leukocyte lysosomal membranes; suppresses the immune response; stimulates bone marrow; and influences protein, fat, and carbohydrate metabolism.

---

*Liquid form contains alcohol.
**May contain tartrazine.
Common reactions are in italics; *life-threatening*, in bold italics.

ONSET, PEAK, DURATION

Onset occurs rapidly after I.V. or oral administration; slowly (6 to 48 hours) after I.M. injection of acetate suspension. Peak effects occur immediately after I.V. injection, within 1 to 2 hours after oral administration, 4 to 8 days after I.M. use, or 7 days after intralesional or intra-articular administration. Effects persist 30 to 36 hours after oral administration, 1 to 4 weeks after I.M. use, or 1 to 5 weeks after intralesional or intra-articular administration.

INDICATIONS & DOSAGE

Severe inflammation or immunosuppression –
Adults: 2 to 60 mg P.O. daily in four divided doses; 40 to 80 mg acetate I.M. daily, or 10 to 250 mg succinate I.M. or I.V. q 4 hours; or 4 to 30 mg acetate into joint or soft tissue, p.r.n.
Children: 0.5 mg/kg succinate I.V. daily in divided doses.
Shock –
Adults: 100 to 250 mg succinate I.V. at 2- to 6-hour intervals; or 30 mg/kg I.V. initially, repeated q 4 to 6 hours p.r.n. Continue therapy for 2 to 3 days or until the patient is stable.
Proctitis –
Adults: 40 mg P.R. (as retention enema) or by continuous I.V. drip three to seven times a week for at least 2 weeks.
Children: 500 mcg to 1 mg/kg or 15 to 30 mg/m² P.R. q 1 to 2 days for at least 2 weeks.

ADVERSE REACTIONS

Most adverse reactions to corticosteroids are dose- or duration-dependent.
CNS: *euphoria, insomnia,* psychotic behavior, pseudotumor cerebri.
CV: *CHF,* hypertension, edema.
EENT: cataracts, glaucoma.
GI: *peptic ulceration,* GI irritation, increased appetite, pancreatitis.

Skin: delayed wound healing, acne, various skin eruptions.
Other: muscle weakness, osteoporosis, hirsutism, susceptibility to infections; hypokalemia, hyperglycemia, and carbohydrate intolerance; growth suppression in children; *acute adrenal insufficiency may occur with increased stress (infection, surgery, or trauma) or abrupt withdrawal after long-term therapy.*
After abrupt withdrawal: rebound inflammation, fatigue, weakness, arthralgia, fever, dizziness, lethargy, depression, fainting, orthostatic hypotension, dyspnea, anorexia, hypoglycemia. *After prolonged use, sudden withdrawal may be fatal.*

INTERACTIONS

Aspirin, indomethacin, and other NSAIDs: increased risk of GI distress and bleeding. Give together cautiously.
Barbiturates, phenytoin, rifampin: decreased corticosteroid effect. Increase corticosteroid dosage, as ordered.
Oral anticoagulants: altered dosage requirements. Monitor PT closely.
Potassium-depleting drugs, such as thiazide diuretics: enhanced potassium-wasting effects of methylprednisolone. Monitor serum potassium levels.
Skin-test antigens: decreased response. Defer skin testing until therapy is completed.
Toxoids and vaccines: decreased antibody response and increased risk of neurologic complications. Avoid concomitant use.

CONTRAINDICATIONS

Contraindicated in patients allergic to any component of the formulation, in those with systemic fungal infections and in premature infants (acetate and succinate).

NURSING CONSIDERATIONS

• Use cautiously in patients with GI

ulceration or renal disease, hypertension, osteoporosis, diabetes mellitus, hypothyroidism, cirrhosis, diverticulitis, nonspecific ulcerative colitis, recent intestinal anastomoses, thromboembolic disorders, seizures, myasthenia gravis, CHF, tuberculosis, ocular herpes simplex, emotional instability, and psychotic tendencies.

• Know that drug may be used for alternate-day therapy.

• For better results and less toxicity, give a once-daily dose in the morning.

• Give oral dose with food when possible. Know that critically ill patients may require concomitant antacid or H_2-receptor antagonist therapy.

• **I.V. use:** Use only methylprednisolone sodium succinate; never use acetate form for I.V. use. Reconstitute according to the manufacturer's directions using the supplied diluent, or use bacteriostatic water for injection with benzyl alcohol.

• When administering as direct injection, inject diluted drug into a vein or free-flowing compatible I.V. solution over at least 1 minute. For treatment of shock, give massive doses over at least 10 minutes to prevent arrhythmias and circulatory collapse. When administering as an intermittent or continuous infusion, dilute solution according to the manufacturer's instructions and give over the prescribed duration. If used for continuous infusion, change solution every 24 hours.

• Compatible solutions include D_5W, 0.9% sodium chloride, and dextrose 5% in 0.9% sodium chloride.

• Do not confuse Solu-Medrol with Solu-Cortef (hydrocortisone sodium succinate).

• The manufacturers of Solu-Medrol state that the drug should not be given intrathecally because severe adverse reactions have been reported.

• Give I.M. injection deeply into gluteal muscle. Avoid S.C. injection because atrophy and sterile abscesses may occur.

• Dermal atrophy may occur with large doses of acetate salt. Use multiple small injections rather than a single large dose and rotate injection sites.

• Don't use acetate salt when immediate onset of action is needed.

• Discard reconstituted solutions after 48 hours.

• Always titrate to lowest effective dose, as ordered.

• Monitor patients' weight, blood pressure, serum electrolyte levels, and sleep patterns. Euphoria may initially interfere with sleep, but patients generally adjust to the medication after 1 to 3 weeks.

• Know that drug may mask or exacerbate infections, including latent amebiasis.

• Watch for depression or psychotic episodes, especially in high-dose therapy.

• Diabetic patients may need increased insulin; monitor blood glucose levels.

• Watch for an enhanced response to drug in patients with hypothyroidism or cirrhosis.

• Unless contraindicated, give low-sodium diet high in potassium and protein. Administer potassium supplements as needed. Watch for additional potassium depletion resulting from diuretic or amphotericin B therapy.

• Know that elderly patients may be more susceptible to osteoporosis.

• Gradually reduce drug dosage after long-term therapy, as ordered.

• Tell patients not to discontinue drug abruptly or without the doctor's consent.

• Teach patients signs of early adrenal insufficiency: fatigue, muscular weakness, joint pain, fever, anorexia, nausea, dyspnea, dizziness, and fainting.

• Instruct patients to carry a card

---

*Liquid form contains alcohol.   *Common* reactions are in italics; *life-threatening*, in bold italics.
**May contain tartrazine.

identifying their need for supplemental systemic glucocorticoids during stress.

• Warn patients on long-term therapy about cushingoid symptoms and to report sudden weight gain or swelling to the doctor.

• Advise patient receiving long-term therapy to consider exercise or physical therapy. Also tell patient to ask doctor about vitamin D or calcium supplements.

prednisolone
Delta-Cortef, Deltasolone‡, Panafcortelone‡, Prelone, Solone‡

prednisolone acetate
Articulose-50, Key-Pred 25, Key-Pred 50, Predaject-50, Predalone 50, Predate 50, Predcor-25, Predcor-50, Predicort-50

prednisolone sodium phosphate
Hydeltrasol, Key-Pred-SP, Pediapred, Predate-S, Predicort RP, Predsol Retention Enema‡, Predsol Suppositories‡

prednisolone steaglate
Sintisone‡

prednisolone tebutate
Hydeltra-TBA, Nor-Pred TBA, Predalone TBA, Predate TBA, Predcor TBA

Pregnancy Risk Category: NR

HOW SUPPLIED
prednisolone
Tablets: 1 mg‡, 5 mg, 25 mg‡
Syrup: 15 mg/5 ml
prednisolone acetate
Injection (suspension): 25 mg/ml, 50 mg/ml, 100 mg/ml
prednisolone acetate and prednisolone sodium phosphate
Injection (suspension): 80 mg acetate and 20 mg sodium phosphate/ml

prednisolone sodium phosphate
Oral solution: 5 mg/5 ml
Injection: 20 mg/ml
Retention enema: 20 mg/100 ml‡
Suppositories: 5 mg‡
prednisolone steaglate
Tablets: 6.65 mg (equal to 3.5 mg prednisolone)‡
prednisolone tebutate
Injection (suspension): 20 mg/ml

ACTION
Not clearly defined. Decreases inflammation, mainly by stabilizing leukocyte lysosomal membranes; suppresses the immune response; stimulates bone marrow; and influences protein, fat, and carbohydrate metabolism.

ONSET, PEAK, DURATION
Onset occurs rapidly after I.V., I.M., or oral administration; 1 to 2 days after intralesional or intra-articular use of tebutate suspension. Peak levels occur within 1 hour of I.M. or I.V. injection or within 1 to 2 hours of oral administration. Effects persist 30 to 36 hours after oral use; up to 4 weeks after I.M. use, or 3 days to 4 weeks after intralesional or intra-articular use.

INDICATIONS & DOSAGE
Severe inflammation or immunosuppression –
Adults: 2.5 to 15 mg P.O. b.i.d., t.i.d., or q.i.d.; 2 to 30 mg I.M. (acetate, phosphate) or I.V. (phosphate) q 12 hours; or 2 to 30 mg (phosphate) into joints, lesions, or soft tissue; or 4 to 40 mg (tebutate) into joints and lesions; or 0.25 to 1 ml (sodium phosphate-acetate suspension) into joints weekly, p.r.n.
Proctitis‡ –
Adults: 1 suppository b.i.d., preferably in the morning and h.s.
Ulcerative colitis‡ –
Adults: 1 retention enema h.s. nightly for 2 to 4 weeks. The contents of the

---

†Available in Canada only.   ‡Available in Australia only.   ◇Available OTC.

enema should be retained overnight.

ADVERSE REACTIONS
Most adverse reactions to corticosteroids are dose- or duration-dependent.
CNS: *euphoria, insomnia,* psychotic behavior, pseudotumor cerebri.
CV: *CHF,* hypertension, edema.
EENT: cataracts, glaucoma.
GI: *peptic ulceration,* GI irritation, increased appetite, pancreatitis.
Skin: delayed wound healing, acne, various skin eruptions.
Other: muscle weakness, osteoporosis, hirsutism, susceptibility to infections; hypokalemia, hyperglycemia, and carbohydrate intolerance; growth suppression in children; *acute adrenal insufficiency may occur with increased stress (infection, surgery, or trauma) or abrupt withdrawal after long-term therapy.*
After abrupt withdrawal: rebound inflammation, fatigue, weakness, arthralgia, fever, dizziness, lethargy, depression, fainting, orthostatic hypotension, dyspnea, anorexia, hypoglycemia. *After prolonged use, sudden withdrawal may be fatal.*

INTERACTIONS
Aspirin, indomethacin, and other NSAIDs: increased risk of GI distress and bleeding. Give together cautiously.
Barbiturates, phenytoin, rifampin: decreased corticosteroid effect. Increase corticosteroid dosage, as ordered.
Oral anticoagulants: altered dosage requirements. Monitor PT closely.
Potassium-depleting drugs, such as thiazide diuretics: enhanced potassium-wasting effects of prednisolone. Monitor serum potassium levels.
Skin-test antigens: decreased response. Defer skin testing until therapy is completed.
Toxoids and vaccines: decreased antibody response and increased risk of

neurologic complications. Avoid concomitant use.

CONTRAINDICATIONS
Contraindicated in patients with hypersensitivity to drug or any of its ingredients and systemic fungal infections.

NURSING CONSIDERATIONS
● Use with extreme caution in a patient with recent MI.
● Use cautiously in patients with GI ulcer, renal disease, hypertension, osteoporosis, diabetes mellitus, hypothyroidism, cirrhosis, diverticulitis, nonspecific ulcerative colitis, recent intestinal anastomoses, thromboembolic disorders, seizures, myasthenia gravis, CHF, tuberculosis, ocular herpes simplex, emotional instability, and psychotic tendencies.
● Don't confuse with prednisone.
● Always titrate to lowest effective dose, as ordered.
● Be aware that prednisolone salts (acetate, sodium phosphate, and tebutate) are used parenterally less often than other corticosteroids that have more potent anti-inflammatory action.
● Know that drug may be used for alternate-day therapy.
● Give oral dose with food when possible to reduce GI irritation.
● Give I.M. injection deeply into gluteal muscle. Rotate injection sites to prevent muscle atrophy. Avoid S.C. injection because atrophy and sterile abscesses may occur.
● **I.V. use:** Use only prednisolone sodium phosphate; never give acetate form I.V. When administering as direct injection, inject undiluted over at least 1 minute. When administering as an intermittent or continuous infusion, dilute solution according to the manufacturer's instructions and give over the prescribed duration. D_5W or 0.9% sodium chloride are recommended as diluents for I.V. infusions.

---

*Liquid form contains alcohol.   *Common* reactions are in italics; *life-threatening,* in bold italics.
**May contain tartrazine.

- Monitor patients' weight, blood pressure, and serum electrolyte levels.
- Watch for depression or psychotic episodes, especially in high-dose therapy.
- Diabetic patients may need increased insulin; monitor blood glucose levels.
- Unless contraindicated, give low-sodium diet high in potassium and protein. Administer potassium supplements as needed. Watch for additional potassium depletion resulting from diuretic or amphotericin B therapy.
- Know that drug may mask or exacerbate infections, including latent amebiasis.
- Know elderly patients may be more susceptible to osteoporosis.
- Gradually reduce drug dosage after long-term therapy as ordered.
- Tell patients not to discontinue drug abruptly or without the doctor's consent.
- Teach patients signs of early adrenal insufficiency: fatigue, muscular weakness, joint pain, fever, anorexia, nausea, dyspnea, dizziness, and fainting.
- Instruct patients to carry a card identifying their need for supplemental systemic glucocorticoids during stress.
- Warn patients on long-term therapy about cushingoid symptoms and to report sudden weight gain or swelling to the doctor.
- Tell patients to report slow healing.
- Advise patient receiving long-term therapy to consider exercise or physical therapy. Also tell patient to ask doctor about vitamin D or calcium supplements.

prednisone

Apo-Prednisone†, Deltasone, Liquid Pred*, Meticorten, Novo-prednisone†, Orasone, Panafcort‡, Panasol, Prednicen-M, Prednisone Intensol*, Sone‡, Sterapred, Winpred†

Pregnancy Risk Category: NR

HOW SUPPLIED
Tablets: 1 mg, 2.5 mg, 5 mg, 10 mg, 20 mg, 25 mg, 50 mg
Oral solution: 5 mg/5 ml*, 5 mg/ml (concentrate)*
Syrup: 5 mg/5 ml*

ACTION
Not clearly defined. Decreases inflammation, mainly by stabilizing leukocyte lysosomal membranes; suppresses the immune response; stimulates bone marrow; and influences protein, fat, and carbohydrate metabolism.

ONSET, PEAK, DURATION
Variable.

INDICATIONS & DOSAGE
Severe inflammation or immunosuppression –
Adults: 2.5 to 15 mg P.O. daily in divided doses. Maintenance dosage given once daily or every other day. Dosage must be individualized.
Acute exacerbations of multiple sclerosis –
Adults: 200 mg P.O. daily for 1 week; then 80 mg P.O. every other day for 1 month.

ADVERSE REACTIONS
Most adverse reactions to corticosteroids are dose- or duration-dependent.
CNS: *euphoria, insomnia,* psychotic behavior, pseudotumor cerebri.
CV: *CHF,* hypertension, edema.
EENT: cataracts, glaucoma.

---

†Available in Canada only.   ‡Available in Australia only.   ◊Available OTC.

GI: *peptic ulceration,* GI irritation, increased appetite, pancreatitis.
Skin: delayed wound healing, acne, various skin eruptions.
Other: muscle weakness, osteoporosis, hirsutism, susceptibility to infections; hypokalemia, hyperglycemia, and carbohydrate intolerance; growth suppression in children; *acute adrenal insufficiency may occur with increased stress (infection, surgery, or trauma) or abrupt withdrawal after long-term therapy.*
After abrupt withdrawal: rebound inflammation, fatigue, weakness, arthralgia, fever, dizziness, lethargy, depression, fainting, orthostatic hypotension, dyspnea, anorexia, hypoglycemia. *After prolonged use, sudden withdrawal may be fatal.*

INTERACTIONS

Aspirin, indomethacin, and other NSAIDs: increased risk of GI distress and bleeding. Give together cautiously.
Barbiturates, phenytoin, rifampin: decreased corticosteroid effect. Increase corticosteroid dosage, as ordered.
Oral anticoagulants: altered dosage requirements. Monitor PT closely.
Potassium-depleting drugs, such as thiazide diuretics: enhanced potassium-wasting effects of prednisone. Monitor serum potassium levels.
Skin-test antigens: decreased response. Defer skin testing until therapy is completed.
Toxoids and vaccines: decreased antibody response and increased risk of neurologic complications. Avoid concomitant use.

CONTRAINDICATIONS

Contraindicated in patients with hypersensitivity to drug or systemic fungal infections.

NURSING CONSIDERATIONS

• Use cautiously in patients with GI ulcer, renal disease, hypertension, osteoporosis, diabetes mellitus, hypothyroidism, cirrhosis, diverticulitis, nonspecific ulcerative colitis, recent intestinal anastomoses, thromboembolic disorders, seizures, myasthenia gravis, CHF, tuberculosis, ocular herpes simplex, emotional instability, and psychotic tendencies.
• Don't confuse with prednisolone.
• Know that drug may be used for alternate-day therapy.
• Always titrate to lowest effective dose as ordered.
• For better results and less toxicity, give a once-daily dose in the morning.
• Unless contraindicated, give oral dose with food when possible to reduce GI irritation.
• Monitor patients' blood pressure, sleep patterns, and serum potassium levels.
• Weigh patients daily; report sudden weight gain to the doctor.
• Watch for depression or psychotic episodes, especially in high-dose therapy.
• Diabetic patients may need increased insulin; monitor blood glucose levels.
• Know elderly patients may be more susceptible to osteoporosis.
• Know that drug may mask or exacerbate infections, including latent amebiasis.
• Unless contraindicated, give low-sodium diet high in potassium and protein. Administer potassium supplements as needed. Watch for additional potassium depletion resulting from diuretic or amphotericin B therapy.
• Gradually reduce drug dosage after long-term therapy, as ordered.
• Tell patients not to discontinue drug abruptly or without the doctor's consent.
• Teach patients signs of early adrenal insufficiency: fatigue, muscular weakness, joint pain, fever, anorexia, nausea, dyspnea, dizziness, and fainting.

---

*Liquid form contains alcohol.
**May contain tartrazine.
Common reactions are in italics; *life-threatening,* in bold italics.

• Instruct patients to carry a card identifying their need for supplemental systemic glucocorticoids during stress.

• Warn patients on long-term therapy about cushingoid symptoms and to report sudden weight gain or swelling to the doctor.

• Advise patient receiving long-term therapy to consider exercise or physical therapy. Also tell patient to ask doctor about vitamin D or calcium supplements.

• Tell patients to report slow healing.

• Advise patients receiving long-term therapy to have periodic ophthalmic examinations.

triamcinolone
Aristocort, Atolone, Kenacort**

triamcinolone acetonide
Cenocort A-40, Cinonide 40, Kenaject-40, Kenalog-10, Kenalog-40, Tac-3, Triam-A, Triamonide 40, Tri-Kort, Trilog

triamcinolone diacetate
Amcort, Aristocort, Aristocort Forte, Aristocort Intralesional, Articulose-L.A., Cenocort Forte, Cinalone 40, Kenacort Diacetate, Triam-Forte, Triamolone 40, Trilone, Tristoject

triamcinolone hexacetonide
Aristospan Intra-articular, Aristospan Intralesional

Pregnancy Risk Category: C

HOW SUPPLIED
triamcinolone
Tablets: 1 mg, 2 mg, 4 mg, 8 mg
Syrup: 2 mg/ml, 4 mg/ml
triamcinolone acetonide
Injection (suspension): 3 mg/ml, 10 mg/ml, 40 mg/ml
triamcinolone diacetate

Injection (suspension): 25 mg/ml, 40 mg/ml
triamcinolone hexacetonide
Injection (suspension): 5 mg/ml, 20 mg/ml

ACTION
Not clearly defined. Decreases inflammation, mainly by stabilizing leukocyte lysosomal membranes; suppresses the immune response; stimulates bone marrow; and influences protein, fat, and carbohydrate metabolism.

ONSET, PEAK, DURATION
Highly variable.

INDICATIONS & DOSAGE
Severe inflammation or immunosuppression –
Adults: 4 to 48 mg P.O. daily in divided doses; 40 mg I.M. (diacetate, acetonide) weekly; 5 to 48 mg (diacetate, acetonide) into lesions; 2 to 40 mg (diacetate, acetonide) into joints or soft tissue; up to 0.5 mg (hexacetonide) per square inch of affected skin intralesionally; or 2 to 20 mg (hexacetonide) by intra-articular or intrasynovial use into soft tissue or into joint or lesion. A local anesthetic often is injected along with triamcinolone into the joint.

ADVERSE REACTIONS
Most adverse reactions to corticosteroids are dose- or duration-dependent.
CNS: *euphoria, insomnia,* psychotic behavior, pseudotumor cerebri.
CV: *CHF,* hypertension, edema.
EENT: cataracts, glaucoma.
GI: *peptic ulceration,* GI irritation, increased appetite, pancreatitis.
Skin: delayed wound healing, acne, various skin eruptions.
Other: muscle weakness, osteoporosis, hirsutism, susceptibility to infections; hypokalemia, hyperglycemia, and carbohydrate intolerance;

growth suppression in children; *acute adrenal insufficiency may occur with increased stress (infection, surgery, or trauma) or abrupt withdrawal after long-term therapy.*

After abrupt withdrawal: rebound inflammation, fatigue, weakness, arthralgia, fever, dizziness, lethargy, depression, fainting, orthostatic hypotension, dyspnea, anorexia, hypoglycemia. *After prolonged use, sudden withdrawal may be fatal.*

INTERACTIONS
Aspirin, indomethacin, and other NSAIDs: increased risk of GI distress and bleeding. Give together cautiously.
Barbiturates, phenytoin, rifampin: decreased corticosteroid effect. Increase corticosteroid dosage, as ordered.
Oral anticoagulants: altered dosage requirements. Monitor PT closely.
Potassium-depleting drugs, such as thiazide diuretics: enhanced potassium-wasting effects of triamcinolone. Monitor serum potassium levels.
Skin-test antigens: decreased response. Defer skin testing until therapy is completed.
Toxoids and vaccines: decreased antibody response and increased risk of neurologic complications. Avoid concomitant use.

CONTRAINDICATIONS
Contraindicated in patients hypersensitive to any component of the formulation or in those with systemic fungal infections.

NURSING CONSIDERATIONS
• Use cautiously in patients with GI ulcer, renal disease, hypertension, osteoporosis, diabetes mellitus, hypothyroidism, cirrhosis, diverticulitis, nonspecific ulcerative colitis, recent intestinal anastomoses, thromboembolic disorders, seizures, myasthenia gravis, CHF, tuberculosis, ocular herpes simplex, emotional instability, and psychotic tendencies.
• Know drug not used for alternate-day therapy.
• Always titrate to lowest effective dose, as ordered.
• For better results and less toxicity, give a once-daily dose in the morning.
• Give oral dose with food when possible to reduce GI irritation.
• Parenteral form is *not* for I.V. use.
• Don't use diluents that contain preservatives; flocculation may occur.
• Give I.M. injection deeply into gluteal muscle. Rotate injection sites to prevent muscle atrophy.
• Monitor patients' weight, blood pressure, and serum electrolyte levels.
• Watch for depression or psychotic episodes, especially in high-dose therapy.
• Diabetic patients may need increased insulin; monitor blood glucose levels.
• Know that drug may mask or exacerbate infections, including latent amebiasis.
• Know elderly patients may be more susceptible to osteoporosis.
• Unless contraindicated, give low-sodium diet high in potassium and protein. Administer potassium supplements as needed. Watch for additional potassium depletion resulting from diuretic or amphotericin B therapy.
• Gradually reduce drug dosage after long-term therapy, as ordered.
• Tell patients not to discontinue drug abruptly or without the doctor's consent.
• Teach patients signs of early adrenal insufficiency: fatigue, muscular weakness, joint pain, fever, anorexia, nausea, dyspnea, dizziness, and fainting.
• Instruct patients to carry a card identifying their need for supplemental systemic glucocorticoids during stress.
• Warn patients on long-term therapy

about cushingoid symptoms and to report sudden weight gain and swelling to the doctor.
• Tell patients to report slow healing.
• Advise patient receiving long-term therapy to consider exercise or physical therapy. Also tell patient to ask doctor about vitamin D or calcium supplements.

54

Androgens and anabolic steroids

danazol
fluoxymesterone
methyltestosterone
nandrolone decanoate
nandrolone phenpropionate
oxandrolone
oxymetholone
stanozolol
testosterone
testosterone cypionate
testosterone enanthate
testosterone propionate
testosterone transdermal system

COMBINATION PRODUCTS

DEPANDROGEN, DEPO-TESTADIOL, DEPOTESTOGEN, DUO-CYP, DURATESTRIN, TEST EST CYP (oil): testosterone cypionate 50 mg and estradiol cypionate 2 mg.
ANDROGYN L.A., DELADUMONE, VALERTEST NO. 1: testosterone enanthate 90 mg/ml and estradiol valerate 4 mg/ml in sesame oil.
ESTRATEST: esterified estrogens 1.25 mg and methyltestosterone 2.5 mg.
ESTRATEST H.S.: esterified estrogens 0.625 mg and methyltestosterone 1.25 mg.
HALODRIN: fluoxymesterone 1 mg with ethinyl estradiol 0.02 mg.
PREMARIN WITH METHYLTESTOSTERONE: conjugated estrogens 0.625 mg and methyltestosterone 5 mg; or conjugated estrogens 1.25 mg and methyltestosterone 10 mg.

danazol
Cyclomen†, Danocrine
Pregnancy Risk Category: X

HOW SUPPLIED
Capsules: 50 mg, 100 mg, 200 mg

ACTION
Not clearly defined. Gonadotropin inhibitor that suppresses the pituitary-ovarian axis and inhibits estrogenic effects.

ONSET, PEAK, DURATION
Onset for pain relief for fibrocystic breast disease occurs within 1 month. Unknown for other indications. Peak effects occur in 6 to 8 weeks when treating endometriosis and in 2 to 3 months when treating fibrocystic breast disease. Unknown for treatment of angioedema. Duration variable.

INDICATIONS & DOSAGE
Mild endometriosis –
Women: initially, 100 to 200 mg P.O. b.i.d. Subsequent dosage based on patient response.
Moderate to severe endometriosis –
Women: 400 mg P.O. b.i.d. uninterrupted for 3 to 6 months; may be continued for 9 months.
Fibrocystic breast disease –
Women: 100 to 400 mg P.O. daily in two divided doses uninterrupted for 2 to 6 months.
Prevention of hereditary angioedema –
Adults: 200 mg P.O. b.i.d to t.i.d., continued until favorable response is achieved. Then dosage decreased 50% at 1- to 3-month intervals.

ADVERSE REACTIONS
CNS: dizziness, headache, sleep disorders, fatigue, tremor, irritability, excitation, lethargy, mental depression, chills, paresthesia.
CV: elevated blood pressure.
EENT: visual disturbances.
GI: gastric irritation, nausea, vomit-

---

*Liquid form contains alcohol.
**May contain tartrazine.

Common reactions are in italics; *life-threatening,* in bold italics.

ing, diarrhea, constipation, change in appetite.
GU: hematuria.
Hematologic: thrombocytopenia, elevated serum lipid levels.
Hepatic: reversible jaundice, peliosis hepatis, elevated liver enzyme levels, *liver cell tumors*.
Other: muscle cramps or spasms; androgenic effects in women *(weight gain, hirsutism,* hoarseness, clitoral enlargement, *decrease in breast size,* changes in libido, *oily skin or hair,* voice deepening); hypoestrogenic effects (flushing, diaphoresis, vaginitis [including itching, dryness, and burning]; vaginal bleeding, nervousness, emotional lability, menstrual irregularities).

INTERACTIONS
None significant.

CONTRAINDICATIONS
Contraindicated in patients with undiagnosed abnormal genital bleeding, porphyria, or impaired renal, cardiac, or hepatic function; during pregnancy; and in breast-feeding patients.

NURSING CONSIDERATIONS
• Use cautiously in patients with seizure disorder or migraine headache.
• Avoid use in women of childbearing age until pregnancy is ruled out.
• Make sure patient understands the importance of using an effective non-hormonal contraceptive during therapy.
• Unless contraindicated, use with diet high in calories and protein.
• Monitor closely for signs of virilization. Some androgenic effects, such as deepening of voice, may not be reversible upon discontinuation of drug.
• Periodically evaluate hepatic function as ordered. Semen evaluation is routinely performed every 3 to 4 months, especially in adolescent males.
• Know that periodic dosage de-

creases or gradual drug withdrawal is best.
• After withdrawal of treatment, ovulation and cyclic menstrual bleeding usually return in 2 to 3 months; fibrocystic disease symptoms return within 1 year for 50% of patients.
• Advise patients taking danazol for fibrocystic breast disease to examine breasts regularly and to call the doctor immediately if breast nodule enlarges during treatment.
• Advise washing after intercourse to decrease the risk of vaginitis. Instruct patients to wear only cotton underwear.

---

fluoxymesterone
Android-F, Halotestin**
Controlled Substance Schedule III
Pregnancy Risk Category: X

HOW SUPPLIED
Tablets: 2 mg, 5 mg, 10 mg

ACTION
Stimulates target tissues to develop normally in androgen-deficient men.

ONSET, PEAK, DURATION
Unknown.

INDICATIONS & DOSAGE
Hypogonadism caused by testicular deficiency –
Adults: 5 to 20 mg P.O. daily.
Delayed puberty –
Adolescent: Highly individualized; duration of therapy 4 to 6 months.
Palliation of breast cancer in women –
Adults: 10 to 40 mg P.O. daily in divided doses. All dosages individualized and reduced to minimum when effect is noted.

ADVERSE REACTIONS
CV: edema.
GI: gastroenteritis, nausea, vomiting, constipation, change in appetite.
GU: bladder irritability.

Hematologic: thrombocytopenia, elevated serum lipid levels.

Hepatic: reversible jaundice, peliosis hepatis, elevated liver enzyme levels, *liver cell tumors*.

Other: hypercalcemia; androgenic effects in women (acne, edema, *weight gain, hirsutism,* hoarseness, clitoral enlargement, *decrease in breast size,* changes in libido, male-pattern baldness, *oily skin or hair); hypoestrogenic effects in women (flushing; diaphoresis; vaginitis, including itching, dryness, and burning; vaginal bleeding; nervousness; emotional lability; menstrual irregularities); excessive hormonal effects in men (prepubertal— premature epiphyseal closure, acne,* priapism, *growth of body and facial hair,* phallic enlargement; postpubertal—testicular atrophy, oligospermia, decreased ejaculatory volume, impotence, gynecomastia, epididymitis).

INTERACTIONS

Hepatotoxic medications: increased risk of hepatotoxicity. Monitor closely.

Insulin, oral antidiabetic agents: altered dosage requirements. Monitor blood glucose levels in diabetic patients.

Oral anticoagulants: altered dosage requirements. Monitor PT.

CONTRAINDICATIONS

Contraindicated in patients with hypersensitivity to drug, in males with breast cancer or prostate cancer, in those with cardiac, hepatic, or renal decompensation; during pregnancy; and in breast-feeding patients.

NURSING CONSIDERATIONS

• Use cautiously in prepubertal males, benign prostatic hypertrophy, and aspirin sensitivity.

• Avoid use in women of childbearing age until pregnancy is ruled out.

• Unless contraindicated, use with diet high in calories and protein. Give small, frequent feedings.

• Watch for symptoms of jaundice and periodically evaluate hepatic function, as ordered. Dosage adjustment may reverse condition. If liver function test results are abnormal, notify doctor as therapy should be stopped.

• Know that edema can be controlled with sodium restriction or diuretics. Monitor weight routinely.

• Monitor male patients for signs of excessive sexual stimulation or priapism.

• Be aware semen evaluation is routinely performed every 3 to 4 months, especially in adolescent males.

• Know that hypercalcemia symptoms may be difficult to distinguish from symptoms associated with condition being treated, unless anticipated and thought of as a symptom cluster. Hypercalcemia is particularly likely to occur in patients with metastatic breast cancer and may indicate bone metastases.

• Observe patients on concomitant anticoagulant therapy for ecchymotic areas, petechiae, or abnormal bleeding. Monitor PT.

• Watch for symptoms of hypoglycemia in diabetic patients. Check blood glucose levels. Dosage of antidiabetic drug may need adjustment.

• Know that when used in breast cancer, subjective effects may not occur for about 1 month; objective effects on clinical symptoms may take 3 months.

• If GI upset occurs, tell patient to take drug with food or meals.

• Make sure patient understands the importance of using an effective nonhormonal contraceptive during therapy.

• Advise washing after intercourse to decrease the risk of vaginitis. Instruct patients to wear only cotton underwear.

• Tell women to report menstrual ir-

---

*Liquid form contains alcohol.   *Common* reactions are in italics; ***life-threatening,*** in bold italics.
**May contain tartrazine.

regularities and to discontinue therapy pending etiologic determination.
• Explain to patients taking drug for palliation of breast cancer that virilization usually occurs. Give emotional support. Tell patients to report androgenic effects immediately. Stopping drug will prevent further androgenic changes but will probably not reverse existing effects.

methyltestosterone

Android, Metandren**, Metandren Linguets, Oreton Methyl, Testomet‡, Testred, Virilon
Controlled Substance Schedule III

Pregnancy Risk Category: X

HOW SUPPLIED
Tablets: 5 mg‡, 10 mg, 25 mg, 50 mg‡
Tablets (buccal): 5 mg, 10 mg
Capsules: 10 mg

ACTION
Stimulates target tissues to develop normally in androgen-deficient men.

ONSET, PEAK, DURATION
Onset and duration unknown. Serum levels peak in 1 hour after buccal administration and 2 hours after oral administration.

INDICATIONS & DOSAGE
Postpartum breast engorgement in non-breast-feeding women–
Adults: 80 mg P.O. daily, or 40 mg buccally daily for 3 to 5 days.
Breast cancer in women 1 to 5 years postmenopausal–
Adults: 50 to 200 mg P.O. daily; or 25 to 100 mg buccally daily.
Male hypogonadism–
Adults: 10 to 50 mg P.O. daily; or 5 to 25 mg buccally daily.
Postpubertal cryptorchidism–
Adults: 30 mg P.O. daily; or 15 mg buccally daily.

ADVERSE REACTIONS
CV: edema.
EENT: irritation of oral mucosa (with buccal administration).
GI: gastroenteritis, constipation, nausea, vomiting, diarrhea, change in appetite.
GU: bladder irritability.
Hepatic: reversible jaundice, cholestatic hepatitis, abnormal liver enzyme levels.
Other: hypercalcemia; muscle cramps or spasms; androgenic effects in women (acne, edema, *weight gain, hirsutism,* hoarseness, clitoral enlargement, *decrease in breast size,* changes in libido, male-pattern baldness, *oily skin or hair); hypoestrogenic effects in women (flushing; diaphoresis; vaginitis, including itching, dryness, and burning; vaginal bleeding; nervousness; emotional lability; menstrual irregularities); excessive hormonal effects in men (prepubertal– premature epiphyseal closure, acne, priapism, growth of body and facial hair,* phallic enlargement; postpubertal – testicular atrophy, oligospermia, decreased ejaculatory volume, impotence, gynecomastia, epididymitis).

INTERACTIONS
Hepatotoxic medications: increased risk of hepatotoxicity. Monitor closely.
Insulin, oral antidiabetic agents: altered dosage requirements. Monitor blood glucose levels in diabetic patients.
Oral anticoagulants: altered dosage requirements. Monitor PT.

CONTRAINDICATIONS
Contraindicated in pregnant and breast-feeding patients or in males with breast cancer or prostate cancer.

NURSING CONSIDERATIONS
• Use cautiously in elderly patients; patients with cardiac, renal, or he-

---

patic disease; or healthy males with delayed puberty.

• Avoid use in women of childbearing age until pregnancy is ruled out.

• In children, X-rays of the wrist bones should be taken before therapy to establish the level of bone maturation. During treatment, bone maturation may proceed more rapidly than linear growth; ensure intermittent dosage and periodically review X-ray results to monitor bone maturation.

• Typically used only for intermittent therapy. Because of potential hepatotoxicity, watch closely for jaundice.

• Watch for ecchymoses, petechiae, and abnormal bleeding in patients receiving concomitant anticoagulants.

• Promptly report signs of virilization in women.

• Unless contraindicated, use with diet high in calories and protein. Give small, frequent feedings.

• Periodically check hemoglobin and hematocrit values, serum cholesterol and calcium levels, and cardiac and liver function test results, as ordered.

• Check weight regularly. Edema can be controlled with sodium restriction or diuretics.

• Therapeutic response in breast cancer is usually apparent within 3 months. Know therapy should be stopped if signs of disease progression appear.

• Report signs of hypercalcemia. In metastatic breast cancer, hypercalcemia may indicate progression of bone metastases.

• Know semen evaluation is routinely performed every 3 to 4 months, especially in adolescent males.

• Make sure patient understands the importance of using an effective non-hormonal contraceptive during therapy.

• Buccal tablets are twice as potent as oral tablets. Tell patients to avoid eating, drinking, chewing, or smoking while buccal tablet is in place and not to swallow tablet. Place in upper or lower buccal pouch between cheek and gum; tablet requires 30 to 60 minutes to dissolve. Instruct patients to change tablet absorption site with each dose to minimize risk of buccal irritation.

• Enhances hypoglycemia; teach patient signs of hypoglycemia and method for checking blood glucose level. Instruct patients to report hypoglycemia immediately.

• Advise washing after intercourse to decrease the risk of vaginitis. Instruct patients to wear only cotton underwear.

nandrolone decanoate
Anabolin LA, Androlone-D, Deca-Durabolin, Decolone, Hybolin Decanoate, Kabolin, Nandrobolic L.A., Neo-Durabolic

nandrolone phenpropionate
Anabolin IM, Androlone, Durabolin, Hybolin Improved, Nandrobolic
Controlled Substance Schedule III

Pregnancy Risk Category: X

HOW SUPPLIED
nandrolone decanoate
Injection (in oil): 50 mg/ml, 100 mg/ml, 200 mg/ml
nandrolone phenpropionate
Injection (in oil): 25 mg/ml, 50 mg/ml

ACTION
Anabolic steroid that promotes tissue-building processes, reverses catabolism, and stimulates erythropoiesis.

ONSET, PEAK, DURATION
Onset and duration unknown. Serum levels peak in 1 to 2 days (phenpropionate) or 3 to 6 days (decanoate).

INDICATIONS & DOSAGE
Severe debility or disease states, refractory anemias –

---

*Liquid form contains alcohol.
May contain tartrazine.   *Common* reactions are in italics; ***life-threatening,* in bold italics.

Adults: 50 to 100 mg decanoate I.M. at 1 to 4 week intervals for females; 50 to 200 mg decanoate I.M. at 1 to 4 week intervals for males. Therapy should be intermittent.

Children 2 to 13 years: 25 to 50 mg decanoate I.M. q 3 to 4 weeks.

Control of metastatic breast cancer –
Adults: 25 to 50 mg phenpropionate I.M. weekly.

ADVERSE REACTIONS
CV: edema.
GI: gastroenteritis, nausea, vomiting, diarrhea, change in appetite.
GU: bladder irritability.
Hematologic: thrombocytopenia, elevated serum lipid levels.
Hepatic: reversible jaundice, peliosis hepatis, elevated liver enzyme levels, *liver cell tumors*.
Skin: pain and induration at injection site.
Other: hypercalcemia; muscle cramps or spasms; androgenic effects in women (acne, edema, *weight gain, hirsutism,* hoarseness, clitoral enlargement, *decrease in breast size,* changes in libido, male-pattern baldness, *oily skin or hair); hypoestrogenic effects in women (flushing; diaphoresis; vaginitis, including itching, dryness, and burning; vaginal bleeding; nervousness; emotional lability; menstrual irregularities); excessive hormonal effects in men (prepubertal – premature epiphyseal closure, acne,* priapism, *growth of body and facial hair,* phallic enlargement; postpubertal – testicular atrophy, oligospermia, decreased ejaculatory volume, impotence, gynecomastia, epididymitis).

INTERACTIONS
Hepatotoxic medications: increased risk of hepatotoxicity. Monitor closely.
Insulin, oral antidiabetic agents: altered dosage requirements. Monitor blood glucose levels in diabetic patients.

Oral anticoagulants: altered dosage requirements. Monitor PT.

CONTRAINDICATIONS
Contraindicated in patients with hypersensitivity to anabolic steroids; in males with breast cancer or prostate cancer; in those with nephrosis; in those experiencing the nephrotic phase of nephritis; in females with carcinoma of the breast and hypercalcemia; during pregnancy; or in breast-feeding patients.

NURSING CONSIDERATIONS
• Use cautiously in patients with diabetes; cardiac, renal, or hepatic disease; epilepsy; or migraine or other conditions that may be aggravated by fluid retention.
• Avoid use in women of childbearing age until pregnancy is ruled out.
• In children, X-rays of the wrist bones should be taken before surgery to establish the level of bone maturation. During treatment, bone maturation may proceed more rapidly than linear growth; ensure intermittent dosage and periodically review X-ray results to monitor bone maturation.
• Inject I.M. drug deeply, preferably into upper outer quadrant of gluteal muscle in adults. Rotate injection sites to prevent muscle atrophy.
• Unless contraindicated, use with diet high in calories and protein. Give small, frequent feedings.
• Watch for signs of virilization, which may be irreversible despite prompt discontinuation of therapy.
• Closely observe boys under 7 years for precocious development of male sexual characteristics.
• Know semen evaluation is routinely performed every 3 to 4 months, especially in adolescent males.
• Periodically evaluate hepatic function, as ordered. Watch for jaundice; dosage adjustment may reverse condition. If liver function test results are abnormal, therapy should be stopped.

• Check weight regularly. Edema generally can be controlled with sodium restrictions or diuretics.
• Watch for symptoms of hypoglycemia in diabetic patients. Check blood glucose levels. Adjust dosage of antidiabetic agent, as ordered.
• Check quantitative urine and serum calcium levels. Hypercalcemia is most likely to occur in patients with breast cancer.
• When used to promote erythropoiesis in refractory anemias, make sure patients have adequate daily iron intake.
• Observe patients receiving concomitant anticoagulant therapy for ecchymotic areas, petechiae, or abnormal bleeding. Monitor PT.
• Be aware anabolic steroids may alter results of laboratory studies performed during therapy and for 2 to 3 weeks after therapy ends.
• Make sure patient understands the importance of using an effective nonhormonal contraceptive during therapy.
• Advise washing after intercourse to decrease the risk of vaginitis. Instruct patients to wear only cotton underwear.
• Tell women to report menstrual irregularities and to discontinue therapy pending etiologic determination.

---

oxandrolone
Anavar, Lonavar‡, Oxandrin
Controlled Substance Schedule III

Pregnancy Risk Category: X

HOW SUPPLIED
Tablets: 2.5 mg

ACTION
Anabolic steroid that promotes tissue-building processes, reverses catabolism, and stimulates erythropoiesis.

ONSET, PEAK, DURATION
Unknown.

INDICATIONS & DOSAGE
To combat catabolic effects of corticosteroid therapy, osteoporosis, prolonged immobilization, and debilitated states —
Adults: 2.5 mg P.O. b.i.d., t.i.d., or q.i.d., up to 20 mg daily.
Children: 0.25 mg/kg P.O. daily

ADVERSE REACTIONS
CV: edema.
GI: gastroenteritis, nausea, vomiting, constipation or diarrhea, change in appetite.
GU: bladder irritability.
Hematologic: thrombocytopenia, elevated serum lipid levels.
Hepatic: reversible jaundice, peliosis hepatis, elevated liver enzyme levels, *liver cell tumors.*
Other: hypercalcemia; muscle cramps or spasms; androgenic effects in women (acne, edema, *weight gain, hirsutism,* hoarseness, clitoral enlargement, *decrease in breast size,* changes in libido, male-pattern baldness, *oily skin or hair); hypoestrogenic effects in women (flushing; diaphoresis; vaginitis, including itching, dryness, and burning; vaginal bleeding; nervousness; emotional lability; menstrual irregularities); excessive hormonal effects in men (prepubertal — premature epiphyseal closure, acne,* priapism, *growth of body and facial hair,* phallic enlargement; postpubertal — testicular atrophy, oligospermia, decreased ejaculatory volume, impotence, gynecomastia, epididymitis).

INTERACTIONS
Hepatotoxic medications: increased risk of hepatotoxicity. Monitor closely.
Insulin, oral antidiabetic agents: altered dosage requirements. Monitor blood glucose levels in diabetic patients.
Oral anticoagulants: altered dosage requirements. Monitor PT.

---

*Liquid form contains alcohol.   *Common* reactions are in italics; *life-threatening*, in bold italics.
**May contain tartrazine.

CONTRAINDICATIONS

Contraindicated in patients with hypersensitivity to anabolic steroids, in males with breast cancer or prostate cancer; in those with nephrosis or nephrotic phase of nephritis; in females with carcinoma of the breast and hypercalcemia; during pregnancy; and in breast-feeding patients.

NURSING CONSIDERATIONS

• Use cautiously in patients with diabetes; cardiac, renal, or hepatic disease, epilepsy; or migraine or other conditions that may be aggravated by fluid retention.
• Avoid use in women of childbearing age until pregnancy is ruled out.
• In children, X-rays of the wrist bones should be taken before therapy to establish the level of bone maturation. During treatment, bone maturation may proceed more rapidly than linear growth; ensure intermittent dosage and review X-ray results periodically to monitor bone maturation.
• Unless contraindicated, use with diet high in calories and protein. Give small, frequent feedings.
• When used to promote erythropoiesis, make sure patients have adequate daily iron intake.
• Watch for signs of virilization, which may be irreversible despite prompt discontinuation of therapy. Doctor must decide if benefits outweigh adverse effects.
• Closely observe boys under 7 years for precocious development of male sexual characteristics.
• Know semen evaluation is routinely performed every 3 to 4 months, especially in adolescent males.
• Monitor weight routinely. Edema generally can be controlled with sodium restriction or diuretics.
• Periodically monitor hepatic function. Watch for jaundice. Dosage adjustment may reverse condition. Periodically check liver function test results.

• Watch for symptoms of hypoglycemia in diabetic patients. Check blood glucose levels. Adjust dosage of antidiabetic agent as necessary.
• Observe patients on concomitant anticoagulant therapy for ecchymotic areas, petechiae, or abnormal bleeding. Monitor PT.
• Know anabolic steroids may alter results of laboratory studies performed during therapy and for 2 to 3 weeks after therapy ends.
• Be aware hypercalcemia symptoms may be difficult to distinguish from symptoms of condition being treated, unless anticipated and thought of as a cluster. Hypercalcemia is most likely to occur with metastatic breast cancer and may indicate bone metastases.
• If GI upset occurs, tell patient to take drug with food or meals.
• Make sure the patient understands the importance of using an effective nonhormonal contraceptive during therapy.
• Advise washing after intercourse to decrease the risk of vaginitis. Instruct patients to wear only cotton underwear.
• Tell women to report menstrual irregularities and to discontinue therapy pending etiologic determination.

oxymetholone

Anadrol-50, Anapolon 50†‡
Controlled Substance Schedule III

Pregnancy Risk Category: X

HOW SUPPLIED

Tablets: 50 mg

ACTION

Anabolic steroid that promotes tissue-building processes, reverses catabolism, and stimulates erythropoiesis.

ONSET, PEAK, DURATION

Unknown.

INDICATIONS & DOSAGE
Aplastic anemia –
Adults and children: 1 to 5 mg/kg
P.O. daily. Dosage is highly individualized; and response is not immediate.
A trial of 3 to 6 months is required.

ADVERSE REACTIONS
CV: edema.
GI: gastroenteritis, nausea, vomiting, constipation, diarrhea, change in appetite.
GU: bladder irritability.
Hematologic: thrombocytopenia, elevated serum lipid levels.
Hepatic: reversible jaundice, peliosis hepatis, elevated liver enzyme levels, *liver cell tumors.*
Other: hypercalcemia; muscle cramps or spasms; androgenic effects in women (acne, edema, *weight gain, hirsutism,* hoarseness, clitoral enlargement, *decrease in breast size,* changes in libido, male-pattern baldness, *oily skin or hair); hypoestrogenic effects in women (flushing; diaphoresis; vaginitis, including itching, dryness, and burning; vaginal bleeding; nervousness; emotional lability; menstrual irregularities); excessive hormonal effects in men (prepubertal – premature epiphyseal closure, acne, priapism, growth of body and facial hair,* phallic enlargement; postpubertal – testicular atrophy, oligospermia, decreased ejaculatory volume, impotence, gynecomastia, epididymitis).

INTERACTIONS
Hepatotoxic medications: increased risk of hepatotoxicity. Monitor closely.
Insulin, oral antidiabetic agents: altered dosage requirements. Monitor blood glucose levels in diabetic patients.
Oral anticoagulants: altered dosage requirements. Monitor PT.

CONTRAINDICATIONS
Contraindicated in patients with hypersensitivity to anabolic steroids; in males with breast cancer or prostate cancer; in nephrosis or nephrotic phase of nephritis; in females with carcinoma of the breast and hypercalcemia; during pregnancy; and in breast-feeding patients.

NURSING CONSIDERATIONS
• Use cautiously in patients with diabetes; cardiac, renal or hepatic disease; epilepsy; or migraine or other conditions that may be aggravated by fluid retention.
• Avoid use in women of childbearing age until pregnancy is ruled out.
• In children, X-rays of the wrist bones should be taken before therapy to establish the level of bone maturation. During treatment, bone maturation may proceed more rapidly than linear growth; ensure intermittent dosage and review X-ray results periodically to monitor bone maturation. Epiphyseal development may continue 6 months after stopping therapy.
• Unless contraindicated, use with diet high in calories and protein. Give small, frequent feedings.
• When used to promote erythropoiesis, make sure patients have adequate daily iron intake.
• Watch for signs of virilization, which may be irreversible despite prompt discontinuation of therapy. Doctor must decide if benefits outweigh adverse effects.
• Closely observe boys under 7 years for precocious development of male sexual characteristics.
• Know semen evaluation is routinely performed every 3 to 4 months, especially in adolescent males.
• Periodically evaluate hepatic function. Watch for symptoms of jaundice; dosage adjustment may reverse condition. If liver function test results are abnormal, therapy should be stopped.
• Monitor weight routinely. Edema

---

*Liquid form contains alcohol.
**May contain tartrazine.

Common reactions are in italics; ***life-threatening,*** in bold italics.

generally can be controlled with sodium restriction or diuretics.
• Watch for symptoms of hypoglycemia in diabetic patients. Check blood glucose levels. Adjust dosage of antidiabetic agent as necessary.
• Observe patients on concomitant anticoagulant therapy for ecchymotic areas, petechiae, or abnormal bleeding. Monitor PT.
• Know that anabolic steroids may alter results of laboratory studies performed during therapy and for 2 to 3 weeks after therapy ends.
• Know that hypercalcemia symptoms may be difficult to distinguish from symptoms of condition being treated, unless anticipated and thought of as a cluster. Hypercalcemia is most likely to occur in metastatic breast cancer and may indicate bone metastases.
• If GI upset occurs, tell patient to take with food or meals.
• Make sure patient understands the importance of using an effective nonhormonal contraceptive during therapy.
• Advise washing after intercourse to decrease the risk of vaginitis. Instruct patients to wear only cotton underwear.
• Tell women to report menstrual irregularities and to discontinue therapy pending etiologic determination.

stanozolol
Winstrol
Controlled Substance Schedule III
Pregnancy Risk Category: X

HOW SUPPLIED
Tablets: 2 mg

ACTION
Anabolic steroid that promotes tissue-building processes, reverses catabolism, and stimulates erythropoiesis.

ONSET, PEAK, DURATION
Unknown.

INDICATIONS & DOSAGE
Prevention of hereditary angio-edema —
Adults: initially, 2 mg P.O. t.i.d. to 4 mg q.i.d for 5 days. Dosage gradually reduced at 1- to 3-month intervals to a dosage of 2 mg P.O. daily.
Children under age 6: 1 mg P.O. daily.
Children ages 6 to 12: up to 2 mg P.O. daily.
   Note: Stanozolol is used in children only during an acute attack.

ADVERSE REACTIONS
CV: edema.
GI: gastroenteritis, nausea, vomiting, constipation, diarrhea, change in appetite.
GU: bladder irritability.
Hematologic: thrombocytopenia, elevated serum lipid levels.
Hepatic: reversible jaundice, peliosis hepatis, elevated liver enzyme levels, *liver cell tumors*.
Other: hypercalcemia; muscle cramps or spasms; androgenic effects in women (acne, edema, *weight gain, hirsutism,* hoarseness, clitoral enlargement, *decrease in breast size,* changes in libido, male-pattern baldness, *oily skin or hair); hypoestrogenic effects in women (flushing; diaphoresis; vaginitis, including itching, dryness, and burning; vaginal bleeding; nervousness; emotional lability; menstrual irregularities); excessive hormonal effects in men (prepubertal — premature epiphyseal closure, acne,* priapism, *growth of body and facial hair,* phallic enlargement; postpubertal — testicular atrophy, oligospermia, decreased ejaculatory volume, impotence, gynecomastia, epididymitis).

INTERACTIONS
Hepatotoxic medications: increased risk of hepatotoxicity. Monitor closely.
Insulin, oral antidiabetic agents: altered dosage requirements. Monitor

blood glucose levels in diabetic patients.

Oral anticoagulants: altered dosage requirements. Monitor PT.

CONTRAINDICATIONS

Contraindicated in patients with hypersensitivity to anabolic steroids; in males with breast cancer or prostate cancer; in nephrosis or nephrotic phase of nephritis; in females with carcinoma of the breast and with hypercalcemia; during pregnancy; and in breast-feeding patients.

NURSING CONSIDERATIONS

• Use cautiously in patients with diabetes; cardiac, renal, or hepatic disease; epilepsy; or migraine or other conditions that may be aggravated by fluid retention.
• Avoid use in women of childbearing age until pregnancy is ruled out.
• In children, X-rays of the wrist bones should be taken before therapy to establish the level of bone maturation. During treatment, bone maturation may proceed more rapidly than linear growth; ensure intermittent dosage and review X-ray results periodically to monitor bone maturation.
• Know that a lower dosage in young women (2 mg b.i.d.) is recommended to avoid virilization. Watch for signs of virilization, which may be irreversible despite prompt discontinuation of therapy. Doctor must decide if benefits of therapy outweigh adverse effects.
• To minimize GI distress, administer before or with meals.
• Unless contraindicated, use with diet high in calories and protein. Give small, frequent feedings.
• Closely observe boys under 7 years for precocious development of male sexual characteristics.
• Know semen evaluation is routinely performed every 3 to 4 months, especially in adolescent males.
• Monitor weight routinely. Edema is generally controllable with sodium restriction or diuretics.
• Periodically evaluate hepatic function. Watch for symptoms of jaundice; dosage adjustment may reverse condition. Check liver function test results regularly; if they are abnormal, therapy should be discontinued.
• Monitor serum cholesterol levels.
• Watch for symptoms of hypoglycemia in diabetic patients. Check blood glucose levels. Adjust dosage of antidiabetic agent, as ordered.
• Observe patients on concomitant anticoagulant therapy for ecchymotic areas, petechiae, or abnormal bleeding. Monitor PT.
• Know anabolic steroids may alter results of laboratory studies performed during therapy and for 2 to 3 weeks after therapy ends.
• Make sure patient understands the importance of using an effective nonhormonal contraceptive during therapy.
• Advise washing after intercourse to decrease the risk of vaginitis. Instruct patients to wear only cotton underwear.
• Tell women to report menstrual irregularities and to discontinue therapy pending etiologic determination.

testosterone
Andro 100, Andronaq-50, Histerone-50, Histerone-100, Testamone 100, Testaqua, Testoject-50

testosterone cypionate
Andro-Cyp 100, Andro-Cyp 200, Andronaq-LA, Andronate 100, Andronate 200, depAndro 100, depAndro 200, Depotest, Depo-Testosterone, Duratest-100, Duratest-200, T-Cypionate, Testa-C, Testoject-LA, Testred Cypionate 200, Virilon IM

---

*Liquid form contains alcohol.   *Common* reactions are in italics; ***life-threatening,*** in bold italics.
**May contain tartrazine.

testosterone enanthate

Andro-L.A. 200, Andropository 100, Andryl 200, Delatest, Delatestryl, Durathate-200, Everone, Malogex†, Testone L.A. 200, Testrin-P.A.

testosterone propionate

Malogen†, Testex

Controlled Substance Schedule III

Pregnancy Risk Category: X

HOW SUPPLIED
testosterone
Injection (aqueous suspension): 25 mg/ml, 50 mg/ml, 100 mg/ml
testosterone cypionate
Injection (in oil): 50 mg/ml, 100 mg/ml, 200 mg/ml
testosterone enanthate
Injection (in oil): 100 mg/ml, 200 mg/ml
testosterone propionate
Injection (in oil): 25 mg/ml, 50 mg/ml, 100 mg/ml

ACTION
Stimulates target tissues to develop normally in androgen-deficient men. Testosterone may have some antiestrogen properties, making it useful to treat certain estrogen-dependent breast cancers. Its action in postpartum breast engorgement is not known because testosterone does not suppress lactation.

ONSET, PEAK, DURATION
Unknown.

INDICATIONS & DOSAGE
Male hypogonadism –
Adults: 10 to 25 mg I.M. two to three times weekly, or 50 to 400 mg (cypionate, enanthate) I.M. q 2 to 4 weeks, or 10 to 25 mg (propionate) I.M. two to four times weekly.
Metastatic breast cancer in women 1 to 5 years post menopausal –
Adults: 100 mg I.M. three times weekly; 50 to 100 mg (propionate)

I.M. three times weekly; or 200 to 400 mg (cypionate, enanthate) I.M. q 2 to 4 weeks.
Postpartum breast pain and engorgement –
Adults: 25 to 50 mg I.M. of testoerone or testosterone propionate daily for 3 to 4 days.

ADVERSE REACTIONS
CV: edema.
GI: gastroenteritis, nausea, vomiting, constipation, diarrhea, change in appetite.
GU: bladder irritability.
Hepatic: reversible jaundice, cholestatic hepatitis, abnormal liver enzyme levels.
Skin: pain and induration at injection site, local edema.
Other: hypercalcemia; androgenic effects in women (*acne, edema, oily skin, weight gain, hirsutism, hoarseness,* clitoral enlargement, decreased or increased libido); hypoestrogenic effects in women (flushing; diaphoresis; vaginitis, including itching, drying, and burning; vaginal bleeding; menstrual irregularities); excessive hormonal effects in men (prepubertal – premature epiphyseal closure, *acne,* priapism, *growth of body and facial hair,* phallic enlargement; postpubertal – testicular atrophy, oligospermia, decreased ejaculatory volume, impotence, gynecomastia, epididymitis).

INTERACTIONS
Hepatotoxic medications: increased risk of hepatotoxicity. Monitor closely.
Insulin, oral antidiabetic agents: altered dosage requirements. Monitor blood glucose levels in diabetic patients.
Oral anticoagulants: altered dosage requirements. Monitor PT.

CONTRAINDICATIONS

Contraindicated in male patients with breast or prostate cancer; in patients with hypercalcemia; in those with cardiac, hepatic, or renal decompensation; during pregnancy, and in breast-feeding patients.

NURSING CONSIDERATIONS

• Use cautiously in elderly patients.
• Avoid use in women of childbearing age until pregnancy is ruled out.
• Administer daily dosage requirement in divided doses for best results.
• Store I.M. preparations at room temperature. If crystals appear, warm and shake the bottle to disperse them.
• Inject deep into upper outer quadrant of gluteal muscle. Rotate injection sites to prevent muscle atrophy. Report soreness at site because of the possibility of postinfection furunculosis.
• Unless contraindicated, use with diet high in calories and protein. Give small, frequent feedings.
• Monitor periodic liver function test results, as ordered.
• In metastatic breast cancer, hypercalcemia usually indicates progression of bone metastases. Report signs of hypercalcemia.
• Report signs of virilization in females; doctor will need to reevaluate treatment.
• Watch for ecchymotic areas, petechiae, or abnormal bleeding in patients on concomitant anticoagulant therapy. Monitor PT.
• Monitor weight routinely. Edema generally can be controlled with sodium restriction or diuretics.
• Monitor prepubertal males by X-ray for rate of bone maturation.
• Therapeutic response in breast cancer is usually apparent within 3 months. Know that therapy should be stopped if signs of disease progression appear.
• Know that androgens may alter results of laboratory studies during therapy and for 2 to 3 weeks after therapy ends.
• Make sure patient understands the importance of using an effective nonhormonal contraceptive during therapy.
• Advise washing after intercourse to decrease the risk of vaginitis. Instruct patients to wear only cotton underwear.
• Instruct men to report priapism, reduced ejaculatory volume, and gynecomastia. Notify doctor if these occur as drug needs to be stopped.
• Enhances hypoglycemia; teach patients to recognize signs of hypoglycemia and immediately report them.

---

testosterone transdermal system

Testoderm
Controlled Substance Schedule III
Pregnancy Risk Category: X

HOW SUPPLIED
Transdermal system: 4 mg/day, 6 mg/day

ACTION
Releases testosterone, which stimulates target tissues to develop normally in androgen-deficient men.

ONSET, PEAK, DURATION
Onset unknown. Serum levels peak within 2 to 4 hours after application. Steady-state levels are reached after 3 to 4 weeks of therapy. Testosterone levels decline toward baseline within 2 hours after removal.

INDICATIONS & DOSAGE
Primary or hypogonadotropic hypogonadism in men ages 18 and older—
Adults: one 6 mg/day patch applied to the scrotal area daily. If scrotal area is too small for the 6 mg/day patch, therapy started with the smaller sized 4 mg/day patch. Patch worn for 22 to 24 hours daily.

ADVERSE REACTIONS
CV: *CVA.*
GU: *gynecomastia,* prostatitis, urinary tract infection, breast tenderness.
Skin: acne.
Other: *itching,* discomfort, irritation.

INTERACTIONS
Antidiabetic agents: altered antidiabetic agent dosage requirements. Monitor blood glucose levels.
Oral anticoagulants: altered anticoagulant dosage requirements. Monitor PT.
Oxyphenbutazone: may elevate serum levels of oxyphenbutazone. Monitor patients for adverse reactions.

CONTRAINDICATIONS
Contraindicated in patients hypersensitive to the drug, in women, and men with known or suspected breast or prostate cancer.

NURSING CONSIDERATIONS
• Use cautiously in elderly men because they may be at greater risk for developing prostatic hyperplasia or prostate cancer. Also use cautiously in patients with preexisting renal, hepatic, or cardiac disease.
• Because chronic use of systemic androgens is associated with polycythemia, monitor hematocrit and hemoglobin values periodically in patients on long-term therapy, as ordered.
• Periodically assess liver function tests, serum lipid profiles, and prostatic acid phosphatase and prostate-specific antigen levels as ordered.
• Teach patients how to apply the transdermal system. Warn patients that adequate serum levels will not be attained if the patch is not applied to genital skin.
• Tell patient topical testosterone preparations used by men have caused virilization in female partners. These women should report acne or changes in body hair distribution.

• Advise patients to report persistent erections, nausea, vomiting, changes in skin color, or ankle edema to the doctor.

---

†Available in Canada only.   ‡Available in Australia only.   ◇Available OTC.

55

Estrogens and progestins

chlorotrianisene
dienestrol
diethylstilbestrol
diethylstilbestrol diphosphate
esterified estrogens
estradiol
estradiol cypionate
estradiol valerate
estrogens, conjugated
estrone
estropipate
ethinyl estradiol
ethinyl estradiol and
    desogestrel
ethinyl estradiol and
    ethynodiol diacetate
ethinyl estradiol and
    levonorgestrel
ethinyl estradiol and
    norethindrone
ethinyl estradiol and
    norethindrone acetate
ethinyl estradiol and
    norgestimate
ethinyl estradiol and
    norgestrel
ethinyl estradiol, norethindrone
    acetate, and ferrous fumarate
mestranol and norethindrone
mestranol and norethynodrel
hydroxyprogesterone caproate
levonorgestrel
medroxyprogesterone acetate
norethindrone
norethindrone acetate
norgestrel
progesterone
quinestrol

COMBINATION PRODUCTS
MENRIUM 5-2: chlordiazepoxide 5
mg and esterified estrogens 0.2 mg.
MENRIUM 5-4: chlordiazepoxide 5
mg and esterified estrogens 0.4 mg.
MENRIUM 10-4: chlordiazepoxide
10 mg and esterified estrogens 0.4 mg.

PMB-200: conjugated estrogens 0.45
mg and meprobamate 200 mg.
PMB-400: conjugated estrogens 0.45
mg and meprobamate 400 mg.

---

chlorotrianisene
TACE**

Pregnancy Risk Category: X

HOW SUPPLIED
Capsules: 12 mg, 25 mg

ACTION
Increases the synthesis of DNA,
RNA, and protein in responsive tissues and reduces release of follicle-
stimulating hormone and luteinizing
hormone from the pituitary gland.

ONSET, PEAK, DURATION
Onset and peak unknown. Effects persist for about 24 hours.

INDICATIONS & DOSAGE
Prostate cancer –
Adults: 12 to 25 mg P.O. daily.
Female hypogonadism –
Adults: 12 to 25 mg P.O. for 21 days,
followed by one dose of progesterone
100 mg I.M. or 5 days of oral proges-
togen concurrently with last 5 days of
chlorotrianisene (for example, medroxyprogesterone 5 to 10 mg).
*Vasomotor symptoms associated with
menopausal symptoms, atrophic vaginitis, kraurosis vulvae –*
Adults: 12 to 25 mg P.O. daily for 30
days or cyclic (3 weeks on, 1 week off).

ADVERSE REACTIONS
CNS: headache, dizziness, chorea,
migraine, depression.
CV: thrombophlebitis; ***thromboembolism;*** hypertension; edema; *increased*

---

*Liquid form contains alcohol.   *Common* reactions are in italics; ***life-threatening,*** in bold italics.
**May contain tartrazine.

risk of CVA, pulmonary embolism, and MI.

EENT: worsening of myopia or astigmatism, intolerance of contact lenses.

GI: *nausea,* vomiting, abdominal cramps, bloating, diarrhea, constipation, anorexia, increased appetite, excessive thirst, weight changes, pancreatitis.

GU: in women—breakthrough bleeding, altered menstrual flow, dysmenorrhea, amenorrhea, cervical erosion or abnormal secretions, enlargement of uterine fibromas, vaginal candidiasis; in men—*gynecomastia, testicular atrophy, impotence.*

Hepatic: cholestatic jaundice.

Skin: melasma, urticaria, acne, seborrhea, oily skin, hirsutism or hair loss.

Other: leg cramps, purpura, breast changes (tenderness, enlargement, secretion), hyperglycemia, hypercalcemia, folic acid deficiency, libido changes.

INTERACTIONS

Bromocriptine: may cause amenorrhea, interfering with bromocriptine's effects. Avoid concomitant use.

Carbamazepine, phenobarbital, rifampin: decreased effectiveness of estrogen therapy. Monitor closely.

Corticosteroids: possible enhanced effects. Monitor closely.

Cyclosporine: increased risk of toxicity. Use together with caution and frequently monitor cyclosporine levels.

Dantrolene, other hepatotoxic medications: increased risk of hepatotoxicity. Monitor closely.

Oral anticoagulants: dosage adjustments may be necessary. Monitor PT.

Tamoxifen: estrogens may interfere with effectiveness of tamoxifen. Avoid concomitant use.

CONTRAINDICATIONS

Contraindicated in patients with thrombophlebitis or thromboembolic disorders; in those with breast, reproductive organ, or genital cancer; in those with undiagnosed abnormal genital bleeding; and during pregnancy.

NURSING CONSIDERATIONS

• Use cautiously in patients with cerebrovascular or coronary artery disease; asthma; bone disease; migraine; seizures; cardiac, hepatic, or renal dysfunction; hypercalcemia from metastatic breast disease; and family history (mother, grandmother, sister) of breast or genital tract cancer, or who have breast nodules, fibrocystic disease, or abnormal mammographic findings.

• Ensure that patients have a thorough physical examination before initiating estrogen therapy. Periodically monitor blood pressure, hepatic function, and serum lipid levels.

• Monitor weight regularly and recommend sodium restriction, as needed. May cause fluid retention and edema.

• Notify the pathologist about any patients receiving estrogen therapy.

• Because of the risk of thromboembolism, know therapy should be stopped at least 1 month before procedures associated with prolonged immobilization or thromboembolism, such as knee or hip surgery.

• Patient package insert that describes estrogen's adverse effects is available; however, also provide verbal explanation.

• Warn patients to immediately report suspected pregnancy; abdominal pain; pain, numbness, or stiffness in legs or buttocks; pressure or pain in chest; shortness of breath; severe headaches; visual disturbances, such as blind spots, flashing lights, or blurriness; vaginal bleeding or discharge; breast lumps; swelling of hands or feet; yellow skin and sclera; dark urine; and light-colored stools.

• Explain to patients on cyclic therapy for postmenopausal symptoms that, although withdrawal bleeding may occur during week off drug, fertility has not been restored. Pregnancy cannot occur because patients have not ovulated.

• Teach women how to perform routine breast self-examination.

• Tell diabetic patients to report elevated blood glucose test results so antidiabetic medication dosage can be adjusted.

• Emphasize the importance of regular physical examinations. Studies suggest that postmenopausal women who use estrogen replacement for more than 5 years to treat menopausal symptoms may be at increased risk for endometrial carcinoma. This risk is reduced by using cyclic rather than continuous therapy and the lowest possible dosages of estrogen. Adding progestins to the regimen decreases the incidence of endometrial hyperplasia; however, it isn't known if progestins affect the incidence of endometrial carcinoma. Most studies show no increased risk of breast cancer.

dienestrol (dienoestrol)
DV, Ortho Dienestrol

Pregnancy Risk Category: X

HOW SUPPLIED
Vaginal cream: 0.01%

ACTION
Unknown. Probably increases the synthesis of DNA, RNA, and protein in responsive tissues. Also reduces release of follicle-stimulating hormone and luteinizing hormone from the pituitary gland.

ONSET, PEAK, DURATION
Unknown.

INDICATIONS & DOSAGE
Atrophic vaginitis and kraurosis vulvae (short-term) –

Postmenopausal women: 1 to 2 intravaginal applications of vaginal cream daily for 1 to 2 weeks (as directed); then half that dose for the same period. Doctor may prescribe a maintenance dosage of 1 applicatorful one to three times a week.

ADVERSE REACTIONS
GU: vaginal discharge, increased intravaginal discomfort, uterine bleeding (with excessive use), burning sensation.
Other: systemic effects (breast tenderness, peripheral edema).

INTERACTIONS
Bromocriptine: may cause amenorrhea, interfering with bromocriptine's effects. Avoid concomitant use.
Carbamazepine, phenobarbital, rifampin: decreased effectiveness of estrogen therapy. Monitor closely.
Corticosteroids: possible enhanced effects. Monitor closely.
Cyclosporine: increased risk of toxicity. Use together with caution and frequently monitor cyclosporine levels.
Dantrolene, other hepatotoxic medications: increased risk of hepatotoxicity. Monitor closely.
Oral anticoagulants: dosage adjustments may be necessary. Monitor PT.
Tamoxifen: estrogens may interfere with effectiveness of tamoxifen. Avoid concomitant use.

CONTRAINDICATIONS
Contraindicated in patients with active thrombophlebitis or thromboembolic disorders associated with estrogen therapy or past history of such events; in those with breast, reproductive organ, or genital cancer; or in those with undiagnosed abnormal genital bleeding; and during pregnancy.

NURSING CONSIDERATIONS
• Use cautiously in patients with cerebral vascular or coronary artery disease, diabetes, hypertension, epilepsy, migraine; strong family history of breast cancer or who have breast

---

*Liquid form contains alcohol.
**May contain tartrazine.
Common reactions are in italics; *life-threatening,* in bold italics.

nodules, fibrocystic disease, or abnormal mammograms; cardiac or renal dysfunction; history of depression; liver dysfunction; metabolic bone diseases; and young patients in whom bone growth is not complete.

• Ensure that patients have a thorough physical examination before initiating estrogen therapy. Patients receiving long-term therapy should have repeat examinations yearly. Periodically monitor body weight, blood pressure, hepatic function, and serum lipid levels as ordered.

• Monitor closely. Systemic reactions may occur with normal intravaginal use.

• Instruct patients to apply drug at bedtime to increase effectiveness.

• Teach patients how to insert suppositories or cream and tell them to wash vaginal area with soap and water before application.

• Instruct patients to remain recumbent for 30 minutes after administration to prevent loss of drug.

• Tell patients not to wear a tampon while receiving vaginal therapy. They may need to wear a sanitary pad to protect clothing.

• Tell patient that patient package insert that describes estrogen's adverse effects is available; however, also provide verbal explanation.

• Instruct patients to report systemic reactions (breast pain or tenderness, swelling of the hands or feet) or vaginal discharge or bleeding.

• Teach women how to perform routine breast self-examination.

• Warn patients not to exceed the prescribed dosage.

• Inform patient withdrawal bleeding may occur if estrogen is suddenly stopped.

diethylstilbestrol (stilboestrol)
DES

diethylstilbestrol diphosphate
DES, Honvol†, Stilphostrol

Pregnancy Risk Category: X

HOW SUPPLIED
diethylstilbestrol
Tablets: 1 mg, 5 mg
diethylstilbestrol diphosphate
Tablets: 50 mg, 83 mg†
Injection: 50 mg/ml†

ACTION
Increases the synthesis of DNA, RNA, and protein in responsive tissues. Also reduces release of follicle-stimulating hormone and luteinizing hormone from the pituitary gland.

ONSET, PEAK, DURATION
Unknown.

INDICATIONS & DOSAGE
Prostate cancer–
Men: initially, 1 to 3 mg P.O. daily; may be reduced to 1 mg daily, or 50 mg P.O. diphosphate t.i.d. Then increased up to 200 mg or more as needed t.i.d. or 0.5 g I.V. followed by 1 g daily for 5 or more days as needed. Maintenance dosage 0.25 to 0.5 g I.V. once or twice weekly.
Metastatic, advanced breast cancer–
Men and postmenopausal women: 15 mg P.O. daily.

ADVERSE REACTIONS
CNS: headache, dizziness, chorea, depression, lethargy.
CV: thrombophlebitis; *thromboembolism;* hypertension; edema; *increased risk of CVA, pulmonary embolism, and MI.*
EENT: worsening of myopia or astigmatism, intolerance of contact lenses.
GI: *nausea,* vomiting, abdominal cramps, bloating, diarrhea, constipation, anorexia, increased appetite, excessive thirst, weight changes, pancreatitis.
GU: in women—breakthrough bleed-

ing, altered menstrual flow, dysmenorrhea, amenorrhea, cervical erosion, altered cervical secretions, enlargement of uterine fibromas, vaginal candidiasis, loss of libido; in men — gynecomastia, testicular atrophy, impotence.

Hepatic: cholestatic jaundice.

Skin: melasma, urticaria, acne, seborrhea, oily skin, hirsutism or hair loss.

Other: leg cramps, breast tenderness or enlargement, hyperglycemia, hypercalcemia, folic acid deficiency.

INTERACTIONS

Bromocriptine: may cause amenorrhea, interfering with bromocriptine's effects. Avoid concomitant use.

Carbamazepine, phenobarbital, rifampin: decreased effectiveness of estrogen therapy. Monitor closely.

Corticosteroids: possible enhanced effects. Monitor closely.

Cyclosporine: increased risk of toxicity. Use together with caution and frequently monitor cyclosporine levels.

Dantrolene, other hepatotoxic medications: increased risk of hepatotoxicity. Monitor closely.

Oral anticoagulants: dosage adjustments may be necessary. Monitor PT.

Tamoxifen: estrogens may interfere with effectiveness of tamoxifen. Avoid concomitant use.

CONTRAINDICATIONS

Contraindicated in men with known or suspected breast cancer except in selected patients being treated for metastatic disease, in patients with active thrombophlebitis or thromboembolic disorders, estrogen-dependent neoplasia, undiagnosed abnormal genital bleeding, during pregnancy, and history of thrombophlebitis, thrombosis, or thromboembolic disorders associated with estrogen use.

NURSING CONSIDERATIONS

• Use cautiously in patients with hypertension, mental depression, bone disease, migraine, seizures, diabetes mellitus, cardiac, hepatic, or renal dysfunction, and cerebrovascular or coronary artery disease.

• Ensure that patients have a thorough physical examination before initiating estrogen therapy. Patients receiving long-term therapy should have repeat examinations yearly. Periodically monitor body weight, blood pressure, hepatic function, and serum lipid levels.

• Be aware high incidence of gross nonmalignant genital changes may occur in offspring of women taking drug during pregnancy. Female offspring have a higher than normal risk of developing cervical and vaginal adenocarcinoma. Male offspring may have a higher than normal risk of developing testicular tumors, epididymal cysts, and impaired fertility.

• If patients experience GI upset, give drug with or immediately after meals.

• **I.V. use:** Mix ordered dose in 250 to 500 ml of D_5W or 0.9% sodium chloride. Infuse at 1 to 2 ml/minute for the first 15 minutes; if no adverse reactions occur, increase infusion rate to administer entire dose within 1 hour.

• To administer I.M., give by deep injection. Rotate injection sites to prevent muscle atrophy.

• Notify the pathologist about any patients receiving estrogen therapy.

• Know that increased number of CV deaths reported in men taking diethylstilbestrol tablet (5 mg daily) for prostate cancer over long time period. This effect is not associated with 1-mg daily dose.

• Tell diabetic patients to report elevated blood glucose test results so antidiabetic medication dosage can be adjusted.

• Because of the risk of thromboembolism, know that therapy should be discontinued at least 1 month before

---

*Liquid form contains alcohol.   *Common* reactions are in italics; *life-threatening,* in bold italics.
**May contain tartrazine.

procedures associated with prolonged immobilization or thromboembolism, such as knee or hip surgery.
• Tell patient not to crush, break, or chew enteric-coated tablets.
• Tell patient that patient package insert that describes estrogen's adverse effects is available; however, also provide verbal explanation.
• Warn patients to immediately report abdominal pain; pain, numbness, or stiffness in legs or buttocks; pressure or pain in chest; shortness of breath; severe headache; visual disturbances, such as blind spots, flashing lights, or blurriness; vaginal bleeding or discharge; breast lumps; sudden weight gain; swelling of hands or feet; yellow sclera or skin; dark urine; and light-colored stools.
• Teach women how to perform routine breast self-examination.

esterified estrogens
Estratab, Menest, Neo-Estrone†

Pregnancy Risk Category: X

HOW SUPPLIED
Tablets: 0.3 mg, 0.625 mg, 1.25 mg, 2.5 mg
Tablets (film-coated): 0.3 mg, 0.625 mg, 1.25 mg, 2.5 mg

ACTION
Increases the synthesis of DNA, RNA, and protein in responsive tissues. Also reduces release of follicle-stimulating hormone and luteinizing hormone from the pituitary gland.

ONSET, PEAK, DURATION
Unknown.

INDICATIONS & DOSAGE
Inoperable prostate cancer –
Men: 1.25 to 2.5 mg P.O. t.i.d.
Breast cancer –
Men and postmenopausal women: 10 mg P.O. t.i.d. for 3 or more months.

Female hypogonadism –
Women: 2.5 mg P.O. daily to t.i.d. in cycles of 20 days, 10 days off.
Castration, primary ovarian failure –
Women: 2.5 mg P.O. daily to t.i.d. in cycles of 3 weeks on, 1 week off.
Vasomotor menopausal symptoms –
Women: average dosage is 1.25 mg P.O. daily in cycles of 3 weeks on, 1 week off.
Atrophic vaginitis and atropic urethritis –
Women: 0.3 to 1.25 mg or more P.O. daily in cycles of 3 weeks on, 1 week off.

ADVERSE REACTIONS
CNS: headache, dizziness, chorea, depression, lethargy.
CV: thrombophlebitis; *thromboembolism;* hypertension; edema; *increased risk of CVA, pulmonary embolism, and MI.*
EENT: worsening of myopia or astigmatism, intolerance of contact lenses.
GI: *nausea,* vomiting, abdominal cramps, bloating, diarrhea, constipation, anorexia, increased appetite, weight changes, pancreatitis.
GU: in women – breakthrough bleeding, altered menstrual flow, dysmenorrhea, amenorrhea, cervical erosion, altered cervical secretions, enlargement of uterine fibromas, vaginal candidiasis; in men – gynecomastia, testicular atrophy, impotence.
Hepatic: cholestatic jaundice.
Skin: melasma, rash, acne, hirsutism or hair loss, seborrhea, oily skin.
Other: breast changes (tenderness, enlargement, secretion), hyperglycemia, hypercalcemia, folic acid deficiency, libido changes.

INTERACTIONS
Bromocriptine: may cause amenorrhea, interfering with bromocriptine's effects. Avoid concomitant use.
Carbamazepine, phenobarbital, rifampin: decreased effectiveness of estrogen therapy. Monitor closely.

Corticosteroids: possible enhanced effects. Monitor closely.

Cyclosporine: increased risk of toxicity. Use together with caution and frequently monitor cyclosporine levels.

Dantrolene, other hepatotoxic medications: increased risk of hepatotoxicity. Monitor closely.

Oral anticoagulants: dosage adjustments may be necessary. Monitor PT.

Tamoxifen: estrogens may interfere with effectiveness of tamoxifen. Avoid concomitant use.

CONTRAINDICATIONS
Contraindicated in patients with breast cancer (except metastatic disease), estrogen-dependent neoplasia, active thrombophlebitis or thromboembolic disorders, undiagnosed abnormal genital bleeding, during pregnancy, hypersensitivity to drug, or history of thromboembolic disease.

NURSING CONSIDERATIONS
• Use cautiously in patients with history of hypertension, mental depression, cardiac or renal dysfunction, liver impairment, or bone diseases, migraine, seizures, or diabetes mellitus.

• Ensure that patients have a thorough physical examination before initiating estrogen therapy. Patients receiving long-term therapy should have repeat examinations yearly. Periodically monitor body weight, blood pressure, serum lipid levels, and hepatic function as ordered.

• Notify the pathologist about any patients receiving estrogen therapy.

• Because of the risk of thromboembolism, know that therapy should be discontinued at least one month before procedures associated with prolonged immobilization or thromboembolism, such as knee or hip surgery.

• Tell patient that patient package insert that describes estrogen's adverse effects is available; however, also provide verbal explanation.

• Emphasize the importance of regular physical examinations. Studies suggest that postmenopausal women who use estrogen replacement for more than 5 years to treat menopausal symptoms may be at increased risk for endometrial carcinoma. This risk is reduced by using cyclic rather than continuous therapy and the lowest possible dosages of estrogen. Adding progestins to the regimen decreases the incidence of endometrial hyperplasia; however, it isn't known if progestins affect the incidence of endometrial carcinoma. Most studies show no increased risk of breast cancer.

• Warn patients to immediately report abdominal pain; pain, numbness, or stiffness in legs or buttocks; pressure or pain in chest; shortness of breath; severe headaches; visual disturbances, such as blind spots, flashing lights, or blurriness; vaginal bleeding or discharge; breast lumps; swelling of hands or feet; yellow skin or sclera; dark urine; and light-colored stools.

• Tell diabetic patients to report elevated blood glucose test results so antidiabetic medication dosage can be adjusted.

• Explain to patients on cyclic therapy for postmenopausal symptoms that, although they may experience withdrawal bleeding during week off drug, fertility has not been restored. Pregnancy cannot occur because patients have not ovulated.

• Teach women how to perform routine breast self-examination.

estradiol (oestradiol)
Estrace**, Estrace Vaginal Cream, Estraderm

estradiol cypionate
depGynogen, Depo-Estradiol, Dura-Estrin, E-Cypionate, Estro-Cyp, Estrofem, Estroject-L.A.

---

estradiol valerate
(oestradiol valerate)
Delestrogen, Dioval, Duragen-10, Duragen-20, Duragen-40, Estradiol L.A., Estra-L 20, Estra-L 40, Estraval, Estraval P.A., Feminate, Femogex, Gynogen L.A., L.A.E., Menaval, Primogyn Depot‡, Ru-Est-Span 20, Ru-Est-Span 40, Valergen-10, Valergen-20, Valergen-40

Pregnancy Risk Category: X

HOW SUPPLIED
estradiol
Tablets (micronized): 0.5 mg, 1 mg, 2 mg
Transdermal: 4 mg/10 cm² (delivers 0.05 mg/24 hours); 8 mg/20 cm² (delivers 0.1 mg/24 hours)
Vaginal cream (in nonliquefying base): 0.1 mg/g
estradiol cypionate
Injection (in oil): 1 mg/ml, 5 mg/ml
estradiol valerate
Injection (in oil): 10 mg/ml, 20 mg/ml, 40 mg/ml

ACTION
Increases the synthesis of DNA, RNA, and protein in responsive tissues. Also reduces release of follicle-stimulating hormone and luteinizing hormone from the pituitary gland.

ONSET, PEAK, DURATION
Unknown.

INDICATIONS & DOSAGE
Vasomotor menopausal symptoms, female hypogonadism, female castration, primary ovarian failure –
Adults: 1 to 2 mg P.O. (estradiol) daily, in cycles of 21 days on and 7 days off or cycles of 5 days on and 2 days off; or 1 transdermal system delivering 0.05 mg/24 hours applied twice weekly in cycles of 3 weeks on and 1 week off. Alternatively, 1 to 5 mg (cypionate) I.M. q 3 to 4 weeks or

10 to 20 mg (valerate) I.M. q 4 weeks p.r.n.
Atrophic vaginitis, kraurosis vulvae –
Adults: 2 to 4 g intravaginal applications of cream daily for 1 to 2 weeks. When vaginal mucosa is restored, maintenance dosage of 1 g one to three times weekly in a cyclic regimen. Alternatively, 10 to 20 mg (valerate) I.M. q 4 weeks p.r.n.
Palliative treatment of advanced, inoperable breast cancer –
Men and postmenopausal women: 10 mg P.O. (estradiol) t.i.d. for 3 months.
Palliative treatment of advanced inoperable prostate cancer –
Men: 30 mg (valerate) I.M. q 1 to 2 weeks, or 1 to 2 mg P.O. (estradiol) t.i.d.

ADVERSE REACTIONS
CV: thrombophlebitis, *thromboembolism,* hypertension, edema.
EENT: worsening of myopia or astigmatism, intolerance of contact lenses.
GI: *nausea,* vomiting, abdominal cramps, bloating, diarrhea, constipation, increased appetite, weight changes, pancreatitis.
GU: in women – breakthrough bleeding, altered menstrual flow, dysmenorrhea, amenorrhea, cervical erosion, altered cervical secretions, enlargement of uterine fibromas, vaginal candidiasis; in men – gynecomastia, testicular atrophy, impotence.
Hepatic: cholestatic jaundice.
Skin: melasma, urticaria, acne, seborrhea, oily skin, hirsutism or hair loss.
Other: breast changes (tenderness, enlargement, secretion), leg cramps, hyperglycemia, hypercalcemia, folic acid deficiency.

INTERACTIONS
Bromocriptine: may cause amenorrhea, interfering with bromocriptine's effects. Avoid concomitant use.
Carbamazepine, phenobarbital, ri-

---

fampin: decreased effectiveness of estrogen therapy. Monitor closely.
Corticosteroids: possible enhanced effects. Monitor closely.
Cyclosporine: increased risk of toxicity. Use together with caution and frequently monitor cyclosporine levels.
Dantrolene, other hepatotoxic medications: increased risk of hepatotoxicity. Monitor closely.
Oral anticoagulants: dosage adjustments may be necessary. Monitor PT.
Tamoxifen: estrogens may interfere with effectiveness of tamoxifen. Avoid concomitant use.

CONTRAINDICATIONS
Contraindicated in patients with thrombophlebitis or thromboembolic disorders, estrogen-dependent neoplasia, breast or reproductive organ cancer (except for palliative treatment), or undiagnosed abnormal genital bleeding and during pregnancy. Also contraindicated in patients with history of thrombophlebitis or thromboembolic disorders associated with previous estrogen use (except for palliative treatment of breast and prostate cancer).

NURSING CONSIDERATIONS
• Use cautiously in patients with cerebrovascular or coronary artery disease; asthma; bone diseases; migraine; seizures; cardiac, hepatic or renal dysfunction; or in women with a strong family history of breast cancer or who have breast nodules, fibrocystic disease, or abnormal mammographic findings.
• Ensure that patients have a thorough physical examination before initiating estrogen therapy. Patients receiving long-term therapy should have repeat examinations yearly. Periodically monitor serum lipid levels, blood pressure, body weight, and hepatic function as ordered.
• Ask patients about allergies, especially to foods or plants. Estradiol is available as an aqueous solution or as a solution in peanut oil; estradiol cypionate, as a solution in cottonseed oil or vegetable oil; estradiol valerate, as a solution in castor oil, sesame oil, or vegetable oil.
• To administer as an I.M. injection, make sure drug is well dispersed in solution by rolling vial between palms. Inject deep I.M. into large muscle. Rotate injection sites to prevent muscle atrophy. Never give drug intravenously.
• Apply the transdermal patch to clean, dry, hairless, intact skin on abdomen or buttocks. Do not apply to breasts, waistline, or other areas where clothing can loosen the patch. When applying, ensure good contact with the skin, especially around the edges, and hold in place with the palm for about 10 seconds. Rotate application sites.
• Know that in women who are currently taking oral estrogen, treatment with the Estraderm transdermal patch can begin 1 week after withdrawal of oral therapy or sooner if menopausal symptoms appear before the end of the week.
• Because of the risk of thromboembolism, know that therapy should be discontinued at least 1 month before procedures associated with prolonged immobilization or thromboembolism, such as knee or hip surgery.
• Notify the pathologist about any patients receiving estrogen therapy.
• Inform patient that patient package insert that describes estrogen's adverse effects is available; however, also provide verbal explanation.
• Emphasize the importance of regular physical examinations. Studies suggest that postmenopausal women who use estrogen replacement for more than 5 years to treat menopausal symptoms may be at increased risk for endometrial carcinoma. This risk is reduced by using cyclic rather than continuous therapy and the lowest

---

*Liquid form contains alcohol.   *Common* reactions are in italics; ***life-threatening***, in bold italics.
**May contain tartrazine.

possible dosages of estrogen. Adding progestins to the regimen decreases the incidence of endometrial hyperplasia; however, it isn't known if progestins affect the incidence of endometrial carcinoma. Most studies show no increased risk of breast cancer.

• Teach patients how to use vaginal cream. Patients should wash vaginal area with soap and water before applying. Tell them to take drug at bedtime or to lie flat for 30 minutes after instillation to minimize drug loss.

• Warn patients to immediately report abdominal pain; pain, numbness, or stiffness in legs or buttocks; pressure or pain in chest; shortness of breath; severe headaches; visual disturbances, such as blind spots, flashing lights, or blurriness; vaginal bleeding or discharge; breast lumps; swelling of hands or feet; yellow skin or sclera; dark urine; and light-colored stools.

• Explain to patients on cyclic therapy for postmenopausal symptoms that, although withdrawal bleeding may occur during week off drug, fertility has not been restored. Pregnancy cannot occur because patients have not ovulated.

• Tell diabetic patients to report elevated blood glucose test results so antidiabetic medication dosage can be adjusted.

• Teach women how to perform routine breast self-examination.

estrogens, conjugated (estrogenic substances, conjugated; oestrogens, conjugated)
C.E.S.†, Premarin, Premarin Intravenous

Pregnancy Risk Category: X

HOW SUPPLIED
Tablets: 0.3 mg, 0.625 mg, 0.9 mg, 1.25 mg, 2.5 mg
Injection: 25 mg/5 ml
Vaginal cream: 0.625 mg/g

ACTION
Increases the synthesis of DNA, RNA, and protein in responsive tissues. Also reduces release of follicle-stimulating hormone and luteinizing hormone from the pituitary gland.

ONSET, PEAK, DURATION
Unknown.

INDICATIONS & DOSAGE
Abnormal uterine bleeding (hormonal imbalance) –
Women: 25 mg I.V. or I.M. Repeated in 6 to 12 hours as needed.
Palliative treatment of breast cancer (at least 5 years after menopause) –
Men and postmenopausal women: 10 mg P.O. t.i.d. for 3 months or more.
Female castration, primary ovarian failure –
Women: 1.25 mg P.O. daily in cycles of 3 weeks on and 1 week off.
Osteoporosis –
Postmenopausal women: 0.625 mg P.O. daily in cyclic regimen (3 weeks on, 1 week off)
Hypogonadism –
Women: 2.5 mg P.O. b.i.d. or t.i.d. for 20 consecutive days each month.
Vasomotor menopausal symptoms –
Women: 0.3 to 1.25 mg P.O. daily in cycles of 3 weeks on and 1 week off.
Atrophic vaginitis, kraurosis vulvae –
Women: 2 to 4 g intravaginally once daily on a cyclical basis (3 weeks on and 1 week off).
Palliative treatment of inoperable prostate cancer –
Men: 1.25 to 2.5 mg P.O. t.i.d.

ADVERSE REACTIONS
CNS: headache, dizziness, chorea, depression, lethargy.
CV: thrombophlebitis; *thromboembolism;* hypertension; edema; *increased risk of CVA, pulmonary embolism, and MI.*
EENT: worsening of myopia or astigmatism, intolerance of contact lenses.

GI: *nausea,* vomiting, abdominal cramps, bloating, diarrhea, constipation, anorexia, increased appetite, weight changes, pancreatitis.

GU: in women — breakthrough bleeding, altered menstrual flow, dysmenorrhea, amenorrhea, cervical erosion, altered cervical secretions, enlargement of uterine fibromas, vaginal candidiasis; in men — gynecomastia, testicular atrophy, impotence.

Hepatic: cholestatic jaundice.

Skin: melasma, urticaria, acne, seborrhea, oily skin, flushing (with rapid I.V. administration), hirsutism or hair loss.

Other: breast changes (tenderness, enlargement, secretion), leg cramps, hyperglycemia, hypercalcemia, folic acid deficiency, libido changes.

INTERACTIONS

Bromocriptine: may cause amenorrhea, interfering with bromocriptine's effects. Avoid concomitant use.

Carbamazepine, phenobarbital, rifampin: decreased effectiveness of estrogen therapy. Monitor closely.

Corticosteroids: possible enhanced effects. Monitor closely.

Cyclosporine: increased risk of toxicity. Use together with caution and frequently monitor cyclosporine levels.

Dantrolene, other hepatotoxic medications: increased risk of hepatotoxicity. Monitor closely.

Oral anticoagulants: dosage adjustments may be necessary. Monitor PT.

Tamoxifen: estrogens may interfere with effectiveness of tamoxifen. Avoid concomitant use.

CONTRAINDICATIONS

Contraindicated in patients with thrombophlebitis or thromboembolic disorders, estrogen-dependent neoplasia, breast or reproductive organ cancer (except for palliative treatment), or undiagnosed abnormal genital bleeding and during pregnancy.

NURSING CONSIDERATIONS

• Use cautiously in patients with cerebrovascular or coronary artery disease; asthma; bone disease; migraine; seizures; cardiac, hepatic, or renal dysfunction; or in women with family history (mother, grandmother, sister) of breast or genital tract cancer or who have breast nodules, fibrocystic disease, or abnormal mammographic findings.

• Ensure that patients have a thorough physical examination before initiating estrogen therapy. Patients receiving long-term therapy should have repeat examinations yearly. Periodically monitor serum lipid levels, blood pressure, body weight, and hepatic function, as ordered.

• Know I.M. or I.V. use preferred for rapid treatment of dysfunctional uterine bleeding or reduction of surgical bleeding.

• Refrigerate before reconstituting. Agitate gently after adding diluent.

• **I.V. use:** When giving by direct I.V. injection, administer slowly to avoid flushing reaction. For infusion, mix with D_5W, 0.9% sodium chloride injection, or invert sugar solutions. Avoid mixing with solutions of acidic pH to prevent incompatibility.

• When administering by I.M. injection, inject deeply into large muscle. Rotate injection sites to prevent muscle atrophy.

• Notify the pathologist about any patients receiving estrogen therapy.

• Because of the risk of thromboembolism, know that therapy should be discontinued at least 1 month before procedures associated with prolonged immobilization or thromboembolism, such as knee or hip surgery.

• Inform patient that patient package insert that describes estrogen's adverse effects is available; however, also provide verbal explanation.

• Emphasize the importance of regular physical examinations. Studies suggest that postmenopausal women

---

*Liquid form contains alcohol.
**May contain tartrazine.

Common reactions are in italics; ***life-threatening,*** in bold italics.

who use estrogen replacement for more than 5 years to treat menopausal symptoms may be at increased risk for endometrial carcinoma. This risk is reduced by using cyclic rather than continuous therapy and the lowest possible dosages of estrogen. Adding progestins to the regimen decreases the incidence of endometrial hyperplasia; however, it isn't known if progestins affect the incidence of endometrial carcinoma. Most studies show no increased risk of breast cancer.

• Teach patients how to use vaginal cream. Patients should wash the vaginal area with soap and water before applying. Tell them to use drug at bedtime or to lie flat for 30 minutes after instillation to minimize drug loss.

• Explain to patients on cyclic therapy for postmenopausal symptoms that, although withdrawal bleeding may occur during week off drug, fertility has not been restored. Pregnancy cannot occur because they have not ovulated.

• Warn patients to immediately report abdominal pain; pain, numbness, or stiffness in legs or buttocks; pressure or pain in chest; shortness of breath; severe headaches; visual disturbances, such as blind spots, flashing lights, or blurriness; vaginal bleeding or discharge; breast lumps; swelling of hands or feet; yellow skin or sclera; dark urine; and light-colored stools.

• Tell diabetic patients to report elevated blood glucose test results so antidiabetic medication dosage can be adjusted.

• Teach women how to perform routine breast self-examination.

estrone (oestrone)
Estroject-2, Estrone A, Estrone 5, Femogen Forte†, Gynogen, Kestrin Aqueous, Kestrone 5, Theelin Aqueous, Unigen, Wehgen-V

Pregnancy Risk Category: X

HOW SUPPLIED
Injection (aqueous suspension): 2 mg/ml, 5 mg/ml

ACTION
Increases the synthesis of DNA, RNA, and protein in responsive tissues. Also reduces release of follicle-stimulating hormone and luteinizing hormone from the pituitary.

ONSET, PEAK, DURATION
Unknown.

INDICATIONS & DOSAGE
Atrophic vaginitis, kraurosis vulvae, and vasomotor menopausal symptoms –
Women: 0.1 to 0.5 mg I.M. two or three times weekly.
Female hypogonadism, castration, and primary ovarian failure –
Women: 0.1 to 1 mg I.M. weekly as a single dose or in divided doses.
Palliative treatment of inoperable prostate cancer –
Men: 2 to 4 mg I.M. two to three times weekly.

ADVERSE REACTIONS
CNS: headache, dizziness, chorea, depression, lethargy.
CV: thrombophlebitis, *thromboembolism,* hypertension, edema.
EENT: worsening of myopia or astigmatism, intolerance of contact lenses.
GI: *nausea,* vomiting, abdominal cramps, bloating, diarrhea, constipation, anorexia, increased appetite, weight changes, pancreatitis.
GU: in women – breakthrough bleeding, altered menstrual flow, dysmen-

---

orrhea, amenorrhea, cervical erosion, altered cervical secretions, enlargement of uterine fibromas, vaginal candidiasis; in men — gynecomastia, testicular atrophy, impotence.
Hepatic: cholestatic jaundice.
Skin: melasma, urticaria, acne, seborrhea, oily skin, hirsutism or hair loss.
Other: breast changes (tenderness, enlargement, secretion), leg cramps, hyperglycemia, hypercalcemia, folic acid deficiency, libido changes.

INTERACTIONS
Bromocriptine: may cause amenorrhea, interfering with bromocriptine's effects. Avoid concomitant use.
Carbamazepine, phenobarbital, rifampin: decreased effectiveness of estrogen therapy. Monitor closely.
Corticosteroids: possible enhanced effects. Monitor closely.
Cyclosporine: increased risk of toxicity. Use together with caution and frequently monitor cyclosporine levels.
Dantrolene, other hepatotoxic medications: increased risk of hepatotoxicity. Monitor closely.
Oral anticoagulants: dosage adjustments may be necessary. Monitor PT.
Tamoxifen: estrogens may interfere with effectiveness of tamoxifen. Avoid concomitant use.

CONTRAINDICATIONS
Contraindicated in patients with thrombophlebitis or thromboembolic disorders, estrogen-dependent neoplasia, breast or reproductive organ cancer (except for palliative treatment), or undiagnosed abnormal genital bleeding and during pregnancy.

NURSING CONSIDERATIONS
• Use cautiously in patients with cerebrovascular or coronary artery disease; asthma; bone diseases; mental depression; migraine; seizures; cardiac, hepatic, or renal dysfunction; or in women with family history

(mother, grandmother, sister) of breast or genital tract cancer or who have breast nodules, fibrocystic disease, or abnormal mammographic findings.
• Ensure that patients have a thorough physical examination before initiating estrogen therapy. Patients receiving long-term therapy should have repeat examinations yearly. Periodically monitor serum lipid levels, blood pressure, body weight, and hepatic function, as ordered.
• Administer estrone I.M. Rotate injection sites to prevent muscle atrophy.
• Notify the pathologist about any patients receiving estrogen therapy.
• Because of the risk of thromboembolism, know that therapy should be discontinued at least 1 month before procedures associated with prolonged immobilization or thromboembolism, such as knee or hip surgery.
• Inform patient that patient package insert that describes estrogen's adverse effects is available; however, also provide verbal explanation.
• Emphasize the importance of regular physical examinations. Studies suggest that postmenopausal women who use estrogen replacement for more than 5 years to treat menopausal symptoms may be at increased risk for endometrial carcinoma. This risk is reduced by using cyclic rather than continuous therapy and the lowest possible dosages of estrogen. Adding progestins to the regimen decreases the incidence of endometrial hyperplasia; however, it isn't known if progestins affect the incidence of endometrial carcinoma. Most studies show no increased risk of breast cancer.
• Explain to patients on cyclic therapy for postmenopausal symptoms that, although withdrawal bleeding may occur during week off drug, fertility has not been restored. Pregnancy cannot occur because patients have not ovulated.

---

*Liquid form contains alcohol.   *Common* reactions are in italics; *life-threatening,* in bold italics.
**May contain tartrazine.

• Warn patients to immediately report abdominal pain; pain, numbness, or stiffness in legs or buttocks; pressure or pain in chest; shortness of breath; severe headaches; visual disturbances, such as blind spots, flashing lights, or blurriness; vaginal bleeding or discharge; breast lumps; swelling of hands or feet; yellow skin and sclera; dark urine; and light-colored stools.

• Tell diabetic patients to report elevated blood glucose test results so antidiabetic medication dosage can be adjusted.

• Teach women how to perform routine breast self-examination.

estropipate (piperazine estrone sulfate)
Ogen, OrthoEST

Pregnancy Risk Category: X

HOW SUPPLIED
Tablets: 0.75 mg, 1.5 mg, 3 mg, 6 mg
Vaginal cream: 1.5 mg/g

ACTION
Increases the synthesis of DNA, RNA, and proteins in responsive tissues. Also reduces release of follicle-stimulating hormone and luteinizing hormone from the pituitary gland.

ONSET, PEAK, DURATION
Unknown.

INDICATIONS & DOSAGE
Vulval and vaginal atrophy –
Women: 0.625 to 5 mg P.O. daily 3 weeks on, 1 week off, or 2 to 4 g of vaginal cream daily. Typically, dosage given on a cyclical, short-term basis.
Primary ovarian failure, female castration, female hypogonadism –
Women: administered on a cyclical basis – 1.25 to 7.5 mg P.O. daily for the first 3 weeks, followed by a rest period of 8 to 10 days. If bleeding does not occur by the end of the rest period, cycle repeated.
Vasomotor menopausal symptoms –
Women: 0.625 mg to 5 mg P.O. daily in cyclic method of 3 weeks on, 1 week off.
Prevention of osteoporosis –
Women: 0.625 mg P.O. daily for 25 days of a 31-day cycle.

ADVERSE REACTIONS
CNS: depression, headache, dizziness, migraine.
CV: edema; thrombophlebitis; *increased risk of CVA, pulmonary embolism, and MI.*
GI: nausea, vomiting, abdominal cramps, bloating, weight changes.
GU: increased size of uterine fibromas, vaginal candidiasis, cystitis-like syndrome, dysmenorrhea, amenorrhea, breakthrough bleeding, condition resembling premenstrual syndrome.
Hepatic: cholestatic jaundice.
Skin: hemorrhagic eruption, erythema nodosum, *erythema multiforme,* hirsutism, melasma, hair loss.
Other: breast engorgement or enlargement, aggravation of porphyria, libido changes.

INTERACTIONS
Bromocriptine: may cause amenorrhea, interfering with bromocriptine's effects. Avoid concomitant use.
Carbamazepine, phenobarbital, rifampin: decreased effectiveness of estrogen therapy. Monitor closely.
Corticosteroids: possible enhanced effects. Monitor closely.
Cyclosporine: increased risk of toxicity. Use together with caution and frequently monitor cyclosporine levels.
Dantrolene, other hepatotoxic medications: increased risk of hepatotoxicity. Monitor closely.
Oral anticoagulants: dosage adjustments may be necessary. Monitor PT.
Tamoxifen: estrogens may interfere

---

†Available in Canada only.   ‡Available in Australia only.   ◊ Available OTC.

with effectiveness of tamoxifen. Avoid concomitant use.

CONTRAINDICATIONS

Contraindicated in patients with active thrombophlebitis or thromboembolic disorders; in those with estrogen-dependent neoplasia, breast, reproductive organ, or genital cancer; in those with undiagnosed genital bleeding; and during pregnancy.

NURSING CONSIDERATIONS

• Use cautiously in patients with cerebrovascular or coronary artery disease; asthma; mental depression; bone disease; migraine; seizures; cardiac, hepatic, or renal dysfunction; and in women with a family history (mother, grandmother, sister) of breast or genital tract cancer or who have breast nodules, fibrocystic disease, or abnormal mammographic findings.

• Ensure that patients have a thorough physical examination before initiating estrogen therapy. Patients receiving long-term therapy should have repeat examinations yearly. Periodically monitor serum lipid levels, blood pressure, body weight, and hepatic function as ordered.

• Know that when used to treat hypogonadism, the duration of therapy necessary to produce withdrawal bleeding depends on the patient's endometrial response to the drug. If satisfactory withdrawal bleeding does not occur, an oral progestin is added to the regimen, as ordered. Explain to the patient that, despite the return of withdrawal bleeding, pregnancy cannot occur because she is not ovulating.

• Be aware of the following estropipate/estrone equivalents:

0.75 mg estropipate	=	0.625 mg estrone
1.5 mg estropipate	=	1.25 mg estrone
3 mg estropipate	=	2.5 mg estrone
6 mg estropipate	=	5 mg estone

• Because of the risk of thromboembolism, know that therapy should be discontinued at least 1 month before procedures associated with prolonged immobilization or thromboembolism, such as knee or hip surgery.

• Tell patient that patient package insert that describes estrogen's adverse effects is available; however, also provide verbal explanation.

• Stress the importance of regular physical examinations. Studies suggest that postmenopausal women who use estrogen replacement for more than 5 years to treat menopausal symptoms may be at increased risk for endometrial carcinoma. This risk is reduced by using cyclic rather than continuous therapy and the lowest possible dosages of estrogen. Adding progestins to the regimen decreases the incidence of endometrial hyperplasia; however, it isn't known if progestins affect the incidence of endometrial carcinoma. Most studies show no increased risk of breast cancer.

• Warn patients to immediately report abdominal pain; pain, stiffness, or numbness in the legs or buttocks; pressure or pain in the chest; shortness of breath; severe headaches; visual disturbances, such as blind spots or flashing lights; vaginal bleeding or discharge; breast lumps; swelling of the hands or feet; yellow skin or sclera; dark urine; and light-colored stools.

• Teach women how to perform routine breast self-examination.

ethinyl estradiol (ethinyloestradiol)

Estinyl**, Feminone

Pregnancy Risk Category: X

HOW SUPPLIED

Tablets: 0.02 mg, 0.05 mg, 0.5 mg

ACTION

Increases the synthesis of DNA, RNA, and protein in responsive tissues. Also reduces release of follicle-

---

*Liquid form contains alcohol.
**May contain tartrazine.

Common reactions are in italics; ***life-threatening,*** in bold italics.

stimulating hormone and luteinizing hormone from the pituitary gland.

ONSET, PEAK, DURATION
Unknown.

INDICATIONS & DOSAGE
Palliative treatment of metastatic breast cancer (at least 5 years after menopause) –
Women: 1 mg P.O. t.i.d. for at least 3 months.
Female hypogonadism –
Women: 0.05 mg P.O. once daily to t.i.d. 2 weeks a month, followed by 2 weeks of progesterone therapy; continued for three to six monthly dosing cycles, followed by 2 months off.
Vasomotor menopausal symptoms –
Women: 0.02 to 0.05 mg P.O. daily for cycles of 3 weeks on and 1 week off.
Palliative treatment of metastatic inoperable prostate cancer –
Men: 0.15 to 2 mg P.O. daily.

ADVERSE REACTIONS
CNS: headache, dizziness, chorea, depression, lethargy.
CV: thrombophlebitis, ***thromboembolism,*** hypertension, edema.
EENT: worsening of myopia or astigmatism, intolerance to contact lenses.
GI: *nausea,* vomiting, abdominal cramps, bloating, diarrhea, constipation, anorexia, increased appetite, weight changes.
GU: in women – breakthrough bleeding, altered menstrual flow, dysmenorrhea, amenorrhea, cervical erosion, altered cervical secretions, enlargement of uterine fibromas, vaginal candidiasis; in men – gynecomastia, testicular atrophy, impotence.
Hepatic: cholestatic jaundice.
Skin: melasma, urticaria, acne, seborrhea, oily skin, hirsutism or hair loss.
Other: breast changes (tenderness, enlargement, secretion), leg cramps, hyperglycemia, hypercalcemia, folic acid deficiency, libido changes.

INTERACTIONS
Bromocriptine: may cause amenorrhea, interfering with bromocriptine's effects. Avoid concomitant use.
Carbamazepine, phenobarbital, rifampin: decreased effectiveness of estrogen therapy. Monitor closely.
Corticosteroids: possible enhanced effects. Monitor closely.
Cyclosporine: increased risk of toxicity. Use together with caution and frequently monitor cyclosporine levels.
Dantrolene, other hepatotoxic medications: increased risk of hepatotoxicity. Monitor closely.
Oral anticoagulants: dosage adjustments may be necessary. Monitor PT.
Tamoxifen: estrogens may interfere with effectiveness of tamoxifen. Avoid concomitant use.

CONTRAINDICATIONS
Contraindicated in patients with thrombophlebitis or thromboembolic disorders, estrogen-dependent neoplasia, breast or reproductive organ cancer (except for palliative treatment), or undiagnosed abnormal genital bleeding and during pregnancy.

NURSING CONSIDERATIONS
• Use cautiously in patients with cerebrovascular or coronary artery disease; asthma; mental depression; bone disease; cardiac, hepatic, or renal dysfunction; or in women with a family history (mother, grandmother, sister) of breast or genital tract cancer, or who have breast nodules, fibrocystic disease, or abnormal mammographic findings.
• Ensure that patients have a thorough physical examination before initiating estrogen therapy. Patients receiving long-term therapy should have repeat examinations yearly. Periodically monitor serum lipid levels, blood pressure,

---

body weight, and hepatic function as ordered.

• Because of the risk of thromboembolism, know that therapy should be discontinued at least 1 month before procedures associated with prolonged immobilization or thromboembolism, such as knee or hip surgery.

• Notify the pathologist about any patients receiving estrogen therapy.

• Tell patient that patient package insert that describes estrogen's adverse effects is available; however, also provide verbal explanation.

• Emphasize the importance of regular physical examinations. Studies suggest that postmenopausal women who use estrogen replacement for more than 5 years to treat menopausal symptoms may be at increased risk for endometrial carcinoma. This risk is reduced by using cyclic rather than continuous therapy and the lowest possible dosages of estrogen. Adding progestins to the regimen decreases the incidence of endometrial hyperplasia; however, it isn't known if progestins affect the incidence of endometrial carcinoma. Most studies show no increased risk of breast cancer.

• Explain to patients on cyclic therapy for postmenopausal symptoms that, although withdrawal bleeding may occur during week off drug, fertility has not been restored. Pregnancy cannot occur because patients have not ovulated.

• Warn patients to immediately report abdominal pain; pain, numbness, or stiffness in legs or buttocks; pressure or pain in chest; shortness of breath; severe headaches; visual disturbances, such as blind spots, flashing lights, or blurriness; vaginal bleeding or discharge; breast lumps; swelling of hands or feet; yellow skin or sclera; dark urine; or light-colored stools.

• Tell diabetic patients to report elevated blood glucose test results so antidiabetic medication dosage can be adjusted.

• Teach women how to perform routine breast self-examination.

---

ethinyl estradiol and desogestrel
monophasic: Desogen

ethinyl estradiol and ethynodiol diacetate
monophasic: Demulen 1/35, Demulen 1/50

ethinyl estradiol and levonorgestrel
monophasic: Levlen, Nordette
triphasic: Tri-Levlen, Triphasil

ethinyl estradiol and norethindrone
monophasic: Brevicon, Genora 0.5/35, Genora 1/35, ModiCon, N.E.E. 1/35, Nelova 0.5/35 E, Nelova 1/35 E, Norcept-E 1/35, Norethin 1/35 E, Norinyl 1 + 35, Ortho-Novum 1/35, Ovcon-35, Ovcon-50
biphasic: Nelova 10/11, Ortho-Novum 10/11
triphasic: Ortho-Novum 7/7/7, Tri-Norinyl

ethinyl estradiol and norethindrone acetate
monophasic: Loestrin 21 1/20, Loestrin 21 1.5/30, Norlestrin 21 1/50, Norlestrin 21 2.5/50

ethinyl estradiol and norgestimate
monophasic: Ortho Cyclen

ethinyl estradiol and norgestrel
monophasic: Lo/Ovral, Ovral

ethinyl estradiol, norethindrone acetate, and ferrous fumarate
monophasic: Loestrin Fe 1/20, Loestrin Fe 1.5/30, Norlestrin Fe 1/50, Norlestrin Fe 2.5/50

---

*Liquid form contains alcohol.   *Common* reactions are in italics; *life-threatening,* in bold italics.
**May contain tartrazine.

mestranol and norethindrone

monophasic: Genora 1/50, Nelova 1/50 M, Norethin 1/50 M, Norinyl 1 + 50, Ortho-Novum 1/50

mestranol and norethynodrel

monophasic: Enovid 5 mg, Enovid 10 mg

Pregnancy Risk Category: X

HOW SUPPLIED

Monophasic oral contraceptives
ethinyl estradiol and desogestrel
Tablets: ethinyl estradiol 30 mcg and desogestrel 0.15 mg (Desogen)
ethinyl estradiol and ethynodiol diacetate
Tablets: ethinyl estradiol 35 mcg and ethynodiol diacetate 1 mg (Demulen 1/35); ethinyl estradiol 50 mcg and ethynodiol diacetate 1 mg (Demulen 1/50)
ethinyl estradiol and levonorgestrel
Tablets: ethinyl estradiol 30 mcg and levonorgestrel 0.15 mg (Levlen, Nordette)
ethinyl estradiol and norethindrone
Tablets: ethinyl estradiol 35 mcg and norethindrone 0.4 mg (Ovcon-35); ethinyl estradiol 35 mcg and norethindrone 0.5 mg (Brevicon, Genora 0.5/35, ModiCon, Nelova 0.5/35 E); ethinyl estradiol 35 mcg and norethindrone 1 mg (Genora 1/35, N.E.E. 1/35, Nelova 1/35 E, Norcept-E 1/35, Norethin 1/35 E, Norinyl 1 + 35, Ortho-Novum 1/35); ethinyl estradiol 50 mcg and norethindrone 1 mg (Ovcon-50)
ethinyl estradiol and norethindrone acetate
Tablets: ethinyl estradiol 20 mcg and norethindrone acetate 1 mg (Loestrin 21 1/20); ethinyl estradiol 30 mcg and norethindrone acetate 1.5 mg (Loestrin 21 1.5/30); ethinyl estradiol 50 mcg and norethindrone acetate 1 mg (Norlestrin 21 1/50); ethinyl estradiol

50 mcg and norethindrone acetate 2.5 mg (Norlestrin 21 2.5/50)
ethinyl estradiol and norgestimate
Tablets: ethinyl estradiol 35 mcg and norgestimate 0.25 mg (Ortho Cyclen)
ethinyl estradiol and norgestrel
Tablets: ethinyl estradiol 30 mcg and norgestrel 0.3 mg (Lo/Ovral); ethinyl estradiol 50 mcg and norgestrel 0.5 mg (Ovral)
ethinyl estradiol, norethindrone acetate, and ferrous fumarate
Tablets: ethinyl estradiol 20 mcg, norethindrone acetate 1 mg, and ferrous fumarate 75 mg (Loestrin Fe 1/20); ethinyl estradiol 30 mcg, norethindrone acetate 1.5 mg, and ferrous fumarate 75 mg (Loestrin Fe 1.5/30); ethinyl estradiol 50 mcg, norethindrone acetate 1 mg, and ferrous fumarate 75 mg (Norlestrin Fe 1/50); ethinyl estradiol 50 mcg, norethindrone acetate 2.5 mg, and ferrous fumarate 75 mg (Norlestrin Fe 2.5/50)
mestranol and norethindrone
Tablets: mestranol 50 mcg and norethindrone 1 mg (Genora 1/50, Nelova 1/50 M, Norethin 1/50 M, Norinyl 1 + 50, Ortho-Novum 1/50)
mestranol and norethynodrel
Tablets: mestranol 75 mg and norethynodrel 5 mg (Enovid 5 mg); mestranol 150 mg and norethynodrel 9.85 mg (Enovid 10 mg).
Biphasic oral contraceptives
ethinyl estradiol and norethindrone
Tablets: ethinyl estradiol 35 mcg and norethindrone 0.5 mg during phase 1 [10 days]; ethinyl estradiol 35 mcg and norethindrone 1 mg during phase 2 [11 days] (Nelova 10/11, Ortho-Novum 10/11)
Triphasic oral contraceptives
ethinyl estradiol and levonorgestrel
Tablets: (Tri-Levlen, Triphasil) ethinyl estradiol 35 mcg and levonorgestrel 0.05 mg during phase 1 [6 days]; ethinyl estradiol 35 mcg and levonorgestrel 0.075 mg during phase 2 [5 days]; ethinyl estradiol 35 mcg and le-

vonorgestrel 0.125 mg during phase 3 [10 days]

ethinyl estradiol and norethindrone
Tablets: (Tri-Norinyl) ethinyl estradiol 35 mcg and norethindrone 0.5 mg during phase 1 [7 days]; ethinyl estradiol 35 mcg and norethindrone 1 mg during phase 2 [9 days]; ethinyl estradiol 35 mcg and norethindrone 0.5 mg during phase 3 [5 days]; (Ortho-Novum 7/7/7) ethinyl estradiol 35 mcg and norethindrone 0.5 mg during phase 1 [7 days]; ethinyl estradiol 35 mcg and norethindrone 0.75 mg during phase 2 [7 days]; ethinyl estradiol 35 mcg and norethindrone 1 mg during phase 3 [7 days]

ACTION
Oral contraceptives inhibit ovulation through a negative feedback mechanism directed at the hypothalamus. They also may prevent transport of the ovum through the fallopian tubes.

Estrogen suppresses secretion of follicle-stimulating hormone, blocking follicular development and ovulation.

Progestin suppresses secretion of luteinizing hormone so ovulation cannot occur even if the follicle develops. Progestin thickens cervical mucus, which interferes with sperm migration, and also causes endometrial changes that prevent implantation of the fertilized ovum.

ONSET, PEAK, DURATION
Onset and duration unknown. Plasma levels of ethinyl estradiol peak within 1 to 2 hours; of norethindrone, within ½ to 4 hours.

INDICATIONS & DOSAGE
Contraception–
Adults: *Monophasic oral contraceptives–* 1 tablet P.O. daily, beginning on day 5 of menstrual cycle (first day of menstrual flow is day 1). With 20- and 21-tablet packages, new dosing cycle begins 7 days after last tablet taken. With 28-tablet packages, dosage is 1 tablet daily without interruption; extra tablets are placebos or contain iron.
Biphasic oral contraceptives–
1 color tablet P.O. daily for 10 days; then next color tablet for 11 days.
Triphasic oral contraceptives–
1 tablet P.O. daily in the sequence specified by the brand.
Endometriosis–
Adults: 1 tablet Enovid 5 mg or 10 mg P.O. daily for 2 weeks starting on day 5 of menstrual cycle. Continued without interruption for 6 to 9 months, increasing dosage by 5 to 10 mg q 2 weeks, up to 20 mg daily; up to 40 mg daily as needed and ordered if breakthrough bleeding occurs.

ADVERSE REACTIONS
CNS: *headache, dizziness,* depression, lethargy, migraine.
CV: ***thromboembolism,*** hypertension, edema.
EENT: worsening of myopia or astigmatism, intolerance of contact lenses.
GI: *nausea,* vomiting, abdominal cramps, bloating, diarrhea, constipation, anorexia, changes in appetite, weight gain, *bowel ischemia,* pancreatitis.
GU: *breakthrough bleeding,* granulomatous colitis, dysmenorrhea, amenorrhea, cervical erosion or abnormal secretions, enlargement of uterine fibromas, vaginal candidiasis.
Hepatic: gallbladder disease, cholestatic jaundice, liver tumors.
Skin: rash, acne, seborrhea, oily skin, ***erythema multiforme,*** hyperpigmentation.
Other: breast changes (*tenderness,* enlargement, secretion); hyperglycemia, hypercalcemia, folic acid deficiency; libido changes.

INTERACTIONS
Bromocriptine: may cause amenorrhea, interfering with bromocriptine's effects. Avoid concomitant use.

---

*Liquid form contains alcohol.   *Common* reactions are in italics; ***life-threatening,*** in bold italics.
**May contain tartrazine.

Carbamazepine, phenobarbital, rifampin: decreased effectiveness of estrogen therapy. Monitor closely.

Corticosteroids: possible enhanced effects. Monitor closely.

Cyclosporine: increased risk of toxicity. Use together with caution and frequently monitor cyclosporine levels.

Dantrolene, other hepatotoxic medications: increased risk of hepatotoxicity. Monitor closely.

Oral anticoagulants: dosage adjustments may be necessary. Monitor PT.

Tamoxifen: estrogens may interfere with effectiveness of tamoxifen. Avoid concomitant use.

CONTRAINDICATIONS

Contraindicated in patients with thromboembolic disorders, cerebrovascular or coronary artery disease, diplopia or any ocular lesion arising from ophthalmic vascular disease, classical migraine, MI, known or suspected breast cancer, known or suspected estrogen-dependent neoplasia, benign or malignant liver tumors, active liver disease or history of cholestatic jaundice with pregnancy or prior use of oral contraceptives, and undiagnosed abnormal vaginal bleeding; in known or suspected pregnancy; and in breast-feeding patients.

NURSING CONSIDERATIONS

● Use cautiously in patients with cardiac, renal, or hepatic insufficiency; hyperlipidemia; hypertension; migraine; seizure disorders; or asthma.

● Be aware that triphasic oral contraceptives may cause fewer adverse reactions, such as breakthrough bleeding and spotting.

● Know that the Centers for Disease Control and Prevention reports that the use of oral contraceptives *may decrease* the incidence of ovarian and endometrial cancers. Also, oral contraceptives do not appear to increase a woman's risk of breast cancer. However, the FDA reports that oral contraceptives may be linked to an increased risk of cervical cancer.

● Periodically monitor serum lipid levels, blood pressure, body weight, and hepatic function as ordered.

● Know that many laboratory tests are affected by oral contraceptives.

● Estrogens and progestins may alter glucose tolerance, thus changing dosage requirements for antidiabetic drugs. Monitor blood glucose levels.

● Discontinue if patients develop granulomatous colitis while on oral contraceptives and notify doctor.

● Know that drug should be discontinued at least 1 week before surgery to decrease risk of thromboembolism. Tell patient to use an alternative method of birth control.

● Tell patients to take tablets at same time each day; nighttime dosing may reduce nausea and headaches.

● Advise patients to use an additional method of birth control, such as condoms or a diaphragm with spermicide, for the first week of administration in the initial cycle.

● Tell patient missed doses in midcycle greatly increase likelihood of pregnancy.

● If one tablet is missed, tell patients to take it as soon as remembered or to take two tablets the next day and continue regular schedule. If patients miss 2 consecutive days, instruct them to take two tablets daily for 2 days and then resume normal schedule. Also advise them to use an additional method of birth control for 7 days after two missed doses. If three or more doses are missed, tell patients to discard remaining tablets in monthly package and to substitute another contraceptive method. If next menstrual period doesn't begin on schedule, warn patients to rule out pregnancy before starting new dosing cycle. If menstrual period begins, have patients start new dosing cycle 7 days after last tablet was taken.

● Warn patients that headache, nausea, dizziness, breast tenderness, spotting, and breakthrough bleeding are common at first. These effects should diminish after three to six dosing cycles (months).

• Instruct patients to weigh themselves at least twice a week and to report any sudden weight gain or edema to the doctor.

• Warn patients to avoid exposure to ultraviolet light or prolonged exposure to sunlight.

• Warn patients to immediately report abdominal pain; numbness, stiffness, or pain in legs or buttocks; pressure or pain in chest; shortness of breath; severe headache; visual disturbances, such as blind spots, blurriness, or flashing lights; undiagnosed vaginal bleeding or discharge; two consecutive missed menstrual periods; lumps in the breast; swelling of hands or feet; or severe pain in the abdomen (tumor rupture in the liver).

• Advise patients of increased risks associated with simultaneous use of cigarettes and oral contraceptives.

• Teach patients how to perform routine breast self-examination.

• If one menstrual period is missed and tablets have been taken on schedule, tell patients to continue taking them. If two consecutive menstrual periods are missed, tell patients to stop drug and have pregnancy test. Progestins may cause birth defects if taken early in pregnancy.

• Advise patients not to take same drug for longer than 12 months without consulting the doctor. Stress importance of Papanicolaou tests and annual gynecologic examinations.

• Advise patients to check with the doctor about how soon pregnancy may be attempted after hormonal therapy is stopped. Many doctors recommend that women not become pregnant within 2 months after stopping drug.

• Warn patients of possible delay in achieving pregnancy when drug is discontinued.

• Tell patient many doctors advise women on prolonged therapy (5 years or longer) to stop drug and use other birth control methods. Periodically reassess patients while off hormone therapy.

hydroxyprogesterone caproate
Delta-Lutin, Duralutin, Gesterol L.A. 250, Hy/Gestrone, Hylutin, Hyprogest 250, Pro-Depo, Prodrox 250, Pro-Span

Pregnancy Risk Category: X

HOW SUPPLIED
Injection: 125 mg/ml, 250 mg/ml

ACTION
Suppresses ovulation, possibly by inhibiting pituitary gonadotropin secretion, and forms thick cervical mucus.

ONSET, PEAK, DURATION
Unknown.

INDICATIONS & DOSAGE
Amenorrhea, uterine bleeding–
Adults: 375 mg I.M. q 4 weeks. Stop after four cycles.
Palliative treatment of advanced inoperable endometrial cancer–
Adults: 1 to 7 g I.M. weekly.

ADVERSE REACTIONS
CNS: dizziness, migraine, lethargy, depression.
CV: hypertension, thrombophlebitis, *pulmonary embolism,* edema.
GI: nausea, vomiting, abdominal cramps.
GU: breakthrough bleeding, dysmenorrhea, amenorrhea, cervical erosion, abnormal secretions, uterine fibromas, vaginal candidiasis.
Hepatic: cholestatic jaundice.
Skin: melasma, rash.

Local: irritation and pain at injection site.
Other: breast tenderness, enlargement, or secretion; decreased libido; hyperglycemia.

INTERACTIONS
Barbiturates, carbamazepine, rifampin: decreased progestin effects. Monitor for diminished therapeutic response.
Bromocriptine: may cause amenorrhea, interfering with bromocriptine's effects. Avoid concomitant use.
Corticosteroids: possible enhanced effects. Monitor closely.
Dantrolene, other hepatotoxic medications: increased risk of hepatotoxicity. Monitor closely.
Oral anticoagulants: dosage adjustments may be necessary. Monitor PT.

CONTRAINDICATIONS
Contraindicated in patients with hypersensitivity to drug, thromboembolic disorders, cerebral apoplexy, breast or genital organ cancer, undiagnosed abnormal vaginal bleeding, severe hepatic disease, or missed abortion and during pregnancy.

NURSING CONSIDERATIONS
• Use cautiously in patients with diabetes mellitus, seizure disorder, migraine, cardiac or renal disease, asthma, mental depression, or impaired liver function.
• Know that drug should not be used to induce withdrawal bleeding or as a test for pregnancy; drug may cause birth defects and masculinization of female fetus.
• Give oil solutions (sesame oil and castor oil) via deep I.M. injection in gluteal muscle. Rotate injection sites to prevent muscle atrophy.
• FDA regulations require that, before receiving first dose, patients read package insert explaining possible adverse effects of progestin. Also provide verbal explanation.

• Tell patients to report any unusual symptoms immediately and to stop drug and call the doctor if visual disturbances or migraine occur.
• Warn patients that edema and weight gain are likely. Tell patient to monitor weight routinely and recommend sodium-restricted diet as needed.
• Instruct patients to report breast pain or tenderness, vaginal discharge or bleeding, and swelling of the hands or feet.
• Teach patients how to perform routine breast self-examination.
• Instruct patients that normal menstrual cycles may not resume for 2 to 3 months after drug is stopped.

---

levonorgestrel
Norplant System

Pregnancy Risk Category: X

HOW SUPPLIED
Implants: 36 mg per capsule; each kit contains six capsules

ACTION
Slowly releases the synthetic progestin levonorgestrel into the bloodstream. How progestins provide contraception is not fully understood, but they alter the mucus covering the cervix, prevent implantation of the egg, and, in some patients, prevent ovulation.

ONSET, PEAK, DURATION
Onset and peak levels occur within 24 hours. Effects persist about 5 years.

INDICATIONS & DOSAGE
Prevention of pregnancy –
Women: six capsules implanted subdermally in the midportion of the upper arm, about 8 cm above the elbow crease, during the first 7 days of the onset of menses. Capsules are placed fanlike, 15 degrees apart (total of 75

---

†Available in Canada only.   ‡Available in Australia only.   ◊ Available OTC.

degrees). Contraceptive efficacy lasts for 5 years.

ADVERSE REACTIONS

CNS: headache, nervousness, dizziness.
GI: nausea, *abdominal discomfort*, appetite change.
GU: *amenorrhea, many days of bleeding or prolonged bleeding, spotting, irregular onset of bleeding, frequent onset of bleeding, scanty bleeding, cervicitis, vaginitis, leukorrhea.*
Skin: dermatitis, acne, hirsutism, hypertrichosis, scalp hair loss, infection at implant site, transient pain or itching at implant site.
Other: adnexal enlargement, mastalgia, weight gain, *musculoskeletal pain, removal difficulty, breast discharge.*

INTERACTIONS

Carbamazepine, phenytoin, rifampin: may reduce the contraceptive efficacy of levonorgestrel implants.

CONTRAINDICATIONS

Contraindicated in patients with active thrombophlebitis or thromboembolic disorders, undiagnosed abnormal genital bleeding, acute liver disease, malignant or benign liver tumors, known or suspected breast cancer, and in known or suspected pregnancy.

NURSING CONSIDERATIONS

• Use cautiously in patients with a history of depression, in diabetic and prediabetic patients, and in patients with hyperlipidemia.
• Know that most patients develop variations in menstrual bleeding patterns, including irregular bleeding, prolonged bleeding, spotting, and amenorrhea. In most patients, these irregularities diminish over time.
• Be aware that irregular bleeding may mask symptoms of cervical or endometrial cancer.

• Closely monitor patients with conditions that may be aggravated by fluid retention because steroid hormones may cause fluid retention.
• Be aware laboratory tests for sex hormone-binding globulin and thyroxine (T_4) concentrations may show decreased values; for triiodothyronine (T_3) uptake, increased values.
• Know implants do not contain estrogen. Levonorgestrel is a totally synthetic progestin.
• Expect implants to be removed if patients develop active thrombophlebitis or thromboembolic disease or will be immobilized for a significant length of time because of illness or some other factor.
• If jaundice develops, expect implants to be removed because steroid hormone metabolism is impaired in patients with liver failure.
• Although retinal thrombosis after use of oral contraceptives has been reported, no similar incidents have been documented after use of the implant system. However, patients with sudden unexplained vision problems, including users of contact lenses who develop vision changes or changes in lens tolerance, should be immediately evaluated by an ophthalmologist.
• Tell patients to report to the doctor immediately if one of the implant capsules falls out (before the skin heals over the implant). Contraceptive efficacy may be impaired.
• Warn patients that missed menstrual periods are not an accurate indicator of early pregnancy because drug may induce amenorrhea. Advise patients that 6 weeks or more of amenorrhea (after a pattern of regular menstrual periods) could indicate pregnancy. If pregnancy is confirmed, the implants must be removed.
• Encourage regular (at least annual) physical examinations.

---

*Liquid form contains alcohol.   *Common* reactions are in italics; ***life-threatening***, in bold italics.
**May contain tartrazine.

medroxyprogesterone acetate

Amen, Curretab, Cycrin, Depo-Provera, Provera

Pregnancy Risk Category: X

HOW SUPPLIED
Tablets: 2.5 mg, 5 mg, 10 mg
Injection (suspension): 100 mg/ml, 150 mg/ml, 400 mg/ml

ACTION
Suppresses ovulation, possibly by inhibiting pituitary gonadotropin secretion, and forms thick cervical mucus.

ONSET, PEAK, DURATION
Unknown.

INDICATIONS & DOSAGE
Abnormal uterine bleeding caused by hormonal imbalance –
Adults: 5 to 10 mg P.O. daily for 5 to 10 days beginning on sixteenth day of menstrual cycle. If the patient also has received estrogen – 10 mg P.O. daily for 10 days beginning on sixteenth day of cycle.
Secondary amenorrhea –
Adults: 5 to 10 mg P.O. daily for 5 to 10 days.
Endometrial or renal carcinoma –
Adults: 400 to 1,000 mg I.M. weekly.
Contraception in women –
Adults: 150 mg I.M. once q 3 months.

ADVERSE REACTIONS
CNS: dizziness, migraine, lethargy, depression.
CV: hypertension, thrombophlebitis, *pulmonary embolism,* edema.
GI: nausea, vomiting, abdominal cramps.
GU: breakthrough bleeding, dysmenorrhea, amenorrhea, cervical erosion, abnormal secretions, uterine fibromas, vaginal candidiasis.
Hepatic: cholestatic jaundice.

Skin: melasma, rash, pain, induration, sterile abscesses.
Other: hyperglycemia; breast tenderness, enlargement, or secretion; decreased libido.

INTERACTIONS
Aminoglutethimide, rifampin: decreased progestin effects. Monitor for diminished therapeutic response. Patient should use a nonhormonal contraceptive during therapy with these drugs.
Bromocriptine: may cause amenorrhea, interfering with bromocriptine's effects. Avoid concomitant use.

CONTRAINDICATIONS
Contraindicated in patients with hypersensitivity to drug, active thromboembolic disorders, or past history of thromboembolic disorders or of cerebral vascular disease or apoplexy, breast cancer, undiagnosed abnormal vaginal bleeding, missed abortion, or hepatic dysfunction and during pregnancy. Tablets are also contraindicated in patients with liver dysfunction or known or suspected malignancy of the genital organs.

NURSING CONSIDERATIONS
• Use cautiously in patients with diabetes mellitus, seizure disorder, migraine, cardiac or renal disease, asthma, and mental depression.
• Know that the drug should not be used as test for pregnancy; drug may cause birth defects and masculinization of female fetus.
• I.M. injection may be painful. Monitor sites for evidence of sterile abscess. Rotate injection sites to prevent muscle atrophy.
• FDA regulations require that, before receiving first dose, patients read package insert explaining possible adverse effects of progestins. Also, provide verbal explanation.
• Tell patients to report any unusual symptoms immediately and to stop

---

drug and call the doctor if visual disturbances or migraine occurs.
• Teach women how to perform routine monthly breast self-examination.

---

norethindrone
Micronor, Norlutin, Nor-Q.D.

norethindrone acetate
Aygestin, Aygestin Cycle Pack, Norlutate

Pregnancy Risk Category: X

HOW SUPPLIED
norethindrone
Tablets: 0.35 mg, 5 mg
norethindrone acetate
Tablets: 5 mg

ACTION
Suppresses ovulation, possibly by inhibiting pituitary gonadotropin secretion, and forms thick cervical mucus.

ONSET, PEAK, DURATION
Unknown.

INDICATIONS & DOSAGE
Amenorrhea, abnormal uterine bleeding –
Adults: 5 to 20 mg norethindrone or 2.5 to 10 mg norethindrone acetate P.O. daily on days 5 to 25 of menstrual cycle.
Endometriosis –
Adults: 10 mg norethindrone P.O. daily for 14 days; then increased by 5 mg daily q 2 weeks up to 30 mg daily. Or 5 mg norethindrone acetate P.O. daily for 14 days; then increased by 2.5 mg daily q 2 weeks up to 15 mg daily.
Contraception in women –
Adults: initially, 0.35 mg norethindrone P.O. on the first day of menstruation; then 0.35 mg daily.

ADVERSE REACTIONS
CNS: dizziness, migraine, lethargy, depression.

CV: hypertension, thrombophlebitis, ***pulmonary embolism,*** edema.
GI: nausea, vomiting, abdominal cramps.
GU: breakthrough bleeding, dysmenorrhea, amenorrhea, cervical erosion, abnormal secretions, uterine fibromas, vaginal candidiasis.
Hepatic: cholestatic jaundice.
Skin: melasma, rash.
Other: breast tenderness, enlargement, or secretion; decreased libido; hyperglycemia.

INTERACTIONS
Barbiturates, carbamazepine, rifampin: decreased progestin effects. Monitor for diminished therapeutic response.
Bromocriptine: may cause amenorrhea, interfering with bromocriptine effects. Avoid concomitant use.

CONTRAINDICATIONS
Contraindicated in patients with thromboembolic disorders, cerebral apoplexy, or history of these conditions; hypersensitivity to drug; breast cancer, undiagnosed abnormal vaginal bleeding, severe hepatic disease, or missed abortion and during pregnancy.

NURSING CONSIDERATIONS
• Use cautiously in patients with diabetes mellitus, seizure disorder, migraine, cardiac or renal disease, asthma, and mental depression.
• Norethindrone acetate is twice as potent as norethindrone. Know that norethindrone acetate should not be used for contraception.
• Know that use as test for pregnancy is not appropriate; drug may cause birth defects and masculinization of female fetus.
• Know that preliminary estrogen treatment is usually needed in menstrual disorders.
• Watch patients carefully for signs of edema.

---

*Liquid form contains alcohol. **May contain tartrazine. *Common* reactions are in italics; ***life-threatening,*** in bold italics.

• FDA regulations require that, before receiving first dose, patients read package insert explaining possible adverse effects of progestin. Also provide verbal explanation.

• Tell patients to report any unusual symptoms immediately and to stop drug and call the doctor if visual disturbances or migraine occurs.

• Teach patients how to perform routine monthly breast self-examination.

---

norgestrel
Ovrette**

Pregnancy Risk Category: X

HOW SUPPLIED
Tablets: 0.075 mg

ACTION
Unknown. Probably suppresses ovulation, possibly by inhibiting pituitary gonadotropin secretion, and forms thick cervical mucus.

ONSET, PEAK, DURATION
Unknown.

INDICATIONS & DOSAGE
Contraception in women –
Adults: 0.075 mg P.O. daily.

ADVERSE REACTIONS
CNS: cerebral thrombosis or hemorrhage, migraine headache, lethargy, depression.
CV: hypertension, thrombophlebitis, *pulmonary embolism,* edema.
GI: nausea, vomiting, abdominal cramps, gallbladder disease.
GU: *breakthrough bleeding, change in menstrual flow,* dysmenorrhea, spotting, amenorrhea, cervical erosion, vaginal candidiasis.
Hepatic: cholestatic jaundice.
Skin: melasma, rash.
Other: breast tenderness, enlargement, or secretion.

INTERACTIONS
Barbiturates, carbamazepine, rifampin: decreased progestin effects. Monitor for diminished therapeutic response.
Bromocriptine: may cause amenorrhea, interfering with bromocriptine's effects. Avoid concomitant use.

CONTRAINDICATIONS
Contraindicated in patients with thromboembolic disorders, cerebral apoplexy, or history of these conditions; hypersensitivity to drug; breast cancer, undiagnosed abnormal vaginal bleeding, severe hepatic disease, and missed abortion, and during pregnancy.

NURSING CONSIDERATIONS
• Use cautiously in patients with diabetes mellitus, seizure disorder, migraine, cardiac or renal disease, asthma, and mental depression.

• Be aware that norgestrel is a progestin-only oral contraceptive known as the "minipill."

• FDA regulations require that, before receiving first dose, patients read package insert explaining possible adverse effects of progestins. Also provide verbal explanation.

• Tell patients to take pill every day, at the same time, even if menstruating.

• Risk of pregnancy increases with each tablet missed. Tell patients who miss one tablet to take it as soon as remembered and then take the next tablet at the regular time. Advise patients who miss two tablets to take one as soon as remembered and then take the next regular dose at the usual time and to use a nonhormonal method of contraception in addition to norgestrel until 14 tablets have been taken. Instruct patients who miss three or more tablets to discontinue drug and use a nonhormonal method of contraception until after menses. If menstrual

---

period does not occur within 45 days, pregnancy testing is necessary.

• Advise women using oral contraceptives of the increased risk of serious adverse CV reactions associated with heavy cigarette smoking (15 or more cigarettes per day). These risks are quite marked in women over age 35.

• Instruct patients to immediately report excessive bleeding or bleeding between menstrual cycles, breast pain or tenderness, vaginal discharge, or swelling of the hands or feet.

• Tell patients to report any unusual symptoms immediately and to stop drug and call the doctor if visual disturbances, migraine, or numbness or tingling in limbs occurs.

• Teach patients how to perform routine breast self-examination.

progesterone
Gesterol 50, Progestilin†

Pregnancy Risk Category: X

HOW SUPPLIED
Injection (in oil): 50 mg/ml

ACTION
Suppresses ovulation, possibly by inhibiting pituitary gonadotropin secretion, and forms thick cervical mucus.

ONSET, PEAK, DURATION
Unknown.

INDICATIONS & DOSAGE
Amenorrhea –
Adults: 5 to 10 mg I.M. daily for 6 to 8 days usually beginning 8 to 10 days before the anticipated start of menstruation.
Dysfunctional uterine bleeding –
Adults: 5 to 10 mg I.M. daily for six doses.

ADVERSE REACTIONS
CNS: dizziness, migraine, lethargy, depression.
CV: hypertension, thrombophlebitis, ***pulmonary embolism***, edema.
GI: nausea, vomiting, abdominal cramps.
GU: breakthrough bleeding, dysmenorrhea, amenorrhea, cervical erosion, abnormal secretions, uterine fibromas, vaginal candidiasis.
Hepatic: cholestatic jaundice.
Local: pain at injection site.
Skin: melasma, rash.
Other: breast tenderness, enlargement, or secretion; decreased libido; hyperglycemia.

INTERACTIONS
Barbiturates, carbamazepine, rifampin: decreased progestin effects. Monitor for diminished therapeutic response.
Bromocriptine: may cause amenorrhea, interfering with bromocriptine's effects. Avoid concomitant use.

CONTRAINDICATIONS
Contraindicated in patients with thromboembolic disorders, cerebral apoplexy, or history of these conditions; hypersensitivity to drug; breast cancer, undiagnosed abnormal vaginal bleeding, severe hepatic disease, and missed abortion.

NURSING CONSIDERATIONS
• Use cautiously in patients with diabetes mellitus, seizure disorder, migraine, cardiac or renal disease, asthma, and mental depression.

• Know preliminary estrogen treatment is usually needed in menstrual disorders.

• Give oil solutions (peanut oil or sesame oil) via deep I.M. injection. Check sites frequently for irritation. Rotate injection sites.

• FDA regulations require that, before receiving first dose, patients read package insert explaining possible adverse effects of progestins. Also provide verbal explanation.

• Tell patients to report any unusual

---

*Liquid form contains alcohol.
May contain tartrazine.*   *Common* reactions are in italics; ***life-threatening*, in bold italics.

symptoms immediately and to stop drug and call the doctor if visual disturbances or migraine occurs.
• Teach patients how to perform routine breast self-examination.

quinestrol
Estrovis

Pregnancy Risk Category: X

HOW SUPPLIED
Tablets: 100 mcg

ACTION
Increases the synthesis of DNA, RNA, and protein in responsive tissues. Also reduces release of follicle-stimulating hormone and luteinizing hormone from the pituitary gland.

ONSET, PEAK, DURATION
Unknown.

INDICATIONS & DOSAGE
Moderate to severe vasomotor symptoms associated with menopause, atrophic vaginitis, kraurosis vulvae, female hypogonadism, female castration, primary ovarian failure –
Adults: 100 mcg P.O. once daily for 7 days, followed by 100 mcg weekly as maintenance dosage beginning 2 weeks after start of treatment. Dosage increased to 200 mcg weekly if necessary.

ADVERSE REACTIONS
CNS: headache, dizziness, chorea, migraine, depression.
CV: thrombophlebitis; *thromboembolism;* hypertension; edema; *increased risk of CVA, pulmonary embolism, and MI.*
EENT: worsening of myopia or astigmatism, intolerance of contact lenses.
GI: *nausea,* vomiting, abdominal cramps, bloating, diarrhea, constipation, anorexia, increased appetite, excessive thirst, weight changes.
GU: breakthrough bleeding, altered

menstrual flow, dysmenorrhea, amenorrhea, cervical erosion or abnormal secretions, enlargement of uterine fibromas, vaginal candidiasis.
Hepatic: cholestatic jaundice.
Skin: melasma, urticaria, acne, seborrhea, oily skin, hirsutism or hair loss.
Other: leg cramps, purpura, breast changes (tenderness, enlargement, secretion), hyperglycemia, hypercalcemia, folic acid deficiency, libido changes.

INTERACTIONS
Bromocriptine: may cause amenorrhea, interfering with bromocriptine's effects. Avoid concomitant use.
Carbamazepine, phenobarbital, rifampin: decreased effectiveness of estrogen therapy. Monitor closely.
Corticosteroids: possible enhanced effects. Monitor closely.
Cyclosporine: increased risk of toxicity. Use together with caution and frequently monitor cyclosporine levels.
Dantrolene, other hepatotoxic medications: increased risk of hepatotoxicity. Monitor closely.
Oral anticoagulants: dosage adjustments may be necessary. Monitor PT.
Tamoxifen: estrogens may interfere with effectiveness of tamoxifen. Avoid concomitant use.

CONTRAINDICATIONS
Contraindicated in patients with thrombophlebitis or thromboembolic disorders, breast or reproductive organ cancer, or undiagnosed abnormal genital bleeding and during pregnancy.

NURSING CONSIDERATIONS
• Use cautiously in patients with asthma; cerebrovascular or coronary artery disease, mental depression; migraine; seizures; bone diseases associated with hypercalcemia; cardiac, hepatic, or renal dysfunction; or in women with family history (mother,

grandmother, sister) of breast or genital tract cancer, or who have breast nodules, fibrocystic disease, or abnormal mammographic findings.

• Ensure that patients have a thorough physical examination before initiating estrogen therapy. Patients receiving long-term therapy should have repeat examinations yearly. Periodically monitor body weight, blood pressure, hepatic function, and serum lipid levels, as ordered.

• Be aware similar in effectiveness to conjugated estrogens in treating postmenopausal symptoms. Biggest advantage is that quinestrol can be taken once a week.

• Notify the pathologist about any patients receiving estrogen therapy.

• Know that attempts to discontinue medication should be made at 3- to 6-month intervals.

• Tell patient that patient package insert that describes estrogen's adverse effects is available; however, also provide verbal explanation.

• Stress the importance of regular physical examinations. Studies suggest that postmenopausal women who use estrogen replacement for more than 5 years to treat menopausal symptoms may be at increased risk for endometrial carcinoma. This risk is reduced by using cyclic rather than continuous therapy and the lowest possible dosages of estrogen. Adding progestins to the regimen decreases the incidence of endometrial hyperplasia; however, it isn't known if progestins affect the incidence of endometrial carcinoma. Most studies show no increased risk of breast cancer.

• Explain to patients on replacement therapy for postmenopausal symptoms that, although menstrual-like bleeding or spotting may occur, fertility has not been restored. Pregnancy cannot occur because patients have not ovulated.

• Warn patients to immediately report abdominal pain; pain, numbness, or

stiffness in legs or buttocks; pressure or pain in chest; shortness of breath; severe headaches; visual disturbances, such as blind spots, flashing lights, or blurriness; vaginal bleeding or discharge; breast lumps; swelling of hands or feet; yellow skin or sclera; dark urine; or light-colored stools.

• Tell diabetic patients to report elevated blood glucose test results so antidiabetic medication dosage can be adjusted.

• Teach women how to perform routine breast self-examination.

56

Gonadotropins

gonadorelin acetate
gonadorelin hydrochloride
gonadotropin, chorionic
histrelin acetate
menotropins
nafarelin acetate

COMBINATION PRODUCTS
None.

---

gonadorelin acetate
Lutrepulse

Pregnancy Risk Category: B

HOW SUPPLIED
Injection: 0.8 mg/10 ml, 3.2 mg/10 ml vials; supplied as a kit with I.V. supplies and ambulatory infusion pump

ACTION
Mimics the action of gonadotropin-releasing hormone (GnRH), which results in the synthesis and release of luteinizing hormone (LH) from the anterior pituitary gland. LH subsequently acts upon the reproductive organs to regulate hormone synthesis.

ONSET, PEAK, DURATION
Unknown.

INDICATIONS & DOSAGE
Induction of ovulation in women with primary hypothalamic amenorrhea —
Adults: 5 mcg I.V. q 90 minutes for 21 days. If no response follows three treatment intervals, increase dosage as ordered.

ADVERSE REACTIONS
Skin: hematoma, local infection, inflammation, mild phlebitis.
Other: multiple pregnancy, ovarian hyperstimulation.

INTERACTIONS
None significant.

CONTRAINDICATIONS
Contraindicated in patients hypersensitive to the drug, in women with conditions that could be complicated by pregnancy (such as prolactinoma), in those who are anovulatory from any cause other than a hypothalamic disorder, and in those with ovarian cysts.

NURSING CONSIDERATIONS
• **I.V. use:** To mimic the naturally occurring hormone, administer gonadorelin in a pulsatile fashion with the available ambulatory infusion pump. Set the pulse period at 1 minute (infuse drug over 1 minute) and the pulse interval at 90 minutes.
• To administer 2.5 mcg/pulse, reconstitute the 0.8-mg vial with 8 ml of supplied diluent and set the pump to deliver 25 microliters/pulse. To administer 5 mcg/pulse, use the same dosage strength and dilution but set the pump to deliver 50 microliters/pulse.
• Some patients may require higher I.V. doses. To administer 10 mcg/pulse, reconstitute the 3.2-mg vial with 8 ml of supplied diluent and set the pump to deliver 25 microliters/pulse. To administer 20 mcg/pulse, use the same dosage strength and dilution but set the pump to deliver 50 microliters/pulse.
• Inspect the I.V. site at each visit.
• Be aware patients usually require pelvic ultrasound on days 7 and 14 after establishment of a baseline scan. Some clinicians prefer shorter intervals between scans.
• Ensure that patients understand a multiple pregnancy is possible (incidence is about 12%). Close monitor-

ing of dosage, as well as ovarian ultrasonography to monitor drug response, is necessary.

• Instruct patients about proper aseptic technique and care of the I.V. site. Cannula and I.V. site should be changed every 48 hours. Written instructions are available for patients.

• Anaphylaxis has been reported with similar drugs. Teach patients how to recognize signs and symptoms of hypersensitivity reactions (hives, wheezing, difficulty breathing) and encourage them to report these as soon as possible.

• Advise patients to report signs of infection, hematoma, inflammation, or phlebitis at the injection site. Patients also should immediately report severe abdominal pain, bloating, swelling of the hands or feet, nausea, vomiting, diarrhea, substantial weight gain, or shortness of breath.

• Encourage patients to adhere to the close monitoring schedule required by the therapy. Regular pelvic examinations, midluteal phase serum progesterone determinations, and multiple ovarian ultrasound scans are necessary.

---

gonadorelin hydrochloride (synthetic luteinizing hormone-releasing hormone, LHRH; synthetic gonadotropin-releasing hormone, GnRH)
Factrel

Pregnancy Risk Category: B

HOW SUPPLIED
Injection: 100 mcg, 500 mcg

ACTION
A synthetic luteinizing hormone that releases LHRH.

ONSET, PEAK, DURATION
Onset and peak unknown. Effects persist for 3 to 5 hours.

INDICATIONS & DOSAGE
Evaluation of the functional capacity and response of gonadotropins –
Adults: 100 mcg S.C. or I.V. In women for whom the menstrual cycle phase can be established, test performed between day 1 and day 7.

ADVERSE REACTIONS
CNS: headache, flushing, light-headedness.
GI: nausea, abdominal discomfort.
Skin: local swelling, occasionally with pain and pruritus when administered S.C.; rash after long-term S.C. administration.

INTERACTIONS
Digoxin, oral contraceptives: may depress gonadotropin levels. Monitor results carefully.
Levodopa, spironolactone: may elevate gonadotropin levels. Monitor results carefully.
Phenothiazines and dopamine antagonists: increase prolactin which may blunt the response to gonadorelin.

CONTRAINDICATIONS
Contraindicated in patients hypersensitive to the drug.

NURSING CONSIDERATIONS
• Use cautiously in patients allergic to other drugs.
• Keep epinephrine readily available when administering gonadorelin to patients allergic to other drugs.
• **I.V. use:** Reconstitute vial with 1 to 2 ml of accompanying sterile diluent. Inject drug directly into vein over 3 to 5 minutes. Alternatively, inject into an I.V. line containing a free-flowing compatible solution. Prepare solution immediately before use. After reconstitution, store at room temperature and use within 1 day. Discard unused reconstituted solution and diluent.
• As a single injection, gonadorelin can be used to evaluate the functional capacity and response of the gonado-

---

*Liquid form contains alcohol.
May contain tartrazine.   *Common* reactions are in italics; ***life-threatening*, in bold italics.

tropins of the anterior pituitary gland. Prolonged or repeated administration may be necessary to measure pituitary gonadotropin reserve.
• Be aware the gonadorelin test can be performed concomitantly with other post-treatment evaluations.
• For specific test methodology and interpretation of test results, refer to the manufacturer's full product information. Ask the pharmacist for a copy.

gonadotropin, chorionic (HCG)
A.P.L., Chorex-5, Chorex-10, Follutein, Gonic, Pregnyl, Profasi HP†

Pregnancy Risk Category: C

HOW SUPPLIED
Injection: 200 units/ml, 500 units/ml, 1,000 units/ml, 2,000 units/ml (after reconstitution)

ACTION
Serves as a substitute for luteinizing hormone to stimulate ovulation of human menopausal gonadotropin-prepared follicle. Also promotes secretion of gonadal steroid hormones by stimulating production of androgen by the interstitial cells of the testes (Leydig cells).

ONSET, PEAK, DURATION
Onset occurs within 2 hours. Serum levels peak within 6 hours. Effects persist at least 36 hours.

INDICATIONS & DOSAGE
Anovulation and infertility in women –
Adults: 5,000 to 10,000 units I.M. 1 day after last dose of menotropins.
Hypogonadotropic hypogonadism –
Adults: 500 to 1,000 units I.M. three times weekly for 3 weeks; then twice weekly for 3 weeks. Or 4,000 units I.M. three times weekly for 6 to 9

months; then 2,000 units three times weekly for 3 more months.
Nonobstructive prepubertal cryptorchidism –
Prepubertal boys: 4000 units I.M. weekly for 3 weeks; or 5,000 units I.M. every other day for 4 doses; or 500 to 1,000 units I.M. for 15 doses given over 6 weeks; or 500 units I.M. 3 times weekly for 4 to 6 weeks.
Stimulation of spermatogenesis –
Men: 5,000 units I.M. 3 times weekly for 4 to 6 months; then 2,000 units twice weekly with menotropin therapy.

ADVERSE REACTIONS
CNS: headache, fatigue, irritability, restlessness, depression.
CV: edema.
Skin: *pain at injection site.*
Other: gynecomastia, early puberty (growth of testes, penis, pubic and axillary hair; voice change; down on upper lip; growth of body hair).

INTERACTIONS
None significant.

CONTRAINDICATIONS
Contraindicated in patients with hypersensitivity to drug, prostate cancer or other androgen-dependent neoplasia, in early puberty (usual onset between ages 10 and 13), and during pregnancy.

NURSING CONSIDERATIONS
• Use cautiously in patients with seizure disorders, migraine, asthma, and cardiac or renal disease.
• Know that usually used only after failure of clomiphene in anovulatory patients.
• Reconstitute with 1 to 2 ml of supplied diluent just before use. Use reconstituted solutions within 24 hours.
• For I.M. use only. Don't inject I.V. Rotate injection sites to prevent muscle atrophy.
• Be alert for symptoms of ectopic

---

pregnancy, which typically are evident between weeks 8 to 12 of gestation.

• Make sure patient understands when used with menotropins to induce ovulation, multiple births are possible.

• In infertility, encourage daily intercourse from day before chorionic gonadotropin is given until ovulation occurs.

• Instruct patients to immediately report severe abdominal pain, bloating, swelling of the hands or feet, nausea, vomiting, diarrhea, substantial weight gain, or shortness of breath.

---

histrelin acetate
Supprelin

Pregnancy Risk Category: X

HOW SUPPLIED
Injection: 120 mcg/0.6 ml, 300 mcg/0.6 ml, 600 mcg/0.6 ml

ACTION
An agonist that mimics the effects of gonadotropin-releasing hormone (GnRH; also called luteinizing hormone-releasing hormone, or LHRH) but is more potent than the naturally occurring hormone. Chronic administration desensitizes responsiveness of the pituitary gonadotropin, decreasing sex hormone production by the testes or ovaries.

ONSET, PEAK, DURATION
Unknown.

INDICATIONS & DOSAGE
Centrally mediated (idiopathic or neurogenic) precocious puberty –
Children (girls 2 to 8 years; boys 2 to 9½ years): 10 mcg/kg S.C. daily.

ADVERSE REACTIONS
CNS: migraine, *visual disturbances, mood changes, nervousness, dizziness, depression, libido changes, insomnia, anxiety,* paresthesia, cognitive changes, syncope, somnolence, lethargy, impaired consciousness, tremor, hyperkinesia, *seizures,* hot flashes, conduct disorder.
CV: *vasodilation,* edema, palpitations, tachycardia, hypertension.
EENT: epistaxis, ear congestion, abnormal pupillary function, otalgia, hearing loss, polyopia, pharyngitis, photophobia, rhinorrhea, sinusitis.
GI: *abdominal pain, nausea, vomiting, diarrhea, flatulence, decreased appetite, dyspepsia,* cramps, constipation, thirst, gastritis.
GU: *menstrual changes, vaginal dryness, leukorrhea, hypermenorrhea,* tenderness of female genitalia, glycosuria.
Hematologic: hyperlipidemia, anemia.
Respiratory: *upper respiratory infection, respiratory congestion, cough,* asthma, breathing disorder, bronchitis, hyperventilation.
Skin: pallor.
Other: urticaria, *fever, arthralgia, muscle stiffness, muscle cramps, breast pain or edema,* breast discharge, decreased breast size, muscle pain, hypotonia, goiter, ***acute hypersensitivity reactions (anaphylaxis, angioedema).***

INTERACTIONS
None significant.

CONTRAINDICATIONS
• Contraindicated in patients hypersensitive to any component of the drug and in pregnant or breast-feeding patients.
• Safety and efficacy have not been established in children under 2 years.

NURSING CONSIDERATIONS
• Be aware drug is indicated only for patients who will comply with the daily administration schedule. Noncompliance or inadequate dosing may result in inadequate control of the

---

Liquid form contains alcohol.   *Common* reactions are in italics; ***life-threatening,*** in bold italics.
**May contain tartrazine.

pubertal process, which can result in recurrence of symptoms, including onset of menses, breast development, or testicular growth; long-term consequences may involve decreased adult height.

• A complete physical and endocrinologic evaluation should be performed before initiating drug therapy; several indices should be reexamined at 3 months, then every 6 to 12 months thereafter. Such evaluations should include determinations of height and weight, hand and wrist X-ray for bone age determination, sex steroid (estradiol or testosterone) levels, and GnRH stimulation test. Monitor these tests periodically to determine effectiveness of therapy.

• Additional tests to rule out other causes of precocious puberty include beta human chorionic gonadotropin levels (to detect chorionic gonadotropin-secreting tumor); pelvic/adrenal/testicular ultrasound (to detect steroid-secreting tumor); and computed tomography scan of the head (to detect any previously undiagnosed intracranial tumor). Workup also establishes baseline of gonad size for serial monitoring.

• Store drug in the refrigerator (36° to 46° F [2° to 8° C]) protected from light and in its original container. Use vials only once because drug does not contain preservatives. Allow medication to reach room temperature before giving.

• Give S.C. and rotate injection sites to minimize local reactions.

• Know decreases in FSH, LH, and sex steroid levels occur within 3 months.

• Patients should be reevaluated if prepubertal levels of sex steroids or GnRH test responses are not achieved within 3 months of therapy.

• Before initiating therapy, make sure that patients and their parents understand the importance of adhering to the daily administration schedules.

Tell them to give drug at about the same time each day to facilitate compliance and ensure adequate dosing.

• Drug is dispensed as a 30-day kit that contains a patient information leaflet. Ensure that caregivers read and understand the leaflet.

• Inform patient because drug is a peptide, it's destroyed in the GI tract and therefore must be administered parenterally.

• Explain to patients the importance of rotating injection sites daily. Sites should include upper arms, thighs, and abdomen.

• Warn patients of the potential risks of therapy and potential adverse effects. During the first month of treatment, girls commonly experience a slight menstrual flow, which probably is related to decreasing estrogen levels brought on by treatment. As estrogen levels drop, menses begins because estrogens support the endometrium.

• Advise patients to seek immediate medical attention if they have any signs of hypersensitivity reactions: sudden development of skin rash, difficulty in breathing or swallowing, or rapid heartbeat. Notify the doctor if severe or persistent swelling, redness, or irritation is present at the injection site.

menotropins
Pergonal

Pregnancy Risk Category: X

HOW SUPPLIED
Injection: 75 international units (IU) of luteinizing hormone (LH) and 75 units of follicle-stimulating hormone (FSH) activity/ampule; 150 units of LH and 150 units of FSH activity/ampule

ACTION
When administered to women who have not had primary ovarian failure, mimics FSH in inducing follicular

growth and LH in aiding follicular maturation.

ONSET, PEAK, DURATION
Onset for follicular growth and maturation, 9 to 12 days. Peak and duration unknown.

INDICATIONS & DOSAGE
Anovulation –
Women: 75 units each of FSH and LH I.M. daily for 7 to 12 days, followed by 5,000 to 10,000 units of human chorionic gonadotropin (HCG) I.M. 1 day after last dose of menotropins. Repeated for one to three menstrual cycles until ovulation occurs.
Infertility with ovulation –
Women: 75 units each of FSH and LH I.M. daily for 7 to 12 days, followed by 5,000 to 10,000 units of HCG I.M. 1 day after last dose of menotropins. Repeated for two menstrual cycles and then increased to 150 units each of FSH and LH daily for 7 to 12 days, followed by 5,000 to 10,000 units of HCG I.M. 1 day after last dose of menotropins. Repeated for two menstrual cycles.
Infertility in men –
Men: Prior treatment with HCG of 5,000 units three times a week for 4 to 6 months; then 75 units each of FSH and LH I.M. three times weekly (given concomitantly with 2,000 units of HCG twice weekly) for at least 4 months. If increased spermatogenesis does not occur, dosage increased to 150 units each of FSH and LH three times weekly (dosage of HCG remains unchanged).

ADVERSE REACTIONS
GI: nausea, vomiting, diarrhea.
GU: *ovarian enlargement with pain and abdominal distention,* multiple births, ovarian hyperstimulation syndrome (sudden ovarian enlargement, ascites with or without pain, or pleural effusion).

Hematologic: hemoconcentration with fluid loss into abdomen.
Other: fever, *gynecomastia.*

INTERACTIONS
None significant.

CONTRAINDICATIONS
Contraindicated in patients hypersensitive to the drug; in women with primary ovarian failure, uncontrolled thyroid or adrenal dysfunction, pituitary tumor, abnormal uterine bleeding, uterine fibromas, or ovarian cysts or enlargement; in pregnant patients; and in men with normal pituitary function, primary testicular failure, or infertility disorders other than hypogonadotropic hypogonadism.

NURSING CONSIDERATIONS
• Close monitoring of patient response is critical to ensure adequate ovarian stimulation without hyperstimulation.
• Reconstitute with 1 to 2 ml of sterile 0.9% sodium chloride injection. Use immediately.
• Rotate injection sites to prevent muscle atrophy.
• Tell patients about possibility of multiple births.
• In infertility, encourage daily intercourse from day before HCG is given until ovulation occurs.
• Tell patient pregnancy usually occurs 4 to 6 weeks after therapy.
• Instruct patients to immediately report severe abdominal pain, bloating, swelling of the hands or feet, nausea, vomiting, diarrhea, substantial weight gain, or shortness of breath.

---

nafarelin acetate
Synarel
Pregnancy Risk Category: X

HOW SUPPLIED
Nasal solution: 200 mcg/spray in metered-dose spray bottle (2 mg/ml)

---

*Liquid form contains alcohol.   *Common* reactions are in italics; ***life-threatening,*** in bold italics.
**May contain tartrazine.

ACTION
A gonadotropin-releasing hormone (GnRH) analog that acts on the pituitary to decrease release of follicle-stimulating hormone and luteinizing hormone, thus decreasing ovarian stimulation, lowering circulating estrogens, and improving symptoms associated with endometriosis.

ONSET, PEAK, DURATION
Decreased levels of sex hormones occur after 4 weeks. Serum levels peak 10 to 40 minutes after dose. Effects persist for up to 3 to 6 months.

INDICATIONS & DOSAGE
Management of endometriosis –
Women 18 years and older: 1 spray in one nostril b.i.d. Treatment begun between days 2 and 4 of the menstrual cycle. Maximum duration of therapy is 6 months.
Central precocious puberty –
Children: 2 sprays in each nostril in the morning and evening. Total daily dosage is 8 sprays (1,600 mcg).

ADVERSE REACTIONS
CNS: *headaches, emotional lability, insomnia,* depression.
CV: edema.
EENT: *nasal irritation.*
Skin: *acne,* seborrhea, hirsutism.
Other: *hot flashes, decreased libido, myalgia,* reduced breast size, weight gain or loss, increased libido, decreased bone density, *vaginal dryness.*

INTERACTIONS
None significant.

CONTRAINDICATIONS
Contraindicated in patients hypersensitive to GnRH analogs or any components of the formulation (benzalkonium chloride, sorbitol, purified water, glacial acetic acid, hydrochloric acid, or sodium hydroxide), in those with undiagnosed vaginal bleeding, in breast-feeding patients, and during pregnancy (because it may harm the fetus).

NURSING CONSIDERATIONS
• Be aware studies have confirmed a small loss in bone density after 6 months of therapy, probably caused by drug-induced hypoestrogenic state. Patients with major risk factors for osteoporosis (chronic alcohol or tobacco use, strong family history of osteoporosis, or use of drugs that may reduce bone mass [such as anticonvulsants or corticosteroids]) should not receive additional courses of therapy and should strongly weigh the risks and benefits before an initial trial of the drug.
• Teach patients that menstruation will stop with regular use of drug and to contact the doctor if menstruation persists or breakthrough bleeding occurs.
• Advise patients to use a nonhormonal form of contraception (such as barrier contraception). Although drug will usually inhibit ovulation and stop menstruation, it's not a reliable contraceptive, particularly if patients miss a few doses. Tell patients to stop the drug immediately and contact the doctor if they believe that they are pregnant.
• Instruct patients to immediately report severe abdominal pain, bloating, swelling of the hands or feet, nausea, vomiting, diarrhea, substantial weight gain, or shortness of breath.
• Tell patients who develop a cold or rhinitis during therapy to notify the doctor. If a topical nasal decongestant is required, the manufacturer suggests that it be used at least 30 minutes after nafarelin treatment to reduce possible interference with nafarelin absorption.

57
Antidiabetic agents and glucagon

acetohexamide
chlorpropamide
glipizide
glucagon
glyburide
insulins
metformin hydrochloride
tolazamide
tolbutamide

COMBINATION PRODUCTS
HUMULIN 50/50◇: isophane insulin
suspension (human) 50% and insulin
injection (human) 50%, 100 units/ml
HUMULIN 70/30◇, MIXTARD HU-
MAN‡, NOVOLIN 70/30◇): isophane
insulin suspension (human) 70% and
insulin injection (human) 30%, 100
units/ml

---

acetohexamide
Dimelor†, Dymelor

Pregnancy Risk Category: NR

HOW SUPPLIED
Tablets: 250 mg, 500 mg

ACTION
Unknown. A sulfonylurea that probably stimulates insulin release from the
pancreatic beta cells and reduces glucose output by the liver. An extrapancreatic effect increases peripheral
sensitivity to insulin.

ONSET, PEAK, DURATION
Onset occurs within 1 hour. Plasma
levels of acetohexamide peak within 2
hours; plasma levels of insulin, within
1 to 2 hours. Effects persist for 12 to
24 hours.

INDICATIONS & DOSAGE
*Adjunct to diet to lower blood glucose
level in patients with type II diabetes
(non-insulin-dependent)* –
Adults: initially, 250 mg P.O. daily
before breakfast; dosage increased q 5
to 7 days (by 250 to 500 mg) as
needed to maximum of 1.5 g daily in
divided doses b.i.d. or t.i.d. before
meals.
*To replace insulin therapy in patients
with type II diabetes* –
Adults: if insulin dosage is less than
20 units daily, insulin is stopped and
oral therapy started with 250 mg P.O.
daily, before breakfast, increased as
above if needed. If insulin dosage is
20 to 40 units daily, oral therapy
started with 250 mg P.O. daily, before
breakfast, while insulin dosage reduced 25% to 30% daily or every
other day, depending on response to
oral therapy.

ADVERSE REACTIONS
GI: *nausea, heartburn,* vomiting.
Skin: *rash, pruritus, facial flushing.*
Other: *hypersensitivity reactions,* so-
dium loss, **hypoglycemia**.

INTERACTIONS
*Anabolic steroids, chloramphenicol,
clofibrate, guanethidine, MAO inhibitors, phenylbutazone, salicylates, sulfonamides:* increased hypoglycemic
activity. Monitor blood glucose level.
Beta blockers, clonidine: prolonged
hypoglycemic effect and masked
symptoms of hypoglycemia. Use together cautiously.
*Corticosteroids, glucagon, rifampin,
thiazide diuretics:* decreased hypoglycemic response. Monitor blood glucose level.
Ethanol: possible disulfiram-like reaction. Avoid concomitant use.

Hydantoins: increased blood levels of hydantoins. Monitor blood levels closely.

Oral anticoagulants: increased hypoglycemic activity or enhanced anticoagulant effect. Monitor blood glucose level and PT.

CONTRAINDICATIONS

Contraindicated for treating patients with type I diabetes (insulin-dependent) or diabetes that can be adequately controlled by diet. Also contraindicated in patients with type II diabetes (non-insulin-dependent) complicated by ketosis, acidosis, diabetic coma; hyperglycemia associated with major renal disease; pregnancy or lactation; major surgery; severe infections; severe trauma; or hypersensitivity to sulfonylureas.

NURSING CONSIDERATIONS

• Use cautiously in patients with a history of porphyria, impaired hepatic or renal function, or in debilitated, malnourished, or geriatric patients.

• Instruct patients about nature of disease, importance of following therapeutic regimen, adhering to specific diet, weight reduction, exercise, and personal hygiene programs and about avoiding infection. Explain how and when to perform self-monitoring of blood glucose level and teach recognition of and intervention for hypoglycemia and hyperglycemia.

• During periods of increased stress, such as infection, fever, surgery, or trauma, patients may require insulin therapy. Monitor patients closely for hyperglycemia in these situations.

• Know patients transferring from another oral agent usually need no transition period.

• Be aware patients transferring from insulin therapy to an oral antidiabetic agent requires blood glucose monitoring at least three times a day before

meals. Patients may require hospitalization during transition.

• Make sure patients understand that therapy relieves symptoms but doesn't cure disease.

• Tell patients not to change drug dosage without the doctor's consent. Report abnormal blood or urine glucose test results.

• Teach patients to carry candy or other simple sugars to treat mild hypoglycemic episodes. Severe episodes may require hospital treatment.

• Advise patients not to take any other medication, including OTC drugs, without first checking with the doctor.

• Advise patients to avoid moderate to large intake of alcohol because of possible disulfiram-like reaction.

• Advise patients to carry medical identification identifying themselves as diabetic patients.

---

chlorpropamide

Apo-Chlorpropamide†, Diabinese, Glucamide, Novo-Propamide†

Pregnancy Risk Category: C

HOW SUPPLIED
Tablets: 100 mg, 250 mg

ACTION
Unknown. A sulfonylurea that probably stimulates insulin release from the pancreatic beta cells and reduces glucose output by the liver. An extrapancreatic effect increases peripheral sensitivity to insulin. Also exerts an antidiuretic effect in patients with diabetes insipidus.

ONSET, PEAK, DURATION
Onset occurs within 1 hour. Peak levels occur in 2 to 4 hours; peak hypoglycemic effect, within 3 to 6 hours. Effects persist up to 60 hours.

INDICATIONS & DOSAGE

Adjunct to diet to lower blood glucose level in patients with type II diabetes (non-insulin-dependent) –

Adults: 250 mg P.O. daily with breakfast or in divided doses if GI disturbances occur. First dosage increased after 5 to 7 days because of extended duration of action; then increased q 3 to 5 days by 50 to 125 mg, if needed, to a maximum of 750 mg daily. On the other hand, some patients with mild diabetes respond well to dosages of 100 mg or less daily.

Adults over 65 years: initially, 100 to 125 mg P.O. daily.

To change from insulin to oral therapy –

Adults: if insulin dosage is less than 40 units daily, insulin stopped and oral therapy started as above. If insulin dosage is 40 units or more daily, oral therapy started as above with insulin reduced 50%. Insulin dosage reduced further according to patient response.

ADVERSE REACTIONS

GI: nausea, heartburn, vomiting.
GU: tea-colored urine.
Skin: rash, pruritus, facial flushing.
Other: *hypersensitivity reactions, prolonged hypoglycemia, dilutional hyponatremia.*

INTERACTIONS

Anabolic steroids, chloramphenicol, clofibrate, guanethidine, MAO inhibitors, phenylbutazone, salicylates, sulfonamides: increased hypoglycemic activity. Monitor blood glucose level.
Beta blockers, clonidine: prolonged hypoglycemic effect and masked symptoms of hypoglycemia. Use together cautiously.
Corticosteroids, glucagon, rifampin, thiazide diuretics: decreased hypoglycemic response. Monitor blood glucose level.
Ethanol: possible disulfiram-like reaction. Avoid concomitant use.

Hydantoins: increased blood levels of hydantoins. Monitor blood levels closely.
Oral anticoagulants: increased hypoglycemic activity or enhanced anticoagulant effect. Monitor blood glucose level and PT.

CONTRAINDICATIONS

Contraindicated for treating type I diabetes (insulin-dependent) or diabetes that can be adequately controlled by diet. Also contraindicated in patients with type II diabetes (non-insulin-dependent) complicated by ketosis, acidosis, diabetic coma, major surgery, severe infections, severe trauma, during pregnancy or breast-feeding; and in patients with hypersensitivity to the drug.

NURSING CONSIDERATIONS

• Use cautiously in patients with porphyria, impaired hepatic or renal function or in debilitated, malnourished or geriatric patients.
• Know elderly patients may be more sensitive to drug's adverse effects.
• Know that drug may accumulate in patients with renal insufficiency.
• Watch for signs of impending renal insufficiency, such as dysuria, anuria, and hematuria, and report them to the doctor immediately.
• Be aware adverse effects of chlorpropamide, especially hypoglycemia, may be more frequent or severe than with some other sulfonylureas because of its long duration of action.
• If hypoglycemia occurs, monitor patients closely for a minimum of 3 to 5 days.
• Monitor serum alkaline phosphatase levels routinely, as ordered. Progressive increases may indicate the need to discontinue drug.
• Patients transferring from another oral antidiabetic agent usually need no transition period.
• Patients may require hospitalization during transition from insulin therapy

---

*Liquid form contains alcohol.
**May contain tartrazine.

Common reactions are in italics; ***life-threatening***, in bold italics.

to an oral antidiabetic agent. Monitor patients' blood glucose levels at least three times a day before meals.

• Instruct patients about nature of the disease, importance of following therapeutic regimen, adhering to specific diet, weight reduction, exercise, and personal hygiene programs, and about avoiding infection. Explain how and when to perform self-monitoring of blood glucose level and teach recognition of and intervention for hypoglycemia and hyperglycemia.

• Make sure patients understand that therapy relieves symptoms but doesn't cure disease.

• Tell patients not to change drug dosage without the doctor's consent. Report abnormal blood or urine glucose test results.

• Teach patients to carry candy or other simple sugars to treat mild hypoglycemic episodes. Severe episodes may require hospital treatment.

• Advise patients not to take any other medication, including OTC drugs, without first checking with the doctor.

• Advise patients to avoid intake of alcohol. Chlorpropamide-alcohol flush is characterized by facial flushing, light-headedness, headache, and occasional breathlessness. Even very small amounts of alcohol can produce this reaction.

• Advise patients to carry medical identification identifying them as diabetic patients.

---

glipizide
Glucotrol, Glucotrol XL, Minidiab‡

Pregnancy Risk Category: C

HOW SUPPLIED
Tablets: 5 mg, 10 mg
Tablets (extended-release): 5 mg, 10 mg

ACTION
Unknown. A sulfonylurea that probably stimulates insulin release from the pancreatic beta cells and reduces glucose output by the liver. An extrapancreatic effect increases peripheral sensitivity to insulin.

ONSET, PEAK, DURATION
Onset occurs within 15 to 30 minutes. Serum drug levels peak 1 to 3 hours after oral dose; peak insulin levels occur in ½ to 2 hours. Effects persist for 10 to 16 hours.

INDICATIONS & DOSAGE
Adjunct to diet to lower blood glucose level in patients with type II diabetes (non-insulin-dependent) –
Adults: initially, 5 mg P.O. daily before breakfast. Elderly patients or those with liver disease may be started on 2.5 mg. Usual maintenance dosage is 10 to 15 mg. Maximum recommended daily dosage is 40 mg.
To replace insulin therapy –
Adults: if insulin dosage is more than 20 units daily, the patient is started at usual dosage in addition to 50% of the insulin. If insulin dosage is less than 20 units, insulin may be discontinued.

ADVERSE REACTIONS
CNS: dizziness.
GI: nausea, vomiting, constipation.
Hepatic: cholestatic jaundice.
Skin: rash, pruritus, facial flushing.
Other: *hypoglycemia.*

INTERACTIONS
Anabolic steroids, chloramphenicol, clofibrate, guanethidine, MAO inhibitors, phenylbutazone, probenecid, salicylates, sulfonamides: increased hypoglycemic activity. Monitor blood glucose level.
Beta blockers, clonidine: prolonged hypoglycemic effect and masked symptoms of hypoglycemia. Use together cautiously.
Corticosteroids, glucagon, rifampin,

---

thiazide diuretics: decreased hypoglycemic response. Monitor blood glucose level.

Ethanol: possible disulfiram-like reaction. Avoid concomitant use.

Hydantoins: increased blood levels of hydantoins. Monitor blood levels closely.

Oral anticoagulants: increased hypoglycemic activity or enhanced anticoagulant effect. Monitor blood glucose levels and PT.

CONTRAINDICATIONS
Contraindicated in patients with hypersensitivity to drug, diabetic ketoacidosis with or without coma, and during pregnancy or breast-feeding.

NURSING CONSIDERATIONS
• Use cautiously in patients with renal and hepatic disease and in debilitated, malnourished, or elderly patients.
• Know elderly patients may be more sensitive to drug's adverse effects.
• Give approximately 30 minutes before meals.
• Know some patients taking glipizide may attain effective control on a once-daily regimen, whereas others show a better response with divided dosing.
• Be aware glipizide is a second-generation sulfonylurea. The frequency of adverse reactions appears to be lower than with first-generation drugs, such as chlorpropamide and tolbutamide.
• During periods of increased stress, such as infection, fever, surgery, or trauma, patients may require insulin therapy. Monitor patients closely for hyperglycemia in these situations.
• Patients transferring from insulin therapy to an oral antidiabetic agent require blood glucose monitoring at least three times daily before meals. Patients may require hospitalization during transition.
• Instruct patients about nature of disease, importance of following therapeutic regimen, adhering to specific diet, weight reduction, exercise, personal hygiene programs, and about avoiding infection. Explain how and when to perform self-monitoring of blood glucose level, and teach recognition of hypoglycemia and hyperglycemia.
• Tell patients not to change drug dosage without the doctor's consent and to report abnormal blood or urine glucose test results.
• Advise patients not to take any other medication, including OTC drugs, without first checking with the doctor.
• Advise patients to carry medical identification identifying them as diabetic patients.

glucagon
Pregnancy Risk Category: B

HOW SUPPLIED
Powder for injection: 1 mg (1 unit)/vial, 10 mg (10 units)/vial

ACTION
Raises blood glucose level by promoting catalytic depolymerization of hepatic glycogen to glucose.

ONSET, PEAK, DURATION
Onset almost immediate after parenteral administration. Peak hyperglycemic effect occurs within 30 minutes. Hyperglycemic effects persist 1 to 2 hours. Onset, peak and duration variable when used to relax GI smooth muscle but occurs more quickly and lasts for shorter duration.

INDICATIONS & DOSAGE
Hypoglycemia –
Adults and children weighing more than 20 kg: 1 mg S.C., I.M., or I.V.
Children weighing 20 kg or less: 0.5 mg S.C., I.M., or I.V.
Note: May repeat in 15 minutes if necessary. I.V. glucose must be given

---

if patient fails to respond. When patient responds, supplemental carbohydrate needs to be given immediately.
Diagnostic aid for radiologic examination –
Adults: 0.25 to 2 mg I.V. or I.M. before initiation of radiologic procedure.

ADVERSE REACTIONS
GI: nausea, vomiting.
Other: hypersensitivity reactions (*bronchospasm,* rash, dizziness, light-headedness).

INTERACTIONS
Phenytoin: inhibited glucagon-induced insulin release. Use cautiously.

CONTRAINDICATIONS
Contraindicated in patients with hypersensitivity to drug or with pheochromocytoma.

NURSING CONSIDERATIONS
• Use cautiously in patients with history of insulinoma or pheochromocytoma.
• **I.V. use:** Reconstitute 1-unit vial with 1 ml of diluent; reconstitute 10-unit vial with 10 ml of diluent. Use only the diluent supplied by the manufacturer when preparing doses of 2 mg or less. For larger doses, dilute with sterile water for injection.
• For I.V. drip infusion, use dextrose solution, which is compatible with glucagon; drug forms a precipitate in chloride solutions. Inject directly into vein or into I.V. tubing of a free-flowing compatible solution over 2 to 5 minutes. Interrupt primary infusion during glucagon injection if using the same I.V. line.
• It is vital to arouse patients from coma as quickly as possible and to give additional carbohydrates orally to prevent secondary hypoglycemic reactions.
• Unstable hypoglycemic diabetic patients may not respond to glucagon; give dextrose I.V. instead as ordered.
• Instruct patients and their family members in proper glucagon administration, recognition of hypoglycemia, and urgency of calling the doctor immediately in emergencies.

glyburide (glibenclamide)
DiaBeta**, Euglucon†, Glynase PresTab, Micronase
Pregnancy Risk Category: B

HOW SUPPLIED
Tablets: 1.25 mg, 2.5 mg, 5 mg
Tablets (micronized): 1.5 mg, 3 mg, 5 mg

ACTION
Unknown. A sulfonylurea that probably stimulates insulin release from the pancreatic beta cells and reduces glucose output by the liver. An extrapancreatic effect increases peripheral sensitivity to insulin and causes a mild diuretic effect.

ONSET, PEAK, DURATION
Onset occurs in 1 hour for micronized form, 2 to 4 hours for nonmicronized form. Peak levels of glyburide occur in 2 to 4 hours; maximum increases in insulin levels are seen in 1 to 2 hours. Effects persist 24 hours.

INDICATIONS & DOSAGE
Adjunct to diet to lower blood glucose level in patients with type II diabetes (non-insulin-dependent) –
Adults: initially, 2.5 to 5 mg regular tablets P.O. once daily with breakfast. Patients who are more sensitive to antidiabetic agents should be started at 1.25 mg daily. Usual maintenance dosage is 1.25 to 20 mg daily as a single dose or in divided doses.
    Alternatively, micronized formulation may be used. Initial dosage is 1.5 to 3 mg daily. Patients who are more

sensitive to antidiabetic agents should be started at 0.75 mg daily.

To replace insulin therapy –

Adults: if insulin dosage is more than 40 units daily, patient started on 5 mg regular tablets or 3 mg micronized formulation P.O. once daily in addition to 50% of the insulin dosage.

ADVERSE REACTIONS
GI: nausea, epigastric fullness, heartburn.
Hepatic: cholestatic jaundice.
Skin: rash, pruritus, facial flushing.
Other: *hypoglycemia.*

INTERACTIONS
Anabolic steroids, chloramphenicol, clofibrate, guanethidine, MAO inhibitors, phenylbutazone, salicylates, sulfonamides: increased hypoglycemic activity. Monitor blood glucose level.
Beta blockers, clonidine: prolonged hypoglycemic effect and masked symptoms of hypoglycemia. Use together cautiously.
Corticosteroids, glucagon, rifampin, thiazide diuretics: decreased hypoglycemic response. Monitor blood glucose level.
Ethanol: possible disulfiram-like reaction. Avoid concomitant use.
Hydantoins: increased blood levels of hydantoins. Monitor blood levels closely.
Oral anticoagulants: increased hypoglycemic activity or enhanced anticoagulant effect. Monitor blood glucose level and PT.

CONTRAINDICATIONS
Contraindicated in patients with hypersensitivity to the drug or diabetic ketoacidosis with or without coma, and during pregnancy or breast-feeding.

NURSING CONSIDERATIONS
• Use cautiously in patients with hepatic or renal impairment, or in debilitated, malnourished, or elderly patients.
• Know elderly patients may be more sensitive to drug's adverse effects.
• Know micronized glyburide (Glynase PresTab) contains drug in a smaller particle size and is not bioequivalent to regular glyburide tablets. Patients who have been taking Micronase or DiaBeta need to be retitrated.
• Be aware that although most patients may take glyburide once daily, patients taking more than 10 mg daily may achieve better results with twice-daily dosage.
• Know glyburide is a second-generation sulfonylurea. The frequency of adverse effects appears to be lower than with first-generation drugs, such as chlorpropamide and tolbutamide.
• During periods of increased stress, such as infection, fever, surgery, or trauma, patients may require insulin therapy. Monitor patients closely for hyperglycemia in these situations.
• Patients transferring from insulin therapy to an oral antidiabetic agent require blood glucose monitoring at least three times a day before meals. Patients may require hospitalization during transition.
• Instruct patients about nature of disease, importance of following therapeutic regimen, adhering to specific diet, weight reduction, exercise, and personal hygiene programs, and about avoiding infection. Explain how and when to perform self-monitoring of blood glucose levels and teach recognition of and intervention for hypoglycemia and hyperglycemia.
• Tell patients not to change drug dosage without the doctor's consent and to report abnormal blood or urine glucose test results.
• Teach patients to carry candy or other simple sugars to treat mild hypoglycemic episodes. Severe episodes may require hospital treatment.
• Advise patients not to take any other

---

*Liquid form contains alcohol.
**May contain tartrazine.

Common reactions are in italics; *life-threatening*, in bold italics.

medication, including OTC drugs, without first checking with the doctor.

• Advise patients to carry medical identification identifying them as diabetic patients.

insulins

insulin injection (regular insulin, crystalline zinc insulin)

Actrapid HM‡, Actrapid HM Penfill‡, Actrapid MC‡, Actrapid MC Penfill‡, Humulin R◇, Hypurin Neutral‡, Insulin 2‡, Novolin R◇, Novolin R PenFill◇, Pork Regular Iletin II◇, Regular (Concentrated) Iletin II◇, Regular Iletin I◇, Regular Purified Pork Insulin◇, Velosulin Human‡, Velosulin Insuject‡

insulin zinc suspension, prompt (semilente)

Semilente MC‡

isophane insulin suspension (neutral protamine Hagedorn insulin, NPH)

Humulin N◇, Humulin NPH‡, Hypurin Isophane‡, Insulatard‡, Insulatard Human†, Isotard MC‡, Novolin N◇, Novolin N PenFill◇, NPH Insulin◇, NPH Purified Pork◇, Pork NPH Iletin II◇, Protaphane HM‡, Protaphane HM Penfill‡, Protaphane MC‡

isophane insulin suspension with insulin injection

Actraphane HM‡, Actraphane HM Penfill‡, Actraphane MC‡, Humulin 50/50◇, Humulin 70/30◇, Novolin 70/30, Novolin 70/30 PenFill◇

insulin zinc suspension (lente)

Humulin L◇, Lente Iletin II◇, Lente Insulin◇, Lente MC‡, Lente Purified Pork Insulin◇, Monotard HM‡, Monotard MC‡, Novolin L◇

protamine zinc suspension (PZI)

Protamine Zinc Insulin MC‡

insulin zinc suspension, extended (ultralente)

Humulin U◇, Ultralente Insulin◇, Ultratard HM‡, Ultratard MC‡

Pregnancy Risk Category: NR

HOW SUPPLIED
insulin injection
Injection (human): 100 units/ml (Actrapid HM‡, Humulin R◇, Novolin R◇, Velosulin Human‡); 100 units/ml in 1.5-ml cartridge system◇ (Actrapid HM Penfill‡, Novolin R PenFill◇)
Injection (from pork): 100 units/ml◇
Injection (purified beef): 100 units/ml (Hypurin Neutral‡, Insulin 2‡)
Injection (purified pork): 100 units/ml (Actrapid MC‡, Pork Regular Iletin II◇, Regular Purified Pork Insulin◇); 100 units/ml in 1.5-ml cartridge system‡ (Actrapid MC Penfill‡); 100 units/ml in 2-ml cartridge system‡; 500 units/ml (Regular [Concentrated] Iletin II)
insulin zinc suspension, prompt
Injection (purified pork): 100 units/ml◇ (Semilente MC‡)
isophane insulin suspension
Injection (from beef): 100 units/ml◇ (NPH Insulin◇)
Injection (human, recombinant): 100 units/ml (Humulin N◇, Humulin NPH‡, Insulatard Human†, Novolin N◇, Protaphane HM‡); 100 units/ml in 1.5-ml cartridge system (Protaphane HM PenFill‡, Novolin N PenFill◇)
Injection (purified beef): 100 units/ml (Hypurin Isophane‡, Isotard MC‡)
Injection (purified pork): 100 units/ml

(Insulatard‡, NPH Purified Pork◊,
Pork NPH Iletin II, Protaphane MC‡)
**isophane insulin suspension 50%
with insulin injection 50%**
Injection (human): 100 units/ml (Humulin 50/50◊)
**isophane insulin suspension 70%
with insulin injection 30%**
Injection (human): 100 units/ml (Actraphane HM‡, Humulin 70/30◊, Novolin 70/30◊); 100 units/ml in 1.5-ml cartridge system (Actraphane HM Penfill‡, Novolin 70/30 PenFill◊)
Injection (purified pork): 100 units/ml
(Actraphane MC‡)
insulin zinc suspension
Injection (from beef): 100 units/ml
(Lente Insulin◊, Lente MC‡)
Injection (purified beef): 100 units/ml
(Lente MC‡)
Injection (purified pork): 100 units/ml
(Lente Iletin II, Monotard MC‡,
Lente Purified Pork Insulin◊)
Injection (human): 100 units/ml◊
(Humulin L◊, Monotard HM‡, Novolin I◊)
protamine zinc suspension
Injection (purified pork): Protamine Zinc Insulin MC‡
insulin zinc suspension, extended
Injection (from beef): 100 units/ml◊
(Ultralente Insulin◊)
Injection (human): 100 units/ml (Ultratard HM‡, Humulin U◊)
Injection (purified pork): 100 units/
ml‡ (Ultratard MC‡)

ACTION
Increases glucose transport across muscle and fat cell membranes to reduce blood glucose level. Promotes conversion of glucose to its storage form, glycogen; triggers amino acid uptake and conversion to protein in muscle cells and inhibits protein degradation; stimulates triglyceride formation and inhibits release of free fatty acids from adipose tissue; and stimulates lipoprotein lipase activity, which converts circulating lipoproteins to fatty acids.

ONSET, PEAK, DURATION
Highly variable. Onset occurs within ½ to 1½ hours with S.C. rapid-acting insulin, 1 to 2½ hours with S.C. intermediate-acting insulins, and 4 to 8 hours with S.C. long-acting insulins. Serum levels peak in 2 to 3 hours with S.C. rapid-acting regular insulins, 4 to 10 hours with S.C. rapid-acting semilente insulin, 4 to 15 hours with S.C. intermediate-acting insulins, and 10 to 30 hours with S.C. long-acting insulins. Effects persist 5 to 7 hours with S.C. rapid-acting regular insulin, 12 to 16 hours with S.C. rapid-acting semilente insulin, 18 to 24 hours with S.C. intermediate-acting insulins, and 36 hours for S.C. long-acting insulins.

INDICATIONS & DOSAGE
Diabetic ketoacidosis (use regular insulin only)–
Adults: 0.33 units/kg as an I.V. bolus, followed by 0.1 units/kg/hour by continuous infusion. Continue infusion until blood glucose level drops to 250 mg/dl; then S.C. insulin begun with dosage and dosage interval adjusted according to patient's blood glucose concentrations.

Alternatively, 50 to 100 units I.V. and 50 to 100 units S.C. stat; then additional doses q 2 to 6 hours based on blood glucose levels.

To prepare infusion, add 100 units of regular insulin and 1 g of albumin to 100 ml of 0.9% sodium chloride solution. Insulin concentration will be 1 unit/ml. (The albumin will adsorb to plastic, preventing loss of the insulin to plastic.)
Children: 0.1 unit/kg as an I.V. bolus, then 0.1 unit/kg hourly by continuous infusion until blood glucose level drops to 250 mg/dl; then S.C. insulin started. Alternatively, 1 to 2 units/kg in two divided doses, one I.V. and the other S.C., followed by 0.5 to 1 unit/kg I.V. q 1 to 2 hours based on blood glucose levels.
Type I diabetes (insulin-dependent),

---

*Liquid form contains alcohol.
**May contain tartrazine.
Common reactions are in italics; *life-threatening*, in **bold italics**.

adjunct to Type II diabetes (nonin-sulin-dependent) inadequately con-trolled by diet and oral antidiabetic agents –

Adults and children: therapeutic regimen is prescribed by the doctor and adjusted according to patient's blood glucose concentrations.

ADVERSE REACTIONS
Skin: urticaria, itching, swelling, redness, stinging, warmth at injection site.
Other: *lipoatrophy, lipohypertrophy,* hypersensitivity reactions (***anaphylaxis,*** rash), ***hypoglycemia,*** hyperglycemia (rebound, or Somogyi, effect).

INTERACTIONS
Anabolic steroids, beta blockers, clofibrate, ethanol, fenfluramine, guanethidine, MAO inhibitors, salicylates, tetracycline: prolonged hypoglycemic effect. Monitor blood glucose level carefully.
Corticosteroids, dextrothyroxine, epinephrine, thiazide diuretics: diminished insulin response. Monitor for hyperglycemia.
Diazoxide, phenytoin (high doses): may inhibit endogenous insulin secretion and may cause hypoglycemia in diabetic patients. Carefully adjust insulin dosage when using with these drugs.
Oral contraceptives: may decrease glucose tolerance in diabetic patients. Monitor blood glucose levels and adjust insulin dosage carefully.

CONTRAINDICATIONS
None known.

NURSING CONSIDERATIONS
• Know that insulin is the drug of choice to treat diabetes during pregnancy.
• Know that regular insulin is used in patients with circulatory collapse, diabetic ketoacidosis, or hyperkalemia. Do not use regular insulin concen-trated (500 units/ml) I.V. Do not use intermediate or long-acting insulins for coma or other emergency requiring rapid drug action.
• Know that insulin requirements increase, sometimes drastically, in pregnant diabetic patients, and then decline immediately postpartum. Monitor patient closely.
• Dosage is always expressed in USP units. Remember to use only the syringes calibrated for the particular concentration of insulin administered. U-500 insulin must be administered with a U-100 syringe because no syringes are made for this strength.
• Be aware some patients may develop insulin resistance and require large insulin doses to control symptoms of diabetes. U-500 insulin is available as Regular (Concentrated) Iletin II for such patients. Although every pharmacy may not normally stock it, it is readily available. Nurses should give the hospital pharmacy sufficient notice before needing to refill in-house prescription. Never store U-500 insulin in same area with other insulin preparations because of danger of severe overdose if given accidentally to other patients.
• To mix insulin suspension, swirl vial gently or rotate between palms or between palm and thigh. Don't shake vigorously: this causes bubbling and air in syringe.
• Know lente, semilente, and ultra-lente insulins may be mixed in any proportion.
• Know regular insulin may be mixed with NPH or lente insulins in any proportion.
• Note that switching from separate injections to a prepared mixture may alter patient response. Whenever NPH or lente is mixed with regular insulin in the same syringe, be sure to administer immediately to avoid loss of potency.
• Don't use insulin that changes color

or becomes clumped or granular in appearance.

• Check expiration date on vial before using contents.

• Know that usual administration route is S.C. For proper S.C. administration, remember to pinch a fold of skin with the fingers at least 3 inches apart and insert the needle at a 45- to 90-degree angle.

• Press but do not rub site after injection. Rotate injection sites and chart to avoid overuse of one area. Know that diabetic patients may achieve better control if injection site is rotated within same anatomic region.

• Know that ketosis-prone type I, severely ill, and newly diagnosed diabetic patients with very high blood glucose levels may require hospitalization and I.V. treatment with regular fast-acting insulin.

• **I.V. use:** Only administer regular insulin I.V. Inject directly at ordered rate into vein, through an intermittent infusion device, or into a port close to I.V. access site. Intermittent infusion is not recommended. If given by continuous infusion, infuse drug diluted in 0.9% sodium chloride at the prescribed rate.

• Store insulin in cool area. Refrigeration is desirable but not essential, except with regular insulin concentrated.

• Make sure patients know that therapy relieves symptoms but doesn't cure disease.

• Instruct patients about nature of disease, importance of following the therapeutic regimen, adhering to specific diet, weight reduction, exercise, and personal hygiene program, and about avoiding infection. Emphasize the importance of the timing of injections and eating and that meals must not be omitted.

• Stress to patient accuracy of measurement is very important, especially with regular insulin concentrated. Aids, such as magnifying

sleeve or dose magnifier may improve accuracy. Instruct patient and family how to measure and administer insulin.

• Advise patient not to alter the order of mixing insulins or change the model or brand of syringe or needle.

• Teach that self-monitoring of blood glucose levels and urine ketone tests are essential guides to dosage and success of therapy. It's important to recognize hypoglycemic symptoms because insulin-induced hypoglycemia is hazardous and may cause brain damage if prolonged; most adverse effects are self-limiting and temporary.

• Instruct patients on proper use of equipment for performing self-monitoring of blood glucose levels.

• Advise patients not to smoke within 30 minutes after insulin injection. Cigarette smoking decreases the amount of absorption of insulin administered subcutaneously.

• Tell patient marijuana use may increase insulin requirements.

• Advise patients to wear a medical identification bracelet at all times, to carry ample insulin supply and syringes on trips, to have carbohydrates (lump of sugar or candy) on hand for emergencies, and to take note of time zone changes for dose schedule when traveling.

---

metformin hydrochloride
Glucophage

Pregnancy Risk Category: B

HOW SUPPLIED
Tablets: 500 mg, 850 mg

ACTION
Decreases hepatic glucose production and intestinal absorption of glucose and improves insulin sensitivity (increases peripheral glucose uptake and utilization).

ONSET, PEAK, DURATION
Not clearly defined, although food does delay the onset and peak of the drug.

INDICATIONS & DOSAGE
Adjunct to diet to lower blood glucose level in patients with Type II diabetes—

Adults: initially, 500 mg P.O. b.i.d. given with morning and evening meals or 850 mg P.O. once daily given with morning meal. When 500-mg dose form used, dosage increased 500 mg weekly to maximum dosage of 2,500 mg P.O. daily as needed. When 850-mg dose form used, dosage increased 850 mg every other week to a maximum dosage of 2,550 mg P.O. daily as needed.

ADVERSE REACTIONS
GI: diarrhea, nausea, vomiting, abdominal bloating, flatulence, anorexia.
Hematologic: megaloblastic anemia.
Skin: rash, dermatitis.
Other: *lactic acidosis,* unpleasant or metallic taste.

INTERACTIONS
Calcium channel blockers, corticosteroids, estrogens, isoniazid, nicotinic acid, oral contraceptives, phenothiazines, phenytoin, sympathomimetics, thiazide and other diuretics, thyroid agents: may produce hyperglycemia. Monitor patient's glycemic control. Metformin dosage may need to be increased.
Cationic drugs, such as amiloride, cimetidine, digoxin, morphine, procainamide, quinidine, quinine, ranitidine, triamterene, trimethoprim, vancomycin: have the potential to compete for common renal tubular transport systems, which may increase metformin plasma levels. Monitor patient's blood glucose level.
Nifedipine: increased metformin plasma levels. Monitor patient

closely. Metformin dosage may need to be decreased.

CONTRAINDICATIONS
Contraindicated in patients with hypersensitivity to the drug, renal disease, or metabolic acidosis. Metformin should be temporarily withheld in patients undergoing radiologic studies involving parenteral administration of iodinated contrast materials because the use of such products may result in acute renal dysfunction. The drug should also be promptly discontinued if the patient enters a hypoxic state. Metformin generally should be avoided in patients with hepatic disease.

NURSING CONSIDERATIONS
• Use caution when administering drug to elderly, debilitated, or malnourished patients and those with adrenal or pituitary insufficiency because of increased risk of hypoglycemia.
• Know that before therapy is begun, the patient's renal function should be assessed and then assessed at least annually thereafter. If renal impairment is detected, expect the doctor to switch the patient to a different antidiabetic agent.
• Administer with meals; once-daily dosage should be administered with breakfast and twice-daily dosage should be administered with breakfast and dinner.
• Know that when transferring patients from standard oral hypoglycemic agents (except chlorpropamide) to metformin, no transition period generally is necessary. When switching patients from chlorpropamide to metformin, care should be exercised during the first 2 weeks of metformin therapy because the prolonged retention of chlorpropamide increases the risk of hypoglycemia during this time.
• Monitor patient's blood glucose levels regularly to evaluate effectiveness

of therapy. Notify doctor if blood glucose levels become elevated despite therapy.

• Be aware that if the patient has not responded to 4 weeks of therapy using the maximum dosage, the doctor may add an oral sulfonylurea while continuing metformin at the maximum dosage. If the patient still does not respond after several months of concomitant therapy at maximum dosages, the doctor may discontinue both agents and institute insulin therapy.

• Monitor patient closely during times of increased stress, such as infection, fever, surgery, or trauma. Insulin therapy may be required in these situations.

• Be aware that the incidence of metformin-induced lactic acidosis is very low. Reported cases have occurred primarily in diabetic patients with significant renal insufficiency, with multiple, concomitant medical or surgical problems, and with multiple, concomitant drug regimens. The risk of lactic acidosis increases with the degree of renal impairment and the patient's age.

• Know that metformin should be discontinued immediately and the doctor notified if the patient develops any condition associated with hypoxemia or dehydration because of the risk of lactic acidosis associated with these conditions.

• Expect metformin therapy to be temporarily suspended for any surgical procedure (except minor procedures not associated with restricted intake of food and fluids) and should not be restarted until the patient's oral intake has resumed and renal function has been evaluated as normal.

• Monitor the patient's hematologic status for evidence of megaloblastic anemia. Patients with inadequate vitamin B_{12} or calcium intake or absorption appear to be predisposed to developing subnormal vitamin B_{12} levels. These patients should have routine serum vitamin B_{12} level determinations every 2 to 3 years.

• Instruct patient to discontinue drug and notify their doctor immediately if they develop unexplained hyperventilation, myalgia, malaise, unusual somnolence, or other nonspecific symptoms of early lactic acidosis.

• Warn patient not to consume excessive amounts of alcohol while taking metformin.

• Instruct patients about nature of diabetes, importance of following therapeutic regimen, adhering to specific diet, weight reduction, exercise, personal hygiene programs, and avoiding infection. Explain how and when to perform self-monitoring of blood glucose level, and teach recognition of hypoglycemia and hyperglycemia.

• Tell patient not to change drug dosage without the doctor's consent. Encourage patient to report abnormal blood glucose results.

• Advise patients not to take any other medication, including OTC drugs, without first checking with the doctor.

• Instruct patient to carry medical identification identifying them as diabetic patients.

---

tolazamide
Tolamide, Tolinase

Pregnancy Risk Category: C

HOW SUPPLIED
Tablets: 100 mg, 250 mg, 500 mg

ACTION
Unknown. A sulfonylurea that probably stimulates insulin release from the pancreatic beta cells and reduces glucose output by the liver. An extrapancreatic effect increases peripheral sensitivity to insulin.

ONSET, PEAK, DURATION
Onset occurs in 4 to 6 hours. Peak hypoglycemic effect within 4 to 6 hours. Effects persist for 12 to 24 hours.

INDICATIONS & DOSAGE
Adjunct to diet to lower blood glucose levels in patients with type II diabetes (non-insulin-dependent) –
Adults: initially, 100 mg P.O. daily with breakfast if fasting blood sugar (FBS) is under 200 mg/dl or 250 mg P.O. if FBS is over 200 mg/dl. Dosage adjusted at weekly intervals by 100 to 250 mg as needed. Maximum daily dosage is 500 mg b.i.d. before meals.
Adults over age 65: 100 mg P.O. once daily.
To change from insulin to oral therapy –
Adults: if insulin dosage is under 20 units daily, insulin stopped and oral therapy started at 100 mg P.O. daily with breakfast. If insulin dosage is 20 to 40 units daily, insulin stopped and oral therapy started at 250 mg P.O. daily with breakfast. If insulin dosage is over 40 units daily, insulin decreased by 50% and oral therapy started at 250 mg P.O. daily with breakfast. Dosage may be adjusted by 100 to 250 mg.

ADVERSE REACTIONS
GI: nausea, vomiting.
Skin: rash, urticaria, facial flushing.
Other: *hypersensitivity reactions, hypoglycemia.*

INTERACTIONS
Anabolic steroids, chloramphenicol, clofibrate, guanethidine, MAO inhibitors, phenylbutazone, salicylates, sulfonamides: increased hypoglycemic activity. Monitor blood glucose level.
Beta blockers, clonidine: prolonged hypoglycemic effect and masked symptoms of hypoglycemia. Use together cautiously.
Corticosteroids, glucagon, rifampin, thiazide diuretics: decreased hypogly-cemic response. Monitor blood glucose level.
Ethanol: possible disulfiram-like reaction. Avoid concomitant use of moderate to large amounts of ethanol.
Hydantoins: increased blood levels of hydantoins. Monitor blood levels closely.
Oral anticoagulants: increased hypoglycemic activity or enhanced anticoagulant effect. Monitor blood glucose levels and PT.

CONTRAINDICATIONS
Contraindicated for treating type I diabetes (insulin-dependent) or diabetes that can be adequately controlled by diet. Also contraindicated in patients with type II diabetes (non-insulin-dependent) complicated by ketosis, acidosis, coma, or other acute complications such as major surgery, severe infection, or severe trauma; in patients with uremia or hypersensitivity to drug; and during pregnancy or breast-feeding.

NURSING CONSIDERATIONS
• Use cautiously in elderly, debilitated, or malnourished patients or patients with impaired hepatic or renal function or porphyria.
• Know elderly patients may be more sensitive to drug's adverse effects.
• Be aware patients transferring from another oral antidiabetic agent usually need no transition period.
• Patients transferring from insulin therapy to an oral antidiabetic agent require blood glucose level testing at least three times a day before meals. Hospitalization may be required during the transition.
• Make sure patients know that therapy relieves symptoms but doesn't cure disease.
• Instruct patients about nature of disease, importance of following therapeutic regimen, adhering to specific diet, weight reduction, exercise, and personal hygiene programs, and about

avoiding infection. Explain how and when to perform self-monitoring of blood glucose levels and teach recognition of and intervention for hypoglycemia and hyperglycemia.

• Tell patients not to change drug dosage without the doctor's consent and to report abnormal blood or urine glucose test results.

• Teach patients to carry candy or other simple sugars to treat mild hypoglycemic episodes. Severe episodes may require hospital treatment.

• Advise patients not to take any other medication, including OTC drugs, without first checking with the doctor.

• Advise patients to avoid moderate to large intake of alcohol because of possible disulfiram-like reaction.

• Advise patients to carry medical identification identifying them as diabetic patients.

---

tolbutamide
Apo-Tolbutamide, Mobenol†, Novo-Butamide†, Oramide, Orinase

Pregnancy Risk Category: C

HOW SUPPLIED
Tablets: 250 mg, 500 mg

ACTION
Unknown. A sulfonylurea that probably stimulates insulin release from the pancreatic beta cells and reduces glucose output by the liver. An extrapancreatic effect increases peripheral sensitivity to insulin.

ONSET, PEAK, DURATION
Onset occurs within 1 hour. Plasma levels peak in 3 to 5 hours; peak hypoglycemic effects within 5 to 8 hours. Effects persist for 6 to 12 hours.

INDICATIONS & DOSAGE
Adjunct to diet to lower blood glucose levels in patients with type II diabetes (non-insulin-dependent)—
Adults: initially, 1 to 2 g P.O. daily as a single dose or in divided doses b.i.d. to t.i.d. Dosage adjusted, if necessary, to maximum of 3 g daily; however, the manufacturer states that little benefit occurs with doses greater than 2 g daily.
To change from insulin to oral therapy—
Adults: if insulin dosage is under 20 units daily, insulin stopped and oral therapy started at 1 to 2 g P.O. daily. If insulin dosage is 20 to 40 units daily, insulin reduced by 30% to 50% and oral therapy started as above. If insulin dosage is over 40 units daily, insulin reduced by 20% and oral therapy started as above. Further reductions in insulin are based on the patient's response to oral therapy.

ADVERSE REACTIONS
GI: nausea, heartburn.
Skin: rash, pruritus, facial flushing.
Other: *hypersensitivity reactions, hypoglycemia, dilutional hyponatremia.*

INTERACTIONS
Anabolic steroids, chloramphenicol, clofibrate, guanethidine, MAO inhibitors, phenylbutazone, salicylates, sulfonamides: increased hypoglycemic activity. Monitor blood glucose level.
Beta blockers, clonidine: prolonged hypoglycemic effect and masked symptoms of hypoglycemia. Use together cautiously.
Corticosteroids, glucagon, rifampin, thiazide diuretics: decreased hypoglycemic response. Monitor blood glucose level.
Ethanol: possible disulfiram-like reaction. Avoid concomitant use of moderate to large amount of ethanol.
Hydantoins: increased blood levels of

---

*Liquid form contains alcohol.   *Common* reactions are in italics; *life-threatening*, in bold italics.
**May contain tartrazine.

hydantoins. Monitor blood levels closely.

Oral anticoagulants: increased hypoglycemic activity or enhanced anticoagulant effect. Monitor blood glucose levels and PT.

CONTRAINDICATIONS

Contraindicated for treating type I diabetes (insulin-dependent) or diabetes that can be adequately controlled by diet. Also contraindicated in patients with type II diabetes (non-insulin-dependent) complicated by fever, ketosis, acidosis, coma, or other acute complications such as major surgery, severe infection, or severe trauma; in patients with hypersensitivity to drug or severe renal insufficiency; and during pregnancy or breast-feeding.

NURSING CONSIDERATIONS

• Use cautiously in elderly, debilitated, or malnourished patients or patients with impaired hepatic or renal function or prophyria.
• Know elderly patients may be more sensitive to drug's adverse effects.
• Know patients transferring from another oral antidiabetic agent usually need no transition period.
• Be aware patients transferring from insulin therapy to an oral antidiabetic agent require blood glucose level testing at least three times a day before meals. Hospitalization may be required during the transition.
• Instruct patients about nature of disease, importance of following therapeutic regimen, adhering to specific diet, weight reduction, exercise, and personal hygiene program, and about avoiding infection. Explain how and when to perform self-monitoring of blood glucose levels and teach recognition of and intervention for hypoglycemia and hyperglycemia.
• Make sure patients know that therapy relieves symptoms but doesn't cure disease.

• Tell patients not to change drug dosage without the doctor's consent and to report abnormal blood or urine glucose test results.
• Teach patients to carry candy or other simple sugars to treat mild hypoglycemic episodes. Severe episodes may require hospital treatment.
• Advise patients not to take any other medication, including OTC drugs, without first checking with the doctor.
• Advise patients to avoid moderate to large intake of alcohol because of possible disulfiram-like reaction.
• Advise patients to carry medical identification identifying them as diabetic patients.

58

Thyroid hormones

levothyroxine sodium
liothyronine sodium
liotrix
thyroid
thyrotropin

COMBINATION PRODUCTS
None.

---

levothyroxine sodium
(T₄ or L-thyroxine sodium)
Eltroxin†, Levoid, Levothroid, Levoxyl, Oroxine‡, Synthroid**

Pregnancy Risk Category: A

HOW SUPPLIED
Tablets: 0.025 mg, 0.05 mg, 0.075 mg, 0.088 mg, 0.1 mg, 0.112 mg, 0.125 mg, 0.137 mg, 0.15 mg, 0.175 mg, 0.2 mg, 0.3 mg.
Injection: 200 mcg/vial, 500 mcg/vial

ACTION
Not completely defined. Stimulates metabolism of all body tissues by accelerating the rate of cellular oxidation.

ONSET, PEAK, DURATION
Onset in 24 hours. Time to peak therapeutic effect is 3 to 4 weeks. Effects persist for 1 to 3 weeks.

INDICATIONS & DOSAGE
Cretinism –
Children under 1 year: initially, 0.025 to 0.05 mg P.O. daily, increased by 0.05 mg P.O. q 4 to 6 weeks as needed.
Myxedema coma –
Adults: 200 to 500 mcg I.V.; then 100 to 300 mcg given on second day followed by parenteral maintenance dosage of 50 to 200 mcg I.V. daily. Patient should be switched to oral maintenance as soon as possible.
Thyroid hormone replacement –
Adults: initially, 0.025 to 0.05 mg P.O. daily, increased by 0.025 mg P.O. q 2 to 4 weeks until desired response occurs. Maintenance dosage is 0.1 to 0.4 mg P.O. daily. May administer I.V. or I.M. when P.O. ingestion is precluded for long periods. However, dosage adjustment may be necessary.
Adults over 65 years: 0.0125 to 0.025 mg P.O. daily. Increased by 0.025 mg at 3- to 8-week intervals depending on response.
Children: initially, 0.025 to 0.05 mg in children younger than 1 year or 3 to 5 mcg/kg in children 1 year and older P.O. daily, gradually increased by 0.025 to 0.05 mg q 2 to 4 weeks until desired response occurs.

ADVERSE REACTIONS
Adverse reactions to thyroid hormones are extensions of their pharmacologic properties and reflect patient sensitivity to them.
CNS: *nervousness, insomnia, tremor.*
CV: *tachycardia, palpitations, **arrhythmias,** angina pectoris,* hypertension.
GI: appetite change, nausea, diarrhea.
Other: headache, leg cramps, weight loss, diaphoresis, heat intolerance, fever, menstrual irregularities.

INTERACTIONS
Cholestyramine, colestipol: impaired levothyroxine absorption. Separate doses by 4 to 5 hours.
Insulin, oral antidiabetic agents: altered serum glucose levels. Monitor blood glucose levels. Dosage adjustments may be necessary.

---

†Liquid form contains alcohol.
***May contain tartrazine.*

*Common reactions are in italics; **life-threatening,** in bold italics.*

I.V. phenytoin: free thyroid released. Monitor for tachycardia.
Oral anticoagulants: altered PT. Monitor PT. Dosage adjustments may be necessary.
Sympathomimetics, such as epinephrine: increased risk of coronary insufficiency. Monitor closely.

CONTRAINDICATIONS
Contraindicated in patients with hypersensitivity to drug, acute MI uncomplicated by hypothyroidism, untreated thyrotoxicosis , or uncorrected adrenal insufficiency.

NURSING CONSIDERATIONS
• Use with extreme caution in elderly patients and patients with angina pectoris, hypertension, or other CV disorders; renal insufficiency; and ischemic states.
• Use cautiously in patients with diabetes mellitus or insipidus, or myxedema.
• Rapid replacement in patients with arteriosclerosis may precipitate angina, coronary occlusion, or CVA. Use cautiously in these patients.
• Know that thyroid hormone replacement requirements are about 25% lower in patients over age 60 than in young adults.
• Also know that patients with adult hypothyroidism are unusually sensitive to thyroid hormone. Patient should be started at lowest dosage and titrated to higher dosages according to patients' symptoms and laboratory data until euthyroid state is reached.
• **I.V. use:** Prepare I.V. dose immediately before injection. Do not mix with other solutions. Inject into vein over 1 to 2 minutes.
• When changing from levothyroxine to liothyronine, levothyroxine should be stopped and liothyronine begun. Dosage increased in small increments after residual effects of levothyroxine have disappeared. When changing from liothyronine to levothyroxine,

levothyroxine is started several days before withdrawing liothyronine to avoid relapse.
• In patients with coronary artery disease who must receive thyroid hormone, observe carefully for possible coronary insufficiency.
• Monitor blood pressure and heart rate closely. High initial I.V dosage is usually well tolerated by patients in myxedema coma. Normal serum levels of T_4 should occur within 24 hours, followed by a threefold increase in serum T_3 in 3 days.
• Know that thyroid hormones alter thyroid function test results. Monitor PT; patients taking these hormones usually require decreased anticoagulant dosage.
• Know that patients taking levothyroxine who need to have radioactive iodine uptake studies performed must discontinue drug 4 weeks before test.
• Make sure patients understand the importance of compliance. Tell patients to take thyroid hormones at the same time each day, preferably before breakfast, to maintain constant hormone levels. Suggest morning dosage to prevent insomnia.
• Warn patients (especially elderly patients) to tell the doctor at once if chest pain, palpitations, sweating, nervousness, shortness of breath, or other signs of overdose or aggravated CV disease occur.
• To avoid problems with bioequivalence, advise patients who have achieved a stable response not to change product brands.
• Tell patients to report unusual bleeding and bruising.

liothyronine sodium (T_3)
Cyronine, Cytomel, Tertroxin‡
Pregnancy Risk Category: A

HOW SUPPLIED
Tablets: 5 mcg, 25 mcg, 50 mcg

ACTION
Not clearly defined. Enhances oxygen consumption by most tissues of the body, increases the basal metabolic rate and the metabolism of carbohydrates, lipids, and proteins.

ONSET, PEAK, DURATION
Onset unknown. Peak effect occurs within 2 to 3 days. Effects persist about 3 days.

INDICATIONS & DOSAGE
Congenital hypothyroidism –
Children: 5 mcg P.O. daily with a 5 mcg increase q 3 to 4 days until desired response achieved.
Myxedema –
Adults: initially, 5 mcg P.O. daily, increased by 5 to 10 mcg q 1 or 2 weeks until daily dosage reaches 25 mcg. Then, increased by 12.5 to 25 mcg daily q 1 to 2 weeks. Maintenance dosage is 50 to 100 mcg daily.
Nontoxic goiter –
Adults: initially, 5 mcg P.O. daily; may increase by 5 to 10 mcg daily q 1 to 2 weeks, until daily dosage reaches 25 mcg. Then, increase by 12.5 to 25 mcg daily q 1 to 2 weeks. Usual maintenance dosage is 75 mcg daily.
Thyroid hormone replacement –
Adults: initially, 25 mcg P.O. daily, increased by 12.5 to 25 mcg q 1 to 2 weeks until satisfactory response. Usual maintenance dosage is 25 to 75 mcg daily.
T_3 suppression test to differentiate hyperthyroidism from euthyroidism –
Adults: 75 to 100 mcg P.O. daily for 7 days.

ADVERSE REACTIONS
Adverse reactions to thyroid hormones are extensions of their pharmacologic properties and reflect patient sensitivity to them.
CNS: hyperirritability, *nervousness, insomnia, tremor,* headache.
CV: *tachycardia,* **arrhythmias,** angina pectoris, increased blood pressure, **cardiac decompensation and collapse.**
GI: diarrhea, abdominal cramps, vomiting.
Other: weight loss, heat intolerance, diaphoresis, accelerated rate of bone maturation in infants and children, menstrual irregularities.

INTERACTIONS
Cholestyramine, colestipol: impaired liothyronine absorption. Separate doses by 4 to 5 hours.
Insulin, oral antidiabetic agents: initial thyroid replacement therapy may cause increases in insulin or oral hypoglycemic requirements. Monitor blood glucose levels. Dosage adjustments may be necessary.
I.V. phenytoin: free thyroid released. Monitor for tachycardia.
Oral anticoagulants: altered PT. Monitor PT. Dosage adjustments may be necessary.
Sympathomimetics, such as epinephrine: increased risk of coronary insufficiency. Monitor closely.

CONTRAINDICATIONS
Contraindicated in patients with hypersensitivity to drug, acute MI uncomplicated by hypothyroidism, untreated thyrotoxicosis, or uncorrected adrenal insufficiency.

NURSING CONSIDERATIONS
● Use with extreme caution in elderly patients and patients with angina pectoris, hypertension, or other CV disorders; renal insufficiency; and ischemic states.
● Use cautiously in patients with diabetes mellitus or insipidus, or myxedema.
● Rapid replacement in patients with arteriosclerosis may precipitate angina, coronary occlusion, or CVA. Use cautiously in these patients.
● Know that levothyroxine is usually the preferred agent for thyroid hormone replacement therapy. Liothyro-

---

*Liquid form contains alcohol.
**May contain tartrazine.

Common reactions are in italics; ***life-threatening,*** in bold italics.

nine may be used when a rapid onset or a rapidly reversible agent is desirable or in patients with impaired peripheral conversion of levothyroxine to liothyronine.

• Be aware in most patients, regulation of liothyronine dosage is difficult.

• Know thyroid hormone replacement requirements are about 25% lower in patients over age 60 than in young adults.

• Monitor pulse and blood pressure.

• In patients with coronary artery disease who must receive thyroid hormones, observe carefully for possible coronary insufficiency.

• Know that thyroid hormones alter thyroid function tests. Monitor PT; patients taking these hormones usually require decreased anticoagulant dosage.

• When changing from levothyroxine to liothyronine, levothyroxine should be stopped and liothyronine begun at a low dosage. Increased in small increments after residual effects of levothyroxine have disappeared. When changing from liothyronine to levothyroxine, levothyroxine is started several days before withdrawing liothyronine to avoid relapse.

• Know that patients taking liothyronine who need to have radioactive iodine uptake studies performed must discontinue drug 7 to 10 days before test.

• Make sure patients understand the importance of compliance. Tell patients to take thyroid hormones at the same time each day, preferably before breakfast, to maintain constant hormone levels. Suggest morning dosage to prevent insomnia.

• To avoid problems with bioequivalence, advise patients who have achieved a stable response not to change product brands.

• Warn patients (especially elderly patients) to tell the doctor at once if chest pain, palpitations, sweating, nervousness, or other signs of overdose occur and to notify the doctor immediately if any signs of aggravated CV disease (chest pain, dyspnea, and tachycardia) develop.

• Tell patients to report unusual bleeding and bruising.

liotrix
Euthroid**, Thyrolar
Pregnancy Risk Category: A

HOW SUPPLIED
Tablets: levothyroxine sodium 30 mcg and liothyronine sodium 7.5 mcg (Euthroid-½); levothyroxine sodium 60 mcg and liothyronine sodium 15 mcg (Euthroid-1); levothyroxine sodium 120 mcg and liothyronine sodium 30 mcg (Euthroid-2); levothyroxine sodium 180 mcg and liothyronine sodium 45 mcg (Euthroid-3); levothyroxine sodium 12.5 mcg and liothyronine sodium 3.1 mcg (Thyrolar-¼); levothyroxine sodium 25 mcg and liothyronine sodium 6.25 mcg (Thyrolar-½); levothyroxine sodium 50 mcg and liothyronine sodium 12.5 mcg (Thyrolar-1); levothyroxine sodium 100 mcg and liothyronine sodium 25 mcg (Thyrolar-2); levothyroxine sodium 150 mcg and liothyronine sodium 37.5 mcg (Thyrolar-3)

ACTION
Not clearly defined. Stimulates metabolism of all body tissues by accelerating the rate of cellular oxidation and provides both T_3 and T_4 to the tissues.

ONSET, PEAK, DURATION
Unknown.

INDICATIONS & DOSAGE
Hypothyroidism –
Dosages are expressed in thyroid equivalents and must be individualized to approximate the deficit in the patient's thyroid secretion.

Adults and children: initially, 12.5 mcg of levothyroxine and 3.1 mcg of liothyronine P.O. daily, or 25 mcg of levothyroxine and 6.25 mcg of liothyronine daily or 30 mcg of levothyroxine and 7.5 mcg of liothyronine daily. Dosage increased in increments of the initial dose at 2-week intervals to achieve desired response.

ADVERSE REACTIONS

Adverse reactions to thyroid hormones are extensions of their pharmacologic properties and reflect patient sensitivity to them.

CNS: hyperirritability, *nervousness, insomnia*, twitching, *tremor*.

CV: increased cardiac output, *tachycardia, **arrhythmias***, angina pectoris, increased blood pressure, ***cardiac decompensation and collapse***.

GI: diarrhea, abdominal cramps, vomiting.

Other: weight loss, heat intolerance, diaphoresis, accelerated rate of bone maturation in infants and children, menstrual irregularities.

INTERACTIONS

Cholestyramine, colestipol: impaired liotrix absorption. Separate doses by 4 to 5 hours.

Insulin, oral antidiabetic agents: altered serum glucose levels. Monitor blood glucose levels. Dosage adjustments may be necessary.

I.V. phenytoin: free thyroid released. Monitor for tachycardia.

Oral anticoagulants: altered PT. Monitor PT. Dosage adjustments may be necessary.

Sympathomimetics, such as epinephrine: increased risk of coronary insufficiency. Monitor closely.

CONTRAINDICATIONS

Contraindicated in patients with hypersensitivity to drug, acute MI uncomplicated by hypothyroidism, untreated thyrotoxicosis, or uncorrected adrenal insufficiency.

NURSING CONSIDERATIONS

• Use with extreme caution in patients with angina pectoris, hypertension, or other CV disorders; renal insufficiency; and ischemic states and in elderly patients.

• Use cautiously in patients with myxedema or diabetes mellitus or insipidus.

• Rapid replacement in arteriosclerosis may precipitate angina, coronary occlusion, or CVA. Use cautiously in these patients.

• Know that thyroid hormone replacement requirements are about 25% lower in patients over age 60 than in young adults.

• In patients with coronary artery disease who must receive thyroid hormones, observe carefully for possible coronary insufficiency. Also observe carefully during surgery because arrhythmias can be precipitated.

• Monitor pulse and blood pressure.

• Know that thyroid hormones alter thyroid function test results. Monitor PT; patients taking these hormones usually require decreased anticoagulant dosage.

• Make sure patients understand the importance of compliance. Tell patients to take thyroid hormones at the same time each day, preferably before breakfast, to maintain constant hormone levels. Suggest morning dosage to prevent insomnia.

• To avoid problems with bioequivalence, advise patients who have achieved a stable response not to change product brands.

• Warn patients (especially elderly patients) to tell the doctor at once if chest pain, palpitations, sweating, nervousness, or other signs of overdose occur. Also notify the doctor immediately if any signs of aggravated CV disease develop (chest pain, dyspnea, and tachycardia).

• The two commercially prepared liotrix drugs contain different amounts of each ingredient; tell patient not to

---

*Liquid form contains alcohol.   *Common* reactions are in italics; ***life-threatening***, in bold italics.
**May contain tartrazine.

change from one brand to the other. Thyrolar-½ contains 25 mcg of T_4 and 6.25 mcg of T_3; Euthroid-½ contains 30 mcg of T_4 and 7.5 mcg of T_3.
• Tell patients to report unusual bleeding and bruising.

---

thyroid
Armour Thyroid, S-P-T, Thyrar, Thyroid Strong, Thyroid USP Enseals, Thyro-Teric, Westhroid

Pregnancy Risk Category: A

HOW SUPPLIED
Tablets: 15 mg, 30 mg, 60 mg, 65 mg, 90 mg, 120 mg, 130 mg, 180 mg, 240 mg, 300 mg
Tablets (bovine origin): 30 mg, 60 mg, 120 mg
Tablets (pork origin): 15 mg, 30 mg, 60 mg, 120 mg, 200 mg, 250 mg, 300 mg
Tablets (enteric-coated): 60 mg, 120 mg
Strong tablets (50% stronger than thyroid USP, and containing 0.3% iodine): 32.5 mg, 65 mg, 130 mg, 200 mg
Capsules (porcine origin): 60 mg, 120 mg, 180 mg, 300 mg

ACTION
Not clearly defined. Stimulates metabolism of all body tissues by accelerating the rate of cellular oxidation.

ONSET, PEAK, DURATION
Unknown.

INDICATIONS & DOSAGE
Mild hypothyroidism —
Adults: initially, 60 mg P.O. daily, increased by 60 mg q 30 days until desired response occurs. Usual maintenance dosage is 60 to 180 mg daily as a single dose.
Severe hypothyroidism —
Adults: initially, 15 mg P.O. daily, increased by 30 mg daily after 2 weeks, and 2 weeks later increased to 60 mg

daily. After 2 months, dosage increased to 120 mg daily as needed for 2 months. Then increased to 180 mg daily as needed.
Congenital or severe hypothyroidism in children —
Children: same as adults with severe hypothyroidism.

ADVERSE REACTIONS
Adverse reactions to thyroid hormones are extensions of their pharmacologic properties and reflect patient sensitivity to them.
CNS: *hyperirritability, nervousness, insomnia,* twitching, tremor, headache.
CV: increased cardiac output, *tachycardia, arrhythmias,* angina pectoris, increased blood pressure, ***cardiac decompensation and collapse.***
GI: diarrhea, abdominal cramps, vomiting.
Other: weight loss, heat intolerance, diaphoresis, accelerated rate of bone maturation in infants and children, menstrual irregularities.

INTERACTIONS
Cholestyramine: impaired thyroid absorption. Separate doses by 4 to 5 hours.
Insulin, oral antidiabetic agents: altered serum glucose levels. Monitor blood glucose levels. Dosage adjustments may be necessary.
I.V. phenytoin: free thyroid released. Monitor for tachycardia.
Oral anticoagulants: altered PT. Monitor PT. Dosage adjustments may be necessary.
Sympathomimetics, such as epinephrine: increased risk of coronary insufficiency. Monitor closely.

CONTRAINDICATIONS
Contraindicated in patients with hypersensitivity to drug, acute MI uncomplicated by hypothyroidism, untreated thyrotoxicosis, or uncorrected adrenal insufficiency.

NURSING CONSIDERATIONS

• Use with extreme caution in patients with angina pectoris, hypertension, or other CV disorders; renal insufficiency; and ischemic states and in elderly patients.
• Use cautiously in patients with myxedema or diabetes mellitus or insipidus.
• Know that thyroid hormone replacement requirements are about 25% lower in patients over age 60 than in young adults.
• Monitor pulse and blood pressure.
• Know that in children, sleeping pulse rate and basal morning temperature are guides to treatment.
• In patients with coronary artery disease who must receive thyroid hormones, observe carefully for possible coronary insufficiency.
• Know that thyroid hormones alter thyroid function test results. Monitor PT; patients taking these hormones usually require decreased anticoagulant dosage.
• Tell patients to take thyroid hormones at the same time each day, preferably before breakfast, to maintain constant hormone levels.
• Suggest morning dosage to prevent insomnia.
• To avoid problems with bioequivalence, advise patients who have achieved a stable response not to change product brands.
• Warn patients (especially elderly patients) to tell the doctor at once if chest pain, palpitations, sweating, nervousness, or other signs of overdose occur and to notify the doctor immediately if any signs of aggravated CV disease develop (chest pain, dyspnea, and tachycardia).
• Tell patients to report unusual bleeding and bruising.

thyrotropin (thyroid-stimulating hormone, or TSH)
Thytropar

Pregnancy Risk Category: C

HOW SUPPLIED
Powder for injection: 10 IU/vial

ACTION
Stimulates uptake of radioactive iodine (^{131}I) in patients with thyroid carcinoma and promotes thyroid hormone production by the anterior pituitary gland.

ONSET, PEAK, DURATION
Onset occurs in minutes. Hypertrophy and hyperplasia of the thyroid gland occur within 24 hours. Effects rapidly reverse after withdrawal.

INDICATIONS & DOSAGE
Diagnosis of thyroid cancer remnant with ^{131}I after surgery –
Adults: 10 IU I.M. or S.C. for 3 to 7 days.
Differential diagnosis of primary and secondary hypothyroidism –
Adults: 10 IU I.M. or S.C. for 1 to 3 days.
In protein-bound iodine or ^{131}I uptake determinations for differential diagnosis of subclinical hypothyroidism or low thyroid reserve –
Adults: 10 IU I.M. or S.C.
Therapy for thyroid carcinoma (local or metastatic) with ^{131}I –
Adults: 10 IU I.M. or S.C. for 3 to 8 days.
To determine thyroid status of patient receiving thyroid hormone –
Adults: 10 units I.M. or S.C. for 1 to 3 days.

ADVERSE REACTIONS
CNS: headache.
CV: *tachycardia,* atrial fibrillation, angina pectoris, **CHF,** hypotension.
GI: nausea, vomiting.

---

*Liquid form contains alcohol.
**May contain tartrazine.

Common reactions are in italics; **life-threatening,** in bold italics.

Other: thyroid hyperplasia (with large doses), fever, hypersensitivity reactions (postinjection flare, urticaria, *anaphylaxis*), menstrual irregularities.

INTERACTIONS
Insulin, oral antidiabetic agents: altered serum glucose levels. Monitor blood glucose levels. Dosage adjustments may be necessary.
Oral anticoagulants: altered PT. Monitor PT. Dosage adjustments may be necessary.
Sympathomimetics such as epinephrine: increased risk of coronary insufficiency. Monitor closely.

CONTRAINDICATIONS
Contraindicated in patients hypersensitive to the drug and in those with coronary thrombosis and untreated Addison's disease.

NURSING CONSIDERATIONS
• Use cautiously in patients with angina pectoris, CHF, hypopituitarism, and adrenocortical suppression.
• Know that three-day dosage schedule may be used in long-standing pituitary myxedema or with prolonged use of thyroid medication.

59

Thyroid hormone antagonists

methimazole
potassium iodide
potassium iodide, saturated
  solution
strong iodine solution
propylthiouracil
radioactive iodine (sodium
  iodide) ^{131}I

COMBINATION PRODUCTS
None.

---

methimazole
Tapazole

Pregnancy Risk Category: D

HOW SUPPLIED
Tablets: 5 mg, 10 mg

ACTION
Inhibits oxidation of iodine in the thyroid gland, blocking iodine's ability to combine with tyrosine to form thyroxine. Also may prevent the coupling of monoiodotyrosine and diiodotyrosine to form thyroxine and triiodothyronine.

ONSET, PEAK, DURATION
Onset occurs within 5 days (for serum levels of T_3 and T_4 to drop). Plasma levels peak in ½ to 1 hour. Duration unknown.

INDICATIONS & DOSAGE
Hyperthyroidism –
Adults: if mild, 15 mg P.O. daily; if moderately severe, 30 to 45 mg daily ; if severe, 60 mg daily. Daily dose divided into 3 doses at 8 hour intervals. Maintenance dosage is 5 to 15 mg daily.
Children: 0.4 mg/kg P.O. daily in divided doses q 8 hours. Maintenance

dosage is 0.2 mg/kg daily in divided doses q 8 hours.

ADVERSE REACTIONS
CNS: headache, drowsiness, vertigo.
EENT: loss of taste.
GI: diarrhea, nausea, vomiting (may be dose-related); salivary gland enlargement.
Hematologic: *agranulocytosis,* leukopenia, thrombocytopenia (appear to be dose-related).
Hepatic: jaundice; hepatic dysfunction (anorexia, pruritus, right upper quadrant pain, yellow skin or sclera).
Skin: rash, urticaria, skin discoloration.
Other: arthralgia, myalgia, drug-induced fever, lymphadenopathy; hypothyroidism (mental depression; cold intolerance; hard, nonpitting edema).

INTERACTIONS
None significant.

CONTRAINDICATIONS
Contraindicated in patients with hypersensitivity to drug and in breast-feeding patients.

NURSING CONSIDERATIONS
• Use with extreme caution in pregnancy.
• Pregnant women may require less drug as pregnancy progresses. Monitor thyroid function studies closely. Thyroid may be added to regimen. Drug may be stopped during last few weeks of pregnancy.
• Monitor CBC periodically as ordered to detect impending leukopenia, thrombocytopenia, and agranulocytosis. Also monitor hepatic function.
• Know that dosages of over 30 mg/

---

*Liquid form contains alcohol.   *Common* reactions are in italics; *life-threatening,* in bold italics.
**May contain tartrazine.

day increase the risk of agranulocytosis.

• Watch for signs of hypothyroidism (mental depression; cold intolerance; hard, nonpitting edema); notify doctor as dosage may need to be adjusted as necessary.

• Discontinue drug if severe rash or enlarged cervical lymph nodes develop and notify doctor.

• Tell patient to take with meals to reduce adverse GI reactions.

• Warn patients to immediately report fever, sore throat, or mouth sores (possible signs of developing agranulocytosis). Agranulocytosis can develop too rapidly to be detected by periodic blood cell counts. Tell patients also to immediately report skin eruptions (sign of hypersensitivity).

• Teach patients to recognize and immediately report signs and symptoms of hepatic dysfunction (anorexia, pruritus, right upper quadrant pain, yellow skin or sclera).

• Tell patients to ask the doctor about using iodized salt and eating shellfish during treatment.

• Warn patients against OTC cough medicines; many contain iodine.

• Instruct patient to store in light-resistant container.

---

potassium iodide
Iostat, Pima, Thyro-Block

potassium iodide, saturated solution (SSKI)

strong iodine solution (Lugol's solution)
Pregnancy Risk Category: D

HOW SUPPLIED
potassium iodide
Tablets: 130 mg
Tablets (enteric-coated): 300 mg
Oral solution: 500 mg/15 ml
Syrup: 325 mg/5 ml

potassium iodide, saturated solution
Oral solution: 1 g/ml
strong iodine solution
Oral solution: iodine 50 mg/ml and potassium iodide 100 mg/ml

ACTION
Inhibits thyroid hormone formation by blocking iodotyrosine and iodothyronine synthesis, limits iodide transport into the thyroid gland, and blocks thyroid hormone release.

ONSET, PEAK, DURATION
Onset occurs within 24 hours. Peak effect on thyroid function occurs within 10 to 15 days. Duration unknown.

INDICATIONS & DOSAGE
Preparation for thyroidectomy –
Adults and children: strong iodine solution, USP, 0.1 to 0.3 ml P.O. t.i.d., or potassium iodide, saturated solution (SSKI), 1 to 5 drops in water P.O. t.i.d., after meals for 10 to 14 days before surgery.
Thyrotoxic crisis –
Adults and children: 500 mg P.O. q 4 hours (approximately 10 drops of SSKI).
Radiation protectant for thyroid gland –
Adults: 130 mg P.O. 24 hours before and for 3 to 14 days after radiation exposure.

ADVERSE REACTIONS
CNS: frontal headache.
EENT: acute rhinitis, inflammation of salivary glands, tooth discoloration, periorbital edema, conjunctivitis, hyperemia.
GI: burning, irritation, *nausea,* vomiting, diarrhea (sometimes bloody), *metallic taste.*
Skin: acneiform rash, mucous membrane ulceration.
Other: fever; *hypersensitivity reac-*

tions, including symptoms resembling serum sickness.

INTERACTIONS
ACE inhibitors, potassium-sparing diuretics: risk of hyperkalemia. Avoid concomitant use.
Antithyroid medications: potassium iodide may potentiate hypothyroid or goitrogenic effects. Monitor closely.
Lithium carbonate: hypothyroidism may occur. Use with caution.

CONTRAINDICATIONS
Contraindicated in patients with tuberculosis, acute bronchitis, iodide hypersensitivity, or hyperkalemia. Some formulations contain sulfites, which may precipitate allergic reactions in certain hypersensitive individuals.

NURSING CONSIDERATIONS
• Use cautiously in patients with hypocomplementemic vasculitis, presence of goiter, or autoimmune thyroid disease.
• Know that usually given with other antithyroid drugs.
• Know that doctor may avoid prescribing enteric-coated tablets, which have been associated with small bowel lesions and can lead to serious complications, including perforation, hemorrhage, or obstruction.
• Dilute oral doses in water, milk, or fruit juice, and give after meals to prevent gastric irritation, to hydrate the patient, and to mask the very salty taste.
• Give iodides through straw to avoid tooth discoloration.
• Know that earliest signs of delayed hypersensitivity reactions caused by iodides are irritation and swelling of the eyelids.
• Store in light-resistant container.
• Know that although drug was once commonly used as an expectorant, clinical studies have failed to demonstrate a clinically significant action.

• Warn patients that sudden withdrawal may precipitate thyroid crisis.
• Tell patients to ask the doctor about using iodized salt and eating shellfish during treatment. Iodine-rich foods may not be permitted.

propylthiouracil (PTU)
Propyl-Thyracil†

Pregnancy Risk Category: D

HOW SUPPLIED
Tablets: 50 mg, 100 mg†

ACTION
Inhibits oxidation of iodine in the thyroid gland, blocking iodine's ability to combine with tyrosine to form thyroxine, and may prevent the coupling of monoiodotyrosine and diiodotyrosine to form thyroxine and triiodothyronine.

ONSET, PEAK, DURATION
Onset and duration unknown. Plasma levels peak 1 to 1.5 hours after oral administration.

INDICATIONS & DOSAGE
Hyperthyroidism –
Adults: 100 to 150 mg P.O. t.i.d.; up to 1200 mg daily have been used in severe cases. Maintenance dosage is 100 to 150 mg once daily in divided doses t.i.d.
Children over 10 years: 150 to 300 mg P.O. daily in divided doses t.i.d. Maintenance dosage determined by patient response.
Children 6 to 10 years: 50 to 150 mg P.O. daily in divided doses t.i.d. Maintenance dosage determined by patient's response.
Preparation for thyroidectomy –
Adults: 200 mg q 4 to 6 hours on first day; once full control of symptoms is achieved, dosage gradually reduced to usual maintenance levels.
Thyrotoxic crisis –
Adults and children: 200 mg P.O.

---

*Liquid form contains alcohol.   *Common* reactions are in italics; *life-threatening*, in bold italics.
**May contain tartrazine.

q 4 to 6 hours on first day; once full control of symptoms is achieved, dosage gradually reduced to usual maintenance levels.

ADVERSE REACTIONS
CNS: headache, drowsiness, vertigo.
CV: vasculitis.
EENT: visual disturbances.
GI: diarrhea, *nausea, vomiting* (may be dose-related), salivary gland enlargement, loss of taste.
Hematologic: *agranulocytosis,* leukopenia, thrombocytopenia (appear to be dose-related).
Hepatic: jaundice, *hepatotoxicity.*
Skin: rash, urticaria, skin discoloration, pruritus.
Other: arthralgia, myalgia, drug-induced fever, lymphadenopathy; dose-related hypothyroidism (mental depression; cold intolerance; hard, nonpitting edema).

INTERACTIONS
None significant.

CONTRAINDICATIONS
Contraindicated in patients with hypersensitivity to drug or in breast-feeding patients.

NURSING CONSIDERATIONS
• Use cautiously in pregnant patients.
• Give with meals to reduce adverse GI reactions.
• Know pregnant women may require less drug as pregnancy progresses. Monitor thyroid function studies closely. Thyroid may be added to regimen. Drug may be stopped during last few weeks of pregnancy.
• Watch for signs of hypothyroidism (mental depression; cold intolerance; hard, nonpitting edema); adjust dosage as ordered.
• Monitor CBC periodically as ordered to detect impending leukopenia, thrombocytopenia, and agranulocytosis.
• Discontinue drug if severe rash or

enlarged cervical lymph nodes develop and notify doctor.
• Store in light-resistant container.
• Warn patients to immediately report fever, sore throat, or mouth sores (possible signs of developing agranulocytosis). Agranulocytosis can develop too rapidly to be detected by periodic blood cell counts. Tell patients to also report skin eruptions (sign of hypersensitivity) immediately.
• Tell patients to ask the doctor about using iodized salt and eating shellfish during treatment.
• Warn patients against OTC cough medicines; many contain iodine.

---

radioactive iodine (sodium iodide) ¹³¹I
Iodotope Therapeutic, Sodium Iodide ¹³¹I Therapeutic

Pregnancy Risk Category: X

HOW SUPPLIED
All radioactivity concentrations are determined at the time of calibration.
Iodotope Therapeutic
Capsules: radioactivity range is 1 to 50 millicuries (mCi)/capsule at time of calibration
Oral solution: radioactivity concentration is 7.05 mCi/ml at time of calibration; in vials containing approximately 7, 14, 28, 70, or 106 mCi at time of calibration
Sodium Iodide ¹³¹I Therapeutic
Capsules: radioactivity range is 0.8 to 100 mCi/capsule at the time of calibration
Oral solution: radioactivity range is 3.5 to 150 mCi/vial at the time of calibration

ACTION
Limits thyroid hormone secretion by destroying thyroid tissue. The affinity of thyroid tissue for radioactive iodine facilitates uptake of drug by cancerous thyroid tissue that has metastasized to other sites in the body.

ONSET, PEAK, DURATION
Onset occurs in 2 to 4 weeks. Peak effect occurs in 2 to 4 months. Duration unknown.

INDICATIONS & DOSAGE
Hyperthyroidism –
Adults: usual dosage is 4 to 10 mCi P.O. Dosage is based on estimated weight of thyroid gland and thyroid uptake. Treatment repeated after 6 weeks, according to serum thyroxine level.
Thyroid cancer –
Adults: 50 to 150 mCi P.O. Dosage is based on estimated malignant thyroid tissue and metastatic tissue as determined by total body scan. Treatment repeated according to clinical status.

ADVERSE REACTIONS
EENT: *feeling of fullness in neck,* metallic taste, "radiation mumps."
Other: hypothyroidism; radiation-induced thyroiditis; possible increased risk of developing **leukemia** later in life after sufficient ^{131}I dose for thyroid ablation following cancer surgery; possible increased risk of birth defects in offspring after sufficient ^{131}I dose for thyroid ablation after cancer surgery.

INTERACTIONS
Lithium carbonate: hypothyroidism may occur. Use with caution.

The following drugs can interfere with the action of ^{131}I and should be withheld the specified time before administering the ^{131}I dose:
Adrenocorticoids: 1 week.
Benzodiazepines: 1 month.
Cholecystographic agents: 6 to 9 months.
Contrast media containing iodine: 1 to 2 months.
Iodine-containing products, including vitamins, expectorants, antitussives, and topical agents: 2 weeks.
Salicylates: 1 to 2 weeks.

CONTRAINDICATIONS
Contraindicated in pregnant patients except to treat thyroid cancer and contraindicated in breast-feeding patients.

NURSING CONSIDERATIONS
● Know that all antithyroid medications and thyroid preparations need to be stopped 1 week before ^{131}I dose. If medications are not stopped, patients may receive thyroid-stimulating hormone for 3 days before ^{131}I dose. When treating women of childbearing age, give dose during menstruation or within 7 days after menstruation.
● Tell patients to fast overnight before administration. Food may delay absorption.
● Know that after therapy for hyperthyroidism, patients should not resume antithyroid drugs, but should continue propranolol or other drugs used to treat symptoms of hyperthyroidism until onset of full ^{131}I effect occurs (usually 6 weeks).
● Monitor thyroid function via serum thyroxine levels, as ordered.
● Institute full radiation precautions during this time. Instruct patients to use appropriate disposal methods when coughing and expectorating. After dose for hyperthyroidism, patients' urine and saliva are slightly radioactive for 24 hours; vomitus is highly radioactive for 6 to 8 hours.
● After dose for thyroid cancer, patients' urine, saliva, and perspiration remain radioactive for 3 days. Isolate patients and observe the following precautions: do not allow pregnant personnel to care for patients, use disposable eating utensils and linens; instruct patients to save all urine in lead containers for 24 to 48 hours so amount of radioactive material excreted can be determined. Tell patients to drink as much fluid as possible for 48 hours after drug administration to facilitate excretion. Limit contact with patients to 30 minutes per

---

*Liquid form contains alcohol.   *Common* reactions are in italics; *life-threatening,* in bold italics.
**May contain tartrazine.

shift per person the first day and increase time, as necessary, to 1 hour second day and longer on third day.

• Warn patients who are discharged less than 7 days after ^{131}I dose for thyroid cancer to avoid close, prolonged contact with small children (for example, holding children on lap) and not to sleep in the same room with spouse for 7 days after treatment because of increased risk of thyroid cancer in persons exposed to [131]I. Tell patients it's okay to use the same bathroom facilities as the rest of the family.

corticotropin
repository corticotropin
cosyntropin
desmopressin acetate
leuprolide acetate
(See Chapter 73, ANTINEOPLASTICS THAT ALTER HORMONE BALANCE.)
lypressin
sermorelin acetate
somatrem
somatropin
vasopressin

COMBINATION PRODUCTS
None.

corticotropin (adrenocorticotropic hormone, ACTH)
ACTH, Acthar

repository corticotropin
Acthar Gel (H.P.)†, ACTH Gel, H.P. Acthar Gel

Pregnancy Risk Category: C

HOW SUPPLIED
Aqueous injection: 25 units/vial, 40 units/vial
Repository injection: 40 units/ml, 80 units/ml

ACTION
By replacing the body's own tropic hormone, stimulates the adrenal cortex to secrete its entire spectrum of hormones.

ONSET, PEAK, DURATION
Variable.

INDICATIONS & DOSAGE
Diagnostic test of adrenocortical function –
Adults: up to 80 units repository form I.M. or S.C. in divided doses or as a single dose; or 10 to 25 units aqueous form in 500 ml of D_5W I.V. over 8 hours, between blood samplings.

Individual dosages generally vary with adrenal glands' sensitivity to stimulation as well as with specific disease. Infants and younger children require larger doses per kilogram than do older children and adults.
For therapeutic use –
Adults: 40 units aqueous form S.C. or I.M. in four divided doses; or 40 to 80 units q 24 to 72 hours (repository form).

ADVERSE REACTIONS
CNS: *seizures, dizziness,* papilledema, headache, *euphoria, insomnia,* mood swings, personality changes, depression, psychosis.
EENT: cataracts, glaucoma.
GI: peptic ulceration with perforation and hemorrhage, pancreatitis, abdominal distention, ulcerative esophagitis, nausea, vomiting.
Skin: impaired wound healing, thin fragile skin, petechiae, ecchymoses, facial erythema, diaphoresis, acne, hyperpigmentation, allergic skin reactions, hirsutism.
Other: muscle weakness, steroid myopathy, loss of muscle mass, osteoporosis, vertebral compression fractures, cushingoid symptoms, suppression of growth in children, activation of latent diabetes mellitus, progressive increase in antibodies, loss of corticotropin stimulatory effect, hypersensitivity reactions (rash, ***bronchospasm***), *sodium and fluid retention,* calcium and potassium loss, hypokalemic alkalosis, negative nitrogen balance, menstrual irregularities.

---

*Liquid form contains alcohol.
**May contain tartrazine.

Common reactions are in italics; *life-threatening,* in bold italics.

INTERACTIONS
Anticonvulsants, barbiturates, rifampin: increased metabolism of corticotropin and decreased effectiveness. Monitor for lack of effect.
Estrogens: may potentiate the effects of cortisol. Dosage adjustments may be necessary.
NSAIDs, salicylates: increased risk of GI bleeding. Avoid concomitant use.
Oral anticoagulants: altered PT. Monitor PT. Dosage adjustments may be necessary.
Potassium-wasting diuretics: increased risk of hypokalemia. Monitor serum potassium levels.

CONTRAINDICATIONS
Contraindicated in patients with peptic ulcer, scleroderma, osteoporosis, systemic fungal infections, ocular herpes simplex, peptic ulceration, CHF, hypertension, sensitivity to pork and pork products, adrenocortical hyperfunction or primary insufficiency, or Cushing's syndrome. Also contraindicated in those who have had recent surgery.

NURSING CONSIDERATIONS
• Use cautiously in pregnant patients and in women of childbearing age. Also use cautiously in patients being immunized and in those patients with latent tuberculosis or tuberculin reactivity, hypothyroidism, cirrhosis, acute gouty arthritis, psychotic tendencies, renal insufficiency, diverticulitis, nonspecific ulcerative colitis, thromboembolic disorders, seizures, uncontrolled hypertension, or myasthenia gravis.
• Know that corticotropin treatment should be preceded by verification of adrenal responsiveness and test for hypersensitivity and allergic reactions.
• Be aware that corticotropin should be adjunctive, not sole, therapy. Oral agents are preferred for long-term therapy.

• **I.V. use:** Use only the aqueous form for I.V. administration. Dilute in 500 ml of D_5W and infuse over 8 hours.
• If administering gel, warm it to room temperature, draw into large needle, and give slowly as deep I.M. injection with 21G or 22G needle. Warn patients that injection is painful.
• Refrigerate reconstituted solution and use within 24 hours.
• Counteract edema by low-sodium, high-potassium intake; nitrogen loss by high-protein diet; and psychotic changes by reducing corticotropin dosage or administering sedatives as ordered.
• Know corticotropin may mask signs of chronic disease and decrease host resistance and ability to localize infection.
• Note and record weight changes, fluid exchange, and resting blood pressures until minimal effective dosage is achieved.
• Watch neonates of corticotropin-treated mothers for signs of hypoadrenalism.
• Unusual stress may require additional use of rapidly acting corticosteroids. When possible, gradually reduce corticotropin dosage to smallest effective dose as ordered to minimize induced adrenocortical insufficiency. Know that therapy can be reinstituted if stressful situation (trauma, surgery, severe illness) occurs shortly after stopping drug.

cosyntropin
Cortrosyn
Pregnancy Risk Category: C

HOW SUPPLIED
Injection: 0.25 mg/vial

ACTION
By replacing the body's own tropic hormone, stimulates the adrenal cor-

---

tex to secrete its entire spectrum of hormones.

ONSET, PEAK, DURATION
Onset occurs within 5 minutes of I.V. use. Peak cortisol levels occur within 1 hour of I.M. or I.V. use. Duration unknown.

INDICATIONS & DOSAGE
Diagnostic test of adrenocortical function –
Adults and children 2 years and older: 0.25 to 1 mg I.M. or I.V. (unless label prohibits I.V. administration) between blood samplings.
Children under 2 years: 0.125 mg I.M. or I.V.

ADVERSE REACTIONS
Skin: pruritus.
Other: flushing, hypersensitivity reactions (*anaphylaxis,* [rare]).

INTERACTIONS
Spironolactone: may interfere with fluorometric analysis of cortisol levels. Avoid concomitant use.

CONTRAINDICATIONS
Contraindicated in patients with hypersensitivity to drug.

NURSING CONSIDERATIONS
• Use cautiously in patients hypersensitive to natural corticotropin.
• **I.V. use:** Reconstitute with 1 ml of supplied diluent. For direct injection, administer over at least 2 minutes. May be further diluted with D₅W or 0.9% sodium chloride and infused over 6 hours. Solution is stable for 12 hours at room temperature.
• Know drug is synthetic duplication of the biologically active part of the corticotropin molecule. It is less likely to produce sensitivity than natural corticotropin derived from animal sources.
• Monitor patients for allergic reac-

tions, rashes, dyspnea, wheezing, or evidence of anaphylaxis.

---

desmopressin acetate
DDAVP, Minirin‡, Stimate

Pregnancy Risk Category: B

HOW SUPPLIED
Nasal solution: 0.1 mg/ml
Injection: 4 mcg/ml

ACTION
Increases the permeability of the renal tubular epithelium to adenosine monophosphate and water; the epithelium promotes reabsorption of water and produces a concentrated urine (ADH effect). Desmopressin also increases factor VIII activity by releasing endogenous factor VIII from plasma storage sites.

ONSET, PEAK, DURATION
Onset occurs within 1 hour for antidiuretic action, within 15 to 30 minutes for antihemorrhagic action. Peak antidiuretic effects occur within 1 to 5 hours, peak antihemorrhagic action in 90 minutes to 2 hours. Antidiuretic effects persist for 8 to 12 hours, antihemorrhagic effects for 4 to 12 hours.

INDICATIONS & DOSAGE
Nonnephrogenic diabetes insipidus, temporary polyuria and polydipsia associated with pituitary trauma –
Adults: 0.1 to 0.4 ml intranasally daily in one to three doses. Morning and evening doses adjusted separately for adequate diurnal rhythm of water turnover. Alternatively, injectable form administered in dosage of 0.5 to 1 ml I.V. or S.C. daily, usually in two divided doses.
Children 3 months to 12 years: 0.05 to 0.3 ml intranasally daily in one or two doses.
Hemophilia A and von Willebrand's disease –
Adults and children: 0.3 mcg/kg di-

---

luted in 0.9% sodium chloride and infused I.V. over 15 to 30 minutes. Dose repeated if necessary as indicated by laboratory response and the patient's clinical condition.

Primary nocturnal enuresis –
Children 6 years and over: initially, 20 mcg intranasally h.s. Dosage adjusted according to response. Maximum recommended dosage is 40 mcg daily.

ADVERSE REACTIONS
CNS: headache.
CV: slight rise in blood pressure at high dosage.
EENT: nasal congestion, rhinitis.
GI: nausea, abdominal cramps.
GU: vulval pain.
Other: flushing.

INTERACTIONS
Clofibrate: enhanced and prolonged effects of desmopressin. Monitor carefully.
Demeclocycline, epinephrine, ethanol, heparin, lithium: increased risk of adverse effects. Monitor closely.

CONTRAINDICATIONS
Contraindicated in patients hypersensitive to the drug, and in patients with Type IIB von Willebrand's disease.

NURSING CONSIDERATIONS
• Use cautiously in patients with coronary artery insufficiency or hypertensive CV disease or in patients with conditions associated with fluid and electrolyte imbalances, such as cystic fibrosis, because these patients are prone to hyponatremia.
• Know that desmopressin injection should not be used to treat hemophilia A with factor VIII levels of 0% to 5% or severe cases of von Willebrand's disease.
• Intranasal use can cause changes in the nasal mucosa resulting in erratic, unreliable absorption. Report a worsening condition to the doctor, who may prescribe injectable DDAVP.
• Adjust fluid intake to reduce risk of water intoxication and sodium depletion, especially in children or elderly patients.
• Overdose may cause oxytocic or vasopressor activity. Withhold drug and notify doctor. Use furosemide if fluid retention is excessive as ordered.
• Instruct patients to clear nasal passages before administering drug.
• Some patients may have difficulty measuring and inhaling drug into nostrils. Teach patients and caregivers correct method of administration.
• Nasal congestion, allergic rhinitis, or upper respiratory infections may impair drug absorption. Advise patients to report such conditions to the doctor; they may require a dosage adjustment.
• Teach patients using S.C. desmopressin to rotate injection sites to prevent tissue damage.
• Warn patients to drink only enough water to satisfy thirst.
• Inform patient that, when treating hemophilia A and von Willebrand's disease, giving desmopressin may avoid the hazards of using blood products.
• Advise patients to wear medical identification indicating their use of this drug.

lypressin
Diapid
Pregnancy Risk Category: B

HOW SUPPLIED
Nasal spray: 0.185 mg/ml

ACTION
Increases the permeability of the renal tubular epithelium to adenosine monophosphate and water; the epithelium promotes reabsorption of water and produces a concentrated urine (ADH effect).

ONSET, PEAK, DURATION
Onset occurs within 1 hour. Serum levels peak in 30 to 120 minutes. Effects persist for 3 to 4 hours.

INDICATIONS & DOSAGE
Nonnephrogenic diabetes insipidus –
Adults and children: 1 or 2 sprays (approximately 2 USP posterior pituitary pressor units/spray) in either or both nostrils q.i.d. and an additional dose h.s., if needed, to prevent nocturia. If usual dosage is inadequate, frequency increased rather than number of sprays.

ADVERSE REACTIONS
CNS: headache, dizziness.
EENT: nasal congestion or ulceration, irritation or pruritus of nasal passages, rhinorrhea, conjunctivitis.
GI: heartburn because of drip of excess spray into pharynx, abdominal cramps, frequent bowel movements.
GU: possible transient fluid retention from overdose.
Skin: hypersensitivity reaction.

INTERACTIONS
None significant.

CONTRAINDICATIONS
Contraindicated in patients hypersensitive to the drug.

NURSING CONSIDERATIONS
● Use cautiously in patients with coronary artery disease, hypertension, allergic rhinitis, or upper airway infection.
● Test patients sensitive to ADH for sensitivity to lypressin as ordered.
● Know particularly useful if diabetes insipidus is unresponsive to other therapy or if ADH of animal origin causes adverse reactions.
● To administer a uniform, well-diffused spray, hold bottle upright with patient in vertical position holding head upright.
● Know nasal congestion, allergic rhi-

nitis, or upper respiratory infections may diminish drug absorption and require larger dose or adjunctive therapy.
● Ensure that patients understand drug is for topical application to the nasal mucosa and should not be inhaled.
● Instruct patients to clear nasal passage before administering drug.
● Warn patient inadvertent inhalation of spray may cause tightness in chest, coughing, and transient dyspnea.
● Instruct patients to wear medical identification indicating their condition.

---

sermorelin acetate
Geref

Pregnancy Risk Category: C

HOW SUPPLIED
Powder for injection: 50 mcg/ampule

ACTION
A synthetic polypeptide that mimics the aminoterminal segment of the naturally occurring human growth hormone (GH).

ONSET, PEAK, DURATION
Onset and duration unknown. Peak levels of GH occur in about 30 minutes after injection in children; 35 minutes after injection in adults.

INDICATIONS & DOSAGE
Diagnostic aid to determine the pituitary gland's ability to secrete GH –
Adults and children: 1 mcg/kg as a single I.V. injection.

ADVERSE REACTIONS
CNS: headache.
EENT: unusual taste in mouth.
GI: nausea.
Skin: pain, redness, or swelling at injection site.
Other: transient warmth or flushing

---

*Liquid form contains alcohol.   *Common* reactions are in italics; *life-threatening*, in bold italics.
**May contain tartrazine.

PITUITARY HORMONES 783

of face, antibody formation, paleness, tightness in chest.

INTERACTIONS
Anticholinergics, antithyroid medications (such as propylthiouracil): decreased response to sermorelin.
Clonidine, insulin-induced hypoglycemia, levodopa: may elevate somatotropin levels.
Corticosteroids, cyclooxygenase inhibitors (for example, acetaminophen, aspirin, or NSAIDs), insulin: altered pituitary gland secretion of somatotropin. Don't perform the test in patients receiving these drugs.

CONTRAINDICATIONS
Contraindicated in patients with hypersensitivity to the drug or any components of the formulation.

NURSING CONSIDERATIONS
• Know that GH therapy should be discontinued 1 week before the test.
• Know response to drug may be blunted in hypothyroid patients.
• Be aware although hypersensitivity reactions have been reported with the administration of other polypeptide hormones, none have been reported with sermorelin. About 25% of patients develop antibody formation with prolonged use; however, no symptomatic allergic reactions have been reported.
• Be aware that baseline GH levels generally are low (< 4 ng/ml). Provocative tests, such as sermorelin, are useful in determining that the pituitary somatotroph can respond. However, a normal response doesn't rule out GH deficiency if the deficit is caused by hypothalamic dysfunction. This test is most easily interpreted if patients have had a subnormal response to conventional provocative testing (such as clonidine, levodopa, or arginine) and a normal response to sermorelin, thus suggesting that the cause of GH deficiency is hypotha-

lamic dysfunction. Abnormal results from both conventional tests and sermorelin can't pinpoint the location of the dysfunction.
• Make sure patients understand that the test must be performed in the morning after an overnight fast. They shouldn't take anything by mouth after midnight.
• Draw venous blood samples for GH determinations 15 minutes before and immediately before injection. Administer bolus injection (1 mcg/kg I.V.) and follow with 3-ml of 0.9% sodium chloride injection flush. Venous samples for GH determinations should be drawn at 15-minute intervals after injection (15 minutes, 30 minutes, 45 minutes, and 60 minutes).
• **I.V. use:** Reconstitute each ampule with a minimum of 0.5 ml of the supplied diluent. One ampule contains 50 mcg of drug, which is sufficient to test a 110-lb (50-kg) subject. Larger subjects require the use of multiple ampules.

somatrem
Protropin
Pregnancy Risk Category: C

HOW SUPPLIED
Injectable lyophilized powder: 5 mg (10 IU)/vial

ACTION
Purified growth hormone (GH) of recombinant DNA origin that stimulates linear, skeletal muscle, and organ growth.

ONSET, PEAK, DURATION
Onset and peak unknown. Effects persist for 12 to 48 hours.

INDICATIONS & DOSAGE
Long-term treatment of children who have growth failure because of lack of adequate endogenous GH secretion —
Children (prepuberty): highly indi-

vidualized; up to 0.1 mg/kg I.M. or S.C. three times weekly.

ADVERSE REACTIONS
Other: hypothyroidism, hyperglycemia, antibodies to GH.

INTERACTIONS
Glucocorticoids: may inhibit growth-promoting action of somatrem. Adjust glucocorticoid dosage as necessary.

CONTRAINDICATIONS
Contraindicated in patients with epiphyseal closure, active neoplasia, or hypersensitivity to benzyl alcohol.

NURSING CONSIDERATIONS
• Use cautiously in patients with hypothyroidism and in those whose GH deficiency results from an intracranial lesion.
• Be sure to check this product's expiration date.
• To prepare the solution, inject the supplied bacteriostatic water for injection into the vial containing the drug. Then swirl the vial with a gentle rotary motion until the contents are completely dissolved. *Don't shake* the vial.
• After reconstitution, vial solution should be clear. Don't inject into the patient if the solution is cloudy or contains any particles.
• If drug is administered to neonates, reconstitute immediately before use with sterile water for injection (without bacteriostat). Use the vial once; then discard.
• Store reconstituted vial in refrigerator; use within 7 days.
• Know that toxicity in newborns has occurred from exposure to benzyl alcohol used in the drug as a preservative.
• Know regular checkups with monitoring of height and of blood and radiologic studies are necessary.
• Observe patients for signs of glucose intolerance and hyperglycemia.

• Monitor periodic thyroid function tests for hypothyroidism as ordered, which may require treatment with a thyroid hormone.
• Reassure patients and their family members that somatrem is *pure* and *safe.* Drug replaces pituitary-derived human GH, which was removed from the market in 1985 because of an association with a rare but fatal viral infection (Jakob-Creutzfeldt disease).

---

somatropin
Humatrope, Nutropin

Pregnancy Risk Category: C

HOW SUPPLIED
Injection: 5 mg/5 ml

ACTION
Purified growth hormone (GH) of recombinant DNA origin that stimulates skeletal, linear, muscle, and organ growth.

ONSET, PEAK, DURATION
Onset and duration unknown. Plasma levels peak in about 7.5 hours.

INDICATIONS & DOSAGE
Long-term treatment of growth failure in children with inadequate secretion of endogenous GH—
Children: up to 0.06 mg/kg body weight S.C. or I.M. three times weekly using Humatrope or 0.30 mg/kg body weight S.C. weekly in daily divided doses using Nutropin.
Growth failure in children associated with chronic renal insufficiency up to the time of renal transplantation (Nutropin only)—
Children: 0.35 mg/kg body weight S.C. weekly in daily divided doses.

ADVERSE REACTIONS
CNS: headache, weakness.
CV: mild, transient edema.
Hematologic: *leukemia.*

Metabolic: mild hyperglycemia, hypothyroidism.
Other: injection site pain, localized muscle pain, antibodies to GH.

INTERACTIONS
None reported.

CONTRAINDICATIONS
Contraindicated in patients with closed epiphyses or an active underlying intracranial lesion. Humatrope should not be reconstituted with the supplied diluent for patients with a known sensitivity to either *m*-cresol or glycerin.

NURSING CONSIDERATIONS
• Use cautiously in children with hypothyroidism and in those whose GH deficiency is caused by an intracranial lesion. Be aware that these children should be examined frequently for progression or recurrence of the underlying disease.
• To prepare the solution, inject the supplied diluent into the vial containing the drug by aiming the stream of the liquid against the glass wall of the vial. Then swirl the vial with a gentle rotary motion until the contents are completely dissolved. *Don't shake the vial.*
• After reconstitution, vial solution should be clear. Don't inject solution if it is cloudy or contains particles.
• Store reconstituted vial in refrigerator; use within 14 days.
• If sensitivity to the diluent should occur, the vials may be reconstituted with sterile water for injection. When drug is reconstituted in this manner, use only 1 reconstituted dose per vial, refrigerate the solution if it is not used immediately after reconstitution, use the reconstituted dose within 24 hours, and discard the unused portion.
• Monitor child's height regularly. Know that regular checkups, including monitoring of blood and radiologic studies, also are necessary.
• Monitor patient's blood glucose levels regularly because GH may induce a state of insulin resistance.
• Know that excessive glucocorticoid therapy will inhibit the growth-promoting effect of somatropin. Patients with a coexisting corticotropin deficiency should have their glucocorticoid replacement dosage carefully adjusted to avoid an inhibitory effect on growth.
• Monitor periodic thyroid function tests, as ordered, for hypothyroidism, which may require treatment with a thyroid hormone.
• Inform parents that children with endocrine disorders (including GH deficiency) may develop slipped capital epiphyses more frequently. Tell them that if they notice a limp in their child, they should notify the doctor.

vasopressin (ADH)
Pitressin

Pregnancy Risk Category: C

HOW SUPPLIED
Injection: 0.5-ml and 1-ml ampules, 20 units/ml

ACTION
Increases the permeability of the renal tubular epithelium to adenosine monophosphate and water; the epithelium promotes reabsorption of water and produces a concentrated urine (ADH effect).

ONSET, PEAK, DURATION
Onset and peak unknown. Effects persist for 2 to 8 hours.

INDICATIONS & DOSAGE
Nonnephrogenic, nonpsychogenic diabetes insipidus –
Adults: 5 to 10 units I.M. or S.C. b.i.d. to q.i.d., p.r.n.; or intranasally (aqueous solution used as spray or ap-

plied to cotton balls) in individualized dosages, based on response.

Children: 2.5 to 10 units I.M. or S.C. b.i.d. to q.i.d., p.r.n.; or intranasally (aqueous solution used as spray or applied to cotton balls) in individualized doses.

Postoperative abdominal distention –
Adults: initially, 5 units (aqueous) I.M.; then q 3 to 4 hours, dose increased to 10 units, if needed. Dosage reduced proportionately for children.

To expel gas before abdominal X-ray –
Adults: 5 to 15 units S.C. at 2 hours; then again at 30 minutes before X-ray.

ADVERSE REACTIONS
CNS: tremor, dizziness, headache.
CV: angina in patients with vascular disease; vasoconstriction. Large doses may cause hypertension; ECG changes; and ***bradycardia, arrhythmias, pulmonary edema*** (with intra-arterial infusion).
GI: abdominal cramps, nausea, vomiting, diarrhea, intestinal hyperactivity.
GU: anuria.
Skin: circumoral pallor.
Other: uterine cramps, water intoxication (drowsiness, listlessness, headache, confusion, weight gain, *seizures, coma),* hypersensitivity reactions (urticaria, angioedema, ***bronchoconstriction,*** fever, rash, wheezing, dyspnea, ***anaphylaxis***), diaphoresis.

INTERACTIONS
Carbamazepine, chlorpropamide, clofibrate, fludrocortisone, tricyclic antidepressants: increased antidiuretic response. Use together cautiously.
Demeclocycline, ethanol, heparin, lithium, norepinephrine: reduced antidiuretic activity. Use together cautiously.

CONTRAINDICATIONS
Contraindicated in patients with chronic nephritis accompanied by nitrogen retention.

NURSING CONSIDERATIONS
● Use cautiously in children, elderly patients, pregnant patients, preoperative and postoperative polyuric patients, and in those with seizure disorders, migraine headache, asthma, CV disease, heart failure, renal disease, goiter with cardiac complications, arteriosclerosis, or fluid overload.
● Know that synthetic desmopressin is sometimes preferred because of its longer duration of action and less frequent adverse reactions. Desmopressin also is commercially available as a nasal solution.
● May be used for transient polyuria resulting from ADH deficiency related to neurosurgery or head injury.
● Never inject during first stage of labor; may cause ruptured uterus.
● Know that minimum effective dosage should be used to reduce adverse reactions.
● Give with 1 to 2 glasses of water to reduce adverse reactions and to improve therapeutic response.
● Monitor specific gravity of urine and fluid intake and output to aid evaluation of drug effectiveness.
● To prevent possible seizures, coma, and death, observe patients closely for early signs of water intoxication.
● Monitor blood pressure of patients on vasopressin twice daily. Watch for excessively elevated blood pressure or lack of response to drug, which may be indicated by hypotension. Also monitor fluid intake and output and daily weight.
● A rectal tube will facilitate gas expulsion after vasopressin injection.
● Instruct patients to rotate injection sites to prevent tissue damage.

---

*Liquid form contains alcohol.   *Common* reactions are in italics; ***life-threatening,*** in bold italics.
**May contain tartrazine.

calcifediol
calcitonin (human)
calcitonin (salmon)
calcitriol
dihydrotachysterol
etidronate disodium

COMBINATION PRODUCTS
None.

calcifediol
Calderol

Pregnancy Risk Category: C

HOW SUPPLIED
Capsules: 20 mcg, 50 mcg

ACTION
A vitamin D analogue that stimulates calcium absorption from the GI tract and promotes secretion of calcium from bone to blood.

ONSET, PEAK, DURATION
Onset unknown. Peak levels occur in 4 hours. Effects persist for 15 to 20 days.

INDICATIONS & DOSAGE
Metabolic bone disease associated with chronic renal failure –
Adults: initially, 300 to 350 mcg P.O. weekly. Dosage increased at 4-week intervals if necessary.

ADVERSE REACTIONS
Vitamin D intoxication associated with hypercalcemia:
CNS: headache, somnolence.
EENT: conjunctivitis, photosensitivity reactions, rhinorrhea.
GI: nausea, vomiting, constipation, metallic taste, dry mouth, anorexia, diarrhea.
GU: polyuria.

Other: weakness, bone and muscle pain.

INTERACTIONS
Cholestyramine, colestipol: decreased absorption of orally administered vitamin D analogues. Avoid concomitant use.
Corticosteroids: counteracts vitamin D analogue effects. Don't use together.
Digitalis glycosides: increased risk of arrhythmias. Avoid concomitant use.
Magnesium-containing antacids: possible hypermagnesemia, especially in patients with chronic renal failure. Avoid concomitant use.
Other vitamin D analogues: increased toxicity. Avoid concomitant use.

CONTRAINDICATIONS
Contraindicated in patients with hypercalcemia or vitamin D toxicity.

NURSING CONSIDERATIONS
• Monitor serum calcium level as ordered; serum calcium level multiplied by serum phosphate level should not exceed 70. During titration, serum calcium level should be determined at least weekly. If hypercalcemia occurs, discontinue calcifediol and notify doctor. Drug may be resumed after serum calcium level returns to normal.
• Provide the patient with adequate daily intake of calcium.
• Teach the patient to report signs and symptoms of hypercalcemia.

calcitonin (human)
Cibacalcin

calcitonin (salmon)
Calcimar, Miacalcin

Pregnancy Risk Category: C

HOW SUPPLIED
calcitonin human
Injection: 0.5 mg/vial
calcitonin salmon
Injection: 100 IU/ml, 1-ml ampules;
200 IU/ml, 2-ml ampules

ACTION
Decreases osteoclastic activity by inhibiting osteocytic osteolysis and decreases mineral release and matrix or collagen breakdown in bone.

ONSET, PEAK, DURATION
Onset immediate after I.V. injection, within 15 minutes after I.M. or S.C. injection. Plasma levels peak immediately after I.V. injection, within 4 hours after I.M. or S.C. injection. Effects persist 30 minutes to 12 hours after I.V. administration, 8 to 24 hours after I.M. or S.C. injection.

INDICATIONS & DOSAGE
Paget's disease of bone (osteitis deformans) –
Adults: initially, 100 IU of calcitonin (salmon) daily S.C. or I.M.; maintenance dosage is 50 to 100 IU daily or every other day. Alternatively, calcitonin (human) 0.5 mg S.C. daily. If the patient improves sufficiently, dosage reduced to 0.25 mg. daily 2 or 3 times per week. Some patients may need as much as 1 mg daily.
Hypercalcemia –
Adults: 4 IU/kg of calcitonin (salmon) q 12 hours I.M. If response inadequate after 1 or 2 days dose increased to 8 IU/kg I.M. q 12 hours. If response remains unsatisfactory after 2 more days, dosage increased to maximum of 8 IU/kg I.M. q 6 hours.
Postmenopausal osteoporosis –
Adults: 100 IU of calcitonin (salmon) daily I.M. or S.C.

ADVERSE REACTIONS
CNS: headache.
GI: *transient nausea,* unusual taste, diarrhea, anorexia.
GU: transient diuresis.
Local: inflammation at injection site, rash.
Other: *facial flushing;* hypocalcemia; hyperglycemia; hand swelling, tingling, and tenderness; hypersensitivity reactions *(anaphylaxis)*.

INTERACTIONS
None significant.

CONTRAINDICATIONS
Contraindicated in patients hypersensitive to calcitonin salmon. Calcitonin human has no contraindications.

NURSING CONSIDERATIONS
• Be aware that skin test is usually done before therapy.
• Systemic allergic reactions possible since hormone is protein. Keep epinephrine handy.
• Know that calcitonin (human) is especially indicated in patients who have developed resistance to calcitonin (salmon). Calcitonin (human) is associated with risk of diminishing efficacy caused by antibody formation or hypersensitivity reactions.
• Administer at bedtime when possible to minimize nausea and vomiting.
• I.M. route is preferred if the volume of the dose to be administered exceeds 2 ml.
• Use freshly reconstituted solution within 2 hours.
• Facial flushing and warmth occur in 20% to 30% of all patients within minutes of injection and usually last about 1 hour. Reassure the patient that this is a transient effect.
• Observe the patient for signs of hypocalcemic tetany during therapy (muscle twitching, tetanic spasms, and seizures if hypocalcemia is severe).
• Monitor serum calcium level

---

*Liquid form contains alcohol.   *Common* reactions are in italics; *life-threatening*, in bold italics.
**May contain tartrazine.

closely. Watch for signs of hypercalcemia relapse: bone pain, renal calculi, polyuria, anorexia, nausea,
vomiting, thirst, constipation, lethargy, bradycardia, muscle hypotonic-
ity, pathologic fracture, psychosis,
and coma.
• Know that periodic examinations of
urine sediment are advisable.
• Monitor periodic serum alkaline
phosphatase and 24-hour urine hydroxyproline levels to evaluate drug
effect as ordered.
• In patients with good initial clinical
response to calcitonin who suffer relapse, expect to evaluate for antibody
response to the hormone protein.
• If symptoms have been relieved after 6 months, know that treatment
may be discontinued until symptoms
or radiologic signs recur.
• Store calcitonin (human) at room
temperature (77° F [25° C]); refrigerate calcitonin (salmon) at 36° to 46° F
(2° to 8° C).
• When administered for postmenopausal osteoporosis, remind the patient to take adequate calcium and vitamin D supplements.
• Tell the patient in whom calcitonin
loses its hypocalcemic activity that
further medication or increased dosages will be of no value.

---

calcitriol (1,25-dihydroxy-cholecalciferol)
Rocaltrol

Pregnancy Risk Category: C

HOW SUPPLIED
Capsules: 0.25 mcg, 0.5 mcg

ACTION
A vitamin D analogue that stimulates
calcium absorption from the GI tract
and promotes secretion of calcium
from bone to blood.

ONSET, PEAK, DURATION
Onset occurs within 2 to 6 hours.
Plasma levels peak in 3 to 6 hours. Ef-
fects persist 3 to 5 days.

INDICATIONS & DOSAGE
*Hypocalcemia in patients undergoing
chronic dialysis* –
Adults: initially, 0.25 mcg P.O. daily.
Dosage may be increased by 0.25 mcg
daily at 4- to 8-week intervals. Maintenance dosage is 0.25 mcg every
other day up to 1.25 mcg daily.
*Hypoparathyroidism and pseudohypo-
parathyroidism* –
**Adults and children 1 year and
older:** initially, 0.25 mcg P.O. daily.
Dosage may be increased at 2- to 4-
week intervals. Maintenance dosage
is 0.25 to 2 mcg daily.

ADVERSE REACTIONS
*Vitamin D intoxication associated with
hypercalcemia:*
CNS: headache, somnolence.
EENT: conjunctivitis, photophobia,
rhinorrhea.
GI: nausea, vomiting, constipation,
metallic taste, dry mouth, anorexia.
GU: polyuria.
Other: weakness, bone and muscle
pain.

INTERACTIONS
*Cholestyramine, colestipol, excessive
use of mineral oil:* decreased absorption of orally administered vitamin D
analogues. Avoid concomitant use.
Corticosteroids: counteracts vitamin
D analogue effects. Don't use together.
Digitalis glycosides: increased risk of
arrhythmias. Avoid concomitant use.
Magnesium-containing antacids: may
induce hypermagnesemia, especially
in patients with chronic renal failure.
Avoid concomitant use.

CONTRAINDICATIONS
Contraindicated in patients with hypercalcemia or vitamin D toxicity.

Withhold all preparations containing vitamin D.

NURSING CONSIDERATIONS

• Monitor serum calcium level; serum calcium level multiplied by the serum phosphate level should not exceed 70. During titration, determine serum calcium twice weekly. Discontinue if hypercalcemia occurs and notify doctor, but resume after serum calcium level returns to normal. The patient should receive adequate daily intake of calcium – 1,000 mg.

• Protect from heat and light.

• Tell the patient to immediately report early symptoms of vitamin D intoxication: weakness, nausea, vomiting, dry mouth, constipation, muscle or bone pain, or metallic taste.

• Instruct the patient to adhere to diet and calcium supplementation and to avoid unapproved OTC drugs and magnesium-containing antacids.

• Tell the patient that this drug must not be taken by anyone for whom it was not prescribed because of its potentially serious toxicities. It is the most potent form of vitamin D available.

---

dihydrotachysterol

AT-10‡, DHT Intensol*, Hytakerol

Pregnancy Risk Category: C

HOW SUPPLIED

Tablets: 0.125 mg, 0.2 mg, 0.4 mg
Capsules: 0.125 mg
Oral solution: 0.2 mg/5 ml, 0.2 mg/ml* (DHT Intensol*), 0.25 mg/ml (in sesame oil)

Note: 1 mg of dihydrotachysterol is equal to 120,000 units ergocalciferol (vitamin D_2)

ACTION

A vitamin D analogue that stimulates calcium absorption from the GI tract and promotes secretion of calcium from bone to blood.

ONSET, PEAK, DURATION

Onset occurs in several hours. Peak effects occur in 1 to 2 weeks. Effects persist up to 9 weeks.

INDICATIONS & DOSAGE

Hypocalcemia associated with hypoparathyroidism and pseudohypoparathyroidism –
Adults: initially, 0.75 to 2.5 mg P.O. daily for several days. Maintenance dosage is 0.2 to 1.5 mg daily.
Children: initially, 1 to 5 mg P.O. for several days. Maintenance dosage is 0.5 to 1.5 mg daily.
Prophylaxis of hypocalcemic tetany following thyroid surgery –
Adults: 0.25 mg P.O. daily (with calcium supplements).

ADVERSE REACTIONS

Vitamin D intoxication associated with hypercalcemia:
CNS: headache, somnolence, vertigo, tinnitus.
EENT: conjunctivitis, photophobia, rhinorrhea.
GI: nausea, vomiting, constipation, metallic taste, dry mouth, anorexia, diarrhea.
GU: polyuria.
Other: weakness, bone and muscle pain, thirst.

INTERACTIONS

Cholestyramine, colestipol, excessive use of mineral oil: decreased absorption of orally administered vitamin D analogues. Avoid concomitant use.
Corticosteroids: counteracts vitamin D analogue effects. Don't use together.
Digitalis glycosides: increased risk of arrhythmias. Avoid concomitant use.
Magnesium-containing antacids: possible hypermagnesemia, especially in patients with chronic renal failure. Avoid concomitant use.
Other vitamin D analogues: increased toxicity. Avoid concomitant use.

---

*Liquid form contains alcohol.   Common reactions are in italics; **life-threatening,** in bold italics.
**May contain tartrazine.

CONTRAINDICATIONS
Contraindicated in patients with hypercalcemia or vitamin D toxicity.

NURSING CONSIDERATIONS
• Monitor serum calcium level as ordered; the serum calcium level multiplied by serum phosphate level should not exceed 70. During titration, determine serum calcium twice weekly. Discontinue if hypercalcemia occurs and notify doctor. Know that drug can be resumed after serum calcium level returns to normal. Adequate daily intake of calcium is 1,000 mg.
• Monitor urine calcium level.
• Report any early signs of hypercalcemia: thirst, headache, vertigo, tinnitus, or anorexia.
• Store in tightly closed, light-resistant container. Don't refrigerate.

etidronate disodium
Didronel

Pregnancy Risk Category: C

HOW SUPPLIED
Tablets: 200 mg, 400 mg
Injection: 50 mg/ml

ACTION
Decreases osteoclastic activity by inhibiting osteocytic osteolysis and decreases mineral release and matrix or collagen breakdown in bone.

ONSET, PEAK, DURATION
Highly variable.

INDICATIONS & DOSAGE
Symptomatic Paget's disease of bone (osteitis deformans) –
Adults: 5 to 10 mg/kg P.O. daily in single dose 2 hours before a meal with water or juice. Maximum dosage is 20 mg/kg P.O. daily.
Heterotopic ossification in spinal cord injuries –
Adults: 20 mg/kg P.O. daily for 2 weeks, then 10 mg/kg daily for 10 weeks. Total treatment period is 12 weeks.
Heterotopic ossification after total hip replacement –
Adults: 20 mg/kg P.O. daily for 1 month before total hip replacement and for 3 months afterward.
Malignancy-associated hypercalcemia –
Adults: 7.5 mg/kg I.V. daily for 3 consecutive days. Maintenance dosage is 20 mg/kg P.O. daily for 30 days. May be used for a maximum of 90 days.

ADVERSE REACTIONS
GI: seen most frequently at dosage of 20 mg/kg daily – diarrhea, increased frequency of bowel movements, nausea.
Other: increased or recurrent bone pain, pain at previously asymptomatic sites, increased risk of fracture, *elevated serum phosphate level.*

INTERACTIONS
None significant.

CONTRAINDICATIONS
None reported.

NURSING CONSIDERATIONS
• Use cautiously in patients with impaired renal function.
• Know that drug should not be given any longer than 3 months at doses above 10 mg/kg daily; can be resumed after 3 months, if needed. Therapy should not exceed 6 months.
• Know that some patients may receive I.V. etidronate for up to 7 days. However, the risk of hypokalemia increases after 3 days of treatment.
• Monitor renal function before and during therapy as ordered.
• Don't give drug with food, milk, or antacids; may reduce absorption.
• **I.V. use:** Dilute daily dose in at least 250 ml 0.9% sodium chloride solution or D$_5$W, and infuse over at least 2 hours.

- To monitor drug effect, review serum alkaline phosphatase and urinary hydroxyproline excretion; both will decrease if therapy is effective.
- Be aware elevated serum phosphate level may occur, especially in patients receiving higher doses. However, serum phosphate level usually returns to normal 2 to 4 weeks after drug is discontinued.
- Stress importance of a diet high in calcium and vitamin D.
- Tell the patient not to eat for 2 hours after daily dose.
- Tell the patient that improvement may not occur for up to 3 months but may continue for months after drug is stopped.

acetazolamide
acetazolamide sodium
amiloride hydrochloride
bendroflumethiazide
bumetanide
chlorothiazide
chlorothiazide sodium
chlorthalidone
dichlorphenamide
ethacrynate sodium
ethacrynic acid
furosemide
hydrochlorothiazide
hydroflumethiazide
indapamide
mannitol
methazolamide
methyclothiazide
metolazone
polythiazide
quinethazone
spironolactone
torsemide
triamterene
trichlormethiazide
urea

COMBINATION PRODUCTS

ALDACTAZIDE 25/25: spironolactone 25 mg and hydrochlorothiazide 25 mg.
ALDACTAZIDE 50/50: spironolactone 50 mg and hydrochlorothiazide 50 mg.
DYAZIDE: triamterene 37.5 mg and hydrochlorothiazide 25 mg.
MAXZIDE: triamterene 75 mg and hydrochlorothiazide 50 mg.
MAXZIDE-25MG: triamterene 37.5 mg and hydrochlorothiazide 25 mg.
MODURETIC: amiloride hydrochloride 5 mg and hydrochlorothiazide 50 mg.
SPIROZIDE: spironolactone 25 mg and hydrochlorothiazide 25 mg.

ZIAC 2.5: bisoprolol fumarate 2.5 mg and hydrochlorthiazide 6.25 mg.
ZIAC 5: bisoprolol fumarate 5 mg and hydrochlorthiazide 6.25 mg.
ZIAC 10: bisoprolol fumarate 10 mg and hydrochlorthiazide 6.25 mg.

---

acetazolamide
Acetazolam†, Apo-Acetazolamide†, Dazamide, Diamox, Diamox Sequels

acetazolamide sodium
Diamox Parenteral, Diamox Sodium†

Pregnancy Risk Category: C

HOW SUPPLIED
acetazolamide
Tablets: 125 mg, 250 mg
Capsules (extended-release): 500 mg
acetazolamide sodium
Injection: 500 mg/vial

ACTION
Blocks the action of carbonic anhydrase, promoting renal excretion of sodium, potassium, bicarbonate, and water, and decreases secretion of aqueous humor in the eye, thereby lowering intraocular pressure. As an anticonvulsant, may inhibit carbonic anhydrase in the CNS and decrease abnormal paroxysmal or excessive neuronal discharge. In acute mountain sickness, carbonic anhydrase inhibitors produce a respiratory and metabolic acidosis that may stimulate ventilation, increase cerebral blood flow, promote the release of oxygen from hemoglobin, and increase ventilation.

ONSET, PEAK, DURATION
Onset occurs 1 to 1½ hours after tablets, 2 hours after capsules, 2 minutes after I.V. injection. Peak effects occur 2 to 4 hours after tablets, 8 to 12 hours after capsules, 15 minutes after I.V. injection. Effects persist for 8 to 12 hours after tablets, 18 to 24 hours after capsules, 4 to 5 hours after I.V. injection.

INDICATIONS & DOSAGE
Secondary glaucoma and preoperative treatment of acute angle-closure glaucoma –
Adults: 250 mg P.O. q 4 hours; or 250 mg P.O. b.i.d. for short-term therapy. To rapidly lower intraocular pressure, 500 mg I.V. q 2 to 4 hours.
Edema in CHF –
Adults: 250 to 375 mg P.O., or I.V. daily in a.m.
Chronic open-angle glaucoma –
Adults: 250 mg to 1 g P.O. daily in divided doses q.i.d., or 500 mg (extended-release) P.O. b.i.d.
Prevention or amelioration of acute mountain sickness –
Adults: 500 mg to 1 g P.O. daily in divided doses q 8 to 12 hours, or 500 mg (extended-release) P.O. b.i.d. Treatment started 24 to 48 hours before ascent, and continued for 48 hours while at high altitude.
Adjunctive treatment of myoclonic, refractory generalized tonic-clonic, absence, or mixed seizures –
Adults and children: 8 to 30 mg/kg P.O. daily in divided doses. For adults, the optimum dosage range is 375 mg to 1 g daily. Usually given with other anticonvulsants.

ADVERSE REACTIONS
CNS: drowsiness, paresthesia, confusion.
EENT: transient myopia.
GI: nausea, vomiting, anorexia, altered taste.
GU: crystalluria, renal calculi, hematuria.

Hematologic: *aplastic anemia,* hemolytic anemia, leukopenia.
Skin: rash.
Other: *pain at injection site,* sterile abscesses, hyperchloremic acidosis, hypokalemia, asymptomatic hyperuricemia.

INTERACTIONS
Amphetamines, anticholinergics, mecamylamine, quinidine: decreased renal clearance of these agents, increasing toxicity. Monitor closely.
Methenamine: reduced effectiveness of acetazolamide. Avoid concomitant use.
Salicylates: possible accumulation and toxicity of acetazolamide, including CNS depression and metabolic acidosis. Monitor closely.

CONTRAINDICATIONS
Contraindicated in patients with hypersensitivity to the drug; in long-term therapy for chronic noncongestive angle-closure glaucoma; and in those with hyponatremia or hypokalemia, renal or hepatic disease or dysfunction, adrenal gland failure, and hyperchloremic acidosis.

NURSING CONSIDERATIONS
• Use cautiously in patients with respiratory acidosis, emphysema, or chronic pulmonary disease, and in patients receiving other diuretics.
• Reconstitute 500-mg vial with at least 5 ml of sterile water for injection. Use within 24 hours of reconstitution.
• **I.V. use:** Inject 100 to 500 mg/minute into a large vein using a 21G or 23G needle. Intermittent or continuous infusion is not recommended.
• If the patient is unable to swallow oral forms, check with a pharmacist. He may make a suspension using crushed acetazolamide tablets in a highly flavored syrup, such as cherry, raspberry, or chocolate. Although concentrations up to 500 mg/5 ml are

---

*Liquid form contains alcohol.
May contain tartrazine.*   *Common* reactions are in italics; ***life-threatening,* in bold italics.

feasible, concentrations of 250 mg/5 ml are more palatable. Refrigeration improves palatability but doesn't improve stability. Suspensions are stable for 1 week.

• Monitor fluid intake and output and electrolytes, especially serum potassium, bicarbonate, and chloride. When used in diuretic therapy, consult the doctor and dietitian to provide high-potassium diet.

• Monitor elderly patients closely because they are especially susceptible to excessive diuresis.

• Weigh the patient daily. Rapid or excessive fluid loss causes weight loss and hypotension.

• Keep in mind that the diuretic effect decreases when acidosis occurs but can be reestablished by withdrawing drug, as ordered, for several days and then restarting, or by using intermittent administration schedules.

• Because bicarbonate ion excretion makes the patient's urine alkaline, be aware that the drug may cause false-positive urine protein tests.

amiloride hydrochloride
Kaluril‡, Midamor

Pregnancy Risk Category: B

HOW SUPPLIED
Tablets: 5 mg

ACTION
A potassium-sparing diuretic that inhibits sodium reabsorption and potassium excretion in the distal tubule.

ONSET, PEAK, DURATION
Onset occurs within 2 hours. Peak effects occur in 6 to 10 hours. Effects persist for 24 hours.

INDICATIONS & DOSAGE
Hypertension; edema associated with CHF, usually in patients also taking thiazide or other potassium-wasting diuretics –

Adults: usual dosage is 5 mg P.O. daily. Increased to 10 mg daily, if necessary. Maximum dosage is 20 mg daily.

ADVERSE REACTIONS
CNS: *headache,* weakness, dizziness.
CV: orthostatic hypotension.
GI: *nausea, anorexia, diarrhea, vomiting,* abdominal pain, constipation.
GU: impotence.
Other: hyperkalemia.

INTERACTIONS
ACE inhibitors, potassium-containing salt substitutes, potassium-sparing diuretics, potassium supplements: possible hyperkalemia. Avoid concomitant use.
Lithium: decreased lithium clearance, increasing risk of lithium toxicity. Monitor lithium level.
NSAIDs: decreased diuretic effectiveness. Avoid concomitant use.

CONTRAINDICATIONS
• Contraindicated in patients with elevated serum potassium level (greater than 5.5 mEq/L). Don't administer to patients receiving other potassium-sparing diuretics, such as spironolactone and triamterene.
• Also contraindicated in patients with anuria, acute or chronic renal insufficiency, diabetic nephropathy, and hypersensitivity to the drug.

NURSING CONSIDERATIONS
• Use with exreme caution, if at all, in patients with diabetes mellitus.
• Use cautiously in patients with severe, existing hepatic insufficiency and in elderly or debilitated patients.
• To prevent nausea, administer amiloride with meals.
• If amiloride is not taken concurrently with a potassium-wasting drug, monitor potassium level daily because of increased risk of hyperkalemia. Alert doctor immediately if potassium

---

level exceeds 6.5 mEq/L and expect drug to be discontinued.
• Advise the patient to avoid sudden posture changes and to rise slowly to avoid orthostatic hypotension.
• Warn the patient to avoid excessive ingestion of potassium-rich foods, potassium-containing salt substitutes, or potassium supplements to prevent serious hyperkalemia.

bendroflumethiazide (bendrofluazide)
Aprinox‡, Aprinox-M‡, Benzide‡, Naturetin

Pregnancy Risk Category: C

HOW SUPPLIED
Tablets: 5 mg, 10 mg

ACTION
A thiazide diuretic that increases sodium and water excretion by inhibiting sodium and chloride reabsorption in the nephron's distal segment.

ONSET, PEAK, DURATION
Onset occurs in 1 to 2 hours. Peak effects occur in 4 hours. Effects persist 6 to 12 hours.

INDICATIONS & DOSAGE
Edema, hypertension –
Adults: initially, 5 to 20 mg P.O. daily or divided b.i.d. Maintenance dosage is 2.5 to 15 mg P.O. daily.
Children: initially, 0.1 to 0.4 mg/kg (3 to 12 mg/m²) P.O. daily or divided b.i.d. Maintenance dosage is 0.05 to 0.1 mg/kg (1.5 to 3 mg/m²) P.O. daily or divided b.i.d.

ADVERSE REACTIONS
CV: volume depletion and dehydration, orthostatic hypotension.
GI: anorexia, nausea, diarrhea, pancreatitis.
GU: nocturia, polyuria, frequent urination.
Hematologic: *aplastic anemia,*

agranulocytosis, leukopenia, thrombocytopenia.
Hepatic: hepatic encephalopathy.
Skin: dermatitis, photosensitivity, rash, ecchymosis; purpura.
Other: impotence, hypokalemia; asymptomatic hyperuricemia; hyperglycemia and impairment of glucose tolerance; fluid and electrolyte imbalances, including dilutional hyponatremia and hypochloremia, metabolic alkalosis (in diabetics), hypercalcemia; gout; hypersensitivity reactions, such as pneumonitis and vasculitis.

INTERACTIONS
Cholestyramine, colestipol: decreased intestinal absorption of thiazides. Separate doses.
Diazoxide: increased antihypertensive, hyperglycemic, and hyperuricemic effects. Use together cautiously.
Digitalis glycosides: increased risk of digitalis toxicity from bendroflumethiazide-induced hypokalemia. Monitor potassium and digitalis levels.
Ethanol, barbiturates, opiates: increased orthostatic hypotensive effect. Monitor closely.
Lithium: decreased lithium clearance, increasing risk of lithium toxicity. Monitor lithium level.
NSAIDs: increased risk of NSAID-induced renal failure. Monitor closely.

CONTRAINDICATIONS
Contraindicated in patients with anuria or hypersensitivity to other thiazides or other sulfonamide-derived drugs.

NURSING CONSIDERATIONS
• Use cautiously in patients with severe renal disease and impaired hepatic function.
• To prevent nocturia, give in the morning.
• Monitor fluid intake and output, weight, serum electrolyte levels, serum creatinine, and BUN regularly.

---

*Liquid form contains alcohol.   *Common* reactions are in italics; **life-threatening,** in bold italics.
**May contain tartrazine.

Drug is not as effective if serum creatinine and BUN are more than twice normal.
• Watch for signs of hypokalemia, such as muscle weakness and cramps. Know that drug may be used with potassium-sparing diuretic to prevent potassium loss.
• Consult the doctor and dietitian to provide high-potassium diet. Foods rich in potassium include citrus fruits, bananas, tomatoes, dates, and apricots.
• Monitor blood glucose levels, and check insulin requirements in diabetic patients.
• Monitor blood uric acid levels, especially in patients with a history of gout.
• Monitor elderly patients, who are especially susceptible to excessive diuresis.
• As ordered, discontinue thiazides and thiazide-like diuretics before parathyroid function tests are performed.
• In hypertension, be aware that therapeutic response may be delayed several days.
• Be aware that drug may produce false-negative results in phentolamine, phenolsulfonphthalein, and tyramine tests.
• Advise the patient to avoid sudden posture changes and to rise slowly to avoid orthostatic hypotension.
• Advise the patient to use a sunblock to prevent photosensitivity reactions.

bumetanide
Bumex, Burinex‡

Pregnancy Risk Category: C

HOW SUPPLIED
Tablets: 0.5 mg, 1 mg, 2 mg
Injection: 0.25 mg/ml

ACTION
A potent loop diuretic that inhibits sodium and chloride reabsorption at the ascending portion of the loop of Henle.

ONSET, PEAK, DURATION
Onset occurs within minutes after I.V. administration, 40 minutes after I.M. injection, 30 to 60 minutes after oral use. Peak effects occur 15 to 30 minutes after I.V. administration, 1 to 2 hours after oral use. Effects persist for 4 to 6 hours after oral use, 3½ to 4 hours after I.V. administration.

INDICATIONS & DOSAGE
Edema in CHF, or hepatic or renal disease–
Adults: 0.5 to 2 mg P.O. once daily. If diuretic response is not adequate, a second or third dose may be given at 4- to 5-hour intervals. Maximum dosage is 10 mg/day. May be administered parenterally if P.O. not feasible. Usual initial dose is 0.5 to 1 mg given I.V. or I.M. If response is not adequate, a second or third dose may be given at 2- to 3-hour intervals. Maximum dosage is 10 mg/day.

ADVERSE REACTIONS
CNS: dizziness, headache.
CV: volume depletion and dehydration, orthostatic hypotension, ECG changes.
EENT: transient deafness.
GI: nausea.
GU: nocturia, polyuria, frequent urination, oliguria.
Hematologic: azotemia.
Skin: rash.
Other: hypokalemia; hypochloremic alkalosis; asymptomatic hyperuricemia; fluid and electrolyte imbalances, including dilutional hyponatremia, hypocalcemia, hypomagnesemia; hyperglycemia and glucose intolerance impairment; muscle pain and tenderness.

INTERACTIONS

Aminoglycoside antibiotics: potentiated ototoxicity. Use together cautiously.

Antihypertensives: increased risk of hypotension. Use together cautiously.

Digitalis glycosides: increased risk of digitalis toxicity from bumetanide-induced hypokalemia. Monitor potassium and digitalis levels.

Indomethacin, NSAIDs, probenicid: inhibited diuretic response. Use together cautiously.

Lithium: decreased lithium clearance, increasing risk of lithium toxicity. Monitor lithium level.

Metolazone: profound diuresis and potential electrolyte loss. Monitor the patient for fluid and electrolyte disorders.

Other potassium-wasting drugs: increased risk of hypokalemia. Use together cautiously.

CONTRAINDICATIONS

Contraindicated in patients with hypersensitivity to the drug or to sulfonamides (possible cross-sensitivity), in those with anuria or hepatic coma, and in patients in states of severe electrolyte depletion.

NURSING CONSIDERATIONS

• Use cautiously in patients with hepatic cirrhosis and ascites and in those with depressed renal function.

• **I.V. use:** Give I.V. doses directly using a 21G or 23G needle over 1 to 2 minutes. For intermittent infusion, give diluted drug through an intermittent infusion device or piggyback into an I.V. line containing a free-flowing, compatible solution. Infuse at ordered rate. Continuous infusion not recommended.

• To prevent nocturia, give in the morning. If second dose is necessary, give in early afternoon.

• Be aware that the safest and most effective dosage schedule for control of edema is intermittent dosage given on alternate days, or for 3 to 4 days with 1 or 2 days of rest periods.

• Monitor fluid intake and output, weight, and serum electrolyte, BUN, and carbon dioxide levels frequently.

• Watch for signs of hypokalemia, such as muscle weakness and cramps.

• Consult the doctor and dietitian to provide high-potassium diet. Foods rich in potassium include citrus fruits, tomatoes, bananas, dates, and apricots.

• Monitor blood glucose levels in diabetic patients.

• Monitor blood uric acid levels, especially in patients with a history of gout.

• Monitor blood pressure and pulse rate during rapid diuresis. Bumetanide can lead to profound water and electrolyte depletion.

• If oliguria or azotemia develops or increases, know that the doctor may stop drug.

• Keep in mind that bumetanide can be safely used in patients allergic to furosemide; 1 mg of bumetanide equals 40 mg of furosemide. May be less ototoxic than furosemide, but the clinical relevance of this has not been determined.

• Advise patients to stand up slowly to prevent dizziness, and to limit alcohol intake and strenuous exercise in hot weather to avoid exacerbating orthostatic hypotension.

---

chlorothiazide
Azide‡, Chlotride‡, Diuret‡, Diurigen, Diuril

chlorothiazide sodium
Sodium Diuril

Pregnancy Risk Category: C

HOW SUPPLIED
Tablets: 250 mg, 500 mg
Oral suspension: 250 mg/5 ml
Injection: 500-mg vial

ACTION
A thiazide diuretic that increases sodium and water excretion by inhibiting sodium reabsorption in the nephron's cortical diluting site.

ONSET, PEAK, DURATION
Onset occurs 2 hours after an oral dose, 15 minutes after I.V. use. Peak effects occur in about 4 hours after an oral dose, 30 minutes after I.V. use. Effects persist for 6 to 12 hours.

INDICATIONS & DOSAGE
Edema, hypertension –
Adults: 500 mg to 2 g P.O. or I.V. daily or in divided doses.
Diuresis, hypertension –
Children 2 to 12 years: 1 g P.O. daily or in divided doses.
Children 6 months to 2 years: 10 to 20 mg/kg P.O. daily or in two divided doses.
Children under 6 months: 10 to 30 mg/kg P.O. daily or in two divided doses.

ADVERSE REACTIONS
CV: volume depletion and dehydration, orthostatic hypotension.
GI: anorexia, nausea, pancreatitis.
GU: nocturia, polyuria, frequent urination.
Hematologic: *aplastic anemia, agranulocytosis,* leukopenia, thrombocytopenia.
Hepatic: hepatic encephalopathy.
Skin: dermatitis, photosensitivity, rash.
Other: impotence, hypersensitivity reactions, such as pneumonitis and vasculitis; hypokalemia; asymptomatic hyperuricemia; hyperglycemia and impairment of glucose tolerance; fluid and electrolyte imbalances, including dilutional hyponatremia and hypochloremia, metabolic alkalosis, hypercalcemia; gout.

INTERACTIONS
Cholestyramine, colestipol: decreased intestinal absorption of thiazides. Separate doses.
Diazoxide: increased antihypertensive, hyperglycemic, and hyperuricemic effects. Use together cautiously.
Digitalis glycosides: increased risk of digitalis toxicity from chlorothiazide-induced hypokalemia. Monitor potassium and digitalis levels.
Ethanol, barbiturates, opiates: increased orthostatic hypotensive effect. Monitor closely.
Lithium: decreased lithium clearance, increasing risk of lithium toxicity. Monitor lithium level.
NSAIDs: increased risk of NSAID-induced renal failure. Monitor the patient for renal failure.

CONTRAINDICATIONS
Contraindicated in patients with anuria or hypersensitivity to other thiazides or other sulfonamide-derived drugs.

NURSING CONSIDERATIONS
• Use cautiously in patients with severe renal disease and impaired hepatic function.
• To prevent nocturia, give in the morning.
• Don't give more than 250 mg P.O. at any one time. Bioavailability studies show that 250 mg P.O. every 6 hours is better absorbed than a single dose of 1 g.
• Administer oral form with food to enhance absorption.
• **I.V. use:** Reconstitute 500 mg with 18 ml of sterile water for injection. Inject reconstituted drug directly into vein, through an I.V. line containing a free-flowing, compatible solution, or through an intermittent infusion device. Store reconstituted solutions at room temperature up to 24 hours. Compatible with I.V. dextrose or sodium chloride solutions.

- Never inject I.M. or S.C.
- Avoid I.V. infiltration; can be very painful.
- Avoid simultaneous administration with whole blood and its derivatives.
- Monitor fluid intake and output, weight, blood pressure, and serum electrolyte levels.
- Watch for signs of hypokalemia, such as muscle weakness and cramps. Drug may be used with potassium-sparing diuretic to prevent potassium loss.
- Consult the doctor and dietitian to provide high-potassium diet. Foods rich in potassium include citrus fruits, tomatoes, bananas, dates, and apricots.
- Monitor blood glucose levels, and check insulin requirements in diabetic patients.
- Monitor serum creatinine and BUN regularly. Drug not as effective if these levels are more than twice normal.
- Monitor blood uric acid level, especially in patients with a history of gout.
- Monitor serum calcium and watch for progressive renal impairment.
- Monitor elderly patients, who are especially susceptible to excessive diuresis.
- As ordered, discontinue thiazides and thiazide-like diuretics before parathyroid function tests are performed.
- In patients with hypertension, be aware that therapeutic response may be delayed several days.
- Advise the patient to avoid sudden posture changes and to rise slowly to avoid orthostatic hypotension.
- Advise the patient to use a sunblock to prevent photosensitivity reactions.

chlorthalidone
Apo-Chlorthalidone†, Hygroton, Novo-Thalidone†, Thalitone, Uridon†

Pregnancy Risk Category: B

HOW SUPPLIED
Tablets: 15 mg, 25 mg, 50 mg, 100 mg

ACTION
Although not a thiazide, chlorthalidone acts similarly, increasing sodium and water excretion by inhibiting sodium and chloride reabsorption in the nephron's distal segment.

ONSET, PEAK, DURATION
Onset occurs in 2 to 3 hours. Peak effects occur in 2 to 6 hours. Effects persist for 2 to 3 days.

INDICATIONS & DOSAGE
Edema, hypertension –
Adults: initially, 25 to 100 mg P.O. daily, or up to 200 mg P.O. on alternate days.
Children: 2 mg/kg or 60 mg/m² P.O. 3 times weekly.

ADVERSE REACTIONS
CV: volume depletion and dehydration, orthostatic hypotension.
GI: anorexia, nausea, pancreatitis.
GU: impotence, nocturia, polyuria, frequent urination.
Hematologic: *aplastic anemia, agranulocytosis,* leukopenia, thrombocytopenia.
Hepatic: hepatic encephalopathy.
Skin: dermatitis, photosensitivity, rash.
Other: hypersensitivity reactions, such as pneumonitis and vasculitis; hypokalemia; asymptomatic hyperuricemia; hyperglycemia and impairment of glucose tolerance; fluid and electrolyte imbalances, including dilutional hyponatremia and hypochlo-

---

*Liquid form contains alcohol.
**May contain tartrazine.

Common reactions are in italics; *life-threatening,* in bold italics.

remia, metabolic alkalosis, hypercalcemia; gout.

INTERACTIONS
Cholestyramine, colestipol: decreased intestinal absorption of thiazides. Separate doses.
Diazoxide: increased antihypertensive, hyperglycemic, and hyperuricemic effects. Use together cautiously.
Digitalis glycosides: increased risk of digitalis toxicity from chlorthalidone-induced hypokalemia. Monitor potassium and digitalis levels.
Ethanol, barbiturates, opiates: increased orthostatic hypotensive effect. Monitor closely.
Lithium: decreased lithium clearance, increasing risk of lithium toxicity. Monitor lithium level.
NSAIDs: increased risk of NSAID-induced renal failure. Monitor closely.

CONTRAINDICATIONS
Contraindicated in patients with anuria or hypersensitivity to thiazides or other sulfonamide-derived drugs.

NURSING CONSIDERATIONS
• Use cautiously in patients with severe renal disease and impaired hepatic function.
• To prevent nocturia, give in the morning.
• Monitor fluid intake and output, weight, blood pressure, and serum electrolyte levels.
• Watch for signs of hypokalemia, such as muscle weakness, and cramps. Know that drug may be used with potassium-sparing diuretic to prevent potassium loss.
• Consult the doctor and dietitian to provide high-potassium diet. Foods rich in potassium include citrus fruits, tomatoes, bananas, dates, and apricots.
• Monitor serum creatinine and BUN levels regularly. Drug is not as effective if these levels are more than twice normal.
• Monitor blood uric acid levels, especially in patients with a history of gout.
• Monitor blood glucose levels, and check insulin requirements in diabetic patients.
• Monitor elderly patients, who are especially susceptible to excessive diuresis.
• As ordered, discontinue thiazides and thiazide-like diuretics before parathyroid function tests are performed.
• In patients with hypertension, be aware that therapeutic response may be delayed several days.
• Do not confuse Uridon tablets (available in Canada only) with the urinary anti-infective Uridon Modified (available in the United States).
• Advise the patient to avoid sudden posture changes and to rise slowly to avoid orthostatic hypotension.
• Advise the patient to use a sunblock to prevent photosensitivity reactions.

---

dichlorphenamide
Daranide

Pregnancy Risk Category: C

HOW SUPPLIED
Tablets: 50 mg

ACTION
Not clearly understood. A carbonic anhydrase inhibitor that appears to decrease secretion of aqueous humor, lowering intraocular pressure.

ONSET, PEAK, DURATION
Onset occurs in ½ to 1 hour. Peak effects occur in 2 to 4 hours. Effects persist for 6 to 12 hours.

INDICATIONS & DOSAGE
Adjunct in glaucoma –
Adults: initially, 100 to 200 mg P.O., followed by 100 mg q 12 hours until

desired response obtained. Maintenance dosage is 25 to 50 mg P.O. daily, b.i.d., or t.i.d., given concomitantly with miotics.

ADVERSE REACTIONS
CNS: drowsiness, paresthesia.
EENT: transient myopia.
GI: nausea, vomiting, anorexia, altered taste.
GU: crystalluria, renal calculi.
Hematologic: *aplastic anemia, hemolytic anemia,* leukopenia.
Skin: rash.
Other: hyperchloremic acidosis, hypokalemia, asymptomatic hyperuricemia.

INTERACTIONS
Amphetamines, anticholinergics, mecamylamine, quinidine: decreased renal clearance of these agents, increasing toxicity. Avoid concomitant use.
Methenamine: reduced effectiveness of dichlorphenamide. Avoid concomitant use.
Salicylates: possible accumulation and toxicity of dichlorphenamide. Monitor closely.

CONTRAINDICATIONS
Contraindicated in patients with hypersensitivity to the drug and in those with hepatic insufficiency, renal failure, adrenocortical insufficiency, hyperchloremic acidosis, depressed sodium or potassium level, and severe pulmonary obstruction with inability to increase alveolar ventilation.

NURSING CONSIDERATIONS
• Use cautiously in patients with respiratory acidosis.
• Monitor electrolyte levels, especially serum potassium, in initial treatment; know that potassium supplements may be necessary.
• In patients with respiratory acidosis, monitor blood pH and blood gases.

• Be aware that drug may cause false-positive results in urine protein tests.
• Evaluate patients for eye pain to determine if drug is effective.

---

ethacrynate sodium
Sodium Edecrin

ethacrynic acid
Edecril‡, Edecrin

Pregnancy Risk Category: B

HOW SUPPLIED
Tablets: 25 mg, 50 mg
Injection: 50 mg (with 62.5 mg of mannitol and 0.1 mg of thimerosal)

ACTION
A potent loop diuretic that inhibits sodium and chloride reabsorption at the proximal and distal tubules and the ascending loop of Henle.

ONSET, PEAK, DURATION
Onset occurs in 5 minutes after I.V. use, 30 minutes after oral use. Peak effects occur 15 to 30 minutes after I.V. use, 2 hours after oral use. Effects persist for 2 hours after I.V use, 6 to 8 hours after oral use.

INDICATIONS & DOSAGE
Acute pulmonary edema –
Adults: 50 mg or 0.5 to 1 mg/kg I.V. Usually only one dose is necessary; occasionally a second dose may be required.
Edema –
Adults: 50 to 200 mg P.O. daily. Refractory cases may require up to 200 mg b.i.d.
Children: initial dose is 25 mg P.O., increased cautiously in 25-mg increments daily until desired effect is achieved.

ADVERSE REACTIONS
CV: volume depletion and dehydration, orthostatic hypotension.

---

*Liquid form contains alcohol.   *Common* reactions are in italics; *life-threatening,* in bold italics.
**May contain tartrazine.

EENT: transient deafness with too-rapid I.V. injection.
GI: abdominal discomfort and pain, diarrhea.
GU: nocturia, polyuria, frequent urination, oliguria.
Hematologic: *agranulocytosis,* neutropenia, thrombocytopenia, azotemia.
Skin: dermatitis.
Other: hypokalemia; hypochloremic alkalosis; asymptomatic hyperuricemia; fluid and electrolyte imbalances, including dilutional hyponatremia, hypocalcemia, hypomagnesemia; hyperglycemia and impairment of glucose tolerance.

INTERACTIONS
Aminoglycoside antibiotics: potentiated ototoxic adverse reactions of both drugs. Use together cautiously.
Antihypertensives: increased risk of hypotension. Use together cautiously.
Cisplatin: increased risk of ototoxicity. Avoid concomitant use.
Digitalis glycosides: increased risk of digitalis toxicity from ethacrynate-induced hypokalemia. Monitor potassium and digitalis levels.
Lithium: decreased lithium clearance, increasing risk of lithium toxicity. Monitor lithium level.
Metolazone: profound diuresis and enhanced electrolyte loss. Use together cautiously.
NSAIDs: decreased diuretic effectiveness. Use together cautiously.
Warfarin: potentiated anticoagulant effect. Use together cautiously.

CONTRAINDICATIONS
Contraindicated in patients with hypersensitivity to the drug, in those with anuria, and in infants.

NURSING CONSIDERATIONS
• Use cautiously in patients with electrolyte abnormalities or hepatic impairment.

• Give with food or milk. Oral use may cause GI upset.
• To prevent nocturia, give oral doses in the morning.
• **I.V. use:** Reconstitute vacuum vial with 50 ml of D_5W or 0.9% sodium chloride solution. Give slowly through tubing of running infusion over several minutes. Discard unused solution after 24 hours. Don't use cloudy or opalescent solutions.
• If more than one I.V. dose is necessary, use a new injection site to avoid thrombophlebitis.
• Don't mix with whole blood or its derivatives.
• Don't give S.C. or I.M. because of local pain and irritation.
• Monitor fluid intake and output, weight, blood pressure, and serum electrolyte levels.
• Watch for signs of hypokalemia, such as muscle weakness and cramps.
• Consult the doctor and dietitian to provide high-potassium diet. Foods rich in potassium include citrus fruits, tomatoes, bananas, dates, and apricots. Know that potassium chloride and sodium supplements may be needed.
• Monitor elderly patients, who are especially susceptible to excessive diuresis.
• Monitor blood uric acid levels, especially in patients with a history of gout.
• Be aware that severe diarrhea may necessitate discontinuing drug.
• Advise patients to avoid sudden posture changes and to rise slowly to avoid orthostatic hypotension.
• Advise diabetic patients to closely monitor blood glucose levels.

furosemide (frusemide†‡)

Apo-Furosemide†, Furoside†,
Lasix*, Lasix Special†,
Myrosemide*, Novosemide†,
Urex‡, Urex-M‡, Uritol†

Pregnancy Risk Category: C

HOW SUPPLIED

Tablets: 20 mg, 40 mg, 80 mg, 500
mg†‡
Oral solution: 8 mg/ml, 10 mg/ml, 40
mg/5 ml
Injection: 10 mg/ml

ACTION

A potent loop diuretic that inhibits sodium and chloride reabsorption at the
proximal and distal tubules and the
ascending loop of Henle.

ONSET, PEAK, DURATION

Onset occurs about 5 minutes after
I.V. administration, about 20 to 60
minutes after oral administration.
Peak effects occur within 30 minutes
of I.V. administration, within 1 to 2
hours of oral administration. Effects
persist about 2 hours after I.V. administration, 6 to 8 hours after oral administration.

INDICATIONS & DOSAGE

Acute pulmonary edema –
Adults: 40 mg I.V. injected slowly
over 1 to 2 minutes; then 80 mg I.V. in
1 to 1½ hours if needed.
Edema –
Adults: 20 to 80 mg P.O. daily in
a.m., second dose in 6 to 8 hours;
carefully titrated up to 600 mg daily if
needed. Or, 20 to 40 mg I.M. or I.V.,
increased by 20 mg q 2 hours until desired response is achieved. Give I.V.
dose slowly over 1 to 2 minutes.
Infants and children: 2 mg/kg P.O.
daily, increased by 1 to 2 mg/kg in 6
to 8 hours if needed; carefully titrated
up to 6 mg/kg daily if needed.
Hypertension –

Adults: 40 mg P.O. b.i.d. Dosage adjusted according to response.

ADVERSE REACTIONS

CV: volume depletion and dehydration, orthostatic hypotension.
EENT: transient deafness with too
rapid I.V. injection.
GI: abdominal discomfort and pain,
diarrhea (with oral solution).
GU: nocturia, polyuria, frequent urination, oliguria.
Hematologic: *agranulocytosis,* leukopenia, thrombocytopenia, azotemia.
Skin: dermatitis.
Other: hypokalemia; hypochloremic
alkalosis; asymptomatic hyperuricemia; fluid and electrolyte imbalances,
including dilutional hyponatremia,
hypocalcemia, hypomagnesemia; hyperglycemia and impairment of glucose tolerance; transient pain at injection site with I.M. administration;
thrombophlebitis with I.V. administration.

INTERACTIONS

Aminoglycoside antibiotics, cisplatin:
potentiated ototoxicity. Use together
cautiously.
Antidiabetic agents: decreased hypoglycemic effects. Monitor blood glucose levels.
Antihypertensives: increased risk of
hypotension. Use together cautiously.
*Corticosteroids, corticotropin, am-
photericin B, metolazone:* increased
risk of hypokalemia. Monitor potassium levels closely.
*Digitalis glycosides, neuromuscular
blocking agents:* increased toxicity of
these agents from furosemide-induced
hypokalemia. Monitor potassium levels closely.
Lithium: decreased lithium excretion,
resulting in lithium toxicity. Monitor
lithium level.
NSAIDs: inhibited diuretic response.
Use together cautiously.

---

*Liquid form contains alcohol.
**May contain tartrazine.

Common reactions are in italics; *life-threatening,* in bold italics.

CONTRAINDICATIONS

Contraindicated in patients with anuria or in patients with a history of hypersensitivity to the drug.

NURSING CONSIDERATIONS

• Use cautiously in patients with hepatic cirrhosis. Know that furosemide should be used in pregnancy only if potential benefits clearly outweigh possible risk to fetus.

• To prevent nocturia, give P.O. and I.M. preparations in the morning. Give second doses in early afternoon.

• **I.V. use:** Given by direct injection over 1 to 2 minutes. Alternatively, dilute with D_5W, 0.9% sodium chloride solution, or lactated Ringer's solution and infuse no faster than 4 mg/minute to avoid ototoxicity. Use prepared infusion solution within 24 hours.

• Monitor weight, blood pressure, and pulse rate routinely with chronic use and during rapid diuresis. Furosemide can lead to profound water and electrolyte depletion.

• Be aware that if oliguria or azotemia develops or increases, it may require stopping drug.

• Monitor fluid intake and output, serum electrolytes, BUN, and carbon dioxide frequently.

• Watch for signs of hypokalemia, such as muscle weakness and cramps.

• Consult the doctor and dietitian to provide high-potassium diet. Foods rich in potassium include citrus fruits, tomatoes, bananas, dates, and apricots.

• Monitor blood glucose levels in diabetic patients.

• Monitor blood uric acid, especially in patients with a history of gout.

• Monitor elderly patients, who are especially susceptible to excessive diuresis, with potential for circulatory collapse and thromboembolic complications.

• Store tablets in light-resistant container to prevent discoloration (doesn't affect potency). Don't use discolored (yellow) injectable preparation. Refrigerate oral furosemide solution to ensure drug stability.

• Advise patients to take the drug with food to prevent GI upset.

• Advise patients to stand slowly to prevent dizziness, and to limit alcohol intake and strenuous exercise in hot weather to avoid exacerbating orthostatic hypotension.

• Advise patients to immediately report ringing in ears, severe abdominal pain, or sore throat and fever; may indicate furosemide toxicity.

• Discourage patients taking furosemide at home from storing different types of medication in the same container, increasing the risk of drug errors. The most popular strengths of furosemide and digoxin are white tablets approximately equal in size.

• Tell patients to check with the doctor or pharmacist before taking any OTC medications.

---

hydrochlorothiazide

Apo-Hydro†, Dichlotride‡, Diuchlor H†, Esidrix, Ezide, Hydro-D, Hydro-Par, HydroDIURIL, Neo-Codema†, Novo-Hydrazide†, Oretic, Urozide†

Pregnancy Risk Category: D

HOW SUPPLIED

Tablets: 25 mg, 50 mg, 100 mg
Oral solution: 10 mg/ml, 50 mg/5 ml, 100 mg/ml

ACTION

A thiazide diuretic that increases sodium and water excretion by inhibiting sodium and chloride reabsorption in the nephron's distal segment.

ONSET, PEAK, DURATION

Onset occurs in 2 hours. Peak effects occur within 4 to 6 hours. Effects persist for 6 to 12 hours.

INDICATIONS & DOSAGE
Edema –
Adults: 25 to 100 mg P.O. daily or intermittently.
Children 2 to 12 years: 37.5 to 100 mg P.O. daily in two divided doses.
Children 6 months to 2 years: 12.5 to 37.5 mg P.O. daily in two divided doses.
Infants under 6 months: up to 3.3 mg/kg P.O. daily in two divided doses. Total daily dosage may range from 12.5 to 37.5 mg.
Hypertension –
Adults: 25 to 50 mg P.O. daily as a single dose or divided b.i.d. Daily dosage increased or decreased according to blood pressure.

Doses greater than 50 mg/day are not required when combined with other antihypertensives.

ADVERSE REACTIONS
CV: volume depletion and dehydration, orthostatic hypotension.
GI: anorexia, nausea, pancreatitis.
GU: nocturia, polyuria, frequent urination.
Hematologic: *aplastic anemia, agranulocytosis,* leukopenia, thrombocytopenia.
Hepatic: hepatic encephalopathy.
Skin: dermatitis, photosensitivity, rash.
Other: hypersensitivity reactions, such as pneumonitis and vasculitis; hypokalemia; asymptomatic hyperuricemia; hyperglycemia and impairment of glucose tolerance; fluid and electrolyte imbalances, including dilutional hyponatremia and hypochloremia, metabolic alkalosis, hypercalcemia; gout.

INTERACTIONS
Antidiabetic agents: decreased effectiveness of hypoglycemic agents; dosage adjustments may be necessary. Monitor blood glucose levels.
Antihypertensive agents: additive antihypertensive effect. Use together cautiously.
Cholestyramine, colestipol: decreased intestinal absorption of thiazides. Separate doses.
Diazoxide: increased antihypertensive, hyperglycemic, and hyperuricemic effects. Use together cautiously.
Digitalis glycosides: increased risk of digitalis toxicity from hydrochlorothiazide-induced hypokalemia. Monitor potassium and digitalis levels.
Ethanol, barbiturates, opiates: increased orthostatic hypotensive effect. Monitor closely.
Lithium: decreased lithium excretion, increasing risk of lithium toxicity. Monitor lithium level.
NSAIDs: increased risk of NSAID-induced renal failure. Monitor closely.

CONTRAINDICATIONS
Contraindicated in patients with anuria or hypersensitivity to other thiazides or other sulfonamide derivatives.

NURSING CONSIDERATIONS
● Use cautiously in patients with severe renal disease, impaired hepatic function, and progressive hepatic disease.
● To prevent nocturia, give in the morning.
● Monitor fluid intake and output, weight, blood pressure, and serum electrolyte levels.
● Watch for signs of hypokalemia, such as muscle weakness and cramps. Drug may be used with potassium-sparing diuretic to prevent potassium loss.
● Consult the doctor and dietitian to provide high-potassium diet. Foods rich in potassium include citrus fruits, tomatoes, bananas, dates, and apricots.
● Monitor serum creatinine and BUN levels regularly. Drug is not as effec-

---

Liquid form contains alcohol.   Common reactions are in italics; ***life-threatening,*** in bold italics.
**May contain tartrazine.

tive if these levels are more than twice normal.
• Monitor blood uric acid levels, especially in patients with a history of gout.
• Check insulin requirements in diabetic patients.
• Monitor elderly patients, who are especially susceptible to excessive diuresis.
• As ordered, discontinue thiazides and thiazide-like diuretics before parathyroid function tests are performed.
• In patients with hypertension, know that therapeutic response may be delayed several days.
• Advise the patient to take the drug with food to minimize GI upset.
• Advise the patient to avoid sudden posture changes and to rise slowly to avoid orthostatic hypotension.
• Advise the patient to use a sunblock to prevent photosensitivity reactions.
• Tell the patient to check with the doctor or pharmacist before taking any OTC medications.

hydroflumethiazide
Diucardin, Saluron

Pregnancy Risk Category: C

HOW SUPPLIED
Tablets: 50 mg

ACTION
A thiazide diuretic that increases sodium and water excretion by inhibiting sodium and chloride reabsorption in the nephron's distal segment.

ONSET, PEAK, DURATION
Onset occurs in 1 to 2 hours. Peak effects occur in 3 to 4 hours. Effects persist for 18 to 24 hours.

INDICATIONS & DOSAGE
Edmea –
Adults: 25 to 200 mg P.O. daily.

Hypertension –
Adults: 50 to 100 mg P.O. daily.

ADVERSE REACTIONS
CV: volume depletion and dehydration, orthostatic hypotension.
GI: anorexia, nausea, pancreatitis.
GU: nocturia, polyuria, frequent urination.
Hematologic: *aplastic anemia, agranulocytosis,* leukopenia, thrombocytopenia.
Hepatic: hepatic encephalopathy.
Skin: dermatitis, photosensitivity, rash.
Other: hypersensitivity reactions, such as pneumonitis and vasculitis; hypokalemia; asymptomatic hyperuricemia; hyperglycemia and impairment of glucose tolerance; fluid and electrolyte imbalances, including dilutional hyponatremia and hypochloremia, metabolic alkalosis, hypercalcemia; gout.

INTERACTIONS
Antihypertensive agents: additive antihypetensive effect. Use together cautiously.
Cholestyramine, colestipol: decreased intestinal absorption of thiazides. Separate doses.
Diazoxide: increased antihypertensive, hyperglycemic, and hyperuricemic effects. Use together cautiously.
Digitalis glycosides: increased risk of digitalis toxicity from hydroflumethiazide-induced hypokalemia. Monitor potassium and digitalis levels.
Ethanol, barbiturates, opiates: increased orthostatic hypotensive effect. Monitor closely.
Lithium: decreased lithium clearance, increasing risk of lithium toxicity. Monitor lithium level.
NSAIDs: increased risk of NSAID-induced renal failure. Monitor the patient for signs of renal failure.

---

†Available in Canada only.   ‡Available in Australia only.   ◇Available OTC.

CONTRAINDICATIONS
Contraindicated in patients with anuria or hypersensitivity to thiazides or other sulfonamide-derived drugs.

NURSING CONSIDERATIONS
• Use cautiously in patients with severe renal disease, impaired hepatic function, and progressive hepatic disease.
• To minimize GI upset, give drug with food or milk.
• To prevent nocturia, give in the morning.
• Monitor fluid intake and output, weight, blood pressure, and serum electrolyte levels.
• Watch for signs of hypokalemia, such as muscle weakness and cramps. Know that drug may be used with potassium-sparing diuretic to prevent potassium loss.
• Consult the doctor and dietitian to provide high-potassium diet. Foods rich in potassium include citrus fruits, tomatoes, bananas, dates, and apricots.
• Monitor serum creatinine and BUN levels regularly. Drug is not as effective if these levels are more than twice normal.
• Monitor blood uric acid levels, especially in patients with a history of gout.
• Check insulin requirements in diabetic patients.
• Monitor elderly patients, who are especially susceptible to excessive diuresis.
• As ordered, discontinue thiazides and thiazide-like diuretics before parathyroid function tests are performed.
• In patients with hypertension, be aware that therapeutic response may be delayed several days.
• Advise the patient to avoid sudden posture changes and to rise slowly to avoid orthostatic hypotension.
• Advise the patient to use a sunblock to prevent photosensitivity reactions.

indapamide
Lozide†, Lozol, Natrilix‡

Pregnancy Risk Category: B

HOW SUPPLIED
Tablets: 1.25 mg, 2.5 mg

ACTION
Unknown. A thiazide-like diuretic that probably inhibits sodium reabsorption in the nephron's distal segment. Also has a direct vasodilating effect that may be a result of calcium channel-blocking action.

ONSET, PEAK, DURATION
Onset occurs in 1 to 2 hours. Peak effects occur within 2 hours. Effects persist for up to 36 hours.

INDICATIONS & DOSAGE
Edema –
Adults: initially, 2.5 mg P.O. daily in a.m. Increased to 5 mg daily after 1 week, if needed.
Hypertension –
Adults: initially, 1.25 mg P.O. daily in a.m. Increased to 2.5 mg daily after 4 weeks, if needed. Increased to 5 mg daily after 4 more weeks, if needed.

ADVERSE REACTIONS
CNS: headache, irritability, nervousness, dizziness, light-headedness, weakness.
CV: volume depletion and dehydration, orthostatic hypotension.
GI: anorexia, nausea, pancreatitis.
GU: nocturia, polyuria, frequent urination.
Skin: dermatitis, photosensitivity, rash.
Other: muscle cramps and spasms; hypokalemia; asymptomatic hyperuricemia; fluid and electrolyte imbalances, including dilutional hyponatremia and hypochloremia, metabolic alkalosis; gout.

---

*Liquid form contains alcohol.   *Common* reactions are in italics; *life-threatening,* in bold italics.
**May contain tartrazine.

INTERACTIONS
Diazoxide: increased antihypertensive, hyperglycemic, and hyperuricemic effects. Use together cautiously.
Digitalis glycosides: increased risk of digitalis toxicity from indapamide-induced hypokalemia. Monitor potassium and digitalis levels.
NSAIDs: increased risk of NSAID-induced renal failure. Monitor the patient for signs of renal failure.

CONTRAINDICATIONS
Contraindicated in patients with anuria or hypersensitivity to other sulfonamide-derived drugs.

NURSING CONSIDERATIONS
• Use cautiously in patients with severe renal disease, impaired hepatic function, and progressive hepatic disease.
• To prevent nocturia, give in the morning.
• Monitor fluid intake and output, weight, blood pressure, and serum electrolyte levels.
• Watch for signs of hypokalemia, such as muscle weakness and cramps. Know that drug may be used with potassium-sparing diuretic to prevent potassium loss.
• Consult the doctor and dietitian to provide high-potassium diet. Foods rich in potassium include citrus fruits, tomatoes, bananas, dates, and apricots.
• Monitor serum creatinine and BUN levels regularly. Drug is not as effective if these levels are more than twice normal.
• Monitor blood uric acid levels, especially in patients with a history of gout.
• Check insulin requirements in diabetic patients.
• Monitor elderly patients, who are especially susceptible to excessive diuresis.
• As ordered, discontinue thiazides and thiazide-like diuretics before parathyroid function tests are performed.
• In patients with hypertension, be aware that therapeutic response may be delayed several days.
• Advise the patient to avoid sudden posture changes and to rise slowly to avoid orthostatic hypotension.
• Advise the patient to use a sunblock to prevent photosensitivity reactions.

mannitol
Osmitrol

Pregnancy Risk Category: C

HOW SUPPLIED
Injection: 5%, 10%, 15%, 20%, 25%

ACTION
An osmotic diuretic that increases the osmotic pressure of glomerular filtrate, inhibiting tubular reabsorption of water and electrolytes, and that elevates blood plasma osmolality, resulting in enhanced water flow into extracellular fluid.

ONSET, PEAK, DURATION
Onset occurs in 30 to 60 minutes. Peak effects occur within 1 hour. Effects persist for 6 to 8 hours.

INDICATIONS & DOSAGE
Test dose for marked oliguria or suspected inadequate renal function –
Adults and children over 12 years: 200 mg/kg or 12.5 g as a 15% or 20% I.V. solution over 3 to 5 minutes. Response is adequate if 30 to 50 ml urine/hour is excreted over 2 to 3 hours; if response is inadequate, a second test dose is given. If still no response after the second dose, mannitol should not be continued.
Oliguria –
Adults and children over 12 years: 100 g I.V. as a 15% to 20% solution over 90 minutes to several hours.

Prevention of oliguria or acute renal failure –

Adults and children over 12 years: 50 to 100 g I.V. of a concentrated solution followed by a 5% to 10% solution. Exact concentration determined by fluid requirements.

Edema; ascites caused by renal, hepatic, or cardiac failure –

Adults and children over 12 years: 100 g I.V. as a 10% to 20% solution over 2 to 6 hours.

Reduction of intraocular or intracranial pressure –

Adults and children over 12 years: 1.5 to 2 g/kg as a 15% to 25% I.V. solution over 30 to 60 minutes.

Diuresis in drug intoxication –

Adults and children over 12 years: 5% to 10% solution continuously up to 200 g I.V., while maintaining 100 to 500 ml urine output/hour and a positive fluid balance.

Irrigating solution during transurethral resection of the prostate –

Adults: 2.5% to 5% solution as needed.

ADVERSE REACTIONS

CNS: rebound increase in intracranial pressure 8 to 12 hours after diuresis; headache, confusion.

CV: transient expansion of plasma volume during infusion causing circulatory overload and ***pulmonary edema,*** tachycardia, angina-like chest pain.

EENT: blurred vision, rhinitis.

GI: thirst, nausea, vomiting, *diarrhea*.

GU: urine retention.

Other: fluid and electrolyte imbalance, water intoxication, cellular dehydration.

INTERACTIONS

Lithium: increased urinary excretion of lithium. Monitor closely.

CONTRAINDICATIONS

Contraindicated in patients with hypersensitivity to the drug and in those with anuria, severe pulmonary congestion, frank pulmonary edema, severe CHF, severe dehydration, metabolic edema, progressive renal disease or dysfunction, or active intracranial bleeding except during craniotomy.

NURSING CONSIDERATIONS

● To redissolve crystallized solution (occurs at low temperatures or in concentrations greater than 15%), warm bottle in hot water bath and shake vigorously. Cool to body temperature before giving. Do not use solution with undissolved crystals.

● **I.V. use:** Administer as intermittent or continuous infusion at prescribed rate, using an in-line filter and an infusion pump. Direct injection is not recommended. Check I.V. line patency at infusion site before and during administration.

● Avoid infiltration; if it occurs, observe for inflammation, edema, and necrosis.

● For maximum intraocular pressure reduction before surgery, give 1 to 1½ hours preoperatively, as ordered.

● Monitor vital signs, including central venous pressure, and fluid intake and output hourly. Report increasing oliguria. Monitor weight, renal function, fluid balance, and serum and urine sodium and potassium levels daily.

● Insert urethral catheter in comatose or incontinent patients because therapy is based on strict evaluation of fluid intake and output. In patients with urethral catheters, use an hourly urometer collection bag to facilitate accurate evaluation of output.

● Be aware that drug can be used to measure glomerular filtration rate.

● To relieve thirst, give frequent mouth care or fluids as permitted.

● When used as an irrigating solution

---

*Liquid form contains alcohol.
**May contain tartrazine.

Common reactions are in italics; *life-threatening,* in bold italics.

for prostate surgery, keep in mind that concentrations of 3.5% or greater are needed to avoid hemolysis.

methazolamide
Neptazane

Pregnancy Risk Category: C

HOW SUPPLIED
Tablets: 25 mg, 50 mg

ACTION
A carbonic anhydrase inhibitor that decreases secretion of aqueous humor, lowering intraocular pressure.

ONSET, PEAK, DURATION
Onset occurs in 2 to 4 hours. Peak effects occur in 6 to 8 hours. Effects persist for 10 to 18 hours.

INDICATIONS & DOSAGE
Glaucoma (chronic open-angle or secondary, or preoperatively in obstructive or acute angle-closure) –
Adults: 50 to 100 mg P.O. b.i.d. or t.i.d.

ADVERSE REACTIONS
CNS: drowsiness, paresthesia.
EENT: transient myopia.
GI: nausea, vomiting, anorexia.
GU: crystalluria, renal calculi.
Hematologic: *aplastic anemia, hemolytic anemia,* leukopenia.
Skin: rash.
Other: hyperchloremic acidosis, hypokalemia, asymptomatic hyperuricemia.

INTERACTIONS
Amphetamines, anticholinergics, mecamylamine, quinidine: decreased renal clearance of these agents, increasing the risk of toxicity. Avoid concomitant use.
Methenamine compounds: reduced methenamine effectiveness. Avoid concomitant use.
Salicylates: accumulation and toxicity

of methazolamide may occur. Monitor closely.

CONTRAINDICATIONS
Contraindicated for long-term use in acute angle-closure glaucoma and in patients with depressed serum sodium or potassium levels, renal or hepatic disease or dysfunction, adrenal gland dysfunction, or hyperchloremic acidosis.

NURSING CONSIDERATIONS
• Use cautiously in patients with emphysema and pulmonary obstruction.
• Monitor fluid intake and output, weight, and serum electrolyte levels.
• Monitor elderly patients, who are especially susceptible to excessive diuresis.
• Know that this drug may cause false-positive urine protein tests by alkalinizing urine.
• Evaluate the patient for eye pain to ensure drug is effective in decreasing intraocular pressure.
• Caution the patient to comply with prescribed dosage to lessen risk of metabolic acidosis. Effects may decrease in acidosis.

methyclothiazide
Aquatensen, Duretic†, Enduron, Enduron M‡

Pregnancy Risk Category: B

HOW SUPPLIED
Tablets: 2.5 mg, 5 mg

ACTION
A thiazide diuretic that increases sodium and water excretion by inhibiting sodium and chloride reabsorption in the nephron's distal segment.

ONSET, PEAK, DURATION
Onset occurs in 2 hours. Peak effects occur in 6 hours. Effects persist for 24 or more hours.

INDICATIONS & DOSAGE
Edema –
Adults: 2.5 to 10 mg P.O daily.
Hypertension –
Adults: 2.5 to 5 mg P.O daily.

ADVERSE REACTIONS
CV: volume depletion and dehydration, orthostatic hypotension.
GI: anorexia, nausea, pancreatitis.
GU: nocturia, polyuria, frequent urination.
Hematologic: *aplastic anemia, agranulocytosis,* leukopenia, thrombocytopenia.
Hepatic: hepatic encephalopathy.
Skin: dermatitis, photosensitivity, rash.
Other: asymptomatic hyperuricemia; gout; hyperglycemia and glucose tolerance impairment; fluid and electrolyte imbalances, including hypokalemia, dilutional hyponatremia and hypochloremia, metabolic alkalosis, hypercalcemia; hypersensitivity reactions, such as pneumonitis and vasculitis.

INTERACTIONS
Cholestyramine, colestipol: decreased intestinal absorption of thiazides. Separate doses.
Diazoxide: increased antihypertensive, hyperglycemic, and hyperuricemic effects. Use together cautiously.
Digitalis glycosides: increased risk of digitalis toxicity from methyclothiazide-induced hypokalemia. Monitor potassium and digitalis levels.
Ethanol, barbiturates, opiates: increased orthostatic hypotensive effect. Monitor closely.
Lithium: decreased lithium clearance, increasing risk of lithium toxicity. Monitor lithium levels.
NSAIDs: increased risk of NSAID-induced renal failure. Monitor closely.

CONTRAINDICATIONS
Contraindicated in patients with anuria or hypersensitivity to thiazides or other sulfonamide-derived drugs.

NURSING CONSIDERATIONS
• Use cautiously in patients with renal disease or dysfunction, impaired hepatic function, and progressive hepatic disease.
• To prevent nocturia, give in the morning.
• Monitor fluid intake and output, weight, blood pressure, and serum electrolyte levels.
• Watch for signs of hypokalemia, such as muscle weakness and cramps. Know that drug may also be used with potassium-sparing diuretic to prevent potassium loss.
• Consult the doctor and dietitian to provide high-potassium diet. Foods rich in potassium include citrus fruits, tomatoes, bananas, dates, and apricots.
• Monitor blood glucose levels.
• Monitor serum creatinine and BUN levels regularly. Drug is not as effective if these levels are more than twice normal.
• Monitor blood uric acid levels, especially in patients with a history of gout.
• As ordered, discontinue thiazides and thiazide-like diuretics before parathyroid function tests are performed.
• Monitor elderly patients, who are especially susceptible to excessive diuresis.
• In patients with hypertension, know that the therapeutic response may be delayed several days.
• Advise the patient to avoid sudden posture changes and to rise slowly to avoid orthostatic hypotension.
• Advise the patient to use a sunblock to prevent photosensitivity reactions.

---

*Liquid form contains alcohol.   *Common* reactions are in italics; *life-threatening,* in bold italics.
**May contain tartrazine.

metolazone

Diulo, Mykrox, Zaroxolyn**

Pregnancy Risk Category: B

HOW SUPPLIED
Tablets (extended): 2.5 mg, 5 mg, 10 mg
Tablets (prompt): 0.5 mg

ACTION
Increases sodium and water excretion by inhibiting sodium reabsorption in the cortical diluting site of the ascending loop of Henle.

ONSET, PEAK, DURATION
Onset occurs in 1 hour. Peak effects occur in about 2 to 4 hours after prompt-release tablets, 8 hours after extended-release tablets. Effects persist for 12 to 24 hours.

INDICATIONS & DOSAGE
Edema in CHF or renal disease –
Adults: 5 to 20 mg (prompt) P.O. daily.
Hypertension –
Adults: 2.5 to 5 mg (prompt) P.O. daily. Maintenance dosage determined by patient's blood pressure. Or 0.5 mg (extended) P.O. once daily in a.m., increased to 1 mg P.O. daily as needed. If response is inadequate, another antihypertensive agent is added.

ADVERSE REACTIONS
CNS: dizziness, headache, fatigue.
CV: volume depletion and dehydration, orthostatic hypotension.
GI: anorexia, nausea, pancreatitis.
GU: nocturia, polyuria, frequent urination.
Hematologic: *aplastic anemia, agranulocytosis,* leukopenia, thrombocytopenia.
Hepatic: hepatic encephalopathy.
Skin: dermatitis, photosensitivity, rash.
Other: asymptomatic hyperuricemia; hyperglycemia and glucose tolerance impairment; fluid and electrolyte imbalances, including hypokalemia, dilutional hyponatremia and hypochloremia, metabolic alkalosis, hypercalcemia; gout; muscle cramps, swelling; hypersensitivity reactions, such as pneumonitis and vasculitis.

INTERACTIONS
Cholestyramine, colestipol: decreased intestinal absorption of thiazides. Separate doses.
Diazoxide: increased antihypertensive, hyperglycemic, and hyperuricemic effects. Use together cautiously.
Digitalis glycosides: increased risk of digitalis toxicity from metolazone-induced hypokalemia. Monitor potassium and digitalis levels.
Ethanol, barbiturates, opiates: increased orthostatic hypotensive effect. Monitor closely.
Lithium: decreased lithium clearance, increasing risk of lithium toxicity. Monitor lithium level.
NSAIDs: increased risk of NSAID-induced renal failure. Monitor the patient for signs of renal failure.

CONTRAINDICATIONS
Contraindicated in patients with anuria, hepatic coma or precoma, or hypersensitivity to thiazides or other sulfonamide-derived drugs.

NURSING CONSIDERATIONS
● Use cautiously in patients with impaired renal or hepatic function.
● To prevent nocturia, give in the morning.
● Keep in mind that Mykrox (prompt) tablets are more rapidly and completely absorbed than other brands mimicking an oral solution. Do not interchange Mykrox with Diulo (extended) or Zaroxolyn (extended) tablets.
● Monitor fluid intake and output, weight, blood pressure, and serum electrolyte levels.

---

†Available in Canada only.   ‡Available in Australia only.   ◇Available OTC.

• Watch for signs of hypokalemia, such as muscle weakness and cramps. Know that drug may be used with potassium-sparing diuretic to prevent potassium loss.
• Consult the doctor and dietitian to provide high-potassium diet. Foods rich in potassium include citrus fruits, tomatoes, bananas, dates, and apricots.
• Monitor blood glucose levels.
• Monitor blood uric acid levels, especially in patients with a history of gout.
• Monitor elderly patients, who are especially susceptible to excessive diuresis.
• In patients with hypertension, know that the therapeutic response may be delayed several days.
• Keep in mind that unlike thiazide diuretics, metolazone is effective in patients with decreased renal function.
• Be aware that drug is used as an adjunct in furosemide-resistant edema.
• As ordered, discontinue thiazides and thiazide-like diuretics before parathyroid function tests are performed.
• Advise the patient to avoid sudden posture changes and to rise slowly to avoid orthostatic hypotension.
• Advise the patient to use a sunblock to prevent photosensitivity reactions.

polythiazide
Renese

Pregnancy Risk Category: C

HOW SUPPLIED
Tablets: 1 mg, 2 mg, 4 mg

ACTION
A thiazide diuretic that increases sodium and water excretion by inhibiting sodium and chloride reabsorption in the nephron's distal segment.

ONSET, PEAK, DURATION
Onset occurs in 2 hours. Peak effects occur in about 6 hours. Effects persist for 24 to 48 hours.

INDICATIONS & DOSAGE
Hypertension –
Adults: 2 to 4 mg P.O. daily.
Edema in heart or renal failure –
Adults: 1 to 4 mg P.O. daily.

ADVERSE REACTIONS
CV: volume depletion and dehydration, orthostatic hypotension.
GI: anorexia, nausea, pancreatitis.
GU: nocturia, polyuria, frequent urination.
Hematologic: *aplastic anemia, agranulocytosis,* leukopenia, thrombocytopenia.
Hepatic: hepatic encephalopathy.
Skin: dermatitis, photosensitivity, rash.
Other: hypokalemia; asymptomatic hyperuricemia; hyperglycemia and glucose tolerance impairment; fluid and electrolyte imbalances, including dilutional hyponatremia and hypochloremia, metabolic alkalosis, hypercalcemia; gout; hypersensitivity reactions, such as pneumonitis and vasculitis.

INTERACTIONS
Cholestyramine, colestipol: decreased intestinal absorption of thiazides. Separate doses.
Diazoxide: increased antihypertensive, hyperglycemic, and hyperuricemic effects. Use together cautiously.
Digitalis glycosides: increased risk of digitalis toxicity from polythiazide-induced hypokalemia.
Ethanol, barbiturates, opiates: increased orthostatic hypotensive effect. Monitor closely.
Lithium: decreased lithium clearance, increasing risk of toxicity. Monitor lithium levels.
NSAIDs: increased risk of NSAID-in-

duced renal failure. Monitor the patient for signs of renal failure.

CONTRAINDICATIONS
Contraindicated in patients wtih anuria or hypersensitivity to thiazides or other sulfonamide-derived drugs.

NURSING CONSIDERATIONS
• Use cautiously in patients with severe renal disease and impaired hepatic function.
• To prevent nocturia, give in the morning.
• Monitor fluid intake and output, weight, blood pressure, and serum electrolytes.
• Watch for signs of hypokalemia, such as muscle weakness and cramps. Know that drug may be used with potassium-sparing diuretic to prevent potassium loss.
• Consult the doctor and dietitian to provide high-potassium diet. Foods rich in potassium include citrus fruits, tomatoes, bananas, dates, and apricots.
• Monitor blood uric acid levels, especially in patients with a history of gout.
• Check insulin requirements in diabetic patients.
• Monitor elderly patients, who are especially susceptible to excessive diuresis.
• As ordered, discontinue thiazides and thiazide-like diuretics before parathyroid function tests are performed.
• In patients with hypertension, know that the therapeutic response may be delayed several days.
• Advise the patient to avoid sudden posture changes and to rise slowly to avoid orthostatic hypotension.
• Advise the patient to use a sunblock to prevent photosensitivity reactions.

quinethazone
Aquamox‡, Hydromox
Pregnancy Risk Category: NR

HOW SUPPLIED
Tablets: 50 mg

ACTION
Although not a thiazide diuretic, quinethazone acts similarly, increasing sodium and water excretion by inhibiting sodium reabsorption in the nephron's cortical diluting site.

ONSET, PEAK, DURATION
Onset occurs in 2 hours. Peak effects occur in 6 hours. Effects persist for 18 to 24 hours.

INDICATIONS & DOSAGE
Management of edema or hypertension –
Adults: 50 to 100 mg P.O. daily or 50 mg P.O. b.i.d. Occasionally, up to 150 to 200 mg P.O. daily may be needed.

ADVERSE REACTIONS
CV: volume depletion and dehydration, orthostatic hypotension.
GI: anorexia, nausea, pancreatitis.
GU: nocturia, polyuria, frequent urination.
Hematologic: *aplastic anemia, agranulocytosis,* leukopenia, thrombocytopenia.
Hepatic: hepatic encephalopathy.
Skin: dermatitis, photosensitivity, rash.
Other: hypokalemia; asymptomatic hyperuricemia; hyperglycemia and glucose tolerance impairment; fluid and electrolyte imbalances, including dilutional hyponatremia and hypochloremia, metabolic alkalosis, hypercalcemia; gout; hypersensitivity reactions, such as pneumonitis and vasculitis.

INTERACTIONS
Cholestyramine, colestipol: decreased intestinal absorption of thiazides. Separate doses.
Diazoxide: increased antihypertensive, hyperglycemic, and hyperuricemic effects. Use together cautiously.
Digitalis glycosides: increased risk of digitalis toxicity from quinethazone-induced hypokalemia. Monitor potassium and digitalis levels.
Ethanol, barbiturates, opiates: increased orthostatic hypotensive effect. Monitor closely.
Lithium: decreased lithium clearance, increasing risk of lithium toxicity. Monitor lithium level.
NSAIDs: increased risk of NSAID-induced renal failure. Monitor the patient for signs of renal failure.

CONTRAINDICATIONS
Contraindicated in patients with anuria or hypersensitivity to quinethazones, thiazides, or other sulfonamide-derived drugs.

NURSING CONSIDERATIONS
• Use cautiously in patients with severe renal disease and impaired hepatic function.
• To prevent nocturia, give in the morning.
• Monitor fluid intake and output, weight, blood pressure, and serum electrolytes.
• Watch for signs of hypokalemia, such as muscle weakness and cramps. Know that drug may be used with potassium-sparing diuretic to prevent potassium loss.
• Consult the doctor and dietitian to provide high-potassium diet. Foods rich in potassium include citrus fruits, tomatoes, bananas, dates, and apricots.
• Monitor serum creatinine, BUN, and blood glucose levels regularly.
• Monitor blood uric acid levels, es-

pecially in patients with a history of gout.
• Monitor elderly patients, who are especially susceptible to excessive diuresis.
• As ordered, discontinue thiazides and thiazide-like diuretics before parathyroid function tests are performed.
• In patients with hypertension, know that the therapeutic response may be delayed several days.
• Advise the patient to avoid sudden posture changes and to rise slowly to avoid orthostatic hypotension.
• Advise the patient to use a sunblock to prevent photosensitivity reactions.

---

spironolactone
Aldactone, Novospiroton†, Spirotone‡

Pregnancy Risk Category: NR

HOW SUPPLIED
Tablets: 25 mg, 50 mg, 100 mg

ACTION
A potassium-sparing diuretic that antagonizes aldosterone in the distal tubule, increasing sodium and water excretion.

ONSET, PEAK, DURATION
Onset occurs in 1 to 2 days. Peak effects occur within 2 to 3 days. Effects persist for 2 to 3 days.

INDICATIONS & DOSAGE
Edema –
Adults: 25 to 200 mg P.O. daily or in divided doses.
Children: 3.3 mg/kg P.O. daily or in divided doses.
Hypertension –
Adults: 50 to 100 mg P.O. daily or in divided doses.
Diuretic-induced hypokalemia –
Adults: 25 to 100 mg P.O. daily when oral potassium supplements are contraindicated.

Detection of primary hyperaldosteronism –

Adults: 400 mg P.O. daily for 4 days (short test) or 3 to 4 weeks (long test). If hypokalemia and hypertension are corrected, a presumptive diagnosis of primary hyperaldosteronism is made.
Management of primary hyperaldosteronism –
Adults: 100 to 400 mg P.O. daily.

ADVERSE REACTIONS
CNS: headache.
GI: anorexia, nausea, diarrhea.
Skin: urticaria.
Other: *hyperkalemia,* dehydration, hyponatremia, transient elevation in BUN, metabolic acidosis, gynecomastia, breast soreness and menstrual disturbances in women.

INTERACTIONS
ACE inhibitors, indomethacin, potassium-containing salt substitutes, potassium-rich foods, potassium supplements: increased risk of hyperkalemia. Don't use together, especially in patients with renal impairment.
Aspirin: possible blocked diuretic effect of spironolactone. Watch for diminished spironolactone response.
Digoxin: may alter digoxin clearance, increasing risk of digoxin toxicity. Monitor digoxin levels.

CONTRAINDICATIONS
Contraindicated in patients with anuria, acute or progressive renal insufficiency, or hyperkalemia.

NURSING CONSIDERATIONS
• Use cautiously in patients with fluid or electrolyte imbalances, impaired renal function, and hepatic disease.
• To enhance absorption, give drug with meals.
• Protect drug from light.
• Monitor serum electrolytes, fluid intake and output, weight, and blood pressure.
• Monitor elderly patients, who are more susceptible to excessive diuresis.
• Inform the laboratory that patient is taking spironolactone because it may interfere with some laboratory tests that measure digoxin levels.
• Be aware that drug is less potent than thiazide and loop diuretics; useful as an adjunct to other diuretic therapy. Diuretic effect delayed 2 to 3 days when used alone.
• Keep in mind that maximum antihypertensive response may be delayed up to 2 weeks.
• Be alert to mild acidosis, which may occur during therapy, because of danger in patients with hepatic cirrhosis.
• Know that breast cancer has been reported in some patients taking spironolactone.
• Warn the patient to avoid excessive ingestion of potassium-rich foods, potassium-containing salt substitutes, and potassium supplements to prevent serious hyperkalemia.

---

torsemide
Demadex

Pregnancy Risk Category: B

HOW SUPPLIED
Injection: 10 mg/ml
Tablets: 5 mg, 10 mg, 20 mg, 100 mg

ACTION
A loop diuretic that enhances excretion of sodium, chloride, and water by acting on the ascending portion of the loop of Henle.

ONSET, PEAK, DURATION
Onset occurs within 10 minutes of I.V. use, 1 hour after oral use. Peak effects occur within 1 hour of I.V. use, 1 to 2 hours after oral use. Effects persist for 6 to 8 hours.

INDICATIONS & DOSAGE

Diuresis in patients with CHF –
Adults: initially, 10 to 20 mg P.O. or I.V. once daily. If response is inadequate, the dose is doubled until a response is obtained. Maximum dosage is 200 mg daily.

Diuresis in patients with chronic renal failure –
Adults: initially, 20 mg P.O. or I.V. once daily. If response is inadequate, the dose is doubled until a response is obtained. Maximum dosage is 200 mg daily.

Diuresis in patients with hepatic cirrhosis –
Adults: initially, 5 to 10 mg P.O. or I.V. once daily with an aldosterone antagonist or a potassium-sparing diuretic. If response is inadequate, the dose is doubled until a response is obtained. Maximum dosage is 40 mg daily.

Hypertension –
Adults: initially, 5 mg P.O. daily. Increased to 10 mg if needed and tolerated. If response is still inadequate, within 4 to 6 weeks another antihypertensive agent should be added.

ADVERSE REACTIONS

CNS: dizziness, headache, nervousness, insomnia.
CV: ECG abnormalitites, chest pain, edema.
EENT: rhinitis, cough, sore throat.
GI: diarrhea, constipation, nausea, dyspepsia.
GU: *excessive urination.*
Other: asthenia, arthralgia, myalgia.

INTERACTIONS

Cholestyramine: decreased absorption of torsemide. Separate administration times by at least 3 hours.
Digoxin: decreased torsemide clearance. No dosage adjustments are necessary.
Indomethacin: decreased diuretic effectiveness in sodium-restricted patients. Avoid concomitant use.

Lithium, ototoxic drugs such as aminoglycosides or ethacrynic acid: possible increased toxicity of these agents. Avoid concomitant use.
NSAIDs: may potentiate nephrotoxicity of NSAIDs. Use together cautiously.
Probenecid: decreased diuretic effectiveness. Avoid concomitant use.
Salicylates: decreased excretion, possibly leading to salicylate toxicity. Avoid concomitant use.
Spironolactone: decreased renal clearance of spironolactone. No dosage adjustments are necessary.

CONTRAINDICATIONS

Contraindicated in patients with anuria or hypersensitivity to the drug or other sulfonylurea derivatives.

NURSING CONSIDERATIONS

• Use cautiously in patients with hepatic disease and associated cirrhosis and ascites; sudden changes in fluid and electrolyte balance may precipitate hepatic coma in these patients.
• To prevent nocturia, give in the morning.
• Inspect ampules for precipitate or discoloration before use.
• **I.V. use:** May be given by direct injection over at least 2 minutes. Rapid injection may cause ototoxicity. Don't give more than 200 mg at a time.
• Monitor fluid intake and output, serum electrolyte levels, blood pressure, weight, and pulse rate during rapid diuresis and routinely with chronic use. Drug can cause profound diuresis and water and electrolyte depletion.
• Watch for signs of hypokalemia, such as muscle weakness and cramps.
• Consult the doctor and dietitian to provide high-potassium diet. Foods rich in potassium include citrus fruits, tomatoes, bananas, dates, and apricots.
• Monitor elderly patients, who are especially susceptible to excessive di-

---

*Liquid form contains alcohol.   *Common* reactions are in italics; ***life-threatening***, in bold italics.
**May contain tartrazine.

uresis, with potential for circulatory collapse and thromboembolic complications.

• Advise the patient to change positions slowly to prevent dizziness, and to limit alcohol intake and strenuous exercise in hot weather to prevent orthostatic hypotension.

• Advise the patient to immediately report ringing in ears. May indicate toxicity.

• Tell the patient to check with the doctor or pharmacist before taking any OTC medications.

triamterene
Dyrenium, Dytac‡

Pregnancy Risk Category: B

HOW SUPPLIED
Tablets†: 50 mg, 100 mg
Capsules: 50 mg, 100 mg

ACTION
A potassium-sparing diuretic that inhibits sodium reabsorption and potassium and hydrogen excretion by direct action on the distal tubule.

ONSET, PEAK, DURATION
Onset occurs in 2 to 4 hours. Peak effects occur in several days. Effects persist for 7 to 9 hours.

INDICATIONS & DOSAGE
Edema –
Adults: initially, 100 mg P.O. b.i.d. after meals. Total dosage should not exceed 300 mg daily.

ADVERSE REACTIONS
CNS: dizziness, weakness, fatigue, headache.
CV: hypotension.
GI: dry mouth, nausea, vomiting, diarrhea.
Hematologic: megaloblastic anemia related to low folic acid levels, thrombocytopenia.
Skin: photosensitivity, rash.

Other: *anaphylaxis, hyperkalemia,* muscle cramps, transient elevation in BUNs or creatinine levels, acidosis, hypokalemia, azotemia, jaundice, increased liver enzyme abnormalities.

INTERACTIONS
ACE inhibitors, potassium-containing salt subtitutes, potassium-rich foods, potassium supplements: increased risk of hyperkalemia. Don't use together.
Amantadine: increased risk of amantadine toxicity. Don't use together.
Lithium: decreased lithium clearance, increasing risk of lithium toxicity. Monitor lithium level.
NSAIDs: may enhance risk of nephrotoxicity. Avoid concomitant use.
Quinidine: may interfere with some laboratory tests that measure quinidine levels. Inform laboratory that patient is taking triamterene.

CONTRAINDICATIONS
Contraindicated in patients with hypersensitivity to the drug and in those with anuria, severe or progressive renal disease or dysfunction, severe hepatic disease, or hyperkalemia.

NURSING CONSIDERATIONS
• Use cautiously in patients with impaired hepatic function or diabetes mellitus and in elderly or debilitated patients.
• To minimize nausea, give medication after meals.
• Monitor blood pressure, BUN, and serum electrolyte levels.
• Watch for blood dyscrasia.
• To minimize excessive rebound potassium excretion, withdraw drug gradually, as ordered.
• Be aware that drug is less potent than thiazides and loop diuretics and is useful as an adjunct to other diuretic therapy. Usually used with potassium-wasting diuretics. Full effect delayed 2 to 3 days when used alone.
• Warn patients to avoid excessive ingestion of potassium-rich foods, po-

tassium-containing salt substitutes, and potassium supplements to prevent serious hyperkalemia.
• Teach the patient to avoid direct sunlight, wear protective clothing, and use a sunblock to prevent photosensitivity reactions.

trichlormethiazide
Diurese, Metahydrin**, Naqua, Trichlorex**

Pregnancy Risk Category: C

HOW SUPPLIED
Tablets: 2 mg, 4 mg

ACTION
A thiazide diuretic that increases sodium and water excretion by inhibiting sodium and chloride reabsorption in the nephron's distal segment.

ONSET, PEAK, DURATION
Onset occurs in 2 hours. Peak effects occur in about 6 hours. Effects persist for 24 hours or longer.

INDICATIONS & DOSAGE
Edema –
Adults: 1 to 4 mg P.O. daily or b.i.d.
Hypertension –
Adults: 2 to 4 mg P.O. daily.

ADVERSE REACTIONS
CV: volume depletion and dehydration, orthostatic hypotension.
GI: anorexia, nausea, pancreatitis.
GU: nocturia, polyuria, frequent urination.
Hematologic: *aplastic anemia, agranulocytosis,* leukopenia, thrombocytopenia.
Hepatic: hepatic encephalopathy.
Skin: dermatitis, photosensitivity, rash.
Other: hypokalemia; asymptomatic hyperuricemia; hyperglycemia and glucose tolerance impairment; fluid and electrolyte imbalances, including dilutional hyponatremia and hypo-

chloremia, metabolic alkalosis, hypercalcemia; gout; hypersensitivity reactions, such as pneumonitis and vasculitis.

INTERACTIONS
Cholestyramine, colestipol: decreased intestinal absorption of thiazides. Separate doses.
Diazoxide: increased antihypertensive, hyperglycemic, and hyperuricemic effects. Use together cautiously.
Digitalis glycosides: increased risk of digitalis toxicity from trichlormethiazide-induced hypokalemia. Monitor potassium and digitalis levels.
Ethanol, barbiturates, opiates: increased orthostatic hypotensive effect. Monitor closely.
Lithium: decreased lithium clearance, increasing risk of lithium toxicity. Monitor lithium level.
NSAIDs: increased risk of NSAID-induced renal failure. Monitor the patient for signs of renal failure.

CONTRAINDICATIONS
Contraindicated in patients with anuria or hypersensitivity to thiazides or other sulfonamide-derived drugs.

NURSING CONSIDERATIONS
• Use cautiously in patients with severe renal disease and impaired hepatic function.
• To prevent nocturia, give in the morning.
• Monitor fluid intake and output, weight, blood pressure, and serum electrolyte levels.
• Watch for signs of hypokalemia, such as muscle weakness and cramps. Know that drug may be used with potassium-sparing diuretic to prevent hypokalemia.
• Consult the doctor and dietitian to provide high-potassium diet. Foods rich in potassium include citrus fruits, tomatoes, bananas, dates, and apricots.

*Liquid form contains alcohol.   *Common* reactions are in italics; *life-threatening,* in bold italics.
**May contain tartrazine.

- Monitor serum creatinine, BUN, and blood glucose levels regularly. Drug is not as effective if these levels are more than twice normal.
- Monitor blood glucose levels and check insulin requirements in patients with diabetes.
- Monitor blood uric acid levels, especially in patients with a history of gout.
- As ordered, discontinue thiazides and thiazide-like diuretics before parathyroid function tests are performed.
- Monitor elderly patients, who are especially susceptible to excessive diuresis.
- In patients with hypertension, know that the therapeutic response may be delayed several days.
- Advise the patient to avoid sudden posture changes and to rise slowly to avoid orthostatic hypotension.
- Advise the patient to use a sunblock to prevent photosensitivity reactions.

urea (carbamide)
Ureaphil

Pregnancy Risk Category: C

HOW SUPPLIED
Injection: 40 g/150 ml

ACTION
An osmotic diuretic that increases the osmotic pressure of glomerular filtrate, inhibiting tubular reabsorption of water and electrolytes. Also elevates blood plasma osmolality, resulting in enhanced water flow into extracellular fluid.

ONSET, PEAK, DURATION
Onset occurs in 30 to 45 minutes. Peak effects occur in 1 to 2 hours. Diuresis and decreased CSF pressure last for 3 to 10 hours; decreased intraocular pressure lasts 5 to 6 hours.

INDICATIONS & DOSAGE
Elevated intracranial or intraocular pressure –
Adults: 1 to 1.5 g/kg as a 30% solution by slow I.V. infusion over 1 to 2½ hours. Rate should not exceed 4 ml/minute. Maximum dosage is 120 g daily.
Children: 0.5 to 1.5 g/kg slow I.V. infusion (rate not to exceed 4 ml/minute) or 35 g/m^2 in 24 hours. Children under 2 years may receive as little as 0.1 g/kg slow I.V. infusion.

ADVERSE REACTIONS
CNS: *headache.*
CV: tachycardia, *CHF.*
GI: *nausea, vomiting.*
Respiratory: *pulmonary edema*
Other: sodium and potassium depletion; irritation or necrotic sloughing with extravasation.

INTERACTIONS
Lithium: increased lithium clearance and decreased lithium effectiveness. Monitor lithium level.

CONTRAINDICATIONS
Contraindicated in patients with severely impaired renal function, marked dehydration, frank hepatic failure, active intracranial bleeding, and sickle-cell disease with CNS involvement.

NURSING CONSIDERATIONS
- Use cautiously in patients with cardiac disease or hepatic or renal impairment and during pregnancy and breast-feeding.
- **I.V. use:** Avoid rapid I.V. infusion; may cause hemolysis or increased capillary bleeding. Maximum infusion rate is 4 ml/minute. Avoid extravasation; may cause reactions ranging from mild irritation to necrosis.
- To prepare 135 ml of 30% solution, mix contents of 40-g vial of urea with 105 ml of D$_5$W or dextrose 10% in water or 10% invert sugar in water.

Each ml of 30% solution provides 300 mg urea.

• Don't give through the same infusion set as blood or blood derivatives.

• Use freshly reconstituted urea only for I.V. infusion; solution becomes ammonia upon standing. Use within minutes of reconstitution and discard within 24 hours.

• Don't infuse into leg veins; may cause phlebitis or thrombosis, especially in elderly patients.

• Assess breath sounds for crackles, indicating pulmonary edema.

• Watch for signs of hyponatremia (nausea, vomiting, tachycardia) or hypokalemia (muscle weakness, lethargy); may indicate electrolyte depletion before serum levels are reduced.

• Maintain adequate hydration; monitor blood pressure, fluid intake and output, and serum electrolyte levels.

• In patients with renal disease, monitor BUN level.

• To ensure bladder emptying in comatose patients, use an indwelling urinary catheter, and use an hourly urometer collection bag for accurate evaluation of diuresis.

• If satisfactory diuresis does not occur in 6 to 12 hours, be aware that urea should be discontinued and renal function reevaluated.

---

*Liquid form contains alcohol.
**May contain tartrazine.

Common reactions are in italics; ***life-threatening,*** in bold italics.

63

Electrolytes and replacement solutions

calcium acetate
calcium carbonate
calcium chloride
calcium citrate
calcium glubionate
calcium gluceptate
calcium gluconate
calcium lactate
calcium phosphate, dibasic
calcium phosphate, tribasic
dextran, low molecular weight
dextran, high molecular weight
hetastarch
magnesium chloride
magnesium sulfate
potassium acetate
potassium bicarbonate
potassium chloride
potassium gluconate
Ringer's injection
Ringer's injection, lactated
sodium chloride

COMBINATION PRODUCTS

KLORVESS*: 20 mEq each potassium and chloride (from potassium chloride, potassium bicarbonate, and l-lysine monohydrochloride).

K-LYTE-CL: 25 mEq potassium, 25 mEq chloride (from potassium chloride, potassium bicarbonate, and lysine hydrochloride).

NEUTRA-PHOS: phosphorus 250 mg, sodium 164 mg, potassium 278 mg (from dibasic and monobasic sodium and potassium phosphate).

TWIN-K: 15 ml supplies 20 mEq of potassium ions as a combination of potassium gluconate and potassium citrate.

---

calcium acetate
Phos-Ex◇, Phos-Lo

calcium carbonate

Apo-Cal†◇, BioCal◇, Calcarb 600◇, Cal-Carb-HD◇, Calci-Chew◇, Calciday 667◇, Calcilac◇, Calci-Mix◇, Calcite 500†◇, Calcium 500†◇, Calcium 600◇, Calglycine◇, Cal-Guard Softgels, Cal-Plus◇, Calsan†◇, Caltrate 300†◇, Caltrate 600†◇, Caltrate Chewable†◇, Chooz◇, Dicarbosil◇, Gencalc 600◇, Mallamint◇, Mega-Cal†◇, Nephro-Calci◇, Nu-Cal†◇, Os-Cal†◇, Os-Cal 500◇, Os-Cal Chewable†◇, Oysco◇, Oysco 500 Chewable◇, Oyst-Cal 500◇, Oyst-Cal 500 Chewable◇, Oystercal 500◇, Oyster Shell Calcium-500◇, Rolaids Calcium Rich◇, Super Calcium 1200◇, Titralac◇, Tums◇, Tums E-X◇

calcium chloride◇
Calciject†

calcium citrate◇
Citrical◇, Citrical Liquitabs†◇

calcium glubionate◇
Calcium-Sandoz†, Neo-Calglucon

calcium gluceptate◇

calcium gluconate
Kalcinate

calcium lactate◇

calcium phosphate, dibasic◇

calcium phosphate, tribasic
Posture◇

Pregnancy Risk Category: C

HOW SUPPLIED
calcium acetate
Contains 253 mg or 12.7 mEq of elemental calcium/g
Tablets: 250 mg◇, 500 mg◇, 667 mg, 668 mg◇, 1,000 mg◇
Injection: 0.5 mEq Ca^{++} per ml
calcium carbonate
Contains 400 mg or 20 mEq of elemental calcium/g
Tablets: 650 mg◇, 667 mg◇, 750 mg◇, 1.25 g◇, 1.5 g◇
Tablets (chewable): 350 mg◇, 420 mg◇, 500 mg◇, 625 mg◇, 750 mg◇, 850 mg◇, 1.25 g◇
Capsules: 600 mg◇, 1.25 g◇
Oral suspension: 1.25 g/5 ml◇
Powder packets: 6.5 g (2,400 mg calcium) per packet◇
calcium chloride
Contains 270 mg or 13.5 mEq of elemental calcium/g
Injection: 10% solution in 10-ml ampules, vials, and syringes
calcium citrate
Contains 211 mg or 10.6 mEq of elemental calcium/g
Tablets: 950 mg◇
Effervescent tablets: 2376 mg◇
calcium glubionate
Contains 64 mg or 3.2 mEq elemental calcium/g
Syrup: 1.8 g/5 ml
calcium glucepate
Contains 82 mg or 4.1 mEq elemental calcium/g
Injection: 1.1 g/5 ml in 5-ml ampules or 10-ml vials
calcium gluconate
Contains 90 mg or 4.5 mEq of elemental calcium/g
Tablets: 500 mg◇, 650 mg◇, 975 mg◇, 1 g◇
Injection: 10% solution in 10-ml ampules and vials, 10-ml or 50-ml vials
Pharmacy bulk vials: 100 ml, 200 ml
calcium lactate
Contains 130 mg or 6.5 mEq of elemental calcium/g
Tablets: 325 mg, 650 mg

calcium phosphate, dibasic
Contains 230 mg or 11.5 mEq of elemental calcium/g
Tablets: 468 mg◇
calcium phosphate, tribasic
Contains 400 mg or 20 mEq of elemental calcium/g
Tablets: 300 mg◇, 600 mg◇

ACTION
Replaces and maintains calcium.

ONSET, PEAK, DURATION
Onset and peak effects occur immediately after I.V. injection, return to normal within ½ to 2 hours.

INDICATIONS & DOSAGE
Hypocalcemic emergency –
Adults: 7 to 14 mEq calcium I.V. May be given as a 10% calcium gluconate solution, 2 to 10% calcium chloride solution, or a 22% calcium glucepate solution.
Children: 1 to 7 mEq calcium I.V.
Infants: up to 1 mEq calcium I.V.
Hypocalcemic tetany –
Adults: 4.5 to 16 mEq calcium I.V. Repeated until tetany is controlled.
Children: 0.5 to 0.7 mEq calcium I.V. 3 to 4 times a day until tetany is controlled.
Neonates: 2.4 mEq I.V. daily in divided doses.
Adjunctive treatment of cardiac arrest –
Adults: 0.027 to 0.054 mEq calcium chloride I.V., 4.5 to 6.3 mEq calcium glucepate I.V., or 2.3 to 3.7 mEq calcium gluconate I.V.
Children: 0.27 mEq/kg calcium chloride I.V. Repeated in 10 minutes if necessary; determine serum calcium levels before administering further doses.
Adjunctive treatment of magnesium intoxication –
Adults: initially, 7 mEq I.V. Subsequent doses must be based upon the patient's response.
During exchange transfusions –

---

*Liquid form contains alcohol. **May contain tartrazine.   *Common* reactions are in italics; ***life-threatening,*** in bold italics.

Adults: 1.35 mEq concurrently with each 100 ml citrated blood.
Neonates: 0.45 mEq after each 100 ml citrated blood.
Hyperphosphatemia –
Adults: 1,334 to 2,000 mg P.O. calcium acetate t.i.d. with meals. Most dialysis patients will require 3 to 4 tablets with each meal.
Dietary supplement –
Adults: 500 mg to 2 g P.O. daily.

ADVERSE REACTIONS
CNS: with I.V. use, tingling sensations, sense of oppression or heat waves; with rapid I.V. injection, syncope.
CV: mild fall in blood pressure; with rapid I.V. injection, vasodilation, bradycardia, *arrhythmias, cardiac arrest.*
GI: with oral use, irritation, hemorrhage, *constipation;* with I.V. use, chalky taste; with oral calcium chloride, hemorrhage, nausea, vomiting, thirst, abdominal pain.
GU: hypercalcemia, polyuria, renal calculi.
Skin: with I.M. use, local reactions including burning, necrosis, tissue sloughing, cellulitis, soft tissue calcification.
Other: with S.C. injection, pain and irritation; with I.V. use, *vein irritation.*

INTERACTIONS
Atenolol, tetracyclines, fluoroquinolones: decreased bioavailability of these agents and calcium when oral preparations are taken together. Separate administration times.
Calcium channel blockers: decreased calcium effectiveness. Avoid concomitant use.
Digitalis glycosides: increased digitalis toxicity; administer calcium cautiously (if at all) to digitalized patients.
Sodium polystyrene sulfonate: risk of

metabolic acidosis in patients with renal disease. Avoid concomitant use.
Thiazide diuretics: risk of hypercalcemia. Avoid concomitant use.
Foods containing oxalic acid (found in rhubarb and spinach), phytic acid (bran and whole cereals), and phosphorus (milk and dairy products): may interfere with calcium absorption.

CONTRAINDICATIONS
Contraindicated in patients with ventricular fibrillation, hypercalcemia, hypophosphatemia, or renal calculi.

NURSING CONSIDERATIONS
● Use all calcium products with exterme caution in patients with sarcoidosis and renal or cardiac disease, and in digitalized patients. Use calcium chloride cautiously in patients with cor pulmonale, respiratory acidosis, and respiratory failure.
● Warm solutions to body temperature before administration.
● **I.V. use (direct injection):** Administer slowly through a small needle into a large vein or through an I.V. line containing a free-flowing, compatible solution at a rate not exceeding 1 ml/minute (1.5 mEq/minute) for calcium chloride, 1.5 to 5 ml/minute for calcium gluconate, and 2 ml/minute for calcium gluceptate. Do not use scalp veins in children.
● **I.V. use (intermittent infusion):** Infuse diluted solution through an I.V. line containing a compatible solution. Maximum rate of 200 mg/minute suggested for calcium gluceptate and calcium gluconate.
● Give calcium chloride I.V. only. When adding to parenteral solutions that contain other additives (especially phosphorus or phosphate), observe closely for precipitate. Use an in-line filter.
● Monitor ECG when giving calcium I.V. Stop if the patient complains of discomfort and notify doctor. Follow-

---

† Available in Canada only.   ‡ Available in Australia only.   ◇ Available OTC.

ing I.V. injection, the patient should remain recumbent for 15 minutes.
• Give I.M. injection in the gluteal region in adults; lateral thigh in infants. I.M. route used only in emergencies when no I.V. route available.
• If GI upset occurs, give oral calcium products 1 to 1½ hours after meals.
• Ensure that the doctor specifies form of calcium he wants administered because crash carts usually contain both calcium gluconate and calcium chloride.
• Monitor blood calcium levels frequently. Hypercalcemia may result after large doses in chronic renal failure. Report abnormalities.
• Be aware that severe necrosis and tissue sloughing can occur after extravasation. Calcium gluconate is less irritating to veins and tissues than calcium chloride.

dextran, low molecular weight (dextran 40)
Dextran 40, Gentran 40, 10% LMD, Rheomacrodex

Pregnancy Risk Category: C

HOW SUPPLIED
Injection: 10% dextran 40 in D_5W or 0.9% sodium chloride solution

ACTION
Expands plasma volume via colloidal osmotic effect, drawing fluid from interstitial to intravascular space, providing fluid replacement.

ONSET, PEAK, DURATION
Onset and peak effects occur immediately after an I.V. infusion. Effects persist up to 3 hours.

INDICATIONS & DOSAGE
Plasma volume expansion—
Adults: dosage by I.V. infusion depends on amount of fluid loss. First 10 ml/kg of dextran infused rapidly with

central venous pressure monitoring, remaining dose slowly. Total dosage not to exceed 20 ml/kg body weight daily. If therapy continued past 24 hours, do not exceed 10 ml/kg daily. Continued for no longer than 5 days.
Prophylaxis of venous thrombosis—
Adults: 10 ml/kg (500 to 1,000 ml) I.V. on the day of the procedure; 500 ml on days 2 and 3.
Hemodiluent in extracorporeal circulation—
Adults: 10 to 20 ml/kg added to the perfusion circuit. Not to exceed total dosage of 20 ml/kg.

ADVERSE REACTIONS
GI: nausea, vomiting.
GU: tubular stasis and blocking, increased urine viscosity.
Hematologic: *decreased hemoglobin and hematocrit levels;* with higher doses, increased bleeding time.
Hepatic: increased AST and ALT levels.
Skin: hypersensitivity reactions, urticaria.
Other: *anaphylaxis.*

INTERACTIONS
None significant.

CONTRAINDICATIONS
Contraindicated in patients with hypersensitivity to the drug and in those with marked hemostatic defects, marked cardiac decompensation, and renal disease with severe oliguria or anuria.

NURSING CONSIDERATIONS
• Use cautiously in patients with active hemorrhage, thrombocytopenia, or diabetes mellitus.
• Assess hydration before starting therapy; otherwise, use urine or serum osmolarity because urine specific gravity is affected by urine dextran concentration.
• **I.V. use:** Observe the patient closely

---

during early phase of infusion, when most anaphylactic reactions occur.

• Watch for circulatory overload and a rise in central venous pressure. Provides plasma expansion slightly greater than volume infused.

• Monitor urine flow rate during administration. If oliguria or anuria occurs or is not relieved by infusion, stop dextran and give loop diuretic as ordered.

• Check hemoglobin and hematocrit levels; if values fall below 30% by volume, notify the doctor.

• As ordered, use D$_5$W solution instead of 0.9% sodium chloride solution because the drug is hazardous for patients with heart failure, especially when given in 0.9% sodium chloride solution.

• Be aware the doctor may order dextran 1 to protect against dextran-induced anaphylaxis. Administer 20 ml of dextran 1 (containing 150 mg/ml) I.V. over 60 seconds, 1 to 2 minutes before the I.V. infusion of dextran.

• Be aware that drug may interfere with analyses of blood grouping, crossmatching, bilirubin, blood glucose, and protein.

• Store at constant 77° F (25° C). May precipitate in storage, but can be heated to dissolve if necessary.

---

dextran, high molecular weight (dextran 70, dextran 75)

Dextran 75, Gentran 70, Gentran 75, Macrodex

Pregnancy Risk Category: C

HOW SUPPLIED
Injection: 6% dextran 70 in 0.9% sodium chloride solution or dextrose 5%; 6% dextran 75 in 0.9% sodium chloride solution or dextrose 5%

ACTION
Expands plasma volume via colloidal osmotic effect, drawing fluid from interstitial to intravascular space, providing fluid replacement.

ONSET, PEAK, DURATION
Onset and peak effects occur immediately after I.V. infusion. Duration of action unknown.

INDICATIONS & DOSAGE
Plasma expander –
Adults: 30 g (500 ml of 6% solution) I.V. In emergencies, may be administered at rate of 1.2 to 2.4 g (20 to 40 ml) per minute. In normovolemic or nearly normovolemic patients, rate of infusion should not exceed 240 mg (4 ml)/minute.

Total dosage during first 24 hours not to exceed 1.2 g/kg; actual dosage depends on amount of fluid loss and resultant hemoconcentration, and must be determined for each patient.

ADVERSE REACTIONS
GI: nausea, vomiting.
GU: increased specific gravity and viscosity of urine, tubular stasis and blocking. oliguria, anuria.
Hematologic: *decreased level of hemoglobin and hematocrit;* with doses of 15 ml/kg body weight, prolonged bleeding time and significant suppression of platelet function.
Hepatic: increased AST and ALT levels.
Skin: hypersensitivity reactions, urticaria.
Other: fever, arthralgia, nasal congestion, *anaphylaxis.*

INTERACTIONS
None significant.

CONTRAINDICATIONS
Contraindicated in patients with hypersensitivity to dextran and in those with marked hemostatic defects, marked cardiac decompensation, renal disease with severe oliguria or anuria, hypervolemic conditions, and severe bleeding disorders.

NURSING CONSIDERATIONS

• Use cautiously in patients with active hemorrhage, thrombocytopenia, impaired renal clearance, chronic liver disease, and abdominal conditions or in patients undergoing bowel surgery.

• Assess hydration before starting therapy; otherwise, use urine or serum osmolarity because urine specific gravity is affected by the urine dextran concentration.

• Have blood samples drawn *before* starting infusion.

• **I.V. use:** Observe the patient closely during early phase of infusion, when most anaphylactic reactions occur.

• As ordered, use D_5W solution instead of 0.9% sodium chloride solution because drug is hazardous for patients with heart failure, especially if given in 0.9% sodium chloride solution.

• Monitor urine flow rate during administration. If oliguria or anuria occurs or is not relieved by infusion, stop dextran and give loop diuretic.

• Watch for circulatory overload. Provides plasma expansion slightly greater than volume infused.

• Monitor hemoglobin and hematocrit levels; if values fall below 30% by volume, notify the doctor.

• Be aware that the doctor may order dextran 1 to protect against dextran-induced anaphylaxis. Administer 20 ml of dextran 1 (containing 150 mg/ml) I.V. over 60 seconds, 1 to 2 minutes before the I.V. infusion of dextran 70.

• Be aware that the drug may interfere with analyses of blood grouping, crossmatching, bilirubin, blood glucose, and protein.

• Know that the drug may precipitate in storage, but can be heated to dissolve if necessary.

hetastarch
Hespan

Pregnancy Risk Category: C

HOW SUPPLIED
Injection: 500 ml (6 g/100 ml in 0.9% sodium chloride solution)

ACTION
Expands plasma volume and provides fluid replacement.

ONSET, PEAK, DURATION
Onset and peak effects occur immediately after I.V. infusion. Duration unknown.

INDICATIONS & DOSAGE
Plasma expander –
Adults: 500 to 1,000 ml I.V., depending on amount of blood lost and resultant hemoconcentration. Total dosage usually not to exceed 1,500 ml/day. Up to 20 ml/kg hourly may be used in hemorrhagic shock.

ADVERSE REACTIONS
CNS: headaches.
CV: peripheral edema of lower extremities.
EENT: periorbital edema.
GI: nausea, vomiting.
Skin: urticaria.
Other: wheezing, mild fever.

INTERACTIONS
None significant.

CONTRAINDICATIONS
Contraindicated in patients with severe bleeding disorders, severe CHF, or renal failure with oliguria and anuria.

NURSING CONSIDERATIONS
• Know that hetastarch is *not* a substitute for blood or plasma.
• To avoid circulatory overload, monitor patients with impaired renal function carefully.

---

*Liquid form contains alcohol.   *Common* reactions are in italics; *life-threatening,* in bold italics.
**May contain tartrazine.

• When used in continuous-flow centrifugation, be aware that leukapheresis ratio is usually 1 part hetastarch to 8 parts venous whole blood.
• Discontinue if allergic or sensitivity reactions occur and notify doctor. If necessary, administer an antihistamine as ordered.
• Discard partially used bottles.

---

magnesium chloride
Slow-Mag◇

magnesium sulfate
Pregnancy Risk Category: NR

HOW SUPPLIED
magnesium chloride
Tablets (delayed-release): 64 mg
magnesium sulfate
Injectable solutions: 10%, 12.5%, 25%, 50% in 2-ml, 5-ml, 10-ml, 20-ml, and 30-ml ampules, vials, and prefilled syringes

ACTION
Replaces and maintains magnesium levels; as an anticonvulsant, reduces muscle contractions by interfering with release of acetylcholine at myoneural junction.

ONSET, PEAK, DURATION
Onset unknown. Serum levels peak within 4 hours of oral dose. Effects persist for 4 to 6 hours.

INDICATIONS & DOSAGE
Mild hypomagnesemia –
Adults: 1 g I.M. q 6 hours for four doses, depending on serum magnesium level.
Severe hypomagnesemia (serum magnesium 0.8 mEq/L or less, with symptoms) –
Adults: 5 g I.V. in 1 liter of solution over 3 hours.
    Subsequent doses depend on serum magnesium levels.
Magnesium supplementation –
Adults: 64 mg (1 tablet) P.O. t.i.d.
Magnesium supplementation in total parenteral nutrition (TPN) –
Adults: 4 to 24 mEq I.V. daily added to TPN solution.
Infants: 2 to 10 mEq I.V. daily added to TPN solution.
    Each 2 ml of 50% solution contains 1 g, or 8.12 mEq, magnesium sulfate.
Acute treatment of preeclampsia and eclampsia –
Adults: loading dose: 2 to 4 g (4 to 8 ml of 50% solution) given by slow I.V. bolus (over 5 minutes). Maintenance dosage is 1 to 2 g hourly by constant infusion. Prepare by adding 8 ml of 50% solution to 250 ml D_5W.
Hypomagnesemic seizures –
Adults: 1 to 2 g of 10% solution I.V. over 15 minutes, then 1 g I.M. q 4 to 6 hours, based on the patient's response and magnesium blood level.
Seizures secondary to hypomagnesemia in acute nephritis –
Children: 0.2 ml/kg of 50% solution I.M. q 4 to 6 hours, p.r.n. or 100 mg/kg of 1% to 3% solution I.V. very slowly. Titrate dosage according to magnesium blood level and seizure response.
Paroxysmal atrial tachycardia unresponsive to other treatments –
Adults: 3 to 4 g I.V. of 10% solution over 30 seconds, with close monitoring of ECG.

ADVERSE REACTIONS
CNS: toxicity – *weak or absent deep tendon reflexes,* flaccid paralysis, hypothermia, drowsiness, hypocalcemia (perioral paresthesia, twitching carpopedal spasm, tetany, and seizures).
CV: slow, weak pulse; arrhythmias (caused by hypocalcemia); *hypotension.*
Respiratory: *respiratory paralysis*
Skin: flushing, diaphoresis.
Other: hypocalcemia.

INTERACTIONS
Digitalis glycosides: possible serious cardiac conduction changes. Administer with extreme caution.
Neuromuscular blocking agents: possible increased neuromuscular blockage. Use cautiously.
Nitrofurantoin, tetracyclines, penicillamine: decreased bioavailability with oral magnesium supplements. Separate administration times by 2 to 3 hours.

CONTRAINDICATIONS
Contraindicated in patients with myocardial damage or heart block and in actively progressing labor.

NURSING CONSIDERATIONS
• Use parenteral magnesium with extreme caution in patients with impaired renal function.
• **I.V. use:** Inject I.V. bolus dose slowly, using infusion pump for continous infusion if available, to avoid respiratory or cardiac arrest. Maximum infusion rate is 150 mg/minute. Rapid drip causes feeling of heat.
• When giving I.V. for severe hypomagnesemia, watch for respiratory depression and signs of heart block. Respirations should be more than 16/minute before dose is given.
• Know that magnesium sulfate may form a precipitate when mixed with solutions containing ethanol, arsenates, barium, calcium, clindamycin, heavy metals, hydrocortisone sodium succinate, phosphates, polymyxin B sulfate, procaine, salicylates, or tartrates. Drug is also incompatible with alkalis, including carbonates and bicarbonates.
• Be aware that undiluted 50% solutions may be given by deep I.M. injection to adults. Dilute solutions to 20% or less for use in children.
• Keep I.V. calcium available to reverse magnesium intoxication.
• Test knee-jerk and patellar reflexes before each additional dose. If absent, notify doctor and give no more magnesium until reflexes return; otherwise, the patient may develop temporary respiratory failure and need cardiopulmonary resuscitation or I.V. administration of calcium.
• Check magnesium level after repeated doses.
• Monitor fluid intake and output. Output should be 100 ml or more during 4-hour period before dose.
• After giving to toxemic patients within 24 hours before delivery, watch neonate for signs of magnesium toxicity, including neuromuscular and respiratory depression.

---

potassium acetate
Pregnancy Risk Category: C

HOW SUPPLIED
Injection: 2 mEq/ml in 20-ml, 30-ml vials.

ACTION
Replaces and maintains potassium level.

ONSET, PEAK, DURATION
Onset and peak levels occur immediately after I.V. infusion. Duration unknown.

INDICATIONS & DOSAGE
Treatment of hypokalemia –
Adults: No more than 20 mEq hourly in concentration of 40 mEq/liter or less. Total 24-hour dosage should not exceed 150 mEq (3 mEq/kg in children). Potassium replacement should be done with ECG monitoring and frequent serum potassium determinations. I.V. should be used only for life-threatening hypokalemia or when oral replacement not feasible.
Prevention of hypokalemia –
Adults: dosage is individualized to the patient's needs, not to exceed 150 mEq/day. Administered as an additive to I.V. infusions. Usual dose is 40

---

*Liquid form contains alcohol.   *Common* reactions are in italics; ***life-threatening,*** in bold italics.
**May contain tartrazine.

mEq/liter infused at a rate not to exceed 20 mEq/hour.
Children: individualized dosage not to exceed 3 mEq/kg/day. Administered as an additive to I.V. infusions.

ADVERSE REACTIONS
Signs of hyperkalemia:
CNS: paresthesia of the extremities, listlessness, mental confusion, weakness or heaviness of legs, flaccid paralysis.
CV: *peripheral vascular collapse with fall in blood pressure, arrhythmias,* heart block, possible cardiac arrest, ECG changes (prolonged PR intervals; widened QRS complex; ST-segment depression; tall, tented T waves).
GI: nausea, vomiting, abdominal pain, diarrhea, bowel ulceration.
GU: oliguria.
Skin: cold skin, gray pallor.
Other: pain and redness at infusion site.

INTERACTIONS
ACE inhibitors, potassium-sparing diuretics: increased risk of hyperkalemia. Use with extreme caution.

CONTRAINDICATIONS
Contraindicated in patients with severe renal impairment with oliguria, anuria, or azotemia; in those with untreated Addison's disease; and in those with acute dehydration, heat cramps, hyperkalemia, hyperkalemic form of familial periodic paralysis, and conditions associated with extensive tissue breakdown.

NURSING CONSIDERATIONS
• Use cautiously in patients with cardiac disease and in those with renal impairment.
• **I.V. use:** Give by I.V. infusion only; never I.V. push or I.M. Observe for pain and redness at infusion site. Large-bore needle reduces local irritation.

• Give slowly as diluted solution; potentially fatal hyperkalemia may result from too-rapid infusion.
• Reconstitute potassium acetate powder with liquids; give after meals with a full glass of water or fruit juice to minimize GI irritation.
• During therapy, monitor ECG, renal function, fluid intake and output, and serum potassium, serum creatinine, and BUN levels. Never give potassium postoperatively until urine flow is established.
• Watch for signs of GI ulceration: obstruction, pain, distention, severe vomiting, and bleeding.

potassium bicarbonate
K+Care ET, K-Gen ET, K-Ide, Klor-Con/EF, K-Lyte
Pregnancy Risk Category: NR

HOW SUPPLIED
Effervescent tablets: 6.5 mEq, 25 mEq

ACTION
Replaces and maintains potassium.

ONSET, PEAK, DURATION
Onset and duration unknown. Peak levels occur within 4 hours.

INDICATIONS & DOSAGE
Hypokalemia –
Adults: 25 to 50 mEq dissolved in one-half to a full glass of water (120 to 240 ml) once daily to q.i.d.

ADVERSE REACTIONS
CNS: paresthesia of the extremities, listlessness, mental confusion, weakness or heaviness of legs, flaccid paralysis.
CV: *arrhythmias,* ECG changes (prolonged PR interval; widened QRS complex; ST-segment depression; tall, tented T waves).
GI: *nausea, vomiting, abdominal*

pain, diarrhea, ulcerations, hemorrhage, obstruction, perforation.

INTERACTIONS
ACE inhibitors, potassium-sparing diuretics: risk of hyperkalemia. Use with extreme caution.

CONTRAINDICATIONS
Contraindicated in patients with severe renal impairment with oliguria, anuria, or azotemia; in those with untreated Addison's disease; and in patients with acute dehydration, heat cramps, hyperkalemia, hyperkalemic form of familial periodic paralysis, and other conditions associated with extensive tissue breakdown.

NURSING CONSIDERATIONS
• Use cautiously in patients with cardiac disease and in those with renal impairment.
• Dissolve potassium bicarbonate tablets completely in 6 to 8 ounces of cold water to minimize GI irritation.
• Ask the patient's flavor preference. Available in lime and orange flavors.
• Have the patient take with meals and sip slowly over 5 to 10 minutes.
• Don't administer potassium supplements postoperatively until urine flow has been established.
• Be aware that potassium bicarbonate does not correct hypochloremic alkalosis.
• Monitor BUN, serum potassium, and creatinine levels, and monitor fluid intake and output.
• Never switch potassium products without a doctor's order. Potassium bicarbonate cannot be given instead of potassium chloride.

---

potassium chloride
Cena-K, K+10, Kaochlor 10%*, Kaochlor S-F 10%*, Kaon-Cl, Kaon-Cl 20%*, Kato Powder, Kay Ciel*, K+Care, K-Dur, K-Lease, K-Lor, Klor-10%*, Klor-Con, Klorvess, Klotrix, K-Lyte/Cl, K-Norm, K-Tab, Micro-K Extencaps, Rum-K, Slow-K, Ten-K

Pregnancy Risk Category: C

HOW SUPPLIED
Tablets: 1.22 mEq (99 mg), 8 mEq (600 mg), 10 mEq (750 mg), 20 mEq (1,500 mg), 25 mEq (1,875 mg)
Tablets (controlled-release): 6.7 mEq (500 mg), 8 mEq (600 mg), 10 mEq (750 mg), 20 mEq (1,500 mg)
Tablets (enteric-coated): 4 mEq (300 mg), 13.4 mEq (1,000 mg)
Capsules (controlled-release): 8 mEq (600 mg), 10 mEq (750 mg)
Oral liquid: 5% (10 mEq/15 ml), 7.5% (15 mEq/15 ml), 10% (20 mEq/15 ml), 15% (30 mEq/15 ml), 20% (40 mEq/15 ml)
Powder for oral use: 15 mEq/packet, 20 mEq/packet, 25 mEq/packet, 25 mEq/dose
Injection: 20 mEq, 40 mEq ampules; additive syringes containing 30 mEq or 40 mEq; 10 mEq, 20 mEq, 30 mEq, 40 mEq, 45 mEq, 60 mEq, 100 mEq, 200 mEq, 400 mEq, or 1,000 mEq vials

ACTION
Replaces and maintains potassium level.

ONSET, PEAK, DURATION
Onset and serum levels peak immediately after I.V. infusion. Duration unknown.

INDICATIONS & DOSAGE
Hypokalemia –
Adults: 40 to 100 mEq P.O. daily in three or four divided doses for treatment; 20 mEq for prevention. Further

---

dosage based on serum potassium level.

Children: 3 mEq/kg daily. Total dosage not to exceed 150 mEq daily or 40 mEq/m^2.

Use I.V. route only when oral replacement is not feasible or when hypokalemia is life-threatening. If serum potassium is less than 2 mEq/ml, maximum infusion rate is 40 mEq/hour; maximum infusion concentration is 80 mEq/L; and maximum 24-hour dose is 400 mEq. If serum potassium level is greater than 2 mEq/ml, maximum infusion rate is 10 mEq/hour; maximum infusion concentration is 40 mEq/L; and maximum 24-hour dose is 200 mEq. For routine supplementation, the usual dose 20 mEq hourly in concentration of 40 mEq/L or less.

ADVERSE REACTIONS
Signs of hyperkalemia –
CNS: paresthesia of the extremities, listlessness, mental confusion, weakness or heaviness of limbs, flaccid paralysis.
CV: *peripheral vascular collapse with fall in blood pressure, arrhythmias, heart block, possible cardiac arrest,* ECG changes (prolonged PR interval; widened QRS complex; ST-segment depression; tall, tented T waves).
GI: *nausea, vomiting, abdominal pain,* diarrhea, GI ulcerations (possible stenosis, hemorrhage, obstruction, perforation).
GU: oliguria.
Skin: cold skin, gray pallor.
Other: *postinfusion phlebitis.*

INTERACTIONS
ACE inhibitors, potassium-sparing diuretics: risk of hyperkalemia. Use with extreme caution.

CONTRAINDICATIONS
Contraindicated in patients with severe renal impairment with oliguria, anuria, or azotemia; in those with untreated Addison's disease; and in patients with acute dehydration, heat cramps, hyperkalemia, hyperkalemic form of familial periodic paralysis, and other conditions associated with extensive tissue breakdown.

NURSING CONSIDERATIONS
• Use cautiously in patients with cardiac disease, and in those with renal impairment.
• **I.V. use:** Give by infusion only; never I.V. push or I.M. Give slowly as dilute solution; potentially fatal hyperkalemia may result from too-rapid infusion.
• Make sure powders are completely dissolved before administering.
• Give with or after meals with full glass of water or fruit juice to lessen GI distress.
• Know that enteric-coated tablets are not recommended because of increased potential for GI bleeding and small-bowel ulcerations.
• Keep in mind that tablets in wax matrix sometimes lodge in esophagus and cause ulceration in cardiac patients who have esophageal compression from enlarged left atrium. Use liquid form in such patients and in those with esophageal stasis or obstruction.
• Know that drug is often used orally with potassium-wasting diuretics to maintain potassium levels.
• Give oral potassium supplements with extreme caution because its many forms deliver varying amounts of potassium. Never switch products without a doctor's order.
• Be aware that sugar-free liquid is available (Kaochlor S-F 10%); use if tablet or capsule passage is likely to be delayed, such as in GI obstruction. Have patients sip slowly to minimize GI irritation.
• Don't crush sustained-release potassium products.

• Monitor ECG and serum electrolyte levels during therapy.
• Monitor renal function. Potassium should not be given during immediate postoperative period until urine flow is established.

potassium gluconate
Glu-K, Kaon Liquid*, Kaon Tablets, Kaylixir*, K-G Elixir*, Potassium-Rougier†

Pregnancy Risk Category: C

HOW SUPPLIED
Tablets: 500 mg (2 mEq K$^+$), 1,170 mg (5 mEq K$^+$)
Elixir: 4.68 g (20 mEq K$^+$)/15 ml*

ACTION
Replaces and maintains intracellular and extracellular potassium.

ONSET, PEAK, DURATION
Onset and duration unknown. Peak levels occur within 4 hours of oral dose.

INDICATIONS & DOSAGE
Hypokalemia –
Adults: 40 to 100 mEq P.O. daily in three or four divided doses for treatment; 20 mEq daily for prevention. Further dosage adjustments are based on serum potassium determinations.

ADVERSE REACTIONS
CNS: paresthesia of the extremities, listlessness, mental confusion, weakness or heaviness of legs, flaccid paralysis.
CV: *arrhythmias,* ECG changes (prolonged PR interval; widened QRS complex; ST-segment depression; tall, tented T waves).
GI: *nausea, vomiting, abdominal pain,* diarrhea, GI ulcerations with oral products (especially enteric-coated tablets); ulcerations may be accompanied by stenosis, hemorrhage, obstruction, perforation.

INTERACTIONS
ACE inhibitors, potassium-sparing diuretics: risk of hyperkalemia. Use with extreme caution.

CONTRAINDICATIONS
Contraindicated in patients with severe renal impairment with oliguria, anuria, or azotemia; in those with untreated Addison's disease; and in patients with acute dehydration, heat cramps, hyperkalemia, hyperkalemic form of familial periodic paralysis, and other conditions associated with extensive tissue breakdown.

NURSING CONSIDERATIONS
• Give oral potassium supplements with extreme caution because their many forms deliver varying amounts of potassium. Never switch products without a doctor's order.
• Use cautiously in patients with cardiac disease and in those with renal impairment.
• To lessen GI distress, give with or after meals with full glass of water or fruit juice.
• Advise the patient to sip liquid potassium slowly to minimize GI irritation.
• Know that enteric-coated tablets are not recommended because of increased potential for GI bleeding and small-bowel ulcerations.
• Don't administer potassium supplements postoperatively until urine flow has been established.
• Monitor ECG, serum potassium and creatinine levels, BUN, and fluid intake and output.
• Keep in mind that therapy with potassium gluconate does not correct hypokalemic hypochloremic alkalosis.

---

*Liquid form contains alcohol.
**May contain tartrazine.

Common reactions are in italics; ***life-threatening,*** in bold italics.

Ringer's injection

Pregnancy Risk Category: NR

HOW SUPPLIED
Injection: 250 ml, 500 ml, 1,000 ml

ACTION
Replaces fluids and electrolytes.

ONSET, PEAK, DURATION
Onset and serum levels peak immediately after I.V. infusion. Duration unknown.

INDICATIONS & DOSAGE
Fluid and electrolyte replacement —
Adults and children: dose highly individualized, but usually 1.5 to 3 liters (2% to 6% body weight) infused I.V. over 18 to 24 hours.

ADVERSE REACTIONS
CV: fluid overload.

INTERACTIONS
None significant.

CONTRAINDICATIONS
Contraindicated in patients with renal failure, except as emergency volume expander.

NURSING CONSIDERATIONS
• Use cautiously in patients with CHF, circulatory insufficiency, renal dysfunction, hypoproteinemia, and pulmonary edema.
• Know that Ringer's injection contains sodium, 147 mEq/liter; potassium, 4 mEq/liter; calcium, 4.5 mEq/liter; and chloride, 155.5 mEq/liter.
• Be aware that electrolyte content is insufficient for treating severe electrolyte deficiencies, but it does provide electrolytes in levels approximately equal to those of the blood.

Ringer's injection, lactated (Hartmann's solution, Ringer's lactate solution)

Pregnancy Risk Category: NR

HOW SUPPLIED
Injection: 150 ml, 250 ml, 500 ml, 1,000 ml

ACTION
Replaces fluids and electrolytes.

ONSET, PEAK, DURATION
Onset and serum levels peak immediately after I.V. infusion. Duration unknown.

INDICATIONS & DOSAGE
Fluid and electrolyte replacement —
Adults and children: dosage highly individualized, but usually 1.5 to 3 liters (2% to 6% body weight) infused I.V. over 18 to 24 hours.

ADVERSE REACTIONS
CV: fluid overload.

INTERACTIONS
None significant.

CONTRAINDICATIONS
Contraindicated in patients with renal failure, except as emergency volume expander.

NURSING CONSIDERATIONS
• Use cautiously in patients with CHF, circulatory insufficiency, renal dysfunction, hypoproteinemia, and pulmonary edema.
• Know that lactated Ringer's injection contains sodium, 130 mEq/liter; potassium, 4 mEq/liter; calcium, 3 mEq/liter; chloride, 109.7 mEq/liter; and lactate, 28 mEq/liter.
• Be aware that lactated Ringer's injection more closely approximates the electrolyte concentration in blood plasma.

sodium chloride

Pregnancy Risk Category: NR

HOW SUPPLIED

Tablets (enteric-coated): 1 g
Tablets (slow-release): 600 mg
Injection: 0.45% sodium chloride solution 500 ml, 1,000 ml; 0.9% sodium chloride solution 50 ml, 100 ml, 150 ml, 250 ml, 500 ml, 1,000 ml; 3% sodium chloride solution 500 ml; 5% sodium chloride solution 500 ml; 14.6% sodium chloride solution 20 ml, 40 ml, 200 ml; 23.4% sodium chloride solution 30 ml, 50 ml, and 200 ml.

ACTION

Replaces and maintains sodium and chloride levels.

ONSET, PEAK, DURATION

Onset and serum levels peak immediately after I.V. infusion. Duration unknown.

INDICATIONS & DOSAGE

Fluid and electrolyte replacement in hyponatremia caused by electrolyte loss or in severe salt depletion –
Adults: dosage is highly individualized. 3% or 5% solution used only with frequent electrolyte determination and given only slow I.V. With 0.45% solution: 3% to 8% of body weight, according to deficiencies, over 18 to 24 hours; with 0.9% solution: 2% to 6% of body weight, according to deficiencies, over 18 to 24 hours.
Management of heat cramp caused by excessive perspiration –
Adults: 1 g P.O. with every glass of water.

ADVERSE REACTIONS

CV: aggravation of CHF; edema if given too rapidly or in excess.
Respiratory: *pulmonary edema* if given too rapidly or in excess.

Other: hypernatremia and aggravation of existing metabolic acidosis with excessive infusion; serious electrolyte disturbances, loss of potassium.

INTERACTIONS

None significant.

CONTRAINDICATIONS

Contraindicated in patients with conditions in which sodium and chloride administration is detrimental. Sodium chloride 3% and 5% injections are contraindicated in patients with increased, normal, or only slightly decreased serum electrolyte concentrations.

NURSING CONSIDERATIONS

• Use cautiously in patients with CHF, circulatory insufficiency, renal dysfunction, and hypoproteinemia and in elderly or post-operative patients.
• **I.V. use:** Infuse 3% and 5% solutions very slowly and cautiously to avoid pulmonary edema. Use only for critical situations, and observe the patient continually.
• Don't confuse concentrates (14.6%, 23.4%) available to add to parenteral nutrient solutions, with 0.9% sodium chloride injection, and never administer without diluting. Read label carefully.
• Monitor serum electrolyte levels.

---

*Liquid form contains alcohol. *Common* reactions are in italics; *life-threatening,* in bold italics.
**May contain tartrazine.

64

Acidifier and alkalinizers

ammonium chloride
sodium bicarbonate
sodium lactate
tromethamine

COMBINATION PRODUCTS
None.

---

ammonium chloride◇

Pregnancy Risk Category: C

HOW SUPPLIED
Tablets: 500 mg◇
Tablets (enteric-coated): 500 mg◇,
1,000 mg◇
Injection: 2.14% (0.4 mEq/ml),
26.75% (5 mEq/ml)

ACTION
Increases free hydrogen ion concentration, resulting in acidosis, and acts as an expectorant by causing reflex stimulation of bronchial mucous glands.

ONSET, PEAK, DURATION
Onset and serum levels peak immediately after I.V. infusion. Duration unknown.

INDICATIONS & DOSAGE
Metabolic alkalosis; chloride replacement —
Adults and children: I.V. dose (in mEq) is equal to the serum chloride deficit (in mEq/ml) multiplied by the extracellular fluid volume (estimated as 20% of the body weight in kilograms). One-half the calculated volume should be given, then the patient reassessed.
Acidifier —
Adults: 4 to 12 g P.O. daily in divided doses q 4 to 6 hours.

Children: 75 mg/kg P.O. daily in four divided doses.

ADVERSE REACTIONS
Adverse reactions usually result from ammonia toxicity or too-rapid I.V. administration.
CNS: headache, confusion, progressive drowsiness, excitement alternating with *coma,* hyperventilation, *calcium-deficient tetany,* twitching, hyperreflexia, EEG abnormalities.
CV: bradycardia.
GI: with oral dose —*gastric irritation, nausea, vomiting,* thirst, anorexia, retching.
GU: glycosuria.
Skin: rash, pallor.
Other: *metabolic acidosis, hyperchloremia, hypokalemia,* hyperglycemia, pain at injection site, irregular respirations with periods of apnea.

INTERACTIONS
Spironolactone: increased systemic acidosis. Use together cautiously.

CONTRAINDICATIONS
Contraindicated in patients with primary respiratory acidosis and high total carbon dioxide (CO_2) and buffer base and in those with severe hepatic or renal dysfunction (as self-medication).

NURSING CONSIDERATIONS
• Use cautiously in patients with pulmonary insufficiency or cardiac edema and in infants.
• Determine CO_2 combining power and serum electrolytes before and during therapy to prevent acidosis. Each gram of ammonium chloride will reduce the CO_2 combining power by 1.1 volume percent.
• **I.V. use:** Dilute concentrated form

(26.75%) before administration. Add 100 to 200 mEq (20 to 40 ml of the 26.75% solution) to 500 or 1,000 ml of 0.9% sodium chloride injection. Administer via infusion pump, not exceeding 5 ml/min in adults.
• Lessen pain of I.V. injection by decreasing infusion rate.
• To decrease GI adverse reactions, give oral form after meals. Enteric-coated tablets may also minimize GI symptoms but are absorbed erratically.
• Do not administer drug with milk or other alkaline solutions; they are not compatible.
• Monitor urine pH and output. Diuresis is normal for first 2 days.
• Monitor rate and depth of respirations frequently.

---

sodium bicarbonate◊
Arm and Hammer Pure Baking Soda, Bell/ans, Citrocarbonate, Soda Mint

Pregnancy Risk Category: NR

HOW SUPPLIED
Tablets◊: 300 mg, 325 mg, 520 mg, 600 mg, 650 mg
Injection: 4% (2.4 mEq/5 ml), 4.2% (5 mEq/10 ml), 5% (297.5 mEq/500 ml), 7.5% (8.92 mEq/10 ml and 44.6 mEq/50 ml), 8.4% (10 mEq/10 ml and 50 mEq/50 ml)

ACTION
Restores body's buffering capacity of the body and neutralizes excess acid.

ONSET, PEAK, DURATION
Onset and peak serum levels occur immediately after I.V. infusion. Duration unknown after I.V. infusion. Onset, peak, and duration unknown after oral administration.

INDICATIONS & DOSAGE
Cardiac arrest–
Adults and children: 1 mEq/kg I.V.

of 7.5% or 8.4% solution followed by 0.5 mEq/kg I.V. every 10 minutes, depending on blood gases. Further dosages based on results of blood gas analysis. If blood gases unavailable, use 0.5 mEq/kg I.V. every 10 minutes until spontaneous circulation returns.
Infants up to 2 years: not to exceed 8 mEq/kg I.V. daily of 4.2% solution.
Metabolic acidosis–
Adults and children: dosage depends on blood CO_2 content, pH, and the patient's clinical condition. Generally, 2 to 5 mEq/kg I.V. infused over 4- to 8-hour period.
Systemic or urinary alkalinization–
Adults: initially, 4 g P.O., followed by 1 to 2 g q 4 hours.
Children: 84 to 840 mg/kg P.O. daily.
Antacid–
Adults: 300 mg to 2 g P.O. up to q.i.d. taken with glass of water.

ADVERSE REACTIONS
GI: gastric distention, belching, flatulence.
GU: renal calculi or crystals.
Other: with overdose – *metabolic alkalosis*, hypernatremia, *hyperkalemia*, hyperosmolarity.

INTERACTIONS
Anorexients, flecainide, mecamylamine, quinidine, sympathomimetics: increased urine alkalinization causes increased renal clearance of these drugs and reduced effectiveness. Monitor closely.
Chlorpropamide, lithium, methotrexate, salicylates, tetracycline: urine alkalinization causes decreased renal clearance of these drugs and increased risk of toxicity. Monitor closely.
Enteric-coated drugs: may be released prematurely in stomach. Avoid concomitant use.

CONTRAINDICATIONS
Contraindicated in patients with metabolic or respiratory alkalosis, in pa-

---

*Liquid form contains alcohol.　　*Common* reactions are in italics; *life-threatening*, in bold italics.
**May contain tartrazine.

tients who are losing chlorides by
vomiting or from continuous GI suction, in those receiving diuretics
known to produce hypochloremic alkalosis; and in those with hypocalcemia in which alkalosis may produce
tetany, hypertension, seizures, or
CHF. Orally administered sodium bicarbonate is contraindicated in patients with acute ingestion of strong
mineral acids.

NURSING CONSIDERATIONS
• Use with extreme caution in patients with CHF or other edematous
or sodium-retaining conditions or
renal insufficiency.
• **I.V. use:** May be added to other I.V.
fluids. Sodium bicarbonate inactivates such catecholamines as norepinephrine and dopamine, and forms
precipitate with calcium. Do not mix
sodium bicarbonate with I.V. solutions of these agents, and flush I.V.
line adequately.
• To avoid risk of alkalosis, obtain
blood pH, PaO_2, $PaCO_2$, and serum
electrolytes. Keep the doctor informed of serum laboratory results.
• If sodium bicarbonate is being used
to produce an alkaline urine, monitor
urine pH every 4 to 6 hours (should be
> 7.0).
• Be aware that sodium bicarbonate is
not routinely recommended for use in
cardiac arrest because it may produce
a paradoxical acidosis from CO_2 production. It should not be routinely administered during the early stages of
resuscitation unless preexisting acidosis is clearly present. May be used
at team leader's discretion after such
interventions as defibrillation, cardiac
compression, and administration of
first-line drugs.
• Tell the patient not to take with
milk. May cause hypercalcemia, alkalosis, and possibly renal calculi.
• Discourage use as an antacid. Offer
a nonabsorbable alternative antacid if
it is to be used repeatedly.

sodium lactate
Pregnancy Risk Category: NR

HOW SUPPLIED
Injection: ⅙ molar solution (167
mEq/liter)
Injection: 5 mEq/ml

ACTION
Metabolized to sodium bicarbonate,
producing buffering effect.

ONSET, PEAK, DURATION
Onset and serum levels peak immediately after I.V. infusion. The conversion of sodium lactate to bicarbonate
requires 1 to 2 hours. Duration unknown.

INDICATIONS & DOSAGE
Alkalinize urine –
Adults: 30 ml of ⅙ molar solution/kg
of body weight I.V. given in divided
doses over 24 hours.
Metabolic acidosis –
Adults: ⅙ molar injection (167 mEq
lactate/L I.V.); dosage depends on degree of bicarbonate deficit.

ADVERSE REACTIONS
Other: fever, infection or thrombophlebitis at injection site; with overdose – *metabolic alkalosis,* hypernatremia, hyperosmolarity.

INTERACTIONS
None significant.

CONTRAINDICATIONS
Contraindicated in patients with hypernatremia, lactic acidosis, or conditions in which sodium administration
is detrimental.

NURSING CONSIDERATIONS
• Use with extreme caution in patients with metabolic or respiratory
alkalosis, severe hepatic or renal disease, shock, hypoxia, or beriberi.
• **I.V. use:** Add sodium lactate to

other I.V. solutions, or give as an isotonic ⅙ molar solution. Drug is compatible with most common I.V. solutions.
• Do not mix with sodium bicarbonate because the drugs are physically incompatible.
• Monitor serum electrolyte levels to avoid alkalosis.

tromethamine
Tham

Pregnancy Risk Category: C

HOW SUPPLIED
Injection: 18 g/500 ml

ACTION
Combines with hydrogen ions and associated acid anions; resulting salts are excreted. Also has osmotic diuretic effect.

ONSET, PEAK, DURATION
Onset and serum levels peak immediately after I.V. infusion. Duration unknown.

INDICATIONS & DOSAGE
Metabolic acidosis associated with cardiac bypass surgery or with cardiac arrest –
Adults: dosage depends on bicarbonate deficit. Calculate as follows: each ml of 0.3 M tromethamine solution required = weight in kg × bicarbonate deficit (mEq/L). Additional therapy based on serial determinations of existing bicarbonate deficit.
Children: calculate dosage as above. Give slowly over 3 to 6 hours. Additional therapy based on degree of acidosis. Total 24-hour dosage should not exceed 33 to 40 ml/kg.

ADVERSE REACTIONS
Respiratory: *respiratory depression.*
Other: hypoglycemia, *hyperkalemia* (with decreased urine output), venospasm; I.V. thrombosis; inflammation,

necrosis, and sloughing if extravasation occurs.

INTERACTIONS
None significant.

CONTRAINDICATIONS
Contraindicated in patients with anuria, uremia, or chronic respiratory acidosis, or during pregnancy (except in acute, life-threatening situations).

NURSING CONSIDERATIONS
• Use cautiously in patients with renal disease and poor urine output. Monitor ECG and serum potassium levels in these patients.
• Make the following determinations before, during and after therapy: blood pH; carbon dioxide tension; bicarbonate, glucose, and electrolyte levels.
• **I.V. use:** Give slowly through 18G to 20G needle into largest antecubital vein, or by indwelling I.V. catheter.
• Be aware that drug should not be used longer than 1 day except in life-threatening situations.
• In patients with associated respiratory acidosis, have mechanical ventilation available.
• To prevent blood pH from rising above normal, be prepared to adjust dosage carefully, as ordered.
• If extravasation occurs, infiltrate area with 1% procaine and 150 units hyaluronidase, as ordered; may reduce vasospasm and dilute remaining drug locally.

---

*Liquid form contains alcohol.   *Common* reactions are in italics; *life-threatening,* in bold italics.
**May contain tartrazine.

65

Hematinics

ferrous fumarate
ferrous gluconate
ferrous sulfate
ferrous sulfate, dried
iron dextran
polysaccharide iron complex

COMBINATION PRODUCTS

FERGON PLUS: ferrous gluconate 58 mg, vitamin B_{12} ½ NF unit with intrinsic factor, and vitamin C 75 mg.
FEROCYL◇: ferrous fumarate 50 mg and docusate sodium 100 mg.
FERRO-DOCUSATE-T.R., FERRO-DOK TR, FERRO-DSS: ferrous fumarate 150 mg and docusate sodium 100 mg.
FERRO-SEQUELS◇: ferrous fumarate 50 mg and docusate sodium 100 mg.

ferrous fumarate

Femiron◇, Feostat◇, Feostat Drops◇, Fumasorb◇, Fumerin◇, Hemocyte◇, Ircon◇, Nephro-Fer◇, Novofumar†, Palafer†, Palafer Pediatric Drops†, Span-FF◇

Pregnancy Risk Category: A

HOW SUPPLIED

Each 100 mg of ferrous fumarate provides 33 mg of elemental iron.
Tablets◇: 60 mg, 195 mg, 200 mg, 300 mg, 324 mg, 325 mg
Tablets (chewable): 100 mg◇
Capsules (extended-release): 325 mg◇
Oral suspension: 100 mg/5 ml◇
Drops: 45 mg/0.6 ml◇

ACTION

Provides elemental iron, an essential component in the formation of hemoglobin.

ONSET, PEAK, DURATION

Onset occurs within 4 days. Peak effects occur in 7 to 10 days. Effects persist for 2 to 4 months.

INDICATIONS & DOSAGE

Iron deficiency –
Adults: 200 mg P.O. t.i.d. or q.i.d.
Children: 3 mg/kg P.O. t.i.d., increased to 6 mg/kg P.O. t.i.d. as needed and tolerated.

ADVERSE REACTIONS

GI: *nausea,* epigastric pain, vomiting, *constipation,* diarrhea, black stools.
Other: suspension and drops may temporarily stain teeth.

INTERACTIONS

Antacids, cholestyramine resin, fluoroquinolones, levodopa, penicillamine, tetracycline, vitamin E: decreased iron absorption. Separate doses by 2 to 4 hours.
Chloramphenicol: delayed response to iron therapy. Watch patient carefully.
L-thyroxine: decreased L-thyroxine absorption. Separate doses by at least 2 hours. Monitor thyroid function.
Vitamin C: may increase iron absorption. Beneficial drug interaction.

CONTRAINDICATIONS

Contraindicated in patients with primary hemochromatosis or hemosiderosis, in patients with hemolytic anemia unless an iron deficiency anemia is also present, in those receiving repeated blood transfusions, and in patients with peptic ulcer disease, regional enteritis, or ulcerative colitis.

†Available in Canada only. ‡Available in Australia only. ◇Available OTC.

NURSING CONSIDERATIONS
- Use cautiously on long-term basis.
- Give tablets with juice (preferably orange juice) or water, but not with milk or antacids.
- To avoid staining teeth, give suspension with straw and place drops at back of throat.
- Do not crush or allow the patient to chew extended-release iron preparations.
- Keep in mind that GI upset may be related to dose. Between-meal dosing preferable, but can be given with some foods, although absorption may be decreased. Enteric-coated products reduce GI upset but also reduce amount of iron absorbed.
- Check for constipation; record color and amount of stool.
- Be aware that oral iron may turn stools black. Although this unabsorbed iron is harmless, it could mask the presence of melena.
- Monitor hemoglobin and hematocrit levels and reticulocyte counts during therapy, as ordered.
- Know that combination products, such as Ferro-Sequels and Ferocyl, contain stool softeners, which help prevent constipation, a common adverse reaction.
- Inform parents that as little as three or four tablets can cause serious poisoning in children.
- If the patient misses a dose, tell him to take it as soon as he remembers but not to double-dose.
- Advise patient to avoid certain foods that may impair oral iron absorption, including yogurt, cheese, eggs, milk, whole-grain breads and cereals, tea, and coffee.
- Teach dietary measures for preventing constipation.

ferrous gluconate
Fergon*◊, Ferralet◊, Fertinic†, Novoferrogluc†

Pregnancy Risk Category: A

HOW SUPPLIED
Each 100 mg of ferrous gluconate provides 11.6 mg of elemental iron.
Tablets: 300 mg◊, 320 mg◊ (contains 37 mg Fe$^+$), 325 mg◊
Capsules: 86 mg◊, 325 mg◊, 435 mg◊
Elixir: 300 mg/5 ml (contains 35 mg Fe$^+$)*◊

ACTION
Provides elemental iron, an essential component in the formation of hemoglobin.

ONSET, PEAK, DURATION
Onset occurs in 4 days. Peak effects occur in 7 to 10 days. Effects persist for 2 to 4 months.

INDICATIONS & DOSAGE
Iron deficiency –
Adults: 300 to 325 mg P.O. q.i.d., increased to 650 mg q.i.d. as needed and tolerated.
Children 2 years or older: 8 mg/kg P.O. daily t.i.d., increased up to 16 mg P.O. t.i.d. as needed and tolerated.

ADVERSE REACTIONS
GI: *nausea,* epigastric pain, vomiting, *constipation,* diarrhea, *black stools.*
Other: elixir may temporarily stain teeth.

INTERACTIONS
Antacids, cholestyramine resin, fluoroquinolones, levodopa, penicillamine, tetracycline, vitamin E: decreased iron absorption. Separate doses by at least 2 hours.
Chloramphenicol: delayed response to

---

*Liquid form contains alcohol.   *Common* reactions are in italics; **life-threatening,** in bold italics.
**May contain tartrazine.

iron therapy. Watch the patient carefully.

L-thyroxine: decreased L-thyroxine absorption. Separate doses by at least 2 hours. Monitor thyroid function.

Vitamin C: may increase iron absorption. Beneficial drug interaction.

CONTRAINDICATIONS

Contraindicated in patients with peptic ulceration, regional enteritis, ulcerative colitis, hemosiderosis, and primary hemochromatosis; in patients with hemolytic anemia unless an iron deficiency anemia is also present; and in patients receiving repeated blood transfusions.

NURSING CONSIDERATIONS

• Use cautiously on long-term basis.
• Dilute liquid preparations in juice (preferably orange juice) or water, but not in milk or antacids. To promote absorption, give tablets with orange juice.
• To avoid staining teeth, give elixirs with straw; the patient may take with water or fruit juice.
• Keep in mind that GI upset may be related to dose. Between-meal dosing preferable, but can be given with some foods, although absorption may be decreased. Enteric-coated products reduce GI upset but also reduce amount of iron absorbed.
• Check for constipation; record color and amount of stool.
• Be aware that oral iron may turn stools black. This unabsorbed iron is harmless; however, it could mask melena.
• Monitor hemoglobin and hematocrit levels and reticulocyte counts during therapy.
• Inform parents that as little as three or four tablets can cause serious iron poisoning in children.
• If the patient misses a dose, tell him

to take it as soon as he remembers but not to double-dose.
• Advise patient to avoid certain foods that may impair oral iron absorption, including yogurt, cheese, eggs, milk, whole-grain breads and cereals, tea, and coffee.
• Teach dietary measures for preventing constipation.

ferrous sulfate

Apo-Ferrous Sulfate†, Feosol*◊, Fer-In-Sol*◊, Fer-In-Sol Drops*◊, Fer-In-Sol Syrup*◊, Fer-Iron Drops◊, Feritard‡, Fero-Grad†, Fero-Gradumet◊, Ferospace◊, Ferralyn Lanacaps◊, Ferra-TD

ferrous sulfate, dried

Mol-Iron*◊, Novoferrosulfa†, PMS Ferrous Sulfate†, Slow-Fe◊

Pregnancy Risk Category: A

HOW SUPPLIED

Ferrous sulfate is 20% elemental iron; dried and powdered, about 32% elemental iron.

Tablets: 195 mg◊, 300 mg◊, 325 mg◊; 200 mg (dried)
Tablets (extended-release): 160 mg (dried)◊, 525 mg
Capsules: 150 mg◊, 159 mg (dried), 190 mg (dried), 250 mg◊, 390 mg◊
Capsules (extended-release): 159 mg (dried)◊, 525 mg◊
Elixir: 220 mg/5 ml*◊
Syrup: 90 mg/5 ml◊
Solution: 300 mg/5 ml
Drops: 125 mg/ml

ACTION

Provides elemental iron, an essential component in the formation of hemoglobin.

ONSET, PEAK, DURATION

Onset occurs within 4 days. Peak effects occur within 7 to 10 days. Effects persist for 2 to 4 months.

INDICATIONS & DOSAGE

Iron deficiency –
Adults: 325 mg P.O. t.i.d. or q.i.d. Alternatively, 1 extended-release capsule (160 to 525 mg) P.O. b.i.d.

Children: 5 to 10 mg/kg P.O. t.i.d.

ADVERSE REACTIONS

GI: *nausea,* epigastric pain, vomiting, *constipation, black stools,* diarrhea.
Other: liquid forms may temporarily stain teeth.

INTERACTIONS

Antacids, cholestyramine resin, fluoroquinolones, levodopa, penicillamine, tetracycline, vitamin E: decreased iron absorption. Separate doses if possible.
Chloramphenicol: delayed response to iron therapy. Watch patient carefully.
L-thyroxine: decreased L-thyroxine absorption. Separate doses by at least 2 hours. Monitor thyroid function.
Vitamin C: may increase iron absorption. Beneficial drug interaction.

CONTRAINDICATIONS

Contraindicated in patients with hemosiderosis and primary hemochromatosis; in those with hemolytic anemia unless iron deficiency anemia is also present; in those with peptic ulceration, ulcerative colitis, and regional enteritis; and in patients receiving repeated blood transfusions.

NURSING CONSIDERATIONS

• Use cautiously on long-term basis.
• Dilute liquid preparations in juice (preferably orange juice) or water, but not in milk or antacids. To promote iron absorption, give tablets with orange juice.
• To avoid staining teeth, give elixirs with straw and place in back of throat.
• Do not crush or allow the patient to chew extended-release preparations.
• Keep in mind that GI upset may be related to dose. Between-meal dosing preferable, but can be given with some foods, although absorption may be decreased. Enteric-coated products reduce GI upset but also reduce amount of iron absorbed.
• Check for constipation; record color and amount of stool.
• Be aware that oral iron may turn stools black. Although this unabsorbed iron is harmless, it could mask melena.
• Monitor hemoglobin and hematocrit levels and reticulocyte counts during therapy, as ordered.
• Be aware that rate and extent of iron absorption varies with need; normal patients absorb only 5% to 10% of dietary iron, whereas patients with iron deficiency can absorb 30% or more of dietary iron.
• Inform parents that as little as three to four tablets can cause serious iron poisoning in children.
• If the patient misses a dose, tell him to take it as soon as he remembers, but not to double-dose.
• Advise patient to avoid certain foods that may impair oral iron absorption, including yogurt, cheese, eggs, milk, whole-grain breads and cereals, tea, and coffee.
• Teach dietary measures for preventing constipation.

iron dextran
Hydextran, Imferon, InFeD, K-FeRON, Proferdex
Pregnancy Risk Category: NR

HOW SUPPLIED
1 ml iron dextran provides 50 mg elemental iron.
Injection: 50 mg elemental iron/ml

ACTION
Provides elemental iron, an essential component in the formation of hemoglobin.

---

*Liquid form contains alcohol.   *Common* reactions are in italics; *life-threatening,* in bold italics.
**May contain tartrazine.

ONSET, PEAK, DURATION
Not clearly defined.

INDICATIONS & DOSAGE
Iron deficiency anemia –
Adults: I.M. or I.V. test dose required before administration.
I.M. (by Z-track method): 0.5 ml test dose injected. If no reactions occur, daily dosage should ordinarily not exceed 0.5 ml (25 mg) for infants under 5 kg; 1 ml (50 mg) for children under 10 kg; 2 ml (100 mg) for heavier children and adults.
I.V.: 0.5 ml test dose injected over 30 seconds. If no reactions occur in 1 hour, remainder of therapeutic dose I.V. is given. Therapeutic dose repeated I.V. daily. Single dose should not exceed 100 mg. Give slowly (1 ml/minute).

ADVERSE REACTIONS
CNS: headache, transitory paresthesia, arthralgia, myalgia, dizziness, malaise, syncope.
CV: chest pain, chest tightness, shock, hypertension, arrhythmias, *hypotensive reaction, peripheral vascular flushing with overly rapid I.V. administration, tachycardia.*
GI: nausea, vomiting, metallic taste, transient loss of taste, abdominal pain, diarrhea.
Respiratory: *bronchospasm.*
Skin: rash, urticaria.
Other: *soreness and inflammation at I.M. injection site; brown skin discoloration at I.M. injection site; local phlebitis at I.V. injection site,* sterile abscess, necrosis, atrophy, fibrosis, *anaphylaxis,* delayed sensitivity reactions.

INTERACTIONS
None significant.

CONTRAINDICATIONS
Contraindicated in patients with hypersensitivity to the drug, in those with all anemias except iron deficiency anemia, and in those with acute infectious renal disease.

NURSING CONSIDERATIONS
• Do not administer iron dextran concomitantly with oral iron preparations.
• Use with extreme caution in patients with serious hepatic impairment, rheumatoid arthritis, and other inflammatory diseases because these patients may be at higher risk for certain delays and reactions.
• Use cautiously in patients with a history of significant allergies and/or asthma.
• **I.V. use:** Check hospital policy before administering I.V.
• Keep in mind that I.M. or I.V. injections of iron are advisable only for patients for whom oral administration is impossible or ineffective. Use I.V. in these situations: Insufficient muscle mass for deep I.M. injection; impaired absorption from muscle due to stasis or edema; possibility of uncontrolled I.M. bleeding from trauma (as may occur in hemophilia); and with massive and prolonged parenteral therapy (as may be necessary in cases of chronic substantial blood loss).
• Upon completion of I.V. dose, flush the vein with 10 ml of 0.9% sodium chloride solution. The patient should rest 15 to 30 minutes after I.V. administration.
• Inject deeply into upper outer quadrant of buttock — never into arm or other exposed area — with a 2- to 3-inch, 19G or 20G needle. Use Z-track method to avoid leakage into S.C. tissue and staining of skin.
• Minimize skin staining by using a separate needle to withdraw the drug from its container.
• Monitor the patient's vital signs for drug reactions, which range from pain, inflammation, and myalgia to hypotension, shock, and death.
• Monitor hemoglobin and hematocrit

---

levels and reticulocyte count, as ordered.
• Be aware that the drug is not removed by hemodialysis.

polysaccharide iron complex
Hytinic, Niferex, Niferex-150, Nu-Iron, Nu-Iron-150

Pregnancy Risk Category: NR

HOW SUPPLIED
Capsules: 150 mg
Solution: 100 mg/5 ml
Tablets (film-coated): 50 mg

ACTION
Provides elemental iron, an essential component in the formation of hemoglobin.

ONSET, PEAK, DURATION
Onset occurs within a few days. Peak reticulocyte effects occur in 5 to 10 days and hemoglobin concentrations rise after 2 to 4 weeks. Normal hemoglobin values are usually attained in 2 months unless blood loss continues.

INDICATIONS & DOSAGE
Treatment of uncomplicated iron deficiency anemia –
Adults and children 12 years and over: 150 to 300 mg P.O. as capsules or tablets daily or 1 to 2 teaspoonsful of elixir P.O. daily.
Children 6 to 12 years: 150 mg to 300 mg P.O. as tablets or 1 teaspoonful of elixir P.O. daily.
Children 2 to 6 years: ½ teaspoonful P.O. daily.

ADVERSE REACTIONS
Although nausea, constipation, black stools, and epigastric pain are common adverse reactions associated with iron therapy, few, if any, occur with polysaccharide iron complex.

INTERACTIONS
Antacids, cholestyramine resin, cimetidine, tetracycline, vitamin E: decreased iron absorption. Separate doses by 2 to 4 hours.
Chloramphenicol: delayed response to iron therapy. Monitor patient carefully.
Fluoroquinolones, levodopa, methyldopa, penicillamine: decreased GI absorption, possibly resulting in decreased serum levels or efficacy.
Vitamin C: may increase iron absorption, a beneficial drug interaction.

CONTRAINDICATIONS
Contraindicated in patients with hypersensitivity to any component of the drug and in those with hemochromatosis and hemosiderosis.

NURSING CONSIDERATIONS
• Give with juice (preferably orange juice) or water but not with milk or antacids.
• Keep in mind that this drug is nontoxic and that relatively few, if any, GI adverse effects associated with other iron preparations occur.
• Check for constipation; record color and amount of stool.
• Be aware that oral iron may turn stools black. This unabsorbed iron is harmless; however, it may mask melena.
• Monitor hemoglobin and hematocrit values and reticulocyte counts during therapy.
• Inform parents that as few as 3 tablets can cause serious iron poisoning in children.
• If the patient misses a dose, tell him to take it as soon as he remembers but not to double-dose.
• Advise patient to avoid certain foods that may impair oral iron absorption, including yogurt, cheese, eggs, milk, whole-grain breads and cereals, tea, and coffee.
• Teach the patient about dietary measures that help prevent constipation.

---

*Liquid form contains alcohol.
**May contain tartrazine.   *Common* reactions are in italics; *life-threatening,* in bold italics.

dalteparin sodium
dicumarol
enoxaparin sodium
heparin calcium
heparin sodium
warfarin sodium

COMBINATION PRODUCTS
None.

dalteparin sodium
Fragmin

Pregnancy Risk Category: B

HOW SUPPLIED
Syringe: 2,500 anti-factor Xa IU/0.2 ml

ACTION
A low-molecular-weight heparin derivative that enhances the inhibition of factor Xa and thrombin by antithrombin.

ONSET, PEAK, DURATION
Onset and duration unknown. Peak anti-factor Xa activity is obtained in about 4 hours.

INDICATIONS & DOSAGE
Prophylaxis against deep vein thrombosis in patients undergoing abdominal surgery who are at risk for thromboembolic complications –
Adults: 2,500 IU S.C. daily, starting 1 to 2 hours prior to surgery and repeated once daily for 5 to 10 days postoperatively.

ADVERSE REACTIONS
Hematologic: thrombocytopenia.
Skin: pruritus, rash.
Local: *hematoma at injection site,* pain or skin necrosis (rare) at injection site.

Other: hemorrhage, ecchymosis, bleeding complications, fever, *anaphylactoid reactions (rare)*.

INTERACTIONS
Oral anticoagulants, antiplatelet agents: May increase risk of bleeding. Use together cautiously.

CONTRAINDICATIONS
Contraindicated in patients with hypersensitivity to the drug, heparin, or pork products; active major bleeding; or thrombocytopenia associated with positive in vitro tests for antiplatelet antibody in the presence of the drug.

NURSING CONSIDERATIONS
• Use with extreme caution in patients with history of heparin-induced thrombocytopenia and in those with increased risk of hemorrhage, such as those with severe uncontrolled hypertension, bacterial endocarditis, congenital or acquired bleeding disorders, active ulceration and angiodysplastic GI disease, or hemorrhagic stroke or shortly after brain, spinal, or ophthalmologic surgery.
• Use with caution in patients with bleeding diathesis, thrombocytopenia, platelet defects, severe liver or kidney insufficiency, hypertensive or diabetic retinopathy, and recent GI bleeding.
• Know that patients who are candidates for dalteparin therapy are those who are at risk for deep vein thrombosis, including patients who are over age 40, obese, undergoing surgery under general anesthesia lasting longer than 30 minutes, or have additional risk factors (such as malignancy or a history of deep vein thrombosis or pulmonary embolism).
• Have patient assume a sitting or su-

pine position when administering the drug. Administer S.C. injection deeply. Injection sites include a U-shaped area around the navel, the upper outer side of the thigh, and the upper outer quadrangle of the buttock. Rotate sites daily. When the area around the navel or the thigh is used, use thumb and forefinger to lift up a fold of skin while giving the injection. The entire length of the needle should be inserted at a 45- to 90-degree angle.

• Never administer the drug I.M.
• Do not mix with other injections or infusions unless specific compatibility data are available that support such mixing.
• Be aware that drug cannot be interchangeable (unit for unit) with unfractionated heparin or other low-molecular-weight heparin.
• Know that periodic, routine CBCs (including platelet count) and fecal occult blood tests are recommended during the course of treatment. Patients do not require regular monitoring of PT or activated partial thromboplastin time.
• Monitor patient closely for thrombocytopenia.
• Be aware that the drug should be discontinued if a thromboembolic event occurs despite dalteparin prophylaxis.
• Instruct the patient and family to watch for signs of bleeding and notify the doctor immediately.
• Tell the patient to avoid OTC medications containing aspirin or other salicylates.

dicumarol
(bishydroxycoumarin)

Pregnancy Risk Category: NR

HOW SUPPLIED
Tablets: 25 mg, 50 mg

ACTION
Inhibits vitamin K-dependent activation of clotting factors II, VII, IX, and X, formed in the liver.

ONSET, PEAK, DURATION
Onset occurs in 1 to 5 days. Peak unknown. Effects persist for 2 to 10 days.

INDICATIONS & DOSAGE
Pulmonary embolism associated with chronic atrial fibrillation, deep vein thrombosis, MI, rheumatic heart disease with heart valve damage, and prosthetic heart valves –
Adults: 200 to 300 mg P.O. on first day, 25 to 200 mg P.O. daily thereafter depending on PT.

ADVERSE REACTIONS
GI: anorexia, nausea, vomiting, cramps, *diarrhea,* mouth ulcerations.
GU: hematuria.
Hematologic: *hemorrhage with excessive dosage,* leukopenia, ***agranulocytosis.***
Hepatic: hepatitis, elevated liver function tests, jaundice.
Skin: dermatitis, urticaria, necrosis, gangrene, alopecia, *rash.*
Other: *fever.*

INTERACTIONS
Acetaminophen: may increase bleeding with chronic (greater than 2 weeks) therapy with high doses (> 2 g/day) of acetaminophen. Monitor very carefully.
Allopurinol, amiodarone, anabolic steroids, cephalosporins, chloramphenicol, cimetidine, ciprofloxacin, clofibrate, danazol, diazoxide, diflunisal, disulfiram, erythromycin, ethacrynic acid, fenoprofen calcium, fluoroquinolones, glucagon, heparin, ibuprofen, influenza virus vaccine, isoniazid, ketoprofen, lovastatin, meclofenamate, methimazole, methylthiouracil, metronidazole, miconazole, nalidixic acid, neomycin (oral),

---

*Liquid form contains alcohol.   *Common* reactions are in italics; ***life-threatening,*** in bold italics.
**May contain tartrazine.

pentoxifylline, propafenone, propoxyphene, propylthiouracil, quinidine, streptokinase, sulfinpyrazone, sulfonamides, sulindac, tamoxifen, tetracyclines, thiazides, thyroid drugs, tricyclic antidepressants, urokinase, vitamin E: increased PT. Monitor the patient carefully for bleeding. Consider anticoagulant dosage reduction.

Barbiturates: inhibited hypoprothrombinemic effect of dicumarol. If barbiturates are withdrawn, reduce anticoagulant dosage; inhibition may last weeks after barbiturate is withdrawn, but fatal hemorrhage can occur when inhibiting effect disappears.

Carbamazepine, corticosteroids, corticotropin, ethchlorvynol, griseofulvin, mercaptopurine, methaqualone, nafcillin, oral contraceptives containing estrogen, rifampin, spironolactone, sulcralfate, trazodone: decreased PT with reduced anticoagulant effect. Monitor patient carefully.

Chloral hydrate, glutethimide, sulfinpyrazone, triclofos sodium: increased or decreased PT. Avoid use if possible, and monitor the patient carefully.

Cholestyramine: decreased response when administered too close together. Administer 6 hours after oral anticoagulants.

Hydantoins: increased serum levels of hydantoin. Monitor closely.

Indomethacin, mefenamic acid, salicylates: increased PT; ulcerogenic effects. Don't use together.

Sulfonylureas (oral antidiabetic agents): increased hypoglycemic response. Monitor blood glucose levels.

Foods or enteral products containing vitamin K: may impair anticoagulation. Patient should maintain consistent daily intake of leafy green vegetables.

CONTRAINDICATIONS

Contraindicated in patients with hemophilia, thrombocytopenic purpura, polycythemia vera, leukemia with pronounced bleeding tendency, open wounds or ulcerations, cerebrovascular hemorrhage, aneurysms, pericarditis, pericardial effusions, vasculitis, diverticulitis, impaired hepatic or renal function, severe hypertension, acute nephritis, subacute bacterial endocarditis, and GI, GU, or respiratory tract ulcerations. Also contraindicated during pregnancy and in patients with recent eye, CNS, or spinal cord surgery.

NURSING CONSIDERATIONS

• Use with extreme caution in psychiatric, debilitated, or cachectic patients. Also use cautiously in breast-feeding patients. Monitor infants carefully; may easily bruise or bleed.

• Use cautiously during menses, during use of any drainage tube, in any patient in whom slight bleeding is dangerous, and in patients with protein C deficiency.

• Use caution when adding or stopping any drug for patients receiving anticoagulants. May change the patient's clotting status and result in hemorrhage.

• Know that dose given depends on PT. Doctors typically try to maintain PT at one and one-half to two times normal. PT values depend on procedure and reagents used in individual laboratory.

• Give drug at same time daily.

• Regularly inspect the patient for bleeding gums, bruises on arms or legs, petechiae, nosebleeds, melena, tarry stools, hematuria, and hematemesis.

• Withhold drug and call the doctor if fever and skin rash (signal severe adverse reactions) occur.

• Be aware that light to moderate alcohol intake does not significantly affect PT.

• Stress importance of complying with recommended dosage and follow-up appointments. The patient should carry a card identifying him as a potential bleeder.

• Instruct the patient and his family to watch for signs of bleeding and notify the doctor immediately.
• Warn the patient to avoid OTC products containing aspirin, other salicylates, or drugs that may interact with dicumarol.
• Tell patients to notify their doctor if menses is heavier than usual; may require dosage adjustment.
• Tell patients to use electric razor when shaving to avoid scratching skin and to use a soft toothbrush.
• Tell patients to eat a consistent amount of leafy green vegetables every day. These contain vitamin K, and eating different amounts daily may alter anticoagulant effect.
• Warn patient that drug may turn alkaline urine red-orange.

enoxaparin sodium
Lovenox

Pregnancy Risk Category: B

HOW SUPPLIED
Injection: 30 mg per 0.3 ml

ACTION
A low-molecular weight heparin derivative that accelerates formation of antithrombin III-thrombin complex and deactivates thrombin, preventing conversion of fibrinogen to fibrin. Enoxaparin has a higher anti-factor Xa-to anti-factor IIa-activity ratio.

ONSET, PEAK, DURATION
Onset unknown. Peak effects occur 3 to 5 hours after S.C. injection. Effects persist up to 24 hours.

INDICATIONS & DOSAGE
Prevent pulmonary embolism and deep vein thrombosis after hip or knee replacement surgery –
Adults: 30 mg S.C. b.i.d. for 7 to 10 days. Initial dose given as soon as possible after surgery, but no later than 24 hours postoperatively.

ADVERSE REACTIONS
CNS: confusion.
CV: edema, peripheral edema.
GI: nausea.
Hematologic: hypochromic anemia, moderate thrombocytopenia.
Other: irritation, pain, hematoma, or erythema at the injection site; fever; pain; hemorrhage; ecchymosis; bleeding complications.

INTERACTIONS
Anticoagulants, antiplatelet agents: increased risk of bleeding. Don't use together.

CONTRAINDICATIONS
Contraindicated in patients with hypersensitivity to the drug or to heparin or pork products; in patients with active, major bleeding or thrombocytopenia; and in those who demonstrate antiplatelet antibodies in the presence of the drug.

NURSING CONSIDERATIONS
• Use with extreme caution in patients with a history of heparin-induced thrombocytopenia.
• Use cautiously in patients with conditions that put them at increased risk for hemorrhage, such as bacterial endocarditis; congenital or acquired bleeding disorders; ulcer disease; angiodysplastic GI disease; hemorrhagic stroke; or recent spinal, eye, or brain surgery.
• Draw blood to establish baseline coagulation parameters before therapy.
• Never administer the drug I.M.
• Don't massage after S.C. injection. Watch for signs of bleeding at injection site. Rotate sites and keep accurate record.
• Avoid excessive I.M. injections of other drugs to prevent or minimize hematomas. If possible, don't give I.M. injections at all.
• Monitor platelet counts regularly. Patients with normal coagulation will

---

*Liquid form contains alcohol.
**May contain tartrazine.

Common reactions are in italics; ***life-threatening,*** in bold italics.

not require regular monitoring of PT or PTT.
- Regularly inspect the patient for bleeding gums, bruises on arms or legs, petechiae, nosebleeds, melena, tarry stools, hematuria, hematemesis.
- To treat severe overdose, give protamine sulfate (a heparin antagonist) by slow I.V. infusion at a concentration of 1% to equal the dosage of enoxaparin injected, as ordered.
- Instruct the patient and his family to watch for signs of bleeding and notify the doctor immediately.
- Tell the patient to avoid OTC medications containing aspirin or other salicylates.

heparin calcium
Calcilean†, Calciparine, Caprin‡, Uniparin-Ca‡

heparin sodium
Hepalean†, Heparin Leo†, Heparin Lock Flush Solution (with Tubex), Hep-Lock, Liquaemin Sodium, Uniparin‡

Pregnancy Risk Category: C

HOW SUPPLIED
Products are derived from beef lung or porcine intestinal mucosa.
heparin calcium
Ampule: 12,500 units/0.5 ml; 20,000 units/0.8 ml
Syringe: 5,000 units/0.2 ml
heparin sodium
Carpuject: 5,000 units/ml
Disposable syringes: 1,000 units/ml, 2,500 units/ml, 5,000 units/ml, 7,500 units/ml, 10,000 units/ml, 15,000 units/ml, 20,000 units/ml, 40,000 units/ml
Premixed I.V. solutions: 1,000 units in 500 ml of 0.9% sodium chloride solution; 2,000 units in 1,000 ml of 0.9% sodium chloride solution; 12,500 units in 250 ml of 0.45% sodium chloride solution; 25,000 units in 250 ml of 0.45% sodium chloride

solution; 25,000 units in 500 ml of 0.45% sodium chloride solution; 10,000 units in 100 ml of D_5W; 12,500 units in 250 ml of D_5W; 25,000 units in 250 ml D_5W; 25,000 units in 500 ml D_5W; 20,000 units in 500 ml of D_5W
Unit-dose ampules: 1,000 units/ml, 5,000 units/ml, 10,000 units/ml
Vials: 1,000 units/ml, 2,500 units/ml, 5,000 units/ml, 7,500 units/ml, 10,000 units/ml, 15,000 units/ml, 20,000 units/ml, 40,000 units/ml
heparin sodium flush
Disposable syringes: 10 units/ml, 100 units/ml
Vials: 10 units/ml, 100 units/ml

ACTION
Accelerates formation of antithrombin III-thrombin complex and deactivates thrombin, preventing conversion of fibrinogen to fibrin.

ONSET, PEAK, DURATION
Onset occurs in 20 to 60 minutes after S.C. administration, immediately after I.V. injection. Plasma levels peak 2 to 4 hours after S.C. injection. Correlation between plasma level and drug effect is poor; heparin is rapidly cleared from plasma within ½ to 3 hours, but its duration of action is dose-dependent.

INDICATIONS & DOSAGE
Heparin dosing is highly individualized, depending upon disease state, age, renal and hepatic status.
Deep vein thrombosis, MI –
Adults: initially, 5,000 to 7,500 units I.V. push, then adjusted according to PTT and given I.V. q 4 hours (usually 4,000 to 5,000 units); or 5,000 to 7,500 units I.V. bolus, then 1,000 units/hour by I.V. infusion pump. Hourly rate adjusted 8 hours after bolus dose according to PTT.
Pulmonary embolism; consumptive coagulopathy (such as disseminated intravascular coagulation) –

Adults: initially, 7,500 to 10,000 units I.V. push, then adjusted according to PTT and given I.V. q 4 hours (usually 4,000 to 5,000 units); or 7,500 to 10,000 units I.V. bolus, then 1,000 units/hour by I.V. infusion pump. Hourly rate adjusted 8 hours after bolus dose according to PTT.

Children: initially, 50 units/kg I.V. drip. Maintenance dosage is 100 units/kg I.V. drip q 4 hours. Constant infusion: 20,000 units/m² daily. Dosages adjusted according to PTT.

Embolism, venous thrombosis, pulmonary embolism, atrial fibrillation with embolism; postoperative deep vein thrombosis –

Adults: 5,000 units S.C. q 12 hours. In surgical patients, first dose given 2 hours before procedure; followed with 5,000 units S.C. q 8 to 12 hours for 5 to 7 days or until patient is fully ambulatory.

Open-heart surgery –

Adults: (total body perfusion) 150 to 300 units/kg continuous I.V infusion.

Patency maintenance of I.V. indwelling catheters –

Adults: 10 to 100 units I.V. flush. Use sufficient volume to fill the device. Not intended for therapeutic use.

ADVERSE REACTIONS

Hematologic: *hemorrhage with excessive dosage, overly prolonged clotting time,* **thrombocytopenia.**

Other: irritation; mild pain; hematoma; ulceration; cutaneous or subcutaneous necrosis; *"white clot" syndrome;* hypersensitivity reactions, including chills, fever, pruritus, rhinitis, burning of feet, conjunctivitis, lacrimation, arthralgia, urticaria.

INTERACTIONS

Anticoagulants, oral: increased additive anticoagulation. Monitor PT and PTT.

Salicylates, other antiplatelet agents: increased anticoagulant effect. Don't use together.

Thrombolytics: increased risk of hemorrhage. Monitor closely.

CONTRAINDICATIONS

Contraindicated in patients hypersensitive to the drug. Conditionally contraindicated in patients with active bleeding; blood dyscrasia; or bleeding tendencies, such as hemophilia, thrombocytopenia, or hepatic disease with hypoprothrombinemia; suspected intracranial hemorrhage; suppurative thrombophlebitis; inaccessible ulcerative lesions (especially of GI tract) and open ulcerative wounds; extensive denudation of skin; ascorbic acid deficiency and other conditions causing increased capillary permeability; during or after brain, eye, or spinal cord surgery; during spinal tap or spinal anesthesia; during continuous tube drainage of stomach or small intestine; in subacute bacterial endocarditis; shock; advanced renal disease; threatened abortion; severe hypertension.

Although use of heparin is clearly hazardous in these conditions, its risk versus its benefits must be evaluated.

NURSING CONSIDERATIONS

• Use cautiously during menses; in patients with mild hepatic or renal disease, alcoholism, occupations with the risk of physical injury; immediately postpartum; and in patients with history of allergies, asthma, or GI ulcerations.

• Draw blood to establish baseline coagulation parameters before therapy.

• Know that when the patient requires anticoagulation during pregnancy, most clinicians use heparin.

• Check order and vial carefully. Heparin comes in various concentrations.

• Give low-dose injections sequentially between iliac crests in lower abdomen deep into S.C. fat. Inject drug S.C. slowly into fat pad. Leave needle in place for 10 seconds after injection;

---

*Liquid form contains alcohol.   *Common* reactions are in italics; **life-threatening,** in bold italics.
**May contain tartrazine.

then withdraw needle. Don't massage after S.C. injection, and watch for signs of bleeding at injection site. Alternate sites every 12 hours — right for morning, left for evening.

• **I.V. use:** Administer I.V. using infusion pump to provide maximum safety because of long-term effect and irregular absorption when given S.C. Check constant I.V. infusions regularly, even when pumps are in good working order, to prevent overdosage or underdosage. Place notice above the patient's bed to inform I.V. team or laboratory personnel to apply pressure dressings after taking blood.

• During intermittent I.V. therapy, always draw blood ½ hour before next scheduled dose to avoid falsely elevated PTT. Blood for PTT may be drawn any time after 8 hours of initiation of continuous I.V. heparin therapy. Blood for PTT should never be drawn from the I.V. tubing of the heparin infusion, or from the infused vein. Falsely elevated PTT will result. Always draw blood from the opposite arm.

• Do not skip a dose or "catch up" with an I.V. containing heparin. If I.V. is out, restart it as soon as possible and reschedule bolus dose immediately.

• Know that concentrated heparin solutions (greater than 100 units/ml) can irritate blood vessels.

• Never piggyback other drugs into an infusion line while the heparin infusion is running. Many antibiotics and other drugs deactivate heparin. Never mix any drug with heparin in syringe when bolus therapy is used.

• Avoid excessive I.M. injections of other drugs to prevent or minimize hematomas. If possible, don't give I.M. injections at all.

• Measure PTT carefully and regularly. Anticoagulation present when PTT values are one and one-half to two times control values.

• Monitor platelet counts regularly.

Thrombocytopenia caused by heparin may be associated with a type of arterial thrombosis known as "white clot" syndrome.

• Regularly inspect the patient for bleeding gums, bruises on arms or legs, petechiae, nosebleeds, melena, tarry stools, hematuria, hematemesis.

• Keep in mind that drug requirements are higher in early phases of thrombogenic diseases and febrile states; lower when the patient's condition stabilizes.

• Be aware that elderly patients should usually start at lower doses.

• To treat severe heparin calcium or heparin sodium overdose, use protamine sulfate, a heparin antagonist, as ordered. Dosage is based on the dose of heparin, its route of administration, and the time elapsed since it was given. As a general rule, 1 to 1.5 units of protamine/100 units of heparin is given if only a few minutes have elapsed; 0.5 to 0.75 mg protamine/100 units heparin if 30 to 60 minutes have elapsed, 0.25 to 0.375 mg protamine/100 units heparin if 2 hours or more have elapsed.

• Be aware that abrupt withdrawal may cause increased coagulability, and heparin therapy is usually followed by oral anticoagulants for prophylaxis.

• Instruct the patient and his family to watch for signs of bleeding and notify the doctor immediately.

• Tell the patient to avoid OTC medications containing aspirin, other salicylates, or drugs that may interact with heparin.

warfarin sodium
Coumadin, Sofarin, Warfilone Sodium†

Pregnancy Risk Category: X

HOW SUPPLIED
Tablets: 1 mg, 2 mg, 2.5 mg, 4 mg, 5 mg, 7.5 mg, 10 mg

ACTION
Inhibits vitamin K-dependent activation of clotting factors II, VII, IX, and X, formed in the liver.

ONSET, PEAK, DURATION
Onset occurs in ½ to 3 days. Peak unknown. Effects persist for 2 to 5 days.

INDICATIONS & DOSAGE
Pulmonary embolism associated with deep vein thrombosis, M.I., rheumatic heart disease with heart valve damage, prosthetic heart valves, chronic atrial fibrillation –
Adults: 10 to 15 mg P.O. for 2 to 4 days, then based on daily PT. Usual maintenance dosage is 2 to 10 mg P.O. daily.

ADVERSE REACTIONS
GI: anorexia, nausea, vomiting, cramps, *diarrhea,* mouth ulcerations.
GU: hematuria.
Hematologic: *hemorrhage with excessive dosage,* leukopenia, *agranulocytosis.*
Hepatic: hepatitis, elevated liver function tests, jaundice.
Skin: dermatitis, urticaria, necrosis, gangrene, alopecia, *rash.*
Other: *fever.*

INTERACTIONS
Acetaminophen: may increase bleeding with chronic (greater than 2 weeks) therapy with high doses (> 2 g/day) of acetaminophen. Monitor very carefully.
Allopurinol, amiodarone, anabolic steroids, cephalosporins, chloramphenicol, cimetidine, ciprofloxacin, clofibrate, danazol, diazoxide, diflunisal, disulfiram, erythromycin, ethacrynic acid, fenoprofen calcium, fluoroquinolones, glucagon, heparin, ibuprofen, influenza virus vaccine, isoniazid, ketoprofen, lovastatin, meclofenamate, methimazole, methylthiouracil, metronidazole, miconazole, nalidixic acid, neomycin (oral),
pentoxifylline, propafenone, propoxyphene, propylthiouracil, quinidine, streptokinase, sulfinpyrazone, sulfonamides, sulindac, tamoxifen, tetracyclines, thiazides, thyroid drugs, tricyclic antidepressants, urokinase, vitamin E: increased PT. Monitor the patient carefully for bleeding. Consider anticoagulant dosage reduction.
Barbiturates: inhibited hypoprothrombinemic effect of dicumarol. If barbiturates are withdrawn, reduce anticoagulant dosage; inhibition may last weeks after barbiturate is withdrawn, but fatal hemorrhage can occur when inhibiting effect disappears.
Carbamazepine, corticosteroids, corticotropin, ethchlorvynol, griseofulvin, mercaptopurine, methaqualone, nafcillin, oral contraceptives containing estrogen, rifampin, spironolactone, sulcralfate, trazodone: decreased PT with reduced anticoagulant effect. Monitor patient carefully.
Chloral hydrate, glutethimide, sulfinpyrazone, triclofos sodium: increased or decreased PT. Avoid use if possible, and monitor the patient carefully.
Cholestyramine: decreased response when administered too close together. Administer 6 hours after oral anticoagulants.
Hydantoins: increased serum levels of hydantoin. Monitor closely.
Indomethacin, mefenamic acid, salicylates: increased PT; ulcerogenic effects. Don't use together.
Sulfonylureas (oral antidiabetic agents): increased hypoglycemic response. Monitor blood glucose levels.
Foods or enteral products containing vitamin K: may impair anticoagulation. Patient should maintain consistent daily intake of leafy green vegetables.

CONTRAINDICATIONS
Contraindicated in pregnancy; in patients with bleeding or hemorrhagic tendencies, GI ulcerations, severe hepatic or renal disease, severe uncon-

---

trolled hypertension, subacute bacterial endocarditis, polycythemia vera, and vitamin K deficiency; and after recent eye, brain, or spinal cord surgery.

NURSING CONSIDERATIONS

• Use cautiously in patients with diverticulitis, colitis, mild or moderate hypertension, mild or moderate hepatic or renal disease, with drainage tubes in any orifice; with regional or lumbar block anesthesia; or in any condition increasing risk of hemorrhage and during lactation.
• Draw blood to establish baseline coagulation parameters before therapy.
• Know that PT determinations essential for proper control. Doctors typically try to maintain PT at 1.5 to 2 times normal; high incidence of bleeding when PT exceeds 2.5 times control values.
• Give warfarin at same time daily.
• Be aware that I.V. form may be obtained from manufacturer in the rare instances that oral therapy cannot be given. Follow manufacturer guidelines carefully regarding preparation and administration.
• Because onset of action is delayed, keep in mind that heparin sodium is often given during first few days of treatment. When heparin is being given simultaneously, blood for PT should not be drawn within 5 hours of intermittent I.V. heparin administration. However, blood for PT may be drawn at any time during continuous heparin infusion.
• Regularly inspect the patient for bleeding gums, bruises on arms or legs, petechiae, nosebleeds, melena, tarry stools, hematuria, and hematemesis.
• Observe breast-feeding infants of patients on drug for unexpected bleeding.
• Withhold drug and call the doctor immediately if fever and skin rash

(signal severe adverse reactions) occur.
• Be aware that half-life of warfarin's anticoagulant effect is 36 to 44 hours. Effect can be neutralized by vitamin K injections.
• Be aware that the drug is the best oral anticoagulant for the patient taking antacids or phenytoin.
• Be aware that elderly patients and patients with renal or hepatic failure are especially sensitive to warfarin effect.
• Be aware that light to moderate alcohol intake does not significantly affect PT.
• Stress importance of complying with prescribed dosage and follow-up appointments. The patient should carry a card that identifies him as a potential bleeder.
• Instruct the patient and his family to watch for signs of bleeding and notify the doctor immediately if they occur.
• Warn the patient to avoid OTC products containing aspirin, other salicylates, or drugs that may interact with warfarin.
• Tell the patient to notify the doctor if menses is heavier than usual; may require dosage adjustment.
• Tell the patient to use electric razor when shaving to avoid scratching skin and to use a soft toothbrush.
• Warn the patient to read food labels. Food and enteral feedings that contain vitamin K may impair anticoagulation.
• Tell the patient to eat a daily, consistent amount of leafy green vegetables, which contain vitamin K. Eating different amounts daily may alter anticoagulant effects.

absorbable gelatin sponge
microfibrillar collagen hemostat
oxidized cellulose
thrombin

COMBINATION PRODUCTS
None.

absorbable gelatin sponge
Gelfoam
Pregnancy Risk Category: NR

HOW SUPPLIED
Sponges: 20 mm × 60 mm × 3 mm,
20 mm × 60 mm × 7 mm, 80 mm ×
62.5 mm × 10 mm, 80 mm × 125
mm × 10 mm, 80 mm × 250 mm ×
10 mm, 80 mm × 125 mm (compressed)
Packs: 40 cm × 2 cm, 40 cm × 6 cm
Dental packs: 10 mm × 20 mm × 7
mm, 20 mm × 20 mm × 7 mm
Prostatectomy cones: 13 cm (5″) diameter, 18 cm (7″) diameter

ACTION
Absorbs and holds many times its
weight in blood, providing a framework for growth of granulation tissue.

ONSET, PEAK, DURATION
Onset immediate. Peak and duration
unknown.

INDICATIONS & DOSAGE
Pressure ulcers –
Adults: place aseptically deep into
wound. Don't disturb or remove; add
extra p.r.n.
Hemostasis in surgery (adjunct) –
Adults: apply saturated with 0.9% so-
dium chloride or thrombin solution.
Hold in place for 10 to 15 seconds.
When oozing is controlled, allow ma-
terial to remain in place.

ADVERSE REACTIONS
CNS: *compression of brain or spinal*
cord, neurologic symptoms, headache, hearing loss.
Other: infection, giant cell granuloma, fever, *toxic shock syndrome.*

INTERACTIONS
None significant.

CONTRAINDICATIONS
Contraindicated in patients with frank
infection, or postpartum bleeding or
hemorrhage; also contraindicated as a
sole hemostatic agent in abnormal
bleeding.

NURSING CONSIDERATIONS
• Do not use to close skin incisions.
• Know that overpacking should be
avoided when placed into body cavities or closed tissue spaces.
• Know that the drug is systemically
absorbed within 4 to 6 weeks; no need
to remove except when used in laminectomy procedures or when used to
pack foramen in bone.

microfibrillar collagen hemostat
Avitene
Pregnancy Risk Category: NR

HOW SUPPLIED
Nonwoven web: 70 mm × 70 mm × 1
mm, 70 mm × 35 mm × 1 mm
Fibrous form: 1-g, 5-g jars

ACTION
Attracts and aggregates platelets.

ONSET, PEAK, DURATION
Onset immediate. Peak and duration
unknown.

---

*Liquid form contains alcohol.   *Common* reactions are in italics; *life-threatening,* in bold italics.
**May contain tartrazine.

INDICATIONS & DOSAGE
Hemostasis in surgery (adjunct) –
Adults and children: amount depends on severity of bleeding. Compress area with dry sponges. Apply web or fibrous form directly to bleeding site for 1 to 5 minutes, gently removing excess. Reapply if needed.

ADVERSE REACTIONS
Hematologic: hematoma.
Other: exacerbation of wound dehiscence, abscess formation, foreign body reaction, adhesion formation, enhanced infection in contaminated wounds, mediastinitis, hypersensitivity reactions, allergic reactions.

INTERACTIONS
None significant.

CONTRAINDICATIONS
Contraindicated in patients with closure of skin incisions; hemostat may interfere with healing. Do not use on bone surfaces where cement is needed to attach prostheses.

NURSING CONSIDERATIONS
• Don't dilute. Always apply dry.
• Handle and apply with smooth, dry forceps. Apply directly to source of bleeding. Adheres to wet gloves, instruments, or tissue surfaces.
• Don't spill on nonbleeding surfaces.
• Know to avoid ethylene oxide sterilization. Autoclaving inactivates product.

oxidized cellulose
Oxycel, Surgicel

Pregnancy Risk Category: NR

HOW SUPPLIED
Pads: 3″ × 3″, 8 ply
Pledgets: 2″ × 1″ × 1″
Strips: ½ × 2″, ½ × 5″, ½ × 36″;
2″ × 3″, 2″ × 14″, 2″ × 18″; 4″ × 8″

ACTION
Absorbs and holds many times its weight in blood.

ONSET, PEAK, DURATION
Onset immediately on contact with blood. Peak and duration unknown.

INDICATIONS & DOSAGE
Hemostasis in surgery (adjunct); external bleeding at tumor sites –
Adults and children: apply loosely against bleeding surface with sterile technique, p.r.n. Remove after hemostasis, if possible, with dry sterile forceps. Leave in place if necessary.

ADVERSE REACTIONS
CNS: headache when used as packing for epistaxis, or after rhinologic procedures or application to surface wounds.
EENT: sneezing, epistaxis, stinging, or burning when used as packing for rhinologic procedures; nasal membrane necrosis or septal perforation.
GI: intestinal obstruction (when used in GI procedures).
GU: difficult urination (when used in GU procedures).
Other: encapsulation of fluid, foreign body reaction, burning or stinging after application to surface wounds, possible prolongation of drainage, *intestinal obstruction following cholecystectomy*.

INTERACTIONS
Thrombin: may decrease blood clotting effectiveness.

CONTRAINDICATIONS
Contraindicated in controlling hemorrhage from large arteries; for use on nonhemorrhagic, serous, oozing surfaces; in implantation in bone defects; or for use around the optic nerve and chiasm.

NURSING CONSIDERATIONS
• Know that only amount needed to produce hemostasis is used, and excess is removed before surgical closure.
• Use minimal amounts in urologic procedures.
• In large wounds, don't overlap skin edges.
• Don't moisten. Hemostatic effect is greater when applied dry.
• Do not pack or wad unless cellulose will be removed after hemostasis. Don't apply too tightly when used as wrap sheet in vascular surgery.
• Keep in mind that drug is not used for permanent packing in fractures because it may result in cyst formation.
• Use sterile technique to remove from open wounds after hemostasis. Don't remove without irrigating material first; otherwise, fresh bleeding may occur.
• Be prepared for removal after hemostasis when used in laminectomies or near optic nerve chiasm.
• Don't autoclave this product.

---

thrombin
Thrombinar, Thrombogen, Thrombostat

Pregnancy Risk Category: C

HOW SUPPLIED
Powder: 1,000-, 5,000-, 10,000-, 20,000-, and 50,000-unit vials
Kit: 10,000-unit or 20,000-unit with sprayer assembly

ACTION
Converts fibrinogen to fibrin.

ONSET, PEAK, DURATION
Onset immediate. Peak and duration unknown.

INDICATIONS & DOSAGE
Bleeding from parenchymatous tissue, cancellous bone, dental sockets, nasal and laryngeal surgery, and in plastic surgery and skin-grafting procedures—
Adults: apply 100 units/ml of sterile isotonic sodium chloride solution or sterile distilled water to area where clotting needed (or may apply dry powder in bone surgery); in major bleeding, apply 1,000 to 2,000 units/ml of sterile 0.9% sodium chloride solution. Sponge blood from area before application, but avoid sponging area after application.

ADVERSE REACTIONS
Other: hypersensitivity reactions and fever from systemic absorption.

INTERACTIONS
None significant.

CONTRAINDICATIONS
• Contraindicated in patients with hypersensitivity to thrombin or bovine products.
• Contraindicated as I.V. injection (of topical thrombin).

NURSING CONSIDERATIONS
• Obtain a patient history of reactions to thrombin or bovine products.
• Have blood typed and crossmatched to treat possible hemorrhage.
• Keep refrigerated (preferably frozen) until ready to use. Unstable in solution. Store away from heat. Use solutions within 3 hours. Refrigerate excess solution at 2° to 8° C or freeze for up to 48 hours.
• Observe patient for allergic reactions, and monitor vital signs regularly.
• Know that injecting topical thrombin or allowing it to enter large blood vessels may cause death because of severe intravascular clotting.
• Keep in mind that drug may be used with absorbable gelatin sponge but not with oxidized cellulose. Check sponge labeling before use.
• Be alert that drug may be broken down by diluted acid, alkali, and salts of heavy metals.

---

*Liquid form contains alcohol.
**May contain tartrazine.

Common reactions are in italics; *life-threatening*, in bold italics.

albumin 5%
albumin 25%
antihemophilic factor
anti-inhibitor coagulant complex
antithrombin III, human
factor IX complex
factor IX (human)
intravascular perfluorochemical emulsion
plasma protein fraction

COMBINATION PRODUCTS
None.

---

albumin 5%
Albuminar 5%, Albutein 5%,
Buminate 5%, Plasbumin 5%

albumin 25%
Albuminar 25%, Albumisol 25%,
Albutein 25%, Buminate 25%,
Plasbumin 25%

Pregnancy Risk Category: C

HOW SUPPLIED
albumin 5%
Injection: 50-ml, 250-ml, 500-ml,
1,000-ml vials
albumin 25%
Injection: 10-ml, 20-ml, 50-ml, 100-
ml vials

ACTION
Albumin 5% supplies colloid to the
blood and expands plasma volume.
Albumin 25% provides intravascular
oncotic pressure in a 5:1 ratio, causing
a fluid shift from interstitial spaces to
the circulation and slightly increasing
plasma protein concentration.

ONSET, PEAK, DURATION
Onset and peak occur immediately to
within 15 minutes if patient well hydrated. Duration of action depends on
the initial blood volume of the patient. If blood volume is reduced, volume expansion persists for many
hours; however, if blood volume is
normal, the effect lasts a shorter time.

INDICATIONS & DOSAGE
Hypovolemic shock –
Adults: initially, 500 to 750 ml 5%
solution by I.V. infusion, repeated
q 30 minutes, p.r.n. Alternatively,
100 to 200 ml I.V. of 25% solution,
repeated after 10 to 30 minutes if
needed. Dosage varies with the patient's condition and response.
Children: 12 to 20 ml 5% solution/kg
body weight by I.V. infusion, repeated
in 15 to 30 minutes if response is not
adequate. Alternatively, 2.5 to 5 ml
I.V. of 25% solution/kg of body
weight, repeated after 10 to 30 minutes if needed.
Hypoproteinemia –
Adults: 1,000 to 1,500 ml 5% solution by I.V. infusion daily, maximum
rate 5 to 10 ml/minute; or 25 to 100 g
25% solution by I.V. infusion daily,
maximum rate 3 ml/minute. Dosage
varies with the patient's condition and
response.
Hyperbilirubinemia –
Infants: 1 g albumin (4 ml 25%)/kg 1
to 2 hours before transfusion.

ADVERSE REACTIONS
CV: *vascular overload after rapid in-
fusion,* hypotension, altered pulse
rate.
GI: increased salivation, nausea,
vomiting.
Respiratory: altered respiration.
Skin: urticaria, rash.
Other: chills, fever.

INTERACTIONS
None significant.

---

†Available in Canada only.　　　‡Available in Australia only.　　　◇Available OTC.

CONTRAINDICATIONS
Contraindicated in patients with hypersensitivity to the drug.

NURSING CONSIDERATIONS
• Use with extreme caution in patients with hypertension, cardiac disease, severe pulmonary infection, severe chronic anemia, or hypoalbuminemia with peripheral edema.
• Make sure the patient is properly hydrated before solution infusion.
• Take care when preparing and administering drug to minimize waste. This product is very expensive, and random supply shortages occur often.
• **I.V. use:** Avoid rapid I.V. infusion. Specific rate is individualized according to the patient's age, condition, and diagnosis. Dilute with sterile water for injection, 0.9% sodium chloride solution, or D_5W injection. Use solution promptly; contains no preservatives. Discard unused solution. Don't use cloudy solutions or those containing sediment. Solution should be clear amber color.
• Do not give more than 250 g in 48 hours.
• Watch for hemorrhage or shock after surgery or injury. Rapid rise in blood pressure may cause bleeding from sites that are not apparent at lower pressures.
• Monitor vital signs carefully.
• Watch for signs of vascular overload (heart failure or pulmonary edema).
• Monitor fluid intake and output, hemoglobin, hematocrit, and serum protein and electrolytes during therapy.
• Know that one volume of 25% albumin is equivalent to five volumes of 5% albumin in producing hemodilution and relative anemia.
• Follow storage instructions on bottle. Freezing may cause bottle to break.

antihemophilic factor (AHF)
Hemofil M, Humate-P, Hyate:C, Koate-HP, Koate-HS, Monoclate, Monoclate-P, Profilate OSD

Pregnancy Risk Category: NR

HOW SUPPLIED
Injection: vials, with diluent. Units specified on label.

ACTION
Directly replaces deficient clotting factor.

ONSET, PEAK, DURATION
Onset immediate after I.V. administration. Time to peak effect is 1 to 2 hours after I.V. administration. Duration unknown.

INDICATIONS & DOSAGE
Spontaneous hemorrhage in patients with hemophilia A (factor VIII deficiency) –
Adults and children: calculate dosage using this formula:

$$\begin{array}{c} \text{AHF} \\ \text{required} \\ \text{(IU)} \end{array} = \begin{array}{c} \text{body weight} \\ \text{(kg)} \end{array} \times \begin{array}{c} \text{desired factor} \\ \text{VIII increase} \\ \text{(\% of normal)} \end{array} \times 0.5$$

To prevent spontaneous hemorrhage, the desired level of factor VIII is 5% of normal; for mild hemorrhage, 30% of normal; for moderate hemorrhage and minor surgery, 30% to 50% of normal; for severe hemorrhage, 80% to 100% of normal.
Treatment of bleeding in patients with hemophilia A (factor VIII deficiency) –
Adults and children: For minor hemorrhage into muscle and joints, 8 to 10 IU/kg I.V. q 8 to 12 hours for 1 or more days. For overt bleeding, an initial dose of 15 to 25 IU/kg I.V., followed by 8 to 15 IU/kg q 8 to 12 hours for 3 to 4 days. To treat massive bleeding or hemorrhage involving major organs, an initial dose of 40 to 50 IU/kg

I.V., followed by 20 to 25 IU/kg I.V.
q 8 to 12 hours.
*Prevention of bleeding in hemophilic
patients requiring surgery –*
Adults: 25 to 30 IU/kg I.V. 1 hour before surgery, followed by one-half of
the initial dosage 5 hours later. Dosage adjusted to achieve a level of AHF
80% to 100% of normal during surgery and maintained at 30% to 60% of
normal for at least 10 to 14 days postoperatively.

ADVERSE REACTIONS
CNS: headache, paresthesia, clouding or loss of consciousness, somnolence, lethargy.
CV: tachycardia, hypotension, *hemolysis* in patients with blood type A, B,
or AB.
EENT: visual disturbances.
GI: nausea, vomiting.
Skin: erythema, *urticaria*.
Other: *chills, fever, backache, flushing,* chest constriction, *hypersensitivity reactions,* rigor, stinging at injection site.

INTERACTIONS
None significant.

CONTRAINDICATIONS
Contraindicated in patients with hypersensitivity to murine (mouse) protein or to the drug.

NURSING CONSIDERATIONS
• Use cautiously in neonates, infants,
and patients with hepatic disease because of susceptibility to hepatitis,
which may be transmitted in antihemophilic factor.
• Monitor coagulation studies before
therapy.
• As ordered, administer hepatitis B
vaccine before administering antihemophilic factor.
• Refrigerate concentrate until ready
to use. Warm concentrate and diluent
bottles to room temperature before re-

constituting. To mix drug, gently roll
vial between hands.
• Use reconstituted solution within 3
hours. Store away from heat and do
not refrigerate. Refrigeration after reconstitution may cause the active ingredient to precipitate. Don't shake or
mix with other I.V. solutions.
• **I.V. use:** Take baseline pulse rate
before I.V. administration. Use plastic
syringe; drug may interact with glass
syringe and bind to its surface. If
pulse rate increases significantly, flow
rate should be reduced or administration stopped.
• Do not use S.C. or I.M.
• Monitor vital signs regularly.
• Monitor coagulation studies frequently during therapy.
• Monitor the patient for allergic reactions.
• Be aware that some patients develop
inhibitors to factor VIII, resulting in
decreased response to the drug.
• Keep in mind that a new porcine
product is now available for patients
with congenital hemophilia A who
have antibodies to human factor
VIII:C.
• Keep in mind that risk of hepatitis,
including non-A and non-B hepatitis,
must be weighed against risk of the
patient not receiving the drug.
• Because of the manufacturing process, be aware that the risk of HIV
transmission is extremely low.

anti-inhibitor coagulant complex
Autoplex T, Feiba VH Immuno
Pregnancy Risk Category: C

HOW SUPPLIED
Injection: number of units of factor
VIII correctional activity indicated on
label of vial

ACTION
Unknown. It has been suggested that
efficacy may be related in part to the

presence of the activated factors, which leads to more complete factor X activation in conjunction with tissue factor, phospholipid, and ionic calcium and allows the coagulation process to proceed beyond those stages where factor VIII is needed.

ONSET, PEAK, DURATION
Onset occurs within 10 to 30 minutes. Peak and duration unknown.

INDICATIONS & DOSAGE
Prevention and control of hemorrhagic episodes in certain patients with hemophilia A who have developed inhibitor antibodies to antihemophilic factor; management of bleeding in patients with acquired hemophilia who have spontaneously acquired inhibitors to factor VIII –

Adults and children: highly individualized and varies among manufacturers. For Autoplex T, 25 to 100 units/kg I.V., depending on the severity of hemorrhage. If no hemostatic improvement occurs within 6 hours after administration, dosage repeated. For Feiba VH Immuno, 50 to 100 units/kg I.V. q 6 or 12 hours until clear signs of improvement.

ADVERSE REACTIONS
CNS: dizziness, headache, lethargy, drowsiness.
CV: hypotension, transient chest discomfort, changes in pulse rate, *acute MI, thromboembolic events*.
GI: nausea, severe abdominal pain (rare).
Hematologic: *disseminated intravascular coagulation (DIC)*.
Respiratory: breathing difficulty.
Skin: flushing, rash, urticaria.
Other: fever, chills, hypersensitivity reactions.

INTERACTIONS
Antifibrinolytic agents: may alter effects of anti-inhibitor coagulant complex. Do not use together.

CONTRAINDICATIONS
Contraindicated in patients with signs of fibrinolysis, in those with DIC, and in those with a normal coagulation mechanism.

NURSING CONSIDERATIONS
• Use with caution in patients with liver disease.
• As ordered, administer hepatitis B vaccine before administering drug.
• Keep epinephrine readily available to treat anaphylaxis.
• **I.V. use:** Warm the drug and diluent to room temperature prior to reconstitution. Reconstitute according to manufacturer's directions. Use the filter needle provided by the manufacturer to withdraw the reconstituted solution from the vial into the syringe; the filter needle should then be replaced with a sterile injection needle for administration. Administer as soon as possible. Autoplex T infusions should be completed within 1 hour after reconstitution; Feiba VH Immuno infusions, within 3 hours.
• The rate of administration should be individualized according to the patient's response. Autoplex T infusions may begin at a rate of 1 ml/minute; if well tolerated, the infusion rate may be increased gradually to 10 ml/minute. Feiba VH Immuno infusion rate should not exceed 2 units/kg.
• If flushing, lethargy, headache, transient chest discomfort, or changes in blood pressure or pulse rate develop because of a rapid rate of infusion, stop the drug and notify the doctor. Know that these symptoms usually disappear with cessation of the infusion. The infusion may then be resumed at a slower rate, as ordered.
• Assess the patient closely for hypersensitivity reactions.
• Monitor vital signs regularly and report significant changes to the doctor.
• Reassure patient that because of the manufacturing process, the risk of HIV transmission is extremely low.

---

*Liquid form contains alcohol.
**May contain tartrazine.

Common reactions are in italics; *life-threatening*, in bold italics.

antithrombin III, human (AT-III, heparin cofactor I)

ATnativ, Thrombate III

Pregnancy Risk Category: C

HOW SUPPLIED

Injection: 500 IU

ACTION

Replaces deficient AT-III in patients with hereditary AT-III deficiency, normalizing coagulation inhibition and inhibiting thromboembolism formation. Also deactivates plasmin (to lesser extent than the clotting factor).

ONSET, PEAK, DURATION

Onset immediate after I.V. administration. Peak unknown. Effects persist about 4 days.

INDICATIONS & DOSAGE

Thromboembolism associated with hereditary AT-III deficiency –

Adults and children: initial dose is individualized to quantity required to increase AT-III activity to 120% of normal activity as determined 30 minutes after administration. Usual dose is 50 to 100 IU/minute I.V., not to exceed 100 IU/minute. Dose is calculated based on anticipated 1% increase in plasma AT-III activity produced by 1 IU/kg of body weight using the formula:

$$\text{Dose (Units)} = \frac{(\text{desired activity [\%]} - \text{baseline activity [\%]}) \times \text{weight (kg)}}{1\% \text{ (IU/kg)}}$$

Maintenance dosage is individualized to quantity required to increase AT-III activity to 80% of normal activity and is administered at 24-hour intervals.

To calculate the dosage, multiply the desired AT-III activity (as % of normal) minus the baseline AT-III activity (as % of normal) by body weight (in kg). Divide by actual increase in AT-III activity (in %) produced by 1 IU/kg as determined 30 minutes after administration of initial dose.

Treatment is usually continued for 2 to 8 days but may be prolonged in pregnancy or when used with surgery or immobilization.

ADVERSE REACTIONS

CV: vasodilation, lowered blood pressure.
GU: diuresis.

INTERACTIONS

Heparin: increased anticoagulant effect of both drugs. Heparin dosage reduction may be necessary.

CONTRAINDICATIONS

None known.

NURSING CONSIDERATIONS

• Use with extreme caution in children and neonates because safety and efficacy have not been established.
• Use drug cautiously. It is prepared from pooled plasma from human donors, and carries with it a minimal risk of transmission of viruses, including hepatitis and HIV.
• Because of the risk of neonatal thromboembolism (sometimes fatal) in children of parents with hereditary AT-III deficiency, anticipate obtaining AT-III levels immediately after birth.
• **I.V. use:** Reconstitute using 10 ml of sterile water (provided), 0.9% sodium chloride solution, or D_5W. *Do not shake vial.* Dilute further in same diluent solution if desired.
• Obtain AT-III activity levels twice daily until the dosage requirement has stabilized, then daily immediately before dose. Functional assays are preferred because quantitative immunologic test results may be normal despite decreased AT-III activity.
• Monitor for dyspnea and increased blood pressure, which may occur if administration rate is too rapid (1,500 IU in 5 minutes).

• Keep in mind that one IU is equivalent to the quantity of endogenous AT-III present in 1 ml of normal human plasma.
• Keep in mind that heparin binds to AT-III lysine binding sites, resulting in increased efficacy of heparin.
• Know that drug is not recommended for long-term prophylaxis of thrombotic episodes.
• Store at 36° to 46° F (2° to 8° C).

factor IX complex
Bebulin VH Immuno, Konyne-80, Profilnine Heat-Treated, Proplex T

factor IX (human)
AlphaNine, AlphaNine SD, Mononine

Pregnancy Risk Category: C

HOW SUPPLIED
Injection: vials, with diluent. Units specified on label.

ACTION
Directly replaces deficient clotting factor.

ONSET, PEAK, DURATION
Onset immediate after I.V. administration. Time to peak effect is 10 to 30 minutes after I.V. administration. Duration unknown.

INDICATIONS & DOSAGE
Factor IX deficiency (hemophilia B or Christmas disease), anticoagulant overdosage –
Adults and children: units required equal 0.8 to 1 × body weight in kg × percentage of desired increase of factor IX level, by slow I.V. infusion or I.V. push. Dosage is highly individualized, depending on degree of deficiency, level of factor IX desired, weight of the patient, and severity of bleeding.

ADVERSE REACTIONS
CNS: somnolence, lethargy, headache.
CV: *thromboembolic reactions; MI; disseminated intravascular coagulation; pulmonary embolism;* possible *hemolysis* in patients with blood types A, B, or AB; changes in blood pressure or heart rate.
GI: nausea, vomiting.
Skin: urticaria.
Other: *transient fever, chills, flushing, tingling, hypersensitivity reactions (anaphylaxis).*

INTERACTIONS
Aminocaproic acid: increased risk of thrombosis. Avoid concomitant use.

CONTRAINDICATIONS
Contraindicated in patients with hepatic disease in whom there is any suspicion of intravascular coagulation or fibrinolysis. Mononine is contraindicated in patients with hypersensitivty to murine protein.

NURSING CONSIDERATIONS
• Use cautiously in neonates and infants because of susceptibility to hepatitis, which may be transmitted with factor IX complex.
• As ordered, administer hepatitis B vaccine before administering factor IX complex.
• Reconstitute with 20 ml of sterile water for injection for each vial of lyophilized drug. Keep refrigerated until ready to use; warm to room temperature before reconstituting. Use within 3 hours of reconstitution. Unstable in solution. Don't shake, refrigerate, or mix solution with other I.V. solutions. Store away from heat.
• **I.V. use:** Avoid rapid infusion. If tingling sensation, fever, chills, or headache develops, decrease flow rate and notify the doctor.
• Observe the patient for allergic reactions, and monitor vital signs regularly.

Liquid form contains alcohol.   *Common* reactions are in italics; *life-threatening*, in bold italics.
**May contain tartrazine.

• Keep in mind that risk of hepatitis, including non-A and non-B hepatitis, must be weighed against risk of not receiving the drug.

• Because of the manufacturing process, be aware that the risk of HIV transmission is extremely low.

intravascular perfluorochemical emulsion (IPE)
Fluosol

Pregnancy Risk Category: B

HOW SUPPLIED
Injection: 20% emulsion; supplied in kit form with additive solutions (1 and 2) and materials to provide continuous oxygenation

ACTION
An emulsion of synthetic perfluorochemicals that acts as an oxygen carrier.

ONSET, PEAK, DURATION
Unknown.

INDICATIONS & DOSAGE
To prevent or decrease myocardial ischemia during percutaneous transluminal coronary angioplasty (PTCA) in patients at high risk for ischemic complications of angioplasty (including patients with a low baseline ejection fraction, patients with large areas of the myocardium at risk, patients with recent MI, and patients with unstable angina or refractory angina requiring hospitalization) –
Adults: A test dose of 0.5 ml is withdrawn from the prepared solution and injected into a peripheral vein. If no adverse reactions occur within 10 minutes, warmed, oxygenated emulsion may be administered by intracoronary injection at a rate of 60 to 90 ml/minute. Administered through the central lumen of an angioplasty balloon catheter without removing the

guide wire. An angiographic power injector with a warming jacket is used.

ADVERSE REACTIONS
CV: *ventricular tachycardia or fibrillation,* bradycardia, chest discomfort, hypotension.
Respiratory: dyspnea, increased respiratory rate, coughing.
Skin: mild pruritus.

INTERACTIONS
Anesthetics: may prolong action of lipid-soluble anesthetics. Monitor the patient carefully.
Hepatotoxic agents: may enhance hepatotoxic effects of hepatotoxic agents. Monitor the patient closely.

CONTRAINDICATIONS
Contraindicated in patients with hypersensitivity to any components of the compound and in those with functionally critical secondary stenosis in areas distal to the site of the lesion being treated.

NURSING CONSIDERATIONS
• Use cautiously in asplenic patients because drug may accumulate.
• Know that breast-feeding is not recommended because drug is excreted in breast milk.
• Be aware that drug should be administered only by doctors familiar with PTCA. Follow institutional policy regarding emergency surgical procedures for coronary artery bypass graft surgery.
• Know not to add anything other than solutions 1 and 2 or carbogen gas (95% oxygen, 5% carbon dioxide) to the emulsion. Do not oxygenate with 100% oxygen because this will adversely affect the solution's final pH.
• **I.V. use:** Do not use an in-line filter when administering because it may damage the emulsion. Never administer any solution that shows evidence of emulsion separation.

• Oxygenate the emulsion and warm to approximately 98.6° F (37° C) before administration. Infusion of solutions at room temperature has been associated with ventricular fibrillation.

• In the unlikely event that the patient reacts adversely to the test dose (1.2% of patients in clinical trials reacted), be prepared not to give the drug. Severe reactions can be managed with methylprednisolone or diphenhydramine.

• Anticipate allowing more than 4 minutes of perfusion time when used with an angiographic power injector reservoir of 260 ml and a flow rate of 60 ml/minute. Perfusion time should be limited by the patient's tolerance and the doctor's judgment.

• Because this drug reportedly accumulates in the body after repeated dosage, know that it should not be given more than once every 6 months.

• Store the container of intravascular perfluorochemical emulsion in the freezer (between 23° and −22° F [−5° and −30° C]). Do not use emulsions that appear to have partially thawed during storage. Use a warming cabinet or water bath set at 98.6° F to thaw the solution, not a microwave oven, because this may cause uneven heating of the solution. Allow at least 30 minutes for thawing of the solution. Do not refreeze thawed solutions, and use within 8 hours.

• Do not freeze the additive solutions (solutions 1 and 2); store at room temperature not exceeding 86° F (30° C).

plasma protein fraction
Plasmanate, Plasma-Plex, Plasmatein, Protenate

Pregnancy Risk Category: C

HOW SUPPLIED
Injection: 5% solution in 50-ml, 250-ml, 500-ml vials

ACTION
Supplies colloid to the blood and expands plasma volume.

ONSET, PEAK, DURATION
Onset and serum levels peak immediately after I.V. infusion. Duration unknown.

INDICATIONS & DOSAGE
Shock –
Adults: varies with the patient's condition and response, but usual dose is 250 to 500 ml I.V. (12.5 to 25 g protein), usually no faster than 10 ml/minute.
Children: 6.6 to 33 ml/kg (0.33 to 1.65 g/kg of protein) I.V., 5 to 10 ml/minute.
Hypoproteinemia –
Adults: 1,000 to 1,500 ml I.V. daily. Maximum infusion rate is 8 ml/minute.

ADVERSE REACTIONS
CNS: headache.
CV: various effects on blood pressure after rapid infusion or intra-arterial administration; *vascular overload after rapid infusion.*
GI: nausea, vomiting, hypersalivation.
Skin: erythema, urticaria.
Other: flushing, chills, fever, back pain, dyspnea.

INTERACTIONS
None significant.

CONTRAINDICATIONS
Contraindicated in patients with severe anemia or heart failure, and in those undergoing cardiac bypass.

NURSING CONSIDERATIONS
• Use cautiously in patients with hepatic or renal failure, low cardiac reserve, and restricted sodium intake.
• **I.V. use:** Check expiration date before using. Don't use solutions that are cloudy, contain sediment, or have

---

*Liquid form contains alcohol.   *Common* reactions are in italics; ***life-threatening,*** in bold italics.
**May contain tartrazine.

been frozen. Discard solutions in containers opened for more than 4 hours because it contains no preservatives.
• If the patient is dehydrated, give additional fluids either P.O. or I.V., as ordered.
• Do not give more than 250 g or 5,000 ml in 48 hours.
• Monitor blood pressure. Be prepared to slow or stop infusion if hypotension suddenly occurs. Vital signs should return to normal gradually; monitor hourly.
• Watch for signs of vascular overload (heart failure or pulmonary edema).
• Monitor intake and output. Watch for and report decreased urine output.
• Keep in mind that drug contains 130 to 160 mEq sodium/liter.

alteplase
anistreplase
streptokinase
urokinase

COMBINATION PRODUCTS
None.

alteplase (tissue plasminogen activator, recombinant; tPA)
Actilyse‡, Activase

Pregnancy Risk Category: C

HOW SUPPLIED
Injection: 20-mg (11.6 million-IU), 50-mg (29 million-IU), 100 mg (58 million-IU) vials

ACTION
Binds to fibrin in a thrombus, and locally converts plasminogen to plasmin, which initiates local fibrinolysis.

ONSET, PEAK, DURATION
Onset immediate. Peak effects occur in about 45 minutes. Effects persist for about 4 hours.

INDICATIONS & DOSAGE
Lysis of thrombi obstructing coronary arteries in acute MI –
Adults: 100 mg I.V. infusion over 3 hours as follows: 60 mg in the first hour, of which 6 to 10 mg is given as a bolus over the first 1 to 2 minutes. Then 20 mg/hour infusion for 2 hours. Smaller adults (< 65 kg) should receive 1.25 mg/kg in a similar fashion (60% in the first hour, 10% as a bolus; then 20% of the total dose per hour for 2 hours).
Management of acute massive pulmonary embolism –
Adults: 100 mg I.V. infusion over 2 hours. Heparin begun at the end of the infusion when PTT or PT returns to twice normal or less.
 Do not exceed 100-mg dose. Higher doses may increase risk of intracranial bleeding.

ADVERSE REACTIONS
CNS: *cerebral hemorrhage,* fever.
CV: hypotension, arrhythmias, edema.
GI: nausea, vomiting.
Hematologic: *severe, spontaneous bleeding (cerebral, retroperitoneal, GU, GI).*
Other: bleeding at puncture sites, hypersensitivity reactions *(anaphylaxis),* urticaria, arthralgias.

INTERACTIONS
Aspirin, coumarin anticoagulants, dipyridamole, heparin: increased risk of bleeding. Monitor the patient carefully.

CONTRAINDICATIONS
Contraindicated in patients with active internal bleeding, intracranial neoplasm, arteriovenous malformation, aneurysm, and severe uncontrolled hypertension. Also contraindicated in patients with a history of CVA, recent (within 2 months) intraspinal or intracranial trauma or surgery, or known bleeding diathesis.

NURSING CONSIDERATIONS
• Use cautiously in patients with recent (within 10 days) major surgery; in pregnancy and first 10 days postpartum; organ biopsy; trauma (including cardiopulmonary resuscitation); GI or GU bleeding; cerebrovascular disease; hypertension (systolic ≥ 180 mm Hg or diastolic ≥ 110 mm Hg); mitral stenosis, atrial fibril-

---

*Liquid form contains alcohol.
**May contain tartrazine.

Common reactions are in italics; *life-threatening,* in bold italics.

lation, or other condition that may lead to left heart thrombus; acute pericarditis or subacute bacterial endocarditis; septic thrombophlebitis; diabetic hemorrhagic retinopathy; in patients receiving anticoagulants; and in patients age 75 and older.

• Know that recanalization of occluded coronary arteries and improvement of heart function require initiation of treatment with alteplase as soon as possible after the onset of symptoms.

• **I.V. use:** Reconstitute drug with sterile water for injection (without preservatives) only. (Check manufacturer's labeling for specific information.) Do not use vial if the vacuum is not present. Reconstitute with a large-bore (18G) needle, directing the stream of sterile water at the lyophilized cake. Do not shake. Slight foaming is common, and solution should be clear or pale yellow.

• Keep in mind that drug may be administered as reconstituted (1 mg/ml) or diluted with an equal volume of 0.9% sodium chloride solution or D_5W to make a 0.5 mg/ml solution. Adding other drugs to the infusion is not recommended.

• Reconstitute alteplase solution immediately before use, and administer it within 8 hours because it contains no preservatives. The drug may be temporarily stored at 35° to 86° F (2° to 30° C), but it is only stable for 8 hours at room temperature. Discard any unused solution.

• Be aware that heparin therapy is frequently initiated after treatment with alteplase to decrease the risk of rethrombosis.

• Have antiarrhythmic agents readily available, and carefully monitor ECG. Coronary thrombolysis is associated with arrhythmias induced by reperfusion of ischemic myocardium. Such arrhythmias do not differ from those commonly associated with MI.

• Avoid invasive procedures during thrombolytic therapy. Carefully monitor the patient for signs of internal bleeding and frequently check all puncture sites. Bleeding is the most common adverse effect and may occur internally and at external puncture sites.

anistreplase (anisoylated plasminogen-streptokinase activator complex; APSAC)
Eminase

Pregnancy Risk Category: C

HOW SUPPLIED
Injection: 30 units/vial

ACTION
Anistreplase, derived from Lys-plasminogen and streptokinase, is formulated into a fibrinolytic enzyme plus activator complex with the activator temporarily blocked by an anisoyl group. The drug is activated in vivo by a nonenzymatic process that removes the anisoyl group. The active Lys-plasminogen-streptokinase activator complex is progressively formed in the bloodstream or within the thrombus.

ONSET, PEAK, DURATION
Onset immediate after I.V. administration. Peak effects occur in about 45 minutes. Effects persist for 6 hours to 2 days.

INDICATIONS & DOSAGE
Lysis of cornary artery thrombi following acute MI –
Adults: 30 units I.V. over 2 to 5 minutes. Administered by direct injection.

ADVERSE REACTIONS
CNS: *intracranial hemorrhage.*
CV: arrhythmias, conduction disorders, hypotension, edema.
EENT: hemoptysis, gum or mouth hemorrhage.

GI: *bleeding.*
GU: hematuria.
Hematologic: *bleeding tendency,* eosinophilia.
Skin: hematomas, urticaria, itching, flushing, delayed (2 weeks after therapy) purpuric rash.
Other: bleeding at puncture sites, *anaphylaxis or anaphylactoid reactions (rare),* arthralgias.

INTERACTIONS
Heparin, oral anticoagulants, drugs that alter platelet function (including aspirin and dipyridamole): may increase the risk of bleeding. Use together cautiously.

CONTRAINDICATIONS
Contraindicated in patients with a history of severe allergic reaction to anistreplase or streptokinase; active internal bleeding, CVA, recent (within the past 2 months) intraspinal or intracranial surgery or trauma, aneurysm, arteriovenous malformation, intracranial neoplasm, uncontrolled hypertension, or known bleeding diathesis.

NURSING CONSIDERATIONS
• Use cautiously in patients with recent (within 10 days) major surgery; trauma (including cardiopulmonary resuscitation); GI or GU bleeding; cerebrovascular disease; hypertension (systolic ≥ 180 mm Hg or diastolic ≥ 110 mm Hg); mitral stenosis, atrial fibrillation, or other conditions that may lead to left heart thrombus; acute pericarditis or subacute bacterial endocarditis; septic thrombophlebitis; diabetic hemorrhagic retinopathy; in pregnancy and first 10 days postpartum; in patients receiving anticoagulants; and in patients 75 years and older.
• **I.V. use:** Unlike other thrombolytics that must be infused, administer anistreplase by direct injection over 2 to 5 minutes.

• Reconstitute the drug by slowly adding 5 ml of sterile water for injection. Direct the stream against the side of the vial, not at the drug itself. Gently roll the vial to mix the dry powder and water. To avoid excessive foaming, don't shake the vial. The reconstituted solution should be colorless to pale yellow. Inspect for precipitate. If the drug is not administered within 30 minutes of reconstituting, discard the vial.
• Do not mix the drug with other medications; do not dilute the solution after reconstitution.
• Carefully monitor ECG during treatment. Be prepared to treat bradycardia or ventricular irritability. Thrombolytic therapy is associated with reperfusion arrhythmias that may signify successful thrombolysis. These arrhythmias are similar to those seen in the course of an acute MI and may include sinus bradycardia, accelerated idioventricular rhythm, ventricular tachycardia, or premature ventricular depolarizations.
• Carefully monitor the patient; avoid I.M. injections and nonessential handling or moving of patient. Bleeding is the most common adverse reaction and may occur internally and at external puncture sites.
• Be aware that heparin therapy is frequently initiated after treatment with anistreplase to decrease the risk of rethrombosis.
• Be aware that anistreplase is derived from human plasma. No cases of hepatitis or HIV infection have been reported to date. The manufacturing process is designed to purify the plasma used in preparation of the drug.
• Keep in mind the efficacy of drug may be limited if antistreptokinase antibodies are present. Antibody levels may be elevated if more than 5 days has elapsed since previous treatment with anistreplase or streptoki-

---

*Liquid form contains alcohol.   *Common* reactions are in italics; *life-threatening,* in bold italics.
**May contain tartrazine.

nase, or if the patient has had a recent streptococcal infection.

• Be aware that in vitro coagulation tests will be affected by the presence of anistreplase. This can be attenuated if blood samples are collected in the presence of aprotinin (150 to 200 units/ml).

• Teach the patient signs of internal bleeding, and tell him to report these immediately. Advise the patient about proper dental care to avoid excessive gum trauma.

---

streptokinase
Kabikinase, Streptase

Pregnancy Risk Category: C

HOW SUPPLIED
Injection: 100,000 IU, 250,000 IU, 600,000 IU, 750,000 IU, 1,500,000 IU in vials for reconstitution

ACTION
Activates plasminogen in two steps: Plasminogen and streptokinase form a complex that exposes the plasminogen-activating site; plasminogen is then converted to plasmin by cleavage of the peptide bond.

ONSET, PEAK, DURATION
Onset immediate after I.V. administration. Peak effects occur in 20 minutes to 2 hours. Effects persist for about 4 hours.

INDICATIONS & DOSAGE
Arteriovenous cannula occlusion –
Adults: 250,000 IU in 2 ml I.V. solution by I.V. pump infusion into each occluded limb of the cannula over 25 to 35 minutes. Clamp off cannula for 2 hours. Then aspirate contents of cannula; flush with sodium chloride solution and reconnect.
Venous thrombosis, pulmonary embolism, and arterial thrombosis and embolism –
Adults: loading dose is 250,000 IU I.V. infusion over 30 minutes. Sustaining dose is 100,000 IU/hour I.V. infusion for 72 hours for deep vein thrombosis and 100,000 IU/hour over 24 to 72 hours by I.V. infusion pump for pulmonary embolism.
Lysis of coronary artery thrombi following acute MI –
Adults: 140,000 units administered as a loading dose followed by maintenance infusion. Loading dose is 20,000 IU via coronary catheter, followed by infusion of maintenance dose of 2,000 IU/minute for 60 minutes. Alternatively, may be administered as an I.V. infusion. Usual adult dose is 1.5 million units infused over 60 minutes.

ADVERSE REACTIONS
CNS: polyradiculoneuropathy.
CV: transient lowering or elevation of blood pressure, reperfusion arrhythmias.
EENT: periorbital edema.
Hematologic: *bleeding,* low hematocrit.
Respiratory: minor breathing difficulty, *bronchospasm.*
Skin: urticaria, pruritus, flushing.
Other: phlebitis at injection site, hypersensitivity reactions *(anaphylaxis),* delayed hypersensitivity reactions (interstitial nephritis, vasculitits, serum sickness-like reactions), musculoskeletal pain, *angioedema,* fever.

INTERACTIONS
Anticoagulants: increased risk of bleeding. Monitor the patient closely.
Antifibrinolytic agents: streptokinase activity is inhibited and reversed by antifibrinolytic agents such as aminocaproic acid.
Aspirin, dipyridamole, indomethacin, phenylbutazone, drugs affecting platelet activity: increased risk of bleeding. Monitor patients closely. Combined therapy with low-dose aspirin (162.5 mg) or dipyridamole has improved acute and long-term results.

CONTRAINDICATIONS

• Contraindicated in patients with ulcerative wounds, active internal bleeding, and recent CVA; recent trauma with possible internal injuries; visceral or intracranial malignant neoplasms; ulcerative colitis; diverticulitis; severe hypertension; acute or chronic hepatic or renal insufficiency; uncontrolled hypocoagulation; chronic pulmonary disease with cavitation; subacute bacterial endocarditis or rheumatic valvular disease; recent cerebral embolism, thrombosis, or hemorrhage.

• Also contraindicated within 10 days after intra-arterial diagnostic procedure or any surgery, including liver or kidney biopsy, lumbar puncture, thoracentesis, paracentesis, or extensive or multiple cutdowns.

• I.M. injections and other invasive procedures are contraindicated during streptokinase therapy.

NURSING CONSIDERATIONS

• Use cautiously when treating arterial embolism that originates from left side of heart because of danger of cerebral infarction.

• Know that only doctors with wide experience in thrombotic disease management where clinical and laboratory monitoring can be performed should use streptokinase.

• Before using streptokinase to clear an occluded arteriovenous cannula, try flushing with heparinized sodium chloride solution, as ordered.

• Keep aminocaproic acid available to treat bleeding, and corticosteroids to treat allergic reactions.

• Have typed and crossmatched packed red cells and whole blood ready to treat possible hemorrhage.

• Before initiating therapy, draw blood to determine PTT and PT. Rate of I.V. infusion depends on thrombin time and streptokinase resistance.

• To check for hypersensitivity reactions, give 100 IU intradermally as ordered; a wheal and flare response within 20 minutes means the patient is probably allergic. Monitor vital signs frequently.

• Be aware that if the patient has had either a recent streptococcal infection or recent treatment with streptokinase, a higher loading dose may be necessary.

• I.V. use: Reconstitute each vial with 5 ml of 0.9% sodium chloride solution for injection. Further dilute to 45 ml. Don't shake; roll gently to mix. Some flocculation may be present after reconstituting; discard if large amounts are present. Filter solution with 0.8 micron or larger filter. Use within 24 hours. Store powder at room temperature and refrigerate after reconstitution.

• Monitor the patient for excessive bleeding every 15 minutes for the first hour, every 30 minutes for the second through eighth hours, then once every shift. If bleeding is evident, stop therapy and notify doctor. Know that pretreatment with heparin or drugs affecting platelets causes high risk of bleeding, but may improve long-term results. Monitor closely.

• Monitor pulses, color, and sensation of extremities every hour.

• Maintain the involved extremity in straight alignment to prevent bleeding from the infusion site.

• Avoid unnecessary handling of patients; pad side rails. Bruising is more likely during therapy.

• Keep a laboratory flow sheet on the patient's chart to monitor PTT, PT, and hemoglobin and hematocrit levels.

• Keep venipuncture sites to a minimum; use pressure dressing on puncture sites for at least 15 minutes.

• Watch for signs of hypersensitivity. Notify the doctor immediately. Antihistamines or corticosteroids may be used to treat mild allergic reactions. If a severe reaction occurs, the infusion

---

*Liquid form contains alcohol.   *Common* reactions are in italics; ***life-threatening***, in bold italics.
**May contain tartrazine.

should be stopped immediately and the doctor notified.

• Be aware that heparin by continuous infusion is usually started within an hour after stopping streptokinase. Use infusion pump to administer heparin.

• Keep in mind that thrombolytic therapy in patients with acute MI may decrease infarct size, improve ventricular function, and decrease incidence of CHF. Streptokinase must be administered within 6 hours of the onset of symptoms for optimal effect.

urokinase

Abbokinase Open-Cath, Ukidan‡, Win-Kinase

Pregnancy Risk Category: B

HOW SUPPLIED

Injection: 5,000 units (IU) per unit-dose vial; 9,000 units (IU) per unit-dose vial; 250,000-IU vial

ACTION

Activates plasminogen by directly cleaving peptide bonds at two different sites.

ONSET, PEAK, DURATION

Onset immediate after I.V. administration. Peak effects occur in 20 minutes to 2 hours. Effects persist for about 4 hours.

INDICATIONS & DOSAGE

Lysis of acute massive pulmonary embolism and lysis of pulmonary embolism accompanied by unstable hemodynamics –

Adults: for I.V. infusion only by constant infusion pump delivering total volume of 195 ml.
Priming dose: 4,400 IU/kg of urokinase-0.9% sodium chloride solution admixture given over 10 minutes. Followed with 4,400 IU/kg hourly for 12 to 24 hours. Total volume should not exceed 200 ml. Therapy followed

with continuous I.V. infusion of heparin, then oral anticoagulants.
Coronary artery thrombosis –
Adults: after a bolus dose of heparin ranging from 2,500 to 10,000 units, 6,000 IU/minute of urokinase is infused into the occluded artery for up to 2 hours. Average total dosage is 500,000 IU.
Venous catheter occlusion –
Adults: 5,000 IU instilled into occluded line and after a 5-minute wait is aspirated. Aspiration attempts repeated q 5 minutes for 30 minutes. If not patent after 30 minutes, the line is capped and urokinase left to work for 30 to 60 minutes before aspirating again. May require second instillation.

ADVERSE REACTIONS

Hematologic: *bleeding,* low hematocrit.
Respiratory: bronchospasm.
Other: phlebitis at injection site, hypersensitivity reactions *(anaphylaxis),* musculoskeletal pain, fever.

INTERACTIONS

Anticoagulants: increased risk of bleeding. Monitor the patient closely.
Aspirin, dipyridamole, indomethacin, phenylbutazone, other drugs affecting platelet activity: increased risk of bleeding.

CONTRAINDICATIONS

• Contraindicated in patients with active internal bleeding, history of CVA, aneurysm, arteriovenous malformation, known bleeding diathesis, recent trauma with possible internal injuries, visceral or intracranial malignancy, pregnancy and first 10 days postpartum, ulcerative colitis, diverticulitis, severe hypertension, hemostatic defects including those secondary to severe hepatic or renal insufficiency, uncontrolled hypocoagulation, chronic pulmonary disease with cavitation, subacute bacterial endocarditis

---

or rheumatic valvular disease, and recent cerebral embolism, thrombosis, or hemorrhage.

• Also contraindicated within 10 days after intra-arterial diagnostic procedure or any surgery (liver or kidney biopsy, lumbar puncture, thoracentesis, paracentesis, or extensive or multiple cutdowns) or within two months after intracranial or intraspinal surgery.

• I.M. injections and other invasive procedures are contraindicated during urokinase therapy.

NURSING CONSIDERATIONS

• Have typed and crossmatched red cells, whole blood, and aminocaproic acid available to treat bleeding, and corticosteroids to treat allergic reactions.

• **I.V. use:** Add 5 ml of sterile water for injection to vial. Dilute further with 0.9% sodium chloride solution or D₅W solution before infusion. The total volume of fluid administered should not exceed 200 ml. Don't use bacteriostatic water for injection to reconstitute; it contains preservatives. Urokinase solutions may be filtered through a 0.45-μm or smaller cellulose-membrane filter before administration.

• Monitor the patient for excessive bleeding every 15 minutes for the first hour; every 30 minutes for the second through eighth hours; then once every shift. Pretreatment with drugs affecting platelets places patient at high risk of bleeding.

• Monitor pulses, color, and sensation of extremities every hour.

• Although the incidence of hypersensitivity reactions is low, watch for signs of this reaction.

• Keep a laboratory flow sheet on the patient's chart to monitor PTT, PT, and hemoglobin and hematocrit levels.

• Monitor vital signs.

• Keep venipuncture sites to a minimum; use pressure dressing on puncture sites for at least 15 minutes.

• Maintain the involved extremity in straight alignment to prevent bleeding from the infusion site.

• Avoid unnecessary handling of patients; pad side rails. Bruising is more likely during therapy.

• Be aware that heparin by continuous infusion is usually started within an hour after urokinase has been stopped to prevent recurrent thrombosis.

• Instruct the patient to report symptoms of bleeding.

---

*Liquid form contains alcohol.   *Common* reactions are in italics; *life-threatening,* in bold italics.
**May contain tartrazine.

busulfan
carboplatin
carmustine
chlorambucil
cisplatin
cyclophosphamide
ifosfamide
lomustine
mechlorethamine hydrochloride
melphalan
streptozocin
thiotepa
uracil mustard

COMBINATION PRODUCTS
None.

busulfan
Myleran
Pregnancy Risk Category: D

HOW SUPPLIED
Tablets: 2 mg

ACTION
Unknown. Thought to cross-link strands of cellular DNA and interferes with RNA transcription, causing an imbalance of growth that leads to cell death. Cell cycle-nonspecific.

ONSET, PEAK, DURATION
Onset occurs in 1 to 2 weeks. Peak and duration unknown.

INDICATIONS & DOSAGE
Chronic myelocytic (granulocytic) leukemia –
Adults: 4 to 8 mg P.O. daily up to 12 mg P.O. daily until WBC count falls to 15,000/mm³; drug stopped until WBC count rises to 50,000/mm³, and then resumed as before; or 4 to 8 mg P.O. daily until WBC count falls to 10,000 to 20,000/mm³, and then daily dosage reduced as needed to maintain WBC count at this level (usually 1 to 3 mg daily).
Children: 0.06 to 0.12 mg/kg/day or 1.8 to 4.6 mg/m²/day P.O.; dosage adjusted to maintain WBC count at 20,000/mm³, but never less than 10,000/mm³.

ADVERSE REACTIONS
CNS: *seizures,* unusual tiredness or weakness.
GI: nausea, vomiting, diarrhea, cheilosis, glossitis.
GU: amenorrhea, testicular atrophy, impotence.
Hematologic: WBC count falling after about 10 days and continuing to fall for 2 weeks after stopping drug; *thrombocytopenia, anemia.*
Respiratory: persistent cough; dyspnea; *irreversible pulmonary fibrosis, commonly termed "busulfan lung."*
Skin: transient hyperpigmentation, rash, urticaria, anhidrosis.
Other: gynecomastia, alopecia, Addison-like wasting syndrome, profound hyperuricemia caused by increased cell lysis.

INTERACTIONS
Anticoagulants, aspirin: increased risk of bleeding. Avoid concomitant use.
Thioguanine: may cause hepatotoxicity, esophageal varices, or portal hypertension. Use together cautiously.

CONTRAINDICATIONS
Contraindicated in patients with chronic myelogenous leukemia, which is known to be resistant to the drug.

NURSING CONSIDERATIONS

• Use cautiously in patients recently given other myelosuppressive drugs or radiation treatment and in those with depressed neutrophil or platelet count. Because high-dose therapy has been associated with seizures, use such therapy cautiously in patients with a history of head trauma or seizures or in patients receiving other drugs that lower the seizure threshold.

• Follow institutional policy regarding preparation and handling of drug. Label as a hazardous drug.

• To prevent bleeding, avoid all I.M. injections when platelet count is below 100,000/mm³.

• Monitor patient response (increased appetite and sense of well-being, decreased total WBC count, reduced size of spleen), which usually begins within 1 to 2 weeks.

• Monitor serum uric acid. To prevent hyperuricemia with resulting uric acid nephropathy, allopurinol may be used with adequate hydration.

• Anticipate need for possible blood transfusion during treatment because of cumulative anemia.

• Know that therapeutic effects are often accompanied by toxicity.

• Be aware that pulmonary fibrosis may occur as late as 4 to 6 months after treatment with busulfan.

• Warn patients to watch for signs of infection (fever, sore throat, fatigue) and bleeding (easy bruising, nosebleeds, bleeding gums, melena). Take temperature daily.

• Instruct patients to report symptoms of toxicity so dosage adjustments can be made. Persistent cough and progressive dyspnea with alveolar exudate, suggestive of pneumonia, may be the result of drug toxicity.

• Instruct patients to avoid any OTC product containing aspirin.

• Advise women of childbearing age to avoid becoming pregnant during therapy. Recommend patient consult with doctor before becoming pregnant.

• Warn breast-feeding patient to discontinue breast-feeding because of the possibility of infant toxicity.

carboplatin
Paraplatin, Paraplatin-AQ†

Pregnancy Risk Category: D

HOW SUPPLIED
Injection: 50-mg, 150-mg, 450-mg vials

ACTION
Unknown. An alkylating agent that probably produces cross-linking of DNA strands. Cell cycle-nonspecific.

ONSET, PEAK, DURATION
Unknown.

INDICATIONS & DOSAGE
Palliative treatment of ovarian cancer—

Adults: 360 mg/m² I.V. on day 1 q 4 weeks; doses should not be repeated until platelet count exceeds 100,000/mm³ and neutrophil count exceeds 2,000/mm³. Subsequent doses are based on blood counts.
For patients with renal dysfunction: Patients with a creatinine clearance of 41 to 59 ml/minute should receive a starting dose of 250 mg/m²; patients with a creatinine clearance of 16 to 40 ml/minute should receive a starting dose of 200 mg/m². Recommended dosage adjustments are not available for patients with a creatinine clearance of 15 ml/minute or less.

ADVERSE REACTIONS
CNS: dizziness, confusion, peripheral neuropathy, ototoxicity, central neurotoxicity.
GI: constipation, diarrhea, *nausea, vomiting.*
Hematologic: *thrombocytopenia,*

---

*Liquid form contains alcohol.
**May contain tartrazine.

Common reactions are in italics; **life-threatening,** in bold italics.

leukopenia, neutropenia, anemia, bone marrow suppression.
Hepatic: hepatotoxicity.
Other: alopecia; hypersensitivity reactions; increased BUN, creatinine, AST, or alkaline phosphatase levels.

INTERACTIONS

Bone marrow depressants (including radiation therapy): increased hematologic toxicity.
Nephrotoxic agents: enhanced nephrotoxicity of carboplatin.

CONTRAINDICATIONS

Contraindicated in patients with a history of hypersensitivity to cisplatin, platinum-containing compounds, or mannitol or with severe bone marrow suppression or bleeding.

NURSING CONSIDERATIONS

• Determine serum electrolyte, creatinine, and BUN levels; CBC; and creatinine clearance before the first infusion and before each course of treatment.
• Follow institutional policy to reduce risks because preparation and administration of parenteral form of this drug is associated with mutagenic, teratogenic, and carcinogenic risks for personnel.
• Check ordered dose against laboratory test results carefully. Only one increase in dosage is recommended. Subsequent doses should not exceed 125% of starting dose.
• Have epinephrine, corticosteroids, and antihistamines available when administering carboplatin because anaphylactoid reactions may occur within minutes of administration.
• **I.V. use:** Reconstitute with D_5W, 0.9% sodium chloride solution, or sterile water for injection to make a concentration of 10 mg/ml. Add 5 ml of diluent to the 50-mg vial, 15 ml of diluent to the 150-mg vial, or 45 ml of diluent to the 450-mg vial. It can then be further diluted for infusion with

0.9% sodium chloride solution or D_5W. A concentration as low as 0.5 mg/ml can be prepared. Give drug by continuous or intermittent infusion over at least 15 minutes.
• Do not use needles or I.V. administration sets containing aluminum to administer carboplatin; precipitation and loss of drug's potency may occur.
• To prevent bleeding, avoid all I.M. injections when platelet count is below 100,000/mm³.
• Monitor vital signs during infusion.
• Monitor CBC and platelet count frequently during therapy and, when indicated, until recovery. WBC and platelet count nadirs usually occur by day 21. Levels usually return to baseline by day 28. Know that dose should not be repeated unless platelet count exceeds 100,000/mm³.
• Know that therapeutic effects are often accompanied by toxicity.
• Administer antiemetic therapy as ordered. Carboplatin can produce severe vomiting.
• Anticipate need for possible blood transfusions during treatment because of cumulative anemia.
• Know that hydration or diuresis before or after treatment is not necessary.
• Keep in mind that bone marrow suppression may be more severe in patients with creatinine clearance below 60 ml/minute; dosage adjustments are recommended for such patients.
• Be aware that patients over age 65 are at greater risk for neurotoxicity.
• Store unopened vials at room temperature. Once reconstituted and diluted as directed, drug is stable at room temperature for 8 hours. Because the drug does not contain antibacterial preservatives, discard unused drug after 8 hours.
• Warn patient to watch for signs of infection (fever, sore throat, fatigue) and bleeding (easy bruising, nose

bleeds, bleeding gums, melena). Take temperature daily.
• Instruct patient to avoid OTC products containing aspirin.
• Advise women of childbearing age to avoid becoming pregnant during therapy. Also recommend consulting with the doctor before becoming pregnant.
• Because of the possibility of infant toxicity, advise breast-feeding patients taking carboplatin to discontinue breast-feeding.

---

carmustine (BCNU)
BiCNU

Pregnancy Risk Category: D

HOW SUPPLIED
Injection: 100-mg vial (lyophilized), with a 3-ml vial of absolute alcohol supplied as a diluent

ACTION
Inhibits enzymatic reactions involved with DNA synthesis, cross-links strands of cellular DNA, and interferes with RNA transcription, causing an imbalance of growth that leads to cell death. Cell cycle-nonspecific.

ONSET, PEAK, DURATION
Unknown.

INDICATIONS & DOSAGE
Brain tumors, Hodgkin's disease, non-Hodgkin's lymphoma, and multiple myeloma—
Adults: 75 to 100 mg/m² I.V. by slow infusion daily for 2 days; repeated q 6 weeks if platelet count is above 100,000/mm³ and WBC count is above 4,000/mm³. Dosage is reduced by 30% when WBC count is 2,000 to 3,000/mm³ and platelet count is 25,000 to 75,000/mm³. Dosage is reduced by 50% when WBC count is less than 2,000/mm³ and platelet count is less than 25,000/mm³.
  Alternative therapy: 150 to 200

mg/m² I.V. by slow infusion as a single dose, repeated q 6 weeks.

ADVERSE REACTIONS
CNS: ataxia, drowsiness.
GI: *nausea beginning in 2 to 6 hours (can be severe), vomiting, anorexia, dysphagia, esophagitis, diarrhea.*
GU: nephrotoxicity.
Hematologic: *cumulative bone marrow suppression,* delayed 4 to 6 weeks, lasting 1 to 2 weeks; *leukopenia; thrombocytopenia; acute leukemia or bone marrow dysplasia* may occur after long-term use.
Hepatic: hepatotoxicity.
Respiratory: *pulmonary fibrosis.*
Skin: facial flushing, hyperpigmentation (if drug contacts skin).
Other: *intense pain at infusion site from venous spasm;* possible hyperuricemia in lymphoma patients when rapid cell lysis occurs.

INTERACTIONS
Anticoagulants, aspirin: increased risk of bleeding. Avoid concomitant use.
Cimetidine: may increase carmustine's bone marrow toxicity. Avoid combination if possible.

CONTRAINDICATIONS
Contraindicated in patients with hypersensitivity to drug.

NURSING CONSIDERATIONS
• Be aware that pulmonary toxicity appears to be dose-related. Obtain baseline pulmonary function tests as ordered before therapy.
• Follow institutional policy to reduce risks because preparation and administration of parenteral form of this drug is associated with carcinogenic, mutagenic, and teratogenic risks for personnel.
• **I.V. use:** To reconstitute, dissolve 100 mg of carmustine in the 3 ml of absolute alcohol provided by the manufacturer. Dilute solution with 27 ml

---

*Liquid form contains alcohol.   *Common* reactions are in italics; **life-threatening,** in bold italics.
**May contain tartrazine.

of sterile water for injection. Resultant solution contains 3.3 mg of carmustine/ml in 10% alcohol. Dilute in 0.9% sodium chloride solution or D₅W for I.V. infusion. Give at least 250 ml over 1 to 2 hours. To reduce pain on infusion, dilute further or slow infusion rate.
• Discard drug if powder liquefies or appears oily (decomposition has occurred).
• Administer only in glass containers. Solution is unstable in plastic I.V. bags.
• Don't mix with other drugs during administration.
• To reduce nausea, give antiemetic before administering drug, as ordered.
• Avoid contact with skin because carmustine will cause a brown stain. If drug comes into contact with skin, wash off thoroughly.
• Perform liver, renal function, and pulmonary function tests periodically.
• Monitor CBC, as ordered.
• Monitor serum uric acid level, as ordered. To prevent hyperuricemia with resulting uric acid nephropathy, know that allopurinol may be used with adequate hydration.
• To prevent bleeding, avoid all I.M. injections when platelet count is below 100,000/mm³.
• Anticipate the need for possible blood transfusions during treatment because of cumulative anemia.
• Be aware that therapeutic effects are often accompanied by toxicity.
• Know that because carmustine crosses the blood-brain barrier, it may be used to treat primary brain tumors.
• Store reconstituted solution in refrigerator for 48 hours. May decompose at temperatures above 80° F (26.6° C).
• Warn patients to watch for signs of infection (fever, sore throat, fatigue) and bleeding (easy bruising, nosebleeds, bleeding gums, melena). Take temperature daily.

• Instruct patients to avoid any OTC product containing aspirin.
• Advise breast-feeding patients to discontinue breast-feeding during therapy because of possible infant toxicity.
• Advise women of childbearing age to avoid becoming pregnant during therapy. Recommend patient consult with doctor before becoming pregnant.

chlorambucil
Leukeran

Pregnancy Risk Category: D

HOW SUPPLIED
Tablets: 2 mg

ACTION
Cross-links strands of cellular DNA and interferes with RNA transcription, causing an imbalance of growth that leads to cell death. Cell cycle-nonspecific.

ONSET, PEAK, DURATION
Clinical onset occurs within 3 to 4 weeks. Peak plasma concentration occurs in 1 hour. Duration unknown.

INDICATIONS & DOSAGE
Chronic lymphocytic leukemia; malignant lymphomas including lymphosarcoma, giant follicular lymphoma, and Hodgkin's disease –
Adults: 0.1 to 0.2 mg/kg P.O. daily for 3 to 6 weeks; then adjusted for maintenance (usually 4 to 10 mg daily).

ADVERSE REACTIONS
CNS: seizures (with overdose).
GI: *nausea, vomiting, stomatitis.*
GU: *azoospermia, infertility.*
Hematologic: *neutropenia,* delayed up to 3 weeks, lasting up to 10 days after last dose; *thrombocytopenia; anemia;* myelosuppression (usually

moderate, gradual, and rapidly reversible).
Hepatic: hepatotoxicity (rare).
Respiratory: interstitial pneumonitis, *pulmonary fibrosis* (rare).
Skin: *exfoliative dermatitis,* rash.
Other: allergic febrile reaction, hyperuricemia.

INTERACTIONS
Anticoagulants, aspirin: increased risk of bleeding. Avoid concomitant use.

CONTRAINDICATIONS
Contraindicated in patients with hypersensitivity or resistance to previous therapy. Patients hypersensitive to other alkylating agents may also be hypersensitive to chlorambucil.

NURSING CONSIDERATIONS
• Use cautiously in patients with a history of head trauma or seizures or in patients receiving other drugs that lower the seizure threshold.
• Monitor CBC, as ordered.
• Monitor serum uric acid level, as ordered. To prevent hyperuricemia with resulting uric acid nephropathy, know that allopurinol may be used with adequate hydration.
• If WBC count falls below 2,000/mm³ or granulocyte count falls below 1,000/mm³, follow institutional policy for infection control in immunocompromised patients. Severe neutropenia is reversible up to cumulative dosage of 6.5 mg/kg in a single course.
• To prevent bleeding, avoid all I.M. injections when platelet count is below 100,000/mm³.
• Be aware that therapeutic effects are often accompanied by toxicity.
• Anticipate the need for possible blood transfusions during treatment because of cumulative anemia.
• Warn patients to watch for signs of infection (fever, sore throat, fatigue) and bleeding (easy bruising, nosebleeds, bleeding gums, melena). Take temperature daily.
• Instruct patients to avoid OTC products containing aspirin.

cisplatin (cis-platinum)
Platamine‡, Platinol, Platinol AQ

Pregnancy Risk Category: D

HOW SUPPLIED
Injection: 0.5 mg/ml†, 1 mg/ml
Powder for injection: 10 mg, 50 mg

ACTION
Unknown. Probably cross-links strands of cellular DNA and interferes with RNA transcription, causing an imbalance of growth that leads to cell death. Cell cycle-nonspecific.

ONSET, PEAK, DURATION
Onset and peak unknown. Effects persist for several days after administration.

INDICATIONS & DOSAGE
Adjunctive therapy in metastatic testicular cancer–
Adults: 20 mg/m² I.V. daily for 5 days. Repeated q 3 weeks for three cycles or longer.
Adjunctive therapy in metastatic ovarian cancer–
Adults: 100 mg/m² I.V.; repeated q 4 weeks. Or 75 to 100 mg/m² I.V. once q 4 weeks in combination with cyclophosphamide.
Advanced bladder cancer–
Adults: 50 to 70 mg/m² I.V. q 3 to 4 weeks. Patients who have received other antineoplastic agents or radiation therapy should receive 50 mg/m² q 4 weeks.
Note: Prehydration and mannitol diuresis may reduce renal toxicity and ototoxicity significantly.

ADVERSE REACTIONS

CNS: *peripheral neuritis,* loss of taste, *seizures.*

EENT: *tinnitus, hearing loss.*

GI: *nausea, vomiting, beginning 1 to 4 hours after dose and lasting 24 hours;* diarrhea; metallic taste.

GU: *more prolonged and severe renal toxicity with repeated courses of therapy.*

Hematologic: *mild myelosuppression in 25% to 30% of patients; leukopenia, thrombocytopenia, anemia;* nadirs in circulating platelet and WBC counts on days 18 to 23, with recovery by day 39.

Other: *anaphylactoid reaction, hypomagnesemia,* hypokalemia, hypocalcemia.

INTERACTIONS

Aminoglycoside antibiotics: additive nephrotoxicity. Monitor renal function studies very carefully.

Bumetanide, ethacrynic acid, furosemide: additive ototoxicity. Avoid concomitant use.

Phenytoin: decreased serum phenytoin levels. Monitor serum levels.

CONTRAINDICATIONS

Contraindicated in patients with hypersensitivity to the drug or to other platinum-containing compounds and in those with severe renal disease, hearing impairment, or myelosuppression.

NURSING CONSIDERATIONS

• Monitor CBC, electrolyte levels (especially potassium and magnesium), platelet count, and renal function studies before initial and subsequent dosages, as ordered.

• To prevent permanent hearing loss, perform audiometry before initial dosage and subsequent courses, as ordered.

• Administer mannitol as 12.5-g I.V. bolus before starting cisplatin infusion, as ordered. Follow, if ordered, by infusion of mannitol at rate of up to 10 g/hour p.r.n. to maintain urine output during and 6 to 24 hours after cisplatin infusion.

• Hydrate patient with 0.9% sodium chloride solution before giving drug, as ordered. Maintain urine output of 100 ml/hour for 4 consecutive hours before therapy and for 24 hours after therapy.

• Follow institutional policy to reduce risks because preparation and administration of parenteral form of this drug is associated with carcinogenic, mutagenic, and teratogenic risks for personnel.

• **I.V. use:** Reconstitute powder using sterile water for injection. Add 10 ml to the 10-mg vial or 50 ml to the 50-mg vial to make a solution containing 1 mg/ml. If necessary, further dilute with dextrose 5% in 0.3% sodium chloride injection or dextrose 5% in 0.45% sodium chloride injection. Solutions are stable for 20 hours at room temperature. Don't refrigerate.

• Keep in mind that infusions are most stable in chloride-containing solutions (such as 0.9% sodium chloride, 0.45% sodium chloride, and 0.22% sodium chloride).

• Be aware that the manufacturer recommends administering the drug as an I.V. infusion in 2 liters of 0.9% sodium chloride solution with 37.5 g of mannitol over 6 to 8 hours.

• Do not use needles or I.V. administration sets that contain aluminum because it will displace the platinum, causing a loss of potency and formation of a black precipitate.

• Know that therapeutic effects are often accompanied by toxicity.

• Check current protocol. Some clinicians use I.V. sodium thiosulfate to minimize toxicity.

• Administer antiemetics as ordered. Nausea and vomiting may be severe and protracted (up to 24 hours). Monitor intake and output. Continue I.V.

---

†Available in Canada only.   ‡Available in Australia only.   ◊Available OTC.

hydration until patient can tolerate adequate oral intake.

• Keep in mind that ondansetron, granisetron, or high-dose metoclopramide has been used very effectively to treat and prevent nausea and vomiting. Some clinicians combine metoclopramide with dexamethasone and antihistamines, or ondansetron or granisetron with dexamethasone.

• Be alert that delayed-onset vomiting (3 to 5 days after treatment) has been reported. Patients may need prolonged antiemetic treatment.

• Know that renal toxicity is cumulative. Renal function must return to normal before next dose can be given.

• Know that dosage should not be repeated unless platelet count is over 100,000/mm³, WBC count is over 4,000/mm³, creatinine level is under 1.5 mg/dl, or BUN level is under 25 mg/dl.

• To prevent bleeding, avoid all I.M. injections when platelet counts are below 100,000/mm³.

• Anticipate the need for possible blood transfusions during treatment because of cumulative anemia.

• To prevent hypokalemia, know that potassium chloride (10 to 20 mEq/L) is frequently added to I.V. fluids before and after cisplatin therapy.

• Immediately administer epinephrine, corticosteroids, or antihistamines for anaphylactoid reactions, as ordered.

• Warn patients to watch for signs of infection (fever, sore throat, fatigue) and bleeding (easy bruising, nosebleeds, bleeding gums, melena). Take temperature daily.

• Tell patients to report tinnitus immediately.

• Instruct patient to avoid any OTC products containing aspirin.

• Advise breast-feeding patients taking this drug to discontinue breast-feeding because of the possibility of infant toxicity.

• Advise women of childbearing age

to avoid becoming pregnant during therapy. Also recommend consulting with doctor before becoming pregnant.

cyclophosphamide
Cycoblastin‡, Cytoxan**, Cytoxan Lyophilized, Endoxan-Asta‡, Neosar, Procytox†

Pregnancy Risk Category: D

HOW SUPPLIED
Tablets: 25 mg, 50 mg
Injection: 100-mg, 200-mg, 500-mg, 1-g, 2-g vials

ACTION
Cross-links strands of cellular DNA and interferes with RNA transcription, causing an imbalance of growth that leads to cell death. Cell cycle-nonspecific.

ONSET, PEAK, DURATION
Unknown.

INDICATIONS & DOSAGE
Breast, head, neck, prostate, lung, and ovarian cancers; Hodgkin's disease; chronic lymphocytic leukemia; chronic myelocytic leukemia; acute lymphoblastic leukemia; acute myelocytic leukemia; neuroblastoma; retinoblastoma; non-Hodgkin's lymphoma; multiple myeloma; mycosis fungoides; sarcoma –
Adults and children: initially, 40 to 50 mg/kg I.V. in divided doses over 2 to 5 days. Alternatively, 10 to 15 mg/kg I.V. q 7 to 10 days, 3 to 5 mg/kg I.V. twice weekly, or 1 to 5 mg/kg P.O. daily, depending on patient tolerance. Subsequent dosages adjusted according to evidence of antitumor activity and/or leukopenia.
Children: same dosage as adults.
"Minimal change" nephrotic syndrome in children –
Children: 2.5 to 3 mg/kg P.O. daily for 60 to 90 days.

ADVERSE REACTIONS

CV: *cardiotoxicity* (with very high doses and in combination with doxorubicin).

GI: anorexia, *nausea and vomiting beginning within 6 hours,* stomatitis, mucositis.

GU: gonadal suppression (may be irreversible), *hemorrhagic cystitis,* bladder fibrosis.

Hematologic: *leukopenia,* nadir between days 8 to 15, recovery in 17 to 28 days; *thrombocytopenia; anemia.*

Respiratory: *pulmonary fibrosis* (high doses).

Other: *reversible alopecia in 50% of patients, especially with high doses;* secondary malignancies, *anaphylaxis,* hyperuricemia, SIADH (with high doses).

INTERACTIONS

Barbiturates: increased pharmacologic effect and enhanced cyclophosphamide toxicity due to induction of hepatic enzymes.

Cardiotoxic drugs: additive adverse cardiac effects.

Chloramphenicol, corticosteroids: reduced activity of cyclophosphamide. Use cautiously.

Digoxin: may decrease serum digoxin levels. Monitor levels closely.

Succinylcholine: prolonged neuromuscular blockade. Don't use together.

CONTRAINDICATIONS

Contraindicated in patients with hypersensitivity to the drug or with severe bone marrow depression.

NURSING CONSIDERATIONS

• Use cautiously in patients with leukopenia, thrombocytopenia, malignant cell infiltration of bone marrow, or hepatic or renal disease and in those who have recently undergone radiation therapy or chemotherapy.

• Follow institutional policy to reduce risks. Preparation and administration of parenteral form of this drug is associated with carcinogenic, mutagenic, and teratogenic risks for personnel.

• **I.V. use:** Reconstitute powder using sterile water for injection or bacteriostatic water for injection containing only parabens. For the nonlyophilized product, add 5 ml to the 100-mg vial, 10 ml to the 200-mg vial, 25 ml to the 500-mg vial, 50 ml to the 1-g vial, or 100 ml to the 2-g vial to produce a solution containing 20 mg/ml. Shake to dissolve; this may take up to 6 minutes and it may be difficult to completely dissolve drug. Lyophilized preparation is much easier to reconstitute; check package insert for quantity of diluent needed to reconstitute drug.

• After reconstitution, administer as ordered by direct I.V. injection or infusion. For I.V. infusion, further dilute with D_5W, dextrose 5% in 0.9% sodium chloride injection, dextrose 5% in Ringer's injection, lactated Ringer's injection, sodium lactate injection, or 0.45% sodium chloride injection.

• Check reconstituted solution for small particles. Filter solution if necessary.

• Know that reconstituted solution is stable for 6 days refrigerated or 24 hours at room temperature. However, use stored solutions cautiously because the drug contains no preservatives.

• Monitor CBC and renal and liver function tests, as ordered.

• Monitor serum uric acid level, as ordered. To prevent hyperuricemia with resulting uric acid nephropathy, know that allopurinol may be used with adequate hydration.

• Monitor for cyclophosphamide toxicity if patient's corticosteroid therapy is discontinued.

• To prevent bleeding, avoid all I.M. injections when platelet count is below 100,000/mm³.

• Anticipate the need for possible

blood transfusions because of cumulative anemia.
• Know that therapeutic effects are often accompanied by toxicity.
• Warn patients that alopecia is likely to occur, but that it is reversible.
• Warn patients to watch for signs of infection (fever, sore throat, fatigue) and bleeding (easy bruising, nosebleeds, bleeding gums, melena). Take temperature daily.
• Instruct patient to avoid OTC products containing aspirin.
• To minimize the risk of hemorrhagic cystitis, encourage patients to void every 1 to 2 hours while awake and to drink at least 3 liters of fluid daily. Don't give the drug at bedtime; infrequent urination during the night may increase the possibility of cystitis. If cystitis occurs, discontinue drug and notify doctor. Cystitis can occur months after therapy ceases. Mesna may be given to lower the incidence and severity of bladder toxicity.
• Advise both male and female patients to practice contraception while taking this drug and for 4 months after; drug is potentially teratogenic.
• Advise breast-feeding patients taking this drug to discontinue breast-feeding because of the possibility of infant toxicity.
• Advise women of childbearing age to avoid becoming pregnant during therapy. Also recommend consulting with doctor before becoming pregnant.

ifosfamide
IFEX

Pregnancy Risk Category: D

HOW SUPPLIED
Injection: 1 g (supplied with 200-mg ampule of mesna), 2 g†, 3 g†

ACTION
Cross-links strands of cellular DNA and interferes with RNA transcription, causing an imbalance of growth that leads to cell death. Cell cycle-nonspecific.

ONSET, PEAK, DURATION
Unknown.

INDICATIONS & DOSAGE
Testicular cancer –
Adults: 1.2 g/m²/day I.V. for 5 consecutive days. Treatment is repeated q 3 weeks or after the patient recovers from hematologic toxicity.

ADVERSE REACTIONS
CNS: *lethargy, somnolence, confusion, depressive psychosis,* **coma, seizures,** *ataxia.*
GI: *nausea, vomiting.*
GU: *hemorrhagic cystitis (dose-limiting, occurring in up to 50% of patients), hematuria,* nephrotoxicity.
Hematologic: *leukopenia,* **thrombocytopenia, myelosuppression.**
Hepatic: elevated liver enzyme levels.
Other: *alopecia.*

INTERACTIONS
Allopurinol: may produce excessive ifosfamide effect by prolonging half-life. Monitor for enhanced toxicity.
Anticoagulants, aspirin: increased risk of bleeding. Avoid concomitant use.
Barbiturates, chloral hydrate, phenytoin: may increase ifosfamide toxicity by inducing hepatic enzymes that hasten the formation of toxic metabolites.
Corticosteroids: may inhibit hepatic enzymes, reducing ifosfamide's effect. Monitor for enhanced ifosfamide toxicity if concurrent steroid dosage is suddenly reduced or discontinued.
Myelosuppressants: enhanced hematologic toxicity. Dosage adjustment may be necessary.

CONTRAINDICATIONS
Contraindicated in patients with hypersensitivity to the drug and in those

---

*Liquid form contains alcohol.   *Common* reactions are in italics; *life-threatening,* in bold italics.
**May contain tartrazine.

with severely depressed bone marrow function.

NURSING CONSIDERATIONS

• Use cautiously in patients with renal impairment or compromised bone marrow reserve as indicated by leukopenia, granulocytopenia, extensive bone marrow metastases, prior radiation therapy, or prior therapy with cytotoxic agents.

• Obtain urinalysis before each dose. If microscopic hematuria is present, patients should be evaluated for hemorrhagic cystitis. Dosage adjustments of mesna may be necessary.

• Administer antiemetics, as ordered, before giving ifosfamide to help decrease nausea.

• Follow institutional policy to reduce risks. Preparation and administration of parenteral form of this drug is associated with carcinogenic, mutagenic, and teratogenic risks for personnel.

• **I.V. use:** Reconstitute each gram of drug with 20 ml of diluent to yield a solution of 50 mg/ml. Use sterile water for injection or bacteriostatic water for injection. Solutions may then be further diluted with sterile water, dextrose 2.5% or 5% in water, 0.45% or 0.9% sodium chloride injection, 5% dextrose and 0.9% sodium chloride injection, or lactated Ringer's injection.

• Infuse each dose over at least 30 minutes.

• As ordered, administer ifosfamide with a protecting agent (mesna) to prevent hemorrhagic cystitis. Mesna must be given concomitantly with or before ifosfamide to prevent cystitis. Adequate fluid intake (2 liters/day, either P.O. or I.V.) is essential.

• Know that ifosfamide and mesna are physically compatible and may be mixed in the same I.V. solution.

• Keep in mind that reconstituted solution is stable for 1 week at room temperature or 6 weeks refrigerated. However, use solution within 6 hours if drug was reconstituted with sterile water without a preservative (such as benzyl alcohol or parabens).

• Don't give the drug at bedtime; infrequent voiding during the night may increase the possibility of cystitis. If cystitis develops, discontinue drug and notify doctor.

• Be aware that bladder irrigation with 0.9% sodium chloride solution may decrease the possibility of cystitis.

• Assess patients for mental status changes; dosage may have to be decreased.

• Monitor CBC and renal and liver function tests, as ordered.

• To prevent bleeding, avoid all I.M. injections when platelet count is below 100,000/mm³.

• Anticipate the need for possible blood transfusions because of cumulative anemia.

• To minimize contact of ifosfamide and its metabolites with the bladder mucosa, remind patients to void frequently.

• Warn patients to watch for signs of infection (fever, sore throat, fatigue) and bleeding (easy bruising, nosebleeds, bleeding gums, melena). Take temperature daily.

• Instruct patients to avoid OTC products containing aspirin.

• Advise breast-feeding patients to discontinue breast-feeding during therapy because of possible infant toxicity.

• Advise women of childbearing age to avoid becoming pregnant during therapy. Also recommend consulting with doctor before becoming pregnant.

lomustine (CCNU)
CeeNU

Pregnancy Risk Category: D

HOW SUPPLIED
Capsules: 10 mg, 40 mg, 100 mg, dose pack (two 10-mg, two 40-mg, two 100-mg capsules)

ACTION
Cross-links strands of cellular DNA and interferes with RNA transcription, causing an imbalance of growth that leads to cell death. Cell cycle-nonspecific.

ONSET, PEAK, DURATION
Unknown.

INDICATIONS & DOSAGE
Brain tumors, Hodgkin's disease—
Adults and children: 100 to 130 mg/m² P.O. as a single dose q 6 weeks. Dosage reduced according to degree of bone marrow suppression. Repeat doses should not be given until WBC count is more than 4,000/mm³ and platelet count is more than 100,000/mm³.

ADVERSE REACTIONS
GI: *nausea and vomiting beginning within 4 to 5 hours;* stomatitis.
GU: nephrotoxicity, progressive azotemia.
Hematologic: *anemia, leukopenia,* delayed up to 6 weeks, lasting 1 to 2 weeks; *thrombocytopenia,* delayed up to 4 weeks, lasting 1 to 2 weeks.

INTERACTIONS
Anticoagulants, aspirin: increased risk of bleeding. Avoid concomitant use.

CONTRAINDICATIONS
Contraindicated in patients with hypersensitivity to the drug.

NURSING CONSIDERATIONS
• Use cautiously in patients with decreased platelet, WBC, or RBC counts and in those receiving other myelosuppressant drugs.

• To avoid nausea, give antiemetic before administering, as ordered.
• Give 2 to 4 hours after meals; drug will be more completely absorbed if taken when the stomach is empty.
• Monitor CBC weekly, as ordered. Usually not administered more often than every 6 weeks; bone marrow toxicity is cumulative and delayed.
• Periodically monitor liver function tests, as ordered.
• To prevent bleeding, avoid all I.M. injections when platelet count is below 100,000/mm³.
• Anticipate the need for possible blood transfusions because of cumulative anemia.
• Know that therapeutic effects are often accompanied by toxicity.
• Be aware that drug may be useful in cancer involving CNS because drug levels in the CSF equal 30% to 50% of plasma level 1 hour after administration.
• Warn patients to watch for signs of infection (fever, sore throat, fatigue) and bleeding (easy bruising, nosebleeds, bleeding gums, melena). Take temperature daily.
• Instruct patients to avoid OTC products containing aspirin.
• Advise breast-feeding patients to discontinue breast-feeding during therapy because of possible infant toxicity.
• Advise women of childbearing age to avoid becoming pregnant during therapy. Also recommend consulting with doctor before becoming pregnant.

mechlorethamine hydrochloride (nitrogen mustard)
Mustargen
Pregnancy Risk Category: D

HOW SUPPLIED
Injection: 10-mg vials

---

*Liquid form contains alcohol.
**May contain tartrazine.

Common reactions are in italics; ***life-threatening***, in bold italics.

ACTION
Cross-links strands of cellular DNA and interferes with RNA transcription, causing an imbalance of growth that leads to cell death. Cell cycle-nonspecific.

ONSET, PEAK, DURATION
Onset occurs in seconds to minutes. Peak and duration unknown.

INDICATIONS & DOSAGE
Polycythemia vera, chronic lymphocytic leukemia, chronic myelocytic leukemia, malignant effusions (pericardial, peritoneal, pleural), mycosis fungoides, Hodgkin's disease, lymphosarcoma, bronchogenic cancer –
Adults: 0.4 mg/kg or 10 mg/m^2 I.V. as a single dose or in divided doses of 0.1 to 0.2 mg/kg/day. Given through running I.V. infusion. Subsequent courses of therapy given when patient has recovered hematologically from previous course (usually 3 to 6 weeks).
Malignant effusions –
Adults: 0.2 to 0.4 mg/kg intracavitarily.

ADVERSE REACTIONS
CNS: headache, weakness, drowsiness, vertigo, light-headedness, *seizures,* progressive paralysis, paresthesia, *cerebral degeneration, coma.*
EENT: tinnitus, *metallic taste* (immediately after dose), deafness with high doses.
GI: *nausea, vomiting, and anorexia* beginning within minutes, lasting 8 to 24 hours.
Hematologic: *thrombocytopenia, agranulocytosis, lymphocytopenia,* nadir of myelosuppression occurring by days 4 to 10 and lasting 10 to 21 days; mild anemia begins in 2 to 3 weeks.
Skin: rash, sloughing, severe irritation if drug extravasates or touches skin.
Other: *alopecia,* precipitation of herpes zoster, *anaphylaxis,* hyperuricemia; *thrombophlebitis.*

INTERACTIONS
Anticoagulants, aspirin: increased risk of bleeding. Avoid concomitant use.

CONTRAINDICATIONS
Contraindicated in patients with hypersensitivity to the drug and with known infectious diseases.

NURSING CONSIDERATIONS
• Use cautiously in patients with severe anemia, depressed neutrophil or platelet count, or in those who have recently undergone radiation therapy or chemotherapy. Monitor CBC.
• Follow institutional policy to reduce risks. Preparation and administration of parenteral form of this drug is associated with carcinogenic, mutagenic, and teratogenic risks for personnel.
• **I.V. use:** Reconstitute the drug using 10 ml of sterile water for injection or 0.9% sodium chloride injection. The resulting solution contains 1 mg/ml of mechlorethamine. Give by direct injection into a vein or into the tubing of a free-flowing I.V. solution.
• Make sure I.V. solution doesn't infiltrate. Mechlorethamine is a potent vesicant. If drug extravasates, apply cold compresses and infiltrate the area with isotonic sodium thiosulfate, as ordered.
• When given intracavitarily for sclerosing effect, dilute using up to 100 ml of 0.9% sodium chloride injection. Turn patient from side to side every 15 minutes to 1 hour to distribute drug.
• Prepare immediately before infusion. Very unstable solution. Visually inspect before using; use within 15 minutes, and discard unused solution.
• Do not use solutions that are discolored or contain particulate matter. Do not use vials that appear to contain droplets of water.

---

†Available in Canada only.　　　　‡Available in Australia only.　　　　◇ Available OTC.

• Dispose of any equipment used in the preparation and administration of mechlorethamine properly and according to institutional policy. Neutralize unused solution with an equal volume of 5% sodium bicarbonate and 5% sodium thiosulfate.

• Monitor serum uric acid level, as ordered. To prevent hyperuricemia with resulting uric acid nephropathy, know that mechlorethamine may be used with adequate hydration.

• Know that therapeutic effects are often accompanied by toxicity.

• Be aware that neurotoxicity increases with dose and patient age.

• To prevent bleeding, avoid all I.M. injections when platelet count is below 100,000/mm³.

• Anticipate the need for possible blood transfusions because of cumulative anemia.

• Warn patients to watch for signs of infection (fever, sore throat, fatigue) and bleeding (easy bruising, nosebleeds, bleeding gums, melena). Take temperature daily.

• Instruct patients to avoid OTC products containing aspirin.

• Advise women of childbearing age to avoid becoming pregnant during therapy. Also recommend consulting with doctor before becoming pregnant.

---

melphalan (L-phenylalanine mustard)
Alkeran

Pregnancy Risk Category: D

HOW SUPPLIED
Tablets (scored): 2 mg
Injection: 50 mg

ACTION
Cross-links strands of cellular DNA and interferes with RNA transcription, causing an imbalance of growth that leads to cell death. Cell cycle-nonspecific.

ONSET, PEAK, DURATION
Unknown.

INDICATIONS & DOSAGE
Multiple myeloma –
Adults: initially, 6 mg P.O. daily for 2 to 3 weeks; then drug stopped for up to 4 weeks or until WBC and platelet counts stop dropping and begin to rise again; maintenance dosage of 2 mg daily then given. Alternative therapy: 0.15 mg/kg P.O. daily for 7 days, or 0.25 mg/kg for 4 days; repeated q 4 to 6 weeks.

Alternatively, administered I.V. to patients who can't tolerate oral therapy. 16 mg/m² given by infusion over 15 to 20 minutes at 2-week intervals for four doses. After patient has recovered from toxicity, drug given at 4-week intervals.
Nonresectable advanced ovarian cancer –
Adults: 0.2 mg/kg P.O. daily for 5 days. Repeated q 4 to 6 weeks, depending on bone marrow recovery.

ADVERSE REACTIONS
Hematologic: *thrombocytopenia, leukopenia, agranulocytosis.*
Respiratory: *pneumonitis, pulmonary fibrosis.*
Skin: dermatitis, pruritus, rash.
Other: *anaphylaxis,* alopecia.

INTERACTIONS
Anticoagulants, aspirin: increased risk of bleeding. Avoid concomitant use.
Antigout agents: decreased effectiveness. Dosage adjustments may be necessary.
Bone marrow suppressants: additive toxicity. Monitor closely.
Vaccines: decreased effectiveness of killed-virus vaccines and increased risk of toxicity from live-virus vaccines. Postpone routine immunization for at least 3 months after last dose of melphalan.

---

*Liquid form contains alcohol.   *Common* reactions are in italics; *life-threatening,* in bold italics.
**May contain tartrazine.

CONTRAINDICATIONS

Contraindicated in patients with hypersensitivity to the drug and in those whose disease is known to be resistant to the drug. Patients hypersensitive to chlorambucil may have cross-sensitivity to melphalan.

NURSING CONSIDERATIONS

• Follow institutional policy to reduce risks. Preparation and administration of parenteral form of the drug is associated with carcinogenic, mutagenic, and teratogenic risks for personnel.
• **I.V. use:** Because drug isn't stable in solution, reconstitute immediately before administering. Reconstitute drug with the 10 ml of sterile diluent supplied by the manufacturer. Shake vigorously until a clear solution is obtained. The resultant solution will contain 5 mg of melphalan/ml. Immediately dilute the required dose in 0.9% sodium chloride injection. Final concentration shouldn't exceed 0.45 mg/ml. Give I.V. infusion over 15 to 20 minutes.
• Promptly dilute and administer; the reconstituted product begins to degrade within 30 minutes. After final dilution, nearly 1% of the drug degrades every 10 minutes. Don't refrigerate the reconstituted product because a precipitate will form.
• Administer on empty stomach. Absorption of drug is decreased by food.
• Know that therapeutic effects are often accompanied by toxicity.
• Monitor serum uric acid level and CBC, as ordered.
• To prevent bleeding, avoid all I.M. injections when platelet count is below 100,000/mm³.
• Anticipate the need for possible blood transfusions because of cumulative anemia.
• Be aware that drug is not recommended in patients with severe leukopenia, thrombocytopenia, or anemia or in those with chronic lymphocytic leukemia.

• Keep in mind that dosage may need to be reduced in patients with renal impairment.
• Be aware that melphalan is the drug of choice in combination with prednisone in patients with multiple myeloma.
• Warn patients to watch for signs of infection (fever, sore throat, fatigue) and bleeding (easy bruising, nosebleeds, bleeding gums, melena). Take temperature daily.
• Instruct patients to avoid OTC products containing aspirin.
• Advise women of childbearing age to avoid becoming pregnant during therapy. Also recommend consulting with the doctor before becoming pregnant.

---

streptozocin
Zanosar

Pregnancy Risk Category: C

HOW SUPPLIED
Injection: 1-g vials

ACTION
Unknown. Probably cross-links strands of cellular DNA and interferes with RNA transcription, causing an imbalance of growth that leads to cell death. Cell cycle-nonspecific.

ONSET, PEAK, DURATION
Unknown.

INDICATIONS & DOSAGE
Metastatic islet cell carcinoma of the pancreas –
Adults and children: 500 mg/m² I.V. for 5 consecutive days q 6 weeks until maximum benefit or toxicity is observed. Alternatively, 1,000 mg/m² at weekly intervals for the first 2 weeks. Not to exceed a single dose of 1,500 mg/m².

ADVERSE REACTIONS
GI: *nausea, vomiting,* diarrhea.
GU: *renal toxicity* (evidenced by azotemia, glycosuria, and renal tubular acidosis), mild proteinuria.
Hematologic: *anemia, leukopenia, thrombocytopenia.*
Hepatic: elevated liver enzyme levels, jaundice.
Other: hyperglycemia, hypoglycemia, diabetes mellitus; *sloughing, severe irritation if extravasation occurs.*

INTERACTIONS
Doxorubicin: prolonged elimination half-life of doxorubicin. Dose of doxorubicin should be reduced.
Other potentially nephrotoxic drugs, such as aminoglycosides: increased risk of renal toxicity. Use cautiously.
Phenytoin: may decrease the effectiveness of streptozocin in patients with pancreatic cancer. Monitor carefully.

CONTRAINDICATIONS
None known.

NURSING CONSIDERATIONS
• Use cautiously in patients with renal disease.
• Obtain renal function tests before therapy, as ordered.
• Follow institutional policy to reduce risks. Preparation and administration of parenteral form of this drug is associated with carcinogenic, mutagenic, and teratogenic risks for personnel.
• **I.V. use:** Reconstitute streptozocin powder with 9.5 ml of D_5W or 0.9% sodium chloride injection. This will produce a pale gold solution. May be further diluted with D_5W or 0.9% sodium chloride injection. Infuse over at least 15 minutes to minimize the risk of phlebitis.
• If extravasation occurs, stop infusion immediately and notify doctor.
• Use within 12 hours of reconstitution. The product contains no preser-

vatives and is not intended as a multiple-dose vial.
• Monitor renal function tests after each course of therapy, as ordered. Renal toxicity resulting from streptozocin therapy is dose-related and cumulative. Urinalysis; BUN, creatinine, and serum electrolyte levels; and creatinine clearance should be obtained at least weekly during drug administration. Weekly monitoring should continue for 4 weeks after each course.
• To minimize risk of renal toxicity, ensure adequate hydration using oral or parenteral fluids, as ordered.
• Test urine for protein and glucose levels each nursing shift. Mild proteinuria is one of the first signs of renal toxicity; notify the doctor if this occurs. Reduction of dosage may be necessary.
• Monitor CBC and liver function studies at least weekly, as ordered.
• Make sure patients are being treated with an antiemetic. Nausea and vomiting occur in most patients.
• Know that therapeutic effects are often accompanied by toxicity.
• Store unopened and unreconstituted vials in the refrigerator.
• Warn patients to watch for signs of infection (fever, sore throat, fatigue) and bleeding (easy bruising, nosebleeds, bleeding gums, melena). Take temperature daily.

thiotepa
Thiotepa
Pregnancy Risk Category: NR

HOW SUPPLIED
Injection: 15-mg vials

ACTION
Cross-links strands of cellular DNA and interferes with RNA transcription, causing an imbalance of growth that leads to cell death. Cell cycle-nonspecific.

---

*Liquid form contains alcohol.   *Common* reactions are in italics; ***life-threatening,*** in bold italics.
**May contain tartrazine.

ONSET, PEAK, DURATION
Unknown.

INDICATIONS & DOSAGE
Breast and ovarian cancers, lymphoma, Hodgkin's disease –
Adults and children over 12 years:
0.3 to 0.4 mg/kg I.V. q 1 to 4 weeks or 0.2 mg/kg 4 to 5 days at intervals of 2 to 4 weeks.
Bladder tumor –
Adults and children over 12 years:
60 mg in 30 to 60 ml of water instilled in bladder for 2 hours once weekly for 4 weeks.
Neoplastic effusions –
Adults and children over 12 years:
0.6 to 0.8 mg/kg intracavitarily.

ADVERSE REACTIONS
CNS: headache, dizziness.
GI: *nausea, vomiting.*
GU: amenorrhea, decreased spermatogenesis.
Hematologic: *leukopenia* begins within 5 to 10 days; *thrombocytopenia; neutropenia; anemia.*
Skin: hives, rash.
Other: fever, tightness of throat, alopecia, hyperuricemia, intense pain at administration site.

INTERACTIONS
Anticoagulants, aspirin: increased risk of bleeding. Avoid concomitant use.

CONTRAINDICATIONS
Contraindicated in patients with hypersensitivity to the drug and in those with severe bone marrow, hepatic, or renal dysfunction.

NURSING CONSIDERATIONS
• Know that use in pregnancy is not recommended except in situations where the benefit to be gained outweighs the risk of teratogenicity involved.
• Use cautiously in patients with mild bone marrow suppression and renal or hepatic dysfunction.
• Follow institutional policy to minimize risks. Preparation and administration of parenteral form of this drug is associated with mutagenic, teratogenic, and carcinogenic risks to personnel.
• **I.V. use:** Reconstitute with 1.5 ml of sterile water for injection. Do not reconstitute with any other solution. Further dilute with 0.9% sodium chloride injection, D_5W, dextrose 5% in 0.9% sodium chloride injection, Ringer's injection, or lactated Ringer's injection. Solutions are stable for up to 5 days if refrigerated.
• Be prepared to use local anesthetic at injection site, as ordered, if intense pain occurs.
• If pain occurs at the insertion site, dilute the drug further or use a local anesthetic, as ordered, to reduce pain. Make sure drug does not infiltrate.
• Discard if solution appears grossly opaque or if a precipitate is present. Solutions should be clear to slightly opaque.
• For neoplastic effusions, mix drug with 2% procaine hydrochloride or epinephrine hydrochloride 1:1,000, as ordered.
• For bladder instillation: Dehydrate patients 8 to 10 hours before therapy. Instill drug into bladder by catheter; ask patients to retain solution for 2 hours. Know that volume may be reduced to 30 ml if discomfort is too great with 60 ml. Reposition patients every 15 minutes for maximum area contact.
• Be aware that drug can be given by all parenteral routes, including direct injection into the tumor.
• Monitor CBC weekly for at least 3 weeks after last dose, as ordered.
• As ordered, discontinue drug if WBC count is below 3,000/mm[3] or if platelet count is below 150,000/mm[3] and notify doctor.

• Monitor serum uric acid levels, as ordered. To prevent hyperuricemia with resulting uric acid nephropathy, know that allopurinol may be used with adequate hydration.
• Know that therapeutic effects are often accompanied by toxicity.
• To prevent bleeding, avoid all I.M. injections when platelet count is below 100,000/mm³.
• Anticipate the need for blood transfusions because of cumulative anemia.
• Be aware that genitourinary adverse reactions are reversible in 6 to 8 months.
• Refrigerate and protect dry powder from direct sunlight to avoid possible drug breakdown.
• Warn patients to watch for signs of infection (fever, sore throat, fatigue) and bleeding (easy bruising, nosebleeds, bleeding gums, melena). Take temperature daily. Tell patients to report even mild infections.
• Instruct patients to avoid OTC products containing aspirin.
• Advise breast-feeding patients to discontinue breast-feeding during therapy because of possible infant toxicity.
• Advise women of childbearing age to avoid becoming pregnant during therapy. Also recommend consulting with doctor before becoming pregnant.

---

uracil mustard
Uracil Mustard Capsules**

Pregnancy Risk Category: NR

HOW SUPPLIED
Capsules: 1 mg

ACTION
Cross-links strands of cellular DNA and interferes with RNA transcription, causing an imbalance of growth that leads to cell death. Cell cycle-nonspecific.

ONSET, PEAK, DURATION
Unknown.

INDICATIONS & DOSAGE
Chronic lymphocytic and myelocytic leukemia, Hodgkin's disease, non-Hodgkin's lymphoma of the histiocytic and lymphocytic types, reticulum cell sarcoma, lymphoma, mycosis fungoides, polycythemia vera —
Adults: 1 to 2 mg P.O. daily for 3 months or until desired response or toxicity; maintenance dosage is 1 mg daily for 3 out of 4 weeks until optimum response or relapse; or 3 to 5 mg P.O. for 7 days not to exceed total dosage of 0.5 mg/kg, then 1 mg daily until response, and then 1 mg daily 3 out of 4 weeks.

ADVERSE REACTIONS
CNS: irritability, nervousness, mental cloudiness, depression.
GI: *nausea, vomiting, diarrhea, epigastric distress,* abdominal pain, anorexia.
Hematologic: bone marrow suppression, delayed 2 to 4 weeks; ***thrombocytopenia; leukopenia; anemia.***
Skin: pruritus, dermatitis, hyperpigmentation.
Other: hyperuricemia, alopecia.

INTERACTIONS
Anticoagulants, aspirin: increased risk of bleeding. Avoid concomitant use.

CONTRAINDICATIONS
Contraindicated in patients with hypersensitivity to the drug and in those with aplastic anemia, thrombocytopenia, or leukopenia.

NURSING CONSIDERATIONS
• Be aware that some commercially available capsules contain tartrazine dye, which may provoke hypersensitivity reactions in certain individuals. This reaction is rare but is more likely to occur in aspirin-sensitive persons.

• Give at bedtime to reduce nausea.
• Monitor platelet count. Check CBC once or twice weekly for 4 weeks; then 4 weeks after stopping drug, as ordered.
• Monitor serum uric acid level, as ordered. To prevent hyperuricemia and resulting uric acid nephropathy, know that allopurinol may be used with adequate hydration.
• Know that therapeutic effects are often accompanied by toxicity.
• To prevent bleeding, avoid all I.M. injections when platelet count is below 100,000/mm^3.
• Anticipate need for possible blood transfusions because of cumulative anemia.
• Warn patients to watch for signs of infection (fever, sore throat, fatigue) and bleeding (easy bruising, nosebleeds, bleeding gums, melena). Take temperature daily.
• Instruct patients to avoid OTC products containing aspirin.
• Advise breast-feeding patients to discontinue breast-feeding during therapy because of possible infant toxicity.
• Advise women of childbearing age to avoid becoming pregnant during therapy. Also recommend consulting with doctor before becoming pregnant. Drug should not be used in pregnancy unless potential benefits outweigh potential risks.

cladribine
cytarabine
floxuridine
fludarabine phosphate
fluorouracil
hydroxyurea
mercaptopurine
methotrexate
methotrexate sodium
thioguanine

COMBINATION PRODUCTS
None.

---

cladribine
(2-chlorodeoxyadenosine)
Leustatin

Pregnancy Risk Category: D

HOW SUPPLIED
Injection: 1 mg/ml

ACTION
Unknown. A purine nucleoside analogue that enters tumor cells, is phosphorylated by deoxycytidine kinase, and is subsequently converted into an active triphosphate deoxynucleotide. This metabolite probably impairs synthesis of new DNA, inhibits repair of existing DNA, and disrupts cellular metabolism.

ONSET, PEAK, DURATION
Onset is approximately a median time of 4 months to response. Peak unknown. Median duration of response is greater than 8 months.

INDICATIONS & DOSAGE
Active hairy cell leukemia –
Adults: 0.09 mg/kg daily by continuous I.V. infusion for 7 days.

ADVERSE REACTIONS
CNS: headache, fatigue, dizziness, insomnia, asthenia.
CV: tachycardia, edema.
EENT: epistaxis.
GI: nausea, decreased appetite, vomiting, diarrhea, constipation, abdominal pain.
GU: acute renal insufficiency.
Hematologic: *neutropenia, anemia, thrombocytopenia.*
Respiratory: abnormal breath or chest sounds, cough, shortness of breath.
Skin: *rash, pruritus, erythema,* purpura, petechiae.
Other: *fever, infection, local reactions at the injection site, chills, diaphoresis, malaise, trunk pain, myalgia, arthralgia,* hyperuricemia.

INTERACTIONS
None significant.

CONTRAINDICATIONS
Contraindicated in patients hypersensitive to the drug.

NURSING CONSIDERATIONS
• Use cautiously in patients with renal or hepatic impairment.
• **I.V. use:** For a 24-hour infusion, add the calculated dose to a 500-ml infusion bag of 0.9% sodium chloride injection. Once diluted, administer promptly or begin administration within 8 hours. Don't use solutions that contain dextrose because studies have shown increased degradation of the drug. Because the drug product doesn't contain any bacteriostatic agents, use strict aseptic technique to prepare the admixture. Repeat daily for 7 consecutive days.
• Alternatively, prepare a 7-day infusion solution, using bacteriostatic so-

---

*Liquid form contains alcohol.
**May contain tartrazine.

Common reactions are in italics; ***life-threatening,*** in bold italics.

dium chloride injection, which contains 0.9% benzyl alcohol. Studies have shown acceptable physical and chemical stability using Pharmacia Deltec medication cassettes. First, pass the calculated amount of drug through a disposable 0.22-micron hydrophilic syringe filter into a sterile infusion reservoir. Next, add sufficient bacteriostatic sodium chloride injection to bring the total volume to 100 ml. Clamp off the line; then disconnect and discard the filter. If necessary, aseptically aspirate air bubbles from the reservoir using a new filter or a sterile vent filter assembly.

• Be aware that because the calculated dose dilutes the benzyl alcohol preservative, 7-day infusion solutions prepared for patients weighing more than 187 lb (85 kg) may have reduced preservative effectiveness.

• Because of the risk of hyperuricemia from tumor lysis, administer allopurinol as ordered during therapy.

• Monitor hematologic function closely as ordered, especially during the first 4 to 8 weeks of therapy. Cladribine is a toxic drug, and some toxicity is expected during treatment. Severe bone marrow suppression, including neutropenia, anemia, and thrombocytopenia, commonly has been observed in patients treated with this drug; many patients also have preexisting hematologic impairment from their disease.

• Keep in mind that fever is commonly observed during the first month of therapy. In clinical trials, virtually all patients received parenteral antibiotics.

• To prevent bleeding, avoid all I.M. injections when platelet count is below 100,000/mm³.

• Anticipate the need for possible blood transfusions because of cumulative anemia.

• Refrigerate unopened vials at 36° to 46° F (2° to 8° C) and protect from light. Although freezing doesn't adversely affect the drug, a precipitate may form; this will disappear if the drug is allowed to warm to room temperature gradually and the vial is vigorously shaken. Don't heat or microwave; don't refreeze.

• Warn patient to watch for signs of infection (fever, sore throat, fatigue) and bleeding (easy bruising, nosebleeds, bleeding gums, melena). Take temperature daily.

• Advise women of childbearing age to avoid becoming pregnant because of the risk of fetal malformations.

cytarabine (ara-C, cytosine arabinoside)
Alexan‡, Cytosar†, Cytosar-U

Pregnancy Risk Category: NR

HOW SUPPLIED
Injection: 40-mg‡, 100-mg, 500-mg, 1-g, 2-g vials

ACTION
Inhibits DNA synthesis.

ONSET, PEAK, DURATION
Onset and duration unknown. Levels peak 20 to 60 minutes after S.C. injection.

INDICATIONS & DOSAGE
Acute non-lymphocytic leukemia, acute lymphocytic leukemia, blast phase of chronic myelocytic leukemia –

Adults and children: 100 mg/m² daily by continuous I.V. infusion or 100 mg/m² I.V. q 12 hours. Given for 7 days and repeated q 2 weeks. For maintenance, 1 mg/kg S.C. once or twice a week.

Meningeal leukemia –

Adults and children: highly variable from 5 mg/m² to 75 mg/m² intrathecally. Frequency also varies from once a day for 4 days to once every 4 days. The most frequently used dosage is 30 mg/m^2, q 4 days until cerebrospinal fluid is normal.

ADVERSE REACTIONS
CNS: neurotoxicity, including ataxia and cerebellar dysfunction, with high doses.
EENT: *keratitis, nystagmus.*
GI: *nausea, vomiting,* diarrhea, dysphagia; reddened area at juncture of lips, followed by sore mouth, oral ulcers in 5 to 10 days; high dose given rapid I.V. may cause projectile vomiting.
Hematologic: *leukopenia,* with initial WBC count nadir 7 to 9 days after drug is stopped and a second (more severe) nadir 15 to 24 days after drug is stopped; anemia; reticulocytopenia; *thrombocytopenia,* with platelet count nadir occurring on day 10; *megaloblastosis.*
Hepatic: hepatotoxicity (usually mild and reversible).
Skin: rash.
Other: flulike syndrome, hyperuricemia, urate nephropathy.

INTERACTIONS
Digoxin: may decrease serum digoxin levels. Monitor closely.

CONTRAINDICATIONS
Contraindicated in patients hypersensitive to the drug.

NURSING CONSIDERATIONS
• Use cautiously in patients with hepatic disease.
• To reduce nausea, give antiemetic before administering, as ordered. Nausea and vomiting are more frequent when large doses are administered rapidly by I.V. push. These reactions are less frequent when given by infusion.
• Follow institutional policy to reduce risks. Preparation and administration of parenteral form of this drug is associated with carcinogenic, mutagenic, and teratogenic risks for personnel.

• **I.V. use:** Reconstitute drug using the provided diluent, which is bacteriostatic water for injection containing benzyl alcohol. Avoid this diluent when preparing drug for neonates or for intrathecal use. Reconstitute 100-mg vial with 5 ml of diluent or 500-mg vial with 10 ml of diluent. Reconstituted solution is stable for 48 hours. Discard cloudy reconstituted solution.
• For I.V. infusion, further dilute using 0.9% sodium chloride injection, D$_5$W, or sterile water for injection.
• For intrathecal administration, use preservative-free 0.9% sodium chloride. Add 5 ml to the 100-mg vial or 10 ml to the 500-mg vial. Use immediately after reconstitution. Discard unused drug.
• Monitor fluid intake and output carefully. Maintain high fluid intake and give allopurinol, if ordered, to avoid urate nephropathy in leukemia induction therapy. Monitor serum uric acid level, as ordered.
• Monitor hepatic and renal function studies and CBC, as ordered.
• Know that therapy may be modified or stopped if granulocyte count is below 1,000/mm^3 or if platelet count is below 50,000/mm^3.
• Know that corticosteroid eye drops are prescribed to prevent drug-induced keratitis.
• Provide diligent mouth care to help prevent stomatitis.
• Assess patients receiving high doses for neurotoxicity, which may first appear as nystagmus, but can progress to ataxia and cerebellar dysfunction.
• To prevent bleeding, avoid all I.M. injections when platelet count is below 100,000/mm^3.
• Anticipate the need for possible blood transfusions because of cumulative anemia.
• Know that therapeutic effects are often accompanied by toxicity.
• Warn patients to watch for signs of infection (fever, sore throat, fatigue) and bleeding (easy bruising, nose-

---

*Liquid form contains alcohol.
**May contain tartrazine.

Common reactions are in italics; ***life-threatening,*** in bold italics.

bleeds, bleeding gums, melena). Take temperature daily.

• Advise breast-feeding patients to discontinue breast-feeding during therapy because of possible infant toxicity.

• Advise women of childbearing age to avoid becoming pregnant during therapy. Also recommend consulting with doctor before becoming pregnant. Drug can cause fetal harm.

floxuridine
FUDR

Pregnancy Risk Category: D

HOW SUPPLIED
Injection: 500-mg vials (50 mg/ml in 10-ml vials or 100 mg/ml in 5-ml vials)

ACTION
Inhibits DNA synthesis.

ONSET, PEAK, DURATION
Unknown.

INDICATIONS & DOSAGE
Gastrointestinal adenocarcinoma metastatic to the liver –
Adults: 0.1 to 0.6 mg/kg daily by intra-arterial infusion for 14 to 21 days or until toxicity occurs; or 0.4 to 0.6 mg/kg daily into hepatic artery.

ADVERSE REACTIONS
CNS: cerebellar ataxia, vertigo, nystagmus, seizures, depression, hemiplegia, hiccups, lethargy.
EENT: blurred vision.
GI: *anorexia, stomatitis, cramps, nausea, vomiting, diarrhea, bleeding, enteritis.*
Hematologic: *leukopenia, anemia, thrombocytopenia.*
Hepatic: cholangitis, jaundice, elevated liver enzyme levels.
Skin: *erythema,* dermatitis, pruritus, rash.
Other: *alopecia.*

INTERACTIONS
None significant.

CONTRAINDICATIONS
Contraindicated in patients with poor nutritional state, bone marrow suppression, or serious infection.

NURSING CONSIDERATIONS
• Use cautiously following high-dose pelvic radiation therapy or use of alkylating agents, and in patients with impaired hepatic or renal function.
• Follow institutional policy to reduce risks. Preparation and administration of parenteral form of this drug is associated with carcinogenic, mutagenic, and teratogenic risks for personnel.
• **IV use:** Reconstitute with sterile water for injection. To prepare infusion, dilute in D_5W or 0.9% sodium chloride solution.
• Use an infusion pump with intra-arterial infusions.
• Check line for bleeding, blockage, displacement, or leakage.
• Monitor fluid intake and output, CBC, and renal and hepatic function, as ordered.
• Know that use of antacid eases but won't prevent GI distress.
• Provide diligent mouth care to help prevent stomatitis.
• Be alert that severe skin and GI adverse reactions require stopping drug.
• Discontinue drug if WBC count falls below 3,500/mm³ or if platelet count falls below 100,000/mm³ and notify doctor.
• Make sure patient knows that therapeutic effect may be delayed 1 to 6 weeks.
• To prevent bleeding, avoid all I.M. injections when platelet count is below 100,000/mm³.
• Anticipate need for possible blood transfusions because of cumulative anemia.
• Warn patient to watch for signs of infection and bleeding.
• Advise breast-feeding patients to

discontinue breast-feeding during therapy because of possible infant toxicity.

• Advise women of childbearing age to avoid becoming pregnant during therapy. Also recommend consulting with the doctor before becoming pregnant.

• Refrigerated solution is stable for no more than 2 weeks.

fludarabine phosphate
Fludara

Pregnancy Risk Category: D

HOW SUPPLIED
Powder for injection: 50 mg

ACTION
Unknown. An antineoplastic antimetabolite that's actions may be multifaceted. After conversion to its active metabolite, fludarabine interferes with DNA synthesis by inhibiting DNA polymerase alpha, ribonucleotide reductase, and DNA primase.

ONSET, PEAK, DURATION
Onset may occur within 7 to 21 hours. Peak and duration unknown.

INDICATIONS & DOSAGE
B-cell chronic lymphocytic leukemia (CLL) in patients who have either not responded or responded inadequately to at least one standard alkylating agent regimen –
Adults: 25 mg/m^2 I.V. over 30 minutes for 5 consecutive days. Cycle repeated q 28 days.

ADVERSE REACTIONS
CNS: *fatigue, malaise, weakness,* paresthesia, headache, sleep disorder, depression, cerebellar syndrome, *CVA,* transient ischemic attack, agitation, *confusion; coma, death* (with very high doses).
CV: *edema,* angina, phlebitis, *arrhythmias, CHF,* supraventricular

tachycardia, deep venous thrombosis, *aneurysm,* hemorrhage.
EENT: *visual disturbances,* hearing loss, delayed blindness (with high doses), sinusitis, pharyngitis, epistaxis.
GI: *nausea, vomiting,* diarrhea, constipation, *anorexia,* stomatitis, GI bleeding, esophagitis, mucositis.
GU: dysuria, urinary infection, urinary hesitancy, proteinuria, hematuria, *renal failure.*
Hematologic: *myelosuppression.*
Hepatic: liver failure, cholelithiasis.
Respiratory: cough, *pneumonia,* dyspnea, upper respiratory infection, allergic pneumonitis, hemoptysis, hypoxia, bronchitis.
Skin: rash, pruritus, seborrhea.
Other: *fever, chills, infection,* pain, myalgia, tumor lysis syndrome, alopecia, *anaphylaxis,* diaphoresis, hyperglycemia, dehydration, hyperuricemia, hyperphosphatemia.

INTERACTIONS
Other myelosuppressants: increased toxicity. Avoid concomitant use.

CONTRAINDICATIONS
Contraindicated in patients hypersensitive to the drug or its components.

NURSING CONSIDERATIONS
• Use cautiously in patients with renal insufficiency.
• Follow institutional policy to reduce risks. Preparation and administration of parenteral form of this drug is associated with mutagenic, teratogenic, and carcinogenic risks for personnel.
• **I.V. use:** To prepare solution, add 2 ml of sterile water for injection to the solid cake of fludarabine. Dissolution should occur within 15 seconds; each milliliter will contain 25 mg of drug. Dilute further in 100 or 125 ml of D$_5$W or 0.9% sodium chloride injection. Use within 8 hours of reconstitution.
• Monitor patients closely and expect

---

*Liquid form contains alcohol.
May contain tartrazine.*   *Common* reactions are in italics; **life-threatening, in bold italics.

dosage modified based on toxicity. Most toxic effects are dose-dependent. Advanced age, renal insufficiency, and bone marrow impairment may predispose patients to increased or excessive toxicity.

• Know that careful hematologic monitoring is required, especially of neutrophil and platelet counts. Bone marrow suppression can be severe.

• To prevent bleeding, avoid all I.M. injections when platelet count is below 100,00/mm³.

• Anticipate the need for possible blood transfusions because of cumulative anemia.

• Know that optimal duration of therapy is not yet determined. Current recommendations suggest three additional cycles after achieving maximal response before discontinuing therapy.

• Store drug in refrigerator at 36° to 46° F (2° to 8° C).

• Warn patient to watch for signs of infection and bleeding.

• Advise women of childbearing age to avoid becoming pregnant during therapy. Also recommend consulting with doctor before becoming pregnant.

---

fluorouracil
(5-fluorouracil, 5-FU)
Adrucil, Efudex, Fluoroplex

Pregnancy Risk Category: D

HOW SUPPLIED
Injection: 50 mg/ml
Cream: 1%, 5%
Topical solution: 1%, 2%, 5%

ACTION
Inhibits DNA synthesis.

ONSET, PEAK, DURATION
Unknown.

INDICATIONS & DOSAGE
Colon, rectal, breast, stomach, and pancreatic cancers –
Adults: 12 mg/kg I.V. daily for 4 days; if no toxicity, dose increased to 6 mg/kg and given on the 6th, 8th, 10th, and 12th day; then a single weekly maintenance dose of 10 to 15 mg/kg I.V. begun after toxicity (if any) from initial course has subsided. (Dosages recommended based on lean body weight.) Maximum single recommended dose is 800 mg.
Palliative treatment of advanced colorectal cancer –
Adults: 425 mg/m² I.V. daily for 5 consecutive days. Given with 20 mg/m² of leucovorin I.V. Repeated at 4-week intervals for two additional courses; then repeated at intervals of 4 to 5 weeks if tolerated.
Multiple actinic (solar) keratoses; superficial basal cell carcinoma –
Adults: apply cream or topical solution b.i.d.

ADVERSE REACTIONS
CNS: acute cerebellar syndrome, ataxia, confusion, disorientation, euphoria, headache, nystagmus, *weakness, malaise.*
GI: *stomatitis, GI ulcer* (may precede leukopenia), *nausea and vomiting in 30% to 50% of patients, diarrhea, anorexia.*
Hematologic: *leukopenia, thrombocytopenia,* anemia; WBC count nadir 9 to 14 days after first dose; platelet count nadir in 7 to 14 days.
Skin: *dermatitis,* hyperpigmentation (especially in blacks), nail changes, pigmented palmar creases; erythematous, desquamative rash of hands and feet with long-term use ("hand-foot syndrome").
Other: *reversible alopecia in 5% to 20% of patients; erythema, pain, burning, scaling, pruritus;* contact dermatitis, soreness, suppuration, swelling (with topical use).

INTERACTIONS

Leucovorin calcium, prior treatment with alkylating agents: increased toxicity of fluorouracil. Use with extreme caution.

CONTRAINDICATIONS

Contraindicated in patients hypersensitive to the drug; patients who are in a poor nutritional state; patients with bone marrow suppression (WBC counts of 5,000/mm^3 or less or platelet counts of 100,000/mm^3 or less); patients with potentially serious infections; and in those who have had major surgery within the previous month.

NURSING CONSIDERATIONS

• Use cautiously after high-dose pelvic radiation therapy or use of alkylating agents or in patients with impaired hepatic or renal function or widespread neoplastic infiltration of bone marrow.
• Follow institutional policy to reduce risks. Preparation and administration of parenteral form of this drug is associated with carcinogenic, mutagenic, and teratogenic risks for personnel.
• Give antiemetic, as ordered, before administering drug to reduce nausea.
• **I.V. use:** Know that drug may be administered by direct injection without dilution. For I.V. infusion, drug may be diluted with D$_5$W, sterile water for injection, or 0.9% sodium chloride injection. Infuse slowly over 2 to 8 hours.
• Don't use cloudy solution. If crystals form, redissolve by warming.
• Use plastic I.V. containers for administering continuous infusions. Solution is more stable in plastic I.V. bags than in glass bottles.
• Don't refrigerate fluorouracil.
• Be aware that the manufacturer recommends using sodium hypochlorite 5% (household bleach) to inactivate the drug in the event of a spill.

• Apply topical form with caution near eyes, nose, and mouth.
• Avoid occlusive dressings with topical dressings because they increase the risk of inflammatory reactions in adjacent normal skin.
• Wash hands immediately after handling topical form of medication.
• Expect to use 1% topical concentration on the face. Higher concentrations are used for thicker-skinned areas or resistant lesions.
• Expect to use 5% topical strength for superficial basal cell carcinoma confirmed by biopsy.
• Be aware that ingestion and systemic absorption of topical form may cause leukopenia, thrombocytopenia, stomatitis, diarrhea, or GI ulceration, bleeding, and hemorrhage. Application to large ulcerated areas may cause systemic toxicity.
• Watch for stomatitis or diarrhea (signs of toxicity). May use topical oral anesthetic to soothe lesions, as ordered. Discontinue drug if diarrhea occurs and notify doctor.
• Encourage diligent oral hygiene to prevent superinfection of denuded mucosa.
• Monitor WBC and platelet counts daily, as ordered. Watch for ecchymoses, petechiae, easy bruising, and anemia.
• Consider protective isolation if WBC count is less than 2,000/mm^3.
• Monitor fluid intake and output, CBC, and renal and hepatic function tests, as ordered.
• Be aware that dermatologic adverse effects are reversible when drug is stopped.
• Be aware that therapeutic concentrations are not reached in CSF.
• To prevent bleeding, avoid all I.M. injections when platelet count is below 100,000/mm^3.
• Anticipate the need for possible blood transfusions because of cumulative anemia.

---

*Liquid form contains alcohol.   *Common* reactions are in italics; **life-threatening,** in bold italics.
**May contain tartrazine.

• Be alert that fluorouracil toxicity may be delayed for 1 to 3 weeks.
• Know that the drug is sometimes ordered as 5-fluorouracil or 5-FU. The numeral 5 is part of the drug name and should not be confused with dosage units.
• Warn patients that alopecia may occur, but that it's reversible.
• Caution patients to avoid prolonged exposure to sunlight or ultraviolet light when topical form is used.
• Tell patients to use highly protective sunblocks to avoid inflammatory erythematous dermatitis. Long-term use of the drug is associated with erythematous, desquamative rash of the hands and feet. May be treated with pyridoxine (50 to 150 mg P.O. daily) for 5 to 7 days.
• Warn patients that topically treated area may be unsightly during therapy and for several weeks after therapy. Complete healing may take 1 or 2 months.

hydroxyurea
Hydrea**

Pregnancy Risk Category: NR

HOW SUPPLIED
Capsules: 500 mg

ACTION
Unknown. Thought to inhibit DNA synthesis.

ONSET, PEAK, DURATION
Onset and duration unknown. Serum levels peak in 2 hours.

INDICATIONS & DOSAGE
Melanoma; resistant chronic myelocytic leukemia; recurrent, metastatic, or inoperable ovarian cancer; head and neck cancers –
Adults: 80 mg/kg P.O. as single dose q 3 days; or 20 to 30 mg/kg P.O. as a single daily dose.

ADVERSE REACTIONS
CNS: drowsiness, hallucinations.
GI: *anorexia, nausea, vomiting, diarrhea,* stomatitis.
GU: increased BUN and serum creatinine levels.
Hematologic: *leukopenia, thrombocytopenia,* anemia, *megaloblastosis; dose-limiting and dose-related bone marrow suppression,* with rapid recovery.
Skin: rash, pruritus.
Other: hyperuricemia.

INTERACTIONS
Cytotoxic drugs, radiation therapy: enhanced toxicity of hydroxyurea. Use together cautiously.

CONTRAINDICATIONS
Contraindicated in patients hypersensitive to the drug and with marked bone marrow depression (leukopenia [less than 2,500 WBC], thrombocytopenia [less than 100,000], or severe anemia).

NURSING CONSIDERATIONS
• Use cautiously in patients with renal dysfunction.
• Routinely measure BUN, uric acid, and serum creatinine levels, as ordered.
• Monitor fluid intake and output; keep patients hydrated.
• To prevent bleeding, avoid all I.M. injections when platelet count is below 100,000/mm^3.
• Anticipate the need for possible blood transfusions because of cumulative anemia.
• Be aware that dosage modification may be required after chemotherapy or radiation therapy.
• Be aware that auditory and visual hallucinations and hematologic toxicity increase when decreased renal function exists.
• Know that the drug crosses blood-brain barrier.
• Be alert that concomitant radiation

---

†Available in Canada only.　　　　‡Available in Australia only.　　　　◊Available OTC.

therapy may increase incidence or severity of GI distress or stomatitis.
• Tell patients who can't swallow capsules that they may empty contents into water and take immediately.
• Warn patients to watch for signs of infection (fever, sore throat, fatigue) and bleeding (easy bruising, nosebleeds, bleeding gums, melena). Take temperature daily.
• Advise women of childbearing age to avoid becoming pregnant during therapy. Also recommend consulting with doctor before becoming pregnant.

---

mercaptopurine
(6-mercaptopurine, 6-MP)
Purinethol

Pregnancy Risk Category: D

HOW SUPPLIED
Tablets (scored): 50 mg

ACTION
Inhibits RNA and DNA synthesis.

ONSET, PEAK, DURATION
Unknown.

INDICATIONS & DOSAGE
Acute myeloblastic leukemia, chronic myelocytic leukemia –
Adults: 80 to 100 mg/m² (rounded to the nearest 25 mg) P.O. daily as a single dose up to 5 mg/kg/day.
Children: 70 mg/m² (rounded to the nearest 25 mg) P.O. daily.
Acute lymphoblastic leukemia –
Children: 70 mg/m² (rounded to the nearest 25 mg) P.O. daily.
   Usual maintenance for adults and children: 1.5 to 2.5 mg/kg/day.

ADVERSE REACTIONS
GI: *nausea, vomiting, and anorexia in 25% of patients;* painful oral ulcers.
Hematologic: *leukopenia,* thrombocytopenia, anemia; all may persist several days after drug is stopped.

Hepatic: biliary stasis, *jaundice,* **hepatic necrosis.**
Skin: rash, hyperpigmentation.
Other: hyperuricemia.

INTERACTIONS
Allopurinol: slowed inactivation of mercaptopurine. Decrease mercaptopurine to ¼ or ⅓ normal dose.
Hepatotoxic drugs: may enhance hepatotoxicity of mercaptopurine.
Nondepolarizing neuromuscular blockers: antagonized muscle relaxant effect. Notify the anesthesiologist that the patient is receiving mercaptopurine.
Warfarin: antagonized anticoagulant effect.

CONTRAINDICATIONS
Contraindicated in patients whose disease has shown resistance to the drug.

NURSING CONSIDERATIONS
• Monitor blood counts and serum transaminase, alkaline phosphatase, and bilirubin levels weekly during induction and monthly during maintenance, as ordered.
• Observe for signs of bleeding and infection.
• Monitor fluid intake and output. Encourage adequate fluid intake (3 liters daily).
• Watch for jaundice, clay-colored stools, and frothy dark urine. Hepatic dysfunction is reversible when drug is stopped. Drug should be stopped if hepatic tenderness occurs and doctor notified.
• Monitor serum uric acid level, as ordered. If allopurinol is ordered, use cautiously.
• To prevent bleeding, avoid all I.M. injections when platelet count is below 100,000/mm³.
• Anticipate the need for possible blood transfusions because of cumulative anemia.
• Be aware that dosage modifications

---

*Liquid form contains alcohol.   *Common* reactions are in italics; ***life-threatening,*** in bold italics.
**May contain tartrazine.

may be required after chemotherapy or radiation therapy, in patients with depressed neutrophil or platelet counts, and in those with impaired hepatic or renal function.
• Be aware that drug is sometimes ordered as 6-mercaptopurine or 6-MP. The numeral 6 is part of drug name and does not signify number of dosage units.
• Be alert that GI adverse reactions are less common in children than in adults.
• Warn patients to watch for signs of infection (fever, sore throat, fatigue) and bleeding (easy bruising, nosebleeds, bleeding gums, melena). Take temperature daily.
• Advise women of childbearing age to avoid becoming pregnant during therapy. Also recommend consulting with the doctor before becoming pregnant.

---

methotrexate

methotrexate sodium
Folex PFS, Mexate-AQ, Rheumatrex

Pregnancy Risk Category: X

HOW SUPPLIED
Tablets (scored): 2.5 mg
Injection: 20-mg, 25-mg, 50-mg, 100-mg, 250-mg vials, lyophilized powder, preservative-free; 25-mg/ml vials, preservative-free solution; 2.5-mg/ml, 25-mg/ml vials, lyophilized powder, preserved

ACTION
Prevents reduction of folic acid to tetrahydrofolate by binding to dihydrofolate reductase.

ONSET, PEAK, DURATION
Onset and duration unknown. Serum concentrations peak immediately after I.V. injection, within ½ to 1 hour after I.M. injection, or 1 to 2 hours after oral dose.

INDICATIONS & DOSAGE
Trophoblastic tumors (choriocarcinoma, hydatidiform mole) –
Adults: 15 to 30 mg P.O. or I.M. daily for 5 days. Repeated after 1 or more weeks, according to response or toxicity.
Acute lymphoblastic and lymphatic leukemia –
Adults and children: 3.3 mg/m^2/day P.O., I.M., or I.V. for 4 to 6 weeks or until remission occurs; then 20 to 30 mg/m^2 P.O. or I.M. twice weekly.
Meningeal leukemia –
Adults and children: 10 to 15 mg/m^2 intrathecally q 2 to 5 days until CSF is normal.
Burkitt's lymphoma (Stage I or Stage II) –
Adults: 10 to 25 mg P.O. daily for 4 to 8 days with 1-week rest intervals.
Lymphosarcoma (Stage III) –
Adults: 0.625 to 2.5 mg/kg daily P.O., I.M., or I.V.
Osteosarcoma –
Adults: initially, 12 g/m^2 I.V. as 4 hour infusion. Subsequent doses 12 to 15 g/m^2 I.V. as 4 hour I.V. infusion given on 4, 5, 6, 7, 11, 12, 15, 16, 29, 30, 44, 45 treatment weeks after surgery. Given with leucovorin, 15 mg P.O., I.M., or I.V. q 6 hours for 10 doses after start of methotrexate infusion.
Mycosis fungoides –
Adults: 2.5 to 10 mg P.O. daily, or 50 mg I.M. weekly, or 25 mg I.M. twice weekly.
Psoriasis –
Adults: 10 to 25 mg P.O., I.M., or I.V. as single weekly dose.
Rheumatoid arthritis –
Adults: initially, 7.5 mg P.O. weekly, either in a single dose or divided as 2.5 mg P.O. q 12 hours for three doses once a week. Dosage may be gradually increased to a maximum of 20 mg weekly.

ADVERSE REACTIONS

CNS: *arachnoiditis* within hours of intrathecal use; subacute neurotoxicity, which may begin a few weeks later; *necrotizing demyelinating leukoencephalopathy* a few years later.
EENT: pharyngitis, gingivitis.
GI: *stomatitis, diarrhea leading to hemorrhagic enteritis and intestinal perforation, nausea, vomiting.*
GU: nephropathy, *tubular necrosis.*
Hematologic: WBC and platelet count nadirs occurring on day 7; *anemia, leukopenia, thrombocytopenia* (all dose-related).
Hepatic: acute toxicity (elevated transaminase level), *chronic toxicity* (cirrhosis, *hepatic fibrosis*).
Respiratory: *pulmonary fibrosis, pulmonary interstitial infiltrates,* pneumonitis.
Skin: *urticaria,* pruritus, hyperpigmentation; exposure to sun may aggravate psoriatic lesions, rash, photosensitivity.
Other: alopecia, osteoporosis (in children, with long-term use), hyperuricemia.

INTERACTIONS

Digoxin: may decrease serum digoxin levels. Monitor closely.
Folic acid derivatives: antagonized methotrexate effect.
NSAIDs, phenylbutazone, probenecid, salicylates, sulfonamides: increased methotrexate toxicity; don't use together if possible.
Phenytoin: may decrease serum phenytoin levels. Monitor closely.
Vaccines: immunizations may be ineffective; risk of disseminated infection with live-virus vaccines.

CONTRAINDICATIONS

Contraindicated in patients hypersensitive to the drug and during pregnancy or lactation. It also is contraindicated in patients with psoriasis or rheumatoid arthritis who also have alcoholism, alcoholic liver, chronic liver disease, immunodeficiency syndromes, or preexisting blood dyscrasias.

NURSING CONSIDERATIONS

• Use cautiously and at modified dosage in patients with impaired hepatic or renal function, bone marrow suppression, aplasia, leukopenia, thrombocytopenia, or anemia. Also use cautiously in patients with infection, peptic ulceration, and ulcerative colitis and in very young, elderly, or debilitated patients.
• Perform baseline pulmonary function tests, as ordered.
• Follow institutional policy to reduce risks. Preparation and administration of parenteral form of this drug is associated with carcinogenic, mutagenic, and teratogenic risks for personnel.
• **I.V. use:** Administer undiluted by direct injection. Alternatively, dilute with up to 25 ml of 0.9% sodium chloride injection (for Folex) or 2 to 10 ml of sterile water for injection, 0.9% sodium chloride injection, or bacteriostatic water for injection containing parabens or benzyl alcohol (for Mexate).
• For intrathecal use, use only 20-, 50-, or 100-mg vials of powder with no preservatives. Reconstitute immediately before using with preservative-free 0.9% sodium chloride injection. Dilute to a maximum concentration of 1 mg/ml. Use only new vials of drug and diluent.
• Reconstitute solutions without preservatives immediately before use, and discard any unused drug.
• Monitor pulmonary function tests periodically, as ordered, and fluid intake and output daily. Encourage fluid intake of 2 to 3 liters daily.
• Monitor serum uric acid level, as ordered.
• Alkalinize urine as ordered by giving sodium bicarbonate tablets to prevent precipitation of drug, especially with high doses. Maintain urine pH at

*Liquid form contains alcohol.   *Common* reactions are in italics; *life-threatening,* in bold italics.
**May contain tartrazine.

more than 6.5. Reduce dosage as ordered if BUN level reaches 20 to 30 mg/dl or creatinine level reaches 1.2 to 2 mg/dl. Stop drug if BUN level is greater than 30 mg/dl or creatinine level is greater than 2 mg/dl and notify doctor.

• Watch for increases in AST, ALT, and alkaline phosphatase levels, which may signal hepatic dysfunction.

• Watch for signs of bleeding (especially GI) and infection.

• Take temperature daily, and watch for cough, dyspnea, and cyanosis.

• To prevent bleeding, avoid all I.M. injections when platelet count is below 100,000/mm³.

• Anticipate the need for blood transfusions because of cumulative anemia.

• Know that rash, redness, or ulcerations in mouth or pulmonary adverse reactions may signal serious complications. Therapy may be discontinued if ulcerative stomatitis or other severe GI adverse reaction occurs, or if pulmonary toxicity is detected.

• Know that leucovorin rescue is necessary with high-dose (greater than 100 mg) protocols. Don't confuse with folic acid. This rescue technique is effective against systemic toxicity but does not interfere with the tumor cells' absorption of methotrexate.

• Teach and encourage diligent mouth care to reduce the risk of superinfection in the mouth.

• Warn patients to use highly protective sunblock when exposed to sunlight.

• Advise patients not to discontinue leucovorin rescue if they experience severe nausea and vomiting. Parenteral leucovorin therapy may be necessary.

• Warn patients to avoid conception during and immediately after therapy because of possible abortion or congenital anomalies.

thioguanine (6-thioguanine, 6-TG)
Lanvis†

Pregnancy Risk Category: D

HOW SUPPLIED
Tablets (scored): 40 mg

ACTION
Inhibits purine synthesis.

ONSET, PEAK, DURATION
Unknown.

INDICATIONS & DOSAGE
Acute nonlymphocytic leukemia, chronic myelogenous leukemia –
Adults and children: initially, 2 mg/kg P.O. daily (usually calculated to nearest 20 mg). If necessary, dose is then increased gradually to 3 mg/kg/day as tolerated.

ADVERSE REACTIONS
GI: nausea, vomiting, stomatitis, diarrhea, anorexia.
Hematologic: *leukopenia, anemia, thrombocytopenia* (occurs slowly over 2 to 4 weeks).
Hepatic: *hepatotoxicity,* jaundice.
Other: hyperuricemia.

INTERACTIONS
Myelosuppressant drugs: increased risk of toxicity, especially myelosuppression and bleeding. Use together cautiously.

CONTRAINDICATIONS
Contraindicated in patients whose disease has shown resistance to the drug.

NURSING CONSIDERATIONS
• Use cautiously and with dosage modification in patients with renal or hepatic dysfunction.
• Monitor CBC daily during induction, and then weekly during maintenance therapy, as ordered.

---

†Available in Canada only.   ‡Available in Australia only.   ◇Available OTC.

• Monitor serum uric acid level, as ordered.
• Watch for jaundice; may be reversible if drug is stopped promptly. Stop drug if hepatotoxicity or hepatic tenderness occurs.
• To prevent bleeding, avoid all I.M. injections when platelet count is below 100,000/mm³.
• Anticipate the need for possible blood transfusions because of cumulative anemia.
• Know that drug is sometimes ordered as 6-thioguanine. The numeral 6 is part of drug name and does not signify dosage units.
• Warn patient to watch for signs of infection and bleeding.
• Advise women of childbearing age to avoid becoming pregnant during therapy. Also recommend consulting with doctor before becoming pregnant.

72

Antibiotic antineoplastic agents

bleomycin sulfate
dactinomycin
daunorubicin hydrochloride
doxorubicin hydrochloride
idarubicin hydrochloride
mitomycin
pentostatin
plicamycin

COMBINATION PRODUCTS
None.

---

bleomycin sulfate
Blenoxane

Pregnancy Risk Category: NR

HOW SUPPLIED
Injection: 15-unit vials (1 unit = 1 mg)

ACTION
Unknown. Thought to inhibit DNA synthesis and cause scission of single- and double-stranded DNA.

ONSET, PEAK, DURATION
Unknown.

INDICATIONS & DOSAGE
Dosage and indications may vary. Check the treatment protocol with the doctor.
Squamous cell carcinoma (head and neck, skin, penis, cervix, and vulva), lymphosarcoma, reticulum cell carcinoma, testicular carcinoma –
Adults: 10 to 20 units/m² I.V., I.M., or S.C. 1 or 2 times weekly to total of 300 to 400 units.
Hodgkin's disease –
Adults: 10 to 20 units/m² I.V., I.M., or S.C. 1 or 2 times weekly. After 50% response, maintenance dosage is 1 unit I.M. or I.V. daily or 5 units I.M. or I.V. weekly.

ADVERSE REACTIONS
CNS: hyperesthesia of scalp and fingers, headache.
GI: *stomatitis, prolonged anorexia in 13% of patients, nausea, vomiting,* diarrhea.
Hematologic: *leukocytosis.*
Respiratory: *pulmonary fibrosis* in 10% of patients, *pulmonary adverse reactions (fine crackles, dyspnea), nonproductive cough.*
Skin: *erythema, vesiculation, and hardening and discoloration of palmar and plantar skin in 8% of patients;* desquamation of hands, feet, and pressure areas; *hyperpigmentation;* acne.
Other: *reversible alopecia,* swelling of interphalangeal joints, hypersensitivity reaction *(fever up to 106° F [41.1° C] with chills up to 5 hours after injection;* **anaphylaxis** in 1% to 6% of patients), fever.

INTERACTIONS
Digitalis glycosides: decreased serum digoxin levels. Monitor closely.
Phenytoin: decreased serum phenytoin levels. Monitor closely.

CONTRAINDICATIONS
Contraindicated in patients hypersensitive to the drug.

NURSING CONSIDERATIONS
• Use cautiously in patients with renal or pulmonary impairment.
• Obtain pulmonary function tests as ordered to establish pretreatment baseline. Know that drug should be stopped if pulmonary function test shows a marked decline.
• Follow institutional policy to reduce risks. Preparation and administration of parenteral form of this drug is asso-

†Available in Canada only.   ‡Available in Australia only.   ◊Available OTC.

ciated with carcinogenic, mutagenic, and teratogenic risks for personnel.
• **I.V. use:** Reconstitute drug with 5 ml or more of D$_5$W or 0.9% sodium chloride injection. For I.V. infusion, dilute with 50 to 100 ml of D$_5$W or 0.9% sodium chloride injection.
• For I.M. use, dilute drug in 1 to 5 ml of sterile water for injection, bacteriostatic water for injection, 0.9% sodium chloride injection, or D$_5$W.
• Monitor injection site for signs of irritation.
• Be aware that pulmonary adverse reactions are common in patients over age 70. Fatal pulmonary fibrosis occurs in 1% of patients, especially when cumulative dosage exceeds 400 units.
• Monitor chest X-ray and pulmonary function tests, as ordered, and listen to lungs regularly.
• Monitor for bleomycin-induced fever which is common and may be treated with antipyretics. This reaction usually occurs within 3 to 6 hours of administration.
• Watch for hypersensitivity reactions which may be delayed for several hours, especially in patients with lymphoma.
• To prevent linear streaking from drug concentrating in keratin of squamous epithelium, don't use adhesive dressings on skin.
• Refrigerate unopened vials containing dry powder.
• Know that refrigerated, reconstituted solution is stable for 4 weeks; at room temperature, it's stable for 2 weeks. Bleomycin may adsorb to plastic I.V. bags. For prolonged stability, use glass containers.
• Warn patients that alopecia may occur, but that it's usually reversible.

dactinomycin (actinomycin D)
Cosmegen
Pregnancy Risk Category: C

HOW SUPPLIED
Injection: 500 mcg/vial

ACTION
Unknown. Thought to interfere with DNA-dependent RNA synthesis by intercalation.

ONSET, PEAK, DURATION
Unknown.

INDICATIONS & DOSAGE
Dosage and indications may vary. Check the treatment protocol with the doctor.
Sarcoma, trophoblastic tumors in women, testicular cancer–
Adults: 500 mcg/m^2 (0.5 mg) I.V. daily for 5 days. Maximum dosage is 15 mcg/kg or 400 to 600 mcg/m^2/day for 5 days. After bone marrow recovery, course may be repeated.
Wilms' tumor, rhabdomyosarcoma, Ewing's sarcoma–
Children: 10 to 15 mcg/kg or 450 mcg/m^2/day I.V. for 5 days. Maximum dosage is 500 mcg/day. Or 2.5 mg/m^2 I.V. in equally divided daily doses over a 7-day period. After bone marrow recovery, course may be repeated.

ADVERSE REACTIONS
GI: *anorexia, nausea, vomiting,* abdominal pain, diarrhea, *stomatitis,* ulceration, proctitis.
Hematologic: *anemia, leukopenia, thrombocytopenia, pancytopenia.*
Hepatic: *hepatotoxicity.*
Skin: *erythema;* desquamation; *hyperpigmentation of skin, especially in previously irradiated areas; acnelike eruptions (reversible).*
Other: phlebitis and severe damage

---

to soft tissue at injection site; reversible alopecia.

INTERACTIONS
Bone marrow suppressants: additive toxicity. Monitor closely.
Vitamin K derivatives: decreased effectiveness. Monitor closely.

CONTRAINDICATIONS
Contraindicated in patients with with chicken pox or herpes zoster.

NURSING CONSIDERATIONS
• To reduce nausea, give antiemetic before administering drug, as ordered.
• Follow institutional policy to reduce risks. Preparation and administration of parenteral form of this drug is associated with carcinogenic, mutagenic, and teratogenic risks for personnel.
• **I.V. use:** Use only sterile water (without preservatives) as diluent for reconstitution. Add 1.1 ml to the vial to yield a gold-colored solution containing 0.5 mg/ml. Give by direct injection into a vein or through the tubing of a free-flowing I.V. solution of 0.9% sodium chloride injection or D_5W.
• For I.V. infusion, dilute with up to 50 ml of D_5W or 0.9% sodium chloride injection and infuse over 15 minutes.
• Administer through a running I.V. line with good blood return. Dactinomycin is a vesicant. If infiltration occurs, apply cold compresses to area and notify doctor.
• If accidental skin contact occurs, irrigate the area with copious amounts of water for at least 15 minutes.
• Be aware that dosage must be reduced in patients who have recently been treated with, or who will receive concomitant treatment with, radiation therapy or other chemotherapy drugs.
• In the event of a spill, keep in mind that the manufacturer recommends

using a solution of trisodium phosphate 5% to inactivate the drug.
• Monitor CBC and platelet counts daily, as ordered.
• Monitor renal and hepatic functions, as ordered.
• Monitor for stomatitis, diarrhea, leukopenia, or thrombocytopenia which may require modifying dosage and schedule.
• Discard unused portions of solutions because they do not contain a preservative.
• Warn patients to watch for signs of infection (fever, sore throat, fatigue) and bleeding (easy bruising, nosebleeds, bleeding gums, melena). Take temperature daily.
• Warn patients that alopecia may occur, but that it's usually reversible.

daunorubicin hydrochloride
Cerubidin‡, Cerubidine
Pregnancy Risk Category: D

HOW SUPPLIED
Injection: 20 mg/vial

ACTION
Unknown. Thought to interfere with DNA-dependent RNA synthesis by intercalation.

ONSET, PEAK, DURATION
Unknown.

INDICATIONS & DOSAGE
Dosage and indications may vary. Check the treatment protocol with the doctor.
Remission induction in acute nonlymphocytic (myelogenous, monocytic, erythroid) leukemia –
Adults: in combination, 30 to 45 mg/m²/day I.V. on days 1, 2, and 3 of the first course and on days 1 and 2 of subsequent courses with cytarabine infusions.

Remission induction in acute lympho-cytic leukemia –
Adults: 45 mg/m^2/day I.V. on days 1, 2, and 3.
Children 2 years and older: 25 mg/m^2 I.V. on day 1 every week for up to 6 weeks, if needed.
Children under 2 years: 0.5 mg/m^2 (1 mg/kg) I.V. on day 1 every week for up to 6 weeks, if needed.

ADVERSE REACTIONS
CV: *irreversible cardiomyopathy* (dose-related), ECG changes, arrhythmias, pericarditis, myocarditis.
GI: *nausea, vomiting, stomatitis, esophagitis,* anorexia, diarrhea.
GU: red urine (transient).
Hematologic: *bone marrow suppression* (lowest blood counts 10 to 14 days after administration).
Hepatic: *hepatotoxicity.*
Skin: rash, pigmentation of fingernails and toenails.
Other: *severe cellulitis or tissue sloughing if drug extravasates, generalized alopecia,* fever, chills, hyperuricemia.

INTERACTIONS
Dexamethasone, heparin: don't mix. May form a precipitate.
Doxorubicin: additive cardiotoxicity. Monitor closely.
Hepatotoxic drugs: increased risk of additive hepatotoxicity. Monitor closely.

CONTRAINDICATIONS
None reported.

NURSING CONSIDERATIONS
• Use cautiously in patients with myelosuppression and in those with impaired cardiac, renal, or hepatic function.
• Check ECG before treatment.
• Follow institutional policy to reduce risks. Preparation and administration of parenteral form of this drug is associated with carcinogenic, mutagenic, and teratogenic risks for personnel.
• **I.V. use:** Reconstitute drug using 4 ml of sterile water for injection to produce a 5 mg/ml solution.
• Withdraw the desired dose into a syringe containing 10 to 15 ml of 0.9% sodium chloride injection. Inject into the tubing of a free-flowing I.V. solution of D$_5$W or 0.9% sodium chloride injection over 2 to 3 minutes. Alternatively, dilute in 50 ml of 0.9% sodium chloride injection and infuse over 10 to 15 minutes, or dilute in 100 ml and infuse over 30 to 45 minutes.
• Avoid extravasation; inject into tubing of free-flowing I.V. line. If extravasation occurs, discontinue I.V. infusion immediately, apply ice to area for 24 to 48 hours and notify doctor.
• Never give drug I.M. or S.C.
• Be aware that cumulative dosage is limited to 500 to 600 mg/m^2 (450 mg/m^2 when patients are also receiving or have received cyclophosphamide or radiation therapy to cardiac area).
• Know that therapeutic effects are often accompanied by toxicity.
• Monitor CBC and hepatic function tests, as ordered; monitor ECG every month during therapy.
• Monitor pulse rate closely. Light resting pulse rate is a sign of cardiac adverse reactions. Notify the doctor if this occurs.
• Stop drug immediately if signs of CHF or cardiomyopathy develop and notify doctor.
• Monitor for nausea and vomiting which may be very severe and may last 24 to 48 hours.
• To prevent bleeding, avoid all I.M. injections when platelet count is below 100,000/mm^3.
• Anticipate the need for possible blood transfusions because of cumulative anemia.
• Know that reddish color is similar to that of doxorubicin. Take care to avoid confusing the two drugs.
• Optimally, use within 8 hours of

---

*Liquid form contains alcohol.   *Common* reactions are in italics; ***life-threatening,*** in bold italics.
**May contain tartrazine.

preparation. Reconstituted solution is stable for 24 hours at room temperature or 48 hours if refrigerated.
• Warn patient to watch for signs of infection and bleeding.
• Advise patients that red urine for 1 to 2 days is normal and does not indicate the presence of blood in urine.
• Advise patients that alopecia may occur, but that it's usually reversible.
• Advise women of childbearing age to avoid becoming pregnant during therapy. Also recommend consulting with doctor before becoming pregnant.

---

doxorubicin hydrochloride
Adriamycin‡, Adriamycin PFS, Adriamycin RDF, Rubex

Pregnancy Risk Category: NR

HOW SUPPLIED
Injection (preservative-free): 2 mg/ml
Powder for injection: 10-mg, 20-mg, 50-mg, 100-mg, 150-mg vials

ACTION
Unknown. Thought to interfere with DNA-dependent RNA synthesis by intercalation.

ONSET, PEAK, DURATION
Unknown.

INDICATIONS & DOSAGE
Dosage and indications may vary. Check the treatment protocol with the doctor.
Bladder, breast, lung, ovarian, stomach, testicular, and thyroid cancers; Hodgkin's disease; acute lymphoblastic and myeloblastic leukemia; Wilms' tumor; neuroblastoma; lymphoma; sarcoma –
Adults: 60 to 75 mg/m² I.V. as single dose q 3 weeks; or 30 mg/m² I.V. in single daily dose, days 1 to 3 of 4-week cycle. Alternatively, 20 mg/m² I.V. once weekly. Maximum cumulative dosage is 550 mg/m².

ADVERSE REACTIONS
CV: cardiac depression, seen in such ECG changes as sinus tachycardia, T-wave flattening, ST-segment depression, voltage reduction; *arrhythmias* in 11% of patients; *irreversible cardiomyopathy (sometimes with pulmonary edema) with mortality of 30% to 75%.*
GI: *nausea, vomiting,* diarrhea, *stomatitis,* esophagitis.
GU: enhancement of cyclophosphamide-induced bladder injury, red urine (transient).
Hematologic: *leukopenia, especially agranulocytosis,* during days 10 to 15, with recovery by day 21; *thrombocytopenia.*
Skin: *hyperpigmentation of nails, dermal creases, or skin,* (especially in previously irradiated areas).
Other: *severe cellulitis or tissue sloughing if drug extravasates;* hyperuricemia; *complete alopecia within 3 to 4 weeks* (hair may regrow 2 to 5 months after drug is stopped).

INTERACTIONS
Aminophylline, cephalothin, dexamethasone, fluorouracil, heparin, hydrocortisone: may form a precipitate. Don't mix together.
Digoxin: may decrease serum digoxin levels. Monitor closely.
Streptozocin: increased and prolonged blood levels. Dosage may have to be adjusted.

CONTRAINDICATIONS
Contraindicated in patients with marked myelosuppression induced by previous treatment with other antitumor agents or by radiotherapy and in patients who have received lifetime cumulative dosage of 550 mg/m².

NURSING CONSIDERATIONS
• Assess ECG before treatment.
• Premedicate with antiemetic, as ordered, to reduce nausea.
• Follow institutional policy to reduce

---

risks. Preparation and administration of parenteral form of this drug is associated with carcinogenic, mutagenic, and teratogenic risks for personnel.

• **I.V. use:** Reconstitute using preservative-free 0.9% sodium chloride injection. Add 5 ml to the 10-mg vial, 10 ml to the 20-mg vial, or 25 ml to the 50-mg vial. Shake vial and allow drug to dissolve; final concentration will be 2 mg/ml. Give by direct injection into the tubing of a free-flowing I.V. solution containing D_5W or 0.9% sodium chloride injection.

• Avoid extravasation; don't place I.V. line over joints or in extremities with poor venous or lymphatic drainage. If extravasation occurs, discontinue I.V. infusion immediately; apply ice to area for 24 to 48 hours and notify doctor. Monitor area closely because the extravasation reaction may be progressive. Early consultation with a plastic surgeon may be advisable.

• If vein streaking occurs, slow administration rate. However, if welts occur, stop administration and report this to the doctor.

• If skin or mucosal contact occurs, immediately wash the area with soap and water.

• In the event of a leak or spill, inactivate drug with 5% sodium hypochlorite solution (household bleach).

• Never give this drug I.M. or S.C.

• Monitor CBC and hepatic function tests, as ordered; monitor ECG monthly during therapy.

• Be prepared to stop drug or slow rate of infusion if tachycardia develops and notify the doctor.

• Stop drug immediately if signs of CHF develop and notify the doctor. Know that in many instances, CHF can be prevented by limiting cumulative dosage to 550 mg/m² (400 mg/m² when patients are also receiving or have received cyclophosphamide or radiation therapy to cardiac area).

• Know that dosage modification may be required in patients with myelosup-pression and in those with impaired cardiac or hepatic function, and in elderly patients.

• Be aware that the alternative dosage schedule (once-weekly dosing) has been found to cause a lower incidence of cardiomyopathy.

• Be prepared to decrease dosage if serum bilirubin is increased: 50% dosage when bilirubin is 1.2 to 3 mg/100 ml; 25% dosage when bilirubin is greater than 3 mg/100 ml.

• Know that reddish color is similar to that of daunorubicin. Take care to avoid confusing the two drugs.

• Keep in mind that esophagitis is very common in patients who have also received radiation therapy.

• Keep in mind that refrigerated, reconstituted solution is stable for 48 hours; at room temperature, it's stable for 24 hours.

• Warn patients to watch for signs of infection (fever, sore throat, fatigue) and bleeding (easy bruising, nosebleeds, bleeding gums, melena). Take temperature daily.

• Advise patients that orange to red urine for 1 to 2 days is normal and does not indicate the presence of blood in urine.

• Warn patients that alopecia may occur, but that it's usually reversible.

---

idarubicin hydrochloride
Idamycin

Pregnancy Risk Category: D

HOW SUPPLIED
Powder for injection: 5 mg, 10 mg

ACTION
Unknown. An antineoplastic antibiotic that probably inhibits nucleic acid synthesis by intercalation and that interacts with the enzyme topoisomerase II. It is highly lipophilic, which results in an increased rate of cellular uptake.

---

*Liquid form contains alcohol.
**May contain tartrazine.

Common reactions are in italics; ***life-threatening,*** in bold italics.

ONSET, PEAK, DURATION
Onset and duration unknown. Intracellular drug levels peak within a few minutes after injection.

INDICATIONS & DOSAGE
Dosage and indications may vary. Check current literature for recommended protocol.

Acute myeloid leukemia, including FAB (French-American-British) classifications M1 through M7, in combination with other approved antileukemic agents –

Adults: 12 mg/m²/day for 3 days by slow I.V. injection (over 10 to 15 minutes) in combination with 100 mg/m²/day of cytarabine for 7 days by continuous I.V. infusion or as a 25 mg/m² bolus followed by 200 mg/m²/day for 5 days by continuous infusion.

A second course may be administered if needed. If patients experience severe mucositis, administration is delayed until recovery is complete. Dosage reduced by 25%. Dosage should also be reduced in patients with hepatic or renal impairment. Idarubicin should not be given if bilirubin level is above 5 mg/dl.

ADVERSE REACTIONS
CNS: headache, changed mental status, peripheral neuropathy, *seizures.*
CV: *CHF,* atrial fibrillation, chest pain, *MI,* asymptomatic decline in left ventricular ejection fraction, *myocardial insufficiency, arrhythmias, hemorrhage, myocardial toxicity.*
GI: *nausea, vomiting,* cramps, diarrhea, *mucositis, severe enterocolitis with perforation* (rare).
GU: decreased renal function.
Hematologic: *myelosuppression.*
Hepatic: changes in hepatic function.
Skin: rash, urticaria, bullous erythrodermatous rash on palms and soles, hives at injection site, erythema at previously irradiated sites, tissue necrosis at injection site (if extravasation occurs).

Other: *infection,* alopecia, fever, hyperuricemia, hypersensitivity reactions.

INTERACTIONS
Alkaline solutions, heparin: incompatible. Idarubicin should not be mixed with other drugs unless specific compatibility data is available.

CONTRAINDICATIONS
None reported.

NURSING CONSIDERATIONS
• Use with extreme caution in patients with bone marrow suppression induced by previous drug therapy or radiotherapy or in patients with hepatic or renal function impairment.
• Take appropriate preventive measures (including adequate hydration) before starting treatment. Hyperuricemia may result from rapid lysis of leukemic cells. Allopurinol may be ordered.
• Assess patient for systemic infection prior to therapy and know that systemic infections should be controlled before therapy.
• Administer antiemetics, as ordered, to prevent or treat nausea and vomiting.
• Follow institutional policy to reduce risks. Preparation and administration of parenteral form of this drug is associated with carcinogenic, mutagenic, and teratogenic risks for personnel.
• **I.V. use:** Reconstitute to a final concentration of 1 mg/ml using 0.9% sodium chloride injection without preservatives. Add 5 ml to the 5-mg vial or 10 ml to the 10-ml vial. *Do not use bacteriostatic sodium chloride.* Vial is under negative pressure.
• Administer over 10 to 15 minutes into a free-flowing I.V. infusion of 0.9% sodium chloride or 5% dextrose solution that is running into a large vein.
• If extravasation occurs, discontinue infusion immediately and notify doc-

tor. Treat with intermittent ice packs—½ hour immediately, and then ½ hour four times daily for 4 days.
• Monitor hepatic and renal function tests and CBC frequently, as ordered.
• To prevent bleeding, avoid all I.M. injections when platelet count is below 100,000/mm³.
• Anticipate the need for possible blood transfusions because of cumulative anemia.
• Know that reconstituted solutions are stable for 3 days (72 hours) at room temperature (59° to 86° F [15° to 30° C]); 7 days if refrigerated. Label any unused solutions with CHEMO-THERAPY HAZARD label.
• Instruct patients to recognize signs and symptoms of extravasation and to call the doctor or nurse if these occur.
• Warn patient to watch for signs of infection and bleeding.
• Advise patients that red urine for several days is normal and does not indicate the presence of blood in urine.
• Advise women of childbearing age to avoid becoming pregnant during therapy. Also recommend consulting with doctor before becoming pregnant.

mitomycin (mitomycin-C)
Mutamycin

Pregnancy Risk Category: NR

HOW SUPPLIED
Injection: 5-mg, 20-mg, 40-mg vials

ACTION
Acts like an alkylating agent, cross-linking strands of DNA. This causes an imbalance of cell growth, leading to cell death.

ONSET, PEAK, DURATION
Unknown.

INDICATIONS & DOSAGE
Dosage and indications may vary. Check the treatment protocol with the doctor.
Breast, colon, head, neck, lung, pancreatic, and stomach cancers; malignant melanoma—
Adults: 20 mg/m² as a I.V. single dose. Cycle repeated after 6 to 8 weeks, when WBC count and platelet count have returned to normal.

ADVERSE REACTIONS
GI: *nausea, vomiting,* anorexia, stomatitis.
Hematologic: ***thrombocytopenia, leukopenia*** (may be delayed up to 8 weeks and may be cumulative with successive doses).
Respiratory: ***interstitial pneumonitis.***
Other: desquamation, induration, pruritus, *pain at injection site;* cellulitis, ulceration, sloughing with extravasation; *reversible alopecia; purple coloration of nail beds;* fever; ***microangiopathic hemolytic anemia, characterized by thrombocytopenia, renal failure, and hypertension.***

INTERACTIONS
None significant.

CONTRAINDICATIONS
Contraindicated in patients hypersensitive to the drug and in those with thrombocytopenia, coagulation disorder, or an increase in bleeding tendency due to other causes.

NURSING CONSIDERATIONS
• Follow institutional policy to reduce risks. Preparation and administration of parenteral form of this drug is associated with mutagenic, teratogenic, and carcinogenic risks to personnel.
• **I.V. use:** Using sterile water for injection, reconstitute the 5-mg vials with 10 ml, the 20-mg vials with 40 ml, and the 40-mg vials with 80 ml.
• For infusion, dilute with 0.9% so-

---

*Liquid form contains alcohol.
**May contain tartrazine.

Common reactions are in italics; ***life-threatening***, in bold italics.

dium chloride injection, D_5W, or sodium lactate for injection. After dilution, drug is stable for 3 hours in D_5W, 12 hours in 0.9% sodium chloride injection, and 24 hours in sodium lactate for injection at room temperature.

• Avoid extravasation. Stop infusion immediately if extravasation occurs because of the potential for severe ulceration and necrosis and notify doctor.

• Never administer this drug I.M. or S.C.

• Continue CBC and blood studies, as ordered, at least 7 weeks after therapy is stopped.

• To prevent bleeding, avoid all I.M. injections when platelet count is below 100,000/mm³.

• Anticipate the need for possible blood transfusions because of cumulative anemia.

• Monitor renal function tests, as ordered.

• Warn patients to watch for signs of infection (fever, sore throat, fatigue) and bleeding (easy bruising, nosebleeds, bleeding gums, melena). Take temperature daily.

• Warn patients that alopecia may occur, but that it's usually reversible.

---

pentostatin (2'-deoxy-coformycin)
Nipent

Pregnancy Risk Category: D

HOW SUPPLIED
Powder for injection: 10 mg/vial

ACTION
Inhibits the enzyme adenosine deaminase (ADA), causing an increase in intracellular levels of deoxyadenosine triphosphate. This leads to cell damage and death. Because the greatest activity of ADA is in cells of the lymphoid system (especially malignant T

cells), pentostatin is useful in treating leukemias.

ONSET, PEAK, DURATION
Unknown.

INDICATIONS & DOSAGE
Alpha-interferon-refractory hairy-cell leukemia –
Adults: 4 mg/m² I.V. every other week.

ADVERSE REACTIONS
CNS: *headache, neurologic symptoms, anxiety, confusion, depression, dizziness, insomnia, nervousness, paresthesia, somnolence, abnormal thinking, fatigue, seizures.*
CV: **arrhythmias,** *abnormal ECG, thrombophlebitis, peripheral edema,* **hemorrhage.**
EENT: abnormal vision, conjunctivitis, ear pain, eye pain, epistaxis, pharyngitis, rhinitis, sinusitis.
GI: *nausea, vomiting, anorexia, diarrhea, constipation, flatulence, stomatitis.*
GU: *hematuria, dysuria, increased BUN and creatinine levels.*
Hematologic: *myelosuppression, leukopenia, anemia, thrombocytopenia, lymphocytopenia, lymphadenopathy.*
Hepatic: *elevated liver enzyme levels.*
Respiratory: *cough, bronchitis, dyspnea, lung edema, pneumonia.*
Skin: photosensitivity, contact dermatitis, *ecchymosis, petechiae, rash, eczema, dry skin, herpes simplex or zoster, maculopapular rash, vesiculobullous rash, pruritus, seborrhea, discoloration, diaphoresis,* **exfoliative dermatitis.**
Other: *fever, infection, pain,* **hypersensitivity reactions,** *chills, sepsis, chest pain, abdominal pain, back pain, flulike syndrome, asthenia, malaise, myalgia, arthralgia, weight loss, increased lactate dehydrogenase level.*

INTERACTIONS
Cytarabine or vidarabine: increased incidence or severity of adverse effects associated with either drug. Avoid concomitant use.
Fludarabine: risk of severe or fatal pulmonary toxicity. Don't use together.

CONTRAINDICATIONS
Contraindicated in patients hypersensitive to the drug.

NURSING CONSIDERATIONS
• Use cautiously and only under the supervision of a doctor qualified and experienced in the use of chemotherapeutic agents. Adverse reactions after pentostatin therapy are common.
• Make sure patients are adequately hydrated before therapy. Administer 500 to 1,000 ml of D_5W in 0.45% sodium chloride injection, as ordered, for hydration.
• Follow institutional policy to reduce risks. Preparation and administration of parenteral form of this drug is associated with mutagenic, teratogenic, and carcinogenic risks to personnel.
• **I.V. use:** Add 5 ml of sterile water for injection to the vial containing pentostatin powder for injection. Mix thoroughly to make a solution of 5 mg/ml. Drug may be administered by I.V. bolus injection or diluted further in 25 or 50 ml of D_5W or 0.9% sodium chloride injection and infused over 20 to 30 minutes.
• Use reconstituted solution within 8 hours because it contains no preservatives.
• Treat all spills and waste products with 5% sodium hypochlorite (household bleach).
• Give an additional 500 ml of D_5W, as ordered, for hydration after drug is administered.
• Know that the optimal duration of therapy is unknown. Current recommendations suggest two additional courses of therapy after a complete re-

sponse. If a partial response is not evident after 6 months of therapy, drug will be discontinued. If a partial response is evident, drug will be continued for another 6 months or for two courses of therapy after a complete response.
• Withhold or discontinue drug in patients with evidence of CNS toxicity, a severe rash, or an active infection and notify the doctor. Drug may be resumed when the infection clears. Know that use in patients with renal damage (creatinine clearance of 60 ml/minute or less) should be avoided.
• Temporarily withhold drug if the absolute neutrophil count falls below 200/mm³ and the pretreatment level was over 500/mm³ and notify the doctor. No recommendations exist regarding dosage adjustments in patients with anemia, neutropenia, or thrombocytopenia.
• Be aware that drug should be used only in patients who have hairy-cell leukemia refractory to alpha-interferon. This is defined as disease that progresses after a minimum of 3 months of treatment with alpha-interferon or disease that does not exhibit a response after 6 months of therapy.

plicamycin (mithramycin)
Mithracin

Pregnancy Risk Category: X

HOW SUPPLIED
Injection: 2.5-mg vials

ACTION
Unknown. Thought to form a complex with DNA, thus inhibiting RNA synthesis. Also inhibits osteocytic activity, blocking calcium and phosphorus resorption from bone.

ONSET, PEAK, DURATION
Onset occurs in 1 to 2 days. Effects peak 3 days after single dose and persist for 7 to 10 days.

INDICATIONS & DOSAGE

Dosage and indications may vary.
Check the treatment protocol with the
doctor.

Hypercalcemia associated with advanced malignancy –

Adults: 15 to 25 mcg/kg/day I.V. for
3 to 4 days. Dosage repeated at
weekly intervals until desired response is obtained.

Testicular cancer –

Adults: 25 to 30 mcg/kg/day I.V. for
8 to 10 days or until toxicity occurs.

ADVERSE REACTIONS

CNS: drowsiness, weakness, lethargy,
headache, dizziness, nervousness, depression.

GI: *nausea, vomiting,* anorexia, diarrhea, stomatitis, metallic taste.

GU: proteinuria; increased BUN and
serum creatinine levels.

Hematologic: *leukopenia, thrombocytopenia; bleeding syndrome from
epistaxis to generalized hemorrhage;
facial flushing.*

Hepatic: *elevated liver enzymes levels.*

Other: *decreased serum calcium,* potassium, and phosphorus levels; irritation, cellulitis with extravasation.

INTERACTIONS

None significant.

CONTRAINDICATIONS

Contraindicated in patients with
thrombocytopenia, bone marrow suppression, in those with coagulation
and bleeding disorders, and in women
who are or who may become pregnant.

NURSING CONSIDERATIONS

• Use with extreme caution in patients with significant renal or hepatic
impairment.
• Obtain baseline platelet count and
PT before therapy, as ordered.
• To reduce nausea, give antiemetic
before administering, as ordered.

• Follow institutional policy to reduce
risks. Preparation and administration
of parenteral form of this drug is associated with carcinogenic, mutagenic,
and teratogenic risks for personnel.
• **I.V. use:** To prepare solution, add
4.9 ml of sterile water for injection to
vial and shake to dissolve. Then dilute
for I.V infusion in 1,000 ml of D_5W or
0.9% sodium chloride. Administer by
infusion over 4 to 6 hours. Discard
unused drug.
• Be aware that slow infusion reduces
nausea that develops with I.V. push.
• Avoid extravasation. Plicamycin is a
vesicant. If I.V. solution infiltrates,
stop immediately, notify doctor, and
use ice packs. Restart I.V. line.
• Monitor platelet count and PT during therapy, as ordered. Discontinue
drug if WBC count is less than 4,000/
mm^3, platelet count falls to less than
150,000/mm^3, or if PT is prolonged
more than 4 seconds longer than control and notify doctor.
• Know that facial flushing is an early
indicator of bleeding.
• To prevent bleeding, avoid all I.M.
injections when platelet count is below 100,000/mm^3.
• Anticipate the need for possible
blood transfusions because of cumulative anemia.
• Monitor lactate dehydrogenase,
AST, ALT, alkaline phosphatase,
BUN, creatinine, potassium, calcium,
and phosphorus levels, as ordered.
• Avoid contact with skin or mucous
membranes.
• Monitor patients for tetany, carpopedal spasm, Chvostek's sign, and
muscle cramps; check serum calcium
level. Preciptious drop in calcium
level is possible.
• Store lyophilized powder in refrigerator and protect from light.
• Warn patients to watch for signs of
infection (fever, sore throat, fatigue)
and bleeding (easy bruising, nosebleeds, bleeding gums, melena). Take
temperature daily.

---

diethylstilbestrol
  (See Chapter 55, ESTROGENS AND
  PROGESTINS)
estramustine phosphate sodium
flutamide
goserelin acetate
leuprolide acetate
megestrol acetate
tamoxifen citrate
testolactone

COMBINATION PRODUCTS
None.

---

estramustine phosphate sodium
Emcyt, Estracyst‡
Pregnancy Risk Category: NR

HOW SUPPLIED
Capsules: 140 mg

ACTION
Unknown. A combination of estrogen
and an alkylating agent; probably acts
by its ability to bind selectively to a
protein present in the human prostate.

ONSET, PEAK, DURATION
Unknown.

INDICATIONS & DOSAGE
*Palliative treatment of metastatic or
progressive prostate cancer –*
Adults: 10 to 16 mg/kg P.O. in three
to four divided doses. Usual dosage is
14 mg/kg daily. Therapy continued
for up to 3 months and, if successful,
maintained as long as the patient responds.

ADVERSE REACTIONS
CV: *MI,* sodium and fluid retention,
thrombophlebitis, *CHF,* hypertension.

GI: *nausea, vomiting,* diarrhea.
GU: loss of libido.
Hematologic: *leukopenia, thrombo-
cytopenia.*
Respiratory: *edema, pulmonary em-
bolism.*
Skin: rash, pruritus.
Other: *painful gynecomastia and
breast tenderness,* thinning of hair,
hyperglycemia, fluid retention.

INTERACTIONS
*Calcium-rich foods (milk and dairy
products):* impaired absorption of estramustine.

CONTRAINDICATIONS
Contraindicated in patients hypersensitive to estradiol and nitrogen mustard. Also contraindicated in those
with active thrombophlebitis or
thromboembolic disorders, except
when the actual tumor mass is the
cause of the thromboembolic phenomenon.

NURSING CONSIDERATIONS
• Use cautiously in patients with history of thrombophlebitis or thromboembolic disorders and cerebrovascular or coronary artery disease.
Monitor weight regularly in these patients. Estramustine may exaggerate
preexisting peripheral edema or CHF.
• Be aware that each 140-mg capsule
contains 12.5 mg of sodium.
• Monitor blood pressure and glucose
tolerance periodically throughout
therapy.
• Keep in mind that estramustine is a
combination of estrogen estradiol and
a nitrogen mustard, shown to be effective in patients refractory to estrogen therapy alone.
• Be aware that patients may continue
therapy as long as response is favor-

---

*Liquid form contains alcohol.   *Common* reactions are in italics; **life-threatening,** in bold italics.
**May contain tartrazine.

able. Some patients have taken the drug for more than 3 years.
• Store capsules in refrigerator.
• Tell patients to take this drug on an empty stomach (2 hours before or 1 hour after meals) and to avoid taking with milk or dairy products.
• Because of the possibility of mutagenic effects, advise patients and their partners to use contraception if woman is of childbearing age.

flutamide
Euflex†, Eulexin

Pregnancy Risk Category: D

HOW SUPPLIED
Capsules: 125 mg, 250 mg†

ACTION
Inhibits androgen uptake or prevents binding of androgens in nucleus of cells within target tissues.

ONSET, PEAK, DURATION
Onset and duration unknown. Plasma levels peak 2 hours after dose.

INDICATIONS & DOSAGE
Metastatic prostatic carcinoma (stage D_2) in combination with luteinizing hormone-releasing hormone analogues such as leuprolide acetate –
Adults: 250 mg P.O. q 8 hours.

ADVERSE REACTIONS
CNS: *drowsiness, confusion, numbness or tingling of hands or feet.*
CV: *peripheral edema, hypertension.*
GI: *diarrhea, nausea, vomiting.*
GU: *impotence, loss of libido.*
Hepatic: elevated liver enzyme levels, hepatitis.
Skin: rash, photosensitivity.
Other: *hot flashes,* gynecomastia.

INTERACTIONS
None significant.

CONTRAINDICATIONS
Contraindicated in patients hypersensitive to the drug.

NURSING CONSIDERATIONS
• Monitor liver function tests periodically, as ordered.
• Make sure patients understand that flutamide must be taken continuously with the agent used for medical castration (such as leuprolide acetate) to allow the full benefit of therapy. Leuprolide suppresses testosterone production while flutamide inhibits testosterone action at the cellular level. Together they can impair the growth of androgen-responsive tumors. Advise patients not to discontinue either drug without consulting their doctor.

goserelin acetate
Zoladex

Pregnancy Risk Category: X

HOW SUPPLIED
Implants: 3.6 mg

ACTION
A luteinizing hormone-releasing hormone (LHRH) analogue that acts on the pituitary to decrease the release of follicle-stimulating hormone and luteinizing hormone, resulting in dramatically lowered serum levels of sex hormones.

ONSET, PEAK, DURATION
Onset occurs in 2 to 4 weeks. Effects peak after 12 to 15 days. Suppression of hormone production to castration levels persists throughout therapy.

INDICATIONS & DOSAGE
Palliative treatment of advanced carcinoma of the prostate; endometriosis –
Adults: 1 implant S.C. q 28 days into the upper abdominal wall. For endometriosis, maximum duration of therapy is 6 months.

ADVERSE REACTIONS

CNS: lethargy, pain (worsened in the first 30 days), dizziness, insomnia, anxiety, depression, headache, chills, emotional lability.

CV: edema, *CHF, arrhythmias, CVA,* hypertension, *MI,* peripheral vascular disorder, chest pain.

GI: nausea, vomiting, diarrhea, constipation, ulcer.

GU: *impotence, sexual dysfunction, lower urinary tract symptoms,* renal insufficiency, urinary obstruction, urinary tract infection, amenorrhea, vaginal dryness.

Hematologic: anemia.

Respiratory: COPD, upper respiratory infection.

Skin: rash, diaphoresis.

Other: *hot flashes,* gout, hyperglycemia, weight increase, breast swelling and tenderness, changes in breast size, loss of bone mineral density in women, fever.

INTERACTIONS

None significant.

CONTRAINDICATIONS

Contraindicated in patients with hypersensitivity to luteinizing hormone-releasing hormone (LHRH), LHRH agonist analogues, or to goserelin acetate. Also contraindicated during pregnancy or breast-feeding.

NURSING CONSIDERATIONS

• Because use of the drug is associated with a loss of bone mineral density in women, use cautiously in patients with other risk factors for osteoporosis, such as family history of osteoporosis, chronic alcohol or tobacco abuse, or the use of drugs such as corticosteroids or anticonvulsants that affect bone density.

• Before administering to female patients, rule out pregnancy.

• Administer drug into the upper abdominal wall using aseptic technique. After cleaning the area with an alcohol swab (and injecting a local anesthetic), stretch the patient's skin with one hand while grasping the barrel of the syringe with the other. Insert the needle into the subcutaneous fat; then change direction of the needle so that it parallels the abdominal wall. The needle should then be pushed in until the hub touches the patient's skin; then withdrawn about 1 cm (this creates a gap for the drug to be injected) before depressing the plunger completely.

• To avoid the need for a new syringe and injection site, do not aspirate after inserting the needle.

• Know that the implant comes in a preloaded syringe. If the package is damaged, do not use the syringe. Make sure that the drug is visible in the translucent chamber of the syringe.

• When used for prostate cancer, be aware that LHRH analogues such as goserelin may initially cause a worsening of prostatic cancer symptoms because the drug initially increases testosterone serum levels. A few patients may experience increased bone pain. Rarely, disease exacerbation (either spinal cord compression or ureteral obstruction) has occurred.

• Advise patients to report every 28 days for a new implant. A delay of a couple of days is permissible.

• Tell women to use a nonhormonal form of contraception during treatment. Caution patients about the significant risks to the fetus should pregnancy occur.

• Tell patients to call the doctor if menstruation persists or if breakthrough bleeding occurs. Menstruation should stop during treatment.

• After therapy ends, inform patient that she may experience a delayed return of menses. Persistent amenorrhea is rare.

---

*Liquid form contains alcohol.   *Common* reactions are in italics; *life-threatening*, in bold italics.
**May contain tartrazine.

leuprolide acetate
Lucrin‡, Lupron, Lupron Depot
Pregnancy Risk Category: X

HOW SUPPLIED
Injection: 1 mg/0.2 ml (5 mg/ml) in
2.8-ml multiple-dose vials
Depot injection: 7.5 mg/ml

ACTION
Initially stimulates but then inhibits
the release of follicle-stimulating hormone and luteinizing hormone, resulting in testosterone suppression.

ONSET, PEAK, DURATION
Testosterone concentrations decline to
castrate levels within 2 to 4 weeks.
Time to peak effect for amenorrhea
usually occurs after 1 to 2 months of
therapy. Normal pituitary-gonadal
system function is usually restored
within 4 to 12 weeks after therapy is
withdrawn. Cyclic bleeding in females usually returns within 60 to 90
days after therapy is withdrawn.

INDICATIONS & DOSAGE
Advanced prostate cancer –
Adults: 1 mg S.C. daily. Alternatively, 7.5 mg I.M. (depot injection)
monthly.
Endometriosis –
Adults: 3.75 mg I.M (depot injection
only) as a single injection once a
month for up to 6 months.

ADVERSE REACTIONS
CNS: dizziness, depression, head-
ache.
CV: arrhythmias, angina, *MI,* pe-
ripheral edema.
GI: nausea, vomiting.
Hepatic: elevated liver enzyme lev-
els.
Respiratory: pulmonary embolism.
Other: transient bone pain during
first week of treatment, *hot flashes,*
decreased libido, skin reactions at in-

jection site, gynecomastia, impotence.

INTERACTIONS
None significant.

CONTRAINDICATIONS
Contraindicated in patients hypersensitive to the drug or other gonadotropin-releasing hormone analogues,
during pregnancy or lactation, and in
women with undiagnosed vaginal
bleeding.

NURSING CONSIDERATIONS
• Use cautiously in patients hypersensitive to benzyl alcohol.
• Never administer by I.V. injection.
• Know that once-monthly depot injection should be administered under
medical supervision. Use supplied
diluent to reconstitute drug. Draw 1
ml into a syringe with a 22G needle
(extra diluent is provided and should
be discarded). Inject into vial; then
shake well. Suspension will appear
milky. Although the suspension is stable for 24 hours after reconstitution, it
contains no bacteriostatic agent. Use
immediately.
• Be aware that studies show leuprolide is therapeutically equivalent to diethylstilbestrol in "medical castration"
palliation treatment but has significantly milder and fewer adverse reactions.
• Know that leuprolide is a nonsurgi-
cal alternative to orchiectomy for
prostate cancer.
• Carefully instruct patients who will
self-administer S.C. injection about
proper administration techniques and
advise them to use only the syringes
provided by the manufacturer.
• Advise patients that if another syringe must be substituted, a low-dose
insulin syringe (U-100, 0.5 ml) may
be an appropriate choice.
• Advise patients to store the drug at
room temperature, protected from
light and sources of heat.

• Reassure patients with history of undesirable effects from other endocrine therapies that leuprolide is much easier to tolerate.
• Reassure patients that these effects are transient and will disappear after about 1 week. Worsening of prostate cancer symptoms may occur when therapy is initiated.

megestrol acetate
Megace, Megostat‡

Pregnancy Risk Category: D

HOW SUPPLIED
Tablets: 20 mg, 40 mg
Oral suspension: 40 mg/ml

ACTION
A progestin that changes the tumor's hormonal environment and alters the neoplastic process. Mechanism responsible for appetite stimulation is unknown.

ONSET, PEAK, DURATION
Unknown.

INDICATIONS & DOSAGE
Breast cancer—
Adults: 40 mg P.O. q.i.d.
Endometrial cancer—
Adults: 40 to 320 mg P.O. daily in divided doses.
Treatment of anorexia, cachexia, or unexplained significant weight loss in patients with AIDS—
Adults: 800 mg P.O. (oral suspension) daily in divided doses.

ADVERSE REACTIONS
CV: hypertension, edema, thrombophlebitis.
GI: nausea, vomiting.
GU: breakthrough menstrual bleeding.
Other: weight gain, increased appetite, carpal tunnel syndrome, alopecia, hirsutism, breast tenderness.

INTERACTIONS
None significant.

CONTRAINDICATIONS
Contraindicated in patients hypersensitive to the drug and during pregnancy.

NURSING CONSIDERATIONS
• Use cautiously in patients with history of thrombophlebitis.
• Know that megestrol is a relatively nontoxic drug with a low incidence of adverse effects.
• Be aware that 2 months is an adequate trial when treating patients with cancer.
• Inform patients that therapeutic response isn't immediate.
• Advise breast-feeding patients to discontinue breast-feeding during therapy because of possible infant toxicity.

tamoxifen citrate
Alpha-Tamoxifen†, Nolvadex, Nolvadex-D†‡, Novo-Tamoxifen†, Tamofen†, Tamone†, Tamoplex†

Pregnancy Risk Category: D

HOW SUPPLIED
Tablets: 10 mg, 20 mg
Tablets (enteric-coated)†: 10 mg, 20 mg

ACTION
Exact antineoplastic action is unknown; acts as an estrogen antagonist.

ONSET, PEAK, DURATION
Onset occurs in 4 to 10 weeks, but may take several months. Peak unknown. Estrogen antagonism may persist for several weeks after drug is discontinued.

INDICATIONS & DOSAGE
Advanced premenopausal and postmenopausal breast cancer—
Adults: 10 mg P.O. b.i.d. to t.i.d.

ADVERSE REACTIONS
GI: *nausea* in 10% of patients, vomiting, anorexia.
GU: vaginal discharge and bleeding.
Hematologic: transient fall in WBC or platelet counts.
Skin: rash.
Other: hypercalcemia, temporary bone or tumor pain, hot flashes in 7% of patients, brief exacerbation of pain from osseous metastases.

INTERACTIONS
None significant.

CONTRAINDICATIONS
Contraindicated in patients hypersensitive to the drug.

NURSING CONSIDERATIONS
• Use cautiously in patients with existing leukopenia or thrombocytopenia. Monitor CBC closely in these patients, as ordered.
• Monitor serum lipid levels, as ordered, during long-term therapy in patients with preexisting hyperlipidemia.
• Monitor serum calcium levels, as ordered. Drug may compound hypercalcemia related to bone metastases during initiation of therapy.
• Know that the drug acts as an "antiestrogen." Best results have been reported in patients with positive estrogen receptors.
• Be aware that adverse reactions are usually minor and well tolerated.
• Tell patients taking enteric-coated tablets (Nolvadex-D†) to swallow the tablets whole without crushing or chewing. Tell them not to take antacids within 2 hours of a dose.
• Reassure patients that acute exacerbation of bone pain during tamoxifen therapy usually indicates drug will produce good response. Use analgesic to relieve pain.
• Strongly encourage women who are taking or have taken tamoxifen to have regular gynecologic examinations because of increased risk of uterine cancer associated with its use.
• Advise patient to use barrier form of contraception because short-term therapy induces ovulation in premenopausal women.
• Advise women of childbearing age to avoid becoming pregnant during therapy. Also recommend consulting with doctor before becoming pregnant.

---

testolactone
Teslac
Controlled Substance Schedule III
Pregnancy Risk Category: C

HOW SUPPLIED
Tablets: 50 mg

ACTION
Exact antineoplastic action is unknown. An androgen that probably changes the tumor's hormonal environment and alters the neoplastic process.

ONSET, PEAK, DURATION
Onset occurs in 6 to 12 weeks. Peak and duration unknown.

INDICATIONS & DOSAGE
Advanced postmenopausal breast cancer—
Women: 250 mg P.O. q.i.d.

ADVERSE REACTIONS
CNS: paresthesia, peripheral neuropathy.
CV: increased blood pressure, edema.
GI: nausea, vomiting, diarrhea.
Other: hypercalcemia, alopecia.

INTERACTIONS
Oral anticoagulants: increased pharmacologic effects. Monitor carefully.

CONTRAINDICATIONS

Contraindicated in patients hypersensitive to the drug and in males with breast cancer.

NURSING CONSIDERATIONS

• Monitor fluid and electrolyte levels, especially calcium level.

• Force fluids to aid calcium excretion and encourage exercise to prevent hypercalcemia. Immobilized patients are prone to hypercalcemia.

• Know that higher-than-recommended doses do not increase incidence of remission.

• Inform patients that therapeutic response isn't immediate. Three months is an adequate trial for this drug.

74

Miscellaneous antineoplastic agents

altretamine
asparaginase
bacillus Calmette-Guérin (BCG),
  live intravesical
dacarbazine
etoposide
mitotane
mitoxantrone hydrochloride
paclitaxel
pegaspargase
procarbazine hydrochloride
teniposide
vinblastine sulfate
vincristine sulfate
vinorelbine

COMBINATION PRODUCTS
None.

---

altretamine (hexamethylmelamine; HMM)

Hexalen

Pregnancy Risk Category: D

HOW SUPPLIED
Capsules: 50 mg

ACTION
Unknown. Structurally similar to the alkylating agent triethylenemelamine but not an alkylating agent. Metabolism is important for antitumor activity; metabolites of the drug are known alkylating agents.

ONSET, PEAK, DURATION
Onset and duration unknown. Plasma levels peak in ½ to 3 hours.

INDICATIONS & DOSAGE
Palliative treatment of patients with persistent or recurrent ovarian cancer after first-line therapy with cisplatin or alkylating agent-based combination therapy –
Adults: 260 mg/m² P.O. daily in four divided doses with meals and h.s. for 14 or 21 consecutive days in a 28-day cycle.

ADVERSE REACTIONS
CNS: *sensory neuropathy,* anorexia, ataxia, paresthesia, hyporeflexia, fatigue, *seizures.*
GI: *nausea and vomiting.*
Hematologic: *leukopenia, thrombocytopenia, anemia.*
Skin: erythematous macropapular eczema.
Other: increased serum creatinine and BUN levels, alopecia.

INTERACTIONS
Cimetidine: may increase the half-life and toxicity of altretamine. Monitor closely for toxicity.
MAO inhibitors: severe orthostatic hypotension. Avoid concomitant use.

CONTRAINDICATIONS
Contraindicated in patients hypersensitive to the drug and in those with preexisting severe bone marrow suppression or severe neurologic toxicity.

NURSING CONSIDERATIONS
• Obtain baseline CBC and platelet count, as ordered, before each course of therapy.
• Perform a careful neurologic assessment before each course of therapy.
• Monitor CBC and platelet count monthly, as ordered. Altretamine causes a mild to moderate dose-related myelosuppression. Nadirs of WBC and platelet counts are reached by 3 to 4 weeks. Normal counts are regained by 6 weeks.

• Know that continuous high-dose daily treatment is associated with a higher incidence of mild to moderate neurotoxicity. It appears to be reversible when therapy is discontinued.

• Be aware that unconfirmed reports suggest that the severity and incidence of neurotoxicity may be decreased by concomitant administration of pyridoxine.

• Be prepared to discontinue drug temporarily for at least 14 days if laboratory tests show a platelet count below 75,000/mm³, WBC count below 2,000/mm³, or granulocyte count below 1,000/mm³, as ordered. Also discontinue temporarily, as ordered, if patients experience severe GI distress that is unresponsive to symptomatic treatment or develop signs of progressive neuropathy. Drug should be discontinued, as ordered, if neurologic symptoms fail to stabilize.

• Continuous daily administration of this drug is associated with nausea and vomiting, which is usually treatable with antiemetics. To minimize nausea and vomiting, tell patients to take the drug with meals. If nausea and vomiting is severe, dosage reduction or temporary discontinuation of the drug may be necessary.

• Advise patients to use contraception; drug may harm a developing fetus.

---

asparaginase
(L-asparaginase)
Elspar, Kidrolase†

Pregnancy Risk Category: C

HOW SUPPLIED
Injection: 10,000-unit vial

ACTION
Destroys the amino acid asparagine, which is needed for protein synthesis in acute lymphocytic leukemia. This leads to death of the leukemic cell.

ONSET, PEAK, DURATION
Onset almost immediate. Time to peak plasma concentration is almost immediate after I.V. administration; 4 to 24 hours after I.M. administration. Effects persist for 23 to 33 days after withdrawal of therapy.

INDICATIONS & DOSAGE
Acute lymphocytic leukemia (in combination with other drugs) –
Adults and children: 1,000 IU/kg I.V. daily for 10 days, injected over 30 minutes or by slow I.V. push; or 6,000 IU/m² I.M. at intervals specified in protocol.
Sole induction agent for acute lymphocytic leukemia –
Adults: 200 IU/kg I.V. daily for 28 days.

ADVERSE REACTIONS
CNS: confusion, drowsiness, depression, hallucinations, nervousness, lethargy, somnolence.
GI: *vomiting* (may last up to 24 hours), *anorexia, nausea,* cramps, weight loss.
GU: *azotemia, **renal failure,*** uric acid nephropathy, glycosuria, polyuria, *increased blood ammonia level.*
Hematologic: *anemia, **hypofibrinogenemia,*** depression of other clotting factors, ***thrombocytopenia, leukopenia,*** depression of serum albumin level.
Hepatic: elevated AST and ALT levels, ***hepatotoxicity.***
Skin: *rash, urticaria.*
Other: ***hemorrhagic pancreatitis and anaphylaxis*** *(common),* chills, fever, elevated alkaline phosphatase and bilirubin (direct and indirect levels), increase or decrease in total lipid level, *hyperuricemia, hyperglycemia.*

INTERACTIONS
Methotrexate: decreased methotrexate effectiveness.
Prednisone, vincristine: increased toxicity.

Liquid form contains alcohol.   Common reactions are in italics; **life-threatening, in bold italics.
**May contain tartrazine.

CONTRAINDICATIONS
Contraindicated in patients with pancreatitis or history of pancreatitis and previous hypersensitivity unless desensitized.

NURSING CONSIDERATIONS
• Use cautiously in patients with pre-existing hepatic dysfunction. Because of the unpredictability of adverse reactions, drug should be administered in hospital setting with close supervision.
• Monitor baseline blood and urine glucose levels before therapy.
• Follow institutional policy to reduce risks. Preparation and administration of parenteral form of this drug is associated with carcinogenic, mutagenic, and teratogenic risks for personnel.
• **I.V. use:** Give I.V. injection over 30 minutes through a running infusion of sodium chloride injection or 5% dextrose injection.
• For I.M. injection, limit dose at single injection site to 2 ml.
• Reconstitute with 2 to 5 ml of either sterile water for injection or sodium chloride injection.
• Don't shake vial; may cause loss of potency. Don't use cloudy solutions.
• If drug comes in contact with skin or mucous membranes, wash with copious amounts of water for at least 15 minutes.
• Keep epinephrine, diphenhydramine, and I.V. corticosteroids available for treating anaphylaxis.
• Monitor CBC and bone marrow function tests, as ordered. Bone marrow regeneration may take 5 to 6 weeks.
• Obtain frequent serum amylase level determinations, as ordered, to check pancreatic status. If elevated, know that asparaginase should be discontinued.
• Prevent occurrence of tumor lysis which can result in uric acid nephropathy by increasing fluid intake. Be aware that allopurinol should be started before therapy begins.
• Monitor blood and urine glucose during therapy. Watch for signs of hyperglycemia, such as polydipsia, polyphagia, and polyuria.
• Because of vomiting, administer parenteral fluids, as ordered, for 24 hours or until oral fluids are tolerated.
• Be aware that some patients may develop hypersensitivity to asparaginase, which is derived from cultures of *Escherichia coli. Erwinia* asparaginase, derived from cultures of *Erwinia carotovora,* has been used in these patients without cross-sensitivity.
• Know that risk of hypersensitivity increases with repeated dosages. Patients may be desensitized, but this doesn't rule out risk of allergic reactions. Be aware that routine administration of 2 IU I.V. test dose may identify high-risk patients.
• Know that drug should not be used as sole agent to induce remission unless combination therapy is inappropriate. Not recommended for maintenance therapy.
• Refrigerate unopened dry powder. Reconstituted solution is stable for 8 hours if refrigerated.
• Warn patients to watch for signs of infection (fever, sore throat, fatigue) and bleeding (easy bruising, nosebleeds, bleeding gums, melena). Take temperature daily.

bacillus Calmette-Guérin (BCG), live intravesical
ImmuCyst†, TheraCys, TICE BCG
Pregnancy Risk Category: C

HOW SUPPLIED
TheraCys
Suspension (freeze-dried) for bladder instillation: 27 mg/vial
TICE BCG
Suspension (freeze-dried) for bladder

instillation: approximately 50 mg/ampule

ACTION
Unknown. Instillation of the live bacterial suspension causes a local inflammatory response. Local infiltration of histiocytes and leukocytes is followed by a decrease in superficial tumors within the bladder.

ONSET, PEAK, DURATION
Unknown.

INDICATIONS & DOSAGE
In situ carcinoma of the urinary bladder (primary and relapsed) –
Adults: 3 reconstituted and diluted vials administered intravesically once weekly for 6 weeks (induction), followed by additional treatments at 3, 6, 12, 18, and 24 months (TheraCys); or, 1 bladder instillation (1 ampule suspended in 50 ml of sterile, preservative-free sodium chloride solution) once weekly for 6 weeks, and then once monthly for 6 to 12 months (TICE BCG).

ADVERSE REACTIONS
GI: nausea, vomiting, anorexia, diarrhea, mild abdominal pain.
GU: *dysuria, urinary frequency, hematuria,* cystitis, urinary urgency, urinary incontinence, urinary tract infection, cramps, pain, decreased bladder capacity, tissue in urine, local infection, renal toxicity, genital pain.
Hematologic: anemia, leukopenia, thrombocytopenia.
Hepatic: elevated liver enzymem levels.
Other: hypersensitivity reaction, malaise, *fever above 101° F (38.3° C),* chills, myalgia, arthralgia, ***disseminated mycobacterial infection.***

INTERACTIONS
Antibiotics: may attenuate the response to BCG intravesical. Avoid concomitant use.

Bone marrow suppressants, immunosuppressants, and radiation therapy: may impair the response to BCG intravesical by decreasing the immune response; may also increase the risk of osteomyelitis or disseminated BCG infection. Avoid concomitant use.

CONTRAINDICATIONS
Contraindicated in immunocompromised patients, in those receiving immunosuppressive therapy (because of the risk of bacterial infection), and in those with urinary tract infection (because of the risk of increased bladder irritation or disseminated BCG infection). Also contraindicated in patients with fever of unknown origin. If fever is caused by an infection, the drug should be withheld until the patient has recovered.

NURSING CONSIDERATIONS
• Determine patients' reactivity to tuberculin before therapy. Tuberculin sensitivity may be rendered positive by BCG intravesical treatment.
• To administer TheraCys, reconstitute only with 1 ml of the provided diluent per vial, just before use. Do not remove the rubber stopper to prepare the solution. Use immediately. Add the contents of the three reconstituted vials to 50 ml of sterile, preservative-free sodium chloride solution (final volume, 53 ml). Instill a urethral catheter into the bladder under aseptic conditions, drain the bladder, and then infuse 53 ml of the prepared solution by gravity feed. Remove the catheter and properly dispose of any unused drug.
• To administer TICE BCG, use thermosetting plastic or sterile glass containers and syringes. Draw 1 ml of sterile, preservative-free sodium chloride solution into a 3-ml syringe. Add to one ampule of the drug; gently expel back into the ampule three times to ensure thorough mixing. Use immediately. Dispense the cloudy sus-

---

*Liquid form contains alcohol.   *Common* reactions are in italics; ***life-threatening,*** in bold italics.
**May contain tartrazine.

pension into the top end of a catheter-tipped syringe that contains 49 ml of sodium chloride solution. Gently rotate the syringe. Properly dispose of any unused drug.

• Handle drug and all material used for instillation of the drug as infectious material because it contains live attenuated mycobacteria. Dispose of all associated materials (syringes, catheters, and containers) as biohazardous waste.

• Use strict aseptic technique to administer the drug to minimize trauma to the GU tract and to prevent introducing other contaminants to the area.

• If there is evidence of traumatic catheterization, do not administer the drug and alert doctor. Subsequent treatment may resume after 1 week as if no interruption of the schedule occurred.

• Carefully monitor patient's urinary status because the drug causes an inflammatory response in the bladder.

• Closely monitor patients for evidence of systemic BCG infection. BCG infections are rarely detected by positive cultures. Know that therapy should be withheld if systemic infection is suspected (short-term high fever above 103° F [39.4° C], or persistent fever above 101° F [38.3° C] over 2 days, or with severe malaise). Contact an infectious disease specialist for initiation of fast-acting antituberculosis therapy, as ordered.

• Know that drug is not used as an immunizing agent for the prevention of cancer or to prevent tuberculosis; the drug should not be confused with BCG vaccine.

• Know that this drug should not be handled or administered by a caregiver with a known immunologic deficiency.

• Be aware that BCG intravesical should not be administered within 7 to 14 days of transurethral resection or biopsy. Fatal disseminated BCG in-

fection has occurred after traumatic catheterization.

• Be aware that patients with a small bladder capacity may experience increased local irritation with the usual dose of BCG intravesical.

• Keep in mind that drug has the potential to cause hypersensitivity. Manage symptomatically.

• Be prepared to treat bladder irritation symptomatically with phenazopyridine, acetaminophen, and propantheline, as ordered. Systemic hypersensitivity can be treated with diphenhydramine. In order to minimize the risk of systemic infection, some clinicians give isoniazid for 3 days starting on the first day of treatment.

• Tell patients to retain the drug in the bladder for 2 hours after instillation (if possible). For the first hour, have patients lie 15 minutes prone, 15 minutes supine, and 15 minutes on each side; the second hour may be spent in the sitting position.

• Instruct patients to sit when voiding.

• Instruct patients to disinfect any urine for 6 hours after instillation of the drug. To disinfect urine, add undiluted household bleach (5% sodium hypochlorite solution) in equal volume to voided urine to the toilet; allow to stand for 15 minutes before flushing.

• Tell patients to call if symptoms worsen or if any of the following symptoms develops: blood in the urine, fever and chills, frequent urge to urinate, painful urination, nausea, vomiting, joint pain, or rash.

• Caution patients that a cough that develops after therapy could indicate a life-threatening BCG infection and to report it to their doctor immediately.

---

dacarbazine (DTIC)
DTIC†, DTIC-Dome

Pregnancy Risk Category: C

HOW SUPPLIED
Injection: 100-mg, 200-mg vials

ACTION
Unknown. Probably cross-links strands of cellular DNA and interferes with RNA transcription, causing an imbalance of growth that leads to cell death. Cell cycle-nonspecific.

ONSET, PEAK, DURATION
Unknown.

INDICATIONS & DOSAGE
Metastatic malignant melanoma –
Adults: 2 to 4.5 mg/kg I.V. daily for 10 days; then repeated q 4 weeks as tolerated. Or 250 mg/m² I.V. daily for 5 days, repeated at 3-week intervals.
Hodgkin's disease –
Adults: 150 mg/m² I.V. daily (in combination with other agents) for 5 days, repeated q 4 weeks; or 375 mg/m² on the first day of a combination regimen, repeated q 15 days.

ADVERSE REACTIONS
GI: *severe nausea and vomiting, anorexia.*
Hematologic: *leukopenia and thrombocytopenia,* nadir between 3 and 4 weeks.
Hepatic: transient increase in liver enzyme levels, hepatotoxicity (rare).
Skin: phototoxicity.
Other: *flulike syndrome* (fever, malaise, myalgia beginning 7 days after treatment stopped and possibly lasting 7 to 21 days), alopecia, *anaphylaxis;* severe pain if I.V. solution infiltrates or if solution is too concentrated; tissue damage; hyperuricemia.

INTERACTIONS
Allopurinol: additive hypouricemic effects. Monitor closely.

Anticoagulants, aspirin: increased risk of bleeding. Avoid concomitant use.
Bone marrow suppressants: additive toxicity. Monitor closely.
Phenobarbital, phenytoin, other drugs that induce hepatic metabolism: enhanced dacarbazine activation and risk of toxicity. Monitor closely.

CONTRAINDICATIONS
Contraindicated in patients hypersensitive to the drug.

NURSING CONSIDERATIONS
• Use cautiously if bone marrow function is impaired.
• Administer antiemetics, as ordered, before giving dacarbazine to help decrease nausea. Nausea and vomiting may sometimes subside after several doses.
• Follow institutional policy to reduce risks. Preparation and administration of parenteral form of this drug is associated with carcinogenic, mutagenic, and teratogenic risks for personnel.
• **I.V. use:** Reconstitute drug using sterile water for injection. Add 9.9 ml to the 100-mg vial or 19.7 ml to the 200-mg vial. The resulting solution will be colorless to clear yellow. For infusion, further dilute using up to 250 ml of 0.9% sodium chloride injection or D₅W; infuse over 30 minutes.
• During infusion, protect bag from direct sunlight to avoid possible drug breakdown. May dilute further or slow infusion to decrease pain at infusion site.
• Take care not to allow extravasation during infusion. If I.V. solution infiltrates, discontinue immediately, apply ice to area for 24 to 48 hours and notify doctor.
• Keep in mind that reconstituted solutions are stable for 8 hours at room temperature and normal lighting conditions, or up to 3 days if refrigerated. Diluted solutions are stable for 8

hours at normal room temperature and light, or up to 24 hours if refrigerated. If solutions turn pink, decomposition has occurred; discard drug.
• Discard refrigerated solution after 72 hours and room temperature solution after 8 hours.
• To prevent bleeding, avoid all I.M. injections when platelet count is below 100,000/mm^3.
• Anticipate the need for possible blood transfusions because of cumulative anemia.
• Know that therapeutic effects are often accompanied by toxicity. Monitor CBC and platelet count, as ordered.
• For Hodgkin's disease, be aware that drug is usually given with bleomycin, vinblastine, and doxorubicin.
• Warn patients to watch for signs of infection (fever, sore throat, fatigue) and bleeding (easy bruising, nosebleeds, bleeding gums, melena). Take temperature daily.
• Instruct patients to avoid OTC products containing aspirin.
• Advise patients to avoid sunlight and sunlamps for first 2 days after treatment.
• Reassure patients that flulike syndrome may be treated with mild antipyretics, such as acetaminophen.

etoposide (VP-16)
VePesid

Pregnancy Risk Category: D

HOW SUPPLIED
Capsules: 50 mg
Injection: 100 mg/5 ml

ACTION
Unknown.

ONSET, PEAK, DURATION
Unknown.

INDICATIONS & DOSAGE
Testicular cancer –
Adults: 50 to 100 mg/m^2 P.O. or I.V. on 5 consecutive days q 3 to 4 weeks; or 100 mg/m^2 on days 1, 3, and 5 q 3 to 4 weeks.
Small-cell carcinoma of the lung –
Adults: 35 mg/m^2/day I.V. for 4 days; 50 mg/m^2/day I.V. for 5 days. Oral dosage is two times the I.V. dose rounded to the nearest 50 mg.

ADVERSE REACTIONS
CNS: occasional headache and fever, peripheral neuropathy.
CV: hypotension from rapid infusion.
GI: nausea and vomiting, anorexia, abdominal pain, *stomatitis.*
Hematologic: *anemia, myelosuppression* (dose-limiting), *leukopenia, thrombocytopenia.*
Other: *reversible alopecia, anaphylaxis* (rare), phlebitis at injection site (infrequent).

INTERACTIONS
Warfarin: may further prolong PT.

CONTRAINDICATIONS
Contraindicated in patients hypersensitive to the drug.

NURSING CONSIDERATIONS
• Use cautiously in patients who have had previous cytotoxic or radiation therapy.
• Obtain baseline blood pressure prior to therapy.
• Have diphenhydramine, hydrocortisone, epinephrine, and necessary emergency equipment available to establish an airway in case of anaphylaxis.
• Follow institutional policy to reduce risks. Preparation and administration of parenteral form of this drug is associated with carcinogenic, mutagenic, and teratogenic risks for personnel.
• I.V. use: Give drug by slow I.V. infusion (over at least 30 minutes) to prevent severe hypotension.

• Dilute the drug for infusion in either D_5W or 0.9% sodium chloride solution to a concentration of 0.2 or 0.4 mg/ml. Higher concentrations may crystallize.
• Do not administer through membrane-type in-line filters because the diluent may dissolve the filter.
• Know that solutions diluted to 0.2 mg/ml are stable for 96 hours at room temperature in plastic or glass unprotected from light; solutions diluted to 0.4 mg/ml are stable for 48 hours under the same conditions.
• Monitor blood pressure at 30-minute intervals during infusion. If systolic blood pressure falls below 90 mm Hg, stop infusion and notify the doctor.
• Monitor CBC, as ordered. Observe patients for signs of bone marrow suppression.
• Store capsules in refrigerator.
• Observe oral cavity for signs of ulceration.
• To prevent bleeding, avoid all I.M. injections when platelet count is below 100,000/mm³.
• Anticipate the need for possible blood transfusion because of cumulative anemia.
• Know that etoposide has produced complete remissions in small-cell lung cancer and testicular cancer.
• Warn patient to watch for signs of infection and bleeding.

mitotane
Lysodren
Pregnancy Risk Category: C

HOW SUPPLIED
Tablets (scored): 500 mg

ACTION
Unknown. Thought to selectively destroy adrenocortical tissue and hinder extra-adrenal metabolism of cortisol.

ONSET, PEAK, DURATION
Steroid levels decrease within 2 to 3 days; tumor response, within 6 months. Levels peak 3 to 5 hours after dose. Duration unknown.

INDICATIONS & DOSAGE
Inoperable adrenocortical cancer –
Adults: initially, 2 to 6 g P.O. daily in divided doses t.i.d. or q.i.d.; increased to 9 to 10 g P.O. daily, in divided doses t.i.d. or q.i.d. Dosage is adjusted until maximum tolerated dosage is achieved (varies from 2 to 16 g/day but is usually 8 to 10 g/day).

ADVERSE REACTIONS
CNS: *depression, somnolence, lethargy, vertigo;* brain damage and dysfunction in long-term, high-dose therapy.
GI: *severe nausea, vomiting,* diarrhea, anorexia.
Skin: dermatitis, maculopapular rash.
Other: hypouricemia, increased serum cholesterol level, adrenal insufficiency, visual disturbances, hemorrhagic cystitis, hypertension.

INTERACTIONS
None significant.

CONTRAINDICATIONS
Contraindicated in patients hypersensitive to the drug. Be aware that drug should not be used in patients in shock or who have suffered trauma.

NURSING CONSIDERATIONS
• Use cautiously in patients with hepatic disease.
• To reduce nausea, give antiemetic before mitotane administration, as ordered.
• Be prepared to reduce dosage if GI or skin adverse reactions are severe.
• Monitor effectiveness according to reduction in pain, weakness, and anorexia.
• Assess and record behavioral and neurologic signs daily throughout

*Liquid form contains alcohol.   *Common* reactions are in italics; *life-threatening,* in bold italics.
**May contain tartrazine.

therapy. Prolonged therapy has been associated with significant neurologic impairment.

• Be aware that use of corticosteroids may avoid acute adrenocorticoid insufficiency and is usually required. Glucocorticoid dosage should be increased in periods of physiologic stress such as infection or trauma, as ordered.

• Because drug distributes mostly to body fat, know that obese patients may need higher dosage and may have longer-lasting adverse reactions.

• Keep in mind that an adequate therapeutic trial is at least 3 months, but treatment can continue if clinical benefits are observed.

• Warn ambulatory patients to avoid activities that require alertness and good motor coordination until CNS effects of the drug are known.

---

mitoxantrone hydrochloride
Novantrone

Pregnancy Risk Category: D

HOW SUPPLIED
Injection: 2 mg/ml in 10-ml, 12.5-ml, 15-ml vials

ACTION
Not fully understood; probably cell cycle-nonspecific. Reacts with DNA, producing cytotoxic effect.

ONSET, PEAK, DURATION
Unknown.

INDICATIONS & DOSAGE
Combination initial therapy for acute nonlymphocytic leukemia –
Adults: induction begins with 12 mg/m² I.V. daily on days 1 through 3, in combination with 100 mg/m² daily of cytarabine on days 1 through 7. A second induction may be given if response is not adequate. Maintenance therapy: 12 mg/m² on days 1 and 2, in combina-

tion with cytarabine on days 1 through 5.

ADVERSE REACTIONS
CNS: *seizures,* headache.
CV: *CHF, arrhythmias,* tachycardia.
EENT: conjunctivitis.
GI: *bleeding, abdominal pain, diarrhea, nausea, mucositis, vomiting, stomatitis.*
GU: uric acid nephropathy.
Hematologic: *myelosuppression.*
Hepatic: jaundice.
Respiratory: dyspnea, cough.
Skin: petechiae, ecchymoses.
Other: alopecia, hyperuricemia.

INTERACTIONS
Heparin: physically incompatible. Do not mix together.

CONTRAINDICATIONS
Contraindicated in patients hypersensitive to mitoxantrone.

NURSING CONSIDERATIONS
• Use cautiously in patients with prior exposure to anthracyclines or other cardiotoxic drugs.

• Follow institutional policy to minimize risks. Preparation and administration of parenteral form of this drug is associated with mutagenic, teratogenic, and carcinogenic risks to personnel.

• **I.V. use:** Dilute dose (available as an aqueous solution of 2 mg/ml in volumes of 10, 12.5, and 15 ml) in at least 50 ml of 0.9% sodium chloride injection or D₅W injection. Administer by direct injection into a free-flowing I.V. line of 0.9% sodium chloride or D₅W injection over at least 3 minutes. Mixing with other drugs is not recommended.

• Although mitoxantrone is not a vesicant; if drug extravasates, discontinue infusion immediately and notify doctor.

• Be prepared to administer allopurinol, as ordered. Uric acid nephropathy can be avoided by adequately hydrating the patient before and during therapy.

• Closely monitor hematologic and laboratory chemistry parameters, as ordered.

• To prevent bleeding, avoid all I.M. injections if platelet count falls below 100,000/mm³.

• Anticipate the need for blood transfusion because of cumulative anemia.

• Be aware that left ventricular ejection fraction should be monitored.

• Be prepared to treat infections with antibiotics, as ordered. If severe nonhematologic toxicity occurs during the first course of therapy.

• Know that the second course should be delayed until patients recover.

• Be aware that patients with significant myelosuppression should not receive mitoxantrone unless the benefits outweigh the risks.

• Store undiluted solution at room temperature. Once diluted, the mixture is stable for 7 days at room temperature.

• Inform patients that urine may appear blue-green within 24 hours after administration and some bluish discoloration of the sclera may occur. These effects are not harmful.

• Warn patient to watch for signs of bleeding and infection.

• Advise women of childbearing age to avoid pregnancy during therapy. Also recommend consulting doctor before becoming pregnant.

paclitaxel
Taxol

Pregnancy Risk Category: D

HOW SUPPLIED
Injection: 30 mg/5 ml

ACTION
Prevents depolymerization of cellular microtubules, thus inhibiting the normal reorganization of the microtubule network necessary for mitosis and other vital cellular functions.

ONSET, PEAK, DURATION
Unknown.

INDICATIONS & DOSAGE
Metastatic ovarian cancer after failure of first-line or subsequent chemotherapy –
Adults: 135 mg/m² or 175 mg/m² I.V. over 3 hours q 3 weeks.
Breast cancer after failure of combination chemotherapy for metastatic disease or relapse within 6 months of adjuvant chemotherapy –
Adults: 175 mg/m² I.V. over 3 hours every 3 weeks.

ADVERSE REACTIONS
CNS: *peripheral neuropathy.*
CV: *bradycardia, hypotension, abnormal ECG.*
GI: *nausea, vomiting, diarrhea, mucositis.*
Hematologic: *neutropenia, leukopenia, thrombocytopenia,* anemia, *bleeding.*
Hepatic: elevated liver enzyme levels.
Other: hypersensitivity reactions *(anaphylaxis),* alopecia, *myalgia, arthralgia,* phlebitis, cellulitis at injection site.

INTERACTIONS
Cisplatin: possible additive myelosuppressive effects. Use together cautiously.
Ketoconazole: inhibited paclitaxel metabolism. Use together cautiously.

CONTRAINDICATIONS
Contraindicated in patients hypersensitive to the drug or to polyoxyethylated castor oil, a vehicle used in drug solution, and in patients with baseline neutrophil counts below 1,500/mm³.

---

*Liquid form contains alcohol.   *Common* reactions are in italics; *life-threatening,* in bold italics.
**May contain tartrazine.

NURSING CONSIDERATIONS

• Use cautiously in patients who have received prior radiation therapy because these patients may display more frequent or more severe myelosuppression.

• Follow institutional protocol for the safe handling, preparation, and administration of chemotherapeutic drugs. Preparation and administration of parenteral form of this drug is associated with carcinogenic, mutagenic, and teratogenic risks for personnel. Mark all waste materials with CHEMOTHERAPY HAZARD labels.

• **I.V. use:** Dilute concentrate before infusion. Compatible solutions include 0.9% sodium chloride injection, D_5W, 5% dextrose in 0.9% sodium chloride injection, and 5% dextrose in Ringer's lactate injection. Dilute to a final concentration of 0.3 to 1.2 mg/ml. Diluted solutions are stable for 27 hours at room temperature.

• Prepare and store infusion solutions in glass containers. The undiluted concentrate shouldn't come in contact with polyvinylchloride I.V. bags or tubing. Store diluted solution in glass or polypropylene bottles, or use polypropylene or polyolefin bags. Administer through polyethylene-lined administration sets, and use an in-line 0.22-micron filter.

• Take care to avoid extravasation.

• To reduce the incidence or severity of severe hypersensitivity, anticipate pretreating patients with corticosteroids, such as dexamethasone, and antihistamines, as ordered. Both histamine$_1$-receptor antagonists, such as diphenhydramine, and histamine$_2$-receptor antagonists, such as cimetidine or ranitidine, may be used. Severe hypersensitivity reactions have occurred in as many as 2% of patients treated in early clinical trials.

• Continuously monitor patients for 30 minutes after initiating the infusion. Continue close monitoring throughout the infusion.

• Frequent monitoring of blood counts is necessary during therapy. Bone marrow toxicity is the most frequent and dose-limiting toxicity. Packed RBC or platelet transfusions may be necessary in severe cases. Institute bleeding precautions as appropriate.

• Avoid all I.M. injections when platelet count is below 100,000/mm^3.

• If patients develop significant cardiac conduction abnormalities during treatment, initiate appropriate therapy and continuous cardiac monitoring during therapy and subsequent infusions.

• Warn patient to watch for signs of bleeding and infection.

• Teach patients the signs and symptoms of peripheral neuropathy, such as a tingling or burning sensation or numbness in the extremities, and advise them to report these symptoms immediately. Although mild symptoms are common, severe symptoms occur infrequently. Dosage reduction may be necessary.

• Warn patients that alopecia is common (up to 82% of patients).

• Advise women of childbearing age to avoid becoming pregnant during therapy. Also recommend consulting with doctor before becoming pregnant.

---

pegaspargase
(PEG-L-asparaginase)
Oncaspar

Pregnancy Risk Category: C

HOW SUPPLIED
Injection: 750 IU/ml

ACTION
A modified version of the enzyme L-asparaginase that exerts its cytotoxic activity by inactivating the amino acid asparagine. Asparagine is required by tumor cells to synthesize proteins. Because the tumor cells cannot syn-

thesize their own asparagine, protein synthesis and, eventually, synthesis of DNA and RNA is inhibited.

ONSET, PEAK, DURATION
Unknown.

INDICATIONS & DOSAGE
Acute lymphoblastic leukemia (ALL) in patients who require L-asparaginase but have developed hypersensitivity to the native forms of L-asparaginase –
Adults and children with body surface area of at least 0.6 m²: 2,500 IU/m² I.M. or I.V. q 14 days.
Children with body surface area less than 0.6 m²: 82.5 IU/kg I.M. or I.V. q 14 days.

ADVERSE REACTIONS
CNS: seizures, headache, paresthesia, *status epilepticus,* somnolence, coma, mental status changes, dizziness, emotional lability, mood changes, parkinsonism, confusion, disorientation, fatigue.
CV: hypotension, tachycardia, chest pain, subacute bacterial endocarditis, hypertension.
EENT: epistaxis.
Endocrine: hyperglycemia, hypoglycemia.
GI: nausea, vomiting, abdominal pain, anorexia, diarrhea, constipation, indigestion, flatulence, GI pain, mucositis, *pancreatitis (sometimes fulminant and fatal),* increased serum amylase and lipase levels, severe colitis.
GU: increased BUN level, increased creatinine level, increased urinary frequency, hematuria, severe hemorrhagic cystitis, renal dysfunction, renal failure.
Hematologic: *thrombosis;* prolonged prothrombin times, prolonged partial thromboplastin times, decreased antithrombin III; disseminated intravascular coagulation; decreased fibrinogen; hemolytic anemia; leukopenia;

pancytopenia; agranulocytosis; thrombocytopenia; increased thromboplastin; easily bruised; ecchymosis; *hemorrhage (may be fatal).*
Hepatic: jaundice, abnormal liver function test results, bilirubinemia, increased ALT and AST, ascites, hypoalbuminemia, fatty changes in liver, *liver failure.*
Metabolic: hyperuricemia, hyponatremia, uric acid nephropathy, hypoproteinemia, proteinuria, weight loss, metabolic acidosis, increased blood ammonia level, hyperglycemia, hypoglycemia.
Musculoskeletal: arthralgia, myalgia, musculoskeletal pain, joint stiffness, cramps.
Respiratory: cough, *severe bronchospasm,* upper respiratory tract infection.
Skin: itching, alopecia, fever blister, purpura, hand whiteness, fungal changes, nail whiteness and ridging, erythema simplex, petechial rash.
Local: injection pain or reaction, localized edema.
Other: hypersensitivity reactions, including *anaphylaxis,* rash, erythema, edema, pain, fever, chills, urticaria, dyspnea, or bronchospasm; pain in extremities; peripheral edema; malaise; nighttime sweating; mouth tenderness; infection; *sepsis, septic shock.*

INTERACTIONS
Aspirin, dipyridamole, heparin, NSAIDs, warfarin: imbalances in coagulation factors may occur, predisposing the patient to bleeding or thrombosis. Use together cautiously.
Methotrexate: during the period of its inhibition of protein synthesis and cell replication, pegaspargase may interfere with the action of such drugs as methotrexate, which require cell replication for their lethal effects. Monitor for decreased effectiveness.
Protein-bound drugs: depletion of serum proteins by pegaspargase may

---

*Liquid form contains alcohol.   *Common* reactions are in italics; *life-threatening,* in bold italics.
**May contain tartrazine.

increase the toxicity of other drugs that bind to proteins. Monitor for toxicity. Pegaspargase also may interfere with the enzymatic detoxification of other drugs, particularly in the liver. Administer concomitantly with caution.

CONTRAINDICATIONS
Contraindicated in patients with pancreatitis or a history of pancreatitis; in those who have had significant hemorrhagic events associated with prior L-asparaginase therapy; and in those with previous serious allergic reactions, such as generalized urticaria, bronchospasm, laryngeal edema, hypotension, or other unacceptable adverse reactions to pegaspargase.

NURSING CONSIDERATIONS
• Use cautiously in pregnant patients and in patients with liver dysfunction.
• Know that use of pegaspargase as the sole induction agent should be undertaken only in an unusual situation when a combined regimen that uses other chemotherapeutic agents is inappropriate because of toxicity or other specific patient-related factors, or in patients refractory to other therapy.
• Be aware that I.M. route is the preferred route of administration because of the lower incidence of hepatotoxicity, coagulopathy, and GI and renal disorders that occur with I.M. administration than with I.V. administration.
• Do not administer if there is any indication that the drug has been frozen. Although there may not be an apparent change in the appearance of the drug, pegaspargase's activity is destroyed after freezing. Obtain new dose from pharmacist.
• Avoid excessive agitation; do *not* shake. Keep refrigerated at 2° to 8° C (36° to 46° F). Do not use if cloudy or if precipitate is present. Do not use if

stored at room temperature for more than 48 hours. Do not freeze. Discard unused portions. Use only one dose per vial; do not reenter the vial. Do not save unused drug for later administration.
• When administering I.M., limit the volume administered at a single injection site to 2 ml. If the volume to be administered is greater than 2 ml, use multiple injection sites.
• When administered I.V., give over a period of 1 to 2 hours in 100 ml of 0.9% sodium chloride or dextrose 5% injection through an infusion that is already running.
• Monitor patient closely for hypersensitivity reactions. Hypersensitivity reactions, including life-threatening anaphylaxis, may occur during therapy, especially in patients with known hypersensitivity to the other forms of L-asparaginase. As a routine precaution, keep patients under observation for 1 hour and have resuscitation equipment and other agents necessary to treat anaphylaxis (such as epinephrine, oxygen, and I.V. steroids) readily available. Know that moderate to life-threatening hypersensitivity reactions require discontinuation of L-asparaginase.
• As a guide to the effects of therapy, monitor the patient's peripheral blood count and bone marrow, as ordered. A fall in circulating lymphoblasts is often noted after initiating therapy. This may be accompanied by a marked rise in serum uric acid levels.
• Obtain frequent serum amylase determinations, as ordered, to detect early evidence of pancreatitis. Monitor patient's blood sugar during therapy because hyperglycemia may occur.
• Monitor patient for liver dysfunction when pegaspargase is used in conjunction with hepatotoxic chemotherapeutic agents.
• Be aware that pegaspargase may affect a number of plasma proteins;

therefore, monitoring of fibrinogen, PT, and PTT may be indicated. Question doctor if not ordered.

• The drug may be a contact irritant, and the solution must be handled and administered with care. Gloves are recommended. Inhalation of vapors and contact with skin or mucous membranes, especially those of the eyes, must be avoided. In case of contact, wash with copious amounts of water for at least 15 minutes.

• Inform the patient of the possibility of hypersensitivity reactions and the importance of alerting the staff immediately if any occur.

• Instruct patient not to take any other drugs, including OTC preparations, until approved by the doctor because risk of bleeding is higher when pegaspargase is given concomitantly with certain drugs, such as aspirin, or because it may increase the toxicity of other medications.

• Instruct the patient to report signs and symptoms of infection (fever, chills, and malaise) to the doctor because drug may have immunosuppressant activity.

---

procarbazine hydrochloride
Matulane, Natulan

Pregnancy Risk Category: D

HOW SUPPLIED
Capsules: 50 mg

ACTION
Unknown. Thought to inhibit DNA, RNA, and protein synthesis.

ONSET, PEAK, DURATION
Unknown.

INDICATIONS & DOSAGE
Dosage and indications may vary. Check the treatment protocol with the doctor.
*Hodgkin's disease, other cancers using MOPP (nitrogen mustard, vincris-*tine, procarbazine, prednisone) regimen –
Adults: 2 to 4 mg/kg P.O. daily in a single dose or divided doses for the first week. Then, 4 to 6 mg/kg/day until WBC count falls below 4,000/mm^3 or platelet count falls below 100,000/mm^3. After bone marrow recovers, maintenance dosage of 1 to 2 mg/kg/day resumed. For the MOPP regimen, 100 mg/m^2/day P.O. for 14 days.
Children: 50 mg/m^2 P.O. daily for first week; then 100 mg/m^2 until response or toxicity occurs. Maintenance dosage is 50 mg/m^2 P.O. daily after bone marrow recovery.

ADVERSE REACTIONS
CNS: nervousness, depression, insomnia, nightmares, paresthesia, neuropathy, *hallucinations,* confusion, *seizures.*
EENT: retinal hemorrhage, nystagmus, photophobia.
GI: *nausea, vomiting,* anorexia, stomatitis, dry mouth, dysphagia, diarrhea, constipation.
Hematologic: *bleeding tendency, thrombocytopenia, leukopenia, anemia.*
Respiratory: *pleural effusion,* pneumonitis.
Skin: dermatitis.
Other: reversible alopecia.

INTERACTIONS
CNS depressants: additive depressant effects. Avoid concomitant use.
Digoxin: may decrease serum digoxin levels. Monitor closely.
Drugs and foods high in tyramine (Chianti wine, cheese), local anesthetics, sympathomimetics, tricyclic antidepressants: possible tremors, palpitations, increased blood pressure. Monitor closely.
Ethanol: mild disulfiram-like reaction. Warn patients not to drink alcoholic beverages.
Meperidine: may cause severe hypo-

---

*Liquid form contains alcohol.   *Common* reactions are in italics; *life-threatening,* in bold italics.
**May contain tartrazine.

tension and possible death. Don't give together.

CONTRAINDICATIONS
Contraindicated in patients hypersensitive to the drug and in those with inadequate bone marrow reserve as documented by bone marrow aspiration.

NURSING CONSIDERATIONS
• Use cautiously in patients with impaired hepatic or renal function.
• Monitor CBC and platelet counts, as ordered.
• To prevent bleeding, avoid all I.M. injections when platelet count is below 100,000/mm³.
• Anticipate the need for possible blood transfusions because of cumulative anemia.
• Be prepared to discontinue drug if patient becomes confused, or if paresthesia or other neuropathies develop. Notify doctor.
• To decrease nausea and vomiting, advise patients to take drug at bedtime and in divided doses.
• Warn patients to watch for signs of infection (fever, sore throat, fatigue) and bleeding (easy bruising, nosebleeds, bleeding gums, melena). Take temperature daily.
• Warn patients to avoid alcohol while taking this drug. Instruct patients to stop medication and check with the doctor immediately if disulfiram-like reaction — chest pains, rapid or irregular heartbeat, severe headache, stiff neck — occurs.
• Warn patients to avoid hazardous activities that require alertness and good motor coordination until the CNS effects are known.
• Advise women of childbearing age to avoid becoming pregnant during therapy. Also recommend consulting with doctor before becoming pregnant.

teniposide (VM-26)
Vumon

Pregnancy Risk Category: D

HOW SUPPLIED
Injection: 10 mg/ml

ACTION
A phase-specific cytotoxic drug that acts in the late S or early G_2 phase of the cell cycle, thus preventing cells from entering mitosis.

ONSET, PEAK, DURATION
Unknown.

INDICATIONS & DOSAGE
Refractory childhood acute lymphoblastic leukemia —
Children: optimum dosage hasn't been established. In clinical trials, dosages ranged from 165 to 250 mg/m² I.V. once or twice weekly for 4 to 6 weeks. Usually used in combination with other agents.

ADVERSE REACTIONS
CV: hypotension from rapid infusion.
GI: nausea and vomiting, mucositis.
Hematologic: *myelosuppression* (dose-limiting), *leukopenia, neutropenia, thrombocytopenia, anemia.*
Other: alopecia (rare), *anaphylaxis* (rare), hypersensitivity reactions (chills, fever, urticaria, tachycardia, *bronchospasm,* dyspnea, hypotension, flushing); mucositis; *phlebitis at injection site with extravasation.*

INTERACTIONS
Heparin: physically incompatible. Don't mix together.

CONTRAINDICATIONS
Contraindicated in patients hypersensitive to the drug or to polyoxyethylated castor oil, an injection vehicle.

NURSING CONSIDERATIONS

• Be aware that some clinicians may decide to use this drug despite a patient's history of hypersensitivity because the therapeutic benefits may outweigh its risks. Such patients should be treated with antihistamines and corticosteroids before the infusion begins and should be closely watched during drug administration.

• Obtain baseline blood counts, renal and hepatic function tests, as ordered.

• Monitor blood pressure before therapy.

• Have on hand diphenhydramine, hydrocortisone, epinephrine, and appropriate emergency equipment to establish an airway in case of anaphylaxis.

• Follow institutional policy to reduce risks. Preparation and administration of parenteral form of this drug is associated with carcinogenic, mutagenic, and teratogenic risks for personnel.

• **I.V. use:** Dilute drug in either D_5W or 0.9% sodium chloride injection to a final concentration of 0.1, 0.2, 0.4, or 1 mg/ml. Don't agitate vigorously; precipitation of drug may occur. Discard cloudy solutions. Prepare and store the drug in glass containers. Infuse over 45 to 90 minutes to prevent hypotension.

• Don't mix with other drugs or solutions.

• Ensure careful placement of the I.V. catheter. Extravasation of the drug can result in local tissue necrosis or sloughing.

• Don't administer through a membrane-type in-line filter because the diluent may dissolve the filter.

• Monitor periodic blood counts and renal and hepatic function tests, as ordered.

• Monitor blood pressure at 30-minute intervals during infusion. If systolic blood pressure falls below 90 mm Hg, stop infusion and notify the doctor.

• Keep in mind that solutions containing 0.5 to 1 mg/ml are stable for 4 hours; those containing 0.1 to 0.2 mg/ml are stable for 6 hours at room temperature.

• Advise women of childbearing age to avoid becoming pregnant during therapy. Also recommend consulting with doctor before becoming pregnant.

---

vinblastine sulfate (VLB)
Alkaban-AQ, Velban, Velbe†‡

Pregnancy Risk Category: NR

HOW SUPPLIED
Injection: 10-mg vials (lyophilized powder), 1 mg/ml in 10-ml vials

ACTION
Arrests mitosis in metaphase, blocking cell division.

ONSET, PEAK, DURATION
Unknown.

INDICATIONS & DOSAGE
Breast or testicular cancer, Hodgkin's and non-Hodgkin's lymphoma, choriocarcinoma, lymphosarcoma, mycosis fungoides, Kaposi's sarcoma, histiocytosis –
Adults: 0.1 mg/kg or 3.7 mg/m² I.V. weekly or q 2 weeks. May be increased to maximum dosage of 0.5 mg/kg or 18.5 mg/m² I.V. weekly according to response. Dosage should not be repeated if WBC count is less than 4,000/mm³.
Children: initial dose, 2.5 mg/m² I.V. Dosage increased by 1.25 mg/m² until WBC count is below 3,000/mm³ or tumor response is seen. Maximum dosage is 12.5 mg/m² I.V. weekly.

ADVERSE REACTIONS
CNS: depression, *paresthesia, peripheral neuropathy and neuritis, numbness, loss of deep tendon reflexes, muscle pain and weakness, seizures,* headache.

CV: hypertension.
EENT: pharyngitis.
GI: *nausea, vomiting,* ulcer, bleeding, *constipation, ileus, anorexia, weight loss,* abdominal pain, *stomatitis.*
GU: oligospermia, aspermia, urine retention.
Hematologic: *anemia, leukopenia* (nadir, days 4 to 10; lasts another 7 to 14 days), *thrombocytopenia.*
Respiratory: *acute bronchospasm,* shortness of breath.
Skin: dermatitis, vesiculation.
Other: reversible alopecia in 5% to 10% of patients, *pain in tumor site,* low-grade fever, hyperuricemia; *irritation, phlebitis,* cellulitis, necrosis with extravasation.

INTERACTIONS
Mitomycin: increased risk of bronchospasm and shortness of breath.
Phenytoin: decreased plasma phenytoin levels.

CONTRAINDICATIONS
Contraindicated in patients with severe leukopenia or bacterial infection.

NURSING CONSIDERATIONS
• Use cautiously in patients with hepatic dysfunction.
• To reduce nausea, give antiemetic before administering drug, as ordered.
• Follow institutional policy to reduce risks. Preparation and administration of parenteral form of this drug is associated with carcinogenic, mutagenic, and teratogenic risks for personnel.
• **I.V. use:** Inject directly into vein or tubing of running I.V. line over 1 minute. May also be given in 50 ml of D₅W or 0.9% sodium chloride solution infused over 15 minutes. If extravasation occurs, stop infusion immediately and notify doctor. The manufacturer recommends that moderate heat be applied to the area of leakage. Local injection of hyaluronidase may help disperse the drug, as ordered. Some clinicians prefer to apply ice packs on and off every 2 hours for 24 hours, with local injection of hydrocortisone or 0.9% sodium chloride.
• Reconstitute 10-mg vial with 10 ml of sodium chloride injection or sterile water. This yields 1 mg/ml. Refrigerate reconstituted solution. Discard after 30 days.
• Do not administer into a limb with compromised circulation.
• After administering, monitor for development of life-threatening acute bronchospasm. If this occurs, notify the doctor immediately. Reaction is most likely to occur in patients who are also receiving mitomycin.
• Monitor patient for stomatitis. Be prepared to stop drug if stomatitis occurs and notify doctor.
• Assess bowel activity. Give laxatives as needed and ordered. May use stool softeners prophylactically.
• Know that dosage should not be repeated more frequently than every 7 days or severe leukopenia will develop.
• Assess for numbness and tingling in hands and feet. Assess gait for early evidence of footdrop.
• Take care to avoid confusing vinblastine with vincristine or vindesine.
• Know that the drug is less neurotoxic than vincristine.
• Anticipate a decrease in dosage by 50% if bilirubin levels are greater than 3 mg/100 ml.
• Warn patients that alopecia may occur, but that it's usually reversible.

---

vincristine sulfate
Oncovin, Vincasar PFS
Pregnancy Risk Category: D

HOW SUPPLIED
Injection: 1 mg/ml in 1-ml, 2-ml, 5-ml multiple-dose vials; 1 mg/ml in 1-ml, 2-ml preservative-free vials

---

ACTION
Arrests mitosis in metaphase, blocking cell division.

ONSET, PEAK, DURATION
Unknown.

INDICATIONS & DOSAGE
Acute lymphoblastic and other leukemias, Hodgkin's disease, non-Hodgkin's lymphoma, neuroblastoma, rhabdomyosarcoma, Wilms' tumor—
Adults: 1.4 mg/m² I.V. weekly. Maximum weekly dosage is 2 mg.
Children over 10 kg: 2 mg/m² I.V. weekly.
Children 10 kg and under: initially, 0.05 mg/kg I.V. weekly. Maximum single dose is 2 mg.

ADVERSE REACTIONS
CNS: *peripheral neuropathy,* sensory loss, *loss of deep tendon reflexes, paresthesia, wristdrop and footdrop,* ataxia, cranial nerve palsies (headache, *jaw pain,* hoarseness, vocal cord paralysis, visual disturbances), *muscle weakness and cramps,* depression, agitation, insomnia; some neurotoxicities may be permanent.
CV: hypotension.
EENT: diplopia, optic and extraocular neuropathy, ptosis.
GI: diarrhea, *constipation, cramps,* ileus that mimics surgical abdomen, *nausea, vomiting,* anorexia, weight loss, dysphagia, *intestinal necrosis, stomatitis.*
GU: urine retention, SIADH, dysuria, polyuria.
Hematologic: rapidly reversible mild anemia and leukopenia.
Respiratory: *acute bronchospasm.*
Other: *reversible alopecia* (up to 71% of patients), fever, severe local reaction with extravasation, *phlebitis,* cellulitis at injection site, hyperuricemia.

INTERACTIONS
Asparaginase: decreased hepatic clearance of vincristine.
Calcium channel blockers: enhanced vincristine accumulation in cells.
Digoxin: decreased digoxin effects. Monitor serum digoxin level.
Mitomycin: possibly increased frequency of bronchospasm and acute pulmonary reactions.

CONTRAINDICATIONS
Contraindicated in patients hypersensitive to the drug or who have the demyelinating form of Charcot-Marie-Tooth syndrome. Do not administer to patients who are concurrently receiving radiation therapy through ports that include the liver.

NURSING CONSIDERATIONS
• Use cautiously in patients with hepatic dysfunction, neuromuscular disease, or infection.
• Follow institutional policy to reduce risks. Preparation and administration of parenteral form of this drug is associated with carcinogenic, mutagenic, and teratogenic risks for personnel.
• **I.V. use:** Inject directly into vein or tubing of running I.V. line slowly over 1 minute. May also be given in 50 ml of D₅W or 0.9% sodium chloride solution infused over 15 minutes. If drug extravasates, stop infusion immediately and notify doctor. Apply heat on and off every 2 hours for 24 hours. Administer 150 units hyalaronidase, as ordered, to area of infiltration.
• Don't administer to one patient as a single dose. The 5-mg vials are for multiple-dose use only.
• After administering, monitor for development of life-threatening acute bronchospasm. If this occurs, notify the doctor immediately. This reaction is most likely to occur in patients who are also receiving mitomycin.
• Monitor for hyperuricemia, especially in patients with leukemia or lymphoma. Maintain good hydration and administer allopurinol, as ordered, to prevent uric acid nephropathy.

---

*Liquid form contains alcohol.
**May contain tartrazine.
Common reactions are in italics; *life-threatening,* in bold italics.

• Monitor fluid intake and output. Fluid restriction may be necessary if SIADH develops.

• Because of the risk of neurotoxicity, know that drug should not be given more than once a week. Children are more resistant to neurotoxicity than adults. Neurotoxicity is dose-related and usually reversible.

• Check for depression of Achilles tendon reflex, numbness, tingling, footdrop or wristdrop, difficulty in walking, ataxia, and slapping gait. Also check ability to walk on heels. Support patients when walking.

• Monitor bowel function. Give stool softener or laxative, as ordered, or water before dosing. Constipation may be an early sign of neurotoxicity.

• Take care to avoid confusing vincristine with vinblastine or vindesine.

• Know that all vials (1-mg, 2-mg, 5-mg) contain 1 mg/ml solution and should be refrigerated.

• Warn patients that alopecia may occur, but that it's usually reversible.

• Advise women of childbearing age to avoid becoming pregnant during therapy. Also recommend consulting with doctor before becoming pregnant.

---

vinorelbine
Navelbine

Pregnancy Risk Category: D

HOW SUPPLIED
Injection: 10 mg/ml, 50 mg/5 ml

ACTION
A semisynthetic vinca alkaloid that exerts its antineoplastic effect by disrupting microtubule assembly, which, in turn, disrupts spindle formation and prevents mitosis.

ONSET, PEAK, DURATION
Unknown.

INDICATIONS & DOSAGE
Alone or as adjunct therapy with cisplatin for first-line treatment of ambulatory patients with nonresectable advanced non-small-cell lung cancer (NSCLC); alone or with cisplatin in stage IV of NSCLC; with cisplatin in stage III of NSCLC –
Adults: 30 mg/m^2 I.V. weekly. In combination treatment, same dosage used along with 120 mg/m^2 of cisplatin, given on days 1 and 29, then every 6 weeks.

ADVERSE REACTIONS
GI: nausea, vomiting, anorexia, abdominal pain, diarrhea, constipation, indigestion, stomatitis.
Hematologic: *bone marrow suppression (agranulocytosis, leukopenia, thrombocytopenia, anemia).*
Hepatic: abnormal liver function test results, bilirubinemia.
Respiratory: dyspnea.
Skin: alopecia, rash.
Local: injection pain or reaction.
Other: peripheral neuropathy, asthenia, jaw pain, fatigue, myalagia, SIADH.

INTERACTIONS
Cisplatin: increased risk of bone marrow suppression when used concomitantly with cisplatin. Monitor patient's hematologic status closely.
Mitomycin: may cause pulmonary reactions. Monitor patient's respiratory status closely.

CONTRAINDICATIONS
Contraindicated in patients with pre-treatment granulocyte counts less than 1,000 cells/mm^3.

NURSING CONSIDERATIONS
• Use with extreme caution in patients whose bone marrow may have been compromised by previous exposure to radiation therapy or chemotherapy or whose bone marrow is still

---

recovering from previous chemotherapy.

• Use cautiously in patients with hepatic impairment.

• Check patient's granulocyte count before administration. The count should be equal to or greater than 1,000 cells/mm³ for drug to be administered. Withhold drug and notify doctor if count is less.

• Know that vinorelbine must be diluted before administration. Administer the drug I.V. over 6 to 10 minutes into the side port of a free-flowing I.V. line that is closest to the I.V. bag, followed by flushing with at least 75 to 125 ml of D_5W or 0.9% sodium chloride solution.

• Take great care to avoid extravasation when administering vinorelbine because drug can cause considerable irritation, localized tissue necrosis, and thrombophlebitis. If extravasation occurs, drug administration should be stopped immediately and any remaining dosage portion injected into a different vein.

• Be aware that dosage adjustments are made according to hematologic toxicity or hepatic insufficiency, whichever results in the lower dosage. Expect dosage to be halved if a patient's granulocyte count falls below 1,500 cells/mm³ but is greater than 1,000 cells/mm³. If 3 consecutive doses are skipped because of agranulocytosis, know that further vinorelbine therapy should not be given.

• Know that the drug may be a contact irritant, and the solution must be handled and administered with care. Gloves are recommended. Inhalation of vapors and contact with skin or mucous membranes, especially those of the eyes, must be avoided. In case of contact, wash with copious amounts of water for at least 15 minutes.

• Monitor patient closely for hypersensitivity reactions.

• As a guide to the effects of therapy, monitor patient's peripheral blood count and bone marrow, as ordered.

• Instruct patient not to take any other drugs, including OTC preparations, until approved by the doctor.

• Instruct patient to report signs and symptoms of infection (fever, chills, malaise) to the doctor because drug may have immunosuppressant activity.

---

*Liquid form contains alcohol.   *Common* reactions are in italics; *life-threatening*, in bold italics.
**May contain tartrazine.

75

Immunosuppressants

azathioprine
cyclosporine
levamisole hydrochloride
lymphocyte immune globulin
muromonab-CD3
tacrolimus

COMBINATION PRODUCTS
None.

---

azathioprine
Imuran, Thioprine‡

Pregnancy Risk Category: D

HOW SUPPLIED
Tablets: 50 mg
Injection: 100 mg

ACTION
Unknown.

ONSET, PEAK, DURATION
Onset occurs in 4 to 8 weeks. Serum levels peak in 1 to 2 hours. Clinical effects may persist for long periods after the drug is eliminated.

INDICATIONS & DOSAGE
Immunosuppression in kidney transplantation –
Adults and children: initially, 3 to 5 mg/kg P.O. or I.V. daily usually beginning on the day of transplantation. Maintained at 1 to 3 mg/kg daily (dosage varies considerably according to patient response).
Severe, refractory rheumatoid arthritis –
Adults: initially, 1 mg/kg P.O. as a single dose or as two doses. If patient response is not satisfactory after 6 to 8 weeks, dosage may be increased by 0.5 mg/kg daily (up to a maximum of 2.5 mg/kg daily) at 4-week intervals.

ADVERSE REACTIONS
EENT: mouth ulceration.
GI: nausea, vomiting, anorexia, *pancreatitis,* steatorrhea, esophagitis.
Hematologic: *leukopenia, bone marrow suppression,* anemia, *pancytopenia, thrombocytopenia.*
Hepatic: *hepatotoxicity,* jaundice.
Skin: rash, pruritus.
Other: *immunosuppression* (possibly profound), arthralgia, muscle wasting, alopecia.

INTERACTIONS
Allopurinol: impaired inactivation of azathioprine. Decrease azathioprine dose to ¼ or ⅓ normal dose.
Angiotensin converting enzyme inhibitors: the combination may cause severe leukopenia. Monitor patient closely.
Nondepolarizing neuromuscular blocking agents: azathioprine may reverse the neuromuscular blockade.
Vaccines: decreased immune response. Postpone routine immunization.

CONTRAINDICATIONS
Contraindicated in patients hypersensitive to the drug.

NURSING CONSIDERATIONS
• Use cautiously in patients with hepatic or renal dysfunction.
• Administer drug in divided doses or after meals to minimize adverse GI effects.
• **I.V. use:** Reconstitute 100-mg vial with 10 ml of sterile water for injection. Visually inspect for particles before giving. Drug may be administered by direct I.V. injection or further diluted in 0.9% sodium chloride injection or D₅W and infused over 30 to

---

60 minutes. Use only for patients unable to tolerate oral medications.
• To prevent bleeding, avoid all I.M. injections when platelet count is below 100,000/mm³.
• Monitor hemoglobin and WBC and platelet counts at least once monthly, as ordered, more often at beginning of treatment. Know that drug should be stopped immediately when WBC count is less than 3,000/mm³ to prevent irreversible bone marrow suppression and doctor notified.
• Watch for early signs of hepatotoxicity: clay-colored stools, dark urine, pruritus, and yellow skin and sclera; and for increased alkaline phosphatase, bilirubin, AST, and ALT levels.
• Be aware that therapeutic response usually occurs within 8 weeks.
• Keep in mind that the benefits must be weighed against the risk with systemic viral infections, such as chicken pox and herpes zoster.
• Be aware that patients with rheumatoid arthritis previously treated with aklylating agents, such as cyclophosphomide, chlorambucil, melphalan, or others may have a prohibitive risk of neoplasia if treated with the drug.
• Know that drug should not be used for treating rheumatoid arthritis in pregnant women.
• Warn patients to report even mild infections (colds, fever, sore throat, and malaise) because drug is a potent immunosuppressant.
• Instruct patients to avoid conception during therapy and for 4 months after stopping therapy.
• Warn patients that some thinning of hair is possible.
• Tell patients taking this drug for refractory rheumatoid arthritis that it may take up to 12 weeks to be effective.

cyclosporine (cyclosporin)
Sandimmun‡, Sandimmune
Pregnancy Risk Category: C

HOW SUPPLIED
Oral solution: 100 mg/ml
Injection: 50 mg/ml
Capsules: 25 mg, 50 mg, 100 mg

ACTION
Unknown. Thought to inhibit the proliferation of T lymphocytes.

ONSET, PEAK, DURATION
Onset and duration unknown. Serum levels peak within 3½ hours after oral dose.

INDICATIONS & DOSAGE
Prophylaxis of organ rejection in kidney, liver, or heart transplantation –
Adults and children: 15 mg/kg P.O. 4 to 12 hours before transplantation and continued daily postoperatively for 1 to 2 weeks. Then dosage reduced by 5% each week to maintenance level of 5 to 10 mg/kg/day. Alternatively, 5 to 6 mg/kg I.V. concentrate 4 to 12 hours before transplantation. Postoperatively, dosage repeated daily until patients can tolerate oral forms.

ADVERSE REACTIONS
CNS: *tremor,* headache.
CV: hypertension.
EENT: *gum hyperplasia,* oral thrush.
GI: nausea, vomiting, diarrhea.
GU: *nephrotoxicity.*
Hematologic: anemia, *leukopenia,* ***thrombocytopenia.***
Hepatic: ***hepatotoxicity.***
Skin: acne.
Other: sinusitis, flushing, increased low-density lipoprotein levels, ***infections,*** *hirsutism.*

INTERACTIONS
Aminoglycosides, amphotericin B, cotrimoxazole, NSAIDs: increased risk of nephrotoxicity.

---

*Liquid form contains alcohol.
**May contain tartrazine.

Common reactions are in italics; ***life-threatening,*** in bold italics.

Amphotericin B, cimetidine, diltiazem, erythromycin, imipenem-cilastatin, ketoconazole, metoclopramide, prednisolone: may increase blood levels of cyclosporine. Monitor for increased toxicity.

Azathioprine, corticosteroids, cyclophosphamide, verapamil: increased immunosuppression.

Carbamazepine, isoniazid, phenobarbital, phenytoin, rifampin: possible decreased immunosuppressant effect. May need to increase cyclosporine dosage.

Vaccines: decreased immune response. Postpone routine immunization.

CONTRAINDICATIONS
Contraindicated in patients hypersensitive to the drug or to polyoxyethylated castor oil (found in injectable form).

NURSING CONSIDERATIONS
• Measure oral doses carefully in an oral syringe. To increase palatability, mix with whole milk, chocolate milk, or fruit juice. Use a glass container to minimize adherence to container walls.
• Give dosage once daily in the morning.
• **I.V. use:** Administer cyclosporine I.V. concentrate at one-third the oral dose and dilute before use. Dilute each milliliter of the concentrate in 20 to 100 ml of D_5W or 0.9% sodium chloride injection. Dilute immediately before administration; infuse over 2 to 6 hours. Usually reserved for patients who cannot tolerate oral medications.
• Always give cyclosporine concomitantly with adrenal corticosteroids as ordered.
• Monitor cyclosporine blood levels at regular intervals. Absorption of cyclosporine oral solution can be erratic.
• Monitor BUN and serum creatinine

levels. Cyclosporine may cause nephrotoxicity. Nephrotoxicity may develop 2 to 3 months after transplant surgery, possibly requiring dosage reduction. Promptly report to the doctor any signs or symptoms that suggest the development of nephrotoxicity.
• Know that doctor must differentiate between transplanted kidney rejection and cyclosporine-induced nephrotoxicity.
• Monitor liver function tests, as ordered, for hepatotoxicity, which usually occurs during first month after transplant.
• Encourage patients to take drug at the same time each day.
• Advise patients to take with meals if drug causes nausea. Anorexia, nausea, and vomiting are usually transient and most frequently occur at the start of therapy.
• Stress to patients that therapy should not be stopped without the doctor's approval.
• To prevent thrush, instruct patients to swish and swallow nystatin four times daily.

---

levamisole hydrochloride
Ergamisol

Pregnancy Risk Category: C

HOW SUPPLIED
Tablets: 50 mg (base)

ACTION
Unknown. It appears to restore depressed immune function and may potentiate the actions of monocytes and macrophages and enhance T-cell responses.

ONSET, PEAK, DURATION
Onset and duration unknown. Plasma levels peak in 1½ to 2 hours.

INDICATIONS & DOSAGE
Adjuvant treatment of Dukes' stage C colon cancer (with fluorouracil) after surgical resection —
Adults: 50 mg P.O. q 8 hours for 3 days. Therapy begun no sooner than 7 days and no later than 30 days after surgery, provided that the patient is out of the hospital, ambulating, and maintaining normal oral nutrition; has well-healed wounds; and has recovered from any postoperative complications. Fluorouracil (450 mg/m²/day I.V.) is given for 5 days concomitant with a 3 day course of levamisole starting 21 to 34 days after surgery.

Maintenance dosage is 50 mg P.O. q 8 hours for 3 days q 2 weeks for 1 year. Given in conjunction with fluorouracil maintenance therapy (450 mg/m²/day by rapid I.V. push, once a week beginning 28 days after the initial 5-day course) for 1 year.

ADVERSE REACTIONS
CNS: *dizziness, headache, paresthesia, somnolence, depression, nervousness, insomnia, anxiety, fatigue, fever.*
CV: chest pain, edema.
EENT: blurred vision, conjunctivitis, *stomatitis, dysgeusia, altered sense of smell.*
GI: *nausea, diarrhea, vomiting, anorexia, abdominal pain, constipation, flatulence, dyspepsia.*
Hematologic: **agranulocytosis, leukopenia, thrombocytopenia.**
Skin: *dermatitis, **exfoliative dermatitis,** pruritus, urticaria.*
Other: hyperbilirubinemia, rigors, *alopecia, infection, arthralgia, myalgia.*

INTERACTIONS
Ethanol: may precipitate a disulfiram-like reaction. Avoid concomitant use.
Phenytoin: plasma levels may be elevated when administered with levamisole and fluorouracil. Monitor phenytoin plasma levels.

CONTRAINDICATIONS
Contraindicated in patients hypersensitive to the drug.

NURSING CONSIDERATIONS
• Use cautiously and with close hematologic monitoring because agranulocytosis, which is sometimes fatal, may occur. Neutropenia is usually reversible when therapy is discontinued.
• Obtain baseline CBC with differential, platelet count, and electrolyte levels, and liver function studies, as ordered, immediately before starting therapy.
• Be aware that if levamisole therapy begins 7 to 20 days after surgery, fluorouracil should be started with the second course of levamisole therapy. It should begin no sooner than 21 days and no later than 35 days after surgery. If levamisole is deferred until 21 to 30 days after surgery, fluorouracil therapy should begin with the first course of levamisole.
• Know that dosage modifications are based on hematologic parameters. If WBC count is 2,500/mm³ to 3,500/mm³, don't administer fluorouracil as ordered until WBC count is above 3,500/mm³. When fluorouracil is restarted, reduce dosage by 20% as ordered. If WBC count stays below 2,500/mm³ for over 10 days after fluorouracil is withdrawn, discontinue levamisole, as ordered.
• Know that recommended doses should not be exceeded. Higher doses are associated with greater incidence of agranulocytosis.
• Obtain CBC with differential and platelet count at weekly intervals, as ordered, before treatment with fluorouracil. Obtain electrolyte levels and liver function studies every 3 months for 1 year, as ordered.
• If platelet count is below 100,000/mm³, know that therapy with both fluorouracil and levamisole

---

*Liquid form contains alcohol.
**May contain tartrazine.

Common reactions are in italics; *life-threatening,* in bold italics.

should be discontinued and doctor notified.

• Tell patients to promptly report the development of stomatitis or diarrhea. If either of these reactions occur during the initial course of fluorouracil therapy, drug is discontinued and then weekly fluorouracil therapy is begun 28 days after the start of the initial course. If stomatitis or diarrhea develops during the weekly doses of fluorouracil, fluorouracil therapy is deferred until these symptoms subside. Then fluorouracil therapy is started at reduced dosages (decrease dose by 20%).

• Advise patients to immediately report any flulike symptoms, such as fever and chills.

---

lymphocyte immune globulin (antithymocyte globulin [equine], ATG)
Atgam

Pregnancy Risk Category: C

HOW SUPPLIED
Injection: 50 mg of equine IgG/ml in 5-ml ampules

ACTION
Unknown. Inhibits cell-mediated immune responses by either altering T-cell function or eliminating antigen-reactive T cells.

ONSET, PEAK, DURATION
Onset and duration unknown. Plasma levels peak after 5 days of therapy.

INDICATIONS & DOSAGE
Prevention of acute renal allograft rejection –
Adults and children: 15 mg/kg I.V. daily for 14 days followed by alternate-day dosing for 14 days; the first dose should be given within 24 hours of transplantation.
Treatment of acute renal allograft rejection –

Adults and children: 10 to 15 mg/kg I.V. daily for 14 days followed by alternate-day dosing for 14 days. Therapy should be initiated when rejection is diagnosed.
Aplastic anemia –
Adults: 10 to 20 mg/kg I.V daily for 8 to 14 days. Additional alternative-day therapy up to a total of 21 doses can be administered.

ADVERSE REACTIONS
CNS: malaise, *seizures,* headache.
CV: *hypotension, chest pain,* thrombophlebitis, tachycardia, edema, iliac vein obstruction, renal artery stenosis.
EENT: *laryngospasm.*
GI: *nausea, vomiting,* diarrhea, hiccups, epigastric pain, abdominal distention, stomatitis.
Hematologic: *leukopenia, thrombocytopenia, hemolysis.*
Hepatic: elevated liver enzyme level.
Respiratory: *dyspnea, pulmonary edema.*
Other: febrile reactions, serum sickness, *anaphylaxis,* rash, infections, arthralgia, night sweats, lymphadenopathy, hyperglycemia.

INTERACTIONS
Muromonab-CD3: increased risk of infection. Monitor closely.

CONTRAINDICATIONS
Contraindicated in patients hypersensitive to the drug. An intradermal skin test is recommended at least 1 hour before the first dose. Marked local swelling or erythema larger than 10 mm indicates an increased potential for severe systemic reaction, such as anaphylaxis. Severe reactions to the skin test, such as hypotension, tachycardia, dyspnea, generalized rash, or anaphylaxis, usually preclude further administration of the drug.

---

†Available in Canada only.   ‡Available in Australia only.   ◊ Available OTC.

NURSING CONSIDERATIONS
• Use cautiously in patients receiving additional immunosuppressive therapy (such as corticosteroids or azathioprine) because of the increased potential for infection. Do not dilute ATG concentrate with dextrose solutions or solutions with a low salt concentration because a precipitate may form. The proteins in ATG can be denatured by air. ATG is unstable in acidic solutions.
• Know that ATG solutions must be filtered during administration; filters with pore sizes of 0.2 to 5 microns have been used.
• **I.V. use:** Dilute concentrated drug for injection before administration. Dilute the required dose in 250 to 1,000 ml of 0.45% or 0.9% sodium chloride injection. The final concentration of drug should not exceed 1 mg/ml. When adding ATG to the infusion solution, make sure the container is inverted so that the drug does not contact air inside the container. Gently rotate or swirl the container to mix contents; do not shake because this may cause excessive foaming or denature the drug protein. Infuse with an in-line filter with a pore size of 0.2 to 1 micron, over no less than 4 hours (most institutions infuse over 4 to 8 hours).
• Do not use solutions that are more than 12 hours old, including actual infusion time.
• Refrigerate at 35° to 47° F (2° to 8° C). Do not freeze. ATG concentrate is heat-sensitive.
• Monitor patients for signs of infection.

---

muromonab-CD3
Orthoclone OKT3

Pregnancy Risk Category: C

HOW SUPPLIED
Injection: 1 mg/1 ml in 5-ml ampules

ACTION
Muromonab-CD3 is an IgG antibody that reacts in the T-lymphocyte membrane with a molecule (CD3) needed for antigen recognition. This drug depletes the blood of CD3-positive T cells, which leads to restoration of allograft function and reversal of rejection.

ONSET, PEAK, DURATION
Onset almost immediate. Peak unknown. Number of cirulating CD3 positive T-cells returns to pretreatment levels within 1 week after drug is withdrawn.

INDICATIONS & DOSAGE
Acute allograft rejection in renal transplant patients; in steroid-resistant hepatic or cardiac allograft rejection –
Adults: 5 mg I.V. bolus once daily for 10 to 14 days.

ADVERSE REACTIONS
CNS: *tremors,* headache, *seizures*.
CV: *chest pain,* tachycardia.
GI: *nausea, vomiting,* diarrhea.
Respiratory: *severe pulmonary edema,* dyspnea.
Other: *fever, chills, tremors, **infection, anaphylaxis**.*

INTERACTIONS
Immunosuppressants: increased risk of infection. Monitor closely.
Indomethacin: increased muromonab-CD3 levels with encephalopathy and other CNS effects. Monitor patient closely.
Live-virus vaccines: may potentiate replication and increase effects of virus vaccine.

CONTRAINDICATIONS
Contraindicated in pregnancy and lactation. Also contraindicated in patients with hypersensitivity to the drug or to any other product of murine origin; who have anti-mouse an-

---

*Liquid form contains alcohol.   *Common* reactions are in italics; ***life-threatening***, in bold italics.
**May contain tartrazine.

tibody titers equal to or greater than 1:1,000; who have fluid overload, as evidenced by chest X-ray or a weight gain greater than 3% within the week before treatment; or who have history of seizures or are predisposed to seizures.

NURSING CONSIDERATIONS
• Obtain chest X-ray within 24 hours before starting drug treatment, as ordered.
• Assess patients for signs of fluid overload before treatment.
• Inform patients of expected adverse reactions, and reassure them that these will be less severe as treatment progresses.
• Keep in mind that treatment should begin in a facility that is equipped and staffed for cardiopulmonary resuscitation and where patients can be monitored closely.
• Be alert that most adverse reactions develop within ½ to 6 hours after the first dose.
• Administer an antipyretic, as ordered, before giving the drug to help lower incidence of expected pyrexia and chills. Corticosteroids may also be administered, as ordered, before first injection to help decrease the incidence of adverse reactions. Methylprednisolone sodium succinate (1 mg/kg) preinjection, followed by hydrocortisone sodium succinate (100 mg) 30 minutes postinjection, have been recommended to alleviate the severity of the first-dose reaction.
• Be aware that muromonab-CD3 is a monoclonal antibody preparation. Patients develop antibodies to this preparation that can lead to loss of effectiveness and more severe adverse reactions if a second course of therapy is attempted. Therefore, experts believe that this drug should be used for only a single course of treatment.

tacrolimus
Prograf

Pregnancy Risk Category: C

HOW SUPPLIED
Capsules: 1 mg, 5 mg
Injection: 5 mg/ml

ACTION
Precise mechanism unknown. Inhibits T-lymphocyte activation, which results in immunosuppression.

ONSET, PEAK, DURATION
Onset and duration unknown. Serum levels peak in 1.5 to 3.5 hours.

INDICATIONS & DOSAGE
Prophylaxis of organ rejection in allogenic liver transplantation –
Adults: 0.05 to 0.1 mg/kg/day I.V. as a continuous infusion administered no sooner than 6 hours after transplantation. Oral therapy should be substituted as soon as possible, with the first oral dose given 8 to 12 hours after discontinuing the I.V. infusion. The recommended initial oral dosage is 0.15 to 0.3 mg/kg/day P.O. in two divided doses q 12 hours. Dosage should be titrated according to clinical response.
Children: initially, 0.1 mg/kg/day I.V., followed by 0.3 mg/kg/day P.O. on a schedule similar to that for adults, adjusted as needed.

ADVERSE REACTIONS
CNS: *headache, tremor,* insomnia, paresthesia.
CV: *hypertension,* peripheral edema.
GI: *diarrhea, nausea,* constipation, abnormal liver function test results, anorexia, vomiting, abdominal pain.
GU: *abnormal renal function,* increased creatinine or BUN, urinary tract infection, oligura.
Hematologic: *anemia,* leukocytosis, thrombocytopenia.
Metabolic: *hyperkalemia,* hypokale-

mia, *hyperglycemia, hypomagnese-mia*.
Respiratory: pleural effusion, atelectasis, dyspnea.
Other: *pain, fever, asthenia,* back pain, ascites.

INTERACTIONS

Bromocriptine, cimetidine, clarithromycin, clotrimazole, cyclosporine, danazol, diltiazem, erythromycin, fluconazole, itraconazole, ketoconazole, methyprednisolone, metoclopramide, nicardipine, verapamil: may increase tacrolimus levels. Monitor for adverse effects.

Carbamazepine, phenobarbital, phenytoin, rifabutin, rifampin: may decrease tacrolimus levels. Monitor effectiveness of tacrolimus.

Cyclosporine: increased risk of excess nephrotoxicity. Do not administer together.

Immunosuppressants (except adrenal corticosteroids): may oversuppress the immune system. Monitor patient closely, especially during times of stress.

Inducers of cytochrome P-450 enzyme system: may increase tacrolimus metabolism and decrease plasma levels. Dosage adjustment may be needed.

Inhibitors of cytochrome P-450 enzyme system: may decrease tacrolimus metabolism and increase plasma levels. Dosage adjustment may be needed.

Nephrotoxic drugs, such as aminoglycosides, amphotericin B, cisplatin, cyclosporine: may cause additive or synergistic effects. Monitor closely.

Viral vaccines: tacrolimus may interfere with the immune response to live virus vaccines.

CONTRAINDICATIONS

Contraindicated in patients with hypersensitivity to the drug. The I.V. form is contraindicated in those who are hypersensitive to castor oil derivatives.

NURSING CONSIDERATIONS

● Know that because of the risk of anaphylaxis, injection should be used only in patients who cannot take the oral form.
● Keep epinephrine 1:1,000 readily available to treat anaphylaxis.
● Be aware that children with normal renal and hepatic function may require higher dosages than adults.
● Also be aware that patients with hepatic or renal dysfunction should receive the lowest dosage possible.
● Expect to administer adrenal corticosteroids concomitantly with this drug.
● **I.V. use:** Dilute drug with 0.9% sodium chloride injection or 5% dextrose injection to a concentration between 0.004 mg/ml and 0.02 mg/ml prior to use. Diluted infusion solution should be stored for no more than 24 hours in glass or polyethylene containers. The drug should not be stored in a polyvinyl chloride container because of decreased stability and the potential for extraction of phthalates.
● Monitor the patient continuously during the first 30 minutes of I.V. administration and frequently thereafter for signs and symptoms of anaphylaxis.
● Monitor the patient for signs of neurotoxicity and nephrotoxicity, especially a patient receiving a high dosage or having renal dysfunction.
● Monitor the patient for signs and symptoms of hyperkalemia and obtain serum potassium levels regularly, as ordered. Know that potassium-sparing diuretics should be avoided during tacrolimus therapy.
● Monitor the patient's blood glucose level regularly, as ordered, and the patient for signs and symptoms of hyperglycemia. Be aware that treatment of hyperglycemia may be necessary.
● Be aware that patients receiving this drug are at increased risk for infections, lymphomas, and other malignancies.

---

*Liquid form contains alcohol.
**May contain tartrazine.

Common reactions are in italics; *life-threatening*, in bold italics.

• Know that other immunosuppressants (except for adrenal corticosteroids) should not be used during tacrolimus therapy.

• Instruct the patient to check with the doctor before taking any other medication during tacrolimus therapy.

76

Vaccines and toxoids

BCG vaccine
cholera vaccine
diphtheria and tetanus toxoids, adsorbed
diphtheria and tetanus toxoids and pertussis vaccine
diphtheria and tetanus toxoids and acellular pertussis vaccine
Haemophilus b conjugate vaccines
hepatitis A vaccine, inactivated
hepatitis B vaccine, recombinant
influenza virus vaccine, 1995-1996 trivalent types A & B (purified surface antigen)
influenza virus vaccine, 1995-1996 trivalent types A & B (subvirion or split virion)
influenza virus vaccine, 1995-1996 trivalent types A & B (whole virion)
Japanese encephalitis virus vaccine, inactivated
measles, mumps, and rubella virus vaccine, live
measles (rubeola) and rubella virus vaccine, live attenuated
measles (rubeola) virus vaccine, live attenuated
meningitis vaccine
mumps virus vaccine, live
plague vaccine
pneumococcal vaccine, polyvalent
poliovirus vaccine, live, oral, trivalent
poliovirus vaccine, inactivated
rabies vaccine, adsorbed
rabies vaccine, human diploid cell
rubella and mumps virus vaccine, live
rubella virus vaccine, live attenuated
tetanus toxoid, adsorbed
tetanus toxoid, fluid
typhoid vaccine
typhoid vaccine, oral
typhoid Vi polysaccharide vaccine
varicella vaccine
yellow fever vaccine

COMBINATION PRODUCTS
TETRAMUNE: 10 mcg purified *Haemophilus* b saccharide and approximately 25 mcg CRM_{197} protein, 12.5 Lf (limit flocculation) units inactivated diphtheria, 5 Lf units inactivated tetanus, and 4 protective units pertussis/0.5 ml.

BCG vaccine
Pregnancy Risk Category: C

HOW SUPPLIED
Percutaneous vaccine: 1 to 8×10^8 CFU/vial (Tice strain)

ACTION
A live, attenuated bacterial vaccine prepared from *Mycobacterium bovis* that promotes active immunity to tuberculosis.

ONSET, PEAK, DURATION
Unknown.

INDICATIONS & DOSAGE
Tuberculosis exposure –
Adults and children 1 month and over: 0.2 to 0.3 ml (percutaneous vaccine) applied to cleaned skin followed by application of multiple-puncture disk.
Children less than 1 month: dosage reduced by one-half by using 2 ml of sterile water when reconstituting.

ADVERSE REACTIONS

Systemic: lymphangitis, urticaria of trunk and limbs, lupus-like syndrome, lymphadenitis, osteomyelitis, flulike syndrome (fever, shivers, chills, nausea, vomiting), *anaphylaxis.*
Other: lymph node and skin abscess, ulceration (2 to 3 weeks after injection) at injection site.

INTERACTIONS

Immunosuppressant therapy: may reduce response to BCG vaccine. Avoid if possible.
Isoniazid, rifampin, streptomycin: inhibited multiplication of BCG. Avoid using together.
Theophylline: may impair theophylline elimination.

CONTRAINDICATIONS

Contraindicated in patients with hypogammaglobulinemia, in the presence of a positive tuberculin reaction (when meant for use as immunoprophylactic after exposure to tuberculosis), in immunosuppressed patients, in those with fresh smallpox vaccinations, in those who have suffered burns, and in patients receiving corticosteroid therapy. Patients should avoid this vaccine during pregnancy.

NURSING CONSIDERATIONS

• Use cautiously in patients with chronic skin disease. Inject in area of healthy skin only.
• Obtain history of allergies and reaction to immunization.
• Keep epinephrine 1:1,000 available to treat anaphylaxis.
• Do not shake vial after reconstitution. Use within 2 hours.
• Keep in mind that recommended injection site is over insertion of deltoid muscle.
• Don't administer to febrile children.
• Know that expected lesion forms in 7 to 14 days. Papules reach a maximum diameter of 3 mm, then start to fade.

• Allow at least 6 to 8 weeks between BCG and live virus vaccines; administer killed virus vaccines 7 days before or 10 days after BCG, as ordered.
• Know that vaccine is of no value as immunoprophylactic in patients with positive tuberculin test.
• Destroy live vaccine by autoclaving or treating with formaldehyde solution before disposal.
• Advise patients to have tuberculin skin test 2 to 3 months after BCG vaccination to determine success of vaccine.

cholera vaccine

Pregnancy Risk Category: C

HOW SUPPLIED

Injection: suspension of killed *Vibrio cholerae* (each milliliter contains 8 units of Inaba and Ogawa serotypes) in 1.5-ml and 20-ml vials

ACTION

Promotes active immunity to cholera.

ONSET, PEAK, DURATION

Although onset and peak are not precisely known, most patients develop immunity after second dose. Effects persist for 3 to 6 months.

INDICATIONS & DOSAGE

Primary immunization –
Adults and children over 10 years: two doses of 0.5 ml I.M. or S.C., 1 week to 1 month apart, before traveling in cholera area. Booster is 0.5 ml q 6 months as long as protection is needed.
Children 6 months to 4 years: 0.2 ml I.M. or S.C. Boosters of same dose should be given q 6 months as long as protection is needed.
Children 5 to 10 years: 0.3 ml I.M. or S.C. Boosters of same dose should be given q 6 months as long as protection is needed.

ADVERSE REACTIONS
Systemic: tachycardia, hypotension, diarrhea, urticaria, malaise, fever, flushing, headache, ***anaphylaxis.***
Other: *erythema, swelling, pain, induration at injection site.*

INTERACTIONS
Plague, typhoid, or other vaccines with systemic adverse reactions: enhanced toxicity. Don't use together.
Yellow fever vaccine: simultaneous administration may interfere with immune response to cholera vaccine and yellow fever vaccine. Administer 3 weeks apart.

CONTRAINDICATIONS
Contraindicated in presence of any acute illness or in patients with a history of severe systemic reaction or allergic response following a prior dose of cholera vaccine.

NURSING CONSIDERATIONS
• Obtain history of allergies and reaction to immunization.
• Keep epinephrine 1:1,000 available to treat anaphylaxis.
• Shake vial vigorously before withdrawing each dose.
• Do not administer I.M. to persons with thrombocytopenia or any coagulation disorder that would contraindicate I.M. injection.
• Administer I.M. in deltoid muscle in adults and children over 3 years.
• Keep in mind that I.M. and S.C. routes give higher levels of protection. May be given intradermally to adults and children over 5 years, but the volume of injection is limited to 0.2 ml.
• Know that vaccine is about 50% effective in reducing clinical illness incidence for 3 to 6 months.
• Advise patients that pain, induration, and swelling are common at the injection site for 24 to 48 hours.

diphtheria and tetanus toxoids, adsorbed
Pregnancy Risk Category: C

HOW SUPPLIED
Available in pediatric (DT) and adult (Td) strengths
Injection (for pediatric use): diphtheria toxoid 6.6 Lf (limit flocculation) units and tetanus toxoid 5 Lf units per 0.5 ml; diphtheria toxoid 7.5 Lf units and tetanus toxoid 7.5 Lf units per 0.5 ml; diphtheria toxoid 10 Lf units and tetanus toxoid 5 Lf units per 0.5 ml; diphtheria toxoid 12.5 Lf units and tetanus toxoid 5 Lf units per 0.5 ml; diphtheria toxoid 15 Lf units and tetanus toxoid 10 Lf units per 0.5 ml
Injection (for adult use): diphtheria toxoid 2 Lf units and tetanus toxoid 5 Lf units per 0.5 ml; diphtheria toxoid 2 Lf units and tetanus toxoid 10 Lf units per 0.5 ml

ACTION
Promotes immunity to diphtheria and tetanus by inducing production of antitoxins.

ONSET, PEAK, DURATION
Onset and peak unknown. Effects persist for 10 years.

INDICATIONS & DOSAGE
Primary immunization–
Adults and children 7 years or older: use adult strength; 0.5 ml I.M. 4 to 8 weeks apart for two doses and a third dose 6 to 12 months after the second dose. Booster is 0.5 ml I.M. q 10 years.
Infants 6 weeks to 1 year: use pediatric strength; 0.5 ml I.M. at least 4 weeks apart for three doses. Give booster dose 6 to 12 months after third injection.
Children 1 to 6 years: use pediatric strength; 0.5 ml I.M. at least 4 weeks apart for two doses. Give booster dosage 6 to 12 months after the second

---

*Liquid form contains alcohol.   *Common* reactions are in italics; *life-threatening,* in bold italics.
**May contain tartrazine.

injection. If the final immunizing dose is given after the seventh birthday, use the adult strength.

ADVERSE REACTIONS
Systemic: *anaphylaxis,* chills, fever, malaise.
Other: stinging, edema, erythema, pain, induration at injection site.

INTERACTIONS
None significant.

CONTRAINDICATIONS
Contraindicated in immunosuppressed patients and in those receiving radiation or corticosteroid therapy. Vaccination should be deferred in patients with respiratory illness and during polio outbreaks; also deferred in those with acute illness except during emergency. When polio is a risk, single antigen is used. Know that in children under 6 years, use only when diphtheria, tetanus, and pertussis combination is contraindicated because of pertussis component.

NURSING CONSIDERATIONS
• Obtain history of allergies and reaction to immunization.
• Before injection, verify strength (pediatric or adult) of toxoid used.
• Keep epinephrine 1:1,000 available to treat anaphylaxis.
• Give in site not recently used for vaccines or toxoids.

---

diphtheria and tetanus toxoids and pertussis vaccine (DTP, DPT)
DTwP, Tri-Immunol

diphtheria and tetanus toxoids and acellular pertussis vaccine
Acel-Imune, Tripedia

HOW SUPPLIED
whole-cell vaccine
Injection: 6.5 Lf (limit flocculation) units inactivated diphtheria, 5 Lf units inactivated tetanus, and 4 protective units pertussis per 0.5 ml, in 2.5, 5, and 7.5-ml vials; 10 Lf units inactivated diptheria, 5.5 Lf units inactivated tetanus, and 4 protective units pertussis per 0.5 ml in 5 ml vials (DTwP); 12.5 Lf units inactivated diphtheria, 5 Lf units inactivated tetanus, and 4 protective units pertussis per 0.5 ml, in 7.5-ml vials (Tri-Immunol)
acellular vaccine
Injection: 5 Lf units inactivated diphtheria, 5 Lf units inactivated tetanus, and 300 hemagglutinating units of acellular pertussis vaccine per 0.5 ml; 66.7 Lf units inactivated diphtheria, 5 Lf units inactivated tetanus, and 46.8 pertussis antigens per 0.5 ml

ACTION
Promotes active immunity to diphtheria, tetanus, and pertussis by inducing production of antitoxins and antibodies.

ONSET, PEAK, DURATION
Onset and peak unknown. Effects persist for 10 years.

INDICATIONS & DOSAGE
Primary immunization –
Children 6 weeks to 6 years: 0.5 ml I.M. 4 to 8 weeks apart for three doses and a fourth dose 1 year later. Booster is 0.5 ml I.M. when starting school.
  Not advised for adults or children over 6 years.
  The acellular vaccine may be used only for the fourth or fifth dose in children 17 months to 7 years who have previously been immunized with three or four doses of the whole-cell vaccine.

ADVERSE REACTIONS
Systemic: *seizures, encephalopathy.*
anorexia, vomiting, slight fever,
chills, malaise, *anaphylaxis, sudden*
infant death syndrome.
Other: *soreness, redness,* expected
nodule remaining several weeks at injection site.

INTERACTIONS
Immunosuppressants: may reduce response to DPT vaccine. Avoid if possible.

CONTRAINDICATIONS
• Contraindicated in immunosuppressed patients, in those on corticosteroid therapy, and in those with a history of seizures. Vaccination should be deferred in patients with acute febrile illness.
• Know that children with preexisting neurologic disorders should not receive pertussis component. Also, children who exhibit neurologic signs after DPT injection shouldn't receive pertussis component in any succeeding injections. Diphtheria and tetanus toxoids (DT) should be given instead.

NURSING CONSIDERATIONS
• Obtain history of allergies and reaction to immunization.
• Keep epinephrine 1:1,000 available to treat anaphylaxis.
• Shake before using. Refrigerate.
• Administer only by deep I.M. injection, preferably in thigh or deltoid muscle. Don't give S.C.
• Keep in mind that DPT injection may be given at same time as trivalent oral polio vaccine.
• Know that acellular vaccine may be associated with a lower incidence of local pain and fever.
• Know that vaccine is not used for active infection.
• Make sure parents read and understand the information booklet available that describes the risks and benefits of this vaccine before vaccine is administered.

Haemophilus b conjugate vaccines

Haemophilus b conjugate vaccine, diphtheria CRM$_{197}$ protein conjugate (HbOC)
HibTITER

Haemophilus b conjugate vaccine, diphtheria toxoid conjugate (PRP-D)
ProHIBiT

Haemophilus b conjugate vaccine, meningococcal protein conjugate (PRP-OMP)
PedvaxHIB

HOW SUPPLIED
***Haemophilus* b conjugate vaccine, diphtheria CRM$_{197}$ protein conjugate**
Injection: 10 mcg purified *Haemophilus* b saccharide and approximately 25 mcg CRM$_{197}$ protein per 0.5 ml
***Haemophilus* b conjugate vaccine, diphtheria toxoid conjugate**
Injection: 25 mcg of *Haemophilus influenzae* type B (HIB) capsular polysaccharide and 18 mcg of diphtheria toxoid protein per 0.5 ml
***Haemophilus* b conjugate vaccine, meningococcal protein conjugate**
Powder for injection: 15 mcg *Haemophilus* b PRP, 250 mcg *Neisseria meningitidis* OMPC per dose

ACTION
Promotes active immunity to HIB; is a polymer of ribose, ribitol, and phosphate (PRP) and is covalently linked to highly antigenic substances, enabling the vaccine to promote an immune response in infants.

---

*Liquid form contains alcohol.   *Common* reactions are in italics; ***life-threatening***, in bold italics.
**May contain tartrazine.

ONSET, PEAK, DURATION
Unknown.

INDICATIONS & DOSAGE
*Immunization against HIB infection –
conjugate vaccine, diphtheria CRM$_{197}$
protein conjugate*
Infants: 0.5 ml I.M. at age 2 months.
Repeated at 4 months and 6 months.
A booster dose is required at age 15
months.
**Previously unvaccinated infants 2 to
6 months:** 0.5 ml I.M. Repeated in 2
months and again in 4 months for a
total of three doses. Booster dose
given at age 15 months.
**Previously unvaccinated infants 7 to
11 months:** 0.5 ml I.M. Repeated in
2 months, for a total of two doses.
Booster dose given at age 15 months
(but no sooner than 2 months after the
last vaccination).
**Previously unvaccinated infants 12
to 14 months:** 0.5 ml I.M. Booster
dose given at age 15 months (but no
sooner than 2 months after the first
vaccination).
**Previously unvaccinated children 15
months to 5 years:** 0.5 ml I.M.
A booster dose is not required.
*conjugate vaccine, diphtheria toxoid
conjugate*
**Previously unvaccinated children 15
months to 5 years:** 0.5 ml I.M.
A booster dose is not required. Not
recommended for use in children under age 15 months.
*conjugate vaccine, meningococcal
protein conjugate*
Infants: 0.5 ml I.M. at age 2 months.
Repeated at age 4 months. Booster
dose is required at age 12 months.
**Previously unvaccinated infants 2 to
6 months:** 0.5 ml I.M. Repeated in 2
months. Booster dose given at age 12
months.
**Previously unvaccinated infants 7 to
11 months:** 0.5 ml I.M. Repeated in
2 months. Booster dose given at 15
months (but no sooner than 2 months
after the last vaccination).

**Previously unvaccinated infants 12
to 14 months:** 0.5 ml I.M. Booster
dose given at age 15 months (but no
sooner than 2 months after the first
vaccination).
**Previously unvaccinated children 15
months to 5 years:** 0.5 ml I.M.
A booster dose is not required.

ADVERSE REACTIONS
Systemic: *anaphylaxis,* fever.
Other: *erythema, pain at injection
site.*

INTERACTIONS
Immunosuppressants: may suppress
antibody response to HIB vaccine.

CONTRAINDICATIONS
Contraindicated in immunosuppressed patients. Immunization
should be deferred in patients with
acute illness.

NURSING CONSIDERATIONS
● Keep epinephrine 1:1,000 available
in case of anaphylaxis.
● Don't administer intradermally or
I.V. Must administer I.M.
● Administer into anterolateral aspect
of the upper thigh in small children.
Injections may be made into the deltoid muscle of larger children if sufficient muscle mass is present.
● Know that vaccine is not routinely
given to adults or children over 5
years unless they are at high risk for
infection (including patients with
chronic conditions such as functional
asplenia, splenectomy, Hodgkin's disease, or sickle cell anemia).
● Don't administer to febrile children.
● Be aware that this vaccine and DPT
may be given simultaneously. A combination product is commercially
available.
● Know that diphtheria toxoid conjugate vaccine (ProHIBiT) is not recommended in children under 15 months.
● Be aware that HIB is an important

cause of meningitis in infants and pre-school children.
• Keep in mind that this vaccine protects against HIB only and will not protect children against any other microorganisms that cause meningitis.
• Know that children vaccinated with nonconjugated vaccine (no longer available in the United States) need not be routinely revaccinated if the primary immunization occurred at 24 months. However, if the first vaccination occurred at 18 to 23 months, revaccinate the child with conjugate vaccine, as ordered, provided at least 2 months has elapsed.

hepatitis A vaccine, inactivated
Havrix

Pregnancy Risk Category: C

HOW SUPPLIED
Injection: 360 ELISA units (EL.U.)/ 0.5 ml; 1,440 EL.U./1 ml

ACTION
Promotes active immunity to hepatitis A virus.

ONSET, PEAK, DURATION
In clinical studies, 80% to 98% of adults vaccinated were seroconverted by day 15 and 96% were seroconverted in 1 month. When a booster was given 6 months after the first dose, 100% of patients were seropositive 1 month later. In clinical studies of children receiving the drug, 99% of those vaccinated were seroconverted following two doses. When a booster (third) dose was administered 6 months after the first dose, 100% of the children were seropositive 1 month later. Effects persist for at least 6 months. Duration beyond 6 months has not been established.

INDICATIONS & DOSAGE
Immunization against hepatitis A virus—
Adults: 1,440 EL.U./1 ml I.M. as a single dose. For booster dose, 1,440 EL. U./1 ml I.M. given 6 to 12 months after initial dosage. Booster dose is recommended to ensure the highest antibody titer.
Children 2 to 18 years: two doses consisting of 360 EL.U./0.5 ml I.M. given 1 month apart. For booster dose, 360 EL.U./0.5 ml I.M. given 6 to 12 months after initial dosage. Booster dose is recommended to ensure the highest antibody titer.

ADVERSE REACTIONS
CNS: episode of hypertonia, insomnia, photophobia, vertigo.
GI: *anorexia, nausea,* abdominal pain, diarrhea, parageusia, vomiting.
Hepatic: jaundice, hepatitis.
Musculoskeletal: arthralgia, elevation of creatine phosphokinase level, myalgia.
Respiratory: pharyngitis, other upper respiratory tract infections.
Skin: pruritus, rash, urticaria.
Local: *induration, redness, swelling,* hematoma.
Other: *fatigue, fever, malaise,* lymphadenopathy.

INTERACTIONS
None significant.

CONTRAINDICATIONS
Contraindicated in patients with hypersensitivity to any component of the vaccine.

NURSING CONSIDERATIONS
• Use with caution in patients with thrombocytopenia or bleeding disorder and in those who are taking an anticoagulant because bleeding may occur following an I.M. injection in these individuals.
• As with any vaccine, administration of hepatitis A vaccine should be de-

---

*Liquid form contains alcohol.   *Common* reactions are in italics; ***life-threatening,*** in bold italics.
**May contain tartrazine.

layed, if possible, in patients with any febrile illness.

• Although anaphylaxis is rare, keep epinephrine readily available to treat an anaphylactoid reaction.

• Be aware that if vaccine is administered to immunosuppressed persons or persons receiving immunosuppressant therapy, the expected immune response may not be obtained.

• Know that persons who should receive the vaccine include people traveling to or living in areas of higher endemicity for hepatitis A (Africa, Asia [except Japan], the Mediterranean basin, Eastern Europe, the Middle East, Central and South America, Mexico, and parts of the Caribbean), military personnel, native peoples of Alaska and the Americas, persons engaging in high-risk sexual activity, and users of illicit injectable drugs. Also, certain institutional workers, employees of child day-care centers, laboratory workers who handle live hepatitis A virus, and handlers of primate animals may benefit from immunization.

• I.M. use: Shake vial or syringe well before withdrawal and use. After it has been agitated thoroughly, the vaccine is an opaque white suspension. Discard if it appears otherwise. No dilution or reconstitution is necessary.

• Administer as an I.M. injection into the deltoid region in adults. It should not be administered in the gluteal region; such injections may result in suboptimal response. Never inject intravenously, intradermally, or subcutaneously.

• Be aware that hepatitis A vaccine will not prevent infection in persons who have an unrecognized hepatitis A infection at the time of vaccination.

• Inform the patient that the vaccine will not prevent hepatitis caused by other agents, such as hepatitis B virus, hepatitis C virus, hepatitis E virus, and other pathogens known to infect the liver.

hepatitis B vaccine, recombinant

Engerix-B, Recombivax HB

Pregnancy Risk Category: C

HOW SUPPLIED

Injection: 5 mcg HB$_s$Ag/0.5 ml (Recombivax HB, pediatric injection); 10 mcg HB$_s$Ag/0.5 ml (Engerix-B, pediatric injection); 10 mcg HB$_s$Ag/ml (Recombivax HB); 20 mcg HB$_s$Ag/ml (Engerix-B); 40 mcg HB$_s$Ag/ml (Recombivax HB Dialysis Formulation)

ACTION

Promotes active immunity to hepatitis B.

ONSET, PEAK, DURATION

Not fully defined.

INDICATIONS & DOSAGE

Immunization against infection from all known subtypes of hepatitis B; primary preexposure prophylaxis against hepatitis B; or postexposure prophylaxis (when given with hepatitis B immune globulin)—
Engerix-B

Adults and children 10 years and over: initially, 20 mcg (1-ml adult formulation) given I.M., followed by a second dose of 20 mcg I.M. 30 days later. A third dose of 20 mcg I.M. is given 6 months after the initial dose.

Neonates and children up to 10 years: initially, 10 mcg (0.5-ml pediatric formulation) I.M., followed by a second dose of 10 mcg I.M. 30 days later. A third dose of 10 mcg I.M. is given 6 months after the initial dose.

Adults undergoing dialysis or receiving immunosuppressants: initially, 40 mcg I.M. (divided into two 20-mcg doses and administered at different sites). Followed with a second dose of 40 mcg I.M. in 30 days, and a final dose of 40 mcg I.M. 6 months after the initial dose.

Note: Certain populations (neonates born to infected mothers, persons recently exposed to the virus, and travelers to high-risk areas) may receive the vaccine on an abbreviated schedule, with the initial dose followed by a second dose in 1 month, and the third dose after 2 months. For prolonged maintenance of protective antibody titers, a booster dose is recommended 12 months after the initial dose.

Recombivax HB

Adults: initially, 10 mcg (1-ml adult formulation) I.M., followed by a second dose of 10 mcg I.M. 30 days later. A third dose of 10 mcg is given I.M. 6 months after the initial dose.

Neonates and children up to 11 years: initially, 2.5 mcg (0.5-ml pediatric formulation) I.M., followed by a second dose of 2.5 mcg I.M. 30 days later. A third dose of 2.5 mcg I.M. is given 6 months after the initial dose.

Children 11 to 19 years: initially, 5 mcg (0.5-ml pediatric formulation) I.M., followed by a second dose of 5 mcg I.M. 30 days later. A third dose of 5 mcg is given I.M. 6 months after the initial dose.

Adults 20 years and older: initially, 10 mcg (1 ml) I.M., followed by a second dose of 10 mcg 30 days later. A third dose of 10 mcg is given I.M. 6 months after the initial dose.

Adults undergoing dialysis or receiving immunosuppressants: initially, 40 mcg I.M. (use dialysis formulation, which contains 40 mcg/ml). Followed with a second dose of 40 mcg I.M. in 30 days, and a final dose of 40 mcg I.M. 6 months after the initial dose.

ADVERSE REACTIONS
Systemic: headache, dizziness, nausea, vomiting, slight fever, transient malaise, flulike symptoms, myalgia.
Other: discomfort and local inflammation at injection site.

INTERACTIONS
None significant.

CONTRAINDICATIONS
Contraindicated in patients hypersensitive to yeast; recombinant vaccines are derived from yeast cultures.

NURSING CONSIDERATIONS
• Use cautiously in patients with any serious, active infections; compromised cardiac or pulmonary status; and in those for whom a febrile or systemic reaction could pose a serious risk.
• Know that the American Academy of Pediatrics recommends hepatitis B vaccination for all neonates and encourages immunization for adolescents when resources allow.
• Although anaphylaxis has not been reported, always keep epinephrine available when administering this vaccine to counteract any possible reaction.
• Thoroughly agitate vial just before administration to restore suspension.
• Give adults the vaccine in the deltoid muscle; give infants and young children the vaccine in the anterolateral aspect of the thigh. Never administer I.V.
• Administer S.C. in persons at risk for hemorrhage, such as hemophiliacs. Otherwise, do not use this route; it may lead to an increased incidence or severity of local reactions.
• Keep in mind that certain health care personnel (especially those working with dialysis patients, in blood banks, and in emergency medicine); selected patients and patient contacts; populations in which the infection is endemic (Inuit [Alaskan], Indo-Chinese, and Haitian refugees); certain military personnel; morticians and embalmers; sexually active homosexual men; prostitutes; prisoners; and users of illicit injectable drugs are at increased risk of infection and should be considered for the vaccine.

---

*Liquid form contains alcohol.   *Common* reactions are in italics; *life-threatening*, in bold italics.
**May contain tartrazine.

• Be aware that recombinant hepatitis B vaccine is not made with any human plasma products.

• Refrigerate both opened and unopened vials. Don't freeze.

---

influenza virus vaccine, 1995-1996 trivalent types A & B (purified surface antigen)
Flu-Imune

influenza virus vaccine, 1995-1996 trivalent types A & B (subvirion or split virion)
Fluogen Split, Flu-Shield, Fluzone Split

influenza virus vaccine, 1995-1996 trivalent types A & B (whole virion)
Fluzone (Whole)

Pregnancy Risk Category: C

HOW SUPPLIED
Injection: 15 mcg A/Texas/36/91-like (H1N1), 15 mcg A/Johannesburg/33/94-like (H3N2), and 15 mcg B/Beijing/184/93-like hemagglutinin antigens per 0.5 ml

ACTION
Promotes immunity to influenza by inducing production of antibodies.

ONSET, PEAK, DURATION
Although onset and peak not precisely known, most patients develop immunity in 2 to 4 weeks. Immunity declines following vaccination, possibly within 6 months.

INDICATIONS & DOSAGE
Influenza prophylaxis–
Adults and children 12 years and over: 0.5 ml whole or split virus I.M. Only one dose is required.
Children 6 to 35 months: 0.25 ml split virus I.M. Repeated in 4 weeks

unless child has been previously vaccinated.
Children 3 to 8 years: 0.5 ml split virus I.M. Repeated in 4 weeks unless child has been previously vaccinated.
Children 9 to 12 years: 0.5 ml split virus I.M. Only one dose is required.

ADVERSE REACTIONS
Systemic: *anaphylaxis,* fever, malaise, myalgia.
Other: erythema, induration, and soreness at injection site.

Fever and malaise reactions occur most often in children and in others not exposed to influenza viruses. Severe reactions in adults are rare.

INTERACTIONS
Theophylline, warfarin: clearance may be impaired.

CONTRAINDICATIONS
Contraindicated in patients with hypersensitivity to eggs. Vaccination should be deferred in patients with acute respiratory or other active infection.

NURSING CONSIDERATIONS
• Use cautiously in patients with a history of sulfite allergy.
• Obtain history of allergies, especially to eggs, and reaction to immunization.
• Keep epinephrine 1:1,000 available to treat anaphylaxis.
• Thoroughly agitate vial just before administration to restore suspension.
• Give injections for adults and older children in deltoid muscle; for infants and children under 3 years, give in anterolateral aspect of thigh.
• Ideally, vaccinations should be performed in November because outbreaks of influenza generally don't occur until December. The vaccine should not be given too early in the season because antibody titers may begin to decline before the flu season.
• Know that children 12 years and un-

der should be given their second dose in December, if possible.

• Vaccines may be given to both children and adults throughout the flu season, even as late as April.

• Do not give children pertussis vaccine within 3 days of influenza virus vaccine. However, they may receive Haemophilus b vaccine; oral polio vaccine; measles, mumps, and rubella vaccine; or pneumococcal vaccine at the same time. Make injections at different sites.

• Know that this vaccine is considered safe in pregnant patients. Vaccination shouldn't be postponed, regardless of the stage of pregnancy, in patients who have high-risk conditions and who will be in the first trimester of pregnancy when the flu season begins.

• Keep in mind that immunodeficient patients may receive two doses 1 month apart; however, little evidence suggests that booster doses improve the immunogenic response to the vaccine. Know that chemoprophylaxis with amantadine may be helpful.

• Note that the combination of antigens used to create influenza vaccine changes annually even though some antigens may be the same as previous years. Do not use leftover supplies of 1994-1995 vaccine to immunize patients for the 1995-1996 flu season.

• Know that vaccine is strongly recommended for anyone over 6 months; for patients with chronic disease, metabolic disorders, or medical conditions that put them at risk for complications from influenza; for health care workers, especially doctors, nurses, employees of nursing homes, volunteer workers, and other personnel in both hospital and outpatient settings; and for household members who may contact persons at high risk for medical complications of influenza. Also recommended for anyone who wishes to reduce the chance of infection.

• Be aware that influenza vaccine is available as whole virus, split virus, and purified surface antigen preparations. Split virus and purified surface antigen vaccines cause somewhat fewer adverse reactions than whole virus in children.

• Keep in mind that allergic reactions, which usually occur immediately, are extremely rare.

• Be alert that paralysis associated with Guillain-Barré syndrome is rare, and has only been associated with the 1976 vaccine.

• Remember that although there is little information regarding influenza in persons with HIV, it is recommended that these patients receive the vaccine. Patients with advanced disease may exhibit a low response; there is no evidence that a booster dose will improve the immune response.

• Advise patients about the risks of vaccination as compared with risk of influenza and its complications.

• Ensure that patients understand that annual vaccination using the current vaccine is necessary because immunity to influenza decreases in the year after the injection.

• Ensure that patients understand that the vaccine cannot cause influenza. Fever, malaise, and myalgia may begin 6 to 12 hours after vaccination and persist 1 to 2 days. These systemic reactions are not common.

Japanese encephalitis virus vaccine, inactivated
JE-VAX

Pregnancy Risk Category: C

HOW SUPPLIED
Injection: 1-ml, 10-ml vials

ACTION
Provides active immunity against Japanese encephalitis (JE), a mosquito-borne arboviral flavivirus infection that's the leading cause of viral encephalitis in Asia.

Liquid form contains alcohol.   *Common* reactions are in italics; *life-threatening*, in bold italics.
**May contain tartrazine.

ONSET, PEAK, DURATION
Not clearly defined. An immune response is thought to occur within 10 days. Duration of protection is thought to be at least 2 years in persons receiving three doses of the vaccine.

INDICATIONS & DOSAGE
Active immunization against JE –
Primary immunization schedule
Adults and children 3 years and over: 1 ml S.C. on days 0, 7, and 30.
Children 1 to 3 years: 0.5 ml S.C. on days 0, 7, and 30.
Booster doses
Adults and children 3 years and over: 1 ml S.C. q 2 years.
Children 1 to 3 years: 0.5 ml S.C. q 2 years.

ADVERSE REACTIONS
Systemic: *headache, dizziness,* hypotension, *nausea, vomiting, abdominal pain,* **respiratory distress, anaphylaxis,** *rash,* generalized urticaria, *fever, malaise, chills, myalgia or* angioedema of the face, oropharynx, extremities, or lips.
Other: *local tenderness and swelling at injection site.*

INTERACTIONS
None significant.

CONTRAINDICATIONS
Contraindicated in patients hypersensitive to the drug or to thimerosal, a preservative, and in patients who exhibited severe adverse reactions, such as generalized urticaria or angioedema, to a prior dose of the vaccine. Because the vaccine is derived from mouse brain, its use is contraindicated in patients hypersensitive to substances of murine or neural origin.

NURSING CONSIDERATIONS
• Use cautiously in pregnant or breast-feeding patients, elderly patients, and those with a history of urticaria after vaccines, drugs, or insect stings. Advanced age may be a risk factor for developing symptomatic illness after JE infection. JE acquired during pregnancy can cause intrauterine infection and fetal death.
• Use vaccine to provide protection against JE in persons planning to travel or reside in areas where the virus is endemic. It's not indicated for all persons traveling to or residing in Asia. For most travelers to Asia, the risk for acquiring JE is extremely low. Contact the Centers for Disease Control and Prevention at (404) 332-4555 for current travel advisories.
• Keep epinephrine 1:1,000 and other resuscitation equipment and drugs available to treat anaphylaxis and other adverse reactions.
• To prepare vaccine for injection, use supplied diluent (sterile water for injection). Add 1.3 ml of diluent to the single-dose vial and 11 ml of diluent to the 10-dose vial. Shake vial thoroughly to ensure dissolution of vaccine. After reconstitution, refrigerate vaccine (36° to 46° F [2° to 8° C]) for up to 8 hours.
• Follow the recommended three-dose schedule for best results. Be aware that when time constraints prohibit the use of this schedule, an abbreviated schedule with injections on days 0, 7, and 14 may be used.
• Know that when it isn't possible to follow usual dose schedule, a two-dose regimen with injections on days 0 and 7 may be used. Antibodies will be induced in about 80% of patients with this schedule. A two-dose regimen should not be used unless circumstances are unusual.
• Monitor patients closely for 30 minutes after injection.
• Be aware that reactions to the first dose have occurred a median of 12 hours after injection (88% happened within 3 days). The delay between the second dose and adverse effects was usually longer, with a median of 3

days and some effects not seen for 2 weeks. Some patients exhibited adverse reactions to the second or third dose, even when the first or second dose was well tolerated.

• Know that the vaccine has been associated with a moderate incidence of local and mild systemic adverse effects. Local tenderness and swelling have been reported in up to 20% of those receiving the vaccine; systemic effects, such as fever, headache, malaise, or rash, in up to 10%. Serious reactions, such as generalized urticaria or angioedema, are uncommon (1% or less of those vaccinated).

• Warn patient about the possibility of delayed generalized urticaria or delayed angioedema of the extremities, face, oropharynx or (especially) the lips. Generalized urticaria or angioedema may occur within minutes of vaccination. Most reactions occur within the first 10 days, with the majority occurring within 48 hours. However, adverse reactions that may be related to the vaccine have occurred as late as 17 days after the injection.

• Because of the possibility of delayed reactions, warn patients to remain in areas where medical care is available for 10 days after injection. Caution against international travel during this time. Advise patients to seek medical assistance as soon as any reaction appears.

• Encourage patients and parents to report adverse effects after vaccination. Health care providers should report these adverse effects to the U.S. Department of Health and Human Services Vaccine Adverse Event Reporting System (VAERS). Contact VAERS at (800) 822-7967 for information about the system and reporting forms.

• Teach patients personal precautions that may avoid exposure to mosquito bites, such as using insect repellents and wearing protective clothing.

Avoiding outdoor activities, especially during twilight periods and in the evening, will further reduce risk.

---

measles, mumps, and rubella virus vaccine, live
M-M-R II

Pregnancy Risk Category: C

HOW SUPPLIED
Injection: single-dose vial containing not less than 1,000 TCID$_{50}$ (tissue culture infective doses) of attenuated measles virus derived from Enders' attenuated Edmonston strain (grown in chick embryo culture), 20,000 TCID$_{50}$ of the Jeryl Lynn (B level) mumps strain (grown in chick embryo culture), and 1,000 TCID$_{50}$ of the Wistar RA 27/3 strain of rubella virus (propagated in human diploid cell culture) per 0.5-ml dose.

ACTION
Promotes immunity to measles, mumps, and rubella virus by inducing production of antibodies.

ONSET, PEAK, DURATION
Although onset and peak are not precisely known, most patients develop immunity in 2 to 6 weeks. Effects have been shown to persist up to 11 years without decline.

INDICATIONS & DOSAGE
Routine vaccination–
Children: one vial S.C. A two-dose schedule is recommended, with the first dose given at 15 months (12 months in high-risk areas) and the second dose given either at 4 to 6 years of age or at 11 to 12 years of age.
Measles outbreak control–
Children: if cases are occurring in children under 1 year, children vaccinated as young as 6 months. All students and their siblings should be re-

---

vaccinated if they are without documentation of measles immunity.

Adults: school workers born in or after 1957 should be revaccinated if they are without proof of measles immunity. If the outbreak is in a medical facility, all workers born in or after 1957 should be revaccinated if they are without proof of immunity. Revaccination should be considered for persons born before 1957 as well.

ADVERSE REACTIONS

Systemic: urticaria, rash, fever, regional lymphadenopathy, *anaphylaxis*.
Other: erythema at injection site.

INTERACTIONS

Immune serum globulin, plasma, whole blood: antibodies in serum may interfere with immune response. Don't use vaccine within 3 months of transfusion.

CONTRAINDICATIONS

Contraindicated in immunosuppressed patients; in those with cancer, blood dyscrasia, gamma globulin disorders, fever, or active untreated tuberculosis, or anaphylactic or anaphylatoid reactions to neomycin, eggs; in those receiving corticosteroid or radiation therapy; and in pregnant patients.

NURSING CONSIDERATIONS

• Obtain history of allergies, especially anaphylactic reactions to antibiotics, or reaction to immunization.
• Keep epinephrine 1:1,000 available to treat anaphylaxis.
• Inject in outer aspect of upper arm. Don't give I.V.
• Use only diluent supplied. Discard 8 hours after reconstituting.
• Refrigerate; protect from light. Solution may be used if red, pink, or yellow, but must be clear.
• Know that incidence of adverse effects is low (0.5% to 4%).

• Treat fever with antipyretics, such as acetaminophen.
• Be aware that presence of maternal antibodies may prevent response in children under 12 months.
• Keep in mind that the Immunization Practices Advisory Committee recommends that colleges and other post-high school educational institutions, as well as medical institutions employing health care providers, obtain documentation of the receipt of two doses of vaccine after age 1 (or other proof of immunity, such as infection, documented by a doctor). Combined measles, mumps, and rubella (MMR) vaccine is preferred.
• Be aware that the Centers for Disease Control and Prevention recommends that, during a measles outbreak in a health care facility, susceptible personnel exposed to the measles virus (whether or not they received measles vaccine or immunoglobulin) avoid patient contact for days 5 through 21 after such exposure. If they become ill, they should avoid patient contact for at least 7 days after developing rash.
• Be aware that clinical trials indicate that vitamin A supplementation reduces morbidity and mortality in children with measles. In these studies, 100,000 to 400,000 IU daily have been used.

measles (rubeola) and rubella virus vaccine, live attenuated

M-R-Vax II

Pregnancy Risk Category: C

HOW SUPPLIED

Injection: single-dose vial containing not less than 1,000 TCID$_{50}$ (tissue culture infective doses) per 0.5 ml of attenuated measles virus derived from Enders' attenuated Edmonston strain (grown in chick embryo culture);

1,000 TCID$_{50}$ of the Wistar RA 27/3 strain of rubella virus

ACTION
Promotes immunity to measles and rubella virus by inducing production of antibodies.

ONSET, PEAK, DURATION
Although onset and peak are not clearly defined, immunity for most patients occurs in 2 to 6 weeks. Effects have been shown to persist up to 11 years without decline.

INDICATIONS & DOSAGE
Immunization—
Children 15 months to puberty: 0.5 ml (1,000 units) S.C.

ADVERSE REACTIONS
Systemic: rash, fever, lymphadenopathy, *anaphylaxis*.

INTERACTIONS
Immune serum globulin, plasma, whole blood: antibodies in serum may interfere with immune response. Don't use vaccine within 3 months of transfusion.
Tuberculin skin test: may temporarily decrease response to test. Defer skin testing.

CONTRAINDICATIONS
Contraindicated in immunosuppressed patients; in those with cancer, blood dyscrasia, gamma globulin disorders, fever, or active untreated tuberculosis; anaphylactic or anaphylactoid reactions to eggs or neomycin; in those receiving corticosteroid or radiation therapy; and in pregnant patients.

NURSING CONSIDERATIONS
• Obtain history of allergies, especially anaphylactic reactions to antibiotics.
• Keep epinephrine 1:1,000 available to treat anaphylaxis.

• Use only diluent supplied. Discard 8 hours after reconstituting.
• Inject in outer upper arm. Don't inject I.V.
• Store in refrigerator and protect from light. Solution may be used if red, pink, or yellow, but must be clear (with no precipitation).
• Know that vaccine should not be given within 1 month of other live virus vaccines, except oral poliovirus vaccine. Know that immunization should be deferred in patients with acute illness.
• Allow at least 3 weeks between BCG and rubella vaccines.

measles (rubeola) virus vaccine, live attenuated
Attenuvax

Pregnancy Risk Category: C

HOW SUPPLIED
Injection: single-dose vial containing not less than 1,000 TCID$_{50}$ (tissue culture infective doses) of attenuated measles virus derived from Enders' attenuated Edmonston strain (grown in chick embryo culture)

ACTION
Promotes immunity to measles virus by inducing production of antibodies.

ONSET, PEAK, DURATION
Although exact onset and peak unknown, most patients develop immunity within 2 to 6 weeks. Vaccine-induced antibody levels have been shown to persist for at least 13 years without substantial decline.

INDICATIONS & DOSAGE
Immunization—
Adults and children age 15 months or over: 0.5 ml (1,000 units) S.C. A two-dose schedule is recommended, with the first dose given at age 15 months (age 12 months in high-risk

areas) and the second dose given at age 4 to 6 or 11 to 12 years of age.
Measles outbreak control –
Children: if cases occur in children under age 1, children vaccinated as young as age 6 months. All students and their siblings should be revaccinated if they are without documentation of measles immunity.
Adults: school personnel born in or after 1957 should be revaccinated if they are without proof of measles immunity. If the outbreak is in a medical facility, all workers born in or after 1957 should be revaccinated if they are without proof of immunity. Revaccination should be considered for persons born before 1957 as well.

ADVERSE REACTIONS
Systemic: febrile seizures in susceptible children, anorexia, leukopenia, fever, rash, lymphadenopathy, *anaphylaxis.*
Other: erythema, swelling, and tenderness at injection site.

INTERACTIONS
Immune serum globulin, plasma, whole blood: antibodies in serum may interfere with immune response. Don't use vaccine within 3 months of transfusion.
Tuberculin skin test: may temporarily decrease response to test. Defer skin testing.

CONTRAINDICATIONS
Contraindicated in immunosuppressed patients; in those with cancer, blood dyscrasia, gamma globulin disorders, fever, or active untreated tuberculosis; anaphylactic or anaphylactoid reactions to neomycin or eggs; in those receiving corticosteroid or radiation therapy; and in pregnant patients.

NURSING CONSIDERATIONS
• Obtain history of allergies, especially anaphylactic reactions to antibi-

otics, or reaction to immunization. Know that immunization should be deferred in patients with acute illness or after administration of blood or plasma.
• Keep epinephrine 1:1,000 available to treat anaphylaxis.
• Use only diluent supplied. Discard 8 hours after reconstituting.
• Do not give I.V.
• Refrigerate and protect from light. Reconstituted solution is clear yellow with no precipitation. Do not use if discolored.
• Know that vaccine may be given with oral poliovirus vaccine.
• Keep in mind that the Immunization Practices Advisory Committee recommends that colleges and other post-high school educational institutions, as well as medical institutions employing health care providers, obtain documentation of the receipt of two doses of vaccine after age 1 (or other proof of immunity, such as infection, documented by a doctor). Combined measles, mumps, and rubella (MMR) vaccine is preferred.
• Be aware that the Centers for Disease Control and Prevention recommends that, during a measles outbreak in a health care facility, susceptible personnel exposed to the measles virus (whether or not they received measles vaccine or immune globulin) avoid patient contact for days 5 through 21 after such exposure. If they become ill, they should avoid patient contact for at least 7 days after developing rash.
• Know that if attenuated measles vaccine is administered immediately after exposure to the disease, some protection may be provided. This level of protection is significantly increased if the vaccine is administered even a few days before exposure.
• Stress the importance of avoiding pregnancy for 3 months after vaccination. Offer to provide contraception information.

meningitis vaccine
Menomune-A/C, Menomune-A/C/
Y/W-135

Pregnancy Risk Category: C

HOW SUPPLIED
Injection: 1-dose, 10-dose, and 50-
dose vials with vial of diluent

ACTION
Promotes active immunity to meningitis.

ONSET, PEAK, DURATION
Although exact onset and peak unknown, most patients develop immunity in 10 to 14 days. Antibody titers
decline within 3 years.

INDICATIONS & DOSAGE
*Meningococcal meningitis prophy-
laxis –*
**Adults and children 2 years and
older:** 0.5 ml S.C.

ADVERSE REACTIONS
Systemic headache, malaise, chills,
fever, muscle cramps, ***anaphylaxis.***
Other: *pain, erythema, and induration at injection site.*

INTERACTIONS
None significant.

CONTRAINDICATIONS
Contraindicated in immunosuppressed and pregnant patients and patients with hypersensitivity to thimerosal. Vaccination should be deferred
in patients with acute illness.

NURSING CONSIDERATIONS
• Obtain history of allergies and reac-
tion to immunization.
• Keep epinephrine 1:1,000 available
to treat anaphylaxis.
• Do not give I.V.
• Know that vaccine may be given
with other immunizations.
• Be aware that some clinicians will

revaccinate children if they are at high
risk and previously received vaccine
before age 4 years.
• Stress to patients the importance of
avoiding pregnancy for 3 months after
vaccination. Offer to provide contraception information.

mumps virus vaccine, live
Mumpsvax

Pregnancy Risk Category: C

HOW SUPPLIED
Injection: single-dose vial containing
not less than 5,000 $TCID_{50}$ (tissue culture infective doses) of attenuated
mumps virus derived from Jeryl Lynn
mumps strain (grown in chick embryo
culture) and vial of diluent

ACTION
Promotes active immunity to mumps.

ONSET, PEAK, DURATION
Although exact onset and peak unknown, most patients develop immunity in 2 to 3 weeks. Effects persist
for at least 20 years; probably lifelong.

INDICATIONS & DOSAGE
Immunization –
**Adults and children 1 year and
older:** 0.5 ml (5,000 units) S.C.

ADVERSE REACTIONS
CNS: febrile seizures (rare).
Other: *slight fever,* rash, malaise,
mild allergic reactions.

INTERACTIONS
*Immune serum globulin, plasma,
whole blood:* antibodies in serum may
interfere with immune response.
Don't use vaccine within 3 months of
transfusion.
Tuberculin skin test: may temporarily
decrease response to test. Defer skin
testing.

---

*Liquid form contains alcohol.   *Common* reactions are in italics; ***life-threatening,*** in bold italics.
**May contain tartrazine.

CONTRAINDICATIONS

Contraindicated in immunosuppressed patients; in those with cancer, blood dyscrasia, gamma globulin disorders, fever, or untreated active tuberculosis; anaphylactic or anaphylactoid reactions to neomycin or eggs; in those receiving corticosteroid or radiation therapy; and in pregnant patients.

NURSING CONSIDERATIONS

• Obtain history of allergies, especially anaphylactic reactions to antibiotics, and reaction to immunization. Defer in patients with acute or febrile illness and for 3 months after transfusions or treatment with immune serum globulin.
• Keep epinephrine 1:1,000 available to treat anaphylaxis.
• Use only diluent supplied. Discard 8 hours after reconstituting.
• Do not give I.V.
• Refrigerate and protect from light. Reconstituted solution is clear yellow; do not use if discolored.
• Treat fever with antipyretics.
• Do not give this vaccine less than 1 month before or after immunization with other live-virus vaccines; however, Attenuvax, Meruvax, or monovalent or trivalent live, oral poliovirus vaccine may be administered simultaneously.
• Know that vaccine is not recommended for infants under 12 months because retained maternal mumps antibodies may interfere with the immune response.
• Stress to patients the importance of avoiding pregnancy for 3 months after vaccination. Offer to provide contraception information.
• Do not use for delayed hypersensitivity (allergy) skin testing. Use mumps skin test antigen, a killed viral product.

plague vaccine

Pregnancy Risk Category: C

HOW SUPPLIED

Injection: 2 billion killed plague bacilli (*Yersinia pestis*)/ml in 20-ml vials

ACTION

Promotes active immunity to plague.

ONSET, PEAK, DURATION

Onset and peak unknown. Effects persist for 6 to 12 months.

INDICATIONS & DOSAGE

Primary immunization and booster –
Adults and children 11 years and older: 1 ml I.M. followed by 0.2 ml in 4 to 12 weeks, then 0.2 ml 3 to 6 months after the second dose. Booster is 0.1 to 0.2 ml q 6 months while in plague area.
Children under 1 year: ⅕ adult primary or booster dose.
Children 1 to 4 years: ⅖ adult primary or booster dose.
Children 5 to 10 years: ⅗ adult primary or booster dose.

ADVERSE REACTIONS

Systemic: headache, malaise, slight fever, lymphadenopathy, *anaphylaxis.*
Other: swelling, *induration, and erythema* at injection site.

INTERACTIONS

Cholera, typhoid vaccine: increased risk of adverse effects. Don't give at the same time.

CONTRAINDICATIONS

Contraindicated in immunosuppressed or pregnant patients and in those hypersensitive to beef, soy, casein, phenol, or formaldehyde. Patients who have had severe local or systemic reactions to plague vaccine should not be revaccinated. Also contraindicated in patients with severe thrombocytopenia or any coagulation disorder that would contraindicate I.M. injections.

NURSING CONSIDERATIONS
• Obtain history of allergies and reaction to immunization. Know that immunization should be deferred in patients with respiratory infection.
• Keep epinephrine 1:1,000 available to treat anaphylaxis.
• Use deltoid area as the preferred injection site.
• Recommended for all laboratory and field personnel working with *Yersinia pestis.*

pneumococcal vaccine, polyvalent
Pneumovax 23, Pnu-Imune 23
Pregnancy Risk Category: C

HOW SUPPLIED
Injection: 25 mcg each of 23 polysaccharide isolates/0.5 ml

ACTION
Promotes active immunity to infections caused by *Streptococcus pneumoniae.*

ONSET, PEAK, DURATION
Onset occurs in 2 to 3 weeks. Peak unknown. Effects persist for 5 to 10 years in most patients.

INDICATIONS & DOSAGE
Pneumococcal immunization –
Adults and children 2 years and older: 0.5 ml I.M. or S.C.

Not recommended for children under 2 years.

ADVERSE REACTIONS
Systemic: *anaphylaxis, slight fever.*
Other: soreness at injection site; severe local reaction can occur when revaccination takes place within 3 years.

INTERACTIONS
None significant.

CONTRAINDICATIONS
Contraindicated in patients hypersensitive to the drug or its components (phenol). Also contraindicated in patients with Hodgkin's disease who have received extensive chemotherapy or nodal irradiation.

NURSING CONSIDERATIONS
• Check immunization history carefully to avoid revaccination within 3 years.
• Obtain history of allergies and reaction to immunization. Eggs and egg protein are not used during the manufacture of the vaccine; contains phenol as a preservative.
• Keep epinephrine 1:1,000 available to treat anaphylaxis.
• Inject in deltoid or midlateral thigh. Don't inject I.V.
• When splenectomy is being considered, know that vaccine should be given at least 2 weeks before procedure to ensure adequate antibody response. This vaccine may be less effective in splenectomized patients.
• Treat fever with mild antipyretics.
• Be aware that vaccine protects against 23 pneumococcal types, accounting for 90% of pneumococcal disease.
• Know that the vaccine may be administered to children 2 years of age and over to prevent pneumococcal otitis media.
• Keep in mind that the vaccine is recommended for all adults over 65 years.
• Be aware that simultaneous administration with influenza virus vaccine is safe and effective.
• Keep refrigerated. Reconstitution or dilution not necessary.

---

*Liquid form contains alcohol.
**May contain tartrazine.

Common reactions are in italics; *life-threatening,* in bold italics.

poliovirus vaccine, live, oral, trivalent (TOPV)
Orimune

poliovirus vaccine, inactivated (IPV)
IPOL, Poliovax

Pregnancy Risk Category: C

HOW SUPPLIED
Oral vaccine: mixture of three live viruses (types 1, 2, and 3), grown in monkey kidney tissue culture, in 0.5-ml single-dose Dispettes
Inactivated virus vaccine injection: mixture of three types of poliovirus (types 1, 2, and 3) grown in tissue culture. IPOL uses monkey kidney cultures; Polivax uses human diploid cell cultures.

ACTION
Promotes immunity to poliomyelitis by inducing humoral antibodies and antibodies in the lymphatic tissue.

ONSET, PEAK, DURATION
An antibody response usually occurs within 7 to 10 days with TOPV; unknown with IPV. Peak effects occur in 21 days with TOPV; unknown for IPV. Duration is thought to last for years.

INDICATIONS & DOSAGE
Poliovirus immunization –
Children and nonimmunized adults: 0.5 ml P.O. (TOPV), followed by a second dose of 0.5 ml in 6 to 8 weeks. A third 0.5-ml dose is given 6 to 12 months after second dose. A reinforcing dose of 0.5 ml should be given before entry to school.
Infants: 0.5 ml P.O. at 2 months, 4 months, and 18 months. Optional dose may be given at 6 months.
Poliovirus immunization in persons who cannot receive TOPV –
Adults: 0.5 ml S.C., followed by a

second dose in 4 to 8 weeks. A third dose is given in 6 to 12 months.
Children: 0.5 ml S.C. at 2 months and 4 months. A third dose is given at 15 to 18 months. A reinforcing dose of 0.5 ml S.C. should be given before entry into school.

ADVERSE REACTIONS
Systemic: *poliomyelitis.*

INTERACTIONS
Immune serum globulin, plasma, whole blood: antibodies in serum may interfere with immune response. Don't use vaccine within 3 months of transfusion.
Tuberculin skin test: may suppress response to skin test. Don't test for 6 weeks.

CONTRAINDICATIONS
Oral vaccine is contraindicated in immunosuppressed patients; in those with cancer or immunoglobulin abnormalities; and in those receiving radiation, antimetabolite, alkylating agent, or corticosteroid therapy. These patients should receive IPV. Injectable vaccine is contraindicated in patients hypersensitive to neomycin, streptomycin, or polymixin B.

NURSING CONSIDERATIONS
• Use with caution in siblings of child with known immunodeficiency syndrome. IPV is preferred.
• Obtain history of allergies and reaction to immunization.
• Check the parents' immunization history when they bring in child for vaccine; this is an excellent time for parents to receive booster immunizations.
• Do not administer oral form of vaccine parenterally.
• Keep frozen until used. Once thawed, if unopened, may refrigerate up to 30 days; if opened, up to 7 days. Thaw before administration.
• Know that color change from pink

to yellow has no effect on efficacy of the vaccine. Yellow color results from vaccine being stored at low temperatures.

• Know that parenteral form should be administered to immunodeficient patients or those with altered immune status because they may be at risk for developing the disease if live-virus vaccine is administered.

• Oral vaccine should be deferred in patients with vomiting or diarrhea. Both forms of vaccine should be deferred in patients with acute illness.

• Do not administer to neonates under 6 weeks.

• Be aware that the highest risk of poliovirus infection occurs after the first dose of the oral vaccine.

• Know that adults at high risk for exposure who have completed a primary course may receive another dose.

• Keep in mind that vaccine is not effective in modifying or preventing existing or incubating poliomyelitis.

• Make sure parents read and understand information booklet available that describes the risks and benefits of this vaccine before vaccine is administered.

rabies vaccine, adsorbed
Pregnancy Risk Category: C

HOW SUPPLIED
Injection: single dose 1-ml vial

ACTION
Promotes active immunity to rabies.

ONSET, PEAK, DURATION
Onset unknown. Antibody levels peak within 2 weeks after the last of the three doses. Duration unknown, although at 9 to 12 months after immunization, 97% of patients continue to have antibody titers at or above a level of 0.1 IU (which is considered by the Centers for Disease Control and Prevention as the minimal acceptable antibody titer for complete rabies virus neutralization).

INDICATIONS & DOSAGE
Preexposure prophylaxis rabies immunization for persons in high-risk groups –
Adults and children: 1 ml I.M. at 0, 7, and 21 or 28 days for a total of three injections. Patients at increased risk for rabies should be checked q 6 months and given a booster vaccination, 1 ml I.M, as needed, to maintain adequate serum titer.
Postexposure rabies prophylaxis –
Adults and children not previously vaccinated against rabies: 20 IU/kg doses of human rabies immune globulin (HRIG) I.M. and five 1-ml injections of rabies vaccine adsorbed I.M. given on days 0, 3, 7, 14, and 28.
Adults and children previously vaccinated against rabies: two 1-ml injections of rabies vaccine absorbed given I.M. given on days 1 and 3. HRIG should not be given.

ADVERSE REACTIONS
Systemic: *headache, nausea, slight fever, fatigue,* reaction resembling serum sickness.
Other: *discomfort at injection site,* aching of the injected muscle, mild inflammatory reaction at injection site.

INTERACTIONS
Antimalarial drugs, corticosteroids, immunosuppressants: decreased response to rabies vaccine. Avoid concomitant use.

CONTRAINDICATIONS
Contraindicated in patients who have experienced life-threatening allergic reactions to previous injections of this vaccine or to components of this vaccine, including thimerosal.

---

*Liquid form contains alcohol.   *Common* reactions are in italics; **life-threatening,** in bold italics.
**May contain tartrazine.

NURSING CONSIDERATIONS
• Use with caution in patients with a history of non-life-threatening allergic reactions to previous injections of the vaccine, in patients with hypersensitivity to monkey-derived proteins, and in children.
• Keep epinephrine 1:1,000 readily available to treat an anaphylactoid reaction.
• Administer as an I.M. injection into the deltoid region in adults and older children. For younger children, the mid-anterolateral aspect of the thigh also is acceptable. Know that this vaccine is not for use by the intradermal route. Take care not to inject the vaccine near a peripheral nerve or into adipose or subcutaneous tissue.
• Know that the vaccine is normally a light pink color because of the presence of phenol red in the suspension.
• Know that preexposure immunization should be delayed in persons with an acute intercurrent illness.
• If patient experiences a serious adverse reaction to the vaccine, report the reaction promptly to the manufacturer: Michigan Department of Public Health, 517-335-8050 during working hours or 517-335-9030 at other times.

---

rabies vaccine, human diploid cell (HDCV)
Imovax, Imovax I.D.

Pregnancy Risk Category: C

HOW SUPPLIED
Intradermal injection: 0.25 IU rabies antigen/dose
I.M. injection: 2.5 IU of rabies antigen/ml, in single-dose vial with diluent

ACTION
Promotes active immunity to rabies.

ONSET, PEAK, DURATION
Onset occurs within 1 week. Antibody levels peak after 1 to 2 months. Effects persist for 2 or more years.

INDICATIONS & DOSAGE
Postexposure antirabies immunization –
Adults and children: five 1-ml doses of HDCV I.M. (for example, in the deltoid region). First dose given as soon as possible after exposure; an additional dose given on each of days 3, 7, 14, and 28 after first dose. If lack of antibody response after this primary series exists, a booster dose is recommended.
Preexposure prophylaxis immunization for persons in high-risk groups –
Adults and children: three 1-ml injections administered I.M. First dose given on day 0 (the first day of therapy), second dose on day 7, and third dose on either day 21 or 28. Alternatively, 0.1 ml intradermally on the same dosage schedule.

ADVERSE REACTIONS
Systemic: headache, dizziness, nausea, abdominal pain, diarrhea, muscle aches, fever, **anaphylaxis,** *serum sickness.*
Other: *pain, erythema, swelling, or itching at injection site.*

INTERACTIONS
Antimalarial drugs, corticosteroids, immunosuppressants: decreased response to rabies vaccine. Avoid concomitant use.

CONTRAINDICATIONS
None reported.

NURSING CONSIDERATIONS
• Use cautiously in patients with a history of hypersensitivity.
• Keep epinephrine 1:1,000 available to treat anaphylaxis.
• Do not use intradermal route for postexposure rabies vaccination.

• Know that the alternative regimen of 0.1-ml doses is only for preexposure prophylaxis. For postexposure prophylaxis, only use the 1-ml doses.
• Be aware that the Centers for Disease Control and Prevention recommends a booster dose with Imovax for all persons who have been potentially exposed to rabies since October 15, 1984, and who have received postexposure prophylaxis with Wyvac unless acceptable titers were proven.
• Be prepared to stop corticosteroid therapy during immunizing period unless therapy is essential for the treatment of other conditions.
• Keep in mind that some patients who receive booster doses experience serum sickness–like hypersensitivity reactions. These reactions usually respond to antihistamines.

---

rubella and mumps virus vaccine, live
Biavax II

Pregnancy Risk Category: C

HOW SUPPLIED
Injection: single-dose vial containing not less than 1,000 TCID$_{50}$ (tissue culture infective doses) of the Wistar RA 27/3 rubella virus (propagated in human diploid cell culture) and not less than 5,000 TCID$_{50}$ of the Jeryl Lynn mumps strain (grown in chick embryo cell culture)

ACTION
Promotes immunity to rubella and mumps by inducing antibody production.

ONSET, PEAK, DURATION
Although onset and peak unknown, most people possess immunity in 2 to 6 weeks. Effects persist for 10 years or longer.

INDICATIONS & DOSAGE
Measles and mumps immunization –
Adults and children 1 year and older: 0.5 ml (1,000 units) S.C.

ADVERSE REACTIONS
Systemic: polyneuritis, rash, thrombocytopenic purpura, urticaria, fever, arthritis, arthralgia, *anaphylaxis,* lymphadenopathy.
Other: pain, erythema, and induration at injection site.

INTERACTIONS
Immune serum globulin, plasma, whole blood: antibodies in serum may interfere with immune response. Don't give vaccine within 3 months of transfusion.
Tuberculin skin test: may temporarily decrease response to test. Defer skin testing.

CONTRAINDICATIONS
Contraindicated in pregnant or immunosuppressed patients; in those with cancer, blood dyscrasia, gamma globulin disorders, fever, or active untreated tuberculosis; history of anaphylaxis or anaphylactoid reactions to neomycin or eggs; and in those receiving corticosteroid (except those receiving corticosteroids as replacement therapy) or radiation therapy.

NURSING CONSIDERATIONS
• Obtain history of allergies, especially anaphylactic reaction to antibiotics, and reaction to immunization.
• Keep epinephrine 1:1,000 available to treat anaphylaxis.
• Know that in patients with acute illness and after administration of immune serum globulin, blood, or plasma, the vaccination should be deferred.
• Use only diluent supplied. Discard 8 hours after reconstituting.
• Inject into outer upper arm. Don't inject I.V.

---

*Liquid form contains alcohol.   *Common* reactions are in italics; *life-threatening,* in bold italics.
**May contain tartrazine.

- Allow an interval of at least 3 weeks between BCG and rubella vaccines.
- Refrigerate and protect from light. Reconstituted solution is clear and yellow; do not use if discolored.
- Stress to patients the importance of avoiding pregnancy for 3 months after vaccination. Offer to provide contraception information.

rubella virus vaccine, live attenuated (RA 27/3)
Meruvax II

Pregnancy Risk Category: C

HOW SUPPLIED
Injection: single-dose vial containing not less than 1,000 TCID$_{50}$ (tissue culture infective doses) of the Wistar RA 27/3 strain of rubella virus (propagated in human diploid cell culture)

ACTION
Promotes immunity to rubella by inducing production of antibodies.

ONSET, PEAK, DURATION
Although the precise onset and peak unknown, most patients develop immunity in 2 to 6 weeks. Effects persist for 10 years or longer.

INDICATIONS & DOSAGE
Measles immunization –
Adults and children 1 year and older: 0.5 ml (1,000 units) S.C.

ADVERSE REACTIONS
Systemic: polyneuritis, rash, thrombocytopenic purpura, urticaria, *joint pain,* fever, arthritis, *anaphylaxis,* lymphadenopathy.
Other: pain, erythema, and induration at injection site.

INTERACTIONS
Immune serum globulin, plasma, whole blood: antibodies in serum may interfere with immune response.

Don't use vaccine within 3 months of transfusion. Immune serum globulin may be given 2 weeks before vaccine. *Tuberculin skin test:* may temporarily decrease response to test. Defer skin testing.

CONTRAINDICATIONS
Contraindicated in pregnant or immunosuppressed patients; in those with cancer, blood dyscrasia, gamma globulin disorders, fever, or active untreated tuberculosis; in those with a history of hypersensitivity to neomycin; and in patients receiving corticosteroid (except those receiving corticosteroids as replacement therapy) or radiation therapy.

NURSING CONSIDERATIONS
- Obtain history of allergies and reaction to immunization.
- Keep epinephrine 1:1,000 available to treat anaphylaxis.
- Immunization should be deferred in patients with acute illness and after administration of human immune serum globulin, blood, or plasma.
- Use only diluent supplied. Discard 8 hours after reconstituting.
- Inject into outer upper arm. Don't inject I.V.
- Refrigerate and protect from light. Reconstituted solution is clear yellow; do not use if discolored.
- Allow at least 3 weeks between BCG and rubella vaccines.
- Stress to patients the importance of avoiding pregnancy for 3 months after vaccination. Offer to provide contraception information.

tetanus toxoid, adsorbed

tetanus toxoid, fluid
Pregnancy Risk Category: C

HOW SUPPLIED
tetanus toxoid, adsorbed
Injection: 5 to 10 Lf (limit floccula-

tion) units of inactivated tetanus/0.5-ml dose, in 0.5-ml syringes and 5-ml vials

tetanus toxoid, fluid
Injection: 4 to 5 Lf units of inactivated tetanus/0.5-ml dose, in 0.5-ml syringes and 7.5-ml vials

ACTION
Promotes immunity to tetanus by inducing antitoxin production.

ONSET, PEAK, DURATION
Although exact onset and peak unknown, most patients possess immunity after two doses. Effects unknown but may persist for 10 years or more.

INDICATIONS & DOSAGE
Primary immunization –
Adults and children 6 years and over: 0.5 ml (adsorbed) I.M. 4 to 8 weeks apart for two doses; then third dose 6 to 12 months after the second. Alternatively, 0.5 ml (fluid) I.M. or S.C. 4 to 8 weeks apart for three doses; then fourth dose of 0.5 ml 6 to 12 months after third dose.
Children 6 weeks to 6 years: 0.5 ml (adsorbed) I.M. at ages 2, 4, and 6 months. A fourth dose is given at age 15 to 18 months. A fifth dose is given at age 4 to 6 years, just before entry into school, if indicated.
Booster doses –
Adults: 0.5 ml I.M. at 10-year intervals.

ADVERSE REACTIONS
Systemic: tachycardia, hypotension, urticaria, pruritus, slight fever, chills, malaise, aches and pains, flushing, *anaphylaxis*.
Other: erythema, induration, and nodule at injection site.

INTERACTIONS
Chloramphenicol: may interfere with response to tetanus toxoid.

CONTRAINDICATIONS
Contraindicated in immunosuppressed patients and in those with immunoglobulin abnormalities or severe hypersensitivity or neurologic reactions to the toxoid or any ingredient in it, such as thimerosal. Also contraindicated in patients with thrombocytopenia or any coagulation disorder that would contraindicate I.M. injection unless the potential benefits outweigh the risk of administration. Vaccination should be deferred in patients with acute illness and during polio outbreaks, except in emergencies.

NURSING CONSIDERATIONS
• Use cautiously (adsorbed) in infants or children with cerebral damage, neurologic disorders, or a history of febrile seizures.
• Obtain history of allergies and reaction to immunization.
• Determine date of last tetanus immunization.
• Keep epinephrine 1:1,000 available to treat anaphylaxis.
• Know that vaccine is used for prevention, not treatment, of tetanus infections.
• Do not confuse this drug with tetanus immune globulin, human.
• Be aware that adsorbed form produces longer duration of immunity. Fluid form provides quicker booster effect in patients actively immunized previously.
• Advise patients to avoid use of hot or cold compresses at injection site; these may increase severity of local reaction.

typhoid vaccine

typhoid vaccine, oral
Vivotif Berna Vaccine
Pregnancy Risk Category: C

HOW SUPPLIED
Injection: suspension of killed Ty-2 strain of *Salmonella typhi;* 8 units/ml in 5-ml, 10-ml, and 20-ml vials
Capsules (enteric-coated): 2 to 6 × 10^9 colony-forming units of viable *Salmonella typhi* Ty^{21}a and 5 to 50 × 10^9 bacterial cells of nonviable Ty^{21}a^2

ACTION
Provides active immunity to typhoid fever.

ONSET, PEAK, DURATION
Immunity occurs at end of primary immunity immunization. Peak unknown. Effects persist for 3 to 5 years.

INDICATIONS & DOSAGE
Primary immunization –
Adults and children over 10 years: 0.5 ml S.C. (injection); repeated in 4 weeks. Protocol repeated as booster q 3 years.
Adults: one capsule (oral vaccine) on alternate days taken 1 hour before meals for four doses. Protocol repeated as booster q 5 years.
Children 6 months to 10 years: 0.25 ml S.C. (injection); repeated in 4 weeks. Protocol repeated as booster q 3 years.

ADVERSE REACTIONS
CNS: headache.
GI: nausea.
Other: *fever,* malaise, *anaphylaxis;* swelling, pain, and inflammation at injection site.

INTERACTIONS
Sulfonamides, other antibiotics: may impair antibody response. Don't use together.

CONTRAINDICATIONS
Contraindicated in immunosuppressed patients and in patients with hypersensitivity to the vaccine. Vacci-

nation should be deferred in patients with acute illness.

NURSING CONSIDERATIONS
● Obtain history of allergies and reaction to immunization.
● Treat fever with antipyretics.
● Keep epinephrine 1:1,000 available to treat anaphylaxis.
● Shake thoroughly before withdrawing from vial.
● Do not give parenteral form intradermally.
● Refrigerate oral vaccine at 35.5° to 50° F (2° to 10° C).
● When administering oral vaccine, ensure that patients understand the importance of taking all four doses. It is imperative to follow the alternate-day regimen.
● Tell patients to take oral vaccine with cold or lukewarm water and not to chew or crush enteric-coated capsules.

typhoid Vi polysaccharide vaccine
Typhim Vi

Pregnancy Risk Category: C

HOW SUPPLIED
Injection: 0.5-ml syringe, 20-dose vial, 50-dose vial

ACTION
Promotes active immunity to typhoid fever.

ONSET, PEAK, DURATION
Unknown.

INDICATIONS & DOSAGE
Active immunization against typhoid fever –
Adults and children 2 years and older: 0.5 ml I.M. as a single dose. Reimmunization every 2 years with 0.5 ml I.M. as a single dose, if needed.

---

†Available in Canada only.   ‡Available in Australia only.   ◊ Available OTC.

ADVERSE REACTIONS
CNS: *headache.*
GI: nausea, diarrhea, vomiting.
Local: *injection site pain or tenderness, induration, erythema at injection site.*
Other: *malaise,* myalgia, fever.

INTERACTIONS
None significant.

CONTRAINDICATIONS
Contraindicated in patients with hypersensitivity to any component of the vaccine. The vaccine should not be used to treat a patient with typhoid fever or given to a patient who is a chronic typhoid carrier.

NURSING CONSIDERATIONS
• Use with caution in patients with thrombocytopenia or a bleeding disorder and those who are taking an anticogulant because bleeding may occur following an I.M. injection in these individuals.
• As with any vaccine, administration should be delayed, if possible, in patients with any febrile illness.
• Although anaphylaxis is rare, keep epinephrine readily available to treat an anaphylactoid reaction.
• Be aware that if vaccine is administered to immunosuppressed persons or persons receiving immunosuppressant therapy, the expected immune response may not be obtained.
• Know that persons who should receive the vaccine include people traveling to or living in areas of higher endemicity for typhoid fever.
• **I.M. use:** Administer as an I.M. injection into the deltoid region in adults and in the deltoid or the vastus lateralis in children. It should not be administered in the gluteal region or areas where there may be a nerve trunk. Never inject I.V.
• Advise patient to take all necessary precautions to avoid contact with or ingestion of contaminated food and water.
• Inform the patient that immunization should be given at least 2 weeks prior to expected exposure. Although an optimal reimmunization schedule has not been established, recommended reimmunization consisting of a single dose for U.S. travelers is every 2 years if exposure to typhoid fever is possible.

---

varicella vaccine
Varivax
Pregnancy risk category: C

HOW SUPPLIED
Injection: single dose vial containing 1350 PFV of Oka/Merck varicella virus (live)

ACTION
Prevents chickenpox by inducing the production of antibodies to varicella-zoster virus.

ONSET, PEAK, DURATION
Although the precise onset and peak unknown, most patients develop immunity in 4 to 6 weeks. Effects persist for at least 2 years.

INDICATIONS & DOSAGE
Prevention of varicella-zoster (chickenpox) infections –
Adults and children 13 years and older: 0.5 ml S.C. followed by 4 to 8 weeks later.
Children 1 to 12 years: 0.5 ml S.C.

ADVERSE REACTIONS
Other: fever, injection site reactions (swelling, *redness, pain,* rash), varicella-like rash.

INTERACTIONS
Blood products, immune globulin: may inactivate vaccine. Defer vaccination for at least 5 months following blood or plasma transfusions or ad-

---

*Liquid form contains alcohol.
**May contain tartrazine.

Common reactions are in italics; ***life-threatening,*** in bold italics.

ministration of immune globulin or varicella-zoster immune globulin.
Immunosuppressants: risk of severe reactions to live-virus vaccines. Postpone routine vaccination.
Salicylates: Reye's syndrome has been reported. Avoid use of salicylates for 6 weeks after varicella infections.

CONTRAINDICATIONS
• Contraindicated in patients hypersensitive to the drug; in those with history of anaphylactoid reaction to neomycin, blood dyscrasia, leukemia, lymphomas, neoplasms affecting bone marrow or lymphatic system, primary and acquired immunosuppressive states, active untreated tuberculosis, or any febrile respiratory illness or other active febrile infection; and in pregnant patients.

NURSING CONSIDERATIONS
• To reconstitute the vaccine, first withdraw 0.7 ml of diluent into the syringe to be used for reconstitution. Inject all the diluent in the syringe into the vial of lyophilized vaccine and gently agitate to mix thoroughly. Administer immediately after reconstitution. Discard if not used within 30 minutes.
• Have epinephrine readily available for potential anaphylaxis reaction.
• Although this drug has been safely and effectively used in combination with measles, mumps, and rubella vaccine, check with the manufacturer for current recommendations.
• Know that in clinical trials, the vaccine was less effective in adults as compared to children.
• Be aware studies are under way to determine the incidence of herpes zoster, which may occur following a latent period.
• Know that the vaccine contains a live attenuated virus. There is some evidence that children who develop a rash may be capable of transmitting the virus.

• A Safety Study protocol program is available for children and adolescents (ages 12 to 17 years) with acute lymphocytic leukemia (ALL). Doctors can enroll patients in this program by contacting Biopharm Clinical Services at (215) 283-0897.

yellow fever vaccine
YF-Vax

Pregnancy Risk Category: C

HOW SUPPLIED
Injection: live, attenuated 17D yellow fever virus in 1- and 5-dose vials, with diluent; supplied only to designated yellow fever vaccination centers authorized to issue yellow fever vaccination certificates

ACTION
Provides active immunity to yellow fever.

ONSET, PEAK, DURATION
Effective immunity occurs in 7 to 10 days. Peak occurs within 28 days of vaccination. Immunity lasts more than 10 years and may persist for life.

INDICATIONS & DOSAGE
Primary vaccination –
Adults and children 9 months and older: 0.5 ml deep S.C.; booster is 0.5 ml S.C. q 10 years.

ADVERSE REACTIONS
Systemic: *anaphylaxis,* fever, malaise.
Other: mild swelling, pain at injection site.

INTERACTIONS
Cholera vaccine: concurrent administration may interfere with immune response to both yellow fever vaccine and cholera vaccine. Administer 3 weeks apart.

---

†Available in Canada only.   ‡Available in Australia only.   ◊ Available OTC.

CONTRAINDICATIONS

Contraindicated in immunosuppressed patients; in those with cancer, gamma globulin deficiency, or hypersensitivity to chickens or eggs; or in those receiving corticosteroid or radiation therapy. Also contraindicated during pregnancy and in infants under 9 months, except in high-risk areas. Information regarding these areas can be obtained from the Centers for Disease Control and Prevention, Division of Vector-Borne Infectious Diseases, at (303) 221-6400.

NURSING CONSIDERATIONS

• Obtain history of allergies, especially to chicken or eggs, and reaction to immunization.
• Keep epinephrine 1:1,000 available to treat anaphylaxis.
• Reconstitute with sodium chloride injection that contains no preservatives (preservatives decrease potency).
• Keep frozen. Don't use unless shipping case contains some dry ice on arrival. Avoid vigorous shaking; carefully swirl mixture until suspension is uniform. Use within 1 hour after reconstituting. Discard remainder.
• Know that yellow fever vaccine should not be given within 1 month of other live-virus vaccines; may be given concurrently with hepatitis B vaccine.

---

*Liquid form contains alcohol.
**May contain tartrazine.

Common reactions are in italics; *life-threatening,* in bold italics.

77

Antitoxins and antivenins

black widow spider antivenin
**botulism antitoxin, bivalent
equine**
Crotalidae antivenin, polyvalent
diphtheria antitoxin, equine
Micrurus fulvius antivenin

COMBINATION PRODUCTS
None.

black widow spider antivenin

Antivenin *(Latrodectus mactans)*
Pregnancy Risk Category: C

HOW SUPPLIED
Injection: combination package — one
vial of antivenin (6,000 units/vial),
one 2.5-ml vial of diluent (sterile
water for injection), and one 1-ml vial
of normal equine (horse) serum (1:10
dilution) for sensitivity testing

ACTION
Unknown.

ONSET, PEAK, DURATION
Unknown.

INDICATIONS & DOSAGE
Black widow spider bite —
Adults and children: 2.5 ml I.M. in
deltoid. Second dose may be needed.
In severe cases, antivenin may be
given I.V.

ADVERSE REACTIONS
Systemic: hypersensitivity reactions,
anaphylaxis, neurotoxicity.

INTERACTIONS
None significant.

CONTRAINDICATIONS
Contraindicated in patients hypersensitive to the drug when desensitization
is not feasible.

NURSING CONSIDERATIONS
• Immobilize the patient; splint the
bitten limb to prevent spread of
venom.
• Obtain accurate patient history of
allergies, especially to horses, and reaction to immunization. Make sure
epinephrine 1:1,000 is available in
case of anaphylaxis.
• For best results, know that antivenin
should be administered as soon as
possible.
• Test for sensitivity before giving the
drug, as ordered. Use 0.2 ml of a 1:10
dilution in 0.9% sodium chloride solution.
• **I.V. use:** Dilute antivenin in 10 to
50 ml of 0.9% sodium chloride solution and infuse over 15 minutes.
• Watch the patient carefully for 2 to
3 days. Venom is neurotoxic and may
cause respiratory paralysis and seizures.

botulism antitoxin, bivalent equine

Pregnancy Risk Category: D

HOW SUPPLIED
Available through your state health
department or the state epidemiolo-
gist's office.

ACTION
Unknown.

ONSET, PEAK, DURATION
Unknown.

INDICATIONS & DOSAGE
Botulism—
Adults and children: one vial I.V. stat and q 4 hours, p.r.n., until the patient's condition improves.

ADVERSE REACTIONS
Systemic: hypersensitivity reactions, *anaphylaxis,* serum sickness (urticaria, pruritus, fever, malaise, arthralgia) may occur in 5 to 13 days.

INTERACTIONS
None significant.

CONTRAINDICATIONS
Contraindicated in patients hypersensitive to the drug.

NURSING CONSIDERATIONS
• Obtain accurate patient history of allergies, especially to horses, and reaction to immunization. Make sure epinephrine 1:1,000 is available in case of hypersensitivity reaction.
• For best results, know antitoxin should be administered as soon as possible.
• Test for sensitivity before giving the drug, as ordered.
• **I.V. use:** Dilute antitoxin 1:10 in D_5W, $D_{10}W$, or 0.9% sodium chloride solution before giving. Give first 10 ml of dilution over 5 minutes; after 15 minutes, rate may be increased.
• Be aware that bivalent antitoxin contains antibodies against types A and B *Clostridium botulinum.* Antitoxins against all other types are available only from Centers for Disease Control and Prevention in Atlanta: Monday through Friday, 8 a.m. to 4:30 p.m. (EST) (404) 639-3670; nights, weekends, and holidays (emergencies only) (404) 639-2888.

Crotalidae antivenin, polyvalent
Pregnancy Risk Category: NR

HOW SUPPLIED
Injection: combination package—one vial of lyophilized serum, one vial of diluent (10 ml of bacteriostatic water for injection), and one 1-ml vial of normal horse serum (diluted 1:10) for sensitivity testing

ACTION
Neutralizes and binds venom of snakes of the species crotalids (pit vipers), including rattlesnakes, water moccasins, and copperheads.

ONSET, PEAK, DURATION
Unknown.

INDICATIONS & DOSAGE
Crotalid (rattlesnake) bites—
Adults and children: initially, 20 to 150 ml I.V., depending on severity of bite and patient response. If large amount of venom, more than 150 ml may be given I.V. directly into superficial vein. Subsequent doses based on patient's response; may need additional 10 to 50 ml if swelling progresses, if systemic symptoms increase in severity, or if new manifestations appear.

ADVERSE REACTIONS
Systemic: *hypersensitivity reactions,* **anaphylaxis, neurotoxicity,** *serum sickness.*

INTERACTIONS
Antihistamines: enhanced toxicity of crotaline venoms. Don't use together.

CONTRAINDICATIONS
Contraindicated in patients hypersensitive to the drug.

NURSING CONSIDERATIONS
• Use cautiously. Studies indicate that 60% of patients treated with this antivenin develop hypersensitivity.
• Immobilize the patient immediately. Splint the bitten extremity.
• Obtain accurate patient history of

---

*Liquid form contains alcohol.   *Common* reactions are in italics; ***life-threatening,*** in bold italics.
**May contain tartrazine.

allergies, especially to horses, and reaction to immunization. Make sure epinephrine 1:1,000 is available in case of hypersensitivity reaction.

• Type and crossmatch blood as soon as possible because hemolysis from venom prevents accurate crossmatching.

• For best results, antivenin should be administered as soon as possible.

• Test for sensitivity before giving drug, as ordered. Give 0.02 to 0.03 ml of a 1:10 dilution in 0.9% sodium chloride solution intradermally. Read results after 5 to 10 minutes. Watch patients carefully for delayed allergic reaction or relapse.

• Be aware that children, who have less resistance and less body fluid to dilute venom, may need twice the adult dose.

• Administer corticosteroids as prescribed. If a large number of vials are administered, serum sickness may result.

• Discard unused portion.

---

diphtheria antitoxin, equine
Pregnancy Risk Category: NR

HOW SUPPLIED
Injection: not less than 500 units/ml in 10,000-unit and 20,000-unit vials

ACTION
Unknown.

ONSET, PEAK, DURATION
Unknown.

INDICATIONS & DOSAGE
Diphtheria prevention —
Adults and children: 5,000 to 10,000 units I.M.
Diphtheria treatment —
Adults and children: 20,000 to 80,000 units or more slow I.V. Additional doses may be given in 24 hours. I.M. route may be used in mild cases.

ADVERSE REACTIONS
Systemic: hypersensitivity reactions, *anaphylaxis,* serum sickness (urticaria, pruritus, fever, malaise, arthralgia) may occur in 7 to 12 days.

INTERACTIONS
None significant.

CONTRAINDICATIONS
Contraindicated in patients hypersensitive to the drug.

NURSING CONSIDERATIONS
• Obtain accurate patient history of allergies, especially to horses, and reaction to immunization. Make sure epinephrine 1:1,000 is available in case of hypersensitivity reaction. Antitoxin should be used with extreme caution in patients with history of allergic disorders.

• Test for sensitivity before giving the drug, as ordered.

• If patient has symptoms of diphtheria (sore throat, fever, tonsillar membrane), therapy should be started immediately, without waiting for culture reports.

• For storage, refrigerate antitoxin at 35.6° to 50° F (2° to 10° C). Before administering, warm to 90° to 95° F (32.2° to 35° C), never higher.

Micrurus fulvius antivenin
Pregnancy Risk Category: NR

HOW SUPPLIED
Injection: combination package with 10 ml of diluent

ACTION
Neutralizes and binds coral snake venom.

ONSET, PEAK, DURATION
Unknown.

INDICATIONS & DOSAGE
Eastern and Texas coral snake bite –
Adults and children: 30 to 50 ml (3 to 5 vials) slow I.V. through running I.V. of 0.9% sodium chloride solution. First 1 to 2 ml given over 3 to 5 minutes, and signs of allergic reaction watched for. If no signs develop, injection is continued. 100 ml or more may be needed.

Not effective for Sonoran or Arizona coral snake bites.

ADVERSE REACTIONS
Systemic: hypersensitivity reactions, *anaphylaxis.*

INTERACTIONS
None significant.

CONTRAINDICATIONS
Contraindicated in patients hypersensitive to the drug.

NURSING CONSIDERATIONS
• Immobilize the patient and splint bitten limb to prevent spread of venom.
• Obtain accurate patient history of allergies, especially to horses, and reaction to immunization. Make sure epinephrine 1:1,000 is available in case of hypersensitivity reaction.
• Test for sensitivity before giving the drug, as ordered.
• For best results, antivenin should be administered as soon as possible (before onset of neurotoxic signs); asymptomatic patients should be treated because systemic signs usually develop late.
• Watch the patient carefully for 24 hours. Venom is neurotoxic and may cause respiratory paralysis.

---

*Liquid form contains alcohol. *Common* reactions are in italics; *life-threatening*, in bold italics.
**May contain tartrazine.

cytomegalovirus immune
  globulin, intravenous
hepatitis B immune globulin,
  human
immune globulin intramuscular
immune globulin intravenous
rabies immune globulin, human
Rh₀(D) immune globulin, human
tetanus immune globulin, human
varicella-zoster immune globulin

COMBINATION PRODUCTS
None.

cytomegalovirus immune globulin, intravenous (CMV-IGIV)
CytoGam

Pregnancy Risk Category: C

HOW SUPPLIED
Powder for injection: 2.5 g with 50 ml sterile water diluent

ACTION
Provides passive immunity by supplying a relatively high concentration of immunoglobulin G (IgG) antibodies against CMV. Increasing these antibody levels in CMV-exposed patients may attenuate or reduce the incidence of serious CMV disease.

ONSET, PEAK, DURATION
Unknown.

INDICATIONS & DOSAGE
To attenuate primary CMV disease in seronegative kidney transplant recipients who receive a kidney from a CMV seropositive donor—
Adults: administered I.V. according to the following schedule.
  —within 72 hours of transplantation: 150 mg/kg

  —2 weeks after transplantation: 100 mg/kg
  —4 weeks after transplantation: 100 mg/kg
  —6 weeks after transplantation: 100 mg/kg
  —8 weeks after transplantation: 100 mg/kg
  —12 weeks after transplantation: 50 mg/kg
  —16 weeks after transplantation: 50 mg/kg.
Initial dose administered at 15 mg/kg/hour. Increased to 30 mg/kg/hour after 30 minutes if no untoward reactions occur, then increased to 60 mg/kg/hour after another 30 minutes if no untoward reactions occur. Volume should not exceed 75 ml/hour. Subsequent doses may be administered at 15 mg/kg/hour for 15 minutes, increasing at 15-minute intervals in a stepwise fashion to 60 mg/kg/hour.

ADVERSE REACTIONS
Systemic: hypotension, nausea, vomiting, wheezing, *anaphylaxis*.
Other: flushing, chills, muscle cramps, back pain, fever.

INTERACTIONS
Live-virus vaccines: may interfere with the immune response to live-virus vaccines. Vaccination should be deferred for at least 3 months.

CONTRAINDICATIONS
Contraindicated in patients with history of sensitivity to other human Ig preparations and in patients with selective IgA deficiency.

NURSING CONSIDERATIONS
• Obtain baseline vital signs prior to beginning therapy.
• **I.V. use:** Reconstitute as follows:

---

†Available in Canada only.   ‡Available in Australia only.   ◊Available OTC.

Remove tab portion of vial cap and clean rubber stopper with 70% alcohol or equivalent. Add 50 ml of sterile water for injection. *To avoid foaming, do not shake vial.* After adding water, release residual vacuum in vial to hasten dissolution. Rotate vial gently to wet all undissolved powder. Allow powder to dissolve for 30 minutes before administration. Inspect vial for clarity and particles.

• If possible, administer through a separate I.V. line using a constant infusion pump. Filters are unnecessary. If unable to administer through separate line, piggyback into preexisting line of sodium chloride injection or one of the following dextrose solutions with or without sodium chloride: dextrose 2.5% in water, D_5W, dextrose 10% in water, or dextrose 20% in water. Do not dilute more than 1:2 with any of the above solutions.

• Begin infusion within 6 hours of reconstitution and finish within 12 hours.

• Monitor the patient's vital signs closely midinfusion, postinfusion, and before any increase in infusion rate.

• If anaphylaxis or drop in blood pressure occurs, discontinue infusion, notify the doctor, and be prepared to administer CPR and such drugs as diphenhydramine and epinephrine.

• Refrigerate powder for injection at 36° to 46° F (2° to 8° C). Do not store reconstituted drug.

hepatitis B immune globulin, human
H-BIG, Hep-B-Gammagee, HyperHep

Pregnancy Risk Category: C

HOW SUPPLIED
Injection: 1-ml, 4-ml, 5-ml vials

ACTION
Provides passive immunity to hepatitis B.

ONSET, PEAK, DURATION
Onset occurs in 1 to 6 days. Peak levels occur 3 to 11 days after I.M. administration. Protective for 2 months or more.

INDICATIONS & DOSAGE
Hepatitis B exposure in high-risk patients –
Adults and children: 0.06 ml/kg I.M. within 7 days after exposure. Dosage repeated 28 days after exposure if patient refuses hepatitis B vaccine.
Neonates born to patients who test positive for hepatitis B surface antigen (HB$_s$Ag): 0.5 ml within 12 hours of birth. Repeated at 1 month and 6 months after the first dose.

ADVERSE REACTIONS
Systemic: *anaphylaxis.*

INTERACTIONS
Live-virus vaccines: may interfere with response to live-virus vaccines. Defer routine immunization for 3 months.

CONTRAINDICATIONS
Contraindicated in patients with a history of anaphylactic reactions to immune serum.

NURSING CONSIDERATIONS
• Obtain history of allergies and reaction to immunizations. Make sure epinephrine 1:1,000 is available in case of anaphylaxis.
• Inject into anterolateral aspect of thigh or deltoid muscle areas in older children and adults; inject into anterolateral aspect of thigh for neonates and children under 3 years.
• For postexposure prophylaxis (for example, needle stick, direct contact), know that drug is usually given with hepatitis B vaccine.

---

*Liquid form contains alcohol.   *Common* reactions are in italics; ***life-threatening,*** in bold italics.
**May contain tartrazine.

immune globulin intramuscular (IGIM, IG, gamma globulin)
Gamastan, Gammar

immune globulin intravenous (IGIV)
Gamimune N, Gammagard S/D, Gammar-IV, Iveegam, Sandoglobulin, Venoglobulin-I

Pregnancy Risk Category: C

HOW SUPPLIED
immune globulin intramuscular
Injection: 2-ml, 10-ml vials
immune globulin intravenous
Injection: 5% in 10-ml, 50-ml, 100-ml vials (Gamimune N)
Powder for injection: 50 mg protein/ml in 0.5-g, 2.5-g, 5-g, 10-g vials (Gammagard); 2.5-g vials (Gammar-IV); 500-mg and 1-g vials (Iveegam); 1-g, 3-g, 6-g vials (Sandoglobulin); 2.5-g, 5-g vials (Venoglobulin-I)

ACTION
Provides passive immunity by increasing antibody titer. The primary component is IgG.

ONSET, PEAK, DURATION
Onset and peak occur immediately after I.V. administration; peak occurs 2 to 5 days after I.M. injection. Duration unknown.

INDICATIONS & DOSAGE
Agammaglobulinemia or hypogammaglobulinemia –
Adults: 30 to 50 ml I.M. monthly. Alternatively, 100 to 200 mg/kg I.V. (Gamimune N) monthly. Infused at 0.01 to 0.02 ml/kg/minute for 30 minutes. If no discomfort, rate increased to maximum of 0.08 ml/kg/minute. For Sandoglobulin, 200 mg/kg I.V. monthly. Infused at 0.5 to 1 ml/minute. After 15 to 30 minutes,

infusion rate increased to 1.5 to 2.5 ml/minute.
Children: 20 to 40 ml I.M. monthly.
Hepatitis A exposure –
Adults and children: 0.02 ml/kg I.M. as soon as possible after exposure. Up to 0.06 ml/kg may be given q 4 to 6 months if exposure will be 3 months or longer.
Measles exposure –
Adults and children: 0.25 ml/kg I.M. within 6 days after exposure.
Modification of measles –
Adults and children: 0.5 ml/kg I.M. within 6 days after exposure.
Prophylaxis in primary immunodeficiencies –
Adults and children: 100 to 200 mg/kg by I.V. infusion monthly (Gamimune only). Infusion rate is 0.01 to 0.02 ml/kg/minute for 30 minutes. If no discomfort, rate increased to maximum of 0.08 ml/kg/minute.
Idiopathic thrombocytopenic purpura –
Adults: 0.4 g/kg Gamimune N or Sandoglobulin I.V. for 5 consecutive days or 1,000 mg/kg Gammagard. Additional doses may be given based on response. Up to three doses given (every other day) if necessary. Or, Venoglobulin-I 500 mg/kg daily for 2 to 7 days.

ADVERSE REACTIONS
Systemic: angioedema, headache, urticaria, malaise, fever, nephrotic syndrome, *anaphylaxis*.
Other: pain, erythema, muscle stiffness at injection site.

INTERACTIONS
Live-virus vaccines: Don't give within 3 months after administration of immune globulin.

CONTRAINDICATIONS
Contraindicated in patients hypersensitive to the drug.

NURSING CONSIDERATIONS

• Obtain history of allergies and reaction to immunizations. Make sure epinephrine 1:1,000 is available in case of anaphylaxis.

• **I.V. use:** Be aware that I.V. products are not interchangeable. Gammagard requires a filter, which is supplied by the manufacturer.

• Know that most adverse effects are related to a rapid infusion rate.

• When giving I.M., use gluteal region. Doses over 10 ml should be divided and injected into several muscle sites to reduce local pain and discomfort.

• Know that immune globulin should not be given for prophylaxis against hepatitis A if 6 weeks or more have elapsed since exposure or after onset of clinical illness.

---

rabies immune globulin, human

Hyperab, Imogam

Pregnancy Risk Category: C

HOW SUPPLIED

Injection: 150 IU/ml in 2-ml, 10-ml vials

ACTION

Provides passive immunity to rabies.

ONSET, PEAK, DURATION

Although onset and peak are not closely defined, an adequate titer of passive antibody is present 24 hours after injection. Exact duration unknown, but it is short.

INDICATIONS & DOSAGE

Rabies exposure –

Adults and children: 20 IU/kg I.M. at time of first dose of rabies vaccine. Half of dose used to infiltrate wound area. Remainder given I.M.

ADVERSE REACTIONS

Systemic: slight fever, *anaphylaxis,* *angioedema.*
Other: pain, redness, induration at injection site.

INTERACTIONS

Corticosteroids and immunosuppressive agents: interferes with response. Avoid during postexposure immunization period.
Live-virus vaccines (measles, mumps, rubella, or polio): interferes with response to vaccine. Delay immunization if possible.

CONTRAINDICATIONS

None known.

NURSING CONSIDERATIONS

• Use with caution in patients with history of prior systemic allergic reactions following the administration of human immunoglobulin preparations or in patients known to be hypersensitive to thimerosal or who have immunoglobulin A deficiency.

• Obtain history of animal bites, allergies, and reaction to immunizations. Have epinephrine 1:1,000 available to treat anaphylaxis.

• Ask patients when last tetanus immunization was received; many doctors order a booster at this time.

• Use only with rabies vaccine and immediate local treatment of wound. Don't give rabies vaccine and rabies immune globulin in same syringe or at same site. Give regardless of interval between exposure and initiation of therapy.

• Don't administer live-virus vaccines within 3 months of rabies immune globulin.

• Don't administer more than 5 ml I.M. at one injection site; divide I.M. doses greater than 5 ml, and administer at different sites.

• Know that this immune serum provides passive immunity. Do not confuse this drug with rabies vaccine,

---

which is a suspension of attenuated or killed microorganisms used to confer active immunity. The two drugs are often given together prophylactically after exposure to known or suspected rabid animals.

Rh₀(D) immune globulin, human

Gamulin Rh, HypRho-D, MICRhoGAM, Mini-Gamulin Rh, Rhesonativ, RhoGAM

Pregnancy Risk Category: C

HOW SUPPLIED
Injection: 300 mcg of $Rh_o(D)$ immune globulin/vial (standard dose); 50 mcg of $Rh_o(D)$ immune globulin/vial (microdose)

ACTION
Suppresses the active antibody response and formation of anti-$Rh_o(D)$ in $Rh_o(D)$-negative, D^u-negative individuals, exposed to Rh-positive blood.

ONSET, PEAK, DURATION
Unknown.

INDICATIONS & DOSAGE
Rh exposure –
Adults (postabortion, postmiscarriage, ectopic pregnancy, or postpartum): transfusion unit or blood bank determines fetal packed RBC volume entering patient's blood; then gives one vial I.M. if fetal packed RBC volume is less than 15 ml. More than one vial I.M. may be required if large fetomaternal hemorrhage occurs. Must be given within 72 hours after delivery or miscarriage.
Transfusion accidents –
Adults and children: consult blood bank or transfusion unit at once. Must be given within 72 hours.
Postabortion or postmiscarriage to prevent Rh antibody formation –
Adults: consult transfusion unit or

blood bank. One microdose vial will suppress immune reaction to 2.5 ml $Rh_o(D)$-positive RBCs. Ideally should be given within 3 hours, but may be given up to 72 hours after abortion or miscarriage.

ADVERSE REACTIONS
Systemic: slight fever, *anaphylaxis*.
Others: discomfort at injection site.

INTERACTIONS
Live-virus vaccines: may interfere with response. Delay immunization if possible.

CONTRAINDICATIONS
Contraindicated in $Rh_o(D)$-positive or D^u-positive patients and those previously immunized to $Rh_o(D)$ blood factor. Also contraindicated in patients with anaphylactic or severe systemic reaction to human globulin.

NURSING CONSIDERATIONS
• Obtain history of allergies and reaction to immunization. Be sure epinephrine 1:1,000 is available in case of anaphylaxis.
• Immediately after delivery, send a sample of neonate's cord blood to laboratory for typing and crossmatching. Confirm if mother is $Rh_o(D)$-negative and D^u-negative. Administer to mother as ordered only if infant is $Rh_o(D)$-positive or D^u-positive.
• Keep in mind that this immune serum provides passive immunity to the patient exposed to Rh_o-positive fetal blood during pregnancy. Prevents formation of maternal antibodies (active immunity), which would endanger future Rh_o-positive pregnancies.
• Know that vaccination with live-virus vaccines should be deferred for 3 months after administration of $Rh_o(D)$ immune globulin.
• Know that MICRhoGAM is recommended for every patient undergoing abortion or miscarriage up to 12 weeks' gestation unless she is $Rh_o(D)$-

positive or D^u-positive or has Rh antibodies, or the father or fetus is Rh-negative.
● Refrigerate at 36° to 46° F (2° to 8° C).
● Explain to patient how drug protects future Rh_o-positive fetuses.

tetanus immune globulin, human
Homo-Tet, Hu-Tet, Hyper-Tet
Pregnancy Risk Category: C

HOW SUPPLIED
Injection: 250 units per vial or syringe

ACTION
Provides passive immunity to tetanus.

ONSET, PEAK, DURATION
Onset unknown. Peak levels occur 2 to 3 days after I.M. injection. Protection lasts about 4 weeks.

INDICATIONS & DOSAGE
Tetanus exposure –
Adults and children: 250 to 500 units I.M.
Tetanus treatment –
Adults and children: single doses of 3,000 to 6,000 units I.M. have been used. Optimal dosage schedules have not been established.

ADVERSE REACTIONS
Systemic: slight fever, hypersensitivity reactions, *anaphylaxis.*
Other: pain, stiffness, erythema at injection site.

INTERACTIONS
None significant.

CONTRAINDICATIONS
Contraindicated in patients with thrombocytopenia or any coagulation disorder that would contraindicate I.M. injection unless potential benefits outweigh the risks.

NURSING CONSIDERATIONS
● Obtain history of injury, tetanus immunizations, last tetanus toxoid injection, allergies, and reaction to immunizations. Have epinephrine 1:1,000 available to treat hypersensitivity reaction.
● Know that tetanus immune globulin is used only if wound is more than 24 hours old or patient has had fewer than two tetanus toxoid injections.
● Thoroughly clean wound and remove all foreign matter.
● Inject into the deltoid muscle for adults and children 3 years and older and into the anterolateral aspect of the thigh in neonates and children under 3 years.
● Do not confuse this drug with tetanus toxoid. Tetanus immune globulin is not a substitute for tetanus toxoid, which should be given at the same time to produce active immunization. Don't give at same site as toxoid.
● Be aware that antibodies remain at effective levels for about 4 weeks, which is several times the duration of antitoxin-induced antibodies. Protects patients for the incubation period of most tetanus cases.

varicella-zoster immune globulin (VZIG)
Pregnancy Risk Category: NR

HOW SUPPLIED
Injection: 10% to 18% solution of the globulin fraction of human plasma containing 125 units of varicella-zoster virus antibody (volume is about 1.25 ml)

ACTION
Provides passive immunity to varicella-zoster virus.

ONSET, PEAK, DURATION
Unknown, although antibodies persist for at least 1 month.

---

*Liquid form contains alcohol.   *Common* reactions are in italics; *life-threatening,* in bold italics.
**May contain tartrazine.

INDICATIONS & DOSAGE

Passive immunization of susceptible immunodeficient patients after exposure to varicella (chicken pox or herpes zoster) –
Children to 10 kg: 125 units I.M.
Children 10.1 to 20 kg: 250 units I.M.
Children 20.1 to 30 kg: 375 units I.M.
Children 30.1 to 40 kg: 500 units I.M.
Adults and children over 40 kg: 625 units I.M.

ADVERSE REACTIONS

Systemic: GI distress, malaise, headache, respiratory distress, ***anaphylaxis.***
Other: discomfort at injection site, rash.

INTERACTIONS

Live-virus vaccines: may interfere with response. Defer vaccination for 3 months after administration of VZIG.

CONTRAINDICATIONS

Contraindicated in patients with a history of severe reaction to human immune serum globulin or thrombocytopenia.

NURSING CONSIDERATIONS

• Obtain accurate patient history of allergies and reaction to immunization. Make sure epinephrine 1:1,000 is available in case of anaphylaxis.
• For maximum benefit, administer as soon as possible after presumed exposure, as ordered. May be of benefit when given as late as 96 hours after exposure.
• Administer only by deep I.M. injection. Never administer I.V.
• Refrigerate vial.
• Although usually restricted to children under 15 years, be aware that VZIG may be administered to adolescents and adults if necessary.
• Know that VZIG is not recommended for nonimmunosuppressed patients.
• Be alert that drug is not commer-cially distributed. Available only from 20 regional U.S. distribution centers. These centers will distribute to Canada and overseas. Call the Centers for Disease Control and Prevention for details Monday through Friday, 8 a.m. to 4:30 p.m. (EST), (404) 639-3670; all other times, (404) 639-2888.

79

Biological response modifiers

aldesleukin
epoetin alfa
filgrastim
interferon alfa-2a, recombinant
interferon alfa-2b, recombinant
interferon alfa-n3
interferon beta-1b, recombinant
interferon gamma-1b
sargramostim

COMBINATION PRODUCTS
None.

---

aldesleukin (interleukin-2, IL-2)
Proleukin

Pregnancy Risk Category: C

HOW SUPPLIED
Powder for injection: 22 million IU/vial

ACTION
Unknown, although it is thought that stimulation of an immunologic host reaction to the tumor is involved.

ONSET, PEAK, DURATION
Unknown, although tumor regression may continue up to 12 months following initiation of therapy.

INDICATIONS & DOSAGE
Metastatic renal cell carcinoma –
Adults: 600,000 IU/kg (0.037 mg/kg) I.V. q 8 hours for 5 days (total of 14 doses). After a 9-day rest, the sequence is repeated for another 14 doses. Repeat courses may be administered after a rest period of at least 7 weeks.

ADVERSE REACTIONS
CNS: headache, *mental status changes, dizziness, sensory dysfunc-* tion, special senses disorders, *syncope, motor dysfunction,* **coma.**
CV: *hypotension, sinus tachycardia, arrhythmias, bradycardia,* **PVCs,** *premature atrial contractions, myocardial ischemia,* **MI, CHF, cardiac arrest,** *myocarditis, endocarditis,* **CVA,** *pericardial effusion, thrombosis,* **capillary leak syndrome (CLS).**
GI: *nausea, vomiting, diarrhea, stomatitis, anorexia, bleeding, dyspepsia, constipation.*
GU: *oliguria,* **anuria,** *proteinuria, hematuria, dysuria,* urine retention, urinary frequency.
Hematologic: *anemia, thrombocytopenia, leukopenia,* coagulation disorders, leukocytosis, eosinophilia.
Hepatic: *jaundice;* ascites; hepatomegaly; *elevated bilirubin, serum transaminase, alkaline phosphatase levels.*
Respiratory: *pulmonary congestion, dyspnea,* **pulmonary edema, respiratory failure, pleural effusion, apnea, pneumothorax,** *tachypnea.*
Skin: *pruritus, erythema, rash, dryness,* **exfoliative dermatitis,** *purpura,* alopecia, petechiae.
Other: *elevated BUN and serum creatinine levels; hypomagnesemia; acidosis; hypocalcemia; hypophosphatemia; hypokalemia; hyperuricemia; hypoalbuminemia;* hypoproteinemia; hyponatremia; hyperkalemia; arthralgia; myalgia; *fever; chills;* abdominal, chest, or back pain; fatigue; weakness; malaise; edema; infections of the catheter tip, urinary tract, or injection site; phlebitis; **sepsis;** weight gain; weight loss; conjunctivitis.

INTERACTIONS
Antihypertensives: increased risk of hypotension. Monitor closely.
Cardiotoxic, hepatotoxic, myelotoxic,

---

*Liquid form contains alcohol.
**May contain tartrazine.

Common reactions are in italics; **life-threatening,** in bold italics.

or nephrotoxic drugs: enhanced toxicity. Avoid concomitant use.
Corticosteroids: decreased antitumor effectiveness of aldesleukin. Avoid concomitant use.
Psychotropic agents: unpredictable interaction. Because aldesleukin can alter CNS function, use together cautiously.

CONTRAINDICATIONS
• Contraindicated in patients hypersensitive to the drug or any component of the formulation and in patients with abnormal cardiac (thallium) stress test or pulmonary function tests or organ allografts.
• Retreatment is contraindicated in patients who experience any of the following adverse effects: pericardial tamponade; disturbances in cardiac rhythm that were uncontrolled or unresponsive to intervention; sustained ventricular tachycardia (five beats or more); chest pain accompanied by ECG changes, indicating MI or angina pectoris; renal dysfunction requiring dialysis for 72 hours or more; coma or toxic psychosis lasting 48 hours or more; seizures that were repetitive or difficult to control; ischemia or perforation of the bowel; GI bleeding requiring surgery.

NURSING CONSIDERATIONS
• Know that this drug should not be used unless the patient has had definitive tests documenting normal cardiac and pulmonary function. Use with extreme caution in patients with normal test results if they have a history of cardiac or pulmonary disease and in patients with a history of seizure disorders because the drug may cause seizures.
• Use cautiously and with close clinical monitoring because severe adverse effects usually accompany therapy at the recommended dosage.
• Use cautiously in patients who re-

quire large volumes of fluid (such as patients with hypercalcemia).
• Know that drug should be administered only in a hospital under the direction of a doctor experienced in the use of chemotherapeutic agents. An intensive care facility and intensive care or cardiopulmonary specialists must be readily available.
• Monitor hematologic tests, including CBC, differential, and platelet counts; serum electrolyte levels; and renal and liver function tests, and obtain chest X-ray before therapy, as ordered. Repeat daily during therapy, as ordered.
• Treat patients with bacterial infections before therapy, as ordered.
• **I.V. use:** To avoid altering the pharmacologic properties of the drug, reconstitute and dilute carefully, and follow manufacturer's recommendations. Do not mix with other drugs or albumin.
• Reconstitute the vial containing 22 million IU (1.3 mg) with 1.2 ml of sterile water for injection. Do not use bacteriostatic water or 0.9% sodium chloride injection; these diluents increase aggregation of drug. Direct the stream at the sides of the vial and gently swirl to reconstitute. Do not shake. The reconstituted solution will have a concentration of 18 million IU (1.1 mg)/ml. It should be particle-free and colorless to slightly yellow.
• Add the ordered dose of reconstituted drug to 50 ml of D_5W and infuse over 15 minutes. Do not use an in-line filter. Plastic infusion bags are preferred because they provide consistent drug delivery.
• Discard unused portion. Vials are for single-dose use and contain no preservatives.
• Be prepared to adjust dosage of other drugs as ordered to compensate for renal and hepatic impairment occurring during treatment. Modify dosage by withholding a dose or inter-

rupting therapy rather than by reducing the dose, as ordered.
• Withhold dose and notify doctor if patient develops moderate to severe lethargy or somnolence; continued administration can result in coma.
• Administer packed RBCs or platelets, as ordered. Severe anemia or thrombocytopenia may occur.
• Know that this drug has been associated with CLS, a condition that results from the loss of vascular tone, in which plasma proteins and fluids escape into the extravascular space. Mean arterial blood pressure begins to drop within 2 to 12 hours of treatment; edema and effusions may be severe, and death can result from hypoperfusion of major organs. Other conditions that accompany CLS include arrhythmias, MI, angina, mental status changes, renal insufficiency, respiratory distress or failure, and GI bleeding or infarction.
• Carefully monitor fluid status, pulse, mental status, urine output, and organ perfusion to treat CLS. Central venous pressure monitoring is necessary.
• Anticipate fluid management or administration of pressor agents to treat CLS.
• Keep in mind that therapy is associated with impaired neutrophil function, which can lead to disseminated infection. Many studies employed prophylactic antibiotic therapy with oxacillin, nafcillin, ciprofloxacin, or vancomycin; check protocol and administer antibiotics, as ordered. Monitor for infection.
• Know that patients should be neurologically stable with a negative computed tomography scan for CNS metastases. Drug may exacerbate symptoms in patients with unrecognized or undiagnosed CNS metastases.
• Refrigerate powder for injection or reconstituted solutions. Return drug to room temperature before administering to patients. After reconstitution and dilution, administer within 48 hours.

---

epoetin alfa (erythropoietin)
Epogen, Procrit
Pregnancy Risk Category: C

HOW SUPPLIED
Injection: 2,000 units/ml, 3,000 units/ml, 4,000 units/ml, 10,000 units/ml

ACTION
Mimics the effects of erythropoietin, a naturally occurring hormone produced by the kidneys. Epoetin alfa is one of the factors controlling the rate of red cell production. It acts on the erythroid tissues in the bone marrow, stimulating the mitotic activity of erythroid progenitor cells and early precursor cells. It functions as a growth factor and as a differentiating factor, enhancing the rate of RBC production.

ONSET, PEAK, DURATION
Increase in reticulocyte count occurs within 7 to 10 days; RBC, hematocrit, and hemoglobin increase in 2 to 6 weeks. Serum levels peak immediately after I.V. infusion or within 4 to 24 hours after S.C. administration. Effects such as the hematocrit may begin to decrease about 2 weeks after treatment has been discontinued.

INDICATIONS & DOSAGE
Anemia due to reduced production of endogenous erythropoietin caused by end-stage renal disease –
Adults: dosage is individualized. Starting dose is 50 to 100 units/kg I.V. three times weekly. (Nondialysis patients with chronic renal failure or patients receiving continuous peritoneal dialysis may receive the drug by S.C. injection or I.V.) Dosage reduced when target hematocrit is reached or if the hematocrit rises more than 4

---

points in any 2-week period. Dosage increased if hematocrit does not increase by 5 to 6 points after 8 weeks of therapy. Maintenance dosage is highly individualized.

Adjunctive treatment of HIV-infected patients with anemia secondary to zidovudine therapy –
Adults: 100 units/kg I.V. or S.C. three times weekly for 8 weeks or until target hemoglobin is reached.

Anemia secondary to cancer chemotherapy –
Adults: 150 units/kg S.C. three times weekly for 8 weeks or until target hemoglobin is reached.

ADVERSE REACTIONS
CNS: headache, *seizures*.
CV: *hypertension,* decreased plasma volume.
GI: nausea, vomiting, diarrhea.
Hematologic: iron deficiency, elevated platelet count.
Skin: rash.
Other: increased clotting of arteriovenous grafts.

INTERACTIONS
None significant.

CONTRAINDICATIONS
Contraindicated in patients with uncontrolled hypertension, hypersensitivity to mammalian cell-derived products or albumin (human).

NURSING CONSIDERATIONS
• Monitor blood pressure before initiating therapy. Up to 80% of patients with chronic renal failure have hypertension. Blood pressure may rise, especially when the hematocrit is increasing in the early part of therapy.
• **I.V. use:** Give by direct injection without dilution. Solution contains no preservatives. Discard unused portion. Do not mix with other drugs.
• When used in HIV-infected patients, be prepared to individualize dosage based on response, as ordered.

Dosage recommendations are for patients with endogenous erythropoietin levels of 500 units/L or less and cumulative zidovudine doses of 4.2 g/week or less.
• After injection (usually within 2 hours), know that some patients complain of pain or discomfort in their limbs (long bones) and pelvis and of coldness and sweating. Symptoms may persist up to 12 hours and then disappear.
• Be aware that patients treated with epoetin alfa may require additional heparin to prevent clotting during dialysis treatments.
• Monitor blood count, as ordered. Hematocrit may rise and cause excessive clotting.
• Institute diet restrictions or drug therapy to control blood pressure. Reduce dosage in patients who exhibit a rapid rise in hematocrit (more than 4 points in any 2-week period), as ordered, because of the risk of hypertension.
• Know that the patient's response to epoetin alfa depends on the amount of endogenous erythropoietin in the plasma. Patients with levels of 500 units/L or more usually have transfusion-dependent anemia and will probably not respond to the drug. Those with levels below 500 units/L usually respond well.
• Keep in mind that patients with end-stage renal disease may experience an improved appetite and enhanced well-being as a result of increased hematocrit.
• Advise patients that blood specimens will be drawn weekly for blood counts and that dosage adjustments may be made based on the results.
• Advise patients to avoid hazardous activities, such as driving or operating heavy machinery, during initiation of therapy. A relationship between excessively rapid hematocrit rise and seizures may exist.

---

filgrastim (granulocyte colony-stimulating factor; G-CSF)
Neupogen

Pregnancy Risk Category: C

HOW SUPPLIED
Injection: 300 mcg/ml

ACTION
A glycoprotein that stimulates proliferation and differentiation of hematopoietic cells. Filgrastim is specific for neutrophils.

ONSET, PEAK, DURATION
Onset occurs with 5 to 60 minutes. Serum levels peak in 24 hours. Effects decline by 50% in first 24 hours after drug discontinued and absolute neutrophil count returns to pretreatment levels within 1 to 7 days.

INDICATIONS & DOSAGE
To decrease the incidence of infection in patients with nonmyeloid malignancies receiving myelosuppressive antineoplastic agents –
Adults and children: 5 mcg/kg/day I.V. or S.C. as a single dose. Doses may be increased in increments of 5 mcg/kg for each chemotherapy cycle depending on the duration and severity of the nadir of the absolute neutrophil count (ANC).
To decrease the incidence of infection in patients with nonmyeloid malignancies receiving myelosuppressive antineoplastic agents followed by bone marrow transplant –
Adults and children: 10 mcg/kg/day I.V. or S.C. at least 24 hours after cytotoxic chemotherapy and bone marrow infusion. Subsequent dosages adjusted according to the neutrophil response.
Congenital neutropenia –
Adults: 6 mcg/kg S.C. b.i.d. Dosage adjusted according to patient's response.

Idiopathic or cyclic neutropenia –
Adults: 5 mcg/kg S.C. daily. Dosage adjusted according to patient's response.

ADVERSE REACTIONS
GU: hematuria, proteinuria.
Hematologic: *thrombocytopenia.*
Skin: alopecia, exacerbation of preexisting conditions (such as psoriasis).
Other: *skeletal pain,* fever, splenomegaly, osteoporosis.

INTERACTIONS
Chemotherapeutic agents: rapidly dividing myeloid cells are potentially sensitive to cytotoxic agents. Do not use filgrastim concomitantly with chemotherapy.

CONTRAINDICATIONS
Contraindicated in patients hypersensitive to proteins derived from *Escherichia coli* or to the drug or its components.

NURSING CONSIDERATIONS
• Obtain baseline CBC and platelet counts before therapy, as ordered.
• **I.V. use:** Dilute in 50 to 100 ml of D_5W and give by intermittent infusion over 15 to 60 minutes or continuous infusion over 24 hours. If the final concentration of the drug is going to be 2 to 15 mcg/ml, add albumin at a concentration of 2 mg/ml (0.2%) to minimize binding of the drug to plastic containers or tubing.
• Do not give the drug within 24 hours of cytotoxic chemotherapy.
• Once a dose is withdrawn, do not reenter vial. Discard unused portion. Vials are for single-dose use and contain no preservatives.
• Obtain CBC and platelet count twice weekly during therapy, as ordered. Patients who receive this drug may potentially receive high doses of chemotherapy, which may increase the risk of chemotherapy-induced toxicities.

---

*Liquid form contains alcohol.   *Common* reactions are in italics; *life-threatening*, in bold italics.
**May contain tartrazine.

• Be aware that a transiently increased neutrophil count is common 1 or 2 days after initiation of therapy. Give daily for up to 2 weeks or until the ANC has returned to 10,000/mm³ after the expected chemotherapy-induced neutrophil nadir, as ordered.

• Refrigerate at 36° to 46° F (2° to 8° C). Do not freeze; avoid shaking. Store at room temperature for a maximum of 6 hours; discard after 6 hours.

• If patients will be self-administering the drug, teach them how to administer it and how to dispose of used needles, syringes, drug containers, and unused medicine. Give them a copy of the "information for patients" included with the product and ensure that they understand the information.

---

interferon alfa-2a, recombinant (rIFN-A)
Roferon-A

Pregnancy Risk Category: C

HOW SUPPLIED
Injection: 3 million IU/vial; 18 and 36 million IU/multiple-dose vial

ACTION
Unknown. Appears to involve direct antiproliferative action against tumor cells or viral cells to inhibit replication and modulation of host immune response by enhancing the phagocytic activity of macrophages and by augmenting specific cytotoxicity of lymphocytes for target cells.

ONSET, PEAK, DURATION
Onset unknown. Peak levels occur 3.8 hours after I.M. administration or 7.3 hours after S.C. administration. Duration unknown.

INDICATIONS & DOSAGE
Hairy-cell leukemia –
Adults: for induction, 3 million units S.C. or I.M. daily for 16 to 24 weeks.

For maintenance, 3 million units S.C. or I.M. three times a week.
AIDS-related Kaposi's sarcoma –
Adults: for induction, 36 million units S.C. or I.M. daily for 10 to 12 weeks. For maintenance, 36 million units S.C. or I.M. three times a week.

ADVERSE REACTIONS
CNS: *dizziness,* confusion, paresthesia, numbness, lethargy, depression, nervousness, difficulty in thinking or concentrating, insomnia, sedation, apathy, anxiety, irritability, fatigue, vertigo, gait disturbances, poor coordination.
CV: hypotension, chest pain, arrhythmias, palpitations, syncope, *CHF,* hypertension, edema.
EENT: visual disturbances, dryness or inflammation of the oropharynx, rhinorrhea, sinusitis, conjunctivitis, earache, eye irritation, rhinitis.
GI: *anorexia, nausea, diarrhea,* vomiting, abdominal fullness, abdominal pain, flatulence, constipation, hypermotility, gastric distress, dysgeusia.
GU: transient impotence.
Hematologic: *leukopenia,* mild thrombocytopenia.
Hepatic: *hepatitis.*
Respiratory: *bronchospasm,* coughing, dyspnea, tachypnea.
Skin: *rash,* dryness, *pruritus,* partial alopecia, urticaria, flushing.
Other: inflammation at injection site (rare), flulike syndrome (fever, fatigue, myalgia, headache, chills, arthralgia), diaphoresis, hot flashes, excessive salivation, cyanosis.

INTERACTIONS
Aminophylline, theophylline: may reduce theophylline clearance. Monitor serum levels.
CNS depressants: enhanced CNS effects. Avoid concomitant use.
Live-virus vaccine: increased risk of adverse reactions and decreased antibody response. Don't use together.

---

†Available in Canada only.   ‡Available in Australia only.   ◊ Available OTC.

CONTRAINDICATIONS

Contraindicated in patients hypersensitive to the drug or to mouse immunoglobulin.

NURSING CONSIDERATIONS

• Use cautiously in patients with severe hepatic or renal function impairment, seizure disorders, compromised CNS function, cardiac disease, or myelosuppression.

• Obtain allergy history. Drug contains phenol as a preservative and serum albumin as a stabilizer.

• Use S.C. administration route in patients whose platelet count is below 50,000/mm³.

• Administer at bedtime to minimize daytime drowsiness.

• Make sure patients are well hydrated, especially during initial stages of treatment.

• At the beginning of therapy, assess patients for flulike symptoms, which tend to diminish with continued therapy. Premedicate with acetaminophen to minimize symptoms.

• Monitor blood studies, as ordered. Interferons may decrease hemoglobin, hematocrit, WBC count, platelet count, and neutrophil count; increase PT and PTT; and increase serum levels of AST, ALT, lactate dehydrogenase, alkaline phosphatase, calcium, phosphorus, and fasting glucose, which are dose-related and reversible. Recovery occurs within several days or weeks after withdrawal of drug.

• Periodically monitor for CNS adverse reactions, such as decreased mental status and dizziness, during therapy.

• For patients who develop thrombocytopenia, exercise extreme care in performing invasive procedures; inspect injection site and skin frequently for signs of bruising; limit frequency of I.M. injections; test urine, emesis fluid, stool, and secretions for occult blood.

• Keep in mind that severe adverse reactions may require dosage reduction to one-half or discontinuation of therapy until reactions subside.

• Know that different brands of interferon may not be equivalent and may require different dosage.

• Be aware that neurotoxicity and cardiotoxicity are more common in elderly patients, especially those with underlying CNS or cardiac impairment.

• Be alert that use with blood dyscrasia-causing medications, bone marrow suppressant, or radiation therapy may increase bone marrow suppressant effects. Dosage reduction may be required.

• Refrigerate the drug.

• Advise patients that laboratory tests will be performed before and periodically during therapy. Tests include a CBC with differential, platelet count, blood chemistry and electrolyte studies, liver function tests, and, if the patient has a preexisting cardiac disorder or advanced stages of cancer, ECGs.

• Instruct patients in proper oral hygiene during treatment because the bone marrow suppressant effects of interferon may lead to microbial infection, delayed healing, and gingival bleeding. This drug may also decrease salivary flow.

• Emphasize need to follow the doctor's instructions about taking and recording temperature, and how and when to take acetaminophen.

• Advise patients to check with the doctor for instructions after missing a dose.

• Tell patients that drug may cause temporary loss of some hair, which should return when drug is withdrawn.

• If patients will be self-administering drug, teach them how to prepare and administer it and how to dispose of used needles, syringes, containers, and unused medication. Give them a copy of the "information for patients"

---

*Liquid form contains alcohol.   *Common* reactions are in italics; *life-threatening*, in bold italics.
**May contain tartrazine.

included with the product and ensure that they understand the information. Also provide information on drug stability.

• Warn patients not to have any immunization without the doctor's approval and to avoid contact with persons who have taken oral polio vaccine. Concurrent use with a live-virus vaccine may potentiate replication of vaccine virus, increase adverse reactions, and decrease patient's antibody response. Patients are at increased risk for infection during therapy.

---

interferon alfa-2b, recombinant (IFN-alpha 2)
Intron A

Pregnancy Risk Category: C

HOW SUPPLIED
Injection: 3 million IU/vial with diluent, 5 million IU/vial with diluent, 10 million IU/vial with diluent, 18 million IU/vial with diluent, 25 million IU/vial with diluent, 50 million IU/vial with diluent

ACTION
Unknown. Appears to involve direct antiproliferative action against tumor cells or viral cells to inhibit replication, and modulation of host immune response by enhancing the phagocytic activity of macrophages and by augmenting specific cytotoxicity of lymphocytes for target cells.

ONSET, PEAK, DURATION
Onset and duration unknown. Serum levels peak in 3 to 12 hours.

INDICATIONS & DOSAGE
Hairy-cell leukemia –
Adults: 2 million units/m² I.M. or S.C., three times a week.
Condylomata acuminata (genital or venereal warts) –
Adults: 1 million units/lesion intrale-

sionally three times a week for 3 weeks.
AIDS-related Kaposi's sarcoma –
Adults: 30 million units/m² S.C. or I.M. three times a week.
Chronic hepatitis B –
Adults: 30 to 35 units weekly I.M. or S.C., administered either as 5 million units daily or 10 million units three times a week, for 16 weeks.
Chronic hepatitis non A, non B/C (NANB/C) –
Adults: 3 million units I.M. or S.C. three times a week.

ADVERSE REACTIONS
CNS: dizziness, confusion, paresthesia, lethargy, depression, difficulty in thinking or concentrating, insomnia, sedation, anxiety, *fatigue,* hypoesthesia, amnesia, agitation, weakness.
CV: hypotension, chest pain.
EENT: visual disturbances, hearing disorders, stye, pharyngitis, nasal congestion, sinusitis, rhinitis.
GI: *anorexia, nausea,* diarrhea, vomiting, abdominal pain, dyspepsia, constipation, loose stools, eructation, dry mouth, dysgeusia, stomatitis, gingivitis.
GU: transient impotence, gynecomastia.
Hematologic: *leukopenia,* mild thrombocytopenia.
Respiratory: dyspnea, coughing.
Skin: rash, dryness, pruritus, partial alopecia, urticaria, moniliasis, flushing, dermatitis.
Other: *flulike symptoms (fever, fatigue, headache, chills, muscle aches), arthralgia,* asthenia, rigors, leg cramps, arthrosis, bone disorders, back pain, increased diaphoresis, decreased libido, hypertonia, migraine, thirst.

INTERACTIONS
Aminophylline, theophylline: may reduce theophylline clearance. Monitor serum concentrations.

CNS depressants: enhanced CNS effects. Avoid concomitant use.

Live-virus vaccines: risk of enhanced adverse reactions to vaccine or decreased antibody response. Postpone immunization.

Zidovudine: may be synergistic adverse effects (higher incidence of neutropenia). Carefully monitor WBC count.

CONTRAINDICATIONS
Contraindicated in patients hypersensitive to the drug.

NURSING CONSIDERATIONS
• Use cautiously in patients with a history of cardiovascular disease, pulmonary disease, diabetes mellitus, coagulation disorders, and severe myelosuppression.
• Use S.C. administration route in patients whose platelet count is below 50,000/mm^3.
• Administer at bedtime to minimize daytime drowsiness.
• When administering interferon for condylomata acuminata, use only 10-million-IU vial because dilution of other strengths required for intralesional use results in a hypertonic solution. Do not reconstitute 10-million-IU vial with more than 1 ml of diluent. Use tuberculin or similar syringe and 25G to 30G needle. Do not inject too deeply beneath lesion or too superficially. As many as five lesions can be treated at one time. To ease discomfort, administer in evening with acetaminophen.
• Make sure patients are well hydrated, especially during initial treatment.
• At the beginning of treatment, monitor most patients for flulike symptoms, which tend to diminish with continued therapy. Premedicate with acetaminophen to minimize flulike symptoms.
• Monitor blood studies, as ordered. Interferons may decrease hemoglo-

bin, hematocrit, WBC count, platelet count, and neutrophil count; increase PT and PTT; and increase serum levels of AST, ALT, lactate dehydrogenase, alkaline phosphatase, calcium, phosphorus, and fasting glucose, which are dose-related and reversible. Recovery occurs within several days or weeks after interferon withdrawal.
• Periodically monitor for adverse CNS reactions, such as decreased mental status and dizziness, during therapy.
• For patients who develop thrombocytopenia: exercise extreme care in performing invasive procedures; inspect injection site and skin frequently for signs of bruising; limit frequency of I.M. injections; test urine, emesis fluid, stool, and secretions for occult blood.
• Keep in mind that severe adverse reactions may require dosage reduction to one-half or discontinuation of therapy until reactions subside.
• Be aware that neurotoxicity and cardiotoxicity are more common in elderly patients, especially those with underlying CNS or cardiac impairment.
• Be alert that use with blood dyscrasia-causing medications, bone marrow suppressants, or radiation therapy may increase bone marrow suppressant effects. Dosage reduction may be required.
• Refrigerate the drug.
• Keep in mind that maximum response usually occurs 4 to 8 weeks after initiation of therapy. If results are not satisfactory after 12 to 16 weeks, a second course may be instituted. Patients with 6 to 10 condylomata may receive a second course of treatment; patients with more than 10 condylomata may receive additional courses.
• Advise patients to avoid contact with persons with viral illness and those who have recently taken oral polio vaccine. Patients are at increased risk for infection during therapy.

---

*Liquid form contains alcohol. *Common* reactions are in italics; *life-threatening,* in bold italics.
**May contain tartrazine.

• Advise patients that laboratory tests will be performed before and periodically during therapy. Tests include a CBC with differential, platelet count, blood chemistry and electrolyte studies, liver function tests, and, if the patient has a preexisting cardiac disorder or advanced stages of cancer, ECGs.

• Instruct patients in proper oral hygiene during treatment because the bone marrow suppressant effects of interferon may lead to microbial infection, delayed healing, and gingival bleeding. This drug may also decrease salivary flow.

• Advise patients to check with the doctor for instructions after missing a dose.

• Emphasize need to follow the doctor's instructions about taking and recording temperature and how and when to take acetaminophen.

• If patients will be self-administering drug, teach them how to prepare the injection and how to use a disposable syringe. Give information on drug stability.

• Tell patients drug may cause temporary loss of some hair, which should return when drug is withdrawn.

interferon alfa-n3
Alferon N

Pregnancy Risk Category: C

HOW SUPPLIED
Injection: 5 million units/ml in 1-ml vials

ACTION
A naturally occurring antiviral agent derived from human leukocytes. It attaches to membrane receptors and causes cellular changes, including increased protein synthesis.

ONSET, PEAK, DURATION
Unknown.

INDICATIONS & DOSAGE
Condylomata acuminata (genital or venereal warts) —
Adults: 0.05 ml/wart by intralesional injection. Treatment usually continues twice weekly for up to 8 weeks. Dosage should not exceed 0.5 ml (2.5 million units) per session.

ADVERSE REACTIONS
CNS: dizziness, light-headedness.
GI: dyspepsia, heartburn, vomiting, nausea.
Other: *acute hypersensitivity reactions with mild to moderate flulike syndrome (myalgia, fever, headache), arthralgia, back pain, malaise.*

INTERACTIONS
None reported.

CONTRAINDICATIONS
Contraindicated in patients hypersensitive to interferon alfa and in those with a history of anaphylactic reactions to murine immunoglobulin, egg protein, or neomycin.

NURSING CONSIDERATIONS
• Use cautiously in patients with debilitating illnesses (uncontrolled CHF, unstable angina, severe pulmonary disease, coagulation disorders, seizure disorders, severe myelosuppression, or diabetes mellitus with ketoacidosis) because of the association of interferon with a flulike syndrome.

• Although anaphylaxis hasn't been reported, be prepared to treat acute hypersensitivity reactions.

• Inject each lesion at the base of the wart, using a 30G needle.

• Administer acetaminophen for flu-like symptoms.

• Teach patients how to recognize symptoms of hypersensitivity: urticaria, tightness of the chest, wheezing, shortness of breath. Tell patients to report such symptoms immediately.

• Explain to patients that warts will continue to disappear after completion of 8 weeks of therapy and discontinuation of drug.

interferon beta-1b, recombinant
Betaseron

Pregnancy Risk Category: C

HOW SUPPLIED
Powder for injection: 9.6 million IU (0.3 mg)

ACTION
A naturally occurring antiviral and immunoregulatory agent derived from human fibroblasts. It attaches to membrane receptors and causes cellular changes, including increased protein synthesis.

ONSET, PEAK, DURATION
Unknown.

INDICATIONS & DOSAGE
To reduce the frequency of exacerbations in patients with relapsing-remitting multiple sclerosis –
Adults: 8 million IU (0.25 mg) S.C. every other day.

ADVERSE REACTIONS
CNS: depression, anxiety, emotional lability, depersonalization, ***suicidal tendencies,*** confusion, somnolence, headache, dizziness.
EENT: laryngitis.
GI: diarrhea, constipation.
GU: *menstrual disorders (bleeding or spotting, early or delayed menses, decreased days of menstrual flow, menorrhagia).*
Hematologic: *decreased WBC and absolute neutrophil counts.*
Respiratory: dyspnea.
Other: *flulike symptoms (fever, chills, malaise, myalgia, diaphoresis),* elevated ALT levels, elevated bilirubin levels, breast pain; *pelvic pain; inflammation, pain, and necrosis at injection site, lymphadenopathy.*

INTERACTIONS
None significant.

CONTRAINDICATIONS
Contraindicated in patients hypersensitive to interferon beta or human albumin.

NURSING CONSIDERATIONS
• Use cautiously in women of childbearing age. Inconclusive evidence exists about the drug's teratogenic effects, but it may be an abortifacient.
• To reconstitute, inject 1.2 ml of the supplied diluent (0.54% sodium chloride injection) into the vial and gently swirl to dissolve drug. Do not shake. Reconstituted solution will contain 8 million IU (0.25 mg)/ml. Discard vials that contain particulate material or discolored solution.
• Inject immediately after preparation.
• Rotate injection sites to minimize local reactions.
• Refrigerate the drug or reconstituted product (up to 3 hours) at 36° to 46° F (2° to 8° C). Do not freeze.
• Warn patients of childbearing age about dangers to the fetus. If a patient becomes pregnant during therapy, tell her to notify the doctor and stop taking the drug.
• Teach the patient how to self-administer S.C. injections, including solution preparation, use of aseptic technique, rotation of injection sites, and equipment disposal. Periodically reevaluate the patient's technique.
• Advise patient to take this drug at bedtime to minimize the mild flulike symptoms that commonly occur.

interferon gamma-1b
Actimmune

Pregnancy Risk Category: C

HOW SUPPLIED
Injection: 100 mcg (3 million units)/ vial

---

*Liquid form contains alcohol.   *Common* reactions are in italics; ***life-threatening,*** in bold italics.
**May contain tartrazine.

ACTION
Acts as an interleukin-type lymphokine. It has potent phagocyte-activating properties and enhances the oxidative metabolism of tissue macrophages.

ONSET, PEAK, DURATION
Onset and duration unknown. Peak levels occur within 7 hours after S.C. use.

INDICATIONS & DOSAGE
Chronic granulomatous disease –
Adults with a body surface area > 0.5 m²: 50 mcg/m² (1.5 million units/m²) S.C. three times weekly, preferably h.s. The preferred injection site is the deltoid or anterior thigh.
Adults with a body surface area ≤ 0.5 m²: 1.5 mcg/kg/dose three times weekly.

ADVERSE REACTIONS
CNS: fatigue, decreased mental status, gait disturbance.
GI: nausea, vomiting, diarrhea.
Hematologic: *myelosuppression* (at high doses).
Metabolic: elevated liver enzyme levels (at high doses).
Skin: rash.
Other: erythema or tenderness at the injection site, *flulike syndrome* (headache, fever, chills, myalgia, arthralgia).

INTERACTIONS
Myelosuppressive agents: possible additive myelosuppression. Monitor closely.
Zidovudine: increased plasma levels of zidovudine. Dosage adjustments are necessary when used at same time.

CONTRAINDICATIONS
Contraindicated in patients hypersensitive to the drug or to genetically engineered products derived from *Escherichia coli*.

NURSING CONSIDERATIONS
• Use cautiously in patients with cardiac disease, including arrhythmias, ischemia, or CHF. The flulike syndrome commonly seen at high doses of the drug can exacerbate these conditions.
• Use cautiously in patients with compromised CNS function or seizure disorders. CNS adverse reactions that may occur at high doses of the drug can exacerbate these conditions.
• Use myelosuppressive agents together with caution.
• Premedicate with acetaminophen to minimize symptoms at the beginning of therapy. Flulike symptoms tend to diminish with continued therapy.
• Discard unused portion. Each vial is for single-dose use only and does not contain a preservative.
• Refrigerate drug immediately. Vials must be stored at 36° to 46° F (2° to 8° C); do not freeze. Do not shake the vial; avoid excessive agitation. Discard vials that have been left at room temperature for more than 12 hours.
• If patients will be self-administering drug, teach them how to administer it and how to dispose of used needles, syringes, containers, and unused medication. Give them a copy of the "information for patients" included with the product and ensure that they understand the information.

---

sargramostim (granulocyte-macrophage colony-stimulating factor, GM-CSF)
Leukine, Prokine

Pregnancy Risk Category: C

HOW SUPPLIED
Powder for injection: 250 mcg, 500 mcg

ACTION
A glycoprotein containing 127 amino acids manufactured by recombinant DNA technology in a yeast expression system. It differs from the natural human granulocyte-macrophage colony-stimulating factor by substitution of leucine for arginine at position 23. The carbohydrate moiety may also be different. Sargramostim induces cellular responses by binding to specific receptors on cell surfaces of target cells.

ONSET, PEAK, DURATION
Onset occurs within 30 minutes. Peak levels occur in 2 hours. Duration unknown.

INDICATIONS & DOSAGE
Acceleration of hematopoietic reconstitution after autologous bone marrow transplantation in patients with non-Hodgkin's lymphoma or acute lymphoblastic leukemia or during autologous bone marrow transplantation in patients with Hodgkin's disease –
Adults: 250 mcg/m² daily for 21 consecutive days given as a 2-hour I.V. infusion beginning 2 to 4 hours after bone marrow transplantation.
Bone marrow transplantation failure or engraftment delay –
Adults: 250 mcg/m²/day for 14 days as a 2-hour I.V. infusion. Dose may be repeated after 7 days off of therapy. If engraftment still has not occurred, a third course of 500 mcg/m²/day I.V. for 14 days may be tried after another 7 days off therapy.

ADVERSE REACTIONS
CNS: malaise, CNS disorder.
CV: *blood dyscrasias,* hemorrhage.
GI: nausea, vomiting, diarrhea, anorexia, hemorrhage, GI disorder, stomatitis.
GU: urinary tract disorder, abnormal kidney function.
Hepatic: liver damage.
Respiratory: dyspnea, lung disorder.

Skin: alopecia, rash.
Other: fever, mucous membrane disorder, asthenia, edema, peripheral edema, *sepsis*.

INTERACTIONS
Corticosteroids, lithium: may potentiate myeloproliferative effects of sargramostim. Use cautiously.

CONTRAINDICATIONS
Contraindicated in patients with excessive leukemic myeloid blasts in bone marrow or peripheral blood and in those with hypersensitivity to the drug or any of its components or to yeast-derived products.

NURSING CONSIDERATIONS
● Use cautiously in patients with pre-existing cardiac disease, hypoxia, preexisting fluid retention, pulmonary infiltrates, CHF, or impaired renal or hepatic function because these conditions may be exacerbated.
● **I.V. use:** Reconstitute with 1 ml of sterile water for injection. Direct stream of sterile water against side of vial and *gently swirl* contents to minimize foaming. Avoid excessive or vigorous agitation or shaking. Dilute in 0.9% sodium chloride solution. If final concentration is below 10 mcg/ml, add human albumin at a final concentration of 0.1% to the sodium chloride solution *before* adding sargramostim to prevent adsorption to components of the delivery system. For a final concentration of 0.1% human albumin, add 1 mg human albumin/1 ml sodium chloride. Administer as soon as possible after mixing and no later than 6 hours after reconstituting.
● Discard any unused portion. Vials are for single-dose use and contain no preservatives. Do not reenter the vial.
● Don't add other medications to infusion solution because no data exist regarding solution compatibility and stability.
● Anticipate reducing dose by half or

---

*Liquid form contains alcohol.
**May contain tartrazine.

Common reactions are in italics; ***life-threatening***, in bold italics.

temporarily discontinue if severe adverse reactions occur and notify doctor. Therapy may be resumed when reactions abate. Transient rashes and local reactions at the injection site may occur; no serious allergic or anaphylactic reactions have been reported.

• Do not administer within 24 hours of last dose of chemotherapy or within 12 hours of last dose of radiotherapy because rapidly dividing progenitor cells may be sensitive to these cytotoxic therapies and drug would be ineffective.

• Monitor CBC with differential, including examination for presence of blast cells biweekly, as ordered. Stimulation of marrow precursors may result in rapid rise of WBC count. If blast cells appear or increase to 10% or more of the WBC count or if progression of the underlying disease occurs, know that therapy should be discontinued. If the absolute neutrophil count is above 20,000/mm^3 or if platelet count is above 50,000/mm^3, know that drug is temporarily discontinued or dose is reduced by half.

• Keep in mind that blood counts return to normal or baseline levels within 3 to 7 days after stopping treatment.

• Know that drug effect may be limited in patients who have received extensive radiotherapy to hematopoietic sites for treatment of primary disease in the abdomen or chest or who have been exposed to multiple agents (alkylating, anthracycline antibiotics, antimetabolites) before autologous bone marrow transplantation.

• Be aware that sargramostim is effective in accelerating myeloid recovery in patients receiving bone marrow purged from monoclonal antibodies.

• Keep in mind that the drug can act as a growth factor for any tumor type, particularly myeloid malignancies.

• Refrigerate the sterile powder, reconstituted solution, and diluted solution for injection. Don't freeze or shake. Don't use after expiration date.

80

Ophthalmic anti-infectives

bacitracin
chloramphenicol
ciprofloxacin hydrochloride
erythromycin
gentamicin sulfate
idoxuridine
natamycin
norfloxacin
ofloxacin 0.3%
polymyxin B sulfate
silver nitrate 1%
sulfacetamide sodium 10%
sulfacetamide sodium 15%
sulfacetamide sodium 30%
sulfisoxazole diolamine
tetracycline hydrochloride
tobramycin
trifluridine
vidarabine

COMBINATION PRODUCTS

BLEPHAMIDE S.O.P. STERILE OPHTHALMIC OINTMENT: sulfacetamide sodium 10% and prednisolone acetate 0.2%.

CETAPRED OINTMENT: sulfacetamide sodium 10% and prednisolone acetate 0.25%.

CHLOROMYCETIN-HYDROCORTISONE OPHTHALMIC: chloramphenicol 0.25% and hydrocortisone acetate 0.5% (as the prepared solution).

CORTISPORIN OPHTHALMIC OINTMENT: polymyxin B sulfate 10,000 units, bacitracin zinc 400 units, neomycin sulfate 0.35%, and hydrocortisone 1%.

CORTISPORIN OPHTHALMIC SUSPENSION: polymyxin B sulfate 10,000 units, neomycin sulfate 0.35%, and hydrocortisone 1%.

ISOPTO CETAPRED: sulfacetamide sodium 10% and prednisolone acetate 0.25%.

MAXITROL OINTMENT/OPHTHALMIC SUSPENSION: dexamethasone 0.1%, neomycin sulfate 0.35%, and polymyxin B sulfate 10,000 units.

METIMYD OPHTHALMIC OINTMENT/SUSPENSION: sulfacetamide sodium 10% and prednisolone acetate 0.5%.

MYCITRACIN OPHTHALMIC OINTMENT: polymyxin B sulfate 5,000 units, neomycin sulfate 3.5 mg, and bacitracin 500 units.

NEOSPORIN OPHTHALMIC: polymyxin B sulfate 10,000 units, neomycin sulfate 1.75 mg, and gramicidin 0.025 mg.

NEOSPORIN OPHTHALMIC OINTMENT: polymyxin B sulfate 10,000 units, neomycin sulfate 3.5 mg, and bacitracin zinc 400 units/g.

NEOTAL: polymyxin B sulfate 5,000 units, neomycin sulfate 5 mg, and bacitracin zinc 400 units.

OPHTHOCORT: chloramphenicol 1.0%, polymyxin B sulfate 10,000 units, and hydrocortisone acetate 0.5%.

OPTIMYD: prednisolone phosphate 0.5% and sulfacetamide sodium 10%.

POLYSPORIN OPHTHALMIC OINTMENT: polymyxin B sulfate 10,000 units and bacitracin zinc 500 units.

POLYTRIM OPHTHALMIC: trimethoprim sulfate 1 mg and polymyxin B sulfate 10,000 units/ml.

PRED G: prednisolone acetate 0.6%, gentamicin sulfate equivalent to gentamicin base 0.3%, chlorobutanol 0.5%, petrolatum, white petrolatum, mineral oil, and lanolin alcohol.

STATROL: neomycin sulfate 3.5 mg and polymyxin B sulfate 10,000 units.

TOBRADEX: dexamethasone 0.1%, tobramycin 0.3%, chlorobutanol 0.5%, mineral oil, and white petrolatum.

VASOCIDIN OPHTHALMIC OINTMENT: sulfacetamide sodium 10%,

---

*Liquid form contains alcohol.
**May contain tartrazine.

*Common reactions are in italics; **life-threatening,** in bold italics.

prednisolone acetate 0.5%, and phenylephrine hydrochloride 0.125%.
VASOCIDIN OPHTHALMIC SOLUTION: sulfacetamide sodium 10% and prednisolone phosphate 0.25%.
VASOSULF: sulfacetamide sodium 15% and phenylephrine hydrochloride 0.125%.

bacitracin
Pregnancy Risk Category: NR

HOW SUPPLIED
Ophthalmic ointment: 500 units/g

ACTION
Inhibits protein synthesis. Bactericidal or bacteriostatic, depending on concentration and infection.

ONSET, PEAK, DURATION
Unknown. Systemic absorption is negligible.

INDICATIONS & DOSAGE
Ocular infections –
Adults and children: small amount of ointment applied into conjunctival sac several times daily or p.r.n. until favorable response is observed.

ADVERSE REACTIONS
EENT: slowed corneal wound healing, temporary visual haze.
Other: overgrowth of nonsusceptible organisms.

INTERACTIONS
Heavy metals (for example, silver nitrate): inactivation of bacitracin. Don't use together.

CONTRAINDICATIONS
Contraindicated in patients hypersensitive to the drug and in atopic patients.

NURSING CONSIDERATIONS
• Ophthalmic ointment may be stored at room temperature.

• Tell patients to clean eye area of excessive exudate before application.
• Teach patients how to apply; tell them only a small amount of ointment is needed and that it may cause blurred vision. Advise patients to wash hands before and after administering and not to touch tip of tube to eye or surrounding tissue.
• Advise patients to watch for signs of sensitivity, such as itching lids, swelling, or constant burning. Tell patients who develop such signs to stop drug and notify doctor immediately.
• Tell patients not to share eye medications, washcloths, or towels with family members. If anyone develops the same symptoms, the doctor should be notified.
• Stress importance of compliance with recommended therapy.

chloramphenicol
AK-Chlor, Chloromycetin
Ophthalmic, Chloroptic, Chloroptic
S.O.P., Chlorsig‡, Fenicol†, Isopto
Fenicol†, Ophthoclor Ophthalmic,
Pentamycetin†

Pregnancy Risk Category: NR

HOW SUPPLIED
Ophthalmic ointment: 1%
Ophthalmic solution: 0.5%
Powder for ophthalmic solution: 25 mg

ACTION
Inhibits protein synthesis. Bacteriostatic or bactericidal, depending on concentration.

ONSET, PEAK, DURATION
Unknown. Systemic absorption occurs, but has not been characterized; higher levels occur with ophthalmic ointment.

INDICATIONS & DOSAGE
Surface bacterial infection involving conjunctiva or cornea –

---
†Available in Canada only.   ‡Available in Australia only.   ◊Available OTC.

Adults and children: 1 or 2 drops of solution instilled in eye q 3 to 6 hours or more frequently, if necessary. Or, a small amount of ointment applied to lower conjunctival sac q 3 to 6 hours or more frequently, if necessary. Continued until condition improves.

ADVERSE REACTIONS
EENT: optic atrophy in children, stinging or burning of eye after instillation, blurred vision (with ointment).
Hematologic: *bone marrow hypoplasia with prolonged use, aplastic anemia.*
Other: overgrowth of nonsusceptible organisms; hypersensitivity reactions, including itching and burning eye, dermatitis, angioedema.

INTERACTIONS
None significant.

CONTRAINDICATIONS
Contraindicated in patients hypersensitive to the drug.

NURSING CONSIDERATIONS
• If chloramphenicol drops are to be given every hour, then tapered, follow order closely to ensure adequate anterior chamber levels.
• Reconstitute powder for ophthalmic solution with supplied diluent. Use 5 ml of diluent to make a 0.5% solution, 10 ml of diluent to make a 0.25% solution, or 15 ml to make a 0.16% solution.
• If patients have more than a superficial infection, anticipate using systemic therapy as well.
• Store in tightly closed, light-resistant container.
• Teach patients how to instill drops or apply ointment. Advise them to wash hands before and after administering ointment or solution, and warn them not to touch tip of applicator to eye or surrounding tissue.
• Tell patients to clean eye area of excessive exudate before application.

• Instruct patients to apply light finger pressure on lacrimal sac for 1 minute after drops are instilled.
• Tell patients not to share eye medications, washcloths, or towels with family members. If anyone develops the same symptoms, the doctor should be notified.
• Tell patients to watch for signs of sensitivity, such as itching lids, swelling, or constant burning. Patients who develop such signs should stop drug and notify the doctor immediately.
• Tell patient to notify the doctor if no improvement occurs in 3 days. Not for long-term use.
• Stress importance of compliance with recommended therapy.

---

ciprofloxacin hydrochloride
Ciloxan

Pregnancy Risk Category: C

HOW SUPPLIED
Ophthalmic solution: 0.3% (base) in 2.5- and 5-ml containers

ACTION
Inhibits bacterial DNA gyrase, an enzyme necessary for bacterial replication. Bacteriostatic or bactericidal, depending on concentration.

ONSET, PEAK, DURATION
Unknown. Systemic absorption is negligible.

INDICATIONS & DOSAGE
Corneal ulcers caused by Pseudomonas aeruginosa, Staphylococcus aureus, S. epidermidis, Streptococcus pneumoniae, *and possibly* Serratia marcescens *and* Streptococcus viridans—
Adults and children over 12 years: 2 drops in the affected eye q 15 minutes for the first 6 hours; then 2 drops q 30 minutes for the remainder of the first day. On day 2, 2 drops hourly. On days 3 to 14, 2 drops q 4 hours.

---

*Liquid form contains alcohol.   *Common* reactions are in italics; *life-threatening,* in bold italics.
**May contain tartrazine.

Bacterial conjunctivitis caused by Staphylococcus aureus *and* S. epidermidis *and possibly* Streptococcus pneumoniae —
Adults and children over 12 years: 1 or 2 drops into the conjunctival sac of the affected eye q 2 hours while awake, for the first 2 days. Then 1 or 2 drops q 4 hours while awake, for the next 5 days.

ADVERSE REACTIONS
EENT: *local burning or discomfort, white crystalline precipitate* (in the superficial portion of the corneal defect in patients with corneal ulcers), *margin crusting, crystals or scales, foreign body sensation, itching, conjunctival hyperemia.*

INTERACTIONS
None significant.

CONTRAINDICATIONS
Contraindicated in patients with a history of hypersensitivity to ciprofloxacin or other fluoroquinolone antibiotics.

NURSING CONSIDERATIONS
• Be aware it's unknown if drug is excreted in breast milk after application to the eye; however, systemically administered ciprofloxacin has been detected in human milk. Use caution.
• Discontinue drug at the first sign of hypersensitivity reactions, such as skin rash, and notify doctor. Serious hypersensitivity reactions, including anaphylaxis, have occurred in patients receiving systemic fluoroquinolone therapy.
• If corneal epithelium is still compromised after 14 days of treatment, be prepared to continue therapy, as ordered.
• Institute appropriate therapy if superinfection occurs. Prolonged use may result in overgrowth of nonsusceptible organisms, including fungi.

• Tell patients to clean eye area of excessive exudate before instilling.
• Teach patients how to instill drops. Advise them to wash hands before and after administering solution and not to touch tip of dropper to eye or surrounding tissues.
• Instruct patient to apply light finger pressure on lacrimal sac for 1 minute after drops are instilled.
• Tell patients not to share eye medications, washcloths, or towels with family members. If anyone develops the same symptoms, the doctor should be notified.
• Stress importance of compliance with recommended therapy.

---

erythromycin
Ilotycin Ophthalmic Ointment
Pregnancy Risk Category: NR

HOW SUPPLIED
Ophthalmic ointment: 0.5%

ACTION
Inhibits protein synthesis. Bacteriostatic, but may be bactericidal in high concentrations or against highly susceptible organisms.

ONSET, PEAK, DURATION
Unknown. Systemic absorption is negligible.

INDICATIONS & DOSAGE
Acute and chronic conjunctivitis, trachoma, other eye infections —
Adults and children: 1 cm in length applied directly to the infected eye up to 6 times daily, depending on severity of infection.
Prophylaxis of ophthalmia neonatorum due to Neisseria gonorrhoeae *or* Chlamydia trachomatis —
Neonates: a ribbon of ointment approximately 1 cm long applied in the lower conjunctival sac of each eye shortly after birth.

Available in Canada only.   ‡Available in Australia only.   ◊ Available OTC.

ADVERSE REACTIONS
Eye: slowed corneal wound healing, blurred vision.
Other: overgrowth of nonsusceptible organisms with long-term use; hypersensitivity reactions, including itching and burning eyes, urticaria, dermatitis.

INTERACTIONS
None significant.

CONTRAINDICATIONS
Contraindicated in patients hypersensitive to the drug.

NURSING CONSIDERATIONS
• For prophylaxis of ophthalmia neonatorum, ointment should be applied no later than 1 hour after birth. Used in neonates born either by vaginal delivery or by cesarean section. Gently massage the eyelids for 1 minute to spread the ointment.
• Be aware that drug has a limited antibacterial spectrum.
• To be used only when sensitivity studies show it is effective against infecting organisms. Not for use in infections of unknown etiology.
• Store at room temperature in tightly closed, light-resistant container.
• Tell patients to clean eye area of excessive exudate before application
• Teach patients how to apply. Advise them to wash hands before and after administering ointment, and warn them not to touch tip of applicator to eye or surrounding tissue.
• Instruct patient to apply light finger pressure on lacrimal sac for 1 minute after administering.
• Warn patients that ointment may cause blurred vision.
• Advise patients to watch for signs of sensitivity, such as itching lids, swelling, or constant burning. Tell patients who develop such signs to stop drug and notify the doctor immediately.
• Tell patients not to share eye medications, washcloths, or towels with family members. If anyone develops the same symptoms, the doctor should be notified.
• Stress importance of compliance with recommended therapy.

---

gentamicin sulfate
Garamycin Ophthalmic, Genoptic, Gentacidin, Gentak, Ocu-Gent

Pregnancy Risk Category: C

HOW SUPPLIED
Ophthalmic ointment: 0.3% (base)
Ophthalmic solution: 0.3% (base)

ACTION
Unknown. Thought to inhibit protein synthesis and is usually bactericidal.

ONSET, PEAK, DURATION
Unknown. Only small amounts of the drug are absorbed systemically.

INDICATIONS & DOSAGE
External ocular infections (conjunctivitis, keratoconjunctivitis, corneal ulcers, blepharitis, blepharoconjunctivitis, meibomianitis, and dacryocystitis) caused by susceptible organisms, especially Pseudomonas aeruginosa, Proteus, Klebsiella pneumoniae, Escherichia coli, *and other gram-negative organisms —*
Adults and children: 1 to 2 drops instilled in eye q 4 hours. In severe infections, up to 2 drops q hour. Alternatively, ointment applied to lower conjunctival sac b.i.d. or t.i.d.

ADVERSE REACTIONS
EENT: burning, stinging, or blurred vision (with ointment), transient irritation (from solution).
Other: hypersensitivity reactions; overgrowth of nonsusceptible organisms with long-term use.
    Systemic absorption from excessive use may cause systemic toxicities.

---

*Liquid form contains alcohol.
**May contain tartrazine.
Common reactions are in italics; **life-threatening,** in bold italics.

INTERACTIONS
None significant.

CONTRAINDICATIONS
Contraindicated in patients hypersensitive to the drug.

NURSING CONSIDERATIONS
• Use cautiously in patients with history of sensitivity to aminoglycosides as cross-sensitivity may occur.
• Have culture taken before giving drug. Therapy may begin before culture results are known.
• If ophthalmic gentamicin is administered concomitantly with systemic gentamicin, carefully monitor serum gentamicin levels.
• Know that solution is not for injection in conjunctiva or anterior chamber of the eye.
• Store away from heat.
• Tell patients to clean eye area of excessive exudate before instilling.
• Teach patients how to instill drops or apply ointment. Advise them to wash hands before and after administering ointment or solution and not to touch tip of dropper or tube to eye or surrounding tissues.
• Instruct patient to apply light finger pressure on lacrimal sac for 1 minute after drops are instilled.
• Tell patients to watch for signs of sensitivity, such as itching lids, swelling, or constant burning. Tell patients who develop such signs to stop drug and notify the doctor immediately.
• Tell patients not to share eye medications, washcloths, or towels with family members. If anyone develops the same symptoms, the doctor should be notified.
• Stress importance of following recommended therapy. *Pseudomonas* infections can cause complete vision loss within 24 hours if infection is not controlled.

idoxuridine (IDU)
Herplex, Stoxil
Pregnancy Risk Category: NR

HOW SUPPLIED
Ophthalmic ointment: 0.5%
Ophthalmic solution: 0.1%

ACTION
Interferes with DNA synthesis.

ONSET, PEAK, DURATION
Unknown. Systemic absorption is unlikely.

INDICATIONS & DOSAGE
Herpes simplex keratitis –
Adults and children: 1 drop of solution instilled into conjunctival sac q hour during day and q 2 hours at night, or 1 cm strip of ointment applied to conjunctival sac q 4 hours or 5 times daily, with last dose h.s.

ADVERSE REACTIONS
EENT: temporary visual haze; blurred vision (with ointment); irritation, pain, burning, or inflammation of eye; mild edema of eyelid or cornea; photophobia; small punctate defects in corneal epithelium; corneal ulceration; slowed corneal wound healing (with ointment).
Other: hypersensitivity reactions.

INTERACTIONS
Boric acid: precipitate formation; increased risk of ocular toxicity. Avoid concomitant use.

CONTRAINDICATIONS
Contraindicated in patients with hypersensitivity to the drug.

NURSING CONSIDERATIONS
• Do not mix idoxuridine with other topical eye medications.
• Keep in mind that drug is not for long-term use. Therapy should not continue longer than 21 days.

• Refrigerate idoxuridine 0.1% solution in a tightly closed, light-resistant container.

• Advise patient not to use old solution; causes ocular burning and has no antiviral activity.

• Tell patient to clean eye area of excessive exudate before application.

• Teach patients how to instill drops or apply ointment. Advise them to wash hands before and after administering, and warn them not to touch tip of dropper to eye or surrounding tissue.

• Instruct patient to apply light finger pressure on lacrimal sac for 1 minute after drops are instilled.

• Advise patients to watch for signs of sensitivity, such as itching lids, swelling, or constant burning. Tell patients who develop such signs to stop drug and notify the doctor immediately.

• Also instruct patients to notify their doctor if symptoms do not improve in 7 days; drug will need to be discontinued and alternative therapy begun.

• Tell patients not to share eye medications, washcloths, or towels with family members. If anyone develops the same symptoms, the doctor should be notified.

• Tell patients to minimize photophobia by wearing sunglasses and avoiding prolonged exposure to sunlight.

• Stress importance of compliance with recommended therapy.

natamycin
Natacyn

Pregnancy Risk Category: NR

HOW SUPPLIED
Ophthalmic suspension: 5%

ACTION
Increases fungal cell-membrane permeability.

ONSET, PEAK, DURATION
Unknown.

INDICATIONS & DOSAGE
Fungal keratitis—
Adults: initially, 1 drop instilled in conjunctival sac q 1 to 2 hours. After 3 to 4 days, dosage reduced to 1 drop six to eight times daily.
Blepharitis or fungal conjunctivitis—
Adults: 1 drop instilled q 4 to 6 hours.

ADVERSE REACTIONS
EENT: ocular edema, hyperemia.

INTERACTIONS
None significant.

CONTRAINDICATIONS
Contraindicated in patients hypersensitive to the drug.

NURSING CONSIDERATIONS
• Administer drug as ordered for 14 to 21 days, or until active disease subsides. Be prepared to reduce dosage gradually at 4- to 7-day intervals to ensure that organism has been eliminated. If infection does not improve within 7 to 10 days of therapy, clinical and laboratory reevaluation is recommended.

• Shake well before use. Refrigerate or store at room temperature.

• Know that drug is the only antifungal available as ophthalmic preparation.

• Tell patient to clean eye area of excessive exudate before application.

• Teach patients how to instill drops. Advise them to wash hands before and after administering solution and not to touch tip of dropper to eye or surrounding tissue.

• Instruct patient to apply light finger pressure on lacrimal sac for 1 minute after drops are instilled.

• Tell patients not to share eye medications, washcloths, or towels with family members. If anyone develops the same symptoms, the doctor should be notified.

---

*Liquid form contains alcohol.
**May contain tartrazine.

Common reactions are in italics; *life-threatening,* in bold italics.

- Stress importance of compliance with recommended therapy.

---

norfloxacin
Chibroxin

Pregnancy Risk Category: C

HOW SUPPLIED
Ophthalmic solution: 0.3% in 5-ml containers

ACTION
Inhibits bacterial DNA gyrase, an enzyme necessary for bacterial replication. Bacteriostatic or bactericidal, depending on concentration.

ONSET, PEAK, DURATION
Unknown. Systemic absorption is negligible.

INDICATIONS & DOSAGE
Conjunctivitis caused by susceptible strains of bacteria —
Adults and children 1 year and over: 1 or 2 drops in the affected eye q.i.d. for up to 7 days. If condition warrants, 2 drops may be applied q 2 hours during the waking hours of the first day of treatment.

ADVERSE REACTIONS
EENT: local burning or discomfort, itching, chemosis, photophobia, conjunctival hyperemia.

INTERACTIONS
Caffeine, cyclosporine, theophylline: impaired metabolism of these drugs with systemic norfloxacin. It's unknown if ophthalmic norfloxacin will have this effect. Monitor closely.
Oral anticoagulants: enhanced activity with systemic norfloxacin. It's unknown if ophthalmic norfloxacin will have this effect. Monitor closely.

CONTRAINDICATIONS
Contraindicated in patients with a history of hypersensitivity to norfloxacin or other fluoroquinolone antibiotics. Drug shouldn't be injected into the eye.

NURSING CONSIDERATIONS
- Be aware that drug is indicated for treating conjunctivitis when caused by susceptible bacteria. Known susceptible strains include *Acinetobacter calcoaceticus, Aeromonas hydrophila, Haemophilus influenzae, Proteus mirabilis, Serratia marcescens, Staphylococcus aureus, S. epidermidis, S. warnerii,* and *Streptococcus pneumoniae.*
- Discontinue drug at the first sign of hypersensitivity, such as skin rash and notify doctor. Serious hypersensitivity reactions, including anaphylaxis, have occurred in patients receiving systemic fluoroquinolone therapy.
- Institute appropriate therapy if superinfection occurs. Prolonged use may result in overgrowth of nonsusceptible organisms, including fungi.
- Know that although systemically administered fluoroquinolones have been shown to cause arthropathy in young animals, ophthalmic norfloxacin has not produced this adverse effect.
- Tell patients to clean eye area of excessive exudate before application.
- Teach patients how to instill drops. Advise them to wash hands before and after administering and not to touch the tip of the tube or dropper to eye or surrounding tissue.
- Tell patients not to share eye medications, washcloths, or towels with family members. If anyone develops the same symptoms, the doctor should be notified.
- Stress the importance of compliance with recommended therapy.

---

ofloxacin 0.3%
Ocuflox

Pregnancy Risk Category: C

HOW SUPPLIED
Ophthalmic solution: 0.3%

ACTION
Bactericidal; inhibits bacterial DNA gyrase, an enzyme necessary for bacterial replication.

ONSET, PEAK, DURATION
Unknown.

INDICATIONS & DOSAGE
Conjunctivitis caused by Staphylococcus aureus, Staph. epidermidis, Streptococcus pneumoniae, Enterobacter cloacae, Haemophilus influenzae, Proteus mirabilis, *and* Pseudomonas aeruginosa —
Adults and children: 1 to 2 drops in the conjunctival sac q 2 to 4 hours daily for the first 2 days, and then four times daily for up to 5 additional days.

ADVERSE REACTIONS
EENT: *transient ocular burning or discomfort,* stinging, redness, itching, photophobia, lacrimation, eye dryness.
Other: dizziness (rare).

INTERACTIONS
None reported.

CONTRAINDICATIONS
Contraindicated in patients with history of hypersensitivity to ofloxacin, to other fluoroquinolones, or to any of the components of this drug and in breast-feeding women.

NURSING CONSIDERATIONS
• Know that the drug should not be injected subconjunctivally or introduced directly into the anterior chamber of the eye.
• Be aware that drug should be discontinued if improvement does not occur within 7 days. Prolonged use may result in overgrowth of nonsusceptible organisms, including fungi.
• If an allergic reaction occurs, tell patient to discontinue the drug and call the doctor. Serious acute hypersensitivity reactions may require emergency treatment.
• Teach patients how to instill drops. Advise them to wash hands before and after instilling solution, and warn them not to touch tip of the dropper to eye or surrounding tissue.
• Advise patients to apply light finger pressure on lacrimal sac for 1 minute after drug instillation.
• Stress the importance of compliance with recommended therapy.
• Warn patient not to use leftover medication for a new eye infection.
• Remind patients to discard drug when no longer needed.

polymyxin B sulfate
Pregnancy Risk Category: NR

HOW SUPPLIED
Ophthalmic sterile powder for solution: 500,000-unit vials to be reconstituted to 20 to 50 ml

ACTION
Bactericidal. Alters the osmotic barrier of the bacteria cell membrane.

ONSET, PEAK, DURATION
Unknown. Systemic absorption is negligible.

INDICATIONS & DOSAGE
Used alone or in combination with other agents to treat superficial eye infections involving the conjunctiva and cornea resulting from infection with Pseudomonas *or other gram-negative organism* —
Adults and children: 1 to 3 drops of 0.1% to 0.25% (10,000 to 25,000 units/ml) instilled q hour. Interval increased according to patient response; or up to 10,000 units subconjunctivally daily. Not to exceed 2 million units daily.

---

*Liquid form contains alcohol.   *Common* reactions are in italics; *life-threatening,* in bold italics.
**May contain tartrazine.

ADVERSE REACTIONS
EENT: eye irritation, conjunctivitis.
Other: overgrowth of nonsusceptible organisms, hypersensitivity reactions (local burning, itching).

INTERACTIONS
None significant.

CONTRAINDICATIONS
Contraindicated in patients hypersensitive to the drug.

NURSING CONSIDERATIONS
• Reconstitute carefully to ensure correct drug concentration in solution.
• Know that drug is often used in combination with neomycin sulfate.
• Be aware that drug is one of the most effective antibiotics against gram-negative organisms, especially *Pseudomonas.*
• In severe, life-threatening *Pseudomonas* infections, know that polymyxin B may be used as an ocular irrigant.
• Tell patients to clean eye area of excessive exudate before application.
• Teach patients how to instill drops . Advise them to wash hands before and after administering solution, and warn them not to touch tip of dropper to eye or surrounding tissue.
• Instruct patient to apply light finger pressure on lacrimal sac for 1 minute after drops are instilled.
• Advise patients to watch for signs of sensitivity, such as itching lids, swelling, or constant burning. Tell patients who develop such signs to stop drug and notify the doctor immediately.
• Tell patients not to share eye medications, washcloths, or towels with family members. If anyone develops the same symptoms, the doctor should be notified.
• Stress importance of compliance with recommended therapy.

---

silver nitrate 1%
Pregnancy Risk Category: NR

HOW SUPPLIED
Ophthalmic solution: 1%

ACTION
Causes protein denaturation, which prevents gonorrheal ophthalmia neonatorum. Bacteriostatic, germicidal, and astringent.

ONSET, PEAK, DURATION
Unknown. Systemic absorption is negligible.

INDICATIONS & DOSAGE
Prevention of gonorrheal ophthalmia neonatorum –
Neonates: clean lids thoroughly; 2 drops of 1% solution instilled into the lower conjunctival sac of each eye at the angle of the nasal bridge and eyes, no later than 1 hour after delivery.

ADVERSE REACTIONS
EENT: periorbital edema, temporary staining of lids and surrounding tissue, *conjunctivitis.*

INTERACTIONS
Bacitracin: inactivation of silver nitrate. Don't use together.

CONTRAINDICATIONS
None.

NURSING CONSIDERATIONS
• Always wash hands before instilling solution.
• Apply within 1 hour of birth, as ordered. Used in neonates born either by vaginal delivery or by cesarean section.
• Be aware that instillation may be delayed slightly to allow neonate to bond with mother.
• Don't use repeatedly.
• Don't irrigate eyes after instillation.

• Never use concentrations greater than 1% in the eye.
• If a concentrated solution is accidentally used in eye, promptly irrigate with 0.9% sodium chloride solution to prevent severe eye irritation or blindness.
• Handle carefully. Solution may stain skin and utensils.
• Know that prophylaxis against gonococcal ophthalmia neonatorum is legally required for neonates in most states. Because of a high incidence of conjunctivitis (> 90%), many clinicians prefer antibiotic ointments such as erythromycin as an alternative.
• Store wax ampules away from light and heat.

---

sulfacetamide sodium 10%
Bleph-10 Liquifilm Ophthalmic, Cetamide Ophthalmic, Sodium Sulamyd 10% Ophthalmic, Sulf-10 Ophthalmic

sulfacetamide sodium 15%
Isopto Cetamide Ophthalmic

sulfacetamide sodium 30%
Sodium Sulamyd 30% Ophthalmic

Pregnancy Risk Category: NR

HOW SUPPLIED
Ophthalmic ointment: 10%
Ophthalmic solution: 10%, 15%, 30%

ACTION
Bacteriostatic although in high concentrations may be bactericidal. Prevents uptake of PABA, a metabolite of bacterial folic acid synthesis.

ONSET, PEAK, DURATION
Unknown. Systemic absorption is negligible.

INDICATIONS & DOSAGE
Inclusion conjunctivitis, corneal ulcers, trachoma, chlamydial infection—

Adults and children: 1 to 2 drops of 10% solution instilled into lower conjunctival sac q 2 to 3 hours during day, less often at night; or 1 to 2 drops of 15% solution instilled into lower conjunctival sac q 1 to 2 hours initially. Interval increased as condition responds; or 1 drop of 30% solution instilled into lower conjunctival sac q 2 hours. 1.25 to 2.5 cm 10% ointment applied into conjunctival sac q.i.d. and h.s. Ointment may be used at night along with drops during the day.

ADVERSE REACTIONS
EENT: slowed corneal wound healing (ointment), *pain on instilling eyedrop,* headache or brow pain, photophobia.
Other: hypersensitivity reactions (including itching or burning), overgrowth of nonsusceptible organisms, **Stevens-Johnson syndrome.**

INTERACTIONS
Gentamicin (ophthalmic): in vitro antagonism. Avoid using together.
Local anesthetics (procaine, tetracaine), PABA derivatives: decreased sulfacetamide sodium action. Wait ½ to 1 hour after instilling anesthetic or PABA derivative before instilling sulfacetamide.
Silver preparations: precipitate formation. Avoid using together.

CONTRAINDICATIONS
• Contraindicated in patients hypersensitive to sulfonamides.
• Not recommended for children under 2 months.

NURSING CONSIDERATIONS
• Keep in mind that drug has been replaced by other antibiotics in treating major ocular infections; still used in minor ocular infections.
• Be aware that drug is often used with oral tetracycline in treating trachoma and inclusion conjunctivitis.

---

*Liquid form contains alcohol.   Common reactions are in italics; **life-threatening,** in bold italics.
**May contain tartrazine.

- Store in tightly closed, light-resistant container away from heat.
- Tell patient to clean eye area of excessive exudate before instilling.
- Teach patients how to instill drops or apply ointment. Advise them to wash hands before and after administering ointment or solution and not to touch tip of dropper to eye or surrounding tissues.
- Instruct patient to apply light finger pressure on lacrimal sac for 1 minute after drops are instilled.
- Warn patients that eyedrops burn slightly.
- Advise patients to watch for signs of sensitivity, such as itching lids, swelling, or constant burning. Tell patients who develop such signs to stop drug and notify the doctor immediately.
- Tell patient to wait at least 5 minutes before administering other eyedrops.
- Warn patients that solution may stain clothing.
- Tell patients to minimize photophobia by wearing sunglasses and avoiding prolonged exposure to sunlight.
- Advise patient not to use discolored solution.
- Tell patients not to share eye medications, washcloths, or towels with family members. If anyone develops the same symptoms, the doctor should be notified.
- Stress importance of compliance with recommended therapy.

sulfisoxazole diolamine
Gantrisin Ophthalmic Solution
Pregnancy Risk Category: C

HOW SUPPLIED
Ophthalmic solution: 4%

ACTION
Inhibits bacterial synthesis of dihydrofolic acid by competing with PABA, thus exerting a bacteriostatic effect.

ONSET, PEAK, DURATION
Unknown.

INDICATIONS & DOSAGE
Conjunctivitis, corneal ulcers, and other superficial ocular infections; adjunct in systemic sulfonamide therapy of trachoma –
Adults and children: 2 to 3 drops instilled in the conjunctival sac three or more times daily.

ADVERSE REACTIONS
EENT: *ocular irritation, itching, chemosis.*

INTERACTIONS
Gentamicin sulfate: antagonism may occur. Do not administer together.
Silver-containing preparations: incompatible. Do not administer together.

CONTRAINDICATIONS
Contraindicated in patients with hypersensitivity to this drug or other sulfonamides, in infants under age 2 months, during pregnancy at term, and in breast-feeding women.

NURSING CONSIDERATIONS
- Teach patients how to instill drops. Advise them to wash hands before and after instilling solution, and warn them not to touch the tip of the dropper to the eye or surrounding tissue.
- Advise patients to apply light finger pressure on lacrimal sac for 1 minute after drug instillation.
- Stress the importance of compliance with recommended therapy.
- Warn patient not to use leftover medication for a new eye infection.
- Remind patients to discard drug when no longer needed.

tetracycline hydrochloride
Achromycin Ophthalmic
Pregnancy Risk Category: B

HOW SUPPLIED
Ophthalmic suspension: 1%
Ophthalmic ointment: 1%

ACTION
Inhibits protein synthesis. Bactericidal or bacteriostatic, depending upon concentration.

ONSET, PEAK, DURATION
Unknown. Systemic absorption is negligible.

INDICATIONS & DOSAGE
Superficial ocular infections–
Adults and children: a small amount of the ointment applied q 2 to 12 hours or 2 drops instilled in eye b.i.d. to q.i.d., or more often, depending on severity of infection.
Inclusive conjunctivitis–
Adults and children: 2 drops instilled in each eye or small amount of ointment applied to each eye b.i.d., t.i.d., or q.i.d. Continued for at least 3 weeks.
Trachoma–
Adults and children: 2 drops instilled in each eye b.i.d., t.i.d., or q.i.d. continued for at least 3 weeks or a small amount of the ointment applied twice daily to each eye for 2 months.
Prophylaxis of ophthalmia neonatorum–
Neonates: 1 to 2 drops of the suspension instilled or 1 to 2 cm of the ointment applied into the lower conjunctival sac of each eye shortly after delivery.

ADVERSE REACTIONS
EENT: itching, blurred vision (with ointment).
Other: hypersensitivity reactions (eye itching and dermatitis); overgrowth of nonsusceptible organisms with long-term use.

INTERACTIONS
None significant.

CONTRAINDICATIONS
Contraindicated in patients hypersensitive to the drug.

NURSING CONSIDERATIONS
• For prophylaxis of ophthalmia neonatorum, apply ointment no later than 1 hour after birth, as ordered. Used in neonates born by either vaginal delivery or cesarean section.
• Know that ophthalmic ointment may be used with suspension to provide prolonged drug contact with affected area at night.
• Although unlikely, be aware drug can cause permanent staining of teeth if used in children under age 8.
• Store in tightly closed, light-resistant container.
• Tell patients or family that trachoma therapy should continue for 1 to 2 months or longer. Trachoma may cause blindness if left untreated or if not treated properly.
• Tell patients that gnats and flies are vectors of *Chlamydia trachomatis.* Warn patients with trachoma not to let gnats or flies settle around eye area. Also explain that infection is spread by direct contact, so handwashing is essential to prevent spread. Severe trachoma may require oral therapy as well.
• Remind patients to shake suspension well before use.
• Tell patients to clean eye area of excessive exudate before applications.
• Teach patients how to instill drops or apply ointment. Advise them to wash hands before and after administering ointment or solution and not to touch tip of dropper to eye or surrounding tissue.
• Instruct patient to apply light finger pressure on lacrimal sac for 1 minute after drops are instilled.
• Tell patients to watch for signs of sensitivity, such as itching lids, swelling, or constant burning. Tell patients who develop such signs to stop drug and notify the doctor immediately.

---

*Liquid form contains alcohol.   *Common* reactions are in italics; ***life-threatening,*** in bold italics.
**May contain tartrazine.

• Tell patients not to share eye medications, washcloths, or towels with family members. If anyone develops the same symptoms, the doctor should be notified.

• Stress importance of compliance with recommended therapy.

---

tobramycin
Tobrex

Pregnancy Risk Category: B

HOW SUPPLIED
Ophthalmic ointment: 0.3%
Ophthalmic solution: 0.3%

ACTION
Unknown. Thought to inhibit protein synthesis. Usually bactericidal.

ONSET, PEAK, DURATION
Unknown. Systemic absorption is negligible.

INDICATIONS & DOSAGE
External ocular infections caused by susceptible bacteria –
Adults and children: in mild to moderate infections, 1 or 2 drops instilled into the affected eye q 4 hours, or a thin strip of ointment applied q 8 to 12 hours. In severe infections, 2 drops instilled into the infected eye q 30 to 60 minutes until condition improves; then frequency reduced. Or, a thin strip of ointment applied q 3 to 4 hours until improvement; then frequency reduced.

ADVERSE REACTIONS
EENT: burning or stinging on instillation, lid itching, lid swelling, blurred vision (with ointment).
Other: hypersensitivity reactions.

INTERACTIONS
Tetracycline-containing eye preparations: incompatible with tyloxapol, an ingredient in Tobrex. Don't use together.

CONTRAINDICATIONS
Contraindicated in patients hypersensitive to the drug.

NURSING CONSIDERATIONS
• When two different ophthalmic solutions are used, allow at least 5 minutes before instillation.

• If topical ocular tobramycin is administered concomitantly with systemic tobramycin, carefully monitor serum levels.

• Stop drug and notify the doctor if symptoms of tobramycin overdose, such as keratitis, erythema, increased lacrimation, edema, and lid itching, occur.

• Know that prolonged use may result in overgrowth of nonsusceptible organisms, including fungi.

• Be aware that drug is often used to combat gram-negative organisms that are resistant to gentamicin.

• Tell patient to clean eye area of excessive exudate before application.

• Teach patients how to instill drops or apply ointment. Advise them to wash hands before and after administering ointment or solution and to avoid touching tip of dropper to eye or surrounding tissue.

• Instruct patient to apply light finger pressure on lacrimal sac for 1 minute after drops are instilled.

• Advise patients to watch for signs of sensitivity, such as itching lids, swelling, or constant burning. Tell patients who develop these signs to discontinue drug and notify the doctor immediately.

• Tell patients not to share eye medications, washcloths, or towels with family members. If anyone develops the same symptoms, the doctor should be notified.

• Stress importance of compliance with recommended therapy.

---

trifluridine
Viroptic Ophthalmic Solution 1%
Pregnancy Risk Category: C

HOW SUPPLIED
Ophthalmic solution: 1%

ACTION
Unknown. Thought to interfere with DNA synthesis.

ONSET, PEAK, DURATION
Unknown.

INDICATIONS & DOSAGE
Primary keratoconjunctivitis and recurrent epithelial keratitis caused by herpes simplex virus, types I and II —
Adults: 1 drop of solution into the affected eye q 2 hours while patient is awake, to a maximum of 9 drops daily until corneal ulcer reepithelialization occurs; then 1 drop q 4 hours (minimum 5 drops daily) for an additional 7 days.

ADVERSE REACTIONS
Eye: *stinging on instillation,* edema of eyelids, increased intraocular pressure.
Other: hypersensitivity reactions.

INTERACTIONS
None significant.

CONTRAINDICATIONS
Contraindicated in patients hypersensitive to the drug.

NURSING CONSIDERATIONS
• Be aware that doctor should consider another form of therapy if improvement doesn't occur after 7 days' treatment or complete reepithelialization after 14 days' treatment. Know that trifluridine should not be used for more than 21 days continuously due to potential ocular toxicity.
• Watch for signs of increased intraocular pressure.
• Continue trifluridine for several days after steroid therapy.
• Know that drug is prescribed only for those patients with clinical diagnosis of herpetic keratitis.
• Be aware that drug is more effective than vidarabine or idoxuridine with fewer adverse reactions.
• Keep refrigerated. Do not use if past the expiration date.
• Tell patients to clean eye area of excessive exudate before application.
• Teach patients how to instill drops. Advise them to wash hands before and after administering, and warn them not to touch tip of dropper to eye or surrounding tissue.
• Instruct patient to apply light finger pressure on lacrimal sac for 1 minute after drops are instilled.
• Reassure patients that mild local irritation of the conjunctiva and cornea that occurs when solution is instilled is usually temporary.
• Tell patients not to share eye medications, washcloths, or towels with family members. If anyone develops the same symptoms, the doctor should be notified.
• Stress importance of complying with recommended therapy.

vidarabine
Vira-A Ophthalmic
Pregnancy Risk Category: C

HOW SUPPLIED
Ophthalmic ointment: 3% in 3.5-g tube (equivalent to 2.8% vidarabine)

ACTION
Unknown. Thought to interfere with DNA synthesis.

ONSET, PEAK, DURATION
Unknown. Systemic absorption is negligible.

INDICATIONS & DOSAGE

Acute keratoconjunctivitis, superficial keratitis, and recurrent epithelial keratitis resulting from herpes simplex types I and II —

Adults and children: 1 cm ointment applied into lower conjunctival sac five times daily at 3-hour intervals.

ADVERSE REACTIONS

EENT: temporary burning, itching, mild irritation, pain, lacrimation, foreign body sensation, conjunctival injection, superficial punctate keratitis, photophobia.

Other: hypersensitivity reactions.

INTERACTIONS

None significant.

CONTRAINDICATIONS

Contraindicated in patients hypersensitive to the drug.

NURSING CONSIDERATIONS

• Use cautiously and with close monitoring with steroids. Vidarabine continued for several days after steroid therapy.

• Be aware that drug is not effective against RNA virus, adenoviral ocular infections, or bacterial, fungal, or chlamydial infections.

• Store in tightly closed, light-resistant container.

• Warn patients not to exceed recommended frequency or duration of dosage. Not for long-term use. Treatment should not exceed 21 days, or 3 to 5 days after healing.

• Tell patients to clean eye area of excessive exudate before application.

• Teach patients how to apply. Advise them to wash hands before and after administering ointment and to avoid touching tip of tube to eye or surrounding tissue.

• Instruct patient to apply light finger pressure on lacrimal sac for 1 minute after drops are instilled.

• Explain to patients that the ointment may produce a temporary visual haze.

• Advise patients to watch for signs of sensitivity, such as itching lids, swelling, or constant burning. Tell patients who develop such signs to stop drug and notify the doctor immediately.

• Tell patients to minimize photophobia by wearing sunglasses and avoiding prolonged exposure to sunlight.

• Tell patients not to share eye medications, washcloths, or towels with family members. If anyone develops the same symptoms, the doctor should be notified.

• Stress importance of complying with recommended therapy.

81

Ophthalmic anti-inflammatory agents

dexamethasone
dexamethasone sodium phosphate
diclofenac sodium 0.1%
fluorometholone
flurbiprofen sodium
ketorolac tromethamine
medrysone
prednisolone acetate (suspension)
prednisolone sodium phosphate (solution)
rimexolone
suprofen

COMBINATION PRODUCTS
Corticosteroids for ophthalmic use are commonly combined with antibiotics and sulfonamides. See Chapter 80, OPHTHALMIC ANTI-INFECTIVES.

---

dexamethasone
Maxidex Ophthalmic Suspension

dexamethasone sodium phosphate
Decadron Phosphate Ophthalmic, Maxidex Ophthalmic

Pregnancy Risk Category: C

HOW SUPPLIED
dexamethasone
Ophthalmic suspension: 0.1%
dexamethasone sodium phosphate
Ophthalmic ointment: 0.05%
Ophthalmic solution: 0.1%

ACTION
Unknown. Thought to decrease the infiltration of WBCs at the site of inflammation.

ONSET, PEAK, DURATION
Unknown.

INDICATIONS & DOSAGE
Uveitis; iridocyclitis; inflammatory conditions of eyelids, conjunctiva, cornea, anterior segment of globe; corneal injury from chemical or thermal burns, or penetration of foreign bodies; allergic conjunctivitis–
Adults and children: 1 to 2 drops of suspension or solution instilled or 1.25 to 2.5 cm of ointment applied into conjunctival sac. In severe disease, drops may be used hourly, tapering to discontinuation as condition improves. In mild conditions, drops may be used up to four to six times daily or ointment applied t.i.d. or q.i.d. As condition improves, dosage tapered to b.i.d., then once daily. Treatment may extend from a few days to several weeks.

ADVERSE REACTIONS
EENT: increased intraocular pressure; thinning of cornea, interference with corneal wound healing, increased susceptibility to viral or fungal corneal infection, corneal ulceration; with excessive or long-term use, glaucoma exacerbations, cataracts, defects in visual acuity and visual field, optic nerve damage; *mild blurred vision; burning, stinging, or redness of eyes; watery eyes.*
Other: systemic effects and adrenal suppression with excessive or long-term use.

INTERACTIONS
None significant.

CONTRAINDICATIONS
Contraindicated in patients with acute superficial herpes simplex (dendritic keratitis), vaccinia, varicella, or other fungal or viral diseases of cornea and conjunctiva; ocular tuberculosis; or

---

*Liquid form contains alcohol. *Common* reactions are in italics; ***life-threatening,*** in bold italics.
**May contain tartrazine.

any acute, purulent, untreated infection of the eye.

NURSING CONSIDERATIONS

• Use cautiously in patients with corneal abrasions that may be infected (especially with herpes).

• Use cautiously in patients with glaucoma (any form), because intraocular pressure may increase. Glaucoma medications may need to be increased to compensate.

• Not for long-term use.

• Watch for corneal ulceration; may require stopping drug.

• Be aware that corneal viral and fungal infections may be exacerbated by steroid application.

• Tell patient to shake suspension well before use.

• Teach patients how to instill drops or apply ointment. Advise them to wash hands before and after administering ointment or solution, and warn them not to touch tip of dropper to eye or surrounding tissue. Tell them to apply light finger pressure on lacrimal sac for 1 minute after instillation.

• Advise patient that he may use eye pad with ointment.

• Warn patients not to use leftover medication for a new eye inflammation; may cause serious problems.

• Warn patients to call the doctor immediately and to stop drug if visual acuity changes or visual field diminishes.

• Tell patients not to share eye medications, washcloths, or towels with family members. If anyone develops similar symptoms, the doctor should be notified.

• Stress the importance of compliance with recommended therapy.

---

diclofenac sodium 0.1%
Voltaren Ophthalmic

Pregnancy Risk Category: B

HOW SUPPLIED
Ophthalmic solution: 0.1%

ACTION
Unknown. Thought to inhibit the enzyme cyclooxygenase, which is essential in the biosynthesis of prostaglandins; prostaglandins may be mediators of certain kinds of intraocular inflammation.

ONSET, PEAK, DURATION
Unknown.

INDICATIONS & DOSAGE
Postoperative inflammation following removal of cataract –
Adults: 1 drop in the conjunctival sac q.i.d., beginning 24 hours after surgery and continuing throughout the first 2 weeks of the postoperative period.

ADVERSE REACTIONS
EENT: *transient stinging and burning, increased intraocular pressure, keratitis.*
Systemic: nausea, vomiting, viral infection.

INTERACTIONS
None known.

CONTRAINDICATIONS
• Contraindicated in patients with hypersensitivity to any component of the drug and in those wearing soft contact lenses.

• Because of the known effects of prostaglandin-inhibiting drugs on the fetal cardiovascular system (closure of the ductus arteriosus), the use of this drug during late pregnancy should be avoided.

NURSING CONSIDERATIONS
• Use cautiously in patients with hypersensitivity to acetylsalicylic acid, phenylacetic acid derivatives, and other NSAIDs; the potential for cross-sensitivity exists. It should also be

---

used cautiously in surgical patients with known bleeding tendencies and in those receiving medications that may prolong bleeding time.

• Be aware that drug may slow or delay healing.

• Know that most cases of increased intraocular pressure have occurred postoperatively and before drug administration.

• Teach patients how to instill drops. Advise them to wash hands before and after instilling solution, and warn them not to touch tip of the dropper to eye or surrounding tissue.

• Advise patients to apply light finger pressure on lacrimal sac for 1 minute after drug instillation.

• Stress the importance of compliance with recommended therapy.

• Warn patient not to use leftover medication for a new eye inflammation; doing so may cause serious problems.

• Remind patients to discard drug when no longer needed.

---

fluorometholone
FML Liquifilm Ophthalmic,
FML S.O.P.

Pregnancy Risk Category: C

HOW SUPPLIED
Ophthalmic ointment: 0.1%
Ophthalmic suspension: 0.1%, 0.25%

ACTION
Unknown. Thought to decrease the infiltration of WBCs at inflammation site.

ONSET, PEAK, DURATION
Unknown.

INDICATIONS & DOSAGE
Inflammatory and allergic conditions of cornea, conjunctiva, sclera, anterior uvea –
Adults and children: 1 to 2 drops instilled in conjunctival sac b.i.d. to

q.i.d. May be given q hour during first 1 to 2 days if needed. Alternatively, 1.25 cm ribbon of ointment applied to conjunctival sac q 4 hours, decreasing to one to three times a day as inflammation subsides.

ADVERSE REACTIONS
EENT: increased intraocular pressure, thinning of cornea, interference with corneal wound healing, corneal ulceration, increased susceptibility to viral or fungal corneal infections; with excessive or long-term use, glaucoma exacerbations, cataracts, decreased visual acuity, diminished visual field, optic nerve damage.
Other: systemic effects and adrenal suppression in excessive or long-term use.

INTERACTIONS
None significant.

CONTRAINDICATIONS
Contraindicated in patients with vaccinia, varicella, acute superficial herpes simplex (dendritic keratitis), or other fungal or viral eye diseases; ocular tuberculosis; or any acute, purulent, untreated eye infection.

NURSING CONSIDERATIONS
• Use cautiously in patients with corneal abrasions that may be contaminated (especially with herpes).

• Safety and efficacy in children under age 2 have not been established.

• Not for long-term use.

• Shake well before using.

• Be aware that drug is less likely to cause increased intraocular pressure with long-term use than other ophthalmic anti-inflammatory drugs (except medrysone).

• Store in tightly covered, light-resistant container.

• Teach patients how to instill drops or apply ointment. Advise them to wash hands before and after administering ointment or solution, and warn

---

*Liquid form contains alcohol.   *Common* reactions are in italics; *life-threatening*, in bold italics.
**May contain tartrazine.

them not to touch tip of dropper to eye or surrounding tissue. Advise patients to apply light finger pressure on lacrimal sac for 1 minute after instillation.
• Advise patients to call the doctor immediately and to stop drug if visual acuity decreases or visual field diminishes.
• Warn patients not to use leftover medication for a new eye inflammation; may cause serious problems.
• Tell patients not to share eye medications, washcloths, or towels with family members. If anyone develops similar symptoms, the doctor should be notified.

flurbiprofen sodium
Ocufen Liquifilm

Pregnancy Risk Category: B

HOW SUPPLIED
Ophthalmic solution: 0.03%

ACTION
Unknown. An NSAID that is thought to inhibit the cyclooxygenase enzyme that is essential in the biosynthesis of prostaglandin.

ONSET, PEAK, DURATION
Unknown.

INDICATIONS & DOSAGE
Inhibition of intraoperative miosis—
Adults: 1 drop instilled into the eye undergoing surgery approximately every ½ hour, beginning 2 hours before surgery. A total of 4 drops is given.

ADVERSE REACTIONS
EENT: transient burning and stinging on instillation, ocular irritation.

INTERACTIONS
Acetylcholine, carbachol: may be rendered ineffective. Avoid concomitant use.
Anticoagulants: increased risk of

bleeding if significant systemic absorption occurs. Monitor closely.

CONTRAINDICATIONS
Contraindicated in patients with hypersensitivity to the drug.

NURSING CONSIDERATIONS
• Use cautiously in patients who may be allergic to aspirin and other NSAIDs.
• Use cautiously in patients with bleeding tendencies and those who are receiving medications that may prolong clotting times.
• Be aware that wound healing may be delayed.
• Advise patients to call the doctor immediately if visual acuity decreases or visual field diminishes.

ketorolac tromethamine
Acular

Pregnancy Risk Category: C

HOW SUPPLIED
Ophthalmic solution: 0.5%

ACTION
Unknown. An NSAID that is thought to inhibit the action of cyclooxygenase, an enzyme responsible for prostaglandin synthesis. Prostaglandins mediate the inflammatory response and also cause miosis.

ONSET, PEAK, DURATION
Unknown. Systemic absorption is negligible.

INDICATIONS & DOSAGE
Relief of ocular itching caused by seasonal allergic conjunctivitis—
Adults: 1 drop into the conjunctival sac instilled in each eye q.i.d.

ADVERSE REACTIONS
EENT: *transient stinging and burning on instillation,* superficial keratitis, superficial ocular infections.

---

†Available in Canada only.   ‡Available in Australia only.   ◇ Available OTC.

Other: allergic reactions.

INTERACTIONS
None reported.

CONTRAINDICATIONS
Contraindicated in patients hypersensitive to any component of the formulation and in wearers of soft contact lenses.

NURSING CONSIDERATIONS
• Use cautiously in patients hypersensitive to other NSAIDs or aspirin and in patients with bleeding disorders.
• Teach patients how to instill drops. Advise them to wash hands before and after instilling solution, and warn them not to touch tip of dropper to eye or surrounding tissue.
• Advise patients to apply light finger pressure on lacrimal sac for 1 minute after instillation.
• Remind patients to store drug away from heat in a dark, tightly closed container and to protect drug from freezing.
• Remind patients to discard drug when it's no longer needed.
• Stress the importance of compliance with recommended therapy.

---

medrysone
HMS Liquifilm Ophthalmic

Pregnancy Risk Category: C

HOW SUPPLIED
Ophthalmic suspension: 1%

ACTION
Unknown. Thought to decrease the infiltration of WBCs at the site of inflammation.

ONSET, PEAK, DURATION
Unknown. Although systemic absorption occurs, plasma levels are very low and systemic effects are negligible.

INDICATIONS & DOSAGE
Allergic conjunctivitis, vernal conjunctivitis, episcleritis, ophthalmic epinephrine sensitivity reaction –
Adults and children: 1 drop instilled in conjunctival sac q 4 hours. May use q hour during first 1 to 2 days if needed.

ADVERSE REACTIONS
EENT: thinning of cornea, interference with corneal wound healing, increased susceptibility to viral or fungal corneal infection, corneal ulceration; with excessive or long-term use, glaucoma exacerbations, cataracts, visual acuity and visual field defects, optic nerve damage.
Other: systemic effects and adrenal suppression with excessive or long-term use.

INTERACTIONS
None significant.

CONTRAINDICATIONS
Contraindicated in patients with vaccinia, varicella, acute superficial herpes simplex (dendritic keratitis), viral diseases of conjunctiva and cornea, ocular tuberculosis, fungal or viral eye diseases, iritis, uveitis, or any acute, purulent, untreated eye infection.

NURSING CONSIDERATIONS
• Use cautiously in patients with corneal abrasions that may be contaminated (especially with herpes).
• Teach patients how to instill drops. Advise them to wash hands before and after instilling solution, and warn them not to touch tip of dropper to eye or surrounding tissue.
• Tell patient to shake well before using. Don't freeze.
• Advise patients to apply light finger pressure on lacrimal sac for 1 minute after instillation.
• Warn patients not to use leftover

---

*Liquid form contains alcohol.   *Common* reactions are in italics; *life-threatening,* in bold italics.
**May contain tartrazine

medication for a new eye inflammation; may cause serious problems.

• Tell patients not to share eye medications, washcloths, or towels with family members. If anyone develops similar symptoms, the doctor should be notified.

• Stress the importance of compliance with recommended therapy.

---

prednisolone acetate (suspension)
Econopred Ophthalmic, Econopred Plus Ophthalmic, Pred-Forte, Pred Mild Ophthalmic

prednisolone sodium phosphate (solution)
AK-Pred, Hydeltrasol Ophthalmic, Inflamase Forte, Inflamase Ophthalmic, Ocu-Pred, Predsol Eye Drops‡

Pregnancy Risk Category: C

HOW SUPPLIED
acetate
Ophthalmic suspension: 0.12%, 0.125%, 1%
sodium phosphate
Ophthalmic solution: 0.125%, 1%

ACTION
Unknown. Thought to decrease the infiltration of WBCs at the site of inflammation.

ONSET, PEAK, DURATION
Unknown. Although systemic absorption occurs, plasma levels are very low and systemic effects are negligible.

INDICATIONS & DOSAGE
Inflammation of palpebral and bulbar conjunctiva, cornea, and anterior segment of globe –
Adults and children: 1 to 2 drops instilled in eye. In severe conditions, may be used hourly, tapering to discontinuation as inflammation sub-

sides. In mild conditions, may be used up to six times daily.

ADVERSE REACTIONS
EENT: increased intraocular pressure; thinning of cornea, interference with corneal wound healing, increased susceptibility to viral or fungal corneal infection, corneal ulceration; with excessive or long-term use, glaucoma exacerbations, cataracts, visual acuity and visual field defects, optic nerve damage.
Other: systemic effects and adrenal suppression with excessive or long-term use.

INTERACTIONS
None significant.

CONTRAINDICATIONS
Contraindicated in patients with acute, untreated, purulent ocular infections; acute superficial herpes simplex (dendritic keratitis); vaccinia, varicella, or other viral or fungal eye diseases; or ocular tuberculosis.

NURSING CONSIDERATIONS
• Use cautiously in patients with corneal abrasions that may be contaminated (especially with herpes).

• Tell patient to shake suspension and check dosage before administering to ensure using the correct strength. Store in tightly covered container.

• Teach patients how to instill drops. Advise them to wash hands before and after applying, and warn them not to touch tip of dropper to eye or surrounding area.

• Advise patients to apply light finger pressure on lacrimal sac for 1 minute after instillation.

• Tell patients on long-term therapy to have frequent tonometric examinations.

• Warn patients not to use leftover medication for a new eye inflammation; may cause serious problems.

• Tell patients not to share eye medi-

---

cations, washcloths, or towels with family members. If anyone develops similar symptoms, the doctor should be notified.

• Stress the importance of compliance with recommended therapy.

---

rimexolone
Vexol 1% Ophthalmic Suspension
Pregnancy Risk Category: C

HOW SUPPLIED
Ophthalmic suspension: 1%

ACTION
Exact mechanism unknown. A corticosteroid, it inhibits edema, cellular infiltration, capillary dilation, fibroblastic proliferation, and deposition of collagen and scar formation associated with inflammation.

ONSET, PEAK, DURATION
Unknown.

INDICATIONS & DOSAGE
Postoperative inflammation following ocular surgery –
Adults: 1 to 2 drops in the conjunctival sac q.i.d., beginning 24 hours after surgery and continuing throughout the first 2 weeks of the postoperative period.
Anterior uveitis –
Adults: 1 to 2 drops in the conjunctival sac q hour during waking hours for the first week, 1 drop q 2 hours during waking hours of the second week, and then tapered until uveitis is resolved.

ADVERSE REACTIONS
EENT: *blurred vision, ocular discharge, ocular pain or discomfort, increased intraocular pressure, foreign-body sensation, ocular hyperemia, ocular pruritus,* sticky sensation, increased fibrin formation, eye dryness, conjunctival edema, corneal staining, keratitis, lacrimation, photophobia, edema, irritation, corneal ulcer, brow pain, crusting at margin of eyelid, corneal edema, infiltrate, corneal erosion.
Other: headache, hypotension, rhinitis, pharyngitis, taste perversion.

INTERACTIONS
None known.

CONTRAINDICATIONS
Contraindicated in patients with hypersensitivity to any component of the drug. Also contraindicated in those with epithelial herpes simplex keratitis, vaccinia, varicella, and most other viral diseases of the cornea and conjunctiva; mycobacterial infection of the eye; and fungal disease of the eye or acute purulent untreated infections that may be masked or enhanced by the presence of a steroid.

NURSING CONSIDERATIONS
• Teach patients how to instill drops. Advise them to shake the dispenser well before using. Also advise them to wash hands before and after instilling suspension, and warn them not to touch tip of the dropper to eye or surrounding tissue.
• Advise patients to apply light finger pressure on lacrimal sac for 1 minute after drug instillation.
• Stress the importance of compliance with recommended therapy.
• Warn patient not to use leftover medication for a new eye inflammation; doing so may cause serious problems.
• Remind patients to discard drug when no longer needed.
• Advise patients to have their intraocular pressure checked frequently.

---

suprofen
Profenal
Pregnancy Risk Category: C

HOW SUPPLIED
Ophthalmic solution: 1%

ACTION
Unknown. An NSAID that inhibits the action of cyclooxygenase, an enzyme responsible for the synthesis of prostaglandins. Prostaglandins mediate the inflammatory response and also cause miosis.

ONSET, PEAK, DURATION
Unknown. Systemic absorption is negligible.

INDICATIONS & DOSAGE
Inhibition of intraoperative miosis –
Adults: 2 drops instilled into the conjunctival sac q 4 hours the day before surgery. On the day of surgery, 2 drops instilled 3 hours, 2 hours, and 1 hour before surgery.

ADVERSE REACTIONS
EENT: *transient stinging and burning on instillation,* discomfort, itching, redness, iritis, pain, chemosis, photophobia, irritation, punctate epithelial staining.
Other: hypersensitivity reaction.

INTERACTIONS
Acetylcholine, carbachol: may be ineffective in patients treated with suprofen.

CONTRAINDICATIONS
Contraindicated in patients hypersensitive to any component of the formulation and in patients with epithelial herpes simplex keratitis.

NURSING CONSIDERATIONS
• Use cautiously in patients hypersensitive to other NSAIDs or aspirin.
• Use cautiously in patients with bleeding disorders.
• Teach patients how to instill drops. Advise them to wash hands before and after administering solution and not to touch tip of dropper to eye or surrounding tissues.
• Tell patients to apply light finger pressure on lacrimal sac for 1 minute after drops are instilled.
• Advise patients to store drug away from heat in a dark, tightly closed container and to protect drug from freezing.
• Remind patients to discard drug when it's no longer needed.
• Stress importance of compliance with recommended therapy.

acetylcholine chloride
carbachol (intraocular)
carbachol (topical)
demecarium bromide
echothiophate iodide
isoflurophate
physostigmine salicylate
physostigmine sulfate
pilocarpine
pilocarpine hydrochloride
pilocarpine nitrate

COMBINATION PRODUCTS
E-PILO: epinephrine bitartrate 1% and pilocarpine hydrochloride 1%, 2%, 3%, 4%, or 6%.
ISOPTO P-ES: pilocarpine hydrochloride 2% and physostigmine salicylate 0.25%.
P_1E_1, P_2E_1, P_3E_1, P_4E_1, P_6E_1: epinephrine bitartrate 1% and pilocarpine hydrochloride 1%, 2%, 3%, 4%, or 6%.

acetylcholine chloride
Miochol

Pregnancy Risk Category: NR

HOW SUPPLIED
Ophthalmic injection: 1%

ACTION
A cholinergic that causes contraction of the sphincter muscles of the iris, resulting in miosis, and that produces ciliary spasm, deepening of the anterior chamber, and vasodilation of conjunctival vessels of the outflow tract.

ONSET, PEAK, DURATION
Onset occurs within seconds. Peak unknown. Effects persist for about 10 minutes.

INDICATIONS & DOSAGE
Anterior segment surgery –
Adults and children: before or after securing sutures, the doctor gently instills 0.5 to 2 ml into anterior chamber.

ADVERSE REACTIONS
CV: bradycardia, hypotension.
EENT: corneal edema, clouding, or decompensation.
Respiratory: breathing difficulties.
Other: flushing, diaphoresis.

INTERACTIONS
None significant.

CONTRAINDICATIONS
Contraindicated in patients with hypersensitivity to the drug or any of its components.

NURSING CONSIDERATIONS
• Reconstitute immediately before using, shaking vial gently until clear solution is obtained.
• Discard any unused solution.
• Don't gas-sterilize vial. Ethylene oxide may produce formic acid.

carbachol (intraocular)
Miostat

carbachol (topical)
Isopto Carbachol

Pregnancy Risk Category: NR

HOW SUPPLIED
Intraocular injection: 0.01%
Topical ophthalmic solution: 0.75%, 1.5%, 2.25%, 3%

ACTION
A cholinergic that causes contraction of the sphincter muscles of the iris, resulting in miosis, and that produces

---

*Liquid form contains alcohol.
**May contain tartrazine.

Common reactions are in italics; *life-threatening,* in bold italics.

ciliary spasm, deepening of the anterior chamber, and vasodilation of conjunctival vessels of the outflow tract.

ONSET, PEAK, DURATION
Onset occurs in 10 to 20 minutes. Peak effect occurs 4 hours after topical application, 2 to 5 minutes after intraocular injection. Effects persist about 8 hours after topical application, 24 hours after intraocular injection.

INDICATIONS & DOSAGE
To produce pupillary miosis in ocular surgery –
Adults: before or after securing sutures, the doctor gently instills 0.5 ml (intraocular form) into anterior chamber.
Open-angle glaucoma –
Adults: 1 to 2 drops instilled (topical form) q 4 to 8 hours.

ADVERSE REACTIONS
CNS: headache.
EENT: spasm of eye accommodation, blurred vision, conjunctival vasodilation, eye and brow pain.
GI: abdominal cramps, diarrhea.
Respiratory: asthma.
Other: diaphoresis, flushing.

INTERACTIONS
Pilocarpine: additive effect. Use together cautiously.

CONTRAINDICATIONS
Contraindicated in patients with hypersensitivity to drug or in patients where cholinergic effects such as constriction are undesirable (i.e. acute iritis, some forms of secondary glaucoma, pupillary block glaucoma, or acute inflammatory disease of the anterior chamber).

NURSING CONSIDERATIONS
• Use cautiously in patients with acute heart failure, bronchial asthma, peptic ulcer, hyperthyroidism, GI

spasm, Parkinson's disease, and urinary tract obstruction.
• In case of toxicity, give atropine parenterally as ordered.
• Be aware that the drug is used in open-angle glaucoma, especially when patients are resistant or allergic to pilocarpine hydrochloride or nitrate.
• Keep in mind that patients with dark eyes (hazel or brown irises) may require stronger solutions or more frequent instillation because eye pigment may absorb the drug.
• If tolerance to the drug develops, know that the doctor may switch to another miotic for a short time.
• Teach patients how to instill. Advise them to wash hands before and after and to apply light finger-pressure on lacrimal sac for 1 minute after drops are instilled. Warn them not to exceed recommended dosage.
• Warn patients to avoid hazardous activities, such as operating machinery or driving, until temporary blurring subsides. Reassure patients that blurred vision usually diminishes with prolonged use.
• Tell glaucoma patients that long-term use may be necessary. Stress compliance. Tell them to remain under medical supervision for periodic tonometric readings.

demecarium bromide
Humorsol

Pregnancy Risk Category: X

HOW SUPPLIED
Ophthalmic solution: 0.125%, 0.25%

ACTION
An anticholinesterase drug that inhibits the enzymatic destruction of acetylcholine by inactivating cholinesterase, leaving acetylcholine free to act on the effector cells of the iridic sphincter and ciliary muscles, causing

pupillary constriction and spasm of accommodation.

ONSET, PEAK, DURATION
Onset occurs in 15 to 60 minutes. Miotic effect peaks within 2 hours; intraocular pressure (IOP) reduction occurs within 24 hours. Miosis persists for 3 to 10 days; IOP reduction, about 9 days.

INDICATIONS & DOSAGE
Acute angle-closure glaucoma after iridectomy, primary open-angle glaucoma –
Adults: 1 drop instilled once or twice daily.
Treatment of convergent strabismus (uncomplicated) –
Adults: 1 drop instilled daily for 2 to 3 weeks, then reduced to 1 drop q 2 days for 3 to 4 weeks. After reevaluation, 1 drop instilled once or twice weekly to once q 2 days as determined by the patient's condition. Reevaluated q 4 to 12 weeks; dosage adjusted as needed. Discontinued after 4 months if dosage required is 1 drop q 2 days.
Diagnosis of convergent strabismus –
Adults: 1 drop instilled daily for 2 weeks, then 1 drop q 2 days for 2 to 4 weeks.

ADVERSE REACTIONS
CNS: browache, unusual fatigue or weakness, headache.
CV: bradycardia, palpitations.
EENT: retinal detachment, iris cysts, conjunctival thickening, lens opacities, paradoxical increase in IOP, *lacrimation,* obstruction of nasolacrimal canals; eye pain, burning, redness, stinging and irritation; twitching eyelids; *blurred vision;* visual disturbances.
GI: nausea, vomiting, diarrhea, abdominal cramps or pain.
GU: loss of bladder control.

INTERACTIONS
Anticholinergics, antimyasthenics, other cholinesterase inhibitors: potential for additive toxicity. Monitor closely.
Carbamate or organophosphate-type insecticides (parathion, malathion): increased risk of systemic effects through respiratory tract or skin. Warn patients to protect themselves.
Cocaine: increased risk of cocaine toxicity; anticholinesterase effects may last weeks or months. Avoid concomitant use.
Epinephrine: additive effect, resulting in better control and lower dosages of both drugs.
Local anesthetics, ophthalmic tetracaine: increased risk of systemic toxicity and prolonged ocular anesthetic effect. Monitor closely.
Ophthalmic adrenocorticoids: increased IOP and decreased antiglaucoma effectiveness. Avoid concomitant use.
Ophthalmic belladonna alkaloids, cyclopentolate: may antagonize miotic effects. Avoid concomitant use.
Succinylcholine: enhanced neuromuscular blockade, possible CV collapse and prolonged respiratory depression or apnea may occur for several weeks or months after demecarium is discontinued. Advise the anesthesiologist that the patient has received demecarium.

CONTRAINDICATIONS
Contraindicated in patients with hypersensitivity to drug, acute angle-closure glaucoma before iridectomy, and other forms of glaucoma (except for primary open-angle glaucoma).

NURSING CONSIDERATIONS
• Use with extreme caution, if at all, in patients with history or risk of retinal detachment, marked vagotonia, bronchial asthma, spastic GI conditions, urinary tract obstruction, peptic ulcer, severe bradycardia, hypoten-

---

*Liquid form contains alcohol.   *Common* reactions are in italics; *life-threatening,* in bold italics.
**May contain tartrazine.

sion, hypertension, hyperthyroidism, acute cardiac failure, recent MI, epilepsy, marked vasomotor instability, or parkinsonism.

• Use with caution in patients with corneal abrasion.

• Administer phenylephrine concurrently, as ordered, to reduce incidence of iris cyst formation.

• If tolerance to the drug develops after prolonged use, know that the doctor may switch to another miotic for a short time.

• Know that toxicity is cumulative; toxic systemic symptoms may not appear for weeks or months after start of therapy. Atropine sulfate S.C., I.M., or I.V. is antidote of choice.

• Teach patients how to instill demecarium. Advise them to wash hands before and after instilling drug, to avoid touching applicator tip to any surface, and to remove excess solution around eyes with clean tissue and without touching eye. Warn them not to exceed recommended dosage.

• If dose is missed, instruct patient not to double dose. If schedule is every other day, tell patient to instill as soon as possible if remembered same day; if remembered later, tell patient not to instill until next day, then skip a day and resume regular schedule. If schedule is once a day, tell patient to instill as soon as possible. If not remembered until next day, tell patient to skip missed dose and resume schedule. If schedule is more than once daily, tell patient to instill as soon as possible. If close to time for next dose, tell patient to skip missed dose and resume regular schedule.

• Tell patients that regular medical supervision is required to check ocular pressure.

• Advise patients to carry medical identification card at all times during therapy.

echothiophate iodide (ecothiopate iodide)
Phospholine Iodide

Pregnancy Risk Category: NR

HOW SUPPLIED
Ophthalmic powder for solution: for reconstitution to make 0.03%, 0.06%, 0.125%, and 0.25% solutions

ACTION
An anticholinesterase drug that inhibits the enzymatic destruction of acetylcholine by inactivating cholinesterase, leaving acetylcholine free to act on the effector cells of the iridic sphincter and ciliary muscles, causing pupillary constriction and spasm of accommodation.

ONSET, PEAK, DURATION
Miosis occurs in 10 to 30 minutes; intraocular pressure (IOP) reduction, 4 to 8 hours. Miotic effect peaks within 30 minutes; IOP reduction occurs within 24 hours. Effects persist for several days to 4 weeks.

INDICATIONS & DOSAGE
Primary open-angle glaucoma, conditions obstructing aqueous outflow –
Adults and children: 1 drop of 0.03% to 0.125% solution instilled into conjunctival sac daily. Maximum dosage is 1 drop b.i.d. Lowest possible dosage used for continuous control of IOP.
Diagnosis of convergent strabismus –
Adults: 1 drop of 0.125% solution instilled daily h.s. for 2 to 3 weeks.
Treatment of convergent strabismus –
Adults: initially, 1 drop of 0.125% solution instilled into each eye daily h.s. for 2 to 3 weeks. Dosage decreased to 1 drop of 0.125% solution every other day or 1 drop of 0.06% solution daily. The 0.03% solution may be used instead for some patients.

ADVERSE REACTIONS
CNS: fatigue, muscle weakness, paresthesia, headache.
CV: bradycardia, hypotension.
EENT: ciliary spasm or spasm of eye accommodation, ciliary or circumcorneal injection, nonreversible cataract formation (time- and dose-related), reversible iris cysts, pupillary block, blurred or dimmed vision, eye or brow pain, twitching of eyelids, hyperemia, photophobia, lens opacities, lacrimation, retinal detachment.
GI: diarrhea, nausea, vomiting, abdominal pain, intestinal cramps, salivation.
GU: frequent urination.
Other: diaphoresis, flushing, ***bronchoconstriction.***

INTERACTIONS
Anticholinergics, ophthalmic belladonna alkaloids (such as atropine), cyclopentolate: antagonized miotic effects. Avoid concomitant use.
Cocaine: increased risk of cocaine toxicity. Avoid concomitant use.
Local anesthetics, ophthalmic tetracaine: increased rate of systemic toxicity and prolonged ocular anesthesia. Monitor closely.
Ophthalmic adrenocorticoids: increased intraocular pressure and decreased antiglaucoma effectiveness. Avoid concomitant use.
Other cholinesterase inhibitors, organophosphate insecticides (parathion, malathion): possible additive effect causing systemic effects. Warn patients exposed to insecticides to protect themselves.
Succinylcholine: respiratory and CV collapse. Don't use together.
Systemic anticholinesterase agents for myasthenia gravis, pilocarpine: effects may be additive. Monitor patients for signs of toxicity.

CONTRAINDICATIONS
Contraindicated in patients with hypersensitivity to drug or iodine, acute angle-closure glaucoma before iridectomy, and other forms of glaucoma (except for primary open-angle glaucoma).

NURSING CONSIDERATIONS
• Use with extreme caution, if at all, in patients with seizure disorders, vasomotor instability, parkinsonism, bronchial asthma, spastic GI conditions, urinary tract obstruction, peptic ulcer, severe bradycardia or hypotension, vascular hypertension, MI, or history or risk of retinal detachment.
• Use with caution in patients with corneal abrasion.
• Reconstitute powder using only diluent provided to avoid contamination. Discard refrigerated, reconstituted solution after 6 months; solution stored at room temperature, after 1 month.
• Stop drug, as ordered, at least 2 weeks preoperatively if succinylcholine is to be used in surgery.
• Know that toxicity is cumulative; toxic systemic symptoms may not appear for weeks or months after start of therapy. Atropine sulfate S.C., I.M., or I.V. is antidote of choice.
• Advise patients to carry medical identification card at all times during therapy. Drug is a potent, long-acting, and irreversible.
• Teach patients how to instill drug. Advise them to wash hands before and after instilling drug, to avoid touching applicator tip to any surface and to apply light finger pressure on lacrimal sac for 1 minute after instillation.
• Tell patients to instill drug at bedtime because it causes transient blurred vision. Warn patients that transient brow pain or dimmed or blurred vision is common at first but usually disappears within 5 to 10 days.
• Warn patients to report salivation, diarrhea, profuse diaphoresis, urinary incontinence, or muscle weakness to the doctor.

---

*Liquid form contains alcohol.   *Common* reactions are in italics; ***life-threatening,*** in bold italics.
**May contain tartrazine.

• Tell patients to remain under constant medical supervision and not to exceed recommended dosage.

isoflurophate
Floropryl

Pregnancy Risk Category: X

HOW SUPPLIED
Ophthalmic ointment: 0.025%

ACTION
An anticholinesterase drug that inhibits the enzymatic destruction of acetylcholine by inactivating cholinesterase, leaving acetylcholine free to act on the effector cells of the iridic sphincter and ciliary muscles, causing pupillary constriction and spasm of accommodation.

ONSET, PEAK, DURATION
Unknown.

INDICATIONS & DOSAGE
Glaucoma –
Adults: 0.5 cm ribbon of ointment applied to conjunctiva q 8 to 72 hours.
Diagnosis of convergent strabismus (uncomplicated) –
Adults: 0.5 cm ribbon of ointment applied to conjunctiva h.s. for 2 weeks.
Treatment of convergent strabismus –
Adults: 0.5 cm ribbon of ointment applied to each eye h.s. for 2 weeks, then once every 2 to 7 days, depending on the patient's condition, for 2 months. If the patient cannot be maintained on a dosage interval of at least 48 hours, the drug should be discontinued.

ADVERSE REACTIONS
CNS: headache, browache, unusual fatigue or weakness.
CV: slow or irregular heartbeat.
EENT: retinal detachment, iris cysts, conjunctival thickening, lens opacities, obstruction of nasolacrimal canals, paradoxical increase in intraocular pressure (IOP); *eye burning,* redness, pain, stinging or irritation; twitching of eyelids; *blurred vision;* visual disturbances.
GI: nausea, vomiting, diarrhea, abdominal cramps or pain.
GU: loss of bladder control.
Other: diaphoresis, flushing.

INTERACTIONS
Anticholinergics, antimyasthenics, other cholinesterase inhibitors: potential for additive toxicity. Monitor closely.
Carbamate or organophosphate-type insecticides (parathion, malathion): increased risk of systemic effects through respiratory tract or skin. Warn patients to protect themselves.
Cocaine: increased risk of cocaine toxicity; anticholinesterase effects may last weeks or months. Avoid concomitant use.
Epinephrine: additive effect, resulting in better control and lower dosages of both drugs.
Local anesthetics, ophthalmic tetracaine: increased risk of systemic toxicity, prolonged ocular anesthesia. Monitor closely.
Ophthalmic adrenocorticoids: increased IOP and decreased antiglaucoma effectiveness. Avoid concomitant use.
Ophthalmic belladonna alkaloids, cyclopentolate: may antagonize miotic effects. Avoid concomitant use.
Ophthalmic physostigmine: may shorten duration of action. Avoid concomitant use.
Succinylcholine: enhanced neuromuscular blockade, possible CV collapse, prolonged respiratory depression, or apnea may occur for several weeks or months after demecarium is discontinued. Advise the anesthesiologist that the patient has received demecarium.

CONTRAINDICATIONS
Contraindicated in patients with hypersensitivity to drug or acute angle-closure glaucoma before iridectomy.

NURSING CONSIDERATIONS
• Use with extreme caution, if at all, in patients with bronchial asthma, pronounced bradycardia and hypotension, seizure disorder, spastic GI disturbances, Parkinson's disease, marked vagotonia, MI, or history of retinal detachment.
• Use with caution in patients with corneal abrasion.
• Administer phenylephrine concurrently, as ordered, to reduce incidence of iris cyst formation.
• If tolerance to the drug develops after prolonged use, know that the doctor may switch to another miotic for a short time.
• Know that toxicity is cumulative; toxic systemic symptoms may not appear for weeks or months after therapy is discontinued. Atropine sulfate S.C., I.M., or I.V. is antidote of choice.
• Teach patients how to apply drug. Advise them to wash hands before and after application, to avoid touching applicator tip to any surface and to wipe tip with clean tissue. Warn them not to exceed recommended dosage.
• If dose is missed, instruct patient not to double dose. If schedule is every other day, tell patient to apply as soon as possible if remembered same day; if remembered later, tell patient not to apply until next day, then skip a day and resume regular schedule. If schedule is once a day, tell patient to apply as soon as possible. If not remembered until next day, tell patient to skip missed dose and resume schedule. If schedule is more than once daily, tell patient to apply as soon as possible. If close to time for next dose, tell patient to skip missed dose and resume regular schedule.
• Tell patients that regular medical

supervision is required to check ocular pressure.
• Advise patients to carry medical identification card at all times during therapy.

---

physostigmine salicylate
Isopto-Eserine

physostigmine sulfate
Eserine Sulfate

Pregnancy Risk Category: NR

HOW SUPPLIED
physostigmine salicylate
Ophthalmic solution: 0.25%, 0.5%
physostigmine sulfate
Ophthalmic ointment: 0.25%

ACTION
Causes contraction of iris sphincter muscles resulting in miosis, and contraction of ciliary muscle, increasing outflow of aqueous humor and decreasing intraocular pressure.

ONSET, PEAK, DURATION
Onset occurs within 30 minutes. Peak unknown. Effects persist for 12 to 48 hours.

INDICATIONS & DOSAGE
Open-angle glaucoma –
Adults and children: 1 to 2 drops of solution instilled 2 to 4 times daily or a thin strip of ointment applied once daily to t.i.d.

ADVERSE REACTIONS
CNS: headache, weakness.
CV: slow or irregular heartbeat.
EENT: blurred vision, eye pain, burning, redness, stinging, eye irritation, twitching of eyelids, watering of eyes.
GI: nausea, vomiting, diarrhea.
GU: loss of bladder control.
Other: diaphoresis, muscle weakness, shortness of breath.

---

*Liquid form contains alcohol.   *Common* reactions are in italics; *life-threatening,* in bold italics.
**May contain tartrazine.

INTERACTIONS
Echothiophate, isoflurophate: duration of action may be shortened. Monitor closely.
Ophthalmic belladonna alkaloids: may antagonize miotic actions. Avoid concomitant use.

CONTRAINDICATIONS
Contraindicated in patients with intolerance to physostigmine, active uveitis, or corneal injury.

NURSING CONSIDERATIONS
• Be aware that ointment may be used at night because of its longer duration of action.
• If tolerance to the drug develops, know that the doctor may switch to another miotic for a short time.
• Teach patients how to instill drug. Advise them to wash hands before and after instilling and to avoid touching applicator tip to any surface. Warn them not to exceed recommended dosage.

---

pilocarpine
Ocusert Pilo

pilocarpine hydrochloride
Adsorbocarpine, Isopto Carpine, Miocarpine†, Ocusert Pilo, Pilocar, Pilocel, Pilomiotin, Pilopine HS, Pilopt‡

pilocarpine nitrate
Ocusert Pilo, P.V. Carpine Liquifilm

Pregnancy Risk Category: NR

HOW SUPPLIED
pilocarpine
Extended-release insert: 20 mcg/hour, 40 mcg/hour for 7 days
pilocarpine hydrochloride
Ophthalmic solution: 0.25%, 0.5%, 1%, 2%, 3%, 4%, 5%, 6%, 8%, 10%
Ophthalmic gel: 4%
pilocarpine nitrate
Ophthalmic solution: 1%, 2%, 4%

ACTION
A cholinergic that causes contraction of iris sphincter muscles, resulting in miosis, and that produces ciliary spasm, deepening of the anterior chamber, and vasodilation of conjunctival vessels of the outflow tract.

ONSET, PEAK, DURATION
Onset of miosis occurs within 30 minutes; intraocular pressure (IOP) reduction, within 60 minutes. Miotic effect peaks within 30 minutes; IOP reduction occurs within 75 minutes. Miosis effects persist up to 8 hours; IOP reduction, 4 to 14 hours with topical solution, up to 24 hours with gel, and up to 7 days with extended-release ocular system.

INDICATIONS & DOSAGE
Primary open-angle glaucoma –
Adults and children: 1 to 2 drops instilled q 4 to 12 hours or 1 cm ribbon of 4% gel (Pilopine HS) applied h.s.
Alternatively, one Ocusert Pilo system (20 or 40 mcg/hour) applied q 7 days.
Emergency treatment of acute angle-closure glaucoma –
Adults and children: 1 drop of 2% solution instilled q 5 to 10 minutes for three to six doses, followed by 1 drop q 1 to 3 hours until pressure is controlled.

ADVERSE REACTIONS
EENT: suborbital headache, *myopia,* ciliary spasm, *blurred vision,* conjunctival irritation, lacrimation, changes in visual field, *brow pain.*
GI: nausea, vomiting, abdominal cramps, diarrhea, salivation.
Respiratory: *bronchoconstriction, pulmonary edema.*
Other: hypersensitivity reactions.

INTERACTIONS
Carbachol, echothiophate: additive effect. Don't use together.
Ophthalmic belladonna alkaloids

---

†Available in Canada only.　　‡Available in Australia only.　　◇Available OTC.

(such as atropine and scopolamine),
cyclopentolate: decreased pilocarpine
antiglaucoma effectiveness and
blocked mydriatic effects of these
agents. Avoid concomitant use.
Phenylephrine: decreased dilation by
phenylephrine. Don't use together.

CONTRAINDICATIONS

Contraindicated in patients with hypersensitivity to drug or when cholinergic effects such as constriction are
undesirable (for example, acute iritis,
some forms of secondary glaucoma,
pupillary block glaucoma, acute inflammatory disease of the anterior
chamber).

NURSING CONSIDERATIONS

• Use cautiously in patients with
acute cardiac failure, bronchial
asthma, peptic ulcer, hyperthyroidism, GI spasm, urinary tract obstruction, and Parkinson's disease.
• Instruct patients to apply gel at bedtime because it will blur vision. Warn
patients to avoid hazardous activities,
such as operating machinery or driving, until temporary blurring subsides.
• Teach patients how to instill pilocarpine. Advise them to wash hands
before and after instilling drug and to
apply light finger pressure on lacrimal
sac for 1 minute after drops are instilled. Warn patients not to touch applicator tip to eye or surrounding tissue.
• If the Ocusert Pilo system falls out
of the eye during sleep, tell patients to
wash hands, rinse the insert in cool
tap water, and reposition it in the eye.
Also tell patients not to use a de-
formed insert.
• Warn patients that transient brow
pain and myopia are common at first
but usually disappear within 10 to 14
days.

---

*Liquid form contains alcohol.   *Common* reactions are in italics; ***life-threatening,*** in bold italics.
**May contain tartrazine.

atropine sulfate
cyclopentolate hydrochloride
epinephrine hydrochloride
epinephryl borate
homatropine hydrobromide
phenylephrine hydrochloride
scopolamine hydrobromide
tropicamide

COMBINATION PRODUCTS
CYCLOMYDRIL OPHTHALMIC: cyclopentolate hydrochloride 0.2% and
phenylephrine hydrochloride 1%.
MUROCOLL-2: scopolamine hydrobromide 0.3% and phenylephrine hydrochloride 10%.

---

atropine sulfate
Atropisol, Atropt‡, BufOpto
Atropine, Isopto Atropine
Pregnancy Risk Category: C

HOW SUPPLIED
Ophthalmic ointment: 0.5%, 1%
Ophthalmic solution: 0.5%, 1%, 2%

ACTION
A potent mydriatic and cycloplegic
whose anticholinergic action leaves
the pupil under unopposed adrenergic
influence, causing it to dilate.

ONSET, PEAK, DURATION
Onset unknown. Mydriatic effect
peaks within 30 to 40 minutes; cycloplegic, within 1 to 3 hours. Effects of
mydriasis persist for 7 to 12 days; of
cycloplegia, 6 to 12 days.

INDICATIONS & DOSAGE
Acute iritis; uveitis –
Adults: 1 to 2 drops instilled into the
eye(s) up to 4 times daily or a small
strip of ointment applied to the conjunctival sac up to 3 times daily.

Children: 1 to 2 drops of 0.5% solution instilled into the eye(s) up to 3
times daily or a small strip of ointment applied to the conjunctival sac
up to 3 times daily.
Cycloplegic refraction –
Adults: 1 to 2 drops of 1% solution
instilled 1 hour before refraction.
Children: 1 to 2 drops of 0.5% solution instilled in each eye b.i.d. for 1
to 3 days before eye examination and
1 hour before refraction.

ADVERSE REACTIONS
CNS: irritability, confusion, somno-
lence, ataxia.
CV: tachycardia.
EENT: ocular congestion with long-
term use, conjunctivitis, contact der-
matitis of eye, ocular edema, *blurred
vision,* eye dryness, *photophobia.*
GI: dry mouth, abdominal distention
in infants.
Skin: dryness.
Other: flushing, fever.

INTERACTIONS
None significant.

CONTRAINDICATIONS
• Contraindicated in patients with
glaucoma, hypersensitivity to drug or
belladonna alkaloids, or who have
adhesions between the iris and lens.
• Do not use atropine during the first
3 months of life because of the possible association between cycloplegia
produced and development of amblyopia.

NURSING CONSIDERATIONS
• Use cautiously in elderly patients
and others where increased intraocular pressure may be encountered.
• Treat drops and ointment as poison
(not for internal use); signs of poison-

---

†Available in Canada only.   ‡Available in Australia only.   ◇Available OTC.

ing are disorientation and confusion. Antidote of choice is physostigmine salicylate I.V. or I.M.

• Watch for signs of glaucoma: increased intraocular pressure, ocular pain, headache, progressive blurring of vision.

• Teach patients how to instill atropine. Advise them to wash hands before and after instilling drug and to apply light finger pressure on lacrimal sac for 1 minute after instillation. Warn patients not to touch tip of dropper or tube to eye or surrounding tissue.

• Warn patients to avoid hazardous activities, such as operating machinery or driving, until temporary blurring subsides.

• Tell patients to use sugarless hard candy or gum for dry mouth.

• Advise patients to ease photophobia by wearing dark glasses.

cyclopentolate hydrochloride
AK-Pentolate, Cyclogyl

Pregnancy Risk Category: NR

HOW SUPPLIED
Ophthalmic solution: 0.5%, 1%, 2%

ACTION
A potent mydriatic and cycloplegic whose anticholinergic action leaves the pupil under unopposed adrenergic influence, causing it to dilate.

ONSET, PEAK, DURATION
Onset rapid. Mydriatic effect peaks within 30 to 60 minutes; cycloplegic, within 25 to 75 minutes. Effects of mydriasis persist for 1 day; of cycloplegia, 0.25 to 1 day.

INDICATIONS & DOSAGE
Diagnostic procedures requiring mydriasis and cycloplegia –
Adults: 1 or 2 drops of 0.5%, 1%, or 2% solution instilled into the eye(s)

followed by 1 or 2 drops in 5 to 10 minutes, if needed.
Children: 1 drop of 0.5%, 1%, or 2% solution instilled in each eye, followed in 5 to 10 minutes with 1 drop 0.5% or 1% solution, if necessary.

ADVERSE REACTIONS
CNS: irritability, confusion, somnolence, hallucinations, ataxia, *seizures,* behavioral disturbances in children.
CV: tachycardia.
EENT: eye burning on instillation, blurred vision, eye dryness, *photophobia,* ocular congestion, contact dermatitis in eye, conjunctivitis.
GU: urine retention.
Skin: dryness.
Other: flushing, fever.

INTERACTIONS
Carbachol, pilocarpine: may counteract mydriatic effect. Avoid concomitant use.
Long-acting cholinergic antiglaucoma agents: miotic actions may be inhibited. Avoid concomitant use.

CONTRAINDICATIONS
Contraindicated in patients with glaucoma, hypersensitivity to drug or belladonna alkaloids, or who have adhesions between the iris and lens.

NURSING CONSIDERATIONS
• Use cautiously in elderly patients and others where increased intraocular pressure may be encountered.

• Know that drug is superior to homatropine hydrobromide, and has a shorter duration of action. Physostigmine is antidote of choice.

• Teach patients how to instill drug. Advise them to wash hands before and after instilling drug and to apply light finger pressure on lacrimal sac for 1 minute after drops are instilled. Warn patients not to touch tip of dropper to eye or surrounding tissue and that drug will burn when instilled.

---

*Liquid form contains alcohol.   *Common* reactions are in italics; *life-threatening,* in bold italics.
**May contain tartrazine.

• Warn patients to avoid hazardous activities, such as operating machinery or driving, until temporary blurring subsides.

• Advise patients to ease photophobia by wearing dark glasses.

---

epinephrine hydrochloride
Epifrin, Glaucon

epinephryl borate
Epinal, Eppy/N

Pregnancy Risk Category: C

HOW SUPPLIED
epinephrine hydrochloride
Ophthalmic solution: 0.1%, 0.25%, 0.5%, 1%, 2%
epinephryl borate
Ophthalmic solution: 0.5%, 1%, 2%

ACTION
An adrenergic that dilates the pupil by contracting the dilator muscle.

ONSET, PEAK, DURATION
Onset of mydriasis occurs within a few minutes; of intraocular pressure (IOP) reduction, within 1 hour. IOP reduction peaks within 4 to 8 hours. Effects of mydriasis persist for several hours; of IOP reduction, 12 to 24 hours.

INDICATIONS & DOSAGE
Open-angle glaucoma –
Adults: 1 or 2 drops of 1 or 2% solution once or twice daily. Dosage adjusted according to tonometric readings. The frequency of instillation may vary from once every 2 to 4 days to 4 times daily.
During ocular surgery –
Adults: 1 or more drops of 0.1% hydrochloride solution up to three times.

ADVERSE REACTIONS
CNS: browache.
CV: palpitations, tachycardia.
EENT: corneal or conjunctival pigmentation or corneal edema in long-term use; follicular hypertrophy; chemosis; conjunctivitis; iritis; hyperemic conjunctiva; maculopapular rash; severe eye stinging, burning, and tearing on instillation.

INTERACTIONS
Cyclopropane, halogenated hydrocarbons: arrhythmias, tachycardia. Use together cautiously, if at all.
Digitalis glycosides: increased risk of arrhythmias. Monitor closely.
Local or systemic sympathomimetics: additive toxic effects. Avoid concomitant use.
MAO inhibitors: exaggerated adrenergic effects. Adjust dose of epinephrine carefully.
Topical miotics, beta-adrenergic blockers, osmotic agents, systemic carbonic anhydrase inhibitors: additive lowering of IOP. Use together cautiously.
Tricyclic antidepressants, antihistamines (diphenhydramine, dexchlorpheniramine): potentiated cardiac effects of epinephrine. Monitor closely.

CONTRAINDICATIONS
Contraindicated in patients with angle-closure glaucoma or glaucoma when nature of the glaucoma has not been established, hypersensitivity to the drug, organic brain syndrome, or cardiac dilation and coronary insufficiency.

NURSING CONSIDERATIONS
• Use cautiously in elderly patients and in those with diabetes mellitus, hypertension, Parkinson's disease, hyperthyroidism, aphakia (eye without lens), cardiac disease, cerebral arteriosclerosis, or bronchial asthma.
• Be aware that drug can also can be injected into anterior chamber to produce rapid mydriasis during cataract removal or can be used to control local bleeding during surgery.
• Don't substitute one salt if another

---

one is ordered; epinephrine salts are not interchangeable.
• Monitor blood pressure and other vital signs.
• Teach patients how to instill drug. Advise them to wash hands before and after instilling drug and to apply light finger pressure on lacrimal sac for 1 minute after drops are instilled. Warn patients not to touch tip of dropper to eye or surrounding tissue.
• Advise patient not to use while wearing soft contact lenses since discoloration of lenses may occur.
• Tell patient not to use darkened solution.

---

homatropine hydrobromide
Homatrine, Homatropine, Isopto Homatropine

Pregnancy Risk Category: C

HOW SUPPLIED
Ophthalmic solution: 2%, 5%

ACTION
Anticholinergic action leaves the pupil under unopposed adrenergic influence, causing it to dilate.

ONSET, PEAK, DURATION
Onset rapid. Mydriatic effect peaks within 40 to 60 minutes; cycloplegic, within 30 to 60 minutes. Effects of mydriasis persist for 1 to 3 days; of cycloplegia, 1 to 3 days.

INDICATIONS & DOSAGE
Cycloplegic refraction –
Adults and children: 1 to 2 drops instilled into the eye(s); if needed, repeated in 5 to 10 minutes, for two or three doses.
Uveitis –
Adults and children: 1 to 2 drops instilled into the eye(s) q 3 to 4 hours.
  Note: Use only 2% solution with children. Patients with heavily pigmented irises may require larger doses.

ADVERSE REACTIONS
CNS: irritability, confusion, somnolence, ataxia.
CV: tachycardia.
EENT: eye irritation, *blurred vision, photophobia.*
GI: dry mouth.
Skin: dryness.
Other: flushing, fever.

INTERACTIONS
None significant.

CONTRAINDICATIONS
Contraindicated in patients with hypersensitivity to the drug or to other belladonna alkaloids, such as atropine, and in those with glaucoma or who have adhesions between the iris and lens.

NURSING CONSIDERATIONS
• Use cautiously in elderly patients and others where increased intraocular pressure may be encountered.
• Be aware that homatropine is similar to atropine but weaker, with a shorter duration of action. May produce symptoms of atropine poisoning, such as severe dryness of mouth or tachycardia.
• Teach patients how to instill drug. Advise them to wash hands before and after instilling drug and to apply light finger pressure on lacrimal sac for 1 minute after drops are instilled. Warn patients not to touch tip of dropper to eye or surrounding tissue.
• Warn patients to avoid hazardous activities, such as operating machinery or driving, until temporary blurring subsides.
• Tell patients to use sugarless hard candy or gum for dry mouth.
• Advise patients to ease photophobia by wearing dark glasses.

---

*Liquid form contains alcohol.   *Common* reactions are in italics; *life-threatening*, in bold italics.
**May contain tartrazine.

phenylephrine hydrochloride

AK-Dilate, AK-Nefrin Ophthalmic◊,
I-Phrine 2.5%, Isopto Frin◊,
Mydfrin, Neo-Synephrine, Prefrin
Liquifilm

Pregnancy Risk Category: C

HOW SUPPLIED
Ophthalmic solution: 0.12%◊, 2.5%,
10%

ACTION
An adrenergic that dilates the pupil by
contracting the dilator muscle.

ONSET, PEAK, DURATION
Onset is rapid. Mydriatic effect peaks
within 15 to 60 minutes after using
the 2.5% solution; 10 to 90 minutes
after using the 10% solution. Effects
of 2.5% solution persist for about 3
hours; of 10% solution, 3 to 7 hours.

INDICATIONS & DOSAGE
Mydriasis without cycloplegia –
Adults and children: 1 or 2 drops of
2.5% or 10% solution instilled before
examination. May be repeated in 10 to
60 minutes, if needed.
Mydriasis and vasoconstriction –
Adults and adolescents: 1 or 2 drops
of 2.5% or 10% solution
Children: 1 drop of 2.5% solution.
Chronic mydriasis –
Adults and adolescents: 1 drop of
2.5% or 10% solution instilled b.i.d.
or t.i.d.
Children: 1 drop of 2.5% solution in-
stilled b.i.d. or t.i.d.
Posterior synechia (adhesion of iris) –
Adults and children: 1 drop of 10%
solution.
    Do not use 10% concentration in
infants.

ADVERSE REACTIONS
CNS: browache, headache.
CV: *hypertension* (with 10% solution), tachycardia, palpitations,
PVCs.
EENT: transient eye burning or stinging on instillation, blurred vision, reactive hyperemia of eye, allergic conjunctivitis, iris floaters, acute angle-
closure glaucoma, rebound miosis.
Other: pallor, trembling, diaphoresis,
dermatitis.

INTERACTIONS
Guanethidine: increased mydriatic
and pressor effects of phenylephrine.
Use together cautiously.
Levodopa (systemic): reduced mydriatic effect of phenylephrine. Use together cautiously.
MAO inhibitors, beta blockers: may
cause arrhythmias because of increased pressor effect. Use together
cautiously.
*Topically applied atropine, cyclopen-
tolate, homatropine, scopolamine:*
may increase dilation of pupil. Use together cautiously.
Tricyclic antidepressants: potentiated
cardiac effects of epinephrine. Use together cautiously.

CONTRAINDICATIONS
Contraindicated in patients with hypersensitivity to drug or angle-closure
glaucoma and in those wearing soft
contact lenses.

NURSING CONSIDERATIONS
• Use cautiously in patients with
marked hypertension, cardiac disorders, advanced arteriosclerotic
changes, Type I diabetes, or hyperthyroidism; in children of low body
weight; and in elderly patients.
• Know that systemic adverse reactions are less likely with 2.5% solution; adverse reactions and toxicity
are much more likely with 10% solution.
• Teach patients how to instill drug.
Advise them to wash hands before and
after instilling drug and to apply light
finger pressure on lacrimal sac for 1

---

minute after drops are instilled. Warn patients not to touch tip of dropper to eye or surrounding tissue.
• Warn patients not to exceed recommended dosage because systemic effects can result. Monitor blood pressure and pulse rate.
• Advise patients to contact the doctor if condition persists longer than 12 hours after discontinuation of the drug.
• Warn patients to avoid hazardous activities, such as operating machinery or driving, until temporary blurring subsides.
• Advise patients to ease photophobia by wearing dark glasses.
• Tell patient not to use brown solutions or solutions that contain precipitate.

---

scopolamine hydrobromide
Isopto Hyoscine

Pregnancy Risk Category: NR

HOW SUPPLIED
Ophthalmic solution: 0.25%

ACTION
Anticholinergic action leaves the pupil under unopposed adrenergic influence, causing it to dilate.

ONSET, PEAK, DURATION
Onset is rapid. Mydriatic effect peaks within 15 to 30 minutes; cycloplegic effect, within 30 to 45 minutes. Effects persist up to 1 week.

INDICATIONS & DOSAGE
Cycloplegic refraction –
Adults: 1 to 2 drops of 0.25% solution 1 hour before refraction.
Children: 1 drop of 0.25% solution b.i.d. for 2 days before refraction.
Iritis, uveitis –
Adults: 1 to 2 drops of 0.25% solution once daily, b.i.d., or t.i.d.
Children: 1 drop once daily to t.i.d.

ADVERSE REACTIONS
CNS: ataxia, irritability, confusion, delirium, somnolence, acute psychotic reactions, hallucinations.
CV: tachycardia.
EENT: ocular congestion with prolonged use, conjunctivitis, *blurred vision,* eye dryness, increased intraocular pressure (IOP), *photophobia.*
GI: dry mouth.
Skin: dryness, contact dermatitis.
Other: flushing, fever.

INTERACTIONS
None significant.

CONTRAINDICATIONS
Contraindicated in patients with shallow anterior chamber and angle-closure glaucoma or hypersensitivity to the drug.

NURSING CONSIDERATIONS
• Use with extreme caution (if at all) in infants and small children.
• Use cautiously in patients with cardiac disease and in elderly patients.
• Observe patients closely for adverse CNS effects (such as disorientation and delirium).
• Know that scopolamine may be used in patients sensitive to atropine because it's faster acting and has a shorter duration of action and fewer adverse reactions.
• Teach patients how to instill drug. Advise them to wash hands before and after instilling drug and to apply light finger pressure on lacrimal sac for 1 minute after drops are instilled. Warn patients to avoid touching tip of dropper to eye or surrounding tissue.
• Warn patients to avoid hazardous activities, such as operating machinery or driving, until temporary blurring subsides.
• Advise patients to ease photophobia by wearing dark glasses.

---

tropicamide
Mydriacyl, Tropicacyl

Pregnancy Risk Category: NR

HOW SUPPLIED
Ophthalmic solution: 0.5%, 1%

ACTION
The shortest-acting cycloplegic available, whose anticholinergic action leaves the pupil under unopposed adrenergic influence, causing it to dilate.

ONSET, PEAK, DURATION
Onset rapid. Mydriatic effect peaks within 20 to 40 minutes; cycloplegic effect, within 20 to 35 minutes. Effects persist up to 7 hours.

INDICATIONS & DOSAGE
Cycloplegic refraction –
Adults: 1 drop of 1% solution; repeated in 5 minutes. If needed, additional drop in 20 to 30 minutes.
Children: 1 drop of 0.5% or 1% solution; repeated in 5 minutes, if needed.
Fundus examinations –
Adults and children: 1 to 2 drops of 0.5% solution in each eye 15 to 20 minutes before examination; instillation may be repeated q 30 minutes as needed.

ADVERSE REACTIONS
CNS: ataxia, irritability, confusion, somnolence, hallucinations, behavioral disturbances in children.
EENT: *transient eye stinging on instillation,* increased intraocular pressure, *blurred vision, photophobia; dry throat.*
GI: dry mouth.
Skin: dryness.
Other: flushing, fever.

INTERACTIONS
None significant.

CONTRAINDICATIONS
Contraindicated in patients with shallow anterior chamber and angle-closure glaucoma or hypersensitivity to drug.

NURSING CONSIDERATIONS
• Use cautiously in elderly patients.
• Know that tropicamide's mydriatic effect is greater than its cycloplegic effect.
• Teach patients how to instill drug. Advise them to wash hands before and after instilling drug and to apply light finger pressure on lacrimal sac for 1 minute after drops are instilled. Warn patients not to touch tip of dropper to eye or surrounding tissue.
• Warn patients that drug causes transient stinging.
• Warn patients to avoid hazardous activities, such as operating machinery or driving, until temporary blurring subsides.
• Advise patients to ease photophobia by wearing dark glasses.

---

†Available in Canada only.   ‡Available in Australia only.   ◇Available OTC.

Ophthalmic vasoconstrictors

naphazoline hydrochloride
oxymetazoline hydrochloride
tetrahydrozoline hydrochloride

COMBINATION PRODUCTS
ALBALON-A LIQUIFILM: naphazoline hydrochloride 0.05% and antazoline phosphate 0.5%.
BLEPHAMIDE LIQUIFILM SUSPENSION: phenylephrine hydrochloride 0.12%, sulfacetamide sodium 10%, and prednisolone acetate 0.2%.
PREFRIN-A: phenylephrine hydrochloride 0.12%, pyrilamine maleate 0.1%, and antipyrine 0.1%.
VASOCIDIN OPHTHALMIC OINTMENT: phenylephrine hydrochloride 0.125%, sulfacetamide sodium 10%, and prednisolone acetate 0.5%.
VASOCIDIN OPHTHALMIC SOLUTION: phenylephrine hydrochloride 0.125%, sulfacetamide sodium 10%, and prednisolone sodium phosphate 0.25%.
VASOCON-A OPHTHALMIC SOLUTION: naphazoline hydrochloride 0.05% and antazoline phosphate 0.5%.
ZINCFRIN◇: phenylephrine hydrochloride 0.12% and zinc sulfate 0.25%.

---

naphazoline hydrochloride
AK-Con, Albalon Liquifilm, Allerest◇, Clear Eyes◇, Degest 2◇, Estivin II, Naphcon◇, Naphcon Forte, Optazine‡, Vasoclear◇, Vasocon Regular

Pregnancy Risk Category: C

HOW SUPPLIED
Ophthalmic solution: 0.012%◇, 0.02%, 0.03%, 0.1%

ACTION
Unknown. Thought to cause vasoconstriction by local adrenergic action on the blood vessels of the conjunctiva.

ONSET, PEAK, DURATION
Local vasoconstriction usually occurs within 10 minutes. Peak unknown. Effects persist for 2 to 6 hours.

INDICATIONS & DOSAGE
Ocular congestion, irritation, itching –
Adults: 1 to 3 drops of 0.1% solution instilled q 3 to 4 hours or 1 to 2 drops of 0.012% to 0.03% solution up to q.i.d.

ADVERSE REACTIONS
CNS: headache, dizziness, nervousness, weakness.
EENT: transient eye stinging, pupillary dilation, eye irritation, photophobia, blurred vision, increased intraocular pressure.
GI: nausea.
Other: diaphoresis.

INTERACTIONS
Tricyclic antidepressants, MAO inhibitors: hypertensive crisis if naphazoline is systemically absorbed. Use together cautiously.

CONTRAINDICATIONS
Contraindicated in patients with hypersensitivity to any of drug's ingredients and in patients with acute angle-closure glaucoma. Use of 0.1% solution is contraindicated in children.

NURSING CONSIDERATIONS
● Use cautiously in patients with hyperthyroidism, cardiac disease, hypertension, or diabetes mellitus.

---

*Liquid form contains alcohol.
**May contain tartrazine.
Common reactions are in italics; *life-threatening,* in bold italics.

• Know that drug is most widely used ocular decongestant.
• Be aware that drug can produce marked sedation and coma in children, especially infants.
• Store in tightly closed container.
• Teach patients how to instill drug. Advise them to wash hands before and after instilling drug and to apply light finger pressure on lacrimal sac for 1 minute after drops are instilled. Warn them not to touch tip of dropper to eye or surrounding tissue.
• Warn patients not to exceed recommended dosage. Rebound congestion and conjunctivitis may occur with frequent or prolonged use.
• Tell patients to notify the doctor if photophobia, blurred vision, pain, or lid edema develops.

oxymetazoline hydrochloride
OcuClear◊, Visine L.R.◊

Pregnancy Risk Category: C

HOW SUPPLIED
Ophthalmic solution: 0.025%

ACTION
A direct-acting sympathomimetic amine that acts on alpha-adrenergic receptors in the arterioles of the conjunctiva to produce vasoconstriction, resulting in decreased conjunctival congestion.

ONSET, PEAK, DURATION
Onset occurs within 5 minutes. Peak unknown. Effects persist for approximately 6 hours.

INDICATIONS & DOSAGE
Relief of eye redness due to minor eye irritations –
Adults and children 6 years and over: 1 to 2 drops in the conjunctival sac two to four times daily (spaced at least 6 hours apart).

ADVERSE REACTIONS
EENT: *transient stinging upon initial instillation,* blurred vision, reactive hyperemia with excessive dosage or prolonged used.
Other: palpitations, tachycardia, irregular heartbeat, headache, lightheadedness, nervousness, trembling, insomnia.

INTERACTIONS
Tricyclic antidepressants, maprotiline: if significant systemic absorption of oxymetazoline occurs, concurrent use may potentiate the pressor effect of oxymetazoline.

CONTRAINDICATIONS
Contraindicated in patients hypersensitive to any component of the drug and in those with angle-closure glaucoma.

NURSING CONSIDERATIONS
• Use cautiously in patients with hyperthyroidism, cardiac disease, hypertension, and eye disease, infection, or injury.
• Tell patients not to use if solution has become cloudy or changes color.
• Teach patients how to instill drops. Advise them to wash hands before and after instilling solution, and warn them not to touch tip of dropper to eye or surrounding tissue.
• Advise patients to apply light finger pressure on lacrimal sac for 1 minute after drug instillation.
• Advise patients to stop the drug and see a doctor if eye pain occurs, if vision changes, or if redness or irritation continues, worsens, or lasts for more than 72 hours.

tetrahydrozoline hydrochloride
Murine Plus◊, Optigene◊, Soothe◊, Tetrasine◊, Visine◊

Pregnancy Risk Category: C

HOW SUPPLIED
Ophthalmic solution: 0.05%◊

ACTION
Unknown. Thought to cause vasoconstriction by local adrenergic action on the blood vessels of the conjunctiva.

ONSET, PEAK, DURATION
Onset occurs within a few minutes. Peak unknown. Effects persist for 4 to 8 hours.

INDICATIONS & DOSAGE
Conjunctival congestion, irritation, and allergic conditions –
Adults and children over 2 years: 1 to 2 drops of 0.05% solution instilled up to four times daily or as directed by the doctor.

ADVERSE REACTIONS
CNS: depression, headache, drowsiness, insomnia, dizziness, tremor.
CV: *cardiac arrhythmias.*
EENT: transient eye stinging, pupillary dilation, increased intraocular pressure, eye irritation, iris floaters in elderly patients.

INTERACTIONS
Guanethidine, MAO inhibitors, tricyclic antidepressants: hypertensive crisis if tetrahydrozoline is systemically absorbed. Don't use together.

CONTRAINDICATIONS
Contraindicated in patients hypersensitive to the drug or any of its components, and in those with angle-closure glaucoma or other serious eye diseases.

NURSING CONSIDERATIONS
• Use cautiously in patients with hyperthyroidism, heart disease, hypertension, or diabetes mellitus.
• Teach patients how to instill drug. Advise them to wash hands before and after instilling drug and to apply light finger pressure on lacrimal sac for 1 minute after drops are instilled. Warn them not to touch tip of dropper to eye or surrounding tissue.
• Warn patients not to exceed recommended dosage. Rebound congestion may occur with frequent or prolonged use.
• Tell patients to stop drug and notify the doctor if redness or irritation persists or increases or if no relief occurs within 2 days.
• Caution patients not to share eye medications with others.

---

*Liquid form contains alcohol.   *Common* reactions are in italics; *life-threatening*, in bold italics.
**May contain tartrazine.

apraclonidine hydrochloride
artificial tears
betaxolol hydrochloride
boric acid
botulinum toxin type A
carteolol hydrochloride
dapiprazole hydrochloride
dipivefrin
dorzolamide hydrochloride
eye irrigation solutions
fluorescein sodium
glycerin, anhydrous
isosorbide
levobunolol hydrochloride
levocabastine hydrochloride
lodoxamide tromethamine
metipranolol hydrochloride
sodium chloride, hypertonic
timolol maleate

COMBINATION PRODUCTS
FLURESS: fluorescein sodium 0.25%
and benoxinate hydrochloride 0.4%.

---

apraclonidine hydrochloride
Iopidine

Pregnancy Risk Category: C

HOW SUPPLIED
Ophthalmic solution: 1%

ACTION
Unknown; an alpha-adrenergic agonist that reduces intraocular pressure
(IOP), possibly by decreasing production of aqueous humor.

ONSET, PEAK, DURATION
Onset occurs within 1 hour. Peak effect occurs within 3 to 5 hours. Effects persist at least 12 hours.

INDICATIONS & DOSAGE
*Prevention or control of IOP elevation
before and after ocular laser surgery —*
Adults: 1 drop of 1% solution instilled 1 hour before initiation of laser
surgery on the anterior segment, followed by 1 drop immediately after
surgery.

ADVERSE REACTIONS
CNS: insomnia, irritability, dream
disturbances, headache.
CV: bradycardia, vasovagal attack,
palpitations, hypotension, or thostatic
hypotension.
EENT: upper eyelid elevation, conjunctival blanching and microhemor-
rhage, mydriasis, eye burning or discomfort, foreign body sensation in
eye, eye dryness and itching, blurred
vision, nasal burning or dryness, or
increased pharyngeal secretions.
GI: abdominal pain, discomfort,
diarrhea, vomiting, taste disturbances, dry mouth.
Skin: pruritus not associated with
rash.
Other: sweaty palms, body heat sensation, decreased libido, extremity
pain or numbness, allergic response.

INTERACTIONS
*Topical pilocarpine or beta-adrenergic
blockers:* additive effects in lowering
IOP. Use together cautiously.

CONTRAINDICATIONS
Contraindicated in patients hypersensitive to apraclonidine or clonidine.

NURSING CONSIDERATIONS
• Use cautiously in patients with severe cardiac disease including hypertension or history of vasovagal attack.
• Closely monitor patients who tend

to develop exaggerated decreases in IOP after drug therapy.
• Observe patients closely for vasovagal attack during laser surgery.
• Closely monitor patients with severe systemic disease, including hypertension, even though drug's systemic effects (altered heart rate and blood pressure) are uncommon after usual dose.

artificial tears

Adsorbotear◇, Hypotears◇, Isopto Alkaline◇, Isopto Plain◇, Isopto Tears◇, Lacril◇, Lacrisert, Liquifilm Forte◇, Liquifilm Tears◇, Lyteers◇, Methulose◇, Moisture Drops◇, Neo-Tears◇, Refresh◇, Tearisol◇, Tears Naturale◇, Tears Plus◇, Ultra Tears◇, Visculose◇

Pregnancy Risk Category: NR

HOW SUPPLIED
Ophthalmic solution: 2 ml◇, 15 ml◇, 30 ml◇
Ocular insert: 5 mg (hydroxypropyl cellulose)

ACTION
Augments insufficient tear production.

ONSET, PEAK, DURATION
Onset occurs immediately. Peak and duration unknown.

INDICATIONS & DOSAGE
Insufficient tear production –
Adults and children: 1 to 2 drops of solution in eye t.i.d., q.i.d., or p.r.n.
Moderate to severe dry eye syndromes, including keratoconjunctivitis sicca –
Adults: 1 Lacrisert rod inserted daily into inferior cul-de-sac. Some patients may require twice-daily use.

ADVERSE REACTIONS
EENT: eye discomfort; eye burning or pain on instillation; blurred vision (especially with Lacrisert); crust formation on eyelids and eyelashes in products with high viscosity, such as Adsorbotear, Isopto Tears, and Tearisol.

INTERACTIONS
Borate external irrigation solutions: may form gummy deposits on the lid when used with artificial tear products containing polyvinyl alcohol (Liquifilm Forte, Liquifilm Tears). Keep the patient's eyelids clean.

CONTRAINDICATIONS
Contraindicated in patients hypersensitive to the drug or any of its components.

NURSING CONSIDERATIONS
• Do not administer with contact lens in place unless product is designated for this use.
• Teach patients how to instill product. Advise them to wash hands before and after instilling and to avoid touching tip of dropper or container to eye, surrounding tissue, or other surface.
• Instruct patients that product should be used by only one person to prevent the spread of infection.
• Familiarize patient with Lacrisert rod insertion and special applicator that is included in the package.
• Tell patients to discontinue use and contact the doctor if condition worsens or does not improve.

betaxolol hydrochloride
Betoptic

Pregnancy Risk Category: C

HOW SUPPLIED
Ophthalmic solution: 0.5%
Ophthalmic suspension: 0.25%

ACTION
Unknown, although as a cardioselective beta blocker it reduces formation

and possibly increases outflow of aqueous humor.

ONSET, PEAK, DURATION
Onset occurs in ½ to 1 hour. Intraocular pressure (IOP) reduction peaks after a single dose within about 2 hours. Effects persist for 12 or more hours.

INDICATIONS & DOSAGE
Chronic open-angle glaucoma and ocular hypertension –
Adults: 1 or 2 drops of 0.5% solution or 0.25% suspension b.i.d.

ADVERSE REACTIONS
CNS: insomnia, confusion.
EENT: *eye stinging upon instillation,* occasional tearing, photophobia.

INTERACTIONS
Calcium channel blockers: AV conduction disturbances, ventricular failure, and hypotension if significant systemic absorption occurs. Monitor closely.
Cocaine: may inhibit betaxolol's effects. Avoid concomitant use.
Digitalis glycosides: excessive bradycardia; patients may require ECG monitoring if significant systemic absorption occurs.
Inhalation hydrocarbon anesthetics: prolonged severe hypotension if significant systemic absorption occurs. Tell the anesthesiologist that the patient is receiving ophthalmic betaxolol.
Ophthalmic epinephrine, dipivefrin: may produce mydriasis. Use together cautiously.
Oral antidiabetic agents, insulin: risk of hypoglycemia or hyperglycemia if significant systemic absorption occurs. Dosage adjustments or hypoglycemic medication may be necessary.
Phenothiazines: additive hypotensive effects; increased risk of adverse effects if significant systemic absorption occurs. Monitor closely.

Reserpine: excessive beta blockade. Monitor closely.
Systemic beta blockers: additive effects. Monitor closely.

CONTRAINDICATIONS
Contraindicated in patients with hypersensitivity to drug, sinus bradycardia, greater-than-first-degree AV block, cardiogenic shock, or overt heart failure.

NURSING CONSIDERATIONS
• Use cautiously in patients with restricted pulmonary function, diabetes mellitus, hyperthyroidism, or a history of heart failure.
• Keep in mind that some patients may need a few weeks' treatment to stabilize IOP-lowering response. Determine IOP after 4 weeks of treatment.
• Teach patients how to instill drug. Advise them to wash hands before and after instilling drug and to apply light finger pressure on lacrimal sac for 1 minute after instillation. Warn patients not to touch tip of dropper to eye or surrounding tissue. Be sure to shake suspension well before instilling.
• Encourage patients to comply with twice-daily dosage regimen.
• Advise patients to ease photophobia by wearing dark glasses.

---

boric acid
Blinx◊, Collyrium◊, Neo-Flo◊
Pregnancy Risk Category: NR

HOW SUPPLIED
Ophthalmic ointment: 5%◊, 10%◊
Ophthalmic solution: 30 ml◊, 120 ml◊, 180 ml◊

ACTION
Unknown. However, drug has fungistatic and bacteriostatic properties.

---

†Available in Canada only.   ‡Available in Australia only.   ◊ Available OTC.

ONSET, PEAK, DURATION
Unknown. Systemic absorption is negligible.

INDICATIONS & DOSAGE
For irrigation after tonometry, gonioscopy, foreign body removal, or use of fluorescein; to soothe and clean the eye –
Adults: eyewash p.r.n.; 1 to 2 eyedrops into affected eye up to q.i.d.; or 5% or 10% ointment one or two times daily.

ADVERSE REACTIONS
Systemic: toxic if absorbed from abraded skin areas, granulating wounds, or ingestion.

INTERACTIONS
Idoxuridine, polyvinyl alcohol (Liquifilm): may form insoluble complex. Check with pharmacy on contents of other eye drugs and contact lens wetting solutions.

CONTRAINDICATIONS
Contraindicated in patients with eye lacerations.

NURSING CONSIDERATIONS
• Don't apply to abraded cornea.
• Teach patients proper way to use eyewash: Fill eyecup half full. Apply the cup tightly to the affected eye and tilt head backward. Open the eye wide and rotate eyeball to thoroughly wash the eye. Always wash hands before and after instilling solution or ointment.
• Advise patient to avoid contaminating solution container. Tell patient not to use cloudy or discolored solutions.
• Tell patients not to share eye solution with family members.
• Tell patients not to use with soft contact lenses.

botulinum toxin type A
Botox
Pregnancy Risk Category: C

HOW SUPPLIED
Powder for injection: 100 units/vial

ACTION
A protein that produces a neuromuscular paralysis by binding to acetylcholine receptors on the motor endplate and that may inhibit the release of acetylcholine from presynaptic nerve endings.

ONSET, PEAK, DURATION
Onset occurs in 1 or 2 days after injection. Peak occurs within 1 to 2 weeks. Effects persist for 2 to 6 weeks.

INDICATIONS & DOSAGE
Strabismus –
Adults and children 12 years and over: injections should be made only by doctors familiar with the technique, which involves surgical exposure of the region as well as electromyographic guidance of the injection needle.

Dosage varies with the degree of deviation (lower doses are used for small deviations). For vertical muscles and for horizontal strabismus of < 20 prism diopters, the usual dosage is 1.25 to 2.5 units injected into any one muscle. For horizontal strabismus of 20 to 50 prism diopters, dosage is 2.5 to 5 units into any one muscle. For persistent (greater than 1 month's duration) palsy of the sixth cranial nerve, dosage is 1.25 to 2.5 units into the medial rectus muscle.

Subsequent injections for recurrent or residual strabismus should not be made until 7 to 14 days after the initial dose and unless substantial function has returned to the injected and adjacent muscles. Dosage may be increased up to twice the initial dose for

*Liquid form contains alcohol.
**May contain tartrazine.
Common reactions are in italics; *life-threatening,* in **bold italics.**

patients experiencing incomplete paralysis; subsequent doses in patients with adequate response should not be increased. The maximum single dose for any one muscle is 25 units.
Blepharospasm—
Adults: initially, 1.25 to 2.5 units injected into the medial and lateral pretarsal orbicularis oculi of the upper lid and into the lateral pretarsal orbicularis oculi of the lower lid. Effects should be apparent within 3 days and peak within 1 to 2 weeks. Dosage may be doubled if inadequate paralysis is achieved; however, exceeding 5 units/site produces no apparent benefit. Each treatment lasts about 3 months and can be repeated indefinitely.

Cumulative dosage should not exceed 200 units/month.

ADVERSE REACTIONS
EENT: double or blurred vision, spacial disorientation, *ptosis, vertical deviation* (after treatment of strabismus), *eye irritation* (after treatment of blepharospasm), *swelling of eyelid.*
Skin: diffuse rash, ecchymosis.

INTERACTIONS
None significant.

CONTRAINDICATIONS
Contraindicated in patients hypersensitive to the drug or any of its components.

NURSING CONSIDERATIONS
• Reconstitute the drug with preservative-free 0.9% sodium chloride solution. The vacuum in the vial should be noticeable when reconstituting. Inject the diluent into the vial gently because severe agitation can denature the protein.
• Keep in mind reconstituting with 1 ml of 0.9% sodium chloride solution produces a concentration of 10 units/0.1 ml; adding 2 ml yields 5 units/0.1 ml. Adding more diluent (such as 4 ml to produce 2.5 units/0.1 ml or 8 ml to

yield 1.25 units/0.1 ml) or using different injection volumes may also be used to adjust dosage.
• Reconstituted drug should be clear, colorless, and free of particulate matter. Record the date and time of reconstitution. Keep reconstituted drug in the refrigerator until use. Drug should be administered within 4 hours of removal from the freezer.
• Prepare the injection by drawing slightly more volume than needed into a sterile 1-ml syringe. Expel air bubbles in the barrel of the syringe and attach an electromyographic injection needle (if treating strabismus), such as a 1.5-inch, 27G needle. Expel excess drug into an appropriate waste container while checking for leakage around the needle. Be sure to use a new needle and syringe for each injection.
• Have epinephrine readily available in case of an anaphylactic reaction.
• Apply several drops of an ocular decongestant and a topical anesthetic as ordered before treating strabismus.
• Freeze at or below 23° F (−5° C).

---

carteolol hydrochloride
Ocupress Ophthalmic Solution, 1%

Pregnancy Risk Category: C

HOW SUPPLIED
Ophthalmic solution: 1%

ACTION
A nonselective beta-adrenergic blocking agent that reduces intraocular pressure, although the exact mechanism of action has not been definitely demonstrated.

ONSET, PEAK, DURATION
Unknown.

INDICATIONS & DOSAGE
Chronic open-angle glaucoma, intraocular hypertension—

Adults: 1 drop in the conjunctival sac of the affected eye b.i.d.

ADVERSE REACTIONS
EENT: *transient eye irritation, burning, tearing, conjunctival hyperemia, ocular edema,* blurred and cloudy vision, photophobia, decreased night vision, ptosis, blepharoconjunctivitis, abnormal corneal staining, corneal sensitivity.
Systemic: bradycardia, hypotension, arrhythmias, palpitations, dyspnea, asthenia, headache, dizziness, insomnia, sinusitis, taste perversion.

INTERACTIONS
Oral beta-adrenergic blocking agents, catecholamine-depleting agents (such as reserpine): may cause additive effects and the development of hypotension or bradycardia. Monitor patient closely.

CONTRAINDICATIONS
Contraindicated in patients hypersensitive to any component of the drug and in those with bronchial asthma, severe COPD, sinus bradycardia, second- or third-degree AV block, overt cardiac failure, or cardiogenic shock.

NURSING CONSIDERATIONS
• Use with caution in patients with nonallergic bronchospastic disease, diabetes mellitus, hyperthyroidism, hypersensitivity to other beta-adrenergic agents, or decreased pulmonary function and in breast-feeding women.
• Discontinue drug at the first sign of cardiac failure and notify the doctor.
• Be aware that when the drug is used to reduce elevated intraocular pressure in angle-closure glaucoma, it should be used in combination with a miotic and should not be used alone.
• Instruct patient that if more than one topical ophthalmic drug is being used, the drugs should be administered at least 10 minutes apart.

• Teach patients how to instill drops. Advise them to wash hands before and after instilling solution, and warn them not to touch tip of the dropper to eye or surrounding tissue.
• Also teach patients to keep bottle tightly closed when not in use and to protect it from light.
• Tell patient that drug is a beta-adrenergic blocker and, although it is administered topically, it has the potential to be absorbed systemically. Advise patient to apply light finger pressure on lacrimal sac for 1 minute after drug instillation to minimize systemic absorption.
• Also tell patient that the same types of adverse reactions that are attributable to beta-adrenergic agent therapy may occur with topical administration. If signs of serious adverse reactions or hypersensitivity occur, tell the patient to discontinue the drug and notify the doctor immediately.
• Advise the patient to ease photophobia by wearing dark glasses.
• Stress the importance of compliance with recommended therapy.

dapiprazole hydrochloride
Rēv-Eyes

Pregnancy Risk Category: B

HOW SUPPLIED
Ophthalmic powder: 25 mg/vial with 5 ml diluent and dropper supplied

ACTION
Blocks alpha-adrenergic receptors in smooth muscle, producing miosis through an effect on the dilator muscle of the iris.

ONSET, PEAK, DURATION
Onset rapid. Peak and duration unknown.

INDICATIONS & DOSAGE
Mydriasis—
Adults: 2 drops instilled into the con-

---

junctiva of each eye, followed in 5 minutes by another 2 drops.

ADVERSE REACTIONS
CNS: headache, browache.
EENT: *conjunctival injection lasting 20 minutes,* eye burning on instillation, ptosis, lid erythema, lid edema, chemosis, eye itching or dryness, punctate keratitis, corneal edema, photophobia, tearing, blurry vision.

INTERACTIONS
None significant.

CONTRAINDICATIONS
Contraindicated in patients hypersensitive to the drug or any of its components; when pupil constriction is undesirable, as in acute iritis; to reduce intraocular pressure (IOP); and to treat open-angle glaucoma.

NURSING CONSIDERATIONS
• To prepare, remove and discard aluminum seals and rubber stoppers from both drug and diluent vials. Pour diluent into drug vial and attach dropper assembly. Shake vial to ensure mixing.
• To avoid contamination, do not touch dropper to any surface.
• Be aware that drug should not be used in same patient more than once per week.
• Be aware that dapiprazole has no significant activity on ciliary muscle contraction, nor does it significantly alter IOP in normotensive eyes or in eyes with increased IOP. Eye color can affect the rate of pupillary constriction, but not the final pupil size.
• Store at room temperature for 21 days. Discard any discolored solution.

dipivefrin
Propine

Pregnancy Risk Category: B

HOW SUPPLIED
Ophthalmic solution: 0.1%

ACTION
A prodrug of epinephrine, dipivefrin is converted to epinephrine in the eye. The liberated epinephrine appears to decrease aqueous production and increase aqueous outflow.

ONSET, PEAK, DURATION
Onset occurs within 30 minutes. Peak effect occurs within 1 hour. Effects persist for 12 hours or more.

INDICATIONS & DOSAGE
Intraocular pressure (IOP) reduction in chronic open-angle glaucoma –
Adults: for initial glaucoma therapy, 1 drop of 0.1% solution q 12 hours. Adjustments in dosage then made based on patient response as determined by tonometric readings.

ADVERSE REACTIONS
CV: tachycardia, hypertension.
EENT: eye burning or stinging.

INTERACTIONS
Digitalis glycosides, inhalation hydrocarbon anesthetics, tricyclic antidepressants: increased risk of adverse cardiac effects if significant systemic absorption occurs. Monitor closely.
Ophthalmic beta blockers, osmotic agents, systemically administered carbonic anhydrase inhibitors: additive lowering of IOP. Use together cautiously. Monitor for potential adverse effects.
Systemic sympathomimetics: possible additive effects if significant systemic absorption occurs. Monitor closely.

CONTRAINDICATIONS
Contraindicated in patients with angle-closure glaucoma or hypersensitivity to drug.

NURSING CONSIDERATIONS

• Use cautiously in patients with aphakia or cardiovascular disease, history of hypersensitivity to epinephrine, and asthma.

• Be aware that drug is often used concomitantly with other antiglaucoma drugs.

• Know that drug may have fewer adverse reactions than conventional epinephrine therapy.

• Teach patients how to instill dipivefrin. Advise them to wash hands before and after instilling drug and to avoid touching tip of dropper to eye or surrounding tissue.

---

dorzolamide hydrochloride
Trusopt

Pregnancy Risk Category: C

HOW SUPPLIED
Ophthalmic solution: 2%

ACTION
Inhibits carbonic anhydrase in the ciliary processes of the eye, which decreases aqueous humor secretion, presumably by slowing the formation of bicarbonate ions with a subsequent reduction in sodium and fluid transport. The result is a reduction in intraocular pressure.

ONSET, PEAK, DURATION
Unknown.

INDICATIONS & DOSAGE
Treatment of elevated intraocular pressure in patients with ocular hypertension or open-angle glaucoma —
Adults: 1 drop in the conjunctival sac of the affected eye t.i.d.

ADVERSE REACTIONS
EENT: *ocular burning, stinging, or discomfort; superficial punctate keratitis; ocular allergic reaction; blurred vision; lacrimation; dryness; photophobia;* iridocyclitis.

Other: bitter taste, headache, nausea, asthenia, fatigue, rash, urolithiasis.

INTERACTIONS
Oral carbonic anhydrase inhibitors: may cause additive effects. Do not administer concomitantly.

CONTRAINDICATIONS
Contraindicated in patients hypersensitive to any component of the drug and in those with renal impairment.

NURSING CONSIDERATIONS

• Use with caution in patients with hepatic impairment.

• Instruct patient that if more than one topical ophthalmic drug is being used, the drugs should be administered at least 10 minutes apart.

• Teach patients how to instill drops. Advise them to wash hands before and after instilling solution, and warn them not to touch tip of the dropper to eye or surrounding tissue.

• Tell patient that the drug is a sulfonamide and, although it is administered topically, it can be absorbed systemically. Advise patient to apply light finger pressure on lacrimal sac for 1 minute after drug instillation to minimize systemic absorption.

• Tell patient that the same types of adverse reactions that are attributable to sulfonamides may occur with topical administration. If signs of serious adverse reactions or hypersensitivity occur, tell the patient to discontinue the drug and notify the doctor immediately.

• Also tell the patient to discontinue the drug and notify the doctor if any ocular reactions, particularly conjunctivitis and eyelid reactions, occur.

• Tell patient not to wear soft contact lenses while using this drug.

• Stress the importance of compliance with recommended therapy.

---

*Liquid form contains alcohol.
**May contain tartrazine.

Common reactions are in italics; ***life-threatening,*** in bold italics.

eye irrigation solutions
Blinx◊, Collyrium◊, Dacriose◊,
Eye-Stream◊, I-Lite Eye Drops◊,
Lauro Eye Wash◊, Lavoptik Eye
Wash◊, Murine Eye Drops◊, Neo-
Flo◊, Sterile 0.9% sodium
chloride◊

Pregnancy Risk Category: NR

HOW SUPPLIED
Ophthalmic solution: 15 ml◊, 30 ml◊,
120 ml◊, 180 ml◊

ACTION
Cleans the eye.

ONSET, PEAK, DURATION
Onset and peak immediate. Effects
persist as long as solution is in contact
with eye.

INDICATIONS & DOSAGE
Eye irrigation –
Adults and children: eye flushed
with 1 to 2 drops t.i.d., q.i.d., or
p.r.n.

ADVERSE REACTIONS
None reported.

INTERACTIONS
*Products containing polyvinyl alco-
hol:* may form gel and gummy deposits on the eye. Keep the patient's eyelids clean.

CONTRAINDICATIONS
Contraindicated in patients hypersensitive to the drug or any of its components.

NURSING CONSIDERATIONS
● Teach patients how to instill solution. Advise them to wash hands before and after instilling solution and to
avoid touching tip of container to eye,
surrounding tissue, or other surface.
Teach patients to turn their head to
side, irrigating from inner to outer
canthus.

● Instruct patients that product
should be used by only one person to
prevent the spread of infection.
● Tell patient to store in tightly
closed, light-resistant container.
Check expiration date.

fluorescein sodium
Fluorescite, Fluor-I-Strip, Fluor-I-
Strip A.T., Ful-Glo, Funduscein
Injections

Pregnancy Risk Category: C

HOW SUPPLIED
Ophthalmic solution: 2%
Ophthalmic strips: 0.6 mg, 1 mg, 9
mg
Parenteral injection: 10%, 25%

ACTION
A water-soluble dye that produces an
intense green fluorescence in alkaline
solution (pH 5.0 or less) or a bright
yellow if viewed under cobalt blue illumination.

ONSET, PEAK, DURATION
Onset immediate. Peak and duration
unknown.

INDICATIONS & DOSAGE
*Diagnostic in corneal abrasions and
foreign bodies; fitting hard contact
lenses; lacrimal patency; fundus pho-
tography; applanation tonometry –*
Adults and children: 1 or 2 drops of
2% solution followed by irrigation; or
strip moistened with sterile water,
then conjunctiva or fornix touched
with moistened tip, and eye flushed
with irrigating solution. Patient
should blink several times after application.
Retinal angiography –
Adults: 5 ml of 10% solution (500
mg) or 3 ml of 25% solution (750 mg)
rapidly injected into antecubital vein.
Children: 0.077 ml of 10% solution
(7.7 mg/kg body weight) or 0.044 ml
of 25% solution (7.5 mg/kg body

weight) rapidly injected into antecubital vein.

ADVERSE REACTIONS
Topical use:
EENT: eye stinging or burning, yellow tears.
Intravenous use:
CNS: headache persisting for 24 to 36 hours, dizziness, syncope, *seizures.*
CV: hypotension, *shock, cardiac arrest, thrombophlebitis.*
GI: nausea, vomiting.
GU: bright yellow urine (persists for 24 to 36 hours).
Skin: yellow skin discoloration (fades in 6 to 12 hours).
Other: hypersensitivity reactions, including urticaria and *anaphylaxis;* extravasation at injection site.

INTERACTIONS
None significant.

CONTRAINDICATIONS
Contraindicated in patients with hypersensitivity to drug; do not use with soft contact lenses (lenses may become discolored).

NURSING CONSIDERATIONS
• Use cautiously in patients with history of allergy or bronchial asthma.
• Always use aseptic technique. Easily contaminated by *Pseudomonas aeruginosa.*
• **I.V. use:** Keep an antihistamine, epinephrine, and oxygen available when giving parenterally. Avoid extravasation during injection.
• Use topical anesthetic as ordered before instilling to relieve burning and irritation.
• Never instill dye while patients are wearing soft contact lenses; fluorescein will ruin them.
• Be aware that defects appear green under normal light or bright yellow under cobalt blue illumination. Foreign bodies are surrounded by a green

ring. Similar lesions of the conjunctiva are delineated in orange-yellow.
• Don't freeze; store below 80° F (26.7° C).
• Warn patients that urine will be bright yellow after injection and that routine urinalysis will be abnormal within 1 hour after injection.

---

glycerin, anhydrous
Ophthalgan

Pregnancy Risk Category: C

HOW SUPPLIED
Ophthalmic solution: 7.5-ml containers

ACTION
Removes excess fluid from the cornea.

ONSET, PEAK, DURATION
Onset and peak immediate. Effect is transient.

INDICATIONS & DOSAGE
Corneal edema before ophthalmoscopy or gonioscopy in acute open-angle glaucoma, bullous keratitis, and Fuchs' endothelial dystrophy–
Adults and children: prior to the examination, 1 to 2 drops after instillation of a local anesthetic.

ADVERSE REACTIONS
EENT: pain if instilled without topical anesthetic.

INTERACTIONS
None significant.

CONTRAINDICATIONS
Contraindicated in patients hypersensitive to the drug.

NURSING CONSIDERATIONS
• Use topical tetracaine or proparacaine, as ordered, before instilling to prevent discomfort.
• Don't touch tip of dropper to eye,

---

*Liquid form contains alcohol.
**May contain tartrazine.
Common reactions are in italics; *life-threatening,* in bold italics.

surrounding tissue, or tear-film; anhydrous glycerin will absorb moisture.
• Be aware that anhydrous glycerin is used to temporarily restore corneal transparency when cornea is too edematous to permit diagnosis.

isosorbide
Ismotic

Pregnancy Risk Category: B

HOW SUPPLIED
Oral solution: 45% (100 g/225 ml) in 220-ml containers

ACTION
Acts as an osmotic agent by promoting redistribution of water and thereby producing diuresis.

ONSET, PEAK, DURATION
Onset occurs within 30 minutes. Peak effects occur in 1 to 1½ hours. Duration unknown.

INDICATIONS & DOSAGE
Short-term reduction of intraocular pressure (IOP) caused by glaucoma –
Adults: initially, 1.5 g/kg P.O. Usual dosage range is 1 to 3 g/kg.

ADVERSE REACTIONS
CNS: vertigo, light-headedness, lethargy, headache, confusion.
GI: gastric discomfort, diarrhea, anorexia, nausea, vomiting.
Other: hypernatremia, hyperosmolality, thirst.

INTERACTIONS
None significant.

CONTRAINDICATIONS
Contraindicated in patients with anuria caused by severe renal disease, severe dehydration, acute pulmonary edema, and hemorrhagic glaucoma.

NURSING CONSIDERATIONS
• Know that additional doses should be used cautiously, especially in patients with diseases associated with sodium retention, such as CHF.
• To improve palatability, pour medication over cracked ice and tell patients to sip it.
• Monitor patients closely for 5 to 10 minutes after administration for adverse effects.
• Keep in mind that isosorbide is especially useful for rapid reduction of IOP. May be used to interrupt acute attack of glaucoma before laser surgery.
• Tell patients that this drug may induce thirst. In patients with diseases associated with sodium retention, carefully monitor fluid and electrolyte balance.

levobunolol hydrochloride
Betagan

Pregnancy Risk Category: C

HOW SUPPLIED
Ophthalmic solution: 0.25%, 0.5%

ACTION
Unknown. A nonselective beta blocker that is thought to reduce formation and possibly increase outflow of aqueous humor.

ONSET, PEAK, DURATION
Onset occurs within 1 hour. Intraocular pressure (IOP) reduction peaks within 2 to 6 hours after a single dose. Effects persist up to 24 hours.

INDICATIONS & DOSAGE
Chronic open-angle glaucoma and ocular hypertension –
Adults: 1 to 2 drops once daily or b.i.d.

ADVERSE REACTIONS
CNS: headache, dizziness, depression.

CV: slight reduction in resting heart rate.
EENT: *transient eye stinging and burning;* decreased corneal sensitivity with long-term use.
GI: nausea.
Skin: urticaria.
Other: evidence of beta blockade and systemic absorption *(hypotension, bradycardia, syncope, **asthmatic attacks in patients with a history of asthma,** and **CHF**).*

INTERACTIONS
Propranolol, metoprolol, and other oral beta-adrenergic blockers: increased ocular and systemic effect. Use together cautiously.
Reserpine and other catecholamine-depleting drugs: enhanced hypotensive and bradycardiac effects. Monitor closely.
Topical miotics, dipivefrin, epinephrine; systemically administered carbonic anhydrase inhibitors: additive lowered IOP. Use together cautiously.

CONTRAINDICATIONS
Contraindicated in patients with hypersensitivity to drug, bronchial asthma, history of bronchial asthma or severe COPD, sinus bradycardia, second- or third-degree AV block, cardiac failure, and cardiogenic shock.

NURSING CONSIDERATIONS
• Use cautiously in patients with chronic bronchitis and emphysema, diabetes mellitus, hyperthyroidism, and myasthenia gravis.
• Teach patients how to instill levobunolol. Advise them to wash hands before and after instilling drug and to apply light finger pressure on lacrimal sac for 1 minute after drops are instilled. Warn patients not to touch dropper to eye or surrounding tissue.

levocabastine hydrochloride
Livostin

Pregnancy Risk Category: C

HOW SUPPLIED
Ophthalmic suspension: 0.05%

ACTION
Selectively blocks ophthalmic histamine H_1 receptors.

ONSET, PEAK, DURATION
Unknown.

INDICATIONS & DOSAGE
Temporary relief of seasonal allergic conjunctivitis –
Adults and children 12 years and older: 1 drop q.i.d. for up to 2 weeks.

ADVERSE REACTIONS
CNS: headache, fatigue, somnolence.
EENT: transient eye discomfort upon instillation (burning, stinging), eye discharge, dryness, pain, or redness; lacrimation; eyelid edema; visual disturbances; pharyngitis.
GI: dry mouth, nausea.
Respiratory: cough, dyspnea.
Skin: rash.

INTERACTIONS
None significant.

CONTRAINDICATIONS
Contraindicated in patients hypersensitive to the drug or any of its components and while soft contacts are worn.

NURSING CONSIDERATIONS
• Teach patients how to instill levocabastine. Advise them to wash hands before and after instilling drug and to avoid touching tip of dropper to eye or surrounding tissue. Be sure to shake suspension well before instilling.
• Warn patient that he may experience transient discomfort or burning

---

upon instillation. Tell him to contact the doctor if pain persists.
- Tell patients not to wear soft contact lenses during therapy.
- Tell patient to store drug at room temperature; avoid freezing. Do not use if solution is discolored.

lodoxamide tromethamine
Alomide

Pregnancy Risk Category: B

HOW SUPPLIED
Ophthalmic solution: 0.1%

ACTION
Stabilizes mast cells and prevents the release of inflammation mediators.

ONSET, PEAK, DURATION
Unknown.

INDICATIONS & DOSAGE
Vernal conjunctivitis, vernal kerato-conjunctivitis, vernal keratitis –
Adults and children 2 years and older: 1 to 2 drops in affected eye q.i.d. for up to 3 months.

ADVERSE REACTIONS
CNS: headache, dizziness, somnolence.
EENT: transient eye discomfort upon instillation (burning, stinging); anterior chamber cells; blepharitis; blurred vision; chemosis; corneal erosion, ulcer, or abrasion; crystalline deposits; epitheliopathy; sensation of foreign body, stickiness, or warmth; hyperemia; keratitis; keratopathy; ocular edema, discharge, swelling, fatigue, itching, or allergy; pruritus; scales on eyelids or eyelash; tearing; dry nose.
GI: nausea, stomach discomfort.
Skin: rash.

INTERACTIONS
None significant.

CONTRAINDICATIONS
Contraindicated in patients hypersensitive to the drug or any of its components.

NURSING CONSIDERATIONS
- Teach patients how to instill lodoxamide. Advise them to wash hands before and after instilling drug and to avoid touching tip of dropper to eye or surrounding tissue.
- Tell patients to contact the doctor if discomfort or burning persists upon instillation.
- Advise patients not to wear soft contact lenses during therapy.

metipranolol hydrochloride
OptiPranolol

Pregnancy Risk Category: C

HOW SUPPLIED
Ophthalmic solution: 0.3% in 5- or 10-ml dropper bottles

ACTION
Unknown. A noncardioselective beta-adrenergic blocker that appears to reduce aqueous production and to reduce elevated and normal intraocular pressure (IOP) with or without glaucoma with little or no effect on pupil size or accommodation. IOP above 24 mm Hg is reduced an average of 20% to 26%.

ONSET, PEAK, DURATION
Onset occurs within 30 minutes. Peak effect occurs within about 2 hours. Effects persist about 12 to 24 hours.

INDICATIONS & DOSAGE
IOP reduction in ocular conditions, including ocular hypertension and chronic open-angle glaucoma –
Adults: 1 drop into affected eye b.i.d. If IOP is not at a satisfactory level, concomitant therapy to lower it may be instituted.

---

†Available in Canada only.   ‡Available in Australia only.   ◇Available OTC.

ADVERSE REACTIONS

CNS: headache, anxiety, dizziness, depression, somnolence, nervousness, asthenia, browache.

CV: hypertension, *MI*, atrial fibrillation, angina, palpitation, bradycardia.

EENT: transient local eye discomfort, tearing, conjunctivitis, eyelid dermatitis, blurred vision, blepharitis, abnormal vision, photophobia, eye edema, rhinitis, epistaxis.

GI: nausea.

Respiratory: dyspnea, bronchitis, cough.

Skin: rash.

Other: hypersensitivity reactions, myalgia.

INTERACTIONS

Calcium channel blockers, digitalis glycosides, quinidine: increased risk of adverse cardiac effects if significant amount of drug is systemically absorbed. Use together cautiously.

Fentanyl, general anesthetics: excessive hypotension. Monitor closely.

Metoprolol tartrate, propranolol, other oral beta-adrenergic blockers: increased ocular and systemic effects. Use together cautiously.

Reserpine and other catecholamine-depleting drugs: enhanced hypotensive and bradycardic effects. Avoid concurrent use.

CONTRAINDICATIONS

Contraindicated in patients hypersensitive to the drug or any of its components and in patients with bronchial asthma, history of bronchial asthma or severe COPD, sinus bradycardia, second- or third-degree AV block, cardiac failure, and cardiogenic shock.

NURSING CONSIDERATIONS

• Use cautiously in patients with non-allergic bronchospasm, chronic bronchitis, emphysema, diabetes mellitus (especially in those subject to spontaneous hypoglycemia), hyperthyroidism, or cerebrovascular insufficiency.

• Anticipate using pilocarpine, other miotics, or systemic carbonic anhydrase inhibitors concomitantly if IOP is not adequately controlled.

• Check expiration date on bottle before use. Do not use if eyedrops have changed color.

• Be aware that a slight increase in outflow facility has been demonstrated with metipranolol. Like other noncardioselective beta-adrenergic blockers, metipranolol does not have significant local anesthetic (membrane-stabilizing) actions or intrinsic sympathomimetic activity.

• Teach patients how to instill metipranolol. Instruct them to first wash hands thoroughly and then tilt head back or lie down and gaze upward. Tell them to gently grasp lower eyelid below eyelashes and pull eyelid away from eye to form a pouch. Then have them place dropper directly over eye, avoiding contact with eye or any surface; look up just before applying drop; and look down for several seconds after instillation and slowly release eyelid.

• Tell patients to close eyes gently for 1 to 2 minutes and to apply gentle pressure to inside corner of eye at bridge of nose to retard draining of solution from intended area. Warn them not to rub eye or rinse dropper.

sodium chloride, hypertonic

Adsorbonac Ophthalmic Solution, Muro-128 Ointment, Sodium Chloride Ointment 5%

Pregnancy Risk Category: NR

HOW SUPPLIED

Ophthalmic ointment: 5%
Ophthalmic solution: 2%, 5%

ACTION

An osmotic agent that removes excess fluid from the cornea.

ONSET, PEAK, DURATION

Unknown.

INDICATIONS & DOSAGE

Temporary relief of corneal edema –
Adults and children: 1 to 2 drops q 3 to 4 hours, or ointment applied h.s.

ADVERSE REACTIONS

EENT: slight eye stinging.
Other: hypersensitivity reactions.

INTERACTIONS

None significant.

CONTRAINDICATIONS

Contraindicated in patients hypersensitive to the drug or any of its components.

NURSING CONSIDERATIONS

• Teach patients how to instill drug. Advise them to wash hands before and after instilling drug and to apply light finger pressure on lacrimal sac for 1 minute after drops are instilled. Warn patients not to touch dropper to eye or surrounding tissue.
• Tell patients to prevent caking on dropper bottle tip by putting a few drops of sterile irrigation solution inside bottle cap.
• Warn patients that ointment may cause blurred vision.
• If patients experience severe headache, pain, rapid change in vision, acute redness of eyes, sudden appearance of floating spots, pain on exposure to light, or double vision, tell them to discontinue the drug and notify doctor.
• Advise patient to store drug in tightly closed container.

timolol maleate

Timoptic Solution

Pregnancy Risk Category: C

HOW SUPPLIED

Ophthalmic solution: 0.25%, 0.5%

ACTION

Unknown. A beta blocker that is thought to reduce aqueous formation and possibly increase aqueous outflow.

ONSET, PEAK, DURATION

Onset occurs within 30 minutes. Peak effects occur within 1 to 2 hours. Effects persist for 12 to 24 hours.

INDICATIONS & DOSAGE

Chronic open-angle, secondary, and aphakic glaucomas; ocular hypertension –
Adults: initially, 1 drop of 0.25% solution in each affected eye b.i.d.; maintenance dosage is 1 drop daily. If no response, 1 drop of 0.5% solution in each affected eye b.i.d. If intraocular pressure (IOP) is controlled, dosage reduced to 1 drop daily.

ADVERSE REACTIONS

CNS: headache, depression, fatigue.
CV: slight reduction in resting heart rate.
Eye: minor eye irritation, decreased corneal sensitivity with long-term use.
GI: anorexia.
Other: apnea in infants, *evidence of beta blockade and systemic absorption (hypotension, bradycardia, syncope, asthmatic attacks in patients with a history of asthma, and CHF).*

INTERACTIONS

Calcium channel blockers, digitalis glycosides, quinidine: increased risk of adverse cardiac effects if significant amounts of timolol are systemi-

cally absorbed. Use together cautiously.
Fentanyl, general anesthetics: excessive hypotension. Monitor closely.
Metoprolol tartrate, propranolol, other oral beta-adrenergic blockers: increased ocular and systemic effects. Use together cautiously.
Reserpine and other catecholamine-depleting drugs: enhanced hypotensive and bradycardiac effects. Avoid concurrent use.

CONTRAINDICATIONS

Contraindicated in patients hypersensitive to the drug and in patients with bronchial asthma, history of bronchial asthma or severe COPD, sinus bradycardia, second- or third-degree AV block, cardiac failure, and cardiogenic shock.

NURSING CONSIDERATIONS

• Use cautiously in patients with non-allergic bronchospasm, chronic bronchitis, emphysema, diabetes mellitus, hyperthyroidism, or cerebrovascular insufficiency.
• Monitor diabetic patients carefully. Systemic beta-blocking effects can mask some signs of hypoglycemia in diabetic patients.
• Be aware that some patients may need a few weeks' treatment to stabilize pressure-lowering response. Determine IOP after 4 weeks of treatment.
• Know that the drug can be used safely in patients with glaucoma who wear conventional hard contact lenses.
• Teach patients how to instill timolol. Advise them to wash hands before and after instilling drug and to apply light finger pressure on lacrimal sac for 1 minute after drops are instilled. Warn patients not to touch dropper to eye or surrounding tissue.

---

acetic acid
boric acid
carbamide peroxide
chloramphenicol
triethanolamine polypeptide
   oleate-condensate

COMBINATION PRODUCTS
BOROFAIR OTIC: acetic acid 2% and
aluminum acetate 2%.

acetic acid
Domeboro Otic, VoSol Otic

Pregnancy Risk Category: NR

HOW SUPPLIED
Otic solution: 2% acetic acid in aluminum acetate solution (Domeboro
Otic), 2% acetic acid with 3% propylene glycol diacetate (VoSol Otic)

ACTION
Inhibits or destroys bacteria in the ear
canal.

ONSET, PEAK, DURATION
Unknown.

INDICATIONS & DOSAGE
External ear canal infection –
Adults and children: 4 to 6 drops
into ear canal t.i.d. or q.i.d.; or insert
saturated wick for first 24 hours, then
continue with instillations.
Prophylaxis of swimmer's ear –
Adults and children: 2 drops in each
ear b.i.d.

ADVERSE REACTIONS
EENT: ear irritation or itching.
Skin: urticaria.
Other: overgrowth of nonsusceptible
organisms.

INTERACTIONS
None significant.

CONTRAINDICATIONS
Contraindicated in patients with perforated eardrum.

NURSING CONSIDERATIONS
• Reculture any persistent drainage.
• Be aware that drug has anti-infective, anti-inflammatory, and antipruritic effects. *Pseudomonas aeruginosa*
is particularly sensitive to this drug.
• Warn patients to avoid touching ear
with dropper to prevent reinfection.

boric acid
Aurocaine 2◇, Auro-Dri◇, Dri/Ear◇,
Ear-Dry◇

Pregnancy Risk Category: NR

HOW SUPPLIED
Otic solution: 2.75% boric acid in iso-
propyl alcohol

ACTION
Weak bacteriostatic that inhibits or
destroys bacteria in the ear canal; also
is a fungistatic agent.

ONSET, PEAK, DURATION
Unknown.

INDICATIONS & DOSAGE
External ear canal infection –
Adults and children: 3 to 6 drops
into ear canal; plug with cotton. Repeated t.i.d. or q.i.d.

ADVERSE REACTIONS
EENT: ear irritation or itching.
Skin: urticaria.
Other: overgrowth of nonsusceptible
organisms.

---

†Available in Canada only.   ‡Available in Australia only.   ◇Available OTC.

INTERACTIONS
None significant.

CONTRAINDICATIONS
Contraindicated in patients with a perforated eardrum or excoriated membranes in ear.

NURSING CONSIDERATIONS
• Watch for signs of superinfection (continual pain, inflammation, fever).
• Warn patients to avoid touching ear with dropper to prevent reinfection.
• Tell patients using cotton plug to always moisten with medication.

carbamide peroxide
Debrox◇

Pregnancy Risk Category: NR

HOW SUPPLIED
Otic solution: 6.5% carbamide in glycerin or glycerin and propylene glycol

ACTION
A ceruminolytic that emulsifies and disperses accumulated cerumen.

ONSET, PEAK, DURATION
Onset and peak unknown. Duration is 15 to 30 minutes.

INDICATIONS & DOSAGE
Impacted cerumen –
Adults and children: 5 to 10 drops into ear canal b.i.d. Allow solution to remain in ear canal for 15 to 30 minutes; remove with warm water.

ADVERSE REACTIONS
None reported.

INTERACTIONS
None significant.

CONTRAINDICATIONS
Contraindicated in patients with a perforated eardrum.

NURSING CONSIDERATIONS
• Use in children under 12 years only under a doctor's direction.
• Warn patients to avoid touching ear with dropper to prevent reinfection.
• Tell patients to flush ear gently with warm water, using a rubber bulb syringe.
• Tell patients to call the doctor if redness, pain, or swelling persists.

chloramphenicol
Chloromycetin Otic, Sopamycetin†

Pregnancy Risk Category: NR

HOW SUPPLIED
Otic solution: 0.5%

ACTION
Inhibits or destroys bacteria in the ear canal.

ONSET, PEAK, DURATION
Unknown.

INDICATIONS & DOSAGE
External ear canal infection –
Adults and children: 2 to 3 drops into ear canal t.i.d.

ADVERSE REACTIONS
EENT: ear itching or burning, sore throat.
Skin: pruritus, urticaria, vesicular or maculopapular dermatitis, angioedema.
Other: overgrowth of nonsusceptible organisms, burning.

INTERACTIONS
None significant.

CONTRAINDICATIONS
Contraindicated in patients with a perforated eardrum.

NURSING CONSIDERATIONS
• Obtain history of use and reaction to drug.
• Watch for signs of superinfection

---

*Liquid form contains alcohol.
**May contain tartrazine.

Common reactions are in italics; ***life-threatening***, in bold italics.

(continued pain, inflammation, fever). Avoid prolonged use.
• Reculture any persistent drainage.
• Watch for signs of sore throat (early sign of toxicity).
• Warn patients to avoid touching ear with dropper to avoid reinfection.

triethanolamine polypeptide oleate-condensate
Cerumenex

Pregnancy Risk Category: NR

HOW SUPPLIED
Otic solution: 10% in 6-ml, 12-ml bottles with droppers

ACTION
A ceruminolytic that emulsifies and disperses accumulated cerumen.

ONSET, PEAK, DURATION
Onset and peak unknown. Duration is 15 to 30 minutes.

INDICATIONS & DOSAGE
Impacted cerumen –
Adults and children: fill ear canal with solution and insert cotton plug. After 15 to 30 minutes, flush ear with warm water.

ADVERSE REACTIONS
EENT: ear erythema or pruritus.
Skin: severe eczema.

INTERACTIONS
None significant.

CONTRAINDICATIONS
Contraindicated in perforated eardrum, otitis media, and otitis externa.

NURSING CONSIDERATIONS
• If hypersensitivity is suspected, anticipate patch test by placing 1 drop of drug on inner forearm; cover with small bandage. Read results in 24 hours. If any reaction (redness, swelling) occurs, know that drug should not be used.
• Teach patients how to apply the drug. Moisten cotton plug with medication before insertion. Leave cotton in place for a maximum of 30 minutes. Flush ear gently with warm water, using a rubber bulb syringe.
• Tell patients not to use drops more often than prescribed.
• Warn patients that this medication is for use only in the ears.
• Advise patients to discontinue the drug if adverse reactions occur and to contact the doctor immediately.
• Tell patient to keep container tightly closed and away from moisture.

Nasal agents

beclomethasone dipropionate
budesonide
dexamethasone sodium
    phosphate
ephedrine sulfate
epinephrine hydrochloride
flunisolide
naphazoline hydrochloride
oxymetazoline hydrochloride
phenylephrine hydrochloride
tetrahydrozoline hydrochloride
triamcinolone acetonide
xylometazoline hydrochloride

COMBINATION PRODUCTS

4-WAY NASAL SPRAY◊: phenylephrine hydrochloride 0.5%, naphazoline
hydrochloride 0.05%, and pyrilamine
maleate 0.2%.

---

beclomethasone dipropionate

Beconase AQ Nasal Spray,
Beconase Nasal Inhaler,
Vancenase AQ Nasal Spray,
Vancenase Nasal Inhaler

Pregnancy Risk Category: C

HOW SUPPLIED

Nasal aerosol: 42 mcg/metered spray,
50 mcg/metered spray‡
Nasal spray: 42 mcg/metered spray,
50 mcg/metered spray‡

ACTION

A corticosteroid that decreases nasal
inflammation, mainly by stabilizing
leukocyte lysosomal membranes.

ONSET, PEAK, DURATION

Onset occurs within 5 to 7 days. Time
to maximal benefit is up to 3 weeks
for some patients. Duration unknown.

INDICATIONS & DOSAGE

*Relief of symptoms of seasonal or pe-
rennial rhinitis; prevention of recurrence of nasal polyps after surgical removal —*
Adults and children over 12 years:
usual dosage is 1 or 2 sprays in each
nostril, b.i.d., t.i.d., or q.i.d.

ADVERSE REACTIONS

CNS: headache.
EENT: *mild transient nasal burning
and stinging,* nasal congestion, sneezing, epistaxis, watery eyes, nasopharyngeal fungal infections.
GI: nausea, vomiting.

INTERACTIONS

None significant.

CONTRAINDICATIONS

Contraindicated in patients hypersensitive to the drug and in patients experiencing status asthmaticus or other
acute episodes of asthma.

NURSING CONSIDERATIONS

• Use cautiously, if at all, in patients
with active or quiescent respiratory
tract tubercular infections or untreated fungal, bacterial, or systemic
viral or ocular herpes simplex infections. Also use cautiously in patients
who have recently had nasal septal ulcers, nasal surgery, or trauma.
• Observe the patient for fungal infections.
• Be aware that beclomethasone is not
effective for acute exacerbations of
rhinitis. Decongestants or antihistamines may be needed.
• To instill, instruct the patient to
shake the container before using; to
blow nose to clear nasal passages; and
to tilt head slightly forward and insert
nozzle into nostril, pointing away

---

from septum. Tell him to hold the other nostril closed and then to inspire gently and spray. Next, have him shake the container again and repeat in the other nostril.
• Advise patient to pump the nasal spray three or four times before the first use, and once or twice before first use each day. The cap and nosepiece of the activator should be cleaned in warm water every day, then allowed to air dry.
• Advise the patient to use drug regularly, as prescribed, because its effectiveness depends on regular use.
• Explain that the drug's therapeutic effects, unlike those of decongestants, are not immediate. Most patients achieve benefit within a few days, but some may require 2 to 3 weeks.
• Warn the patient not to exceed recommended dosages because of the risk of hypothalamic-pituitary-adrenal function suppression.
• Tell the patient to notify the doctor if symptoms don't improve within 3 weeks or if nasal irritation persists.
• Teach the patient good nasal and oral hygiene.

---

budesonide
Rhinocort

Pregnancy Risk Category: C

HOW SUPPLIED
Nasal spray: 32 mcg/metered spray (7-g canister)

ACTION
Unknown. A corticosteroid that probably decreases nasal inflammation, mainly by inhibiting the activities of specific cells and the mediators involved in the allergic response.

ONSET, PEAK, DURATION
Not clearly defined.

INDICATIONS & DOSAGE
Symptoms of seasonal or perennial allergic rhinitis –
Adults and children 6 years and older: 2 sprays in each nostril in the morning and evening or 4 sprays in each nostril in the morning. Maintenance dosage should be the fewest number of sprays needed to control symptoms.

ADVERSE REACTIONS
CNS: nervousness.
EENT: *nasal irritation, epistaxis, pharyngitis,* reduced sense of smell, nasal pain, hoarseness.
GI: bad taste, dry mouth, dyspepsia, nausea.
Respiratory: *cough,* moniliasis, wheezing, dyspnea.
Skin: facial edema, rash, pruritus, contact dermatitis.
Other: myalgia, hypersensitivity reactions.

INTERACTIONS
None significant.

CONTRAINDICATIONS
Contraindicated in patients hypersensitive to the drug or any of its components and in those who have had recent septal ulcers, nasal surgery, or nasal trauma until total healing has occurred.

NURSING CONSIDERATIONS
• Use cautiously in patients with tuberculous infections; untreated fungal, bacterial, or systemic viral infections; or ocular herpes simplex.
• To instill, instruct the patient to shake the container before using; to blow nose to clear nasal passages; and to tilt head slightly forward and insert nozzle into nostril, pointing away from septum. Tell him to hold the other nostril closed and then to inspire gently and spray. Next, have him shake container again and repeat in the other nostril.

• Instruct the patient that the product should be used by one person only to prevent the spread of infection.

• Advise the patient not to break, incinerate, or store canister in extreme heat; contents under pressure.

• Warn the patient not to exceed prescribed dosage or use for long periods of time because of the risk of hypothalamic-pituitary-adrenal axis suppression.

• Tell the patient to contact the doctor if symptoms do not improve in 3 weeks or if condition worsens.

• Teach the patient good nasal and oral hygiene.

dexamethasone sodium phosphate
Decadron Phosphate Turbinaire

Pregnancy Risk Category: C

HOW SUPPLIED
Nasal aerosol: 84 mcg/metered spray, 170 doses/canister

ACTION
Decreases nasal inflammation, mainly by stabilizing leukocyte lysosomal membranes.

ONSET, PEAK, DURATION
Not clearly defined.

INDICATIONS & DOSAGE
Allergic or inflammatory conditions, nasal polyps –
Adults: 2 sprays in each nostril b.i.d. or t.i.d. Maximum dosage is 12 sprays daily.
Children 6 to 12 years: 1 or 2 sprays in each nostril b.i.d. Maximum 8 sprays daily.

Each spray delivers 0.1 mg dexamethasone sodium phosphate equal to 0.084 mg dexamethasone.

ADVERSE REACTIONS
EENT: nasal irritation, dryness, rebound nasal congestion.

Other: hypersensitivity reactions, systemic effects with prolonged use (pituitary-adrenal suppression, sodium retention, *CHF,* hypertension, hypokalemia, headaches, *seizures,* peptic ulceration, ecchymoses, petechiae, masking of infection).

INTERACTIONS
None significant.

CONTRAINDICATIONS
Contraindicated in patients with hypersensitivity to drug or in patients with systemic fungal infections, tuberculosis, viral and fungal nasal conditions, or ocular herpes simplex.

NURSING CONSIDERATIONS
• Use cautiously in patients with diabetes mellitus, peptic ulcer, ulcerative colitis, abscess or other pyrogenic infection, diverticulitis, fresh intestinal anastomosis, renal insufficiency, hypertension, osteoporosis, and myasthenia gravis.

• Frequently monitor blood pressure and serum potassium level. Hypertension and hypokalemia can occur with systemic absorption.

• Monitor for fluid retention which can occur from systemic absorption.

• Be prepared to gradually reduce dosage as nasal condition improves.

• Notify the doctor if you suspect underlying bacterial infection which should be controlled with anti-infectives.

• Know that irritation or sensitivity may require stopping drug.

• To instill, instruct the patient to shake the container before using; to blow nose to clear nasal passages; and to tilt head slightly forward and insert nozzle into nostril, pointing away from septum. Tell him to hold the other nostril closed and then to inspire gently and spray. Next, have him shake container again and repeat in the other nostril.

---

*Liquid form contains alcohol.   *Common* reactions are in italics; *life-threatening,* in bold italics.
**May contain tartrazine.

- Teach the patient good nasal and oral hygiene.
- Warn the patient that product should be used by only one person to prevent spread of infection.
- Warn the patient to avoid prolonged use because of the risk of hypothalamic-pituitary-adrenal-axis suppression.
- Advise the patient to contact the doctor if he experiences fever, joint or muscle aches, or extreme tiredness.
- Advise the patient not to break, incinerate, or store canister in extreme heat; contents under pressure.

ephedrine sulfate
Vicks Vatronol Nose Drops◇

Pregnancy Risk Category: NR

HOW SUPPLIED
Nasal solution: 0.5%◇

ACTION
Causes local vasoconstriction of dilated arterioles, reducing blood flow and nasal congestion.

ONSET, PEAK, DURATION
Unknown.

INDICATIONS & DOSAGE
Nasal congestion–
Adults and children: 2 to 3 drops of 0.5% solution into each nostril. Used no more frequently than q 4 hours.

ADVERSE REACTIONS
CNS: nervousness, excitation.
CV: *tachycardia.*
EENT: rebound nasal congestion with long-term or excessive use.
Other: mucosal irritation.

INTERACTIONS
MAO inhibitors: hypertensive crisis if ephedrine is absorbed. Don't use together.

CONTRAINDICATIONS
Contraindicated in patients with angle-closure glaucoma, psychoneurosis, angina pectoris, substantial organic heart disease, cardiovascular disease, and hypersensitivity to the drug or other sympathomimetics.

NURSING CONSIDERATIONS
- Use cautiously in patients with hyperthyroidism, hypertension, diabetes mellitus, or prostatic hypertrophy.
- Teach patients how to instill nosedrops.
- Instruct patients that product should be used by only one person to prevent spread of infection.
- Tell patients not to exceed recommended dosage and use only when needed.

epinephrine hydrochloride
Adrenalin Chloride

Pregnancy Risk Category: NR

HOW SUPPLIED
Nasal solution: 0.1%

ACTION
Causes local vasoconstriction of dilated arterioles, reducing blood flow and nasal congestion.

ONSET, PEAK, DURATION
Onset occurs within 1 minute. Peak and duration unknown.

INDICATIONS & DOSAGE
Nasal congestion, local superficial bleeding–
Adults and children: instill 1 or 2 drops of solution.

ADVERSE REACTIONS
CNS: nervousness, excitation.
CV: *tachycardia.*
EENT: rebound nasal congestion, slight sting upon application.

---

†Available in Canada only.   ‡Available in Australia only.   ◇Available OTC.

INTERACTIONS
None significant.

CONTRAINDICATIONS
Contraindicated in patients with hypersensitivity to the drug.

NURSING CONSIDERATIONS
• Use cautiously in patients with hyperthyroidism, coronary artery disease, hypertension, or diabetes mellitus.
• Teach patients how to instill nosedrops.
• Instruct patients that product should be used by only one person to prevent spread of infection.
• Tell patients not to exceed recommended dosage and to use only when needed.

---

flunisolide
Nasalide, Rhinalar Nasal Mist‡

Pregnancy Risk Category: C

HOW SUPPLIED
Nasal inhalant: 25 mcg/metered spray, 200 doses/bottle‡
Nasal solution: 0.25 mg/ml in pump spray bottle

ACTION
Decreases nasal inflammation, mainly by stabilizing leukocyte lysosomal membranes by unknown mechanism.

ONSET, PEAK, DURATION
Unknown.

INDICATIONS & DOSAGE
Symptoms of seasonal or perennial rhinitis –
Adults: starting dose is 2 sprays (50 mcg) in each nostril b.i.d. Total daily dosage is 200 mcg. If necessary, dosage may be increased to 2 sprays in each nostril t.i.d. Maximum total daily dosage is 8 sprays in each nostril (400 mcg daily).

Children 6 to 14 years: starting dose is 1 spray (25 mcg) in each nostril t.i.d. or 2 sprays (50 mcg) in each nostril b.i.d. Total daily dosage is 150 to 200 mcg. Maximum total daily dosage is 4 sprays in each nostril (200 mcg daily).

ADVERSE REACTIONS
CNS: headache.
EENT: *mild, transient nasal burning and stinging,* nasal congestion, nasopharyngeal fungal infection, sneezing, epistaxis, watery eyes.
GI: nausea, vomiting.

INTERACTIONS
None significant.

CONTRAINDICATIONS
Contraindicated in patients hypersensitive to the drug. Also, drug should not be used in the presence of untreated localized infection involving nasal mucosa.

NURSING CONSIDERATIONS
• Use cautiously, if at all, in patients with active or quiescent respiratory tract tubercular infections or in untreated fungal, bacterial, or systemic viral or ocular herpes simplex infections. Also use cautiously in patients who have recently had nasal septal ulcers, nasal surgery, or nasal trauma.
• Be aware that flunisolide is not effective for acute exacerbations of rhinitis. Decongestants or antihistamines may be needed.
• To instill, instruct patients to shake the container before using; to blow nose to clear nasal passages; and to tilt head slightly forward and insert nozzle into nostril, pointing away from septum. Tell them to hold the other nostril closed, and then to inspire gently and spray. Next, have them shake container again and repeat in the other nostril. Tell patients to clean nosepiece with warm water if it becomes clogged.

---

*Liquid form contains alcohol.
**May contain tartrazine.

Common reactions are in italics; *life-threatening,* in bold italics.

• Explain that the drug's therapeutic effects, unlike those of decongestants, are not immediate. Most patients achieve benefit within a few days, but some may require 2 to 3 weeks.
• Advise patients to use drug regularly, as prescribed, because its effectiveness depends on regular use.
• Warn patients not to exceed recommended dosage to avoid suppression of hypothalamic-pituitary-adrenal function.
• Tell patients to stop drug and notify the doctor if symptoms don't improve within 3 weeks or if nasal irritation persists.

naphazoline hydrochloride
Privine◇

Pregnancy Risk Category: NR

HOW SUPPLIED
Nasal drops: 0.05% solution
Nasal spray: 0.05% solution

ACTION
Causes local vasoconstriction of dilated arterioles, reducing blood flow and nasal congestion.

ONSET, PEAK, DURATION
Onset occurs within 10 minutes. Peak unknown. Effects persist 2 to 6 hours.

INDICATIONS & DOSAGE
Nasal congestion –
Adults and children 12 years and older: 2 drops or sprays instilled in each nostril q 3 to 4 hours.
Children 6 to 12 years: 1 to 2 drops or sprays instilled in each nostril q 3 to 6 hours, p.r.n. Not to be used longer than 3 to 5 days.

ADVERSE REACTIONS
EENT: rebound nasal congestion with excessive or long-term use, sneezing, stinging, dryness of mucosa.
Other: systemic effects in children

after excessive or long-term use, marked sedation.

INTERACTIONS
None significant.

CONTRAINDICATIONS
Contraindicated in patients with hypersensitivity to drug.

NURSING CONSIDERATIONS
• Use cautiously in patients with hyperthyroidism, heart disease, hypertension, or diabetes mellitus.
• Teach patients how to apply. For nasal drops, instruct patients to tilt head back as far as possible, instill drops, then lean head forward while inhaling and to repeat procedure for other nostril. For nasal spray, instruct patients to hold spray container and head upright. Tell patients not to shake the container.
• Instruct patients that product should be used by only one person to prevent spread of infection.
• Warn patients not to exceed recommended dosage.
• Tell patients to contact the doctor if nasal congestion persists after 5 days.

oxymetazoline hydrochloride
Afrin◇, Afrin Children's Strength Nose Drops◇, Allerest 12-Hour Nasal◇, Chlorphed-LA◇, Coricidin Nasal Mist◇, Dristan Long Lasting◇, Drixine Nasal‡, Duramist Plus◇, Duration◇, 4-Way Long-Acting Nasal, Genasal Spray◇, Neo-Synephrine 12 Hour◇, Nostrilla◇, NTZ Long Acting Nasal◇, Sinarest 12-Hour◇, Sinex Long-Acting◇, Twice-A-Day Nasal◇

Pregnancy Risk Category: NR

HOW SUPPLIED
Nasal solution: 0.025%◇, 0.05%◇

ACTION

Unknown. Thought to cause local vasoconstriction of dilated arterioles, reducing blood flow and nasal congestion.

ONSET, PEAK, DURATION

Onset occurs in 5 to 10 minutes. Peak effect occurs within 6 hours. Effects persist less than 12 hours.

INDICATIONS & DOSAGE

Nasal congestion –
Adults and children 6 years and older: 2 to 3 drops or sprays of 0.05% solution in each nostril b.i.d.
Children 2 to 6 years: 2 to 3 drops of 0.025% solution in each nostril b.i.d. Use no longer than 3 to 5 days.

ADVERSE REACTIONS

CNS: headache, drowsiness, dizziness, insomnia, possible sedation.
CV: palpitations, *CV collapse,* hypertension.
EENT: rebound nasal congestion or irritation with excessive or long-term use, dryness of nose and throat, increased nasal discharge, stinging, sneezing.
Other: systemic effects in children with excessive or long-term use.

INTERACTIONS

None significant.

CONTRAINDICATIONS

Contraindicated in patients with hypersensitivity to drug.

NURSING CONSIDERATIONS

• Use cautiously in patients with hyperthyroidism, cardiac disease, hypertension, or diabetes mellitus.
• Teach patients how to apply oxymetazoline. Tell them to hold head upright to minimize swallowing of medication, then sniff spray briskly.
• Instruct patients that product should be used by only one person to prevent spread of infection.

• Tell patients not to exceed recommended dosage and to use only when needed.
• Warn patients that excessive use may cause bradycardia, hypotension, dizziness, and weakness.

phenylephrine hydrochloride

Alconefrin 12◇, Alconefrin 25◇, Alconefrin 50◇, Doktors◇, Duration◇, Neo-Synephrine◇, Nostril◇, Rhinall◇, Rhinall-10◇, Sinex◇, St. Joseph Measured Dose Nasal Decongestant◇

Pregnancy Risk Category: NR

HOW SUPPLIED

Nasal jelly: 0.5%
Nasal solution: 0.125%, 0.16%, 0.2%, 0.25%, 0.5%, 1%

ACTION

Causes local vasoconstriction of dilated arterioles, reducing blood flow and nasal congestion.

ONSET, PEAK, DURATION

Onset is rapid. Peak unknown. Effects persist for ½ to 4 hours.

INDICATIONS & DOSAGE

Nasal congestion –
Adults and children 12 years and older: 2 to 3 drops or 1 to 2 sprays instilled in each nostril or small amount of jelly to nasal mucosa q 4 hours, p.r.n.
Children 6 to 12 years: 2 to 3 drops or 1 to 2 sprays of a 0.25% solution instilled in each nostril.
Children under 6 years: 2 to 3 drops of 0.125% solution q 4 hours, p.r.n.

ADVERSE REACTIONS

CNS: headache, tremor, dizziness, nervousness.
CV: *palpitations, tachycardia, PVCs,* hypertension, pallor.
EENT: transient burning or stinging,

---

*Liquid form contains alcohol.   *Common* reactions are in italics; ***life-threatening***, in bold italics.
**May contain tartrazine.

dryness of nasal mucosa, rebound nasal congestion with continued use.
GI: nausea.

INTERACTIONS
None significant.

CONTRAINDICATIONS
Contraindicated in patients with hypersensitivity to drug.

NURSING CONSIDERATIONS
• Use cautiously in patients with hyperthyroidism, marked hypertension, Type I diabetes mellitus, cardiac disease, or advanced arteriosclerotic changes; in children of low body weight; and in elderly patients.
• Teach patients how to apply phenylephrine. Tell them to hold head upright to minimize swallowing of medication, then sniff spray briskly.
• Instruct patients that product should be used by only one person to prevent spread of infection.
• Tell patients not to exceed recommended dosage and to use only when needed.
• Advise patients to contact the doctor if symptoms persist beyond 3 days.

---

tetrahydrozoline hydrochloride
Tyzine Drops, Tyzine Pediatric Drops

Pregnancy Risk Category: C

HOW SUPPLIED
Nasal solution: 0.05%, 0.1%

ACTION
Unknown. Thought to cause local vasoconstriction of dilated arterioles, reducing blood flow and nasal congestion.

ONSET, PEAK, DURATION
Onset occurs within a few minutes. Peak unknown. Effects persist for 4 to 8 hours.

INDICATIONS & DOSAGE
Nasal congestion –
Adults and children over 6 years: 2 to 4 drops of 0.1% solution or spray into each nostril q 4 to 6 hours, p.r.n.
Children 2 to 6 years: 2 to 3 drops of 0.05% solution into each nostril q 4 to 6 hours, p.r.n.

ADVERSE REACTIONS
EENT: transient burning, stinging; sneezing, rebound nasal congestion in excessive or long-term use.

INTERACTIONS
None significant.

CONTRAINDICATIONS
Contraindicated in patients with hypersensitivity to drug and in those with angle-closure glaucoma or other serious eye diseases. Also contraindicated in chilren under 2 years. The 0.1% solution is contraindicated in children under 6 years.

NURSING CONSIDERATIONS
• Use cautiously in patients with hyperthyroidism, hypertension, and diabetes mellitus.
• Teach patients how to apply tetrahydrozoline. Tell them to hold head upright to minimize swallowing of medication, then sniff spray briskly.
• Instruct patients that product should be used by only one person to prevent spread of infection.
• Tell patients not to exceed recommended dosage and to use only as needed for 3 to 5 days.

---

triamcinolone acetonide
Nasacort

Pregnancy Risk Category: C

HOW SUPPLIED
Nasal aerosol: 55 mcg/metered spray

ACTION
Unknown. A glucocorticoid with anti-inflammatory properties.

ONSET, PEAK, DURATION
A decrease in symptoms may occur within 12 hours after therapy is started. Effects peak within 3 to 4 days and may last for several days after drug is discontinued.

INDICATIONS & DOSAGE
Relief of symptoms of seasonal or perennial allergic rhinitis –
Adults and children 12 years and over: initially, 2 sprays (110 mcg) in each nostril once daily. Increased as needed up to 440 mcg daily either as once-daily dosage or in divided doses up to four times daily. After desired effect is obtained, dosage decreased, if possible, to as little as one spray (55 mcg) in each nostril daily.

ADVERSE REACTIONS
EENT: *nasal irritation,* dry mucous membranes, nasal and sinus congestion, throat discomfort, sneezing, epistaxis.
Other: *headache.*

INTERACTIONS
None known.

CONTRAINDICATIONS
Contraindicated in patients hypersensitive to any component of the drug.

NURSING CONSIDERATIONS
• Use with extreme caution, if at all, in patients with active or quiescent tuberculosis infection of the respiratory tract and in patients with untreated fungal, bacterial, or systemic viral infection or ocular herpes simplex.
• Use cautiously in patients who are already receiving systemic corticosteroids because of the increased likelihood of hypothalamic-pituitary-adrenal suppression compared with a therapeutic dosage of either one alone.

Also use cautiously in patients with recent nasal septal ulcers, nasal surgery, or trauma because of the inhibitory effect on wound healing. Also use with caution in breast-feeding women.
• Be aware that when excessive doses are used, signs and symptoms of hyperadrenocorticism and adrenal suppression may occur; the drug should be discontinued slowly.
• Urge patient to read the patient-instruction sheet contained in each package before using drug for the first time.
• To instill, instruct the patient to shake the container before using; to blow nose to clear nasal passages; and to tilt head slightly forward and insert nozzle into nostril, pointing away from the septum. Tell him to hold the other nostril closed and then to inspire gently and spray. Next, have patient shake container again and repeat this procedure in the other nostril.
• Tell the patient to discard the canister after 100 actuations.
• Stress the importance of using the drug on a regular schedule because its effectiveness depends on regular use. However, caution the patient not to exceed the dosage prescribed because serious adverse reactions may occur.
• Tell the patient to notify the doctor if symptoms do not improve within 2 to 3 weeks or if condition worsens.
• Warn patients to avoid exposure to chicken pox or measles and, if exposed to either, to obtain medical advice.
• Instruct patient to watch for signs and symptoms of nasal infection. If symptoms occur, tell the patient to notify the doctor because the drug may need to be discontinued and appropriate local therapy given.
• Advise the patient not to break canister, to incinerate canister, or to store canister in extreme heat; contents are under pressure and may explode.

---

xylometazoline hydrochloride

4-Way Long Acting, Neo-Synephrine II, Otrivin, Sine-Off Nasal Spray, Sinex-L.A.

Pregnancy Risk Category: NR

HOW SUPPLIED
Nasal solution: 0.05%, 0.1%

ACTION
Unknown. Thought to cause local vasoconstriction of dilated arterioles, reducing blood flow and nasal congestion.

ONSET, PEAK, DURATION
Onset occurs in 5 to 10 minutes. Peak unknown. Effects persist for 5 to 6 hours.

INDICATIONS & DOSAGE
Nasal congestion –
Adults and children 12 years and over: 2 to 3 drops or sprays of 0.1% solution in each nostril q 8 to 10 hours.
Children 2 to 12 years: 2 to 3 drops of 0.05% solution in each nostril q 8 to 10 hours.
Children 6 months to 2 years: 1 drop of 0.05% solution instilled into each nostril q 6 hours, p.r.n.

ADVERSE REACTIONS
EENT: transient burning, stinging; dryness or ulceration of nasal mucosa; sneezing; rebound nasal congestion or irritation with excessive or long-term use.

INTERACTIONS
None significant.

CONTRAINDICATIONS
Contraindicated in patients with hypersensitivity to drug or angle-closure glaucoma.

NURSING CONSIDERATIONS
• Use cautiously in patients with hyperthyroidism, cardiac disease, hypertension, diabetes mellitus, and advanced arteriosclerosis.
• Teach patients how to apply xylometazoline. Have patients hold head upright to minimize swallowing of medication, then sniff spray briskly.
• Instruct patients that product should be used by only one person to prevent spread of infection.
• Tell patients not to exceed recommended dose and to use only as needed for 3 to 5 days.

88

Local anti-infectives

acyclovir
amphotericin B
bacitracin
butoconazole nitrate
chloramphenicol
chlortetracycline hydrochloride
ciclopirox olamine
clindamycin phosphate
clotrimazole
econazole nitrate
erythromycin
gentamicin sulfate
gentian violet
haloprogin
iodochlorhydroxyquin
ketoconazole
mafenide acetate
metronidazole (topical)
miconazole nitrate
mupirocin
naftifine
neomycin sulfate
nitrofurazone
nystatin
oxiconazole nitrate
podofilox
silver sulfadiazine
sulconazole nitrate
terbinafine hydrochloride
terconazole
tetracycline hydrochloride
tioconazole
tolnaftate
undecylenic acid and zinc
   undecylenate

COMBINATION PRODUCTS
BENZAMYCIN GEL: erythromycin 3%
and benzoyl peroxide 5%.
LANABIOTIC◇: polymyxin B sulfate
5,000 units, neomycin sulfate 5 mg,
bacitracin 500 units, and lidocaine 40
mg/g.
LOTRISONE CREAM: clotrimazole
1% and betamethasone dipropionate
0.05%.

MYCITRACIN OINTMENT◇: polymyxin B sulfate 5,000 units, bacitracin 500 units, and neomycin sulfate
3.5 mg/g.
MYCOLOG II CREAM, OINTMENT:
triamcinolone acetonide 0.1% and
nystatin 100,000 units/g.
NEO-CORTEF OINTMENT: hydrocortisone acetate 1% and neomycin sulfate 0.5%.
NEODECADRON CREAM: dexamethasone phosphate 0.1% and neomycin
sulfate 0.5%.
NEOSPORIN CREAM†◇: polymyxin B
sulfate 10,000 units and neomycin
sulfate 5 mg.
NEOSPORIN OINTMENT◇: polymyxin
B sulfate 5,000 units, bacitracin zinc
400 units, and neomycin sulfate
5 mg/g.
POLYSPORIN OINTMENT◇: polymyxin B sulfate 10,000 units and bacitracin zinc 500 units/g.
VIOFORM-HYDROCORTISONE MILD
CREAM: iodochlorhydroxyquin 3%
and hydrocortisone 0.5%.

acyclovir
Zovirax

Pregnancy Risk Category: C

HOW SUPPLIED
Ointment: 5%

ACTION
Inhibits herpes simplex and varicella-
zoster viral DNA synthesis by interfering with viral DNA polymerase action.

ONSET, PEAK, DURATION
Not applicable.

*Liquid form contains alcohol. *Common* reactions are in italics; *life-threatening,* in bold italics.
**May contain tartrazine.

INDICATIONS & DOSAGE

Initial herpes genitalis; limited, non-life-threatening mucocutaneous herpes simplex virus infections in immunocompromised patients —

Adults and children: thoroughly cover all lesions q 3 hours six times daily for 7 days. Although dosage will vary depending on the total lesion area, use approximately a ½″ ribbon of ointment on each 4″ square of surface area.

ADVERSE REACTIONS

Skin: transient burning and stinging, rash, pruritus, vulvitis.

INTERACTIONS

None significant.

CONTRAINDICATIONS

Contraindicated in patients with hypersensitivity or chemical intolerance to the drug.

NURSING CONSIDERATIONS

• Know that most studies show that topically applied acyclovir is not effective when used to treat recurrent genital herpes.
• As ordered, initiate therapy as early as possible after onset of signs and symptoms of herpes.
• Apply with a finger cot or rubber glove to prevent autoinoculation of other body sites and transmission of infection to other persons.
• Know that the drug is for cutaneous use only; don't apply to the eye.
• Teach the patient that virus transmission can occur during treatment.
• Emphasize importance of compliance for successful therapy.

amphotericin B
Fungizone

Pregnancy Risk Category: B

HOW SUPPLIED

Cream: 3%
Lotion: 3%
Ointment: 3%

ACTION

Usually fungistatic; binds to sterols in the fungal cell membrane, resulting in increased membrane permeability and subsequent cell leakage.

ONSET, PEAK, DURATION

Not applicable.

INDICATIONS & DOSAGE

Cutaneous or mucocutaneous candidal infections —

Adults and children: apply liberally b.i.d. to q.i.d. for 1 to 3 weeks; interdigital lesions and paronychias treated for 2 to 4 weeks, and onychomycoses for several months because relapses are common.

ADVERSE REACTIONS

Skin: possible drying, contact sensitivity, erythema, burning, pruritus.

INTERACTIONS

None significant.

CONTRAINDICATIONS

Contraindicated in patients hypersensitive to the drug.

NURSING CONSIDERATIONS

• Clean area before applying.
• Watch for and report signs of local irritation. Cream may dry the skin; ointment may irritate if applied to moist hairy areas.
• Avoid using occlusive dressings.
• Be aware that cream or lotion is preferred for such areas as groin folds, armpit, and neck creases.
• Be prepared to discontinue drug if irritation or hypersensitivity occurs, and notify the doctor.
• Keep in mind that drug is well tolerated, even by infants, for long periods.

• Store at room temperature; avoid freezing.
• Tell the patient to continue using medication for full length of time prescribed, even if condition has improved.
• Inform patient that cream discolors skin slightly when rubbed in; lotion or ointment may stain nail lesions but not skin if thoroughly rubbed in.
• Tell the patient that discoloration of fabric caused by cream or lotion can usually be removed by washing; discoloration by ointment, with cleaning fluid.

---

bacitracin
Baciguent◊, Bacitin†

Pregnancy Risk Category: NR

HOW SUPPLIED
Ointment: 500 units/g

ACTION
Bactericidal or bacteriostatic, depending on organism and concentration of drug; inhibits bacterial cell wall synthesis.

ONSET, PEAK, DURATION
Not applicable.

INDICATIONS & DOSAGE
Topical infections, impetigo, abrasions, cuts, and minor burns or wounds –
Adults and children: apply thin film b.i.d., t.i.d., or p.r.n., depending on severity of condition.

ADVERSE REACTIONS
Skin: stinging, rashes, other allergic reactions; pruritus, burning, or swelling of lips or face.
Systemic: *possible systemic adverse reactions when used over large areas for prolonged periods, including potential nephrotoxicity and ototoxicity; hypersensitivity reactions;* tightness in chest, hypotension.

INTERACTIONS
None significant.

CONTRAINDICATIONS
Contraindicated in patients hypersensitive to the drug and in atopic patients.

NURSING CONSIDERATIONS
• Clean area before applying, especially areas with crusted or suppurative lesions.
• Anticipate alternative treatment for burns that cover more than 20% of body surface, especially if the patient suffers impaired renal function.
• Be aware that prolonged use may result in overgrowth of nonsusceptible organisms, particularly *Candida* species.
• If no improvement occurs or condition worsens, tell the patient to stop using and notify the doctor.

---

butoconazole nitrate
Femstat

Pregnancy Risk Category: C

HOW SUPPLIED
Vaginal cream: 2% supplied with applicators

ACTION
Unknown. Thought to control or destroy fungus by disrupting cell membrane permeability, causing osmotic instability.

ONSET, PEAK, DURATION
Not known.

INDICATIONS & DOSAGE
Vulvovaginal mycotic infections caused by Candida *species –*
Adults: for nonpregnant patient, 1 applicatorful intravaginally h.s. for 3 days. If necessary, treatment can be extended for another 3 days. For pregnant patient during second or third

---

*Liquid form contains alcohol.
**May contain tartrazine.

Common reactions are in italics; *life-threatening*, in bold italics.

trimester, 1 applicatorful intravaginally h.s. for 6 days.

ADVERSE REACTIONS
GU: vulvovaginal itching, soreness, and swelling.
Skin: finger itching.

INTERACTIONS
None significant.

CONTRAINDICATIONS
Contraindicated in patients hypersensitive to the drug.

NURSING CONSIDERATIONS
• Confirm diagnosis of *Candida* vulvovaginal infection by smears or cultures, as ordered.
• Be aware that symptom resolution is comparable to 7-day miconazole cream therapy.
• Be aware that butoconazole may be used with oral contraceptive and antibiotic therapy.
• Know that drug should be used in the first trimester of pregnancy only when the potential benefits justify the possible risks to the fetus.
• Teach the patient how to apply, and tell her not to use tampons during treatment.
• Advise the patient to keep affected area cool and dry, wear loose-fitting cotton clothing, avoid feminine hygiene sprays, wash daily with unscented soap, dry thoroughly with a clean towel, and maintain proper hygiene by wiping perineum from front to back to prevent reinfection.
• Tell the patient's sexual partner to wear a condom during intercourse until treatment is complete. He should consult the doctor if he experiences penile itching, redness, or discomfort.

chloramphenicol
Chloromycetin
Pregnancy Risk Category: NR

HOW SUPPLIED
Cream: 1%

ACTION
Usually bacteriostatic but may be bactericidal in high concentrations; inhibits bacterial protein synthesis.

ONSET, PEAK, DURATION
Not applicable.

INDICATIONS & DOSAGE
Superficial skin infections caused by susceptible bacteria –
Adults and children: after thoroughly cleaning the skin, apply t.i.d. or q.i.d.

ADVERSE REACTIONS
Skin: possible contact sensitivity; burning, urticaria, pruritus, angioedema in hypersensitive patients.

INTERACTIONS
None significant.

CONTRAINDICATIONS
Contraindicated in patients hypersensitive to the drug or any components of the formulation.

NURSING CONSIDERATIONS
• Be aware that prolonged use may result in overgrowth of fungi or other nonsusceptible organisms.
• Know that topical use of this drug should be supplemented by appropriate systemic medication for all but very superficial infections.
• Discontinue if hypersensitivity reactions develop, and notify the doctor.
• Tell the patient to avoid prolonged or frequent intermittent use. Systemically administered chloramphenicol has been linked to serious adverse reactions and toxicity.

†Available in Canada only.   ‡Available in Australia only.   ◇Available OTC.

• If no improvement occurs or if condition worsens, advise patient to discontinue drug and notify the doctor.
• Tell the patient to continue using for full treatment period prescribed, even if condition has improved.

chlortetracycline hydrochloride
Aureomycin 3%◇

Pregnancy Risk Category: NR

HOW SUPPLIED
Ointment: 3%

ACTION
Usually bacteriostatic; disrupts protein synthesis in susceptible organisms.

ONSET, PEAK, DURATION
Not applicable.

INDICATIONS & DOSAGE
Superficial skin infections caused by susceptible bacteria –
Adults and children: rub into affected area b.i.d. or t.i.d.

ADVERSE REACTIONS
Skin: *dermatitis,* drying.

INTERACTIONS
Abrasive or medicated soaps or cleansers; acne preparations or other preparations containing peeling agents (benzoyl peroxide, resorcinol, salicylic acid, sulfur, tretinoin); alcohol-containing products (after-shave, cosmetics, perfumed toiletries, shaving creams or lotions); astringent soaps or cosmetics; isotretinoin; medicated cosmetics or cover-ups: may cause cumulative drying or irritation, resulting in excessive skin irritation. Use together cautiously.

CONTRAINDICATIONS
Contraindicated in patients hypersensitive to the drug.

NURSING CONSIDERATIONS
• Don't use in patients allergic to wool. Drug has lanolin base.
• Be aware that prolonged use may result in overgrowth of nonsusceptible organisms.
• Know that treated skin fluoresces under ultraviolet light.
• If no improvement occurs or if condition worsens, advise patient to stop using and report to the doctor.

ciclopirox olamine
Loprox

Pregnancy Risk Category: B

HOW SUPPLIED
Cream: 1%
Lotion: 1%

ACTION
Unknown. Thought to deplete essential fungal intracellular substrates by blocking amino acid transport and alters cell membrane integrity.

ONSET, PEAK, DURATION
Not applicable.

INDICATIONS & DOSAGE
Tinea pedis, cruris, corporis, and versicolor; cutaneous candidiasis –
Adults and children over 10 years: massage gently into the affected and surrounding areas b.i.d., in the morning and evening for 2 to 4 weeks.

ADVERSE REACTIONS
Skin: pruritus, burning.

INTERACTIONS
None significant.

CONTRAINDICATIONS
Contraindicated in patients hypersensitive to the drug.

---

*Liquid form contains alcohol. *Common* reactions are in italics; *life-threatening*, in bold italics.
**May contain tartrazine.

NURSING CONSIDERATIONS
• Don't use occlusive dressings.
• Know that hypopigmentation from tinea versicolor will resolve gradually.
• If hypersensitivity reaction occurs, advise patient to discontinue treatment and notify the doctor.
• Tell patient to continue using drug for the full treatment period even though symptoms may have improved, usually 1 week after clearing.
• Tell the patient to notify the doctor if no improvement occurs after 4 weeks.

---

clindamycin phosphate
Cleocin T Gel, Lotion, Solution; Cleocin Vaginal Cream

Pregnancy Risk Category: B

HOW SUPPLIED
Gel: 1%
Lotion: 1%
Topical solution: 1%
Vaginal cream: 2%

ACTION
Bacteriostatic or bactericidal, depending on concentration of drug and susceptibility of organism; suppresses growth of susceptible organisms in sebaceous glands by blocking protein synthesis.

ONSET, PEAK, DURATION
Not applicable for gel, lotion, or solution. Unknown for vaginal cream.

INDICATIONS & DOSAGE
Inflammatory acne vulgaris, grades II and III –
Adults and adolescents: apply to skin b.i.d., morning and evening.
Bacterial vaginosis –
Adults: 1 applicatorful intravaginally h.s. for 7 consecutive days.

ADVERSE REACTIONS
GI: upset, diarrhea, bloody diarrhea, abdominal pain, colitis (including pseudomembranous colitis).
GU: *cervicitis or vaginitis,* Candida albicans overgrowth, *vulvar irritation.*
Skin: *dryness,* rash, redness, pruritus, swelling, irritation, contact dermatitis.

INTERACTIONS
Abrasive or medicated soaps or cleansers; acne preparations or other preparations containing peeling agents (benzoyl peroxide, resorcinol, salicylic acid, sulfur, tretinoin); alcohol-containing products (after-shave, cosmetics, perfumed toiletries, shaving creams or lotions); astringent soaps or cosmetics; isotretinoin; medicated cosmetics or cover-ups: potential cumulative drying or irritation, resulting in excessive skin irritation. Use cautiously.

CONTRAINDICATIONS
Contraindicated in patients hypersensitive to the drug; in those with a history of ulcerative colitis, regional enteritis, or antibiotic-associated colitis; and in those with a history of atopic reactions.

NURSING CONSIDERATIONS
• For treating acne, know that drug may be used concurrently with tretinoin or benzoyl peroxide as well as systemic antibiotics.
• Instruct the patient to wash area with warm water and soap, rinse, and pat dry before application and to wait 30 minutes after washing or shaving to apply.
• Warn the patient to avoid too frequent washing of area. Tell him to cover entire affected area, but to avoid contact with eyes, nose, mouth, and other mucous membranes.
• Tell the patient to use only as prescribed.

---

†Available in Canada only.   ‡Available in Australia only.   ◊ Available OTC.

• Tell the patient to dab, not roll, applicator-tipped bottle. If tip becomes dry, the patient should invert bottle and depress tip several times to moisten.
• Caution the patient to notify the doctor if skin becomes excessively dry.
• Warn the patient not to smoke while applying topical solution.
• When used intravaginally, ensure that the patient understands how to use the applicators that come with the drug.
• If diarrhea occurs, tell the patient to check with the doctor or pharmacist before using antidiarrheal medication because it may worsen the condition.

---

clotrimazole
Canesten†, Gyne-Lotrimin◇, Lotrimin, Mycelex, Mycelex-7◇, Mycelex-G, Mycelex-OTC◇

Pregnancy Risk Category: B

HOW SUPPLIED
Lozenges: 1%
Cream: 1%
Topical lotion: 1%
Topical solution: 1%
Vaginal cream: 1%◇
Vaginal tablets: 100 mg◇, 500 mg
Combination pack: vaginal inserts 100 mg and vulvar cream 1%◇

ACTION
Fungistatic but may be fungicidal, depending on concentrations. Alters fungal cell wall permeability and produces osmotic instability.

ONSET, PEAK, DURATION
Onset and peak unknown for lozenges. Effects persist for 3 hours with lozenges. Not applicable for other forms.

INDICATIONS & DOSAGE
Superficial fungal infections (tinea pedis, tinea cruris, tinea corporis, or tinea versicolor; candidiasis) –
Adults and children: apply thinly and massage into affected and surrounding area, morning and evening, for 2 to 8 weeks.
Vulvovaginal candidiasis –
Adults: two 100-mg vaginal tablets inserted daily h.s. for 3 consecutive days, or one 500-mg vaginal tablet daily h.s. for 3 days; or 1 applicatorful vaginal cream daily h.s. for 7 to 14 days.
Oropharyngeal candidiasis –
Adults and children: dissolve lozenge over 15 to 30 minutes in mouth five times daily for 14 consecutive days.

ADVERSE REACTIONS
GI: nausea and vomiting (with lozenges).
GU: *mild vaginal burning or irritation with vaginal use.*
Hepatic: elevated AST levels (from lozenges).
Skin: blistering, *erythema,* edema, pruritus, burning, stinging, peeling, urticaria, skin fissures, general irritation.

INTERACTIONS
None significant.

CONTRAINDICATIONS
• Contraindicated in patients hypersensitive to the drug.
• Also contraindicated for ophthalmic use.

NURSING CONSIDERATIONS
• Clean area before applying.
• Watch for and report irritation or sensitivity; discontinue if irritation occurs and notify doctor.
• Know that improvement usually demonstrated within a week; if no improvement occurs in 4 weeks, diagnosis should be reviewed.

---

*Liquid form contains alcohol.
May contain tartrazine.   *Common* reactions are in italics; **life-threatening, in bold italics.

• When compliance is a problem, be aware that mild to moderate vaginal candidiasis may be treated with a single 500-mg tablet.
• Know that hypopigmentation from tinea versicolor will resolve gradually.
• Warn the patient not to use occlusive wrappings or dressings.
• Ensure that the patient understands that frequent or persistent yeast infections may be a symptom of a more serious medical problem, such as immunodeficiency or AIDS.
• Warn patient that topical preparation may stain clothing.
• Emphasize the need to continue treatment for full course even if symptoms have improved.

econazole nitrate
Ecostatin†, Spectazole

Pregnancy Risk Category: C

HOW SUPPLIED
Cream: 1%

ACTION
Fungistatic; may be fungicidal, depending on concentration. Alters fungal cell-wall permeability and promotes osmotic instability.

ONSET, PEAK, DURATION
Not applicable.

INDICATIONS & DOSAGE
Tinea pedis, tinea cruris, and tinea corporis; cutaneous candidiasis –
Adults and children: rub into affected areas once daily for at least 2 weeks.
Cutaneous candidiasis –
Adults and children: rub into affected areas b.i.d.

ADVERSE REACTIONS
Skin: burning, pruritus, stinging, erythema.

INTERACTIONS
Topical corticosteroids: may inhibit antifungal effect.

CONTRAINDICATIONS
Contraindicated in patients hypersensitive to the drug.

NURSING CONSIDERATIONS
• Clean affected area before applying.
• Don't use occlusive dressings.
• Know that hypopigmentation from tinea versicolor will resolve gradually.
• If condition persists or worsens or if irritation (burning, pruritus, stinging, redness) occurs, tell patient to discontinue use and report this to doctor.
• Warn patient that drug may stain clothing.
• Tell the patient to use medication for entire treatment period, even though symptoms may have improved. Instruct him to notify the doctor if no improvement occurs after 2 weeks (tinea cruris, tinea corporis, and tinea versicolor) or 4 weeks (tinea pedis).

erythromycin
Akne-mycin, A/T/S, Del-Mycin, Erycette, EryDerm, EryGel, Ery-Sol†, ETS†, Sans-Acne†, Staticin, T-Stat†

Pregnancy Risk Category: B

HOW SUPPLIED
Ointment: 2%
Topical gel: 2%
Topical solution: 1.5%*, 2%*
Pledgets: 2%

ACTION
Usually bacteriostatic but may be bactericidal in high concentrations or against highly susceptible organisms. Disrupts protein synthesis in susceptible bacteria.

ONSET, PEAK, DURATION
Not applicable.

INDICATIONS & DOSAGE

Inflammatory acne vulgaris –
Adults and children: apply to affected area b.i.d.

ADVERSE REACTIONS

Skin: sensitivity reactions, erythema, burning, *dryness, pruritus.*

INTERACTIONS

Abrasive or medicated soaps or cleansers; acne preparations or other preparations containing peeling agents (benzoyl peroxide, resorcinol, salicylic acid, sulfur, tretinoin); alcohol-containing products (after-shave, cosmetics, perfumed toiletries, shaving creams or lotions); astringent soaps or cosmetics; isotretinoin; medicated cosmetics or cover-ups: may cause cumulative drying or irritation, resulting in excessive skin irritation. Use cautiously.

CONTRAINDICATIONS

Contraindicated in patients hypersensitive to the drug.

NURSING CONSIDERATIONS

• Wash, rinse, and dry affected areas before application.
• Know that prolonged use may be necessary when treating acne vulgaris; such use may result in overgrowth of nonsusceptible organisms.
• Advise patient not to use near eyes, nose, mouth, or other mucous membranes.
• If no improvement occurs or if condition worsens, tell patient to stop using and notify the doctor.

---

gentamicin sulfate

Garamycin, G-Myticin

Pregnancy Risk Category: NR

HOW SUPPLIED

Cream: 0.1%
Ointment: 0.1%

ACTION

A bactericidal agent that disrupts bacterial protein synthesis by binding to ribosomes although its exact mechanism is unknown.

ONSET, PEAK, DURATION

Not applicable.

INDICATIONS & DOSAGE

Superficial infections of the skin caused by susceptible bacteria –
Adults and children over 1 year: rub in small amount gently t.i.d. or q.i.d., with or without gauze dressing.

ADVERSE REACTIONS

Skin: minor skin irritation, possible photosensitivity, allergic contact dermatitis.

INTERACTIONS

None significant.

CONTRAINDICATIONS

Contraindicated in patients hypersensitive to the drug or in those who may exhibit cross-sensitivity with other aminoglycosides, such as neomycin.

NURSING CONSIDERATIONS

• Clean affected area before applying.
• Remove crusts before application of gentamicin in impetigo contagiosa to enhance absorption.
• Avoid use on large skin lesions or over a wide area because of possible systemic toxic effects.
• Use only in selected patients; widespread use may lead to resistant organisms.
• Know that prolonged use may result in overgrowth of nonsusceptible organisms.
• Be aware that drug may be used to treat bacterial infections that have not responded to other antibacterial agents.
• Store in cool place.
• If no improvement occurs or if con-

---

*Liquid form contains alcohol.   *Common* reactions are in italics; **life-threatening,** in bold italics.
**May contain tartrazine.

dition worsens, tell patient to stop using and notify the doctor.

---

gentian violet (methylrosaniline chloride, crystal violet)
Genapax

Pregnancy Risk Category: NR

HOW SUPPLIED
Topical solution: 1%◊, 2%◊
Tampons: 5 mg

ACTION
Unknown, although drug has fungistatic and antibacterial activity.

ONSET, PEAK, DURATION
Not applicable.

INDICATIONS & DOSAGE
Superficial skin infections –
Adults and children: apply with swab b.i.d.
Vaginal fungal infections –
Adults: 1 tampon inserted for 3 to 4 hours daily or b.i.d. for 12 days. For resistant infections, an additional tampon inserted h.s.

ADVERSE REACTIONS
Skin: *permanent discoloration if applied to granulation tissue;* irritation or ulceration of mucous membranes.

INTERACTIONS
None significant.

CONTRAINDICATIONS
Contraindicated in patients hypersensitive to the drug.

NURSING CONSIDERATIONS
• Apply carefully to avoid undue staining.
• Keep affected area clean, dry, and exposed to air to prevent spread of infection.
• Do not use on ulcerative facial lesions.

• Do not use occlusive dressings.
• Be aware that tattooing of the skin may occur if applied to granulation tissue.
• Be alert that toxicity has occurred after ingestion or with excessive use.
• Inform patient that drug will stain skin and clothing.

---

haloprogin
Halotex

Pregnancy Risk Category: B

HOW SUPPLIED
Cream: 1%
Topical solution: 1%

ACTION
Unknown, although drug has fungistatic and fungicidal activity.

ONSET, PEAK, DURATION
Not applicable.

INDICATIONS & DOSAGE
Superficial fungal infections (tinea pedis, tinea cruris, tinea corporis, tinea manuum, and tinea versicolor) –
Adults: apply liberally b.i.d. for 2 to 3 weeks. Intertriginous lesions may require 4 weeks of therapy.

ADVERSE REACTIONS
Skin: burning sensation, irritation, vesicle formation, increased maceration, *pruritus, or exacerbation of preexisting lesions.*

INTERACTIONS
None significant.

CONTRAINDICATIONS
Contraindicated in patients hypersensitive to the drug.

NURSING CONSIDERATIONS
• Don't allow drug to come in contact with the eyes.
• Be aware that diagnosis should be

---

reconsidered if no improvement occurs after 4 weeks of therapy.
• Tell the patient to continue using for full treatment period prescribed, even if condition has improved.
• Tell the patient to notify the doctor if increased irritation occurs.

iodochlorhydroxyquin (clioquinol)
Ala-Quin, Corque, Cortin, Torofor◇, Vioform◇

Pregnancy Risk Category: NR

HOW SUPPLIED
Cream: 3%
Ointment: 3%

ACTION
Unknown, although drug has fungistatic and fungicidal activity.

ONSET, PEAK, DURATION
Not applicable.

INDICATIONS & DOSAGE
Inflamed skin conditions –
Adults and children over 2 years: apply a thin layer b.i.d. or t.i.d. Should not be used for more than 1 week.

ADVERSE REACTIONS
CNS: neurotoxicity (with systemic absorption).
Skin: *possible burning, pruritus, acneiform eruptions,* allergic contact dermatitis.
Other: altered protein-bound iodine levels (with systemic absorption).

INTERACTIONS
Systemic corticosteroids: possible increased absorption. Use together cautiously.

CONTRAINDICATIONS
Contraindicated in patients hypersensitive to the drug.

NURSING CONSIDERATIONS
• Know that drug should not be used to treat diaper rash. Drug is also not effective in the treatment of fungal infections of the scalp or nails.
• Note all adverse reactions and precautions related to each component of combination antifungal products.
• Presence of drug in urine may cause false-positive result for phenylketonuria or inaccurate thyroid function tests; discontinue drug at least 1 month before such tests, as ordered.
• Warn patient that drug will stain fabric and hair.

ketoconazole
Nizoral

Pregnancy Risk Category: C

HOW SUPPLIED
Cream: 2%
Shampoo: 2%

ACTION
Unknown. An imidazole that probably inhibits yeast growth by altering the permeability of the cell membrane.

ONSET, PEAK, DURATION
Not applicable.

INDICATIONS & DOSAGE
Tinea corporis, tinea cruris, and tinea versicolor caused by susceptible organisms; seborrheic dermatitis; cutaneous candidiasis –
Adults: cover the affected and immediate surrounding area once daily for at least 2 weeks; for seborrheic dermatitis apply b.i.d. for 4 weeks. When using shampoo, wet hair, lather, and massage for 1 minute. Rinse and repeat, but leave drug on scalp for 3 minutes before rinsing. Shampoo twice weekly for 4 weeks, with at least 3 days between shampooing.

---

*Liquid form contains alcohol.   *Common* reactions are in italics; ***life-threatening***, in bold italics.
**May contain tartrazine.

ADVERSE REACTIONS
Skin: severe irritation, pruritus, stinging.
Other: swelling, inflammation.

INTERACTIONS
None significant.

CONTRAINDICATIONS
Contraindicated in patients hypersensitive to the drug.

NURSING CONSIDERATIONS
• Be aware that most patients show improvement soon after treatment begins. However, treatment of tinea cruris or tinea corporis should continue for at least 2 weeks to reduce the possibility of recurrence.
• Tell patient to discontinue drug and notify doctor if hypersensitivity reaction occurs.
• Advise patient to check with the doctor if condition worsens; drug may have to be discontinued and diagnosis redetermined.

---

mafenide acetate
Sulfamylon

Pregnancy Risk Category: C

HOW SUPPLIED
Cream: 8.5%

ACTION
Unknown, although it interferes with bacterial cellular metabolism.

ONSET, PEAK, DURATION
Not applicable.

INDICATIONS & DOSAGE
Adjunctive treatment of second- and third-degree burns to prevent infection caused by susceptible organisms (especially Pseudomonas aeruginosa*) —*
Adults and children: apply ¹⁄₁₆″ thickness of cream daily or b.i.d. to clean, debrided wounds. Reapply p.r.n. to keep burned area covered.

ADVERSE REACTIONS
Hematologic: eosinophilia.
Skin: pain, *burning sensation,* rash, pruritus, swelling, hives, blisters, erythema.
Other: *metabolic acidosis,* facial edema.

INTERACTIONS
None significant.

CONTRAINDICATIONS
None reported.

NURSING CONSIDERATIONS
• Use cautiously in patients with acute renal failure and in those with known hypersensitivity to the drug or to sulfonamides.
• Clean area before applying, bathing patient daily, if possible.
• Use sterile gloves and instruments when applying cream to minimize risk of further wound contamination.
• Keep burn areas medicated at all times.
• Know that mafenide can cause pain and burning at application site; if either occurs, notify the doctor. Severe and prolonged pain may indicate allergy; if these or other allergic reactions occur, treatment may have to be temporarily discontinued.
• Closely monitor acid-base balance, especially in patients with pulmonary and renal dysfunction. If acidosis occurs, discontinue use for 24 to 48 hours and notify doctor.
• Be aware that sometimes it is difficult to distinguish between adverse reactions and effects of severe burn.

---

metronidazole (topical)
MetroGel, MetroGel-Vaginal

Pregnancy Risk Category: B

HOW SUPPLIED
Topical gel: 0.75%
Vaginal gel: 0.75%

ACTION
Unknown; may cause bactericidal effect by interacting with bacterial DNA. Active against many anaerobic gram-negative bacilli, anaerobic gram-positive cocci, *Gardnerella vaginalis,* and *Campylobacter fetus.*

ONSET, PEAK, DURATION
Not applicable for topical gel. Onset and duration unknown for vaginal gel; peak effects occur in 6 to 12 hours after intravaginal use.

INDICATIONS & DOSAGE
Acne rosacea –
Adults: apply a thin film to affected area b.i.d., morning and evening. Frequency and duration of therapy is adjusted after response is seen.
Bacterial vaginosis –
Adults: 1 applicatorful b.i.d., morning and evening, for 5 days.

ADVERSE REACTIONS
Topical gel
EENT: lacrimation (if drug applied around the eyes).
Vaginal form
CNS: dizziness, light-headedness, headache.
GI: cramps, pain, nausea, diarrhea, constipation, metallic or bad taste in mouth.
GU: *cervicitis, vaginitis.*
Skin: rash, *transient redness, dryness, mild burning, stinging.*
Other: overgrowth of nonsusceptible organisms, decreased appetite.

INTERACTIONS
Oral anticoagulants: may potentiate anticoagulant effect. Monitor the patient for potential adverse reactions.

CONTRAINDICATIONS
Contraindicated in patients hypersensitive to drug or its ingredients (such as parabens) and other nitromidazole derivatives.

NURSING CONSIDERATIONS
• Use cautiously in patients with history or evidence of blood dyscrasia; chemically related compounds are associated with blood dyscrasia.
• Use vaginal gel cautiously in patients with history of CNS diseases; a theoretical risk of seizures and peripheral neuropathy exist because these adverse reactions are associated with the oral form. However, plasma levels after typical doses of vaginal gel are usually less than 5% of those seen after a 500-mg oral dose.
• Be aware that topical metronidazole therapy has not been associated with the adverse effects observed with parenteral or oral metronidazole therapy (including disulfiram-like reactions after alcohol ingestion). However, some of the drug can be absorbed after topical use.
• Instruct the patient using topical gel to avoid use of drug around the eyes. Also advise the patient to clean area thoroughly before use, but wait 15 to 20 minutes after cleaning the skin before applying drug to minimize risk of local irritation. Cosmetics may be used after applying drug.
• If local reactions occur, advise the patient to apply less frequently or to discontinue and contact the doctor.

---

miconazole nitrate
Micatin◇, Monistat-Derm Cream and Lotion, Monistat 3 Vaginal Suppository, Monistat 7 Vaginal Cream◇, Monistat 7 Vaginal Suppository◇

Pregnancy Risk Category: C

HOW SUPPLIED
Cream: 2%◇
Powder: 2%◇
Spray: 2%◇
Vaginal cream: 2%◇
Vaginal suppositories: 100 mg◇, 200 mg

ACTION
A fungicidal imidazole that disrupts fungal cell membrane permeability.

ONSET, PEAK, DURATION
Not applicable for spray or cream form. Onset, peak, and duration unknown for suppositories.

INDICATIONS & DOSAGE
Tinea pedis, tinea cruris, tinea corporis; cutaneous candidiasis (moniliasis); common dermatophyte infections –
Adults and children: apply or spray sparingly b.i.d. for 2 to 4 weeks.
Tinea versicolor –
Adults and children: apply sparingly once daily for 2 weeks.
Vulvovaginal candidiasis –
Adults: 1 applicatorful or 100 mg suppository (Monistat 7) inserted intravaginally h.s. for 7 days; course repeated if necessary. Alternatively, 200 mg suppository (Monistat 3) intravaginally h.s. for 3 days.

ADVERSE REACTIONS
GU: vulvovaginal burning, pruritus, or irritation with vaginal cream.
Skin: irritation, burning, maceration.

INTERACTIONS
None significant.

CONTRAINDICATIONS
Contraindicated in patients hypersensitive to the drug.

NURSING CONSIDERATIONS
• Know that concurrent use of intravaginal forms and certain latex products, such as vaginal contraceptive diaphragms, are not recommended because of possible interaction.
• Advise patient that drug is for perineal or intravaginal use only. Keep out of eyes.
• Ensure that the patient understands that frequent or persistent yeast infections may be a symptom of a more serious medical problem, such as immunodeficiency or AIDS.
• Tell the patient to cautiously insert intravaginal forms high into the vagina with applicator provided.
• Warn patient not to use occlusive dressings.
• Tell patient drug may stain clothing.
• Warn patient to discontinue if sensitivity or chemical irritation occurs.
• Tell the patient to continue using for full treatment period prescribed, even if condition has improved.

---

mupirocin
Bactroban

Pregnancy Risk Category: B

HOW SUPPLIED
Ointment: 2%

ACTION
Unknown. Thought to inhibit bacterial protein and RNA synthesis.

ONSET, PEAK, DURATION
Not applicable.

INDICATIONS & DOSAGE
Impetigo –
Adults and children: apply to affected areas t.i.d. for 1 to 2 weeks.

ADVERSE REACTIONS
Skin: burning, pruritus, stinging, rash.

INTERACTIONS
None significant.

CONTRAINDICATIONS
Contraindicated in patients hypersensitive to the drug.

NURSING CONSIDERATIONS
• Use cautiously in patients with burns or impaired renal function.
• Not for ophthalmic use.
• Know that prolonged use may cause

overgrowth of nonsusceptible bacteria and fungi.
• Be aware that local reactions appear to be caused by the polyethylene glycol vehicle.
• If no improvement occurs in 3 to 5 days or if condition worsens, tell patient to notify the doctor immediately.

naftifine
Naftin

Pregnancy Risk Category: B

HOW SUPPLIED
Cream: 1%
Gel: 1%

ACTION
Unknown. A broad-spectrum fungicidal agent that is thought to inhibit sterol biosynthesis in susceptible fungi by blocking the enzyme squalene 2,3 epoxidase.

ONSET, PEAK, DURATION
Not applicable.

INDICATIONS & DOSAGE
Tinea corporis or tinea cruris –
Adults: apply to affected area once daily with the cream, or b.i.d. in the morning and evening with the gel.

ADVERSE REACTIONS
Skin: *burning, stinging,* dryness, pruritus, local irritation.

INTERACTIONS
None significant.

CONTRAINDICATIONS
Contraindicated in patients hypersensitive to the drug.

NURSING CONSIDERATIONS
• Obtain cultures, as ordered, to confirm diagnosis before therapy.
• Keep in mind that therapy should be reevaluated if no improvement occurs after 4 weeks.

• Instruct the patient to keep cream away from mucous membranes (eyes, nose, and mouth). Not for ophthalmic use.
• Tell patient not to use occlusive dressings unless directed otherwise by the doctor.
• Instruct the patient to wash hands after application.
• Instruct the patient to discontinue therapy and notify the doctor if irritation or sensitivity develops.

neomycin sulfate
Mycifradin†, Myciguent◇, Neo-Rx

Pregnancy Risk Category: NR

HOW SUPPLIED
Cream: 0.5%◇
Ointment: 0.5%◇

ACTION
Unknown. Thought to disrupt bacterial protein synthesis by binding to bacterial ribosomes.

ONSET, PEAK, DURATION
Not applicable.

INDICATIONS & DOSAGE
Prevention or treatment of superficial bacterial infections –
Adults and children: rub into affected area one to three times daily.

ADVERSE REACTIONS
Skin: *rashes, contact dermatitis,* urticaria.
Systemic: *possible nephrotoxicity, ototoxicity, and **neuromuscular blockade**.*

INTERACTIONS
None significant.

CONTRAINDICATIONS
Contraindicated in patients hypersensitive to the drug.

*Liquid form contains alcohol.   *Common* reactions are in italics; *life-threatening*, in bold italics.
**May contain tartrazine.

NURSING CONSIDERATIONS
• Use cautiously in patients with extensive dermatologic conditions. Don't use on more than 20% of the body surface.
• Know that prolonged use may result in overgrowth of nonsusceptible organisms.
• In combination products containing corticosteroids, be aware that use of occlusive dressings increases corticosteroid absorption and the likelihood of systemic effects.
• Keep in mind that enhanced systemic absorption occurs on denuded or abraded areas.
• Watch for signs of hypersensitivity and contact dermatitis.
• Evaluate patients for signs of ototoxicity with prolonged or extended use.
• If no improvement occurs or if condition worsens, tell patient to stop using and notify the doctor.

nitrofurazone
Furacin

Pregnancy Risk Category: C

HOW SUPPLIED
Cream: 0.2%
Ointment: 0.2% (soluble dressing)
Topical solution: 0.2%

ACTION
Unknown. A broad-spectrum antibiotic that probably inhibits bacterial enzymes involved in carbohydrate metabolism.

ONSET, PEAK, DURATION
Not applicable.

INDICATIONS & DOSAGE
Adjunctive treatment of second- and third-degree burns (especially when resistance to other antibiotics and sulfonamides occurs); prevention of skin allograft rejection –
Adults and children: apply directly

to lesion daily or every few days, depending on severity of burn. May also be applied to dressings used to cover affected area.

ADVERSE REACTIONS
GU: possible renal toxicity.
Skin: *erythema, pruritus,* burning, edema, severe reactions (vesiculation, denudation, ulceration), *allergic contact dermatitis.*

INTERACTIONS
None significant.

CONTRAINDICATIONS
Contraindicated in patients hypersensitive to the drug.

NURSING CONSIDERATIONS
• Use cautiously in patients with known or suspected renal impairment. Monitor serum creatinine levels regularly, as ordered.
• Clean wound, as indicated by the doctor, before reapplying dressings.
• Use sterile application technique to prevent further wound contamination.
• When using wet dressing, protect skin around wound with zinc oxide ointment.
• Be aware that drug may discolor in light but still retains its potency.
• Discard cloudy solutions if warming to 55° to 60° C (131° to 140° F) does not restore clarity.
• Store solution in tight, light-resistant containers (brown bottles). Avoid exposure to direct light, prolonged heat, and alkaline materials.
• If irritation, sensitization, or infection occurs, advise patient to discontinue use and notify doctor.

nystatin
Mycostatin, Nadostine†, Nilstat

Pregnancy Risk Category: NR

HOW SUPPLIED
Cream: 100,000 units/g
Ointment: 100,000 units/g
Powder: 100,000 units/g
Vaginal tablets: 100,000 units

ACTION
Disrupts integrity of fungal cell wall, promoting osmotic instability.

ONSET, PEAK, DURATION
Not applicable for cream, ointment, or powder. Unknown for vaginal tablets.

INDICATIONS & DOSAGE
Cutaneous and mucocutaneous infections caused by Candida albicans —
Adults and children: apply to affected area up to several times a day.
Vulvovaginal candidiasis —
Adults: 1 vaginal tablet daily or b.i.d. for 14 days.

ADVERSE REACTIONS
Skin: occasional contact dermatitis from preservatives in some formulations.

INTERACTIONS
None significant.

CONTRAINDICATIONS
Contraindicated in patients hypersensitive to the drug.

NURSING CONSIDERATIONS
• Do not use occlusive dressings.
• Know that drug is generally well tolerated by all age groups, including debilitated infants.
• Keep in mind that preparation does not stain skin or mucous membranes.
• Be aware that cream is recommended for intertriginous areas; powder, for very moist areas; ointment, for dry areas.
• Refrigerate vaginal tablets.
• Tell the female patient to continue using the vaginal tablets during her menstrual period.

• Tell the patient to use drug for the full prescribed period, even if condition has improved. Immunosuppressed patients may use the drug chronically.

oxiconazole nitrate
Oxistat

Pregnancy Risk Category: B

HOW SUPPLIED
Cream: 1%
Lotion: 1%

ACTION
Unknown. Thought to inhibit ergosterol synthesis in fungal cell walls, causing osmotic instability and cell lysis.

ONSET, PEAK, DURATION
Not applicable.

INDICATIONS & DOSAGE
Tinea pedis, cruris, and tinea corporis caused by Trichophyton rubrum or T. mentagrophytes —
Adults: apply to affected area once daily in the evening. Treat tinea cruris and tinea corporis for 2 weeks, and tinea pedis for 1 month, to minimize risk of recurrence.

ADVERSE REACTIONS
Skin: pruritus, burning, stinging, contact dermatitis, irritation, scaling, tingling, pain.

INTERACTIONS
None significant.

CONTRAINDICATIONS
Contraindicated in patients hypersensitive to the drug or any component of the formulation.

NURSING CONSIDERATIONS
• Ensure that the patient understands that drug is for external use only.

---

*Liquid form contains alcohol.   Common *reactions are in italics; ***life-threatening,*** in bold italics.
**May contain tartrazine.

- Inform patient that drug shouldn't touch the eyes or vagina.
- Tell the patient to discontinue drug and contact the doctor if local irritation occurs.

podofilox
Condylox*

Pregnancy Risk Category: C

HOW SUPPLIED
Topical solution: 0.5%*

ACTION
Unknown; a keratolytic agent that probably causes local necrosis of wart tissue.

ONSET, PEAK, DURATION
Not applicable.

INDICATIONS & DOSAGE
External genital warts (condylomata acuminata) –
Adults: apply to affected areas q 12 hours for 3 consecutive days; then withhold for 4 consecutive days. Repeated as needed up to 4 weeks until warts disappear.

ADVERSE REACTIONS
CNS: insomnia, dizziness.
GI: vomiting.
GU: foreskin retraction, dyspareunia, hematuria.
Skin: burning, pain, inflammation, erosion, pruritus, tingling, *tenderness,* chafing, scarring, vesicle formation, crusting edema, dryness and peeling.

INTERACTIONS
None significant.

CONTRAINDICATIONS
Contraindicated in patients with hypersensitivity to or intolerance of any component of the medication (contains 95% alcohol).

NURSING CONSIDERATIONS
- Know that drug should not be used to treat genital warts in the perianal area or on mucous membranes of the genital area, including the urethra, rectum, and vagina.
- If no response occurs after 4 weeks of therapy, anticipate using alternative therapy.
- Tell the patient that the drug is for external use only. Systemic administration has caused hematologic toxicity, hematuria, seizures, and GI disturbances.
- Teach the patient how to apply the drug:
   - Dampen the supplied cotton-tipped applicator with drug and touch it to the wart.
   - Apply least amount needed to cover the lesion; 0.5 ml or less, and covering less than 10 cm^2 (4″) of wart tissue.
   - Allow the area to dry before allowing skin to retract.
   - Dispose of used applicator properly and wash hands thoroughly afterward.
- Tell the patient to avoid contact with eyes. If eye contact occurs, the patient should flush the area with plenty of water and contact the doctor immediately.
- Tell the patient that additional applications will not improve efficacy but can increase adverse reactions and the risk of systemic absorption, which is associated with substantial toxicity.

silver sulfadiazine
Flamazine†, Flint SSD, Silvadene, SSD-AF, Thermazene

Pregnancy Risk Category: B

HOW SUPPLIED
Cream: 1%

ACTION
Broad-spectrum sulfonamide that acts on cell membrane and cell wall; bac-

tericidal for many gram-positive and gram-negative organisms.

ONSET, PEAK, DURATION
Not applicable.

INDICATIONS & DOSAGE
Prevention and treatment of wound infection in second- and third-degree burns—
Adults and children: apply 1/16″ thickness to clean debrided burn wound daily or b.i.d.

ADVERSE REACTIONS
Hematologic: *neutropenia* (in 3% to 5% of those receiving extensive applications).
Skin: pain, burning, rashes, itching.

INTERACTIONS
Topical proteolytic enzymes: inactivation of enzymes. Do not use together.

CONTRAINDICATIONS
Contraindicated in premature and full-term neonates during first 2 months of life. Drug may increase possibility of kernicterus. Also contraindicated in patients with hypersensitivity to the drug or in pregnant women at or near term.

NURSING CONSIDERATIONS
• Use with caution in patients hypersensitive to sulfonamides.
• Use sterile application technique to prevent wound contamination.
• Use only on affected areas. Keep these areas medicated at all times.
• Bathe the patient daily, if possible.
• Inspect the patient's skin daily, and note any changes. Notify the doctor if burning or excessive pain develops.
• Monitor serum sulfadiazine concentrations and renal function, as ordered, and check urine for sulfa crystals in patients with extensive burns.
• If hepatic or renal dysfunction occurs, notify doctor as drug may need to be discontinued.

• Discard darkened cream, which indicates drug is ineffective.

---

sulconazole nitrate
Exelderm

Pregnancy Risk Category: C

HOW SUPPLIED
Topical solution: 1%
Cream: 1%

ACTION
Unknown. A broad-spectrum antifungal imidazole derivative that inhibits the growth of both fungi and yeast.

ONSET, PEAK, DURATION
Not applicable.

INDICATIONS & DOSAGE
Tinea cruris, tinea corporis, tinea pedis, or tinea versicolor—
Adults: massage a small amount of drug into affected area daily to b.i.d. for 3 weeks. Treat tinea pedis with cream b.i.d. for 4 weeks.

ADVERSE REACTIONS
Skin: pruritus, burning, stinging.

INTERACTIONS
None significant.

CONTRAINDICATIONS
Contraindicated in patients hypersensitive to any component of the formulation.

NURSING CONSIDERATIONS
• Use only cream for tinea pedia. Efficacy against tinea pedis (athlete's foot) has not been proven with the topical solution.
• Know that if no improvement occurs after 4 weeks, diagnosis should be reconsidered.
• Tell the patient to avoid touching the eyes with the drug and to wash hands thoroughly after applying.
• Explain to the patient the necessity

---

*Liquid form contains alcohol. *Common* reactions are in italics; *life-threatening*, in bold italics.
**May contain tartrazine.

of completing the full course of therapy, even after symptoms subside, to prevent recurrence. Clinical improvement is usually apparent within 1 week, with symptomatic relief in just a few days.
• If irritation develops during treatment, tell the patient to discontinue drug and contact the doctor.

terbinafine hydrochloride
Lamisil

Pregnancy Risk Category: B

HOW SUPPLIED
Cream: 1%

ACTION
Fungicidal; selectively inhibits an early step in synthesis of sterols used by fungi for cell wall synthesis.

ONSET, PEAK, DURATION
Not applicable.

INDICATIONS & DOSAGE
Interdigital tinea pedis, tinea cruris, and tinea corporis –
Adults: cover affected area and immediate surrounding area daily or b.i.d. for at least 1 week.

ADVERSE REACTIONS
Skin: irritation, burning, pruritus, dryness.

INTERACTIONS
None significant.

CONTRAINDICATIONS
Contraindicated in patients hypersensitive to the drug.

NURSING CONSIDERATIONS
• Observe patients for 2 to 4 weeks after therapy is complete to determine if treatment was successful; review the diagnosis if the condition persists beyond this observation period.

• Be aware that therapy shouldn't exceed 4 weeks.
• Teach the patient proper use of drug. Tell the patient to use only as directed for the full recommended course, even if symptoms disappear; and not to apply near the eyes, mouth, or mucous membranes or use occlusive dressings unless so directed.
• Tell the patient to discontinue drug and contact the doctor if irritation or sensitivity develops.

terconazole
Terazol 3 Vaginal Suppositories,
Terazol 7 Vaginal Cream

Pregnancy Risk Category: C

HOW SUPPLIED
Vaginal cream: 0.4%, 0.8%
Vaginal suppositories: 80 mg

ACTION
Unknown; may increase fungal cell membrane permeability (*Candida* species only).

ONSET, PEAK, DURATION
Unknown.

INDICATIONS & DOSAGE
Vulvovaginal candidiasis –
Adults: 1 applicatorful of cream or 1 suppository inserted into vagina h.s. 0.4% cream used for 7 consecutive days; 0.8% cream or 80-mg suppository for 3 consecutive days. Course repeated, if necessary, after reconfirmation by smear or culture.

ADVERSE REACTIONS
CNS: headache.
Skin: vulvovaginal burning, irritation, *pruritus.*
Other: fever, chills, body aches.

INTERACTIONS
None significant.

CONTRAINDICATIONS

Contraindicated in patients with known sensitivity to terconazole or any inactive ingredients in formulation.

NURSING CONSIDERATIONS

• Discontinue if the patient develops fever, chills, other flulike symptoms, or sensitivity and notify doctor

• Keep in mind that vaginal burning or pruritus is reportedly less frequent with terconazole than with miconazole or clotrimazole.

• Advise patient to continue treatment during the menstrual period; therapeutic effect of terconazole is unaffected by menstruation. However, tell the patient not to use tampons.

• Tell the patient to use for full treatment period prescribed. Explain how to prevent reinfection.

---

tetracycline hydrochloride
Achromycin, Topicycline

Pregnancy Risk Category: B

HOW SUPPLIED
Ointment: 3%
Topical solution: 2.2 mg/ml

ACTION
Unknown. A broad-spectrum antibiotic that probably disrupts bacterial protein synthesis; usually bacteriostatic.

ONSET, PEAK, DURATION
Unknown.

INDICATIONS & DOSAGE
Acne vulgaris –
Adults and children over 12 years: rub generously into affected areas b.i.d. until skin is thoroughly covered.
Prevention or treatment of superficial skin infections caused by susceptible bacteria –
Adults: apply to affected area b.i.d. in morning and evening or t.i.d.

ADVERSE REACTIONS
Skin: temporary stinging or burning on application; slight yellowing of treated skin, especially in patients with light complexions; severe dermatitis.

INTERACTIONS
Abrasive or medicated soaps or cleansers; acne preparations or other preparations containing peeling agents (benzoyl peroxide, resorcinol, salicylic acid, sulfur, tretinoin); alcohol-containing products (after-shave, cosmetics, perfumed toiletries, shaving creams or lotions); astringent soaps or cosmetics; isotretinoin; medicated cosmetics or cover-ups: may cause cumulative drying or irritation, resulting in excessive skin irritation. Use cautiously.

CONTRAINDICATIONS
Contraindicated in patients hypersensitive to the drug.

NURSING CONSIDERATIONS
• Use cautiously in patients with hepatic or renal impairment.

• Know that prolonged use may result in overgrowth of nonsusceptible organisms.

• Store at room temperature, away from excessive heat.

• Be aware that significant systemic effects are unlikely because serum levels of topical tetracycline hydrochloride are much lower than those of orally administered drug.

• Tell patient to wash area before applying.

• Explain that floating plug in bottle of Topicycline – an inert and harmless result of proper reconstitution of the preparation – shouldn't be removed.

• Instruct patient how to increase or decrease applicator pressure against the skin to control flow rate of solution.

• Tell the patient that she may continue normal use of cosmetics.

---

*Liquid form contains alcohol.   *Common* reactions are in italics; *life-threatening,* in bold italics.
**May contain tartrazine.

• Tell the patient not to share medication with family members.
• Advise the patient to use or discard the drug within 2 months.
• If no improvement occurs or if condition worsens, advise patient to stop using and notify the doctor.

tioconazole
Vagistat

Pregnancy Risk Category: C

HOW SUPPLIED
Vaginal ointment: 6.5%

ACTION
A fungicidal imidazole that alters cell wall permeability.

ONSET, PEAK, DURATION
Unknown.

INDICATIONS & DOSAGE
Vulvovaginal candidiasis –
Adults: 1 applicatorful (about 4.6 g) inserted intravaginally h.s.

ADVERSE REACTIONS
GU: *burning, pruritus,* discharge, vulvar edema and swelling, irritation.

INTERACTIONS
None significant.

CONTRAINDICATIONS
Contraindicated in patients hypersensitive to the drug or other imidazole antifungal agents (miconazole, ketoconazole).

NURSING CONSIDERATIONS
• Review proper use of the drug with the patient. Written instructions for the patient are available with the product. Tell the patient to insert drug high into the vagina.
• To avoid contamination of the ointment, tell patient to open the applicator just before using it.

• Tell the patient to use a sanitary napkin to avoid staining her clothing.
• Advise the patient to avoid sexual intercourse during therapy, or advise partner to use a condom to prevent reinfection.
• Emphasize the need to complete the full course of therapy, even after symptoms have improved. The patient should continue using the drug during her menstrual period.
• If irritation or sensitivity occurs, tell the patient to discontinue drug and report adverse reaction to the doctor.

tolnaftate
Aftate for Athlete's Foot◇, Aftate for Jock Itch◇, Dr. Scholl's Athlete's Foot Powder◇, Dr. Scholl's Athlete's Foot Spray◇, Footwork◇, Fungatin◇, Genaspor◇, NP-27◇, Tinactin◇, Ting◇, Zeasorb-AF◇

Pregnancy Risk Category: NR

HOW SUPPLIED
Aerosol liquid: 1% (36% alcohol)◇
Aerosol powder: 1% (14% alcohol)◇
Cream: 1%◇
Gel: 1%◇
Powder: 1%◇
Pump spray liquid: 1% (36% alcohol)◇
Topical solution: 1%◇

ACTION
Unknown, although drug has been demonstrated to distort the hyphae and stunt mycelial growth in susceptible fungi.

ONSET, PEAK, DURATION
Not applicable.

INDICATIONS & DOSAGE
Superficial fungal infections of the skin; infections due to common pathogenic fungi; tinea pedis, tinea cruris, tinea corporis, and tinea versicolor –
Adults and children: apply ¼″ to ½″

---

†Available in Canada only.   ‡Available in Australia only.   ◇ Available OTC.

ribbon of cream or 2 to 3 drops of solution to cover area about the size of one hand; same amount of cream or 2 to 3 drops of solution to cover toes and interdigital webs of one foot; or gel, powder, or spray to cover affected area. Apply and massage gently into skin b.i.d. for 2 to 6 weeks.

ADVERSE REACTIONS
Skin: possible irritation.

INTERACTIONS
None significant.

CONTRAINDICATIONS
Contraindicated in patients hypersensitive to the drug.

NURSING CONSIDERATIONS
• Be aware that drug is not used to treat fungal infections of the hair or nails; tolnaftate is ineffective against these fungi.
• Know that drug is odorless and greaseless; it won't stain or discolor skin, hair, nails, or clothing.
• Know that powder or aerosol may be used inside socks and shoes of persons susceptible to tinea infections.
• Advise patient to use only a small quantity of cream or lotion; treated area should not be wet with solution.
• If no improvement occurs after 10 days, advise patient to consult the doctor.
• Tell the patient to continue using for full treatment period prescribed, even if condition has improved. Treatment should continue for at least 2 weeks after symptoms have resolved to prevent reinfection.
• Tell patient to discontinue if condition worsens and to check with the doctor.

undecylenic acid and zinc undecylenate
Cruex◇, Desenex◇, Desenex Aerosol◇, Quinsana Plus◇

Pregnancy Risk Category: NR

HOW SUPPLIED
Cream: 15 g
Ointment: 15 g, 30 g
Powder: 2% undecylenic acid and 20% zinc undecylenate◇

ACTION
Unknown, although drug has fungistatic and fungicidal activity.

ONSET, PEAK, DURATION
Not applicable.

INDICATIONS & DOSAGE
Tinea pedis, tinea cruris, and tinea corporis (except nails and hairy areas) —
Adults and children: apply b.i.d. to thoroughly clean area. Treat tinea cruris for 2 weeks, tinea pedis or tinea corporis for 4 weeks.

ADVERSE REACTIONS
Skin: possible irritation.

INTERACTIONS
None significant.

CONTRAINDICATIONS
Contraindicated in patients hypersensitive to the drug.

NURSING CONSIDERATIONS
• Know that liquids are preferable for hairy areas; powders in moist areas such as skin folds. Ointment or cream should be used at night, but the powder may be used during the day.
• Instruct patient to apply for at least 2 weeks to minimize risk of relapse.
• Tell the patient to continue using for full treatment period prescribed, even if condition has improved.

---

*Liquid form contains alcohol.
**May contain tartrazine.

Common reactions are in italics; ***life-threatening,*** in bold italics.

89

Scabicides and pediculicides

benzyl benzoate lotion
crotamiton
lindane
permethrin
pyrethrins

COMBINATION PRODUCTS
None.

---

benzyl benzoate lotion
Scabanca

Pregnancy Risk Category: C

HOW SUPPLIED
Lotion: 14% (with benzocaine 2%)
Emulsion: 50%

ACTION
Unknown.

ONSET, PEAK, DURATION
Unknown.

INDICATIONS & DOSAGE
Parasitic infestation (scabies, Phthirus pubis, Pediculus humanus capitis)—
Adults and children: scrub entire body with soap and water. Remove scales or crusts. Then apply the lotion undiluted over affected area (include whole body for scabies), except the face and scalp, while still damp. Be sure to apply around nails. Let dry. Apply second coat on the most involved areas. Bathe after 24 hours.

Treatment may be repeated in 7 to 10 days if mites appear or new lesions develop.

ADVERSE REACTIONS
Skin: *irritation, pruritus; contact dermatitis with repeated applications.*

INTERACTIONS
None significant.

CONTRAINDICATIONS
Contraindicated when skin is raw or inflamed or in patients hypersensitive to drug.

NURSING CONSIDERATIONS
• Do not apply to face, eyes, mucous membranes, or urethral meatus. If accidental contact with eyes occurs, flush with water and notify the doctor.
• Apply topical corticosteroids as prescribed if dermatitis develops from scratching.
• Do not apply to infants' or small children's hands because they put hands in their mouths.
• Make sure hospitalized patients are placed in isolation, with linen-handling precautions, until treatment is completed.
• Store drug in light-resistant container; avoid exposure to excessive heat.
• Be aware that drug is preferred over lindane for treatment of infants, young children, and pregnant or breast-feeding patients.
• Tell the patient to discontinue drug and to wash it off skin and notify the doctor immediately if skin irritation or hypersensitivity develops.
• Instruct the patient to change and sterilize (boil, launder, dry clean, or apply very hot iron) all clothing and bed linen after drug is washed off.
• Instruct the patient to reapply drug if it is washed off during treatment time.
• After application for lice infestation, tell patient to use a fine-tooth comb dipped in white vinegar to remove nits from hairy areas.

• Tell the patient to warn other family members and sexual contacts about infestation. Sexual contacts should be treated simultaneously.

• Reassure the patient that although itching may continue for several weeks, it will cease; continued itching does not indicate that therapy is ineffective.

crotamiton
Eurax
Pregnancy Risk Category: C

HOW SUPPLIED
Cream: 10%
Lotion: 10%

ACTION
Unknown.

ONSET, PEAK, DURATION
Unknown.

INDICATIONS & DOSAGE
Parasitic infestation (scabies) –
Adults and children: scrub entire body with soap and water. Remove scales or crusts. Then apply a thin layer of cream over entire body, from chin down (with special attention to folds, creases, interdigital spaces, and genital area). Apply second coat in 24 hours. Wait additional 48 hours, then wash off.

Treatment repeated in 7 to 10 days if mites reappear or new lesions develop.
Itching –
Adults and children: applied locally and repeated p.r.n.

ADVERSE REACTIONS
Skin: *irritation.*

INTERACTIONS
None significant.

CONTRAINDICATIONS
Contraindicated when skin is raw or inflamed and in patients hypersensitive to drug.

NURSING CONSIDERATIONS
• Estimate amount of cream needed per application; most patients have a tendency to overuse scabicides. For most adults, a single tube of cream provides a sufficient amount for two applications.

• Apply topical corticosteroids, as prescribed, if dermatitis develops from scratching.

• Make sure hospitalized patients are placed in isolation, with special linen-handling precautions, until treatment is completed.

• Be aware that monthly maintenance treatments may be necessary in long-term care facilities, where infestation is a problem.

• Instruct patient not to apply to face, eyes, mucous membranes, or urethral meatus. If accidental contact with eyes occurs, flush with water and notify the doctor.

• Tell the patient to discontinue drug and to wash it off skin and to notify the doctor immediately if skin irritation or hypersensitivity develops.

• Instruct the patient to change and sterilize (boil, launder, dry clean, or apply very hot iron) all clothing and bed linen after drug is washed off.

• After application for lice infestation, tell patient to use a fine-tooth comb dipped in white vinegar to remove nits from hairy areas.

• Instruct the patient to reapply drug if it is washed off during treatment time.

• Tell the patient to warn other family members and sexual contacts about infestation. Sexual contacts should be treated simultaneously.

---

*Liquid form contains alcohol.   *Common* reactions are in italics; ***life-threatening,*** in bold italics.
**May contain tartrazine.

lindane
Gamma Benzene, gBh†, Kildane, Kwell, Kwellada†, Scabene

Pregnancy Risk Category: B

HOW SUPPLIED
Cream: 1%
Lotion: 1%
Shampoo: 1%

ACTION
Unknown. Appears to inhibit neuronal membrane function in arthropods, causing neuronal hyperactivity, seizures, and death after penetrating the parasites' exoskeleton.

ONSET, PEAK, DURATION
Unknown.

INDICATIONS & DOSAGE
Parasitic infestation (scabies, pediculosis) –
Adults and children: scrub entire body with soap and water; let skin dry thoroughly before using.

Apply thin layer of cream or lotion over entire skin surface (with special attention to folds, creases, interdigital spaces, and genital area) for scabies, or to hairy areas for pediculosis. After 8 to 12 hours, wash off drug. Repeat process in 1 week if mites appear or new lesions develop.

Apply shampoo undiluted to affected area and work into lather for 4 to 5 minutes; small amounts of water may enhance formation of lather. Apply 30 ml of shampoo for short hair, 45 ml for medium length hair, or 60 ml for long hair. Rinse thoroughly and rub dry with towel.

ADVERSE REACTIONS
CNS: *dizziness, seizures.*
Skin: *irritation with repeated use.*

INTERACTIONS
None significant.

CONTRAINDICATIONS
Contraindicated in patients hypersensitive to the drug and when skin is raw or inflamed.

NURSING CONSIDERATIONS
• Use cautiously in infants and young children; there is a greater risk for CNS toxicity in this group.
• Apply topical corticosteroids or administer oral antihistamines, as prescribed, for pruritus.
• Make sure that hospitalized patients are placed in isolation, with special linen-handling precautions, until treatment is completed.
• Know that modest amounts (6% to 13%) are absorbed through intact skin. Absorption is increased if used with creams, oils, or lotions or if applied to face, scalp, axillae, neck, scrotum, or irritated or broken skin.
• Warn patient not to apply to open areas, acutely inflamed skin, or to face, eyes, mucous membranes, or urethral meatus. If accidental contact with eyes occurs, flush with water and notify the doctor. Avoid inhaling vapors.
• Tell patient to wash it off skin and to notify the doctor immediately if skin irritation or hypersensitivity develops.
• Discourage repeated use, which can lead to skin irritation, systemic toxicity, or seizures. Repeat use only if live lice or nits are found after 1 week.
• Instruct the patient to change and sterilize (boil, launder, dry clean, or apply very hot iron) all clothing and bed linen after drug is washed off.
• After application for lice infestation, tell patient to use a fine-tooth comb dipped in white vinegar to remove nits from hairy areas.
• Advise patient to use shampoo to clean combs or brushes; wash them thoroughly afterward. Warn the patient not to use routinely.
• Warn the patient that itching may continue for several weeks after effective treatment, especially in scabies.

---

†Available in Canada only.   ‡Available in Australia only.   ◊Available OTC.

• Instruct the patient to reapply drug if it is washed off during treatment time.
• Tell patients to warn other family members and sexual contacts about infestation. Sexual contacts should be treated simultaneously.

permethrin
Elimite, Nix

Pregnancy Risk Category: B

HOW SUPPLIED
Topical liquid (cream-rinse): 1%

ACTION
Acts on the parasites' nerve cells to disrupt the sodium channel current, causing paralysis of the parasite.

ONSET, PEAK, DURATION
Onset and peak unknown. Residual activity persists for about 10 days.

INDICATIONS & DOSAGE
Infestation with Pediculus humanus capitis *(head lice) and its nits* —
Adults and children: use after hair has been washed with shampoo, rinsed with water, and towel-dried. Apply 25 to 50 ml of liquid to saturate the hair and scalp. Allow to remain on hair for 10 minutes before rinsing off with water.

ADVERSE REACTIONS
Skin: pruritus, burning, stinging, tingling, numbness or scalp discomfort, mild erythema, scalp rash.

INTERACTIONS
None significant.

CONTRAINDICATIONS
Contraindicated in patients hypersensitive to pyrethrins or chrysanthemums.

NURSING CONSIDERATIONS
• Be aware that a single treatment is usually all that is necessary. Combing of nits is not required for effectiveness but drug package supplies a fine-tooth comb for cosmetic use as desired.
• Retreat, as prescribed, if lice are observed 7 days after the initial application.
• Explain to the patient that treatment with permethrin may temporarily worsen the symptoms of head lice infestation, such as pruritus, erythema, and edema.
• Tell the patient that headgear, scarves, coats, and bed linens should be disinfected by machine washing using hot water and machine drying for at least 20 minutes, using the hot cycle. Dry-clean nonwashable items and seal in a plastic bag for 2 weeks, or spray with a product designed to eliminate lice and their nits.
• Tell the patient to warn other family members and sexual contacts about infestation. Sexual contacts should be treated simultaneously.

pyrethrins
A-200 Pyrinate◇, Barc◇, Blue Gel, Pronto, Pyrinyl◇, R&C, RID◇, TISIT◇, Triple X◇

Pregnancy Risk Category: NR

HOW SUPPLIED
Shampoo: pyrethrins 0.17% and piperonyl butoxide 2%; pyrethrins 0.3% and piperonyl butoxide 3%
Topical gel: pyrethrins 0.18% and piperonyl butoxide 2.2%; pyrethrins 0.33% and piperonyl butoxide 3%; pyrethrins 0.3% and piperonyl butoxide 4%
Topical solution: pyrethrins 0.18% and piperonyl butoxide 2%; pyrethrins 0.2%, piperonyl butoxide 2%, and deodorized kerosene 0.8%; pyrethrins 0.3% and piperonyl butoxide 3%

---

*Liquid form contains alcohol.
**May contain tartrazine.

Common reactions are in italics; **life-threatening,** in bold italics.

ACTION
Acts as contact poison that disrupts parasite's nervous system, causing parasite paralysis and death.

ONSET, PEAK, DURATION
Not applicable.

INDICATIONS & DOSAGE
Infestations of head, body, and pubic (crab) lice and their eggs –
Adults and children: apply to hair, scalp, or other infested areas until entirely wet. Allow to remain for 10 minutes but no longer. Wash thoroughly with warm water and soap or shampoo. Remove dead lice and eggs with fine-tooth comb. Treatment repeated, if necessary, in 7 to 10 days to kill newly hatched lice. Not to exceed two applications within 24 hours.

ADVERSE REACTIONS
Skin: *irritation with repeated use.*

INTERACTIONS
None significant.

CONTRAINDICATIONS
Contraindicated in patients hypersensitive to the drug or ragweed.

NURSING CONSIDERATIONS
• Use cautiously in infants and small children.
• Apply topical corticosteroids or oral antihistamines as prescribed if dermatitis develops from scratching.
• Know that pyrethrins and lindane may be equally effective for lice infestation, but pyrethrins may be less hazardous.
• Be aware that drug is not effective against scabies.
• Instruct patient not to apply to open areas or acutely inflamed skin or to face, eyes, mucous membranes, or urethral meatus. If accidental contact with eyes occurs, flush with water and notify the doctor.
• Discourage repeated use, which can lead to skin irritation and possible systemic toxicity.
• Tell the patient to discontinue drug and to wash it off skin and to notify the doctor immediately if skin irritation develops. All preparations contain petroleum distillates.
• Instruct the patient to change and sterilize (boil, launder, dry clean, or apply very hot iron) all clothing and bed linen after drug is washed off.
• Teach the patient to remove dead parasites with a fine-tooth comb.
• Tell the patient to warn other family members and sexual contacts about infestation. Sexual contacts should be treated simultaneously.

---

alclometasone dipropionate
amcinonide
betamethasone benzoate
betamethasone dipropionate
betamethasone valerate
clobetasol propionate
clocortolone pivalate
desonide
desoximetasone
dexamethasone
dexamethasone sodium
  phosphate
diflorasone diacetate
fluocinolone acetonide
fluocinonide
flurandrenolide
fluticasone propionate
halcinonide
halobetasol propionate
hydrocortisone
hydrocortisone acetate
hydrocortisone butyrate
hydrocortisone valerate
mometasone furoate
triamcinolone acetonide

COMBINATION PRODUCTS
Corticosteroids for topical use are commonly combined with antibiotics and antifungals. (See Chapter 88, LOCAL ANTI-INFECTIVES.)

---

alclometasone dipropionate
Alclovate, Logoderm‡

Pregnancy Risk Category: C

HOW SUPPLIED
Cream: 0.05%
Ointment: 0.05%

ACTION
Unknown. Diffuses across cell membranes to form complexes with specific cytoplasmic receptors. Exhibits anti-inflammatory, antipruritic, vasoconstrictive, and antiproliferative activity. Considered a group IV (low-potency) agent, according to vasoconstrictive properties.

ONSET, PEAK, DURATION
Onset and duration unknown. Plasma levels are highest when applied to inflamed or damaged skin, eyelids, or scrotal area; lowest when applied to intact normal skin, palms of hands, or soles of feet.

INDICATIONS & DOSAGE
Inflammation associated with corticosteroid-responsive dermatoses –
Adults: apply a thin film to affected areas b.i.d. or t.i.d. Gently massage until the medication disappears.

ADVERSE REACTIONS
Skin: burning, pruritus, irritation, dryness, erythema, folliculitis, striae, acneiform eruptions, perioral dermatitis, hypopigmentation, hypertrichosis, allergic contact dermatitis; *secondary infection, maceration, atrophy, striae, miliaria* (with occlusive dressings).
Systemic: *hypothalamic-pituitary-adrenal (HPA) axis suppression,* Cushing's syndrome, hyperglycemia, glucosuria.

INTERACTIONS
None significant.

CONTRAINDICATIONS
Contraindicated in patients hypersensitive to the drug or other corticosteroids.

NURSING CONSIDERATIONS
• Gently wash skin before applying. To prevent skin damage, rub medica-

---

*Liquid form contains alcohol.   *Common* reactions are in italics; ***life-threatening,*** in bold italics.
**May contain tartrazine.

tion in gently, leaving a thin coat. When treating hairy sites, part hair and apply directly to lesions.

• Avoid application near eyes or mucous membranes. Do not apply to face, armpits, groin, or under breasts, unless specifically ordered.

• If an occlusive dressing is ordered, advise patient not to leave it in place longer than 16 hours each day or use it on infected or exudative lesions.

• Change dressings as ordered by the doctor. Discontinue drug and notify the doctor if skin infection, striae, or atrophy occurs.

• Notify the doctor and remove occlusive dressing if fever develops.

• If antifungal agents or antibiotics are used concomitantly, discontinue corticosteroids until infection is controlled, as ordered.

• Monitor the patient for systemic adverse reactions. Systemic absorption likely with use of occlusive dressings, prolonged treatment, or application to extensive body surface.

• To prevent recurrence, know that treatment should be continued for a few days after lesions clear, as ordered.

• Know that children may absorb larger amounts of drug and be more prone to systemic toxicity.

• Know that repeated application can result in diminished effectiveness.

• Warn the patient not to use for more than 14 consecutive days; potential for systemic absorption and HPA axis suppression exists.

• Instruct patient how to apply drug.

• Tell patient to stop drug and notify the doctor if the patient develops signs of systemic absorption, skin irritation or ulceration, hypersensitivity, or infection.

---

amcinonide
Cyclocort
Pregnancy Risk Category: C

HOW SUPPLIED
Cream: 0.1%
Lotion: 0.1%
Ointment: 0.1%

ACTION
Unknown. Diffuses across cell membranes to form complexes with specific cytoplasmic receptors. Exhibits anti-inflammatory, antipruritic, vasoconstrictive, and antiproliferative activity. Considered a group II (high-potency) agent according to vasoconstrictive properties.

ONSET, PEAK, DURATION
Onset and duration unknown. Plasma levels are highest when applied to inflamed or damaged skin, eyelids, or scrotal area; lowest when applied to intact normal skin, palms of hands, or soles of feet.

INDICATIONS & DOSAGE
Inflammation associated with corticosteroid-responsive dermatoses –
Adults and children: apply a light film to affected areas b.i.d. or t.i.d. Rub cream in gently and thoroughly until it disappears.

ADVERSE REACTIONS
Skin: burning, pruritus, irritation, dryness, erythema, folliculitis, striae, acneiform eruptions, perioral dermatitis, hypopigmentation, hypertrichosis, allergic contact dermatitis; *secondary infection, maceration, atrophy, striae, miliaria* (with occlusive dressings).
Systemic: *hypothalamic-pituitary-adrenal (HPA) axis suppression,* Cushing's syndrome, hyperglycemia, glucosuria.

INTERACTIONS
None significant.

CONTRAINDICATIONS
Contraindicated in patients hypersensitive to the drug.

---

†Available in Canada only.   ‡Available in Australia only.   ◊ Available OTC.

NURSING CONSIDERATIONS
• Avoid application near eyes or mucous membranes. Do not use on face, armpits, groin, in ear canal, or under breasts unless specifically ordered.
• Gently wash skin before applying. To prevent skin damage, rub medication in gently, leaving a thin coat. Part hair and apply directly to lesion when treating hairy sites.
• If an occlusive dressing is ordered, do not leave it in place longer than 16 hours each day or use it on infected or exudative lesions.
• For patients with eczematous dermatitis whose skin may be irritated by adhesive material, hold dressing in place with gauze, elastic bandages, stockings, or stockinette.
• Change dressings as ordered. Discontinue drug and notify the doctor if skin infection, striae, or atrophy occurs.
• Notify the doctor and remove occlusive dressing if fever develops.
• If antifungal agents or antibiotics are being used concomitantly, stop corticosteroids until infection is controlled, as ordered.
• Avoid using plastic pants or tight-fitting diapers on treated areas in young children. Children may absorb larger amounts of drug and be more prone to systemic toxicity.
• Monitor patients for systemic adverse reactions. Systemic absorption likely with use of occlusive dressings, prolonged treatment, or extensive body-surface treatment.
• To prevent recurrence, continue treatment for a few days after lesions clear, as ordered.
• Stop drug and notify the doctor if the patient develops signs of systemic absorption, skin irritation or ulceration, hypersensitivity, or infection.
• Instruct patient how to apply drug.

betamethasone benzoate
Benisone, Uticort

betamethasone dipropionate
Alphatrex, Diprolene, Diprolene AF, Diprosone, Maxivate, Psorion

betamethasone valerate
Betatrex, Beta-Val, Betnovate†‡, Valisone

Pregnancy Risk Category: C

HOW SUPPLIED
betamethasone benzoate
Cream: 0.025%
Gel: 0.025%
Lotion: 0.025%
Ointment: 0.025%
betamethasone dipropionate
Aerosol: 0.1%
Cream: 0.05%
Lotion: 0.05%
Ointment: 0.05%
betamethasone valerate
Aerosol: 0.1%
Cream: 0.01%, 0.1%
Lotion: 0.1%
Ointment: 0.1%

ACTION
Unknown. Diffuses across cell membranes to form complexes with specific cytoplasmic receptors. Exhibits anti-inflammatory, antipruritic, vasoconstrictive, and antiproliferative activity. Considered a group III (medium-potency) agent according to vasoconstrictive properties.

ONSET, PEAK, DURATION
Onset and duration unknown. Plasma levels are highest when applied to inflamed or damaged skin, eyelids, or scrotal area; lowest when applied to intact normal skin, palms of hands, or soles of feet.

INDICATIONS & DOSAGE
Inflammation associated with corticosteroid-responsive dermatoses –
Adults and children: clean area; apply cream, ointment, lotion, aerosol spray, or gel sparingly daily to b.i.d.

*Liquid form contains alcohol.
**May contain tartrazine.

Common reactions are in italics; *life-threatening*, in **bold italics**.

ADVERSE REACTIONS
Skin: burning, pruritus, irritation, dryness, erythema, folliculitis, striae, acneiform eruptions, perioral dermatitis, hypopigmentation, hypertrichosis, allergic contact dermatitis; *secondary infection, maceration, atrophy, striae, miliaria* (with occlusive dressings).
Systemic: *hypothalamic-pituitary-adrenal (HPA) axis suppression,* Cushing's syndrome, hyperglycemia, and glucosuria (with betamethasone dipropionate).

INTERACTIONS
None significant.

CONTRAINDICATIONS
Contraindicated in patients hypersensitive to the drug or to other corticosteroids.

NURSING CONSIDERATIONS
• Gently wash skin before applying. To prevent skin damage, rub medication in gently, leaving a thin coat. When treating hairy sites, part hair and apply directly to lesions.
• Avoid application near eyes, mucous membranes, or in ear canal.
• Because of alcohol content of vehicle, be aware that gel preparations may cause mild, transient stinging, especially if used on or near excoriated skin.
• If an occlusive dressing is ordered, do not leave it in place longer than 16 hours each day. Do not use occlusive dressings on infected or exudative lesions.
• For patients with eczematous dermatitis whose skin may be irritated by adhesive material, hold dressing in place with gauze, elastic bandages, stockings, or stockinette.
• Change dressings as ordered. Discontinue drug and notify the doctor if infection, striae, or atrophy occurs.
• Notify the doctor and remove occlusive dressing if fever develops.

• If antifungal agents or antibiotics are used concomitantly, stop corticosteroids until infection is controlled, as ordered.
• Monitor the patient for systemic adverse reactions. Systemic absorption likely with use of occlusive dressings, prolonged treatment, or extensive body-surface treatment.
• Avoid the use of plastic pants or tight-fitting diapers on treated areas when used in young children. Children may absorb larger amounts of drug and be more prone to systemic toxicity.
• To prevent recurrence, know that treatment should be continued for a few days after lesions clear.
• Stop drug and notify the doctor if the patient develops signs of systemic absorption, skin irritation or ulceration, hypersensitivity, or infection.
• Note that Diprolene and Diprolene AF may not be substituted generically because other products have different potencies.
• Instruct patient how to apply drug.

---

clobetasol propionate
Dermovate†, Temovate
Pregnancy Risk Category: C

HOW SUPPLIED
Cream: 0.05%
Lotion: 0.05%
Ointment: 0.05%

ACTION
Unknown. Diffuses across cell membranes to form complexes with specific cytoplasmic receptors. Exhibits anti-inflammatory, antipruritic, vasoconstrictive, and antiproliferative activity. Considered a group I (very high-potency) agent according to vasoconstrictive properties.

ONSET, PEAK, DURATION
Onset and duration unknown. Plasma levels are highest when applied to in-

flamed or damaged skin, eyelids, or scrotal area; lowest when applied to intact normal skin, palms of hands, or soles of feet.

INDICATIONS & DOSAGE
Inflammation associated with corticosteroid-responsive dermatoses –
Adults: apply a thin layer to affected skin areas b.i.d., in the morning and evening for a maximum of 14 days. Total dosage should not exceed 50 g weekly.

ADVERSE REACTIONS
Skin: burning, pruritus, irritation, dryness, erythema, folliculitis, perioral dermatitis, allergic contact dermatitis, hypopigmentation, hypertrichosis, acneiform eruptions.
Systemic: *hypothalamic-pituitary-adrenal (HPA) axis suppression,* Cushing's syndrome, hyperglycemia, glucosuria.

INTERACTIONS
None significant.

CONTRAINDICATIONS
Contraindicated in patients hypersensitive to the drug or to other corticosteroids.

NURSING CONSIDERATIONS
• Gently wash skin before applying. To prevent skin damage, rub medication in gently, leaving a thin coat. When treating hairy sites, part hair and apply directly to lesions.
• Avoid application near eyes, mucous membranes, or in ear canal.
• Don't use occlusive dressings or bandage, cover, or wrap treated areas.
• If antifungal agents or antibiotics are used concomitantly, stop corticosteroids until infection is controlled, as ordered.
• Know that repeated application can result in diminished effectiveness.
• Stop drug and notify the doctor if the patient develops signs of systemic

absorption, skin irritation or ulceration, hypersensitivity, or infection.
• Discontinue drug and notify the doctor if skin infection, striae, or atrophy occurs.
• Do not refrigerate.
• Warn the patient not to use for longer than 14 consecutive days; risk of systemic absorption and HPA axis suppression.
• Instruct patient how to apply drug.

clocortolone pivalate
Cloderm

Pregnancy Risk Category: C

HOW SUPPLIED
Cream: 0.1%

ACTION
Unknown. Diffuses across cell membranes to form complexes with specific cytoplasmic receptors. Exhibits anti-inflammatory, antipruritic, vasoconstrictive, and antiproliferative activity. Considered a group III (medium-potency) agent according to vasoconstrictive properties.

ONSET, PEAK, DURATION
Onset and duration unknown. Plasma levels are highest when applied to inflamed or damaged skin, eyelids, or scrotal area; lowest when applied to intact normal skin, palms of hands, or soles of feet.

INDICATIONS & DOSAGE
Inflammation associated with corticosteroid-responsive dermatoses –
Adults and children: apply cream sparingly to affected areas t.i.d. and rub in gently.

ADVERSE REACTIONS
Skin: burning, pruritus, irritation, dryness, erythema, folliculitis, striae, acneiform eruptions, perioral dermatitis, hypertrichosis, hypopigmentation, allergic contact dermatitis; *sec-*

---

*Liquid form contains alcohol.   *Common* reactions are in italics; *life-threatening,* in bold italics.
**May contain tartrazine.

ondary infection, maceration, atrophy, striae, miliaria (with occlusive dressings).
Systemic: *hypothalamic-pituitary-adrenal (HPA) axis suppression,* Cushing's syndrome, hyperglycemia, glucosuria.

INTERACTIONS
None significant.

CONTRAINDICATIONS
Contraindicated in patients hypersensitive to the drug.

NURSING CONSIDERATIONS
• Gently wash skin before applying. To prevent skin damage, rub medication in gently, leaving a thin coat. When treating hairy sites, part hair and apply directly to lesions.
• Avoid application near eyes or mucous membranes.
• If an occlusive dressing is ordered, don't leave it in place longer than 16 hours each day; don't use occlusive dressings on infected or exudative lesions.
• For patients with eczematous dermatitis whose skin may be irritated by adhesive material, hold dressing in place with gauze, elastic bandages, or stockinette.
• Change dressings as ordered. Discontinue drug and notify the doctor if skin infection, striae, or atrophy occurs.
• Notify the doctor and remove occlusive dressing if fever develops.
• If antifungal agents or antibiotics are being used concomitantly, stop corticosteroids until infection is controlled, as ordered.
• Monitor the patient for systemic adverse reactions. Systemic absorption likely with use of occlusive dressings, prolonged treatment, or extensive body-surface treatment.
• Avoid using plastic pants or tight-fitting diapers on treated areas in young children. Children may absorb

larger amounts of drug and be more prone to systemic toxicity.
• To prevent recurrence, continue treatment for a few days after lesions clear.
• Stop drug and notify the doctor if the patient develops signs of systemic absorption, skin irritation or ulceration, hypersensitivity, or infection.
• Instruct patient how to apply drug.

---

desonide
DesOwen, Tridesilon
Pregnancy Risk Category: C

HOW SUPPLIED
Cream: 0.05%
Ointment: 0.05%
Lotion: 0.05%

ACTION
Unknown. Diffuses across cell membranes to form complexes with specific cytoplasmic receptors. Exhibits anti-inflammatory, antipruritic, vasoconstrictive, and antiproliferative activity. Considered a group IV (low-potency) agent according to vasoconstrictive properties.

ONSET, PEAK, DURATION
Onset and duration unknown. Plasma levels are highest when applied to inflamed or damaged skin, eyelids, or scrotal area; lowest when applied to intact normal skin, palms of hands, or soles of feet.

INDICATIONS & DOSAGE
Inflammation associated with corticosteroid-responsive dermatoses—
Adults and children: clean area; apply cream or ointment sparingly b.i.d. to t.i.d.

ADVERSE REACTIONS
Skin: burning, pruritus, irritation, dryness, erythema, folliculitis, perioral dermatitis, allergic contact dermatitis, hypertrichosis, hypopigmen-

tation, acneiform eruptions; *maceration of skin, secondary infection, atrophy, striae, miliaria* (with occlusive dressings).
Systemic: *hypothalamic-pituitary-adrenal (HPA) axis suppression,* Cushing's syndrome, hyperglycemia, glucosuria.

INTERACTIONS
None significant.

CONTRAINDICATIONS
Contraindicated in patients hypersensitive to the drug.

NURSING CONSIDERATIONS
• Gently wash skin before applying. To prevent skin damage, rub medication in gently, leaving a thin coat. When treating hairy sites, part hair and apply directly to lesions.
• Avoid application near eyes, mucous membranes, or in ear canal.
• If an occlusive dressing is ordered, don't leave dressing in place longer than 16 hours each day; don't use occlusive dressings on infected or exudative lesions.
• For patients with eczematous dermatitis whose skin may be irritated by adhesive material, hold dressing in place with gauze, elastic bandages, stockings, or stockinette.
• Change dressing as ordered. Discontinue drug and notify doctor if skin infection, striae, or atrophy occurs.
• Notify the doctor and remove occlusive dressing if fever develops.
• If antifungal agents or antibiotics are used concomitantly, stop corticosteroids until infection is controlled, as ordered.
• Monitor the patient for systemic adverse reactions. Systemic absorption likely with use of occlusive dressings, prolonged treatment, or extensive body-surface treatment.
• Avoid using plastic pants or tight-fitting diapers on treated areas in

young children. Children may absorb larger amounts of drug and be more prone to systemic toxicity.
• To prevent recurrence, continue treatment for a few days after lesions clear.
• Stop drug and notify the doctor if patient develops signs of systemic absorption, skin irritation or ulceration, hypersensitivity, or infection.
• Instruct patient how to apply drug.

---

desoximetasone
Topicort
Pregnancy Risk Category: C

HOW SUPPLIED
Cream: 0.05%, 0.25%
Gel: 0.05%
Ointment: 0.25%

ACTION
Unknown. Diffuses across cell membranes to form complexes with specific cytoplasmic receptors. Exhibits anti-inflammatory, antipruritic, vasoconstrictive, and antiproliferative activity. Considered a group III (medium-potency) agent according to vasoconstrictive properties.

ONSET, PEAK, DURATION
Onset and duration unknown. Plasma levels are highest when applied to inflamed or damaged skin, eyelids, or scrotal area; lowest when applied to intact, normal skin, palms of hands, or soles of feet.

INDICATIONS & DOSAGE
Inflammation associated with corticosteroid-responsive dermatoses –
Adults and children: clean area; apply cream, gel, or ointment sparingly b.i.d.

ADVERSE REACTIONS
Skin: burning, pruritus, irritation, dryness, erythema, folliculitis, hypertrichosis, acneiform eruptions, peri-

---

*Liquid form contains alcohol.   *Common* reactions are in italics; *life-threatening,* in bold italics.
**May contain tartrazine.

oral dermatitis, hypopigmentation, allergic contact dermatitis; *maceration, secondary infection, atrophy, striae, miliaria* (with occlusive dressings). **Systemic: *hypothalamic-pituitary-adrenal (HPA) axis suppression,*** Cushing's syndrome, hyperglycemia, glucosuria.

INTERACTIONS
None significant.

CONTRAINDICATIONS
Contraindicated in patients hypersensitive to the drug.

NURSING CONSIDERATIONS
• Gently wash skin before applying. To prevent skin damage, rub medication in gently, leaving a thin coat. When treating hairy sites, part hair and apply directly to lesions.
• Avoid application near eyes, mucous membranes, or in ear canal.
• If an occlusive dressing is ordered, don't leave dressing in place longer than 16 hours each day; don't use occlusive dressings on infected or exudative lesions.
• For patients with eczematous dermatitis whose skin may be irritated by adhesive material, hold dressing in place with gauze, elastic bandages, stockings, or stockinette.
• Change dressing as ordered. Discontinue drug and notify doctor if skin infection, stiae, or atrophy occurs.
• Notify the doctor and remove occlusive dressing if fever develops.
• If antifungal agents or antibiotics are used concomitantly, stop corticosteroids until infection is controlled, as ordered.
• Monitor patients for systemic adverse reactions. Systemic absorption likely with use of occlusive dressings, prolonged treatment, or extensive body-surface treatment.
• Avoid using plastic pants or tight-fitting diapers on treated areas in young children. Children may absorb larger amounts of drug and be more prone to systemic toxicity.
• To prevent recurrence, continue treatment for a few days after lesions clear as ordered.
• Be aware that gel contains alcohol and may cause burning or irritation in open lesions.
• Stop drug and notify the doctor if the patient develops signs of systemic absorption, skin irritation or ulceration, hypersensitivity, or infection.
• Store in tightly sealed containers.
• Instruct patient how to apply drug.

---

dexamethasone
Aeroseb-Dex, Decaderm, Decaspray

dexamethasone sodium phosphate
Decadron Phosphate

Pregnancy Risk Category: C

HOW SUPPLIED
dexamethasone
Aerosol: 0.01%, 0.04%
Gel: 0.1%
dexamethasone sodium phosphate
Cream: 0.1%

ACTION
Unknown. Diffuses across cell membranes to form complexes with specific cytoplasmic receptors. Exhibits anti-inflammatory, antipruritic, vasoconstrictive, and antiproliferative activity. Considered a group IV (low-potency) agent according to vasoconstrictive properties.

ONSET, PEAK, DURATION
Onset and duration unknown. Plasma levels are highest when applied to inflamed or damaged skin, eyelids, or scrotal area; lowest when applied to intact normal skin, palms of hands, or soles of feet.

INDICATIONS & DOSAGE
Inflammation associated with cortico-steroid-responsive dermatoses –
Adults and children: clean area; apply cream, gel, or aerosol sparingly t.i.d. to q.i.d.

For aerosol use on scalp, shake can well but gently and apply to dry scalp after shampooing. Hold can upright. Slide applicator tube under hair so that it touches scalp. Spray while moving tube to all affected areas, keeping tube under hair and in contact with scalp throughout spraying, which should take about 2 seconds. Spot spray inadequately covered areas by sliding applicator tube through hair to touch scalp, then pressing and immediately releasing spray button. Don't massage medication into scalp or spray forehead or near eyes.

ADVERSE REACTIONS
Skin: burning, pruritus, irritation, dryness, erythema, folliculitis, hypertrichosis, acneiform eruptions, perioral dermatitis, hypopigmentation, allergic contact dermatitis; *maceration, secondary infection, atrophy, striae, miliaria* (with occlusive dressings).
Systemic: *hypothalamic-pituitary-adrenal (HPA) axis suppression,* Cushing's syndrome, hyperglycemia, glucosuria.

INTERACTIONS
None significant.

CONTRAINDICATIONS
Contraindicated in patients hypersensitive to the drug.

NURSING CONSIDERATIONS
• Gently wash skin before applying. To prevent skin damage, rub medication in gently, leaving a thin coat. When treating hairy sites, part hair and apply directly to lesions.
• Avoid application near eyes, mucous membranes, or in ear canal.
• If an occlusive dressing is ordered, don't leave it in place longer than 16 hours each day; don't use occlusive dressings on infected or exudative lesions.
• For patients with eczematous dermatitis whose skin may be irritated by adhesive material, hold dressing in place with gauze, elastic bandages, stockings, or stockinette.
• Change dressing as ordered. Discontinue drug and notify doctor if skin infection, striae, or atrophy occurs.
• Notify the doctor and remove occlusive dressing if fever develops.
• When using aerosol around the face, cover the patient's eyes and warn against inhalation of the spray. Aerosol preparation contains alcohol and may produce irritation or burning in open lesions. To avoid freezing tissues, do not spray longer than 3 seconds or closer than 6″ (15 cm).
• If antifungal agents or antibiotics are used concomitantly, stop corticosteroids until infection is controlled, as ordered.
• Monitor the patient for systemic adverse reactions. Systemic absorption likely with use of occlusive dressings, prolonged treatment, or extensive body-surface treatment.
• Avoid using plastic pants or tight-fitting diapers on treated areas in young children. Children may absorb larger amounts of drug and be more prone to systemic toxicity.
• To prevent recurrence, continue treatment for a few days after lesions clear, as ordered.
• Stop drug and notify the doctor if the patient develops signs of systemic absorption, skin irritation or ulceration, hypersensitivity, or infection.
• Instruct patient how to apply drug.

---

diflorasone diacetate
Florone, Flutone, Maxiflor, Psorcon
Pregnancy Risk Category: C

---

*Liquid form contains alcohol. *Common* reactions are in italics; **life-threatening,** in bold italics.
**May contain tartrazine.

HOW SUPPLIED
Cream: 0.05%
Ointment: 0.05%

ACTION
Unknown. Diffuses across cell membranes to form complexes with specific cytoplasmic receptors. Exhibits anti-inflammatory, antipruritic, vasoconstrictive, and antiproliferative activity. Considered a group II (high-potency) agent according to vasoconstrictive properties.

ONSET, PEAK, DURATION
Onset and duration unknown. Plasma levels are highest when applied to inflamed or damaged skin, eyelids, or scrotal area; lowest when applied to intact normal skin, palms of hands, or soles of feet.

INDICATIONS & DOSAGE
Inflammation associated with corticosteroid-responsive dermatoses –
Adults and children: clean area; apply sparingly in a thin film. Apply daily to q.i.d. as determined by severity of condition.

ADVERSE REACTIONS
Skin: burning, pruritus, irritation, dryness, erythema, folliculitis, perioral dermatitis, hypertrichosis, hypopigmentation, acneiform eruptions; *maceration, secondary infection, atrophy, striae, miliaria* (with occlusive dressings).
Systemic: *hypothalamic-pituitary-adrenal (HPA) axis suppression*, Cushing's syndrome, hyperglycemia, glucosuria.

INTERACTIONS
None significant.

CONTRAINDICATIONS
Contraindicated in patients hypersensitive to the drug.

NURSING CONSIDERATIONS
• Before applying, gently wash skin. To prevent skin damage, rub medication in gently, leaving a thin coat. When treating hairy sites, part hair and apply directly to lesions.
• Avoid application near eyes, mucous membranes, or in ear canal.
• If an occlusive dressing is ordered, don't leave it in place longer than 16 hours each day; don't use occlusive dressings on infected or exudative lesions on in combination with Psorcon.
• For patients with eczematous dermatitis whose skin may be irritated by adhesive material, hold dressing in place with gauze, elastic bandages, stockings, or stockinette.
• Change dressing as ordered. Discontinue drug and notify the doctor if skin infection, striae, or atrophy occurs.
• Notify the doctor and remove occlusive dressing if fever develops.
• If antifungal agents or antibiotics are used concomitantly, stop corticosteroids until infection is controlled, as ordered.
• Monitor the patient for systemic adverse reactions. Systemic absorption likely with use of occlusive dressings, prolonged treatment, or extensive body-surface treatment.
• Avoid using plastic pants or tight-fitting diapers on treated areas in young children. Children may absorb larger amounts of drug and be more prone to systemic toxicity.
• Stop drug and notify the doctor if the patient develops signs of systemic absorption, skin irritation or ulceration, hypersensitivity, or infection.
• Instruct patient how to apply drug.

fluocinolone acetonide
Fluocet, Fluonid, Flurosyn, Synalar, Synemol

Pregnancy Risk Category: C

HOW SUPPLIED
Cream: 0.01%, 0.025%, 0.2%
Ointment: 0.025%
Topical solution: 0.01%

ACTION
Unknown. Diffuses across cell membranes to form complexes with specific cytoplasmic receptors. Exhibits anti-inflammatory, antipruritic, vasoconstrictive, and antiproliferative activity. Considered a group III (medium-potency) agent according to vasoconstrictive properties.

ONSET, PEAK, DURATION
Onset and duration unknown. Plasma levels are highest when applied to inflamed or damaged skin, eyelids, or scrotal area; lowest when applied to intact normal skin, palms of hands, or soles of feet.

INDICATIONS & DOSAGE
Inflammation associated with corticosteroid-responsive dermatoses –
Adults and children: clean area; apply cream, ointment, or topical solution sparingly b.i.d. to q.i.d.

ADVERSE REACTIONS
Skin: burning, pruritus, irritation, dryness, erythema, folliculitis, hypertrichosis, hypopigmentation, acneiform eruptions, perioral dermatitis, allergic contact dermatitis; *maceration, secondary infection, atrophy, striae, miliaria* (with occlusive dressings).
Systemic: *hypothalamic-pituitary-adrenal (HPA) axis suppression,* Cushing's syndrome, hyperglycemia, glucosuria.

INTERACTIONS
None significant.

CONTRAINDICATIONS
Contraindicated in patients hypersensitive to the drug.

NURSING CONSIDERATIONS
• Gently wash skin before applying. To prevent skin damage, rub medication in gently, leaving a thin coat. When treating hairy sites, part hair and apply directly to lesions.
• Avoid application near eyes, mucous membranes, or in ear canal.
• If an occlusive dressing is ordered, don't leave it in place longer than 16 hours each day; don't use occlusive dressings on infected or exudative lesions.
• For patients with eczematous dermatitis whose skin may be irritated by adhesive material, hold dressing in place with gauze, elastic bandages, stockings, or stockinette.
• Change dressing as ordered. Discontinue drug and notify the doctor if skin infection, striae, or atrophy occurs.
• Notify the doctor and remove occlusive dressing if fever develops.
• If antifungal agents or antibiotics are used concomitantly, stop corticosteroids until infection is controlled, as ordered.
• Monitor the patient for systemic adverse reactions. Systemic absorption likely with use of occlusive dressings, prolonged treatment, or extensive body-surface treatment.
• In young children, avoid using plastic pants or tight-fitting diapers on treated areas. Children may absorb larger amounts of drug and be more prone to systemic toxicity.
• Be aware that fluonid solution on dry lesions may increase dryness, scaling, or pruritus; on denuded or fissured areas, may produce burning or stinging. If burning or stinging persists and dermatitis has not improved, discontinue use of solution and notify doctor.
• Stop drug and notify the doctor if the patient develops signs of systemic absorption, skin irritation or ulceration, hypersensitivity, or infection.
• Instruct patient how to apply drug.

---

*Liquid form contains alcohol.
**May contain tartrazine.   *Common* reactions are in italics; *life-threatening*, in bold italics.

fluocinonide

Lidemol†, Lidex, Lidex-E, Topsyn

Pregnancy Risk Category: C

HOW SUPPLIED

Cream: 0.05%
Gel: 0.05%
Ointment: 0.05%
Topical solution: 0.05%

ACTION

Unknown. Diffuses across cell membranes to form complexes with specific cytoplasmic receptors. Exhibits anti-inflammatory, antipruritic, vasoconstrictive, and antiproliferative activity. Considered a group II (high-potency) agent according to vasoconstrictive properties.

ONSET, PEAK, DURATION

Onset and duration unknown. Plasma levels are highest when applied to inflamed or damaged skin, eyelids, or scrotal area; lowest when applied to intact, normal skin, palms of hands, or soles of feet.

INDICATIONS & DOSAGE

Inflammation associated with corticosteroid-responsive dermatoses –
Adults and children: clean area; apply cream, gel, ointment, or topical solution sparingly b.i.d. or q.i.d.

ADVERSE REACTIONS

Skin: burning, pruritus, irritation, dryness, erythema, folliculitis, hypertrichosis, hypopigmentation, acneiform eruptions, perioral dermatitis, allergic contact dermatitis; *maceration, secondary infection, atrophy, striae, miliaria* (with occlusive dressings).
Systemic: *hypothalamic-pituitary-adrenal (HPA) axis suppression,* Cushing's syndrome, hyperglycemia, glucosuria.

INTERACTIONS

None significant.

CONTRAINDICATIONS

Contraindicated in patients hypersensitive to the drug.

NURSING CONSIDERATIONS

• Gently wash skin before applying. To prevent skin damage, rub medication in gently, leaving a thin coat. When treating hairy sites, part hair and apply directly to lesion.
• Avoid application near eyes, mucous membranes, or in ear canal.
• If an occlusive dressing is ordered, don't leave it in place longer than 16 hours each day; don't use occlusive dressings on infected or exudative lesions.
• For patients with eczematous dermatitis whose skin may be irritated by adhesive material, hold dressing in place with gauze, elastic bandages, stockings, or stockinette.
• Change dressing as ordered. Discontinue drug and notify the doctor if skin infection, striae, or atrophy occurs.
• Notify the doctor and remove occlusive dressing if fever develops.
• If antifungal agents or antibiotics are used concomitantly, stop corticosteroids until infection is controlled, as ordered.
• Monitor the patient for systemic adverse reactions. Systemic absorption likely with use of occlusive dressings, prolonged treatment, or extensive body-surface treatment.
• In young children, avoid using plastic pants or tight-fitting diapers on treated areas. Children may absorb larger amounts of drug and be more prone to systemic toxicity.
• To prevent recurrence, continue treatment for a few days after lesions clear, as ordered.
• Stop drug and notify the doctor if patient develops signs of systemic ab-

---

sorption, skin irritation or ulceration, hypersensitivity, or infection.
● Instruct patient how to apply drug.

---

flurandrenolide
Cordran, Cordran SP, Cordran Tape, Drenison†, Drenison ¼†, Drenison Tape†

Pregnancy Risk Category: C

HOW SUPPLIED
Cream: 0.025%, 0.05%
Lotion: 0.05%
Ointment: 0.025%, 0.05%
Tape: 4 mcg/cm²

ACTION
Unknown. Diffuses across cell membranes to form complexes with specific cytoplasmic receptors. Exhibits anti-inflammatory, antipruritic, vasoconstrictive, and antiproliferative activity. Considered a group III (medium-potency) agent according to vasoconstrictive properties.

ONSET, PEAK, DURATION
Onset and duration unknown. Plasma levels are highest when applied to inflamed or damaged skin, eyelids, or scrotal area; lowest when applied to intact normal skin, palms of hands, or soles of feet.

INDICATIONS & DOSAGE
Inflammation associated with corticosteroid-responsive dermatoses –
Adults and children: clean area; apply cream, lotion, or ointment sparingly b.i.d. or t.i.d.

Apply Cordran tape q 12 to 24 hours. Before applying tape, clean skin carefully, removing scales, crust, and dried exudate. Allow skin to dry for 1 hour before applying new tape. Shave or clip hair to allow good contact with skin and comfortable removal. If tape ends loosen prematurely, trim off and replace with fresh tape.

ADVERSE REACTIONS
Skin: burning, pruritus, irritation, dryness, erythema, folliculitis, hypertrichosis, hypopigmentation, acneiform eruptions, allergic contact dermatitis; *maceration, secondary infection, atrophy, striae, miliaria* (with occlusive dressings); purpura, stripping of epidermis, furunculosis (with tape).
Systemic: *hypothalamic-pituitary-adrenal (HPA) axis suppression,* Cushing's syndrome, hyperglycemia, glucosuria.

INTERACTIONS
None significant.

CONTRAINDICATIONS
Contraindicated in patients hypersensitive to the drug.

NURSING CONSIDERATIONS
● Gently wash skin before applying. To prevent skin damage, rub medication in gently, leaving a thin coat. When treating hairy sites, part hair and apply directly to lesions.
● Avoid application near eyes, mucous membranes, or in ear canal.
● If an occlusive dressing is ordered, don't leave it in place longer than 16 hours each day; don't use occlusive dressings on infected or exudative lesions.
● For patients with eczematous dermatitis whose skin may be irritated by adhesive material, hold dressing in place with gauze, elastic bandages, stockings, or stockinette.
● Discontinue drug and notify the doctor if skin infection, striae, or atrophy occurs.
● Notify the doctor and remove occlusive dressing if fever develops.
● Know that tape not advised for exudative lesions or lesions in intertriginous areas.
● Replace tape every 12 hours or, if well tolerated and adherence is satis-

---

factory, every 24 hours. Do not tear Cordran tape; cut it with scissors.
• If antifungal agents or antibiotics are used concomitantly, stop corticosteroids until infection is controlled, as ordered.
• Monitor the patient for systemic adverse reactions. Systemic absorption likely with use of occlusive dressings, prolonged treatment, or extensive body-surface treatment.
• Avoid using plastic pants or tight-fitting diapers on treated areas in young children. Children may absorb larger amounts of drug and be more prone to systemic toxicity.
• To prevent recurrence, continue treatment for a few days after lesions clear, as ordered.
• Stop drug and notify the doctor if the patient develops signs of systemic absorption, skin irritation or ulceration, hypersensitivity, or infection.
• Instruct patient how to apply drug.

---

fluticasone propionate
Cutivate

Pregnancy Risk Category: C

HOW SUPPLIED
Cream: 0.05%
Ointment: 0.005%

ACTION
Unknown. Diffuses across cell membranes to form complexes with specific cytoplasmic receptors. Exhibits anti-inflammatory, antipruritic, vasoconstrictive, and antiproliferative activity. Considered a group III (medium-potency) agent according to vasoconstrictive properties.

ONSET, PEAK, DURATION
Onset and duration unknown. Plasma levels are highest when applied to inflamed or damaged skin, eyelids, or scrotal area; lowest when applied to intact normal skin, palms of hands, or soles of feet.

INDICATIONS & DOSAGE
Inflammation associated with corticosteroid-responsive dermatoses –
Adults and children: apply cream or ointment sparingly to affected area b.i.d. and rub in gently and completely.

ADVERSE REACTIONS
Skin: stinging, burning, pruritus, irritation, dryness, erythema, folliculitis, skin atrophy, leukoderma, vesicles, rash, hypertrichosis, acneiform eruptions, hypopigmentation, perioral dermatitis, allergic contact dermatitis, secondary infection, striae, miliaria.
Significant systemic absorption can produce the following reactions:
CNS: euphoria, insomnia, headache, psychotic behavior, pseudotumor cerebri, mental changes, nervousness, restlessness.
CV: *CHF,* hypertension, edema.
EENT: cataracts, glaucoma, thrush.
GI: peptic ulceration, irritation, increased appetite.
Other: immunosuppression, increased susceptibility to infection, hypokalemia, sodium retention, fluid retention, weight gain, ***hypothalamic-pituitary-adrenal (HPA) axis suppression,*** Cushing's syndrome, hyperglycemia, glucosuria, osteoporosis, muscle atrophy, growth suppression in children, withdrawal syndrome.

INTERACTIONS
None significant.

CONTRAINDICATIONS
Contraindicated in patients hypersensitive to the drug or any of its components and in patients with viral, fungal, herpetic, or tubercular skin lesions.

NURSING CONSIDERATIONS
• Do not mix drug with other bases or vehicles; this may affect potency.
• If adverse reactions occur, be aware

---

that doctor may order a less potent agent.

• Know that one-time coverage of the adult body requires 12 to 26 g. Use of more than 50 g weekly is not recommended.

• Discontinue drug if local irritation or systemic infection, absorption, or hypersensitivity occurs, as ordered.

• Instruct patient how to apply drug.

• Tell the patient to avoid prolonged use and contact with eyes. Warn the patient not to apply around eyes, genitals, or rectum; on face; and in skin creases.

• Tell the patient to notify the doctor if the condition persists or worsens or if burning or irritation develops.

---

halcinonide
Halciderm, Halog

Pregnancy Risk Category: C

HOW SUPPLIED
Cream: 0.025%, 0.1%
Ointment: 0.1%
Topical solution: 0.1%

ACTION
Unknown. Diffuses across cell membranes to form complexes with specific cytoplasmic receptors. Exhibits anti-inflammatory, antipruritic, vasoconstrictive, and antiproliferative activity. Considered a group II (high-potency) agent according to vasoconstrictive properties.

ONSET, PEAK, DURATION
Onset and duration unknown. Plasma levels are highest when applied to inflamed or damaged skin, eyelids, or scrotal area; lowest when applied to intact normal skin, palms of hands, or soles of feet.

INDICATIONS & DOSAGE
Inflammation associated with corticosteroid-responsive dermatoses –
Adults and children: clean area; apply cream, ointment, or topical solution sparingly b.i.d. or t.i.d.

ADVERSE REACTIONS
Skin: burning, pruritus, irritation, dryness, erythema, folliculitis, hypertrichosis, hypopigmentation, acneiform eruptions, allergic contact dermatitis; *maceration, secondary infection, atrophy, striae, miliaria* (with occlusive dressings).
Systemic: ***hypothalamic-pituitary-adrenal (HPA) axis suppression,*** Cushing's syndrome, hyperglycemia, glucosuria.

INTERACTIONS
None significant.

CONTRAINDICATIONS
Contraindicated in patients hypersensitive to the drug.

NURSING CONSIDERATIONS
• Gently wash skin before applying. To prevent skin damage, rub medication in gently, leaving a thin coat. When treating hairy sites, part hair and apply directly to lesions.

• Avoid application near eyes, mucous membranes, or in ear canal.

• Gently rub small amount of cream into lesion until it disappears. Reapply, leaving a thin coating on lesion, and cover with occlusive dressing, if ordered. Apply ointment to lesion and cover with occlusive dressing, if ordered. Do not leave dressing in place longer than 16 hours each day.

• Don't use occlusive dressings on infected or exudative lesions.

• For patients with eczematous dermatitis whose skin may be irritated by adhesive material, hold dressing in place with gauze, elastic bandages, stockings, or stockinette.

• Change dressing as ordered. Discontinue drug and notify doctor if skin infection, striae, or atrophy occurs.

• Be aware that good results have

---

*Liquid form contains alcohol. *Common* reactions are in italics; *life-threatening*, in bold italics.
**May contain tartrazine.

been obtained by applying occlusive dressings in evening and removing them in morning, providing 12-hour occlusion. Medication should then be reapplied in the morning, without use of occlusive dressings during the day.

• Notify the doctor and remove occlusive dressing if fever develops.

• If antifungal agents or antibiotics are used concomitantly, stop corticosteroids until infection is controlled, as ordered.

• Monitor the patient for systemic adverse reactions. Systemic absorption especially likely with use of occlusive dressings, prolonged treatment, or extensive body-surface treatment.

• Avoid using plastic pants or tight-fitting diapers on treated areas in young children. Children may absorb larger amounts of drug and be more prone to systemic toxicity.

• To prevent recurrence, continue treatment for a few days after lesions clear, as ordered.

• Stop drug and notify the doctor if the patient develops signs of systemic absorption, skin irritation or ulceration, hypersensitivity, or infection.

• Instruct patient how to apply drug.

halobetasol propionate
Ultravate

Pregnancy Risk Category: C

HOW SUPPLIED
Cream: 0.05%
Ointment: 0.05%

ACTION
Unknown. Diffuses across cell membranes to form complexes with specific cytoplasmic receptors. Exhibits anti-inflammatory, antipruritic, vasoconstrictive, and antiproliferative activity. Considered a group I (very high-potency) agent according to vasoconstrictive properties.

ONSET, PEAK, DURATION
Onset and duration unknown. Plasma levels are highest when applied to inflamed or damaged skin, eyelids, or scrotal area; lowest when applied to intact normal skin, palms of hands, or soles of feet.

INDICATIONS & DOSAGE
Inflammation associated with corticosteroid-responsive dermatoses –
Adults: apply cream or ointment sparingly to affected area once daily or b.i.d. and rub in gently and completely. Treatment beyond 2 consecutive weeks is not recommended. Total dosage should not exceed 50 g weekly.

ADVERSE REACTIONS
Skin: stinging, burning, pruritus, irritation, dryness, erythema, folliculitis, skin atrophy, leukoderma, vesicles, rash, hypertrichosis, acneiform eruptions, hypopigmentation, perioral dermatitis, allergic contact dermatitis, secondary infection, striae, miliaria.
Significant systemic absorption can produce the following reactions:
CNS: euphoria, insomnia, headache, mental changes, nervousness, psychotic behavior, restlessness, pseudotumor cerebri, fatigue, dizziness, syncope.
CV: *CHF,* hypertension, hypotension.
EENT: cataracts, glaucoma, thrush.
GI: peptic ulceration, GI irritation, increased appetite, nausea, anorexia.
Other: edema, hypokalemia, weight gain, *hypothalamic-pituitary-adrenal (HPA) axis suppression,* Cushing's syndrome, hyperglycemia, glucosuria, fluid retention, osteoporosis, muscle atrophy, myalgia, arthralgia, fever, growth suppression in children.

INTERACTIONS
None significant.

---

†Available in Canada only.   ‡Available in Australia only.   ◊ Available OTC.

CONTRAINDICATIONS
Contraindicated in patients hypersensitive to the drug or any of its components.

NURSING CONSIDERATIONS
• Do not use occlusive dressings with this drug.
• Avoid use on face, groin, or axilla.
• Be alert that some systemic absorption usually occurs and may cause HPA axis suppression, Cushing's syndrome, hyperglycemia, and glucosuria, which are reversible after discontinuation of therapy.
• Keep in mind that corticotropin stimulation, morning plasma cortisol, and urinary cortisol tests are useful in determining the extent of HPA axis suppression.
• If HPA axis suppression occurs, discontinue drug, reduce frequency of application, or substitute a less potent corticosteroid, as prescribed.
• Discontinue if infection occurs and notify the doctor.
• Instruct patient how to apply drug.
• Tell the patient that drug is for external use only, as directed by the doctor. Tell him to avoid contact with eyes and not to cover, bandage, or wrap treated area unless directed by the doctor. Tell the patient not to use more often or for any condition other than prescribed.
• Tell the patient to notify the doctor of any signs of stinging, burning, or irritation.

hydrocortisone
Acticort, Aeroseb-HC, Bactine HC◊, CaldeCort, Carmol HC, Cetacort, Cort-Dome, Cortef◊, Cortenema, Cortinal, Cortizone 5◊, Cortril, Cremesone, Delacort, DermaCort◊, Dermolate◊, Dermtex HC, Durel-Cort, Ecosone, HC Cream, HI-Cor-2.5, Hycortole, Hydrocortex, HydroTex, Hytone, Ivocort, Maso-Cort, Microcort, Nutracort, Orabase HCA, Penecort, Proctocort, Rhus Tox HC, Rocort, Squibb-HC‡, Synacort, T/Scalp, Unicort

hydrocortisone acetate
CortaGel, Cortaid◊, Cortamed†, Cortef, Corticaine, Corticreme†, Cortifoam, Dermacort‡, Dermacort Ointment‡, Epifoam, Gynecort, Hydrocortisone Acetate, Lanacort, MyCort Lotion, Proctofoam-HC

hydrocortisone butyrate
Locoid

hydrocortisone valerate
Westcort Cream

Pregnancy Risk Category: C

HOW SUPPLIED
hydrocortisone
Aerosol: 0.5%
Cream: 0.25%◊, 0.5%◊, 1%◊, 2.5%
Gel: 1%
Lotion: 0.125%, 0.25%, 0.5%◊, 1%, 2%, 2.5%
Ointment: 0.5%◊, 1%◊, 2.5%
Topical solution: 1%
hydrocortisone acetate
Cream: 0.5%◊
Lotion: 0.5%◊
Ointment: 0.5%◊, 1%
Rectal foam: 90 mg/application
hydrocortisone butyrate
Cream: 0.1%
Ointment: 0.1%
hydrocortisone valerate
Cream: 0.2%

---

*Liquid form contains alcohol.
**May contain tartrazine.

Common reactions are in italics; ***life-threatening,*** in bold italics.

Ointment: 0.2%

ACTION
Unknown. Diffuses across cell membranes to form complexes with specific cytoplasmic receptors. Exhibits anti-inflammatory, antipruritic, vasoconstrictive, and antiproliferative activity. Considered a group IV (low-potency) agent according to vasoconstrictive properties.

ONSET, PEAK, DURATION
Onset atnd duration unknown. Plasma levels are highest when applied to inflamed or damaged skin, eyelids, or scrotal area; lowest when applied to intact normal skin, palms of hands, or soles of feet.

INDICATIONS & DOSAGE
Inflammation associated with corticosteroid-responsive dermatoses; adjunctive topical management of seborrheic dermatitis of scalp –
Adults and children: clean area; apply cream, gel, lotion, ointment, or topical solution sparingly daily to q.i.d. Spray aerosol onto affected area daily to q.i.d. until acute phase is controlled; then reduce dosage to one to three times weekly as needed.
Inflammation associated with proctitis –
Adults: 1 applicatorful of rectal foam P.R. daily or b.i.d. for 2 to 3 weeks, then every other day as necessary.

ADVERSE REACTIONS
Skin: burning, pruritus, irritation, dryness, erythema, folliculitis, hypertrichosis, hypopigmentation, acneiform eruptions, allergic contact dermatitis; *maceration, secondary infection, atrophy, striae, miliaria* (with occlusive dressings).
Systemic: *hypothalamic-pituitary-adrenal (HPA) axis suppression,* Cushing's syndrome, hyperglycemia, glucosuria.

INTERACTIONS
None significant.

CONTRAINDICATIONS
Contraindicated in patients hypersensitive to the drug.

NURSING CONSIDERATIONS
• Gently wash skin before applying. To prevent skin damage, rub medication in gently, leaving a thin coat. When treating hairy sites, part hair and apply directly to lesions.
• Avoid application near eyes, mucous membranes, or in ear canal; may be safely used on face, groin, armpits, and under breasts.
• If an occlusive dressing is ordered, don't leave it in place longer than 16 hours each day; don't use occlusive dressings on infected or exudative lesions.
• For patients with eczematous dermatitis whose skin may be irritated by adhesive material, hold dressing in place with gauze, elastic bandages, stockings, or stockinette.
• Notify the doctor and remove occlusive dressing if fever develops.
• Change dressing as ordered. Discontinue drug and notify doctor if skin infection, striae, or atrophy occurs.
• When using aerosol around the face, cover the patient's eyes and warn against inhalation of the spray. Aerosol preparation contains alcohol and may produce irritation or burning in open lesions. Do not spray longer than 3 seconds or closer than 6″ (15 cm) to avoid freezing of tissues. Apply to dry scalp after shampooing; no need to massage medication into scalp after spraying.
• If antifungal agents or antibiotics are used concomitantly, stop corticosteroids until infection is controlled, as ordered.
• Monitor patient for systemic adverse reactions. Systemic absorption likely with use of occlusive dressings,

---

prolonged treatment, or extensive body-surface treatment.

• Avoid using plastic pants or tight-fitting diapers on treated areas in young children. Children may absorb larger amounts of drug and be more prone to systemic toxicity.

• To prevent recurrence, continue treatment for a few days after lesions clear, as ordered.

• Stop drug and notify the doctor if the patient develops signs of systemic absorption, skin irritation or ulceration, hypersensitivity, or infection.

• Instruct patient how to apply drug.

mometasone furoate
Elocon

Pregnancy Risk Category: C

HOW SUPPLIED
Cream: 0.1%
Ointment: 0.1%
Lotion: 0.1%

ACTION
Unknown. Diffuses across cell membranes to form complexes with specific cytoplasmic receptors. Exhibits anti-inflammatory, antipruritic, vasoconstrictive, and antiproliferative activity. Considered a group III (medium-potency) agent according to vasoconstrictive properties.

ONSET, PEAK, DURATION
Onset and duration unknown. Plasma levels are highest when applied to inflamed or damaged skin, eyelids, or scrotal area; lowest when applied to intact normal skin, palms of hands, or soles of feet.

INDICATIONS & DOSAGE
Inflammation associated with corticosteroid-responsive dermatoses —
Adults: apply cream or ointment to affected areas once daily.

ADVERSE REACTIONS
Skin: burning, erythema, pruritus, atrophy, irritation, acneiform eruptions, hypopigmentation, allergic contact dermatitis.
Systemic: *hypothalamic-pituitary-adrenal (HPA) axis suppression,* Cushing's syndrome, hyperglycemia, glucosuria.

INTERACTIONS
None significant.

CONTRAINDICATIONS
Contraindicated in patients hypersensitive to the drug or to other corticosteroids.

NURSING CONSIDERATIONS
• Use cautiously in young children.
• Gently wash skin before applying. To prevent skin damage, rub medication in gently, leaving a thin coat. When treating hairy sites, part hair and apply directly to lesions.
• Avoid application near eyes, mucous membranes, or in ear canal.
• Do not use occlusive dressings with this drug.
• If antimicrobial agents are used concomitantly, stop corticosteroids until infection is controlled, as ordered.
• Monitor the patient for systemic adverse reactions. Systemic absorption likely with use of occlusive dressings, prolonged treatment, or extensive body-surface treatment.
• Be aware that children may absorb larger amounts of drug and be more prone to systemic toxicity. Avoid using plastic pants or tight fitting diapers on treated areas in young children.
• Stop drug and notify the doctor if the patient develops signs of systemic absorption, skin irritation or ulceration, hypersensitivity, or infection.
• Instruct patient how to apply drug.

---

*Liquid form contains alcohol.
May contain tartrazine.   *Common* reactions are in italics; ***life-threatening*, in bold italics.

triamcinolone acetonide
Aristocort, Flutex, Kenalog, Kenalone‡, Triacet

Pregnancy Risk Category: C

HOW SUPPLIED
Aerosol: 0.2 mg/2-second spray
Cream: 0.02%‡, 0.025%, 0.1%, 0.5%
Lotion: 0.025%, 0.1%
Ointment: 0.02%‡, 0.025%, 0.1%, 0.5%
Paste: 0.1%

ACTION
Unknown. Diffuses across cell membranes to form complexes with specific cytoplasmic receptors. Exhibits anti-inflammatory, antipruritic, vasoconstrictive, and antiproliferative activity. Considered a group III (medium-potency) agent according to vasoconstrictive properties.

ONSET, PEAK, DURATION
Onset and duration unknown. Plasma levels are highest when applied to inflamed or damaged skin, eyelids, or scrotal area; low levels result when applied to intact, normal skin, palms of hands, or soles of feet.

INDICATIONS & DOSAGE
Inflammation associated with corticosteroid-responsive dermatoses –
Adults and children: clean area; apply aerosol, cream, lotion, or ointment sparingly t.i.d. to q.i.d.
Inflammation associated with oral lesions –
Adults and children: apply paste h.s. and, if needed, 2 or 3 times daily, preferably after meals. Apply a small amount without rubbing and press to lesion in mouth until a thin film develops.

ADVERSE REACTIONS
Skin: burning, pruritus, irritation, dryness, erythema, folliculitis, hyper-trichosis, hypopigmentation, acneiform eruptions, perioral dermatitis, allergic contact dermatitis; *maceration, secondary infection, atrophy, striae, miliaria* (with occlusive dressings).
Systemic: *hypothalmic-pituitary-adrenal (HPA) axis suppression,* Cushing's syndrome, hyperglycemia, glucosuria.

INTERACTIONS
None significant.

CONTRAINDICATIONS
Contraindicated in patients hypersensitive to the drug.

NURSING CONSIDERATIONS
• Gently wash skin before applying. To avoid skin damage, rub medication in gently, leaving a thin coat. When treating hairy sites, part hair and apply directly to lesions.
• Avoid application near eyes or in ear canal.
• If an occlusive dressing is ordered, don't leave it in place longer than 16 hours each day; don't use occlusive dressings on infected or exudative lesions.
• Change dressing as ordered. Discontinue drug and notify the doctor if skin infection, striae, or atrophy occurs.
• When using aerosol about the face, cover the patient's eyes and warn against inhalation of the spray. Aerosol preparation contains alcohol and may produce irritation or burning in open lesions. Do not spray longer than 3 seconds or closer than 6" (15 cm) to avoid freezing of tissues.
• If antifungal agents or antibiotics are used concomitantly, stop corticosteroids until infection is controlled, as ordered.
• Monitor the patient for systemic adverse reactions. Systemic absorption likely with use of occlusive dressings,

---

†Available in Canada only.   ‡Available in Australia only.   ◇ Available OTC.

prolonged treatment, or extensive body-surface treatment.

• Avoid using plastic pants or tight-fitting diapers on treated areas in young children. Children may absorb larger amounts of drug and be more prone to systemic toxicity.

• Stop drug and notify the doctor if the patient develops signs of systemic absorption, skin irritation or ulceration, hypersensitivity, or infection.

• Instruct patient how to apply drug.

---

*Liquid form contains alcohol.   *Common* reactions are in italics; ***life-threatening,*** in bold italics.
**May contain tartrazine.

91
Vitamins and minerals

vitamin A

vitamin B complex
cyanocobalamin
hydroxocobalamin
folic acid
leucovorin calcium
niacin
niacinamide
pyridoxine hydrochloride
riboflavin
thiamine hydrochloride

vitamin C

vitamin D
cholecalciferol
ergocalciferol

vitamin E

vitamin K analogue
phytonadione

sodium fluoride
sodium fluoride, topical

trace elements
chromium
copper
iodine
manganese
selenium
zinc

TRACE ELEMENT COMBINATION PRODUCTS

M.T.E.-4: zinc sulfate 1 mg, copper sulfate 0.4 mg, manganese sulfate 0.1 mg, and chromium chloride 4 mcg per ml.
M.T.E.-4 CONCENTRATED: zinc sulfate 5 mg, copper sulfate 1 mg, manganese sulfate 0.5 mg, and chromium chloride 10 mcg per ml.

M.T.E.-5: zinc sulfate 1 mg, copper sulfate 0.4 mg, manganese sulfate 0.1 mg, chromium chloride 4 mcg, and selenium (as selenious acid) 20 mcg per ml.
M.T.E.-5 CONCENTRATED: zinc sulfate 5 mg, copper sulfate 1 mg, manganese sulfate 0.5 mg, chromium chloride 10 mcg, and selenium (as selenious acid) 60 mcg per ml.
M.T.E.-6: zinc sulfate 1 mg, copper sulfate 0.4 mg, manganese sulfate 0.1 mg, chromium chloride 4 mcg, selenium (as selenious acid) 20 mcg, and sodium iodide 25 mcg per ml.
M.T.E.-6 CONCENTRATED: zinc sulfate 5 mg, copper sulfate 1 mg, manganese sulfate 0.5 mg, chromium chloride 10 mcg, selenium (as selenious acid) 60 mcg, and sodium iodide 75 mcg per ml.
M.T.E.-7: zinc sulfate 1 mg, copper sulfate 0.4 mg, manganese sulfate 0.1 mg, chromium chloride 4 mcg, selenium (as selenious acid) 20 mcg, and sodium iodide 25 mcg per ml.
MULTIPLE TRACE ELEMENT CONCENTRATED: zinc sulfate 5 mg, copper sulfate 1 mg, manganese sulfate 0.5 mg, and chromium chloride 10 mcg per ml.
MULTIPLE TRACE ELEMENT NEONATAL: zinc sulfate 0.5 mg, copper sulfate 0.1 mg, manganese sulfate 0.025 mg, chromium chloride 0.85 mcg.
MULTIPLE TRACE ELEMENT WITH SELENIUM: zinc sulfate 1 mg, copper sulfate 0.4 mg, manganese sulfate 0.1 mg, chromium chloride 4 mcg, and selenious acid 20 mcg.
MULTITRACE 5 CONCENTRATE: zinc chloride 5 mg, copper chloride 1 mg, manganese chloride 0.5 mg, chromium chloride 10 mcg per ml, and selenious acid 60 mcg.

NEOTRACE-4: zinc sulfate 1.5 mg, copper sulfate 0.1 mg, manganese sulfate 0.025 mg, and chromium chloride 0.85 mcg per ml.
PEDIATRIC MULTIPLE TRACE ELEMENT: zinc sulfate 0.5 mg, copper sulfate 0.1 mg, manganese sulfate 0.03 mg, and chromium chloride 1 mcg per ml.
PEDTRACE-4: zinc sulfate 0.5 mg, copper sulfate 0.1 mg, manganese sulfate 0.025 mg, and chromium chloride 0.85 mcg per ml.
P.T.E.-4: zinc sulfate 1 mg, copper sulfate 0.1 mg, manganese sulfate 0.025 mg, and chromium chloride 1 mcg per ml.
P.T.E.-5: zinc sulfate 1 mg, copper sulfate 0.1 mg, manganese sulfate 0.025 mg, chromium chloride 1 mcg, and selenium (as selenious acid) 15 mcg per ml.
TRACE METALS ADDITIVE: zinc chloride 0.8 mg, copper chloride 0.2 mg, manganese chloride 0.16 mg, and chromium chloride 2 mcg per ml.

VITAMIN COMBINATION PRODUCTS
B complex vitamins◊
B complex vitamins with iron◊
B complex with vitamin C◊
B vitamin combinations◊
Calcium and vitamin products◊
Fluoride with vitamins◊
Geriatric supplements with multivitamins and minerals◊
Miscellaneous vitamins and minerals◊
Multivitamins◊
Multivitamins and minerals with hormones◊
Multivitamins with B$_{12}$◊
Vitamin A and D combinations◊

---

vitamin A (retinol)
Acon, Aquasol A, Del-Vi-A

Pregnancy Risk Category: NR

HOW SUPPLIED
Tablets: 10,000 IU
Capsules: 10,000 IU◊, 25,000 IU, 50,000 IU
Drops: 30 ml with dropper (50,000 IU/0.1 ml)
Injection: 2-ml vials (50,000 IU/ml with 0.5% chlorobutanol, polysorbate 80, butylated hydroxyanisol, and butylated hydroxytoluene)

ACTION
Coenzyme that stimulates retinal function, bone growth, reproduction, and integrity of epithelial and mucosal tissues.

ONSET, PEAK, DURATION
Onset and duration unknown. Peak levels occur in 3 to 5 hours.

INDICATIONS & DOSAGE
Recommended daily allowance (RDA) –
Note: RDAs have been converted to retinol equivalents (RE). One RE has the activity of 1mcg all-*trans* retinol, 6 mcg beta carotene, or 12 mcg carotenoid provitamins.
Neonates and infants to 1 year: 375 mcg RE or 1,250 IU.
Children 1 to 3 years: 400 mcg RE or 1,330 IU.
Children 4 to 6 years: 500 mcg RE or 1,665 IU.
Children 7 to 10 years: 700 mcg RE or 2,330 IU.
Males over 11 years: 1,000 mcg RE or 3,330 IU.
Females over 11 years: 800 mcg RE or 2,665 IU.
Pregnant women: 800 mcg RE or 2,665 IU.
Lactating women (first 6 months): 1,300 mcg RE or 4,330 IU.
Lactating women (second 6 months): 1,200 mcg RE or 4,000 IU.
Severe vitamin A deficiency –
Adults and children over 8 years: 50,000 to 100,000 IU I.M. or 100,000 to 500,000 IU P.O. for 3

---

*Liquid form contains alcohol.   *Common* reactions are in italics; **life-threatening,** in bold italics.
**May contain tartrazine.

days, followed by 50,000 IU I.M. or P.O. for 2 weeks; then 10,000 to 20,000 IU P.O. for 2 months. Follow with adequate dietary nutrition and RDA vitamin A supplements.
Infants under 1 year: 7,500 to 15,000 IU I.M. daily for 10 days.
Children 1 to 8 years: 17,500 to 35,000 IU I.M. daily for 10 days.
Maintenance dosage to prevent recurrence of vitamin A deficiency –
Children 1 to 8 years: 5,000 to 10,000 IU P.O. daily for 2 months, then adequate dietary nutrition and RDA vitamin A supplements.

ADVERSE REACTIONS
Adverse reactions are usually seen only with toxicity.
CNS: irritability, headache, *increased intracranial pressure,* fatigue, lethargy, malaise, vertigo, visual disturbances.
EENT: miosis, papilledema, exophthalmos.
GI: anorexia, epigastric pain, diarrhea, nausea, vomiting.
GU: hypomenorrhea.
Hematologic: leukopenia.
Hepatic: jaundice, hepatomegaly, *cirrhosis,* elevated liver enzymes.
Skin: alopecia; drying, cracking, scaling of skin; pruritus; lip fissures; massive desquamation; increased pigmentation; night sweating.
Other: skeletal – slow growth, decalcification of bone, hypercalcemia, hypercalciuria, hyperostosis, periostitis, premature closure of epiphyses, migratory arthralgia, cortical thickening over the radius and tibia, bulging fontanelles; splenomegaly.

INTERACTIONS
Cholestyramine resin, mineral oil: reduced GI absorption of fat-soluble vitamins. If needed, give mineral oil at bedtime.
Isotretinoin, multivitamins containing vitamin A: increased risk of toxicity. Avoid concomitant use.
Warfarin: increased risk of bleeding. Monitor PT closely.

CONTRAINDICATIONS
• Contraindicated for oral administration in patients with malabsorption syndrome; if malabsorption is from inadequate bile secretion, oral route may be used with concurrent administration of bile salts (dehydrocholic acid). Also contraindicated in hypervitaminosis A and hypersensitivity to any ingredient in product.
• I.V. administration contraindicated except for special water-miscible forms intended for infusion with large parenteral volumes. I.V. push of vitamin A of any type is also contraindicated (anaphylaxis or anaphylactoid reactions and death have resulted).

NURSING CONSIDERATIONS
• Use cautiously in pregnant patients, avoiding doses exceeding RDA.
• Assess the patient's vitamin A intake from fortified foods, dietary supplements, self-administered drugs, and prescription drug sources.
• Liquid preparations available if nasogastric administration is necessary. May be mixed with cereal or fruit juice.
• Know that adequate vitamin A absorption requires suitable protein, vitamin E, and zinc intake and bile secretion; give supplemental salts if necessary and ordered. Zinc supplements may be necessary in patients receiving long-term total parenteral nutrition.
• Monitor for adverse reactions if dosage is high.
• Monitor the patient closely for skin disorders; high dosages may induce chronic toxicity.
• Record dietary and bowel habits, and report abnormalities to doctor.
• Be aware that acute toxicity has resulted from single doses of 25,000 IU/kg of body weight; 350,000 IU in infants and over 2 million IU in adults

have also proved acutely toxic. Doses that do not exceed the RDA are usually nontoxic.

• Be aware that chronic toxicity in infants (3 to 6 months) has resulted from doses of 18,500 IU daily for 1 to 3 months. In adults, chronic toxicity has resulted from doses of 50,000 IU daily for over 18 months; 500,000 IU daily for 2 months, and 1 million IU daily for 3 days.

• Keep in mind absorption is fastest and most complete with water-miscible preparations, intermediate with emulsions, and slowest with oil suspensions.

• Protect from light.

• To avoid toxicity, advise the patient against self-administration of megadoses of vitamins without specific indications. Also stress that the patient should not share prescribed vitamins with family members or others.

cyanocobalamin (vitamin B₁₂)
Anacobin†, Bedoz†, Bioglan B₁₂ Plus‡, Crystamine, Crysti-12, Cyanabin†, Cyanocobalamin, Cyanoject, Cyomin, Rubesol-1000, Rubion†, Rubramin

hydroxocobalamin (vitamin B₁₂ₐ)
Codroxomin, Hydrobexan, Hydro-Cobex, Hydro-Crysti-12, LA-12

Pregnancy Risk Category: NR

HOW SUPPLIED
cyanocobalamin
Tablets: 25 mcg◊, 50 mcg◊, 100 mcg◊, 250 mcg◊, 500 mcg◊, 1,000 mcg◊
Injection: 1,000 mcg/ml
hydroxocobalamin
Injection: 1,000 mcg/ml

ACTION
Coenzyme that stimulates metabolic functions. Necessary for cell replica-tion, hematopoiesis, and nucleoprotein and myelin synthesis.

ONSET, PEAK, DURATION
Onset and duration unknown. Time to peak plasma levels after oral administration is 8 to 12 hours; after intramuscular administration, 60 minutes.

INDICATIONS & DOSAGE
Recommended daily allowance (RDA) for cyanocobalamin –
Neonates and infants to 6 months: 0.3 mcg.
Infants 6 months to 1 year: 0.5 mcg.
Children over 1 year to 3 years: 0.7 mcg.
Children 4 to 6 years: 1 mcg.
Children 7 to 10 years: 1.4 mcg.
Adults and children 11 years and over: 2 mcg.
Pregnant women: 2.2 mcg.
Lactating women: 2.6 mcg.
Vitamin B₁₂ deficiency caused by inadequate diet, subtotal gastrectomy, or any other condition, disorder, or disease except malabsorption related to pernicious anemia or other GI disease –
Adults: 30 mcg hydroxocobalamin I.M. daily for 5 to 10 days, depending on severity of deficiency. Maintenance dosage is 100 to 200 mcg I.M. once monthly. For subsequent prophylaxis, advise adequate nutrition and daily RDA vitamin B₁₂ supplements.
Children: 1 to 5 mg hydroxocobalamin spread over 2 or more weeks in doses of 100 mcg I.M., depending on severity of deficiency. Maintenance dosage is 30 to 50 mcg/month I.M. For subsequent prophylaxis, advise adequate nutrition and daily RDA vitamin B₁₂ supplements.
Pernicious anemia or vitamin B₁₂ malabsorption –
Adults: initially, 100 mcg cyanocobalamin I.M. or S.C. daily for 6 to 7 days, then 100 mcg I.M. or S.C. once monthly.
Children: 30 to 50 mcg I.M. or S.C.

---

daily over 2 or more weeks; then 100 mcg I.M. or S.C. monthly for life.
Methylmalonic aciduria –
Neonates: 1,000 mcg cyanocobalamin I.M. daily.
Schilling test flushing dose –
Adults and children: 1,000 mcg hydroxocobalamin I.M. in a single dose.

ADVERSE REACTIONS
CV: peripheral vascular thrombosis, pulmonary edema, CHF.
GI: transient diarrhea.
Skin: itching, transitory exanthema, urticaria.
Other: *anaphylaxis, anaphylactoid reactions with parenteral administration*, pain or burning at S.C. or I.M. injection sites.

INTERACTIONS
Aminoglycosides, chloramphenicol, colchicine, para-aminosalicylic acid and salts: malabsorption of vitamin B₁₂. Don't use concomitantly.

CONTRAINDICATIONS
Contraindicated in patients hypersensitive to vitamin B₁₂ or cobalt and in patients with early Leber's disease.

NURSING CONSIDERATIONS
• Use cautiously in anemic patients with coexisting cardiac, pulmonary, or hypertensive disease; and in patients with severe vitamin B₁₂-dependent deficiencies.
• Use cautiously in premature infants. Some products contain benzyl alcohol which mauy cause a "gasping syndrome."
• Determine reticulocyte count, hematocrit, B₁₂, iron, and folate levels before beginning therapy, as ordered.
• Don't mix parenteral liquids in same syringe with other medications.
• Keep in mind that drug is physically incompatible with dextrose solutions, alkaline or strongly acidic solutions, oxidizing or reducing agents, heavy metals, chlorpromazine, phytona-

dione, prochlorperazine, and many other drugs.
• Know that hydroxocobalamin is approved for I.M. use only. Its only advantage over cyanocobalamin is its longer duration.
• Do not administer large oral doses of vitamin B₁₂ routinely as the drug is lost through excretion.
• Monitor reticulocyte count, hematocrit, B₁₂, iron, and folate levels between the fifth and seventh day of therapy and periodically thereafter, as ordered.
• Closely monitor serum potassium levels for first 48 hours. Give potassium supplement if necessary, as ordered.
• Be aware that drug may cause false-positive intrinsic factor antibody test.
• Know that vitamin B₁₂ is usually nontoxic.
• Be aware that infection, tumors, or renal, hepatic, and other debilitating diseases may reduce therapeutic response.
• Keep in mind that deficiencies are more common in strict vegetarians and their breast-fed infants.
• Be aware B₁₂ deficiency may suppress the symptoms of polycythemia vera.
• Protect from light. Do not refrigerate or freeze.
• Stress need for patients with pernicious anemia to return for monthly injections. Although total body stores may last 3 to 6 years, anemia will recur if not treated monthly.

folic acid (vitamin B₉)
Folvite, Novofolacid†
Pregnancy Risk Category: NR

HOW SUPPLIED
Tablets: 0.4 mg, 0.8 mg, 1 mg
Injection: 10-ml vials (5 mg/ml with 1.5% benzyl alcohol or 10 mg/ml with 1.5% benzyl alcohol and 0.2% EDTA)

ACTION
Stimulates normal erythropoiesis and nucleoprotein synthesis.

ONSET, PEAK, DURATION
Onset and duration unknown. Serum levels peak in 30 to 60 minutes.

INDICATIONS & DOSAGE
Recommended daily allowance (RDA) –
Neonates and infants to 6 months: 25 mcg.
Infants 6 months to 1 year: 35 mcg.
Children over 1 year to 3 years: 50 mcg.
Children 4 to 6 years: 75 mcg.
Children 7 to 11 years: 100 mcg.
Children 11 to 14 years: 150 mcg.
Males 15 years and over: 200 mcg.
Females 15 years and over: 180 mcg.
Pregnant women: 400 mcg.
Lactating women (first 6 months): 280 mcg.
Lactating women (second 6 months): 260 mcg.
Megaloblastic or macrocytic anemia secondary to folic acid or other nutritional deficiency, hepatic disease, alcoholism, intestinal obstruction, excessive hemolysis –
Adults and children over 4 years: 0.4 mg to 1 mg P.O., S.C., or I.M. daily. After anemia secondary to folic acid deficiency is corrected, proper diet and RDA supplements are necessary to prevent recurrence.
Children under 4 years: up to 0.3 mg P.O., S.C., or I.M. daily.
Pregnant and lactating women: 0.8 mg P.O., S.C., or I.M. daily.
Prevention of megaloblastic anemia in pregnancy and fetal damage –
Adults: up to 1 mg P.O., S.C., or I.M. daily throughout pregnancy.
Nutritional supplement –
Adults: 0.1 mg P.O., S.C., or I.M. daily.
Children: 0.05 mg P.O. daily.
To test folic acid deficiency in patients

with megaloblastic anemia without masking pernicious anemia –
Adults and children: 0.1 to 0.2 mg P.O. or I.M. for 10 days while maintaining a diet low in folate and vitamin B_{12}.
Tropical sprue –
Adults: 3 to 15 mg P.O. daily.

ADVERSE REACTIONS
Respiratory: *bronchospasm*.
Skin: allergic reactions (rash, pruritus, erythema).
Other: general malaise.

INTERACTIONS
Aminosalicylic acid, chloramphenicol, methotrexate, sulfasalazine, trimethoprim: antagonism of folic acid. Monitor for decreased folic acid effect. Use together cautiously.
Anticonvulsants such as phenobarbital and phenytoin: increased anticonvulsant metabolism and decreased blood levels of the anticonvulsants. Monitor closely.

CONTRAINDICATIONS
Contraindicated in patients with undiagnosed anemia because it may mask pernicious anemia. Also contraindicated in those with B_{12} deficiency.

NURSING CONSIDERATIONS
• Don't mix with other medications in same syringe for I.M. injections.
• Be aware that concurrent folic acid and vitamin B_{12} therapy may be used if supported by diagnosis.
• Be alert that patients with small-bowel resections and intestinal malabsorption may require parenteral administration routes.
• Be aware that reticulosis, reversion to normoblastic hematopoiesis, and return to normal hemoglobin indicate folic acid deficiency.
• Protect from light and heat; store at room temperature.
• Know that safety in pregnancy has not been established but pregnant

---

Liquid form contains alcohol.
**May contain tartrazine.
Common reactions are in italics; ***life-threatening,*** in bold italics.

women are more prone to develop folate deficiency. Folate deficient mothers may be more prone to pregnancy-related complications and fetal abnormalities.

• Teach patient about proper nutrition necessary to prevent recurrence of anemia.

---

leucovorin calcium (citrovorum factor, folinic acid)
Wellcovorin

Pregnancy Risk Category: C

HOW SUPPLIED
Tablets: 5 mg, 10 mg, 15 mg, 25 mg
Injection: 1-ml ampule (3 mg/ml with 0.9% benzyl alcohol)
Powder for injection: 50 mg/vial, 100 mg/vial, 350 mg/vial

ACTION
A reduced form of folic acid that is readily converted to other folic acid derivatives.

ONSET, PEAK, DURATION
Onset occurs in 5 minutes after I.V. administration, 10 to 20 minutes after I.M. administration, 20 to 30 minutes after oral administration. Levels peak within 10 minutes after I.V. administration, less than 1 hour after I.M. administration, or 2 to 3 hours after oral administration. Effects persist for 3 to 6 hours regardless of administration route.

INDICATIONS & DOSAGE
Overdose of folic acid antagonist –
Adults and children: P.O., I.M., or I.V. dose equivalent to weight of antagonist given.
Leucovorin rescue after high methotrexate dose in treatment of malignancy –
Adults and children: 10 mg/m² P.O., I.M., or I.V. q 6 hours until methotrexate levels fall below 5×10^{-8} M.

Megaloblastic anemia caused by congenital enzyme deficiency –
Adults and children: 3 to 6 mg I.M., then 1 mg P.O. or I.M. daily for life.
Folate-deficient megaloblastic anemia –
Adults and children: up to 1 mg of leucovorin I.M daily. Duration of treatment depends on hematologic response.
Prevention of hematologic toxicity caused by pyrimethamine or trimethoprim therapy –
Adults and children: 400 mcg to 5 mg I.M. with each dose of the folic acid antagonist.
Treatment of hematologic toxicity caused by pyrimethamine or trimethoprim therapy –
Adults and children: 5 to 15 mg I.M. daily.
Palliative treatment of advanced colorectal carcinoma –
Adults: 20 mg/m² I.V., followed by fluorouracil 425 mg/m² I.V. daily for 5 consecutive days. Repeated at 4-week intervals for two additional courses; then at intervals of 4 to 5 weeks if tolerated.

ADVERSE REACTIONS
Respiratory: *bronchospasm.*
Skin: hypersensitivity reactions (rash, pruritus, erythema).

INTERACTIONS
Fluorouracil: may enhance fluorouracil toxicity. Avoid concomitant use.

CONTRAINDICATIONS
Contraindicated in patients with pernicious anemia and other megaloblastic anemias secondary to the lack of vitamin B_{12}.

NURSING CONSIDERATIONS
• **I.V. use:** When using powder for injection, reconstitute 50-mg vial with 5 ml, 100-mg vial with 10 ml, or 350-mg vial with 17 ml of sterile water or bacteriostatic water for injection.

When doses are greater than 10 mg/m², don't use diluents containing benzyl alcohol.

• Don't exceed 160 mg/minute when giving by direct injection.

• Do not confuse leucovorin (folinic acid) with folic acid.

• Follow leucovorin rescue schedule and protocol closely to maximize therapeutic response.

• Do not administer leucovorin simultaneously with systemic methotrexate. Time intervals have ranged from 0 to 72 hours after methotrexate.

• Protect from light and heat, especially reconstituted parenteral preparations.

• Tell patient why drug is necessary.

niacin (vitamin B₃, nicotinic acid)

Niac, Niacor, Nico-400, Nicobid◊, Nicolar**, Nicotinex

niacinamide (nicotinamide)◊

Pregnancy Risk Category: C

HOW SUPPLIED
niacin
Tablets: 25 mg◊, 50 mg◊, 100 mg◊, 250 mg◊, 500 mg
Tablets (timed-release): 150 mg◊, 250 mg◊, 500 mg◊, 750 mg◊
Capsules (timed-release): 125 mg◊, 250 mg◊, 300 mg◊, 400 mg◊, 500 mg
Elixir: 50 mg/5 ml◊
Injection: 100 mg/ml in 30-ml vials
niacinamide
Tablets: 50 mg◊, 100 mg◊, 125 mg◊, 250 mg◊, 500 mg◊

ACTION
Niacin and niacinamide stimulate lipid metabolism, tissue respiration, and glycogenolysis; niacin decreases synthesis of low-density lipoproteins and inhibits lipolysis in adipose tissue.

ONSET, PEAK, DURATION
Onset of vitamin effects unknown. Triglyceride levels begin to decrease within several hours; cholesterol levels, within several days. Serum levels peak 45 minutes after oral administration. Duration unknown.

INDICATIONS & DOSAGE
Recommended daily allowance (RDA) –
Neonates and infants to 6 months: 5 mg.
Infants 6 months to 1 year: 6 mg.
Children 1 to 3 years: 9 mg.
Children 4 to 6 years: 12 mg.
Children 7 to 10 years: 13 mg.
Males 11 to 14 years: 17 mg.
Males 15 to 18 years: 20 mg.
Males 19 to 50 years: 19 mg.
Males 51 years and over: 15 mg.
Females 11 to 50 years: 15 mg.
Females 51 years and over: 13 mg.
Pregnant women: 17 mg.
Lactating women: 20 mg.
Pellagra –
Adults: 300 to 500 mg P.O., S.C., I.M., or I.V. daily in divided doses, depending on severity of niacin deficiency.
Children: up to 300 mg P.O. or 100 mg I.V. daily, depending on severity of niacin deficiency.
    After symptoms subside, advise adequate nutrition and RDA supplements to prevent recurrence.
Hartnup disease –
Adults: 50 to 200 mg P.O. daily
Niacin deficiency –
Adults: up to 100 mg P.O. daily.
Hyperlipidemias, especially with hypercholesterolemia –
Adults: 1 to 2 g P.O. three times a day with or after meals, increased at intervals to 6 g daily.

ADVERSE REACTIONS
Most adverse reactions are dose-dependent.
CNS: dizziness, transient headache.

CV: *excessive peripheral vasodilation (especially niacin).*
GI: *nausea, vomiting, diarrhea,* possible activation of peptic ulceration, epigastric or substernal pain.
Hepatic: *hepatic dysfunction.*
Skin: *flushing,* pruritus, dryness, tingling.
Other: hyperglycemia, hyperuricemia.

INTERACTIONS
Antihypertensive drugs (sympathetic or ganglionic blockers): potential additive vasodilating effect, causing postural hypotension. Use together cautiously; also warn the patient about postural hypotension.

CONTRAINDICATIONS
Contraindicated in patients with hepatic dysfunction, active peptic ulcers, severe hypotension, arterial hemorrhage, or hypersensitivity to the drug.

NURSING CONSIDERATIONS
• Use cautiously in patients with gallbladder disease, diabetes mellitus, or coronary artery disease and in patients with a history of liver disease, peptic ulcer, allergy, or gout.
• **I.V. use:** Give slow I.V. (no faster than 2 mg/minute). Explain harmlessness of flushing syndrome to ease anxiety.
• To minimize GI side effects, give with meals.
• Administer aspirin (325 mg P.O. 30 minutes before niacin dose) as ordered to possibly reduce the flushing response to niacin.
• Be aware that timed-release niacin or niacinamide may prevent excessive flushing that occurs with large doses. However, timed-release niacin has been associated with hepatic dysfunction, even at doses as low as 1 g/day.
• Monitor hepatic function and blood glucose early in therapy, as ordered.
• Stress that this substance is a potent medication, not just a vitamin, and may cause serious adverse effects. Explain importance of adhering to therapeutic regimen.
• Advise patient against self-medicating for hyperlipidemia.

---

pyridoxine hydrochloride (vitamin B₆)

Beesix, Hexa-Betalin, Nestrex◊, Rodex

Pregnancy Risk Category: A

HOW SUPPLIED
Tablets: 10 mg◊, 25 mg◊, 50 mg◊, 100 mg◊, 200 mg◊, 250 mg◊, 500 mg◊
Capsules (timed-release): 100 mg
Capsules: 500 mg
Tablets (timed-release): 100 mg
Injection: 100 mg/ml

ACTION
Acts as a coenzyme that stimulates various metabolic functions, including amino acid metabolism.

ONSET, PEAK, DURATION
Unknown.

INDICATIONS & DOSAGE
Recommended daily allowance (RDA) –
Neonates and infants to 6 months: 0.3 mg.
Infants 6 months to 1 year: 0.6 mg.
Children 1 year to 3 years: 1 mg.
Children 4 to 6 years: 1.1 mg.
Children 7 to 10 years: 1.4 mg.
Males 11 to 14 years: 1.7 mg.
Males 15 years and over: 2 mg.
Females 11 to 14 years: 1.4 mg.
Females 15 to 18 years: 1.5 mg.
Females 19 years and over: 1.6 mg.
Pregnant women: 2.2 mg.
Lactating women: 2.1 mg.
Dietary vitamin B₆ deficiency –
Adults: 10 to 20 mg P.O., I.M., or I.V. daily for 3 weeks, then 2 to 5 mg daily as a supplement to a proper diet.

Seizures related to vitamin B₆ deficiency or dependency –
Adults and children: 100 mg I.M. or I.V. in single dose.
Vitamin B₆-responsive anemias or dependency syndrome (inborn errors of metabolism) –
Adults: up to 600 mg P.O., I.M., or I.V. daily until symptoms subside, then 30 mg daily for life.
Prevention of vitamin B₆ deficiency during drug therapy –
Adults: 6 to 100 mg P.O. daily for isoniazid therapy.
Drug-induced vitamin B₆ deficiency –
Adults and children: 50 to 200 mg P.O., I.M., or I.V. daily for 3 weeks, followed by 25 to 100 mg P.O., I.M., or I.V. daily to prevent relapse.
Antidote for isoniazid poisoning –
Adults: 4 g I.V., followed by 1 g I.M. q 30 minutes until the amount of pyridoxine administered equals the amount of isoniazid ingested.

ADVERSE REACTIONS
CNS: drowsiness, paresthesia, unstable gait.

INTERACTIONS
Levodopa: decreased levodopa effect. Avoid concomitant use.
Phenobarbital, phenytoin: decreased anticonvulsant serum levels, increasing risk of seizures. Avoid concomitant use.

CONTRAINDICATIONS
Contraindicated in patients hypersensitive to pyridoxine.

NURSING CONSIDERATIONS
• **I.V. use:** Inject undiluted drug into I.V. line containing a free-flowing compatible solution. Alternatively, infuse diluted drug over prescribed duration for intermittent infusions. Do not use for continuous infusion.
• Protect from light. Do not use solution if it contains a precipitate, although slight darkening is acceptable.

• When used to treat isoniazid toxicity, expect to also administer anticonvulsants.
• If sodium bicarbonate is required to control acidosis in isoniazid toxicity, do not mix in same syringe with pyridoxine.
• Be aware that patients taking high doses (2 to 6 g/day) may experience difficulty walking because of diminished proprioceptive and sensory function.
• Carefully monitor the patient's diet and snacking habits. Excessive protein intake increases daily pyridoxine requirements.
• Advise patients taking levodopa alone to avoid multivitamins containing pyridoxine because of decreased levodopa effect.
• Stress importance of compliance and of good nutrition if prescribed for maintenance therapy to prevent recurrence of deficiency. Explain that pyridoxine in combination therapy with isoniazid has a specific therapeutic purpose and is not just a vitamin. Explain importance of adhering to therapeutic regimen.

riboflavin (vitamin B₂)◊
Pregnancy Risk Category: NR

HOW SUPPLIED
Tablets: 10 mg◊, 25 mg◊, 50 mg◊, 100 mg◊
Tablets (sugar-free): 50 mg◊, 100 mg◊

ACTION
Converts to two other coenzymes that are necessary for normal tissue respiration.

ONSET, PEAK, DURATION
Unknown.

INDICATIONS & DOSAGE
Recommended daily allowance (RDA) –

---

*Liquid form contains alcohol.   *Common* reactions are in italics; *life-threatening*, in bold italics.
**May contain tartrazine.

Neonates and infants to 6 months:
0.4 mg.
Infants 6 months to 1 year: 0.5 mg.
Children 1 year to 3 years: 0.8 mg.
Children 4 to 6 years: 1.1 mg.
Children 7 to 10 years: 1.2 mg.
Males 11 to 14 years: 1.5 mg.
Males 15 to 18 years: 1.8 mg.
Males 19 to 50 years: 1.7 mg.
Males 51 years and over: 1.4 mg.
Females 11 to 50 years: 1.3 mg.
Females 51 years and over: 1.2 mg.
Pregnant women: 1.6 mg.
Lactating women (first 6 months):
1.8 mg.
**Lactating women (second 6
months):** 1.7 mg.
*Riboflavin deficiency or adjunct to
thiamine treatment for polyneuritis or
cheilosis secondary to pellagra* –
Adults and children over 12 years: 5
to 30 mg P.O. daily, depending on se-
verity.
Children under 12 years: 3 to 10 mg
P.O. daily, depending on severity.
  For maintenance, increase nutri-
tional intake and supplement with vitamin B complex.

ADVERSE REACTIONS
GU: bright yellow urine (with high
doses).

INTERACTIONS
Propantheline, other anticholinergics:
decreased rate and extent of absorption. Avoid concomitant use.

CONTRAINDICATIONS
None reported.

NURSING CONSIDERATIONS
• Keep in mind that drug may be
given I.M. or I.V. as a component of
multiple vitamins.
• Know that riboflavin deficiency
usually accompanies other vitamin B
complex deficiencies and may require
multivitamin therapy.
• Protect from air and light.
• Encourage patient to take riboflavin

with meals because food increases its
absorption.
• Stress proper nutritional habits to
prevent recurrence of deficiency.

---

thiamine hydrochloride (vitamin B₁)
Betamin‡, Beta-Sol‡, Biamine,
Thiamilate

Pregnancy Risk Category: A

HOW SUPPLIED
Tablets: 5 mg◊, 10 mg◊, 25 mg◊, 50
mg◊, 100 mg◊, 250 mg◊, 500 mg◊
Tablet (enteric-coated): 20 mg
Elixir†: 250 mcg/5 ml
Injection: 100 mg/ml, 200 mg/ml

ACTION
Combines with adenosine triphosphate to form a coenzyme necessary
for carbohydrate metabolism.

ONSET, PEAK, DURATION
Unknown.

INDICATIONS & DOSAGE
*Recommended daily allowance
(RDA)* –
Neonates and infants to 6 months:
0.3 mg.
Infants 6 months to 1 year: 0.4 mg.
Children over 1 year to 3 years: 0.7
mg.
Children 4 to 6 years: 0.9 mg.
Children 7 to 10 years: 1 mg.
Males 11 to 14 years: 1.3 mg.
Males 15 to 50 years: 1.5 mg.
Males 51 years and over: 1.2 mg.
Females 11 to 50 years: 1.1 mg.
Females 51 years and over: 1 mg.
Pregnant women: 1.5 mg.
Lactating women: 1.6 mg.
Beriberi –
Adults: depending on severity, 10 to
20 mg I.M. t.i.d. for 2 weeks, fol-
lowed by dietary correction and mul-
tivitamin supplement containing 5 to
10 mg thiamine daily for 1 month.
Children: depending on severity, 10

to 50 mg I.M. daily for several weeks with adequate diet.
Wet beriberi with myocardial failure –
Adults and children: 10 to 30 mg I.V. t.i.d.
Wernicke's encephalopathy –
Adults: initially 100 mg I.V., followed by 50 to 100 mg I.V. or I.M. daily until patient is consuming a regular balanced diet.

ADVERSE REACTIONS
CNS: restlessness.
CV: *hypotension after rapid I.V. injection, angioedema,* cyanosis.
EENT: tightness of throat (allergic reaction).
GI: nausea, hemorrhage, diarrhea.
Respiratory: pulmonary edema.
Skin: feeling of warmth, pruritus, urticaria, sweating.
Other: *anaphylactoid reactions,* weakness.

INTERACTIONS
None significant.

CONTRAINDICATIONS
Contraindicated in patients hypersensitive to thiamine products.

NURSING CONSIDERATIONS
• Know that parenteral administration should be used only when P.O. route is not feasible.
• **I.V. use:** Dilute before administration.
• Administer large I.V. doses cautiously; give the patient a skin test before therapy if he has a history of hypersensitivity reactions. Have epinephrine on hand to treat anaphylaxis should it occur.
• Do not use with materials that yield alkaline solutions. Unstable in alkaline solutions.
• Know that thiamine malabsorption is most likely in alcoholism, cirrhosis, or GI disease.
• Be aware that clinically significant deficiency can occur in approximately

3 weeks of totally thiamine-free diet. Thiamine deficiency usually requires concurrent treatment for multiple deficiencies.
• Keep in mind that doses larger than 30 mg t.i.d. may not be fully utilized. After tissue saturation with thiamine, it is excreted in urine as pyrimidine.
• Be aware that if beriberi occurs in a breast-fed infant, both mother and child should be treated with thiamine.
• Stress proper nutritional habits to prevent recurrence of deficiency.

---

vitamin C (ascorbic acid)
Ascorbicap◇, Cebid Timecelles◇, Cecon◇, Cee-1000 T.D.◇, Cenolate◇, Cetane◇, Cevalin◇, Cevi-Bid, Ce-Vi-Sol*, Cevita◇, C-Span◇, Dull-C◇, Flavettes‡, Flavorcee◇, N'ice Vitamin C Drops◇, Redoxon†, Vita C Crystals◇

Pregnancy Risk Category: C

HOW SUPPLIED
Tablets: 25 mg◇, 50 mg◇, 100 mg◇, 250 mg◇, 500 mg◇, 1,000 mg◇
Tablets (chewable): 50 mg, 100 mg◇, 250 mg◇, 500 mg◇, 1,000 mg◇
Tablets (effervescent): 1,000 mg sugar-free◇
Tablets (timed-release): 500 mg◇, 1,000 mg◇, 1,500 mg
Capsules (timed-release): 500 mg◇
Crystals: 100 g (4 g/tsp)◇, 500 g (4 g/tsp)◇
Lozenges: 60 mg◇
Oral liquid: 50 ml (35 mg/0.6 ml)*◇
Oral solution: 60 mg/ml◇, 100 mg/ml◇
Powder: 100 g (4 g/tsp)◇, 500 g (4 g/tsp)◇
Syrup: 20 mg/ml in 120 ml, 480 ml◇; 500 mg/5 ml in 5 ml◇, 120 ml◇, 480 ml◇
Injection: 100 mg/ml; 250 mg/ml; 500 mg/ml

---

*Liquid form contains alcohol.   *Common* reactions are in italics; **life-threatening,** in bold italics.
**May contain tartrazine.

ACTION
Stimulates collagen formation and tissue repair; involved in oxidation-reduction reactions throughout the body.

ONSET, PEAK, DURATION
Unknown.

INDICATIONS & DOSAGE
Recommended daily allowance (RDA) –
Neonates and infants to 6 months: 30 mg.
Infants 6 months to 1 year: 35 mg.
Children 1 to 3 years: 40 mg.
Children 4 to 10 years: 45 mg.
Children 11 to 14 years: 50 mg.
Children 15 years and over, adults: 60 mg.
Pregnant women: 70 mg.
Lactating women (first 6 months): 95 mg.
Lactating women (second 6 months): 90 mg.
Frank and subclinical scurvy –
Adults: depending on severity, 300 mg to 1 g P.O., S.C., I.M., or I.V. daily, then at least 50 mg daily for maintenance.
Children: depending on severity, 100 to 300 mg P.O., S.C., I.M., or I.V. daily, then at least 30 mg daily for maintenance.
Premature infants: 75 to 100 mg P.O., I.M., I.V., or S.C. daily.
Extensive burns, delayed fracture or wound healing, postoperative wound healing, severe febrile or chronic disease states –
Adults: 300 to 500 mg S.C., I.M., or I.V. daily for 7 to 10 days. 1 to 2 g daily for extensive burns.
Children: 100 to 200 mg P.O., S.C., I.M., or I.V. daily.
Prevention of vitamin C deficiency in patients with poor nutritional habits or increased requirements –
Adults: 70 to 150 mg P.O., S.C., I.M., or I.V. daily.
Pregnant and lactating women: at least 70 to 150 mg P.O., S.C., I.M., or I.V. daily.
Children: at least 40 mg P.O., S.C., I.M., or I.V. daily.
Infants: at least 35 mg P.O., S.C., I.M., or I.V. daily.
Potentiation of methenamine in urine acidification –
Adults: 4 to 12 g P.O. daily in divided doses.

ADVERSE REACTIONS
CNS: faintness or dizziness with fast I.V. administration.
GI: nausea, vomiting, diarrhea, epigastric burning, esophagitis, intestinal obstruction.
GU: acid urine, oxaluria, renal calculi, *renal failure.*
Hematologic: hemolysis.
Other: discomfort at injection site.

INTERACTIONS
Aspirin (high doses): increased risk of ascorbic acid deficiency. Monitor the patient closely.
Oral iron supplements: increased iron absorption (a beneficial drug interaction).
Warfarin: decreased anticoagulant effect. Monitor closely.

CONTRAINDICATIONS
None reported.

NURSING CONSIDERATIONS
• **I.V. use:** Administer I.V. infusion cautiously in patients with renal insufficiency.
• Avoid rapid I.V. administration.
• Know that utilization of vitamin may be better with I.M. route, the preferred parenteral route.
• When administering for urine acidification, check urine pH to ensure efficacy.
• Protect solution from light, and refrigerate ampules.
• Stress proper nutritional habits to prevent recurrence of deficiency.

vitamin D

cholecalciferol (vitamin D₃)
Delta-D◊, Vitamin D₃◊

ergocalciferol (vitamin D₂)
Calciferol, Deltalin Gelseals,
Drisdol, Radiostol†, Radiostol
Forte†, Vitamin D

Pregnancy Risk Category: C

HOW SUPPLIED
Tablets: 1.25 mg (50,000 IU)
Capsules: 1.25 mg (50,000 IU)
Oral liquid: 8,000 IU/ml in 60-ml
dropper bottle◊
Injection: 12.5 mg (500,000 IU)/ml

ACTION
Promotes absorption and utilization of
calcium and phosphate, helping to
regulate calcium homeostasis.

ONSET, PEAK, DURATION
According to metabolites formed or
derivative, onset is as follows: oral
calcitriol, 2 to 6 hours; dihydrotachysterol, several hours to 1 day; ergocalciferol, 12 to 24 hours although therapeutic onset may take 10 to 14 days.
Time to peak as follows: alfacalcidol,
about 12 hours; calcifediol, about 4
hours; calcitriol, about 3 to 6 hours.
Duration as follows: alfacalcidol, up
to 48 hours; calcifediol, 15 to 20 days;
calcitriol, 3 to 5 days; dihydrotachysterol, up to 9 weeks; ergocalciferol,
up to 6 months.

INDICATIONS & DOSAGE
*Recommended daily allowance (RDA)
for cholecalciferol –*
Neonates and infants to 6 months:
300 IU.
Infants 6 months to adults 24 years:
400 IU.
Adults 25 years and over: 200 IU.
Pregnant or lactating women: 400
IU.

*Rickets and other vitamin D deficiency
diseases; renal osteodystrophy –*
Adults: initially, 12,000 IU P.O. or
I.M. daily, usually increased as indicated by response up to 500,000 IU
daily.
Children: 1,500 to 5,000 IU P.O. or
I.M. daily for 2 to 4 weeks, repeated
after 2 weeks, if necessary. Alternatively, give single dose of 600,000 IU.
   After correction of deficiency,
maintenance includes adequate diet
and RDA supplements.
Hypoparathyroidism –
Adults and children: 50,000 to
200,000 IU P.O. or I.M. daily, with
calcium supplement.
Familial hypophosphatemia –
Adults: 50,000 to 200,000 IU daily
with phosphorus supplement.

ADVERSE REACTIONS
Adverse reactions listed are usually
seen only in vitamin D toxicity.
CNS: headache, dizziness, ataxia,
weakness, somnolence, decreased libido, overt psychosis, *seizures.*
CV: *calcifications of soft tissues, including the heart.*
EENT: rhinorrhea, conjunctivitis
(calcific), photophobia, tinnitus.
GI: anorexia, nausea, vomiting, constipation, diarrhea, dry mouth, metallic taste.
GU: polyuria, albuminuria, hypercalciuria, nocturia, *impaired renal function,* renal calculi.
Skin: pruritus.
Other: bone and muscle pain, bone
demineralization, weight loss, *hypercalcemia,* hyperphosphatemia.

INTERACTIONS
Cholestyramine resin, mineral oil: inhibited GI absorption of oral vitamin
D. Space doses. Use together cautiously.
Corticosteroids: antagonized effect of
vitamin D. Monitor vitamin D levels
closely.
Digitalis glycosides: increased risk of

---

*Liquid form contains alcohol.   *Common* reactions are in italics; *life-threatening,* in bold italics.
**May contain tartrazine.

arrhythmias. Monitor serum calcium levels.

Magnesium-containing antacids: possible hypermagnesemia, especially in patients with chronic renal failure. Monitor serum magnesium levels.

Phenobarbital, phenytoin: increased vitamin D metabolism and decreased effectiveness. Monitor closely.

Thiazide diuretics: may cause hypercalcemia in patients with hypoparathyroidism. Monitor closely.

CONTRAINDICATIONS

Contraindicated in patients with hypercalcemia, hypervitaminosis A, or renal osteodystrophy with hyperphosphatemia.

NURSING CONSIDERATIONS

• Ergocalciferol should be administered with extreme caution, if at all, to patients with impaired renal function, heart disease, renal stones, or arteriosclerosis.

• Use cautiously in cardiac patients, especially those receiving digitalis glycosides. Also use cautiously in patients with increased sensitivity to these drugs.

• Use I.M. injection of vitamin D dispersed in oil for patients unable to absorb the oral form, as ordered.

• Monitor the patient's eating and bowel habits; dry mouth, nausea, vomiting, metallic taste, and constipation may be early signs and symptoms of toxicity.

• Monitor serum and urine calcium, potassium, and urea levels when high therapeutic dosages are used.

• Keep in mind that dosages of 60,000 IU/day can cause hypercalcemia.

• Be aware that malabsorption from inadequate bile or hepatic dysfunction may require addition of exogenous bile salts to oral form.

• Know that patients with hyperphosphatemia require dietary phosphate restrictions and binding agents to

avoid metastatic calcifications and renal calculi.

• Warn the patient of the dangers of increasing dosage without consulting the doctor. This vitamin is fat-soluble.

• Tell patients taking vitamin D to restrict their intake of magnesium-containing antacids.

---

vitamin E (tocopherol)

Amino-Opti-E◇, Aquasol E◇, E-Complex-600◇, E-200 I.U. Softgels◇, E-400 I.U. Softgels◇, E Vitamin Succinate◇, Vita-Plus E Softgels◇

Pregnancy Risk Category: NR

HOW SUPPLIED

Tablets (chewable): 200 IU◇, 400 IU◇
Capsules: 200 IU◇, 400 IU◇, 500 IU◇, 600 IU◇, 1,000 IU◇, 330 mg, 147 mg, 73.5 mg
Oral solution: 50 mg/ml◇

ACTION

Unknown. Thought to act as an antioxidant and protect RBC membranes against hemolysis.

ONSET, PEAK, DURATION

Unknown.

INDICATIONS & DOSAGE

Recommended daily allowance (RDA) –
Note: RDAs for vitamin E have been converted to alpha-tocopherol equivalents (α-TE). One α-TE equals 1 mg of D-alpha tocopherol or 1.49 IU.
Neonates and infants to 6 months: 3 α-TE or 4 IU.
Infants 6 months to 1 year: 4 α-TE or 6 IU.
Children over 1 year to 3 years: 6 α-TE or 9 IU.
Children 4 to 10 years: 7 α-TE or 10 IU.
Males 11 years and over: 10 α-TE or 15 IU.

Females 11 years and over: 8 α-TE or 12 IU.
Pregnant women: 10 α-TE or 15 IU.
Lactating women (first 6 months): 12 α-TE or 18 IU.
Lactating women (second 6 months): 11 α-TE or 16 IU.
Vitamin E deficiency in premature neonates and in patients with impaired fat absorption –
Adults: depending on severity, 60 to 75 IU P.O. daily.
Children: 1 IU/kg daily.

ADVERSE REACTIONS
None reported with recommended dosages.

INTERACTIONS
Anticoagulants (oral): hypoprothrombinemic effects may be increased, possibly causing bleeding. Monitor closely.
Cholestyramine resin, mineral oil: inhibited GI absorption of oral vitamin E. Space doses. Use together cautiously.
Vitamin K: antagonized effects of vitamin K possible with large doses of vitamin E. Avoid concurrent use.

CONTRAINDICATIONS
None reported.

NURSING CONSIDERATIONS
• Monitor the patient with liver or gallbladder disease for response to therapy. Adequate bile is essential for vitamin E absorption.
• Be aware that water-miscible forms more completely absorbed in GI tract.
• Know that requirements increase with rise in dietary polyunsaturated acids.
• Keep in mind that vitamin E may protect other vitamins against oxidation.
• Tell the patient that tablets should not be crushed and capsules should not be opened. An oral solution and chewable tablets are commercially available.
• Discourage the patient from self-medication with megadoses, which can cause thrombophlebitis. This vitamin is fat-soluble.

phytonadione (vitamin K₁)
AquaMEPHYTON, Konakion, Mephyton

Pregnancy Risk Category: C

HOW SUPPLIED
Tablets: 5 mg
Injection (aqueous colloidal solution): 2 mg/ml, 10 mg/ml
Injection (aqueous dispersion): 2 mg/ml, 10 mg/ml

ACTION
An antihemorrhagic factor that promotes hepatic formation of active prothrombin.

ONSET, PEAK, DURATION
Onset occurs in 6 to 12 hours after oral administration, 1 to 2 hours (with hemorrhage controlled in 3 to 6 hours) after parenteral administration. Peak unknown. Normal prothrombin concentrations are often obtained in 12 to 14 hours.

INDICATIONS & DOSAGE
Recommended daily allowance (RDA) –
Neonates and infants to 6 months: 5 mcg.
Infants 6 months to 1 year: 10 mcg.
Children 1 year to 3 years: 15 mcg.
Children 4 to 6 years: 20 mcg.
Children 7 to 10 years: 30 mcg.
Children 11 to 14 years: 45 mcg.
Males 15 to 18 years: 65 mcg.
Males 19 to 24 years: 70 mcg.
Males 25 years and over: 80 mcg.
Females 15 to 18 years: 55 mcg.
Females 19 to 24 years: 60 mcg.

Females 25 years and over; pregnant or lactating women: 65 mcg.
Hypoprothrombinemia secondary to vitamin K malabsorption, drug therapy, or excessive vitamin A dosage –
Adults: depending on severity, 2.5 to 10 mg P.O., S.C., or I.M. repeated and increased up to 50 mg if necessary.
Infants: 2 mg P.O. or parenterally.
Children: 5 to 10 mg P.O. or parenterally.

I.V. injection rate for infants and children should not exceed 3 mg/m²/minute or a total of 5 mg.
Hypoprothrombinemia secondary to effect of oral anticoagulants –
Adults: 2.5 to 10 mg P.O., S.C., or I.M. based on PT, repeated if necessary within 12 to 48 hours after oral dose or within 6 to 8 hours after parenteral dose. In emergency, 10 to 50 mg slow I.V., rate not to exceed 1 mg/minute, repeated q 4 hours, p.r.n.
Prevention of hemorrhagic disease of newborn –
Neonates: 0.5 to 1 mg I.M. within 1 hour after birth.
Treatment of hemorrhagic disease of newborn –
Neonates: 1 mg S.C. or I.M. Higher doses may be necessary if mother has been receiving oral anticoagulants.
To differentiate between hepatocellular disease or biliary obstruction as source of hypoprothrombinemia –
Adults and children: 10 mg I.M. or S.C.
Prevention of hypoprothrombinemia related to vitamin K deficiency in long-term parenteral nutrition –
Adults: 5 to 10 mg I.M. weekly.
Children: 2 to 5 mg I.M. weekly.
Prevention of hypoprothrombinemia in infants receiving less than 0.1 mg/liter vitamin K in breast milk or milk substitutes –
Infants: 1 mg I.M. monthly.

ADVERSE REACTIONS
CNS: dizziness, seizurelike movements.
CV: transient hypotension after I.V. administration, rapid and weak pulse, cardiac irregularities.
GI: nausea, vomiting.
Respiratory: *bronchospasm,* dyspnea.
Skin: diaphoresis, flushing, erythema.
Other: cramp-like pain, *anaphylaxis and anaphylactoid reactions* (usually after rapid I.V. administration); pain, swelling, and hematoma at injection site.

INTERACTIONS
Anticoagulants: temporary resistance to prothrombin-depressing anticoagulants may result, especially when larger doses of phytonadione are used. Monitor closely.
Cholestyramine resin, mineral oil: inhibited GI absorption of oral vitamin K. Space doses. Use together cautiously.

CONTRAINDICATIONS
Contraindicated in patients with hypersensitivity to drug.

NURSING CONSIDERATIONS
• Check brand name labels for administration route restrictions.
• Effects of I.V. injection are more rapid but shorter-lived than S.C. or I.M. injections.
• **I.V. use:** Dilute with 0.9% sodium chloride injection, D₅W, or D₅W in 0.9% sodium chloride injection. Administer I.V. by slow infusion over 2 to 3 hours. Infusion rate shouldn't exceed 1 mg/minute in adults or 3 mg/m²/minute in children.
• Protect parenteral products from light. Wrap infusion container with aluminum foil.
• For I.M. administration in adults and older children, administer in upper outer quadrant of buttocks; for in-

fants, administer in the anterolateral aspect of the thigh or deltoid region.
• Anticipate order of weekly addition of 5 to 10 mg of phytonadione to total parenteral nutrition solutions.
• Monitor PT to determine dosage effectiveness, as ordered.
• If severe bleeding occurs, don't delay other measures, such as fresh frozen plasma or whole blood.
• Observe the patient closely for signs of flushing, weakness, tachycardia, and hypotension; may progress to shock.
• This vitamin is fat-soluble.
• Be aware that phytonadione therapy for hemorrhagic disease in infants causes fewer adverse reactions than do other vitamin K analogues.
• Be aware that failure to respond to vitamin K may indicate coagulation defects.
• Explain to patient why drug is being given.

---

sodium fluoride
Fluor-A-Day†, Fluoritab, Fluorodex, Fluotic†, Flura, Flura-Drops, Flura-Loz, Karidium, Luride, Luride Lozi-Tabs, Luride-SF, Luride-SF Lozi-Tabs, Pediaflor, Pedi-Dent†, Pharmaflur, Pharmaflur df, Pharmaflur 1.1, Phos-Flur, Solu-Flur†

sodium fluoride, topical
ACT◊, Fluorigard◊, Fluorinse, Gel Kam, Gel-Tin◊, Karigel, Karigel-N, Listermint with Fluoride, Minute Gel, Point-Two, PreviDent, Stop◊, Thera-Flur, Thera-Flur-N

Pregnancy Risk Category: NR

HOW SUPPLIED
sodium fluoride
Tablets: 1 mg
Tablets (chewable): 0.5 mg, 1 mg
Drops: 0.125 mg/drop, 0.25 mg/drop, 0.2 mg/ml, 0.5 mg/ml
Lozenges: 1 mg

sodium fluoride, topical
Gel: 0.1%, 0.5%, 1.23%
Gel drops: 0.5%
Rinse: 0.01%◊, 0.02%◊, 0.09%

ACTION
Stabilizes the apatite crystal of bone and teeth.

ONSET, PEAK, DURATION
Onset and duration unknown. Peaks in 30 to 60 minutes.

INDICATIONS & DOSAGE
Prevention of dental caries –
Adults and children over 12 years: 5 to 10 ml of rinse or thin ribbon of gel applied to teeth with toothbrush or mouth trays for at least 1 minute h.s.
Children under 2 years: 0.25 mg P.O. (tablet or drops) daily.
Children 2 to 3 years: 0.5 mg P.O. (tablet or drops) daily.
Children 3 to 6 years: 1 mg P.O. (tablet or lozenge) daily.
Children 6 to 12 years: 5 to 10 ml of rinse or thin ribbon of gel applied to teeth with toothbrush or mouth trays for at least 1 minute h.s.

ADVERSE REACTIONS
CNS: headache, weakness.
GI: gastric distress, nausea, vomiting, bad taste (salty, soapy).
Skin: hypersensitivity reactions, such as atopic dermatitis, eczema, and urticaria.
Other: staining of teeth.

INTERACTIONS
Dairy products: incompatibility may occur due to formation of calcium fluoride, which is poorly absorbed.

CONTRAINDICATIONS
Contraindicated in patients hypersensitive to fluoride or when fluoride intake from drinking water exceeds 0.7 ppm.

---

*Liquid form contains alcohol.   *Common* reactions are in italics; *life-threatening,* in bold italics.
**May contain tartrazine.

NURSING CONSIDERATIONS

- Administer oral drops undiluted or mixed with fluids or food.
- Know that chronic toxicity (fluorosis) may result from prolonged use of higher-than-recommended doses.
- Know that fluoride in prenatal vitamins has produced healthier teeth in infants.
- Tell patient that tablets may be dissolved in mouth, chewed, or swallowed whole.
- Advise patient that topical rinses and gels should not be swallowed by children under 3 years or used if water supply is fluorinated. Most effective when used immediately after brushing teeth. Tell the patient to rinse around and between teeth for 1 minute, then spit out.
- Tell the patient to dilute drops or rinses in plastic rather than glass containers.
- Advise the patient to notify the dentist if tooth mottling occurs.

---

trace elements

chromium (chromic chloride)
Chroma-Pak, Chromic Chloride, Chromium Chloride

copper (cupric chloride, cupric sulfate)
Cupric Sulfate

iodine (sodium iodide)
Iodopen

manganese (manganese chloride, manganese sulfate)

selenium (selenious acid)
Sele-Pak, Selepen

zinc (zinc chloride, zinc sulfate)
Zinca-Pak

Pregnancy Risk Category: C

HOW SUPPLIED
chromium
Injection: 4 mcg/ml, 20 mcg/ml
copper
Injection: 0.4 mg/ml, 2 mg/ml
iodine
Injection: 100 mcg/ml
manganese
Injection: 0.1 mg/ml
selenium
Injection: 40 mcg/ml
zinc
Injection: 1 mg/ml, 5 mg/ml

ACTION
Participates in synthesis and stabilization of proteins and nucleic acids in subcellular and membrane transport systems.

ONSET, PEAK, DURATION
Onset and peak occur immediately after an I.V. infusion. Duration unknown.

INDICATIONS & DOSAGE
Prevention of individual trace element deficiencies in patients receiving long-term total parenteral nutrition—
Chromium—
Adults: 10 to 15 mcg I.V. daily.
Children: 0.14 to 0.20 mcg/kg I.V. daily.
Copper—
Adults: 0.5 to 1.5 mg I.V. daily.
Children: 20 mcg/kg I.V. daily.
Iodine—
Adults: 1 to 2 mcg/kg I.V. daily.
Manganese—
Adults: 0.15 to 0.8 mg I.V. daily.
Children: 2 to 10 mcg/kg I.V. daily.
Selenium—
Adults: 20 to 40 mcg I.V. daily.
Children: 3 mcg/kg I.V. daily.
Zinc—
Adults: 2.5 to 4 mg I.V. daily.

Children: 0.05 to 0.1 mg/kg I.V. daily.

ADVERSE REACTIONS
None reported when used at recommended dosages except for hypersensitivity to iodides.

INTERACTIONS
None significant at recommended dosages.

CONTRAINDICATIONS
None.

NURSING CONSIDERATIONS
• **I.V. use:** Cautiously infuse diluted solution through a patent I.V. line over the ordered duration.
• Do not administer undiluted due to potential for phlebitis.
• Check serum levels of trace elements in patients who have received total parenteral nutrition (TPN) for 2 months or longer, as ordered. Give supplement, if ordered. Call the doctor's attention to low serum levels of these elements.
• Keep in mind that normal serum levels are 0.85 ng/ml chromium; 0.07 to 0.15 mg/ml copper; 4 to 20 mcg/100 ml manganese; 0.1 to 0.19 mcg/ml selenium; and 0.05 to 0.15 mg/100 ml zinc.
• Be aware that solutions of trace elements are compounded by pharmacy for addition to TPN solutions according to various formulas. One common trace element solution is Shil's solution, which contains copper 1 mg/ml, iodide 0.06 mg/ml, manganese 0.4 mg/ml, and zinc 2 mg/ml.

---

*Liquid form contains alcohol.   *Common* reactions are in italics; ***life-threatening,*** in bold italics.
**May contain tartrazine.

amino acid infusions, crystalline
amino acid infusions in dextrose
amino acid infusions with
  electrolytes
amino acid infusions with
  electrolytes in dextrose
amino acid infusions for hepatic
  failure
amino acid infusions for high
  metabolic stress
amino acid infusions for renal
  failure
corn oil
dextrose
fat emulsions
invert sugar
medium-chain triglycerides

COMBINATION PRODUCTS
Various products contain dextrose or
invert sugar in combination with electrolytes.

---

amino acid infusions, crystalline
Aminosyn, Aminosyn II, Aminosyn-
PF, FreAmine III, Novamine,
Travasol, TrophAmine

amino acid infusions in dextrose
Aminosyn II with dextrose

amino acid infusions with electrolytes
Aminosyn with electrolytes,
Aminosyn II with electrolytes,
FreAmine III with electrolytes,
ProcalAmine with electrolytes,
Travasol with electrolytes

amino acid infusions with electrolytes in dextrose
Aminosyn II with electrolytes in
dextrose

amino acid infusions for hepatic failure
HepatAmine

amino acid infusions for high metabolic stress
Aminosyn-HBC, BranchAmin,
FreAmine HBC

amino acid infusions for renal failure
Aminess, Aminosyn-RF,
NephrAmine, RenAmin

Pregnancy Risk Category: C

HOW SUPPLIED
Injection: 250 ml, 500 ml, 1,000 ml,
2,000 ml containing amino acids in
varying concentrations
amino acid infusions, crystalline
Aminosyn: 3.5%, 5%, 7%, 8.5%,
10%
Aminosyn II: 3.5%, 5%, 7%, 8.5%,
10%
Aminosyn-PF: 7%, 10%
FreAmine III: 8.5%, 10%
Novamine: 11.4%, 15%
Travasol: 5.5%, 8.5%, 10%
TrophAmine: 6%, 10%
amino acid infusions in dextrose
Aminosyn II: 3.5% in 5% dextrose,
3.5% in 25% dextrose, 4.25% in 10%
dextrose, 4.25% in 20% dextrose,
4.25% in 25% dextrose, 5% in 25%
dextrose
**amino acid infusions with electro-
lytes**
Aminosyn: 3.5%, 7%, 8.5%
Aminosyn II: 3.5%, 7%, 8.5%, 10%
FreAmine III: 3%, 8.5%
ProcalAmine: 3%
Travasol: 3.5%, 5.5%, 8.5%
**amino acid infusions with electro-
lytes in dextrose**
Aminosyn II: 3.5% with electrolytes

---

in 5% dextrose, 4.25% with electro-lytes in 10% dextrose
amino acid infusions for hepatic failure
HepatAmine: 8%
amino acid infusions for high metabolic stress
Aminosyn-HBC: 7%
BranchAmin: 4%
FreAmine HBC: 6.9%
amino acid infusions for renal failure
Aminess: 5.2%
Aminosyn-RF: 5.2%
NephrAmine: 5.4%
RenAmin: 6.5%

ACTION

Provides a substrate for protein synthesis or enhances conservation of existing body protein. Formulations for hepatic failure and high metabolic stress contain essential and nonessential amino acids, with high concentrations of the branched chain amino acids isoleucine, leucine, and valine. Formulations for patients with renal failure contain histidine and minimal amounts of essential amino acids; nonessential amino acids are synthesized from excess ammonia in the blood of the uremic patient, thus lowering azotemia.

ONSET, PEAK, DURATION

Onset and peak occur immediately after an I.V. infusion. Duration unknown.

INDICATIONS & DOSAGE

Total parenteral nutrition in patients who cannot or will not eat –
Adults: 1 to 1.5 g/kg I.V. daily.
Children under 10 kg: 2 to 4 g/kg I.V. daily.
Children over 10 kg: 20 to 25 g/kg I.V. daily for the first 10 kg, then 1 to 1.25 g/kg I.V. daily for each kg over 10 kg.

Nutritional support in patients with cirrhosis, hepatitis, and hepatic encephalopathy –
Adults: 80 to 120 g of amino acids (12 to 18 g of nitrogen) I.V. daily of the formulation for hepatic failure.
Nutritional support in patients with high metabolic stress –
Adults: 1.5 g/kg I.V. daily of the formulation for high metabolic stress.
Nutritional support in patients with renal failure –
Adults: 0.3 to 0.5 g/kg I.V. daily (up to total of 26 g daily). Patients on dialysis may require 1 to 1.2 g/kg daily.

ADVERSE REACTIONS

CNS: mental confusion, unconsciousness, headache, dizziness.
CV: hypervolemia, *CHF* (in susceptible patients), *pulmonary edema,* exacerbation of hypertension (in predisposed patients), thrombophlebitis.
GI: nausea, vomiting.
GU: glycosuria, osmotic diuresis.
Hepatic: fatty liver.
Skin: chills, flushing, feeling of warmth.
Other: hypersensitivity reactions, tissue sloughing at infusion site caused by extravasation, *catheter sepsis,* thrombosis, *rebound hypoglycemia* (when long-term infusions are abruptly stopped), hyperglycemia, metabolic acidosis, alkalosis, hypophosphatemia, *hyperosmolar nonketotic syndrome,* hyperammonemia, *electrolyte imbalances,* dehydration (if hyperosmolar solutions are used).

INTERACTIONS

Tetracycline: may reduce the protein sparing effects of infused amino acids because of its antianabolic activity.

CONTRAINDICATIONS

Contraindicated in patients with anuria and in patients with inborn errors of amino acid metabolism, such as maple syrup urine disease and isovaleric acidemia. Also contraindicated in

---

*Liquid form contains alcohol.
**May contain tartrazine.

Common reactions are in italics; *life-threatening*, in bold italics.

patients with severe uncorrected electrolyte or acid-base imbalances, hyperammonemia, and decreased circulating blood volume.

NURSING CONSIDERATIONS
• Use with extreme caution in pediatric patients and in neonates, especially those with low birth weight.
• Use cautiously in patients with renal insufficiency or failure, cardiac disease, or hepatic impairment.
• Administer cautiously to diabetic patients; insulin may be required to prevent hyperglycemia. Administer cautiously in cardiac insufficiency; may cause circulatory overload. Patients with fluid restriction may tolerate only 1 to 2 liters.
• Obtain baseline serum electrolytes, glucose, BUN, calcium and phosphorus levels before therapy, as ordered.
• **I.V. use:** Control infusion rate carefully with infusion pump. If infusion rate falls behind, notify the doctor; do not increase the rate to catch up.
• Know that peripheral infusions should be limited to 2.5% amino acids and dextrose 10%. Check infusion site frequently for erythema, inflammation, irritation, tissue sloughing, necrosis, and phlebitis. Change peripheral I.V. sites routinely to prevent irritation and infection. If a subclavian catheter is used, administer solution into the midsuperior vena cava.
• Add vitamins, electrolytes, and trace elements, as ordered.
• Monitor serum electrolytes, glucose and BUN levels, and hepatic function, as ordered. Also monitor serum calcium and phosphorus levels frequently, as ordered.
• Check fractional urine every 6 hours for glycosuria initially, then every 12 to 24 hours in stable patients. Abrupt onset of glycosuria may be an early sign of impending sepsis.
• Assess body temperature every 4 hours; elevation may indicate sepsis or infection.

• Monitor for extraordinary electrolyte losses that may occur during nasogastric suction, vomiting, diarrhea, or drainage from GI fistula.
• Be prepared to individualize dosage to metabolic and clinical response as determined by nitrogen balance and body weight corrected for fluid balance.
• If the patient has chills, fever, or other signs of sepsis, replace I.V. tubing and bottle and send them to the laboratory to be cultured.
• Know that safe and effective use of parenteral nutrition requires a knowledge of nutrition as well as clinical expertise in the recognition and treatment of potential complications. Frequent evaluation of the patient and laboratory determinations are necessary.

---

corn oil
Lipomul

Pregnancy Risk Category: NR

HOW SUPPLIED
Liquid: 473-ml container with 10 g corn oil/15 ml (sugar-free)

ACTION
Source of calories and fatty acids.

ONSET, PEAK, DURATION
Unknown.

INDICATIONS & DOSAGE
To increase caloric intake –
Adults: 45 ml P.O. b.i.d. to q.i.d. after or between meals, alone or with proteins, milk, or other nutritional energy sources.
Children: 30 ml P.O. daily to q.i.d. after or between meals, alone or with proteins, milk, or other nutritional energy sources.

ADVERSE REACTIONS
GI: nausea, vomiting, diarrhea.

INTERACTIONS
Griseofulvin: increased GI absorption of griseofulvin. A beneficial interaction.

CONTRAINDICATIONS
Contraindicated in patients with gallbladder calculi or complete GI obstruction.

NURSING CONSIDERATIONS
• Use cautiously in patients with diabetes mellitus, steatorrhea, partial GI obstruction, or enterostomies.
• To minimize nausea, diarrhea, and vomiting, give more frequent, smaller doses with meals or mixed with milk.
• Be aware that dosage varies greatly with individual requirements; 30 ml of the emulsion provides 180 calories.

---

dextrose (D-glucose)

Pregnancy Risk Category: C

HOW SUPPLIED
Injection: 3-ml ampule (10%); 5-ml ampule (10%); 10 ml (25%); 50 ml (5% and 50% available in vial, ampule, and Bristoject); 70-ml pin-top vial (70% for additive use only); 100 ml (5%); 250 ml (5%, 10%); 400 ml (5%); 500 ml (5%, 10%, 20%, 30%, 40%, 50%, 60%, 70%); 650 ml (38.5%); 1,000 ml (2.5%, 5%, 10%, 20%, 30%, 40%, 50%, 60%, 70%)

ACTION
A simple water-soluble sugar that minimizes glyconeogenesis and promotes anabolism in patients who can't receive sufficient oral caloric intake.

ONSET, PEAK, DURATION
Onset and serum levels peak immediately after I.V. infusion. Duration unknown.

INDICATIONS & DOSAGE
Fluid replacement and caloric supplementation in patients who can't maintain adequate oral intake or who are restricted from doing so—
Adults and children: dosage depends on fluid and caloric requirements. Peripheral I.V. infusion of 2.5%, 5%, or 10% solution or central I.V. infusion of 20% solution is used for minimal fluid needs. 25% solution is used to treat acute hypoglycemia in neonate or older infant. 50% solution is used to treat insulin-induced hypoglycemia. 10%, 20%, 30%, 40%, 50%, 60%, and 70% solutions diluted in admixtures, normally amino acid solutions, for total parenteral nutrition (TPN) given through a central vein.

ADVERSE REACTIONS
CNS: confusion, *unconsciousness in hyperosmolar nonketotic syndrome.*
CV: with fluid overload—*pulmonary edema, exacerbated hypertension, and CHF* in susceptible patients. Prolonged or concentrated infusions may cause *phlebitis and venous sclerosis,* especially when administered peripherally.
GU: glycosuria, osmotic diuresis.
Skin: sloughing and tissue necrosis, if extravasation occurs with concentrated solutions.
Other: with rapid infusion of concentrated solution or prolonged infusion—hyperglycemia, hypervolemia, hyperosmolarity. Rapid termination of long-term infusions may cause hypoglycemia from rebound hyperinsulinemia.

INTERACTIONS
None significant.

CONTRAINDICATIONS
Contraindicated in patients in diabetic coma, while blood glucose remains excessively high. Use of concentrated solutions contraindicated in patients with intracranial or intraspinal hemorrhage, or in dehydrated patients with delirium tremens or in patients with severe dehydration, anuria, he-

---

*Liquid form contains alcohol. *Common* reactions are in italics; *life-threatening*, in bold italics.
**May contain tartrazine.

patic coma, or glucose-galactose malabsorption syndrome.

NURSING CONSIDERATIONS
• Use cautiously in patients with cardiac or pulmonary disease, hypertension, renal insufficiency, urinary obstruction, or hypovolemia.
• **I.V. use:** Control infusion rate carefully; maximal rate is 0.5 g/kg/hour. Use infusion pump when infusing with amino acids for TPN. Never infuse concentrated solutions rapidly; may cause hyperglycemia and fluid shift.
• Monitor serum glucose levels carefully. Prolonged therapy with D_5W can cause depletion of pancreatic insulin production and secretion.
• Never stop hypertonic solutions abruptly. If necessary, have dextrose 10% in water solution available to treat hypoglycemia if rebound hyperinsulinemia occurs.
• Don't give dextrose solutions without sodium chloride solution in blood transfusions; may cause clumping of RBCs. Use central veins to infuse dextrose solutions with concentrations greater than 10%.
• Take care to prevent extravasation. Check injection site frequently to prevent irritation, tissue sloughing, necrosis, and phlebitis.
• Check vital signs frequently. Report adverse effects promptly.
• Monitor fluid intake and output and weight carefully, especially patients with renal function impairment.
• Watch closely for signs of fluid overload, especially if fluid intake is restricted.

---

fat emulsions
Intralipid 10%, Intralipid 20%, Liposyn II 10%, Liposyn II 20%, Liposyn III 10%, Liposyn III 20%

Pregnancy Risk Category: C

HOW SUPPLIED
Injection: 50 ml (10%, 20%), 100 ml (10%, 20%), 200 ml (10%, 20%), 250 ml (10%, 20%), 500 ml (10%, 20%)

ACTION
Provides neutral triglycerides, predominantly unsaturated fatty acids; acts as a source of calories; and prevents fatty acid deficiency. When substituted for dextrose as a source of calories, fat emulsions decrease carbon dioxide production.

ONSET, PEAK, DURATION
Onset and serum levels peak immediately after I.V. infusion. Duration unknown.

INDICATIONS & DOSAGE
Intralipid:
Source of calories as adjunct to total parenteral nutrition (TPN) –
Adults: 1 ml/minute I.V. for 15 to 30 minutes (10% emulsion); 0.5 ml/minute I.V. for 15 to 30 minutes (20% emulsion). If no adverse reactions occur, rate increased to deliver 500 ml over 4 to 8 hours; total daily dosage should not exceed 2.5 g/kg.
Children: 0.1 ml/minute for 10 to 15 minutes (10% emulsion), 0.05 ml/minute I.V. for 10 to 15 minutes (20% emulsion). If no adverse reactions occur, rate increased to deliver 1 g/kg over 4 hours; daily dosage should not exceed 4 g/kg. Equals 60% of daily caloric intake; protein-carbohydrate TPN should supply remaining 40%.
Fatty acid deficiency –
Adults and children: 8% to 10% of total caloric intake I.V.
Liposyn:
Prevention of fatty acid deficiency –
Adults: 500 ml (10% emulsion) I.V. twice weekly. Infused initially at a rate of 1 ml/minute for 30 minutes. Rate may be increased but should not exceed 500 ml over 4 to 6 hours.
Children: 5 to 10 ml/kg (10% emul-

sion) I.V. daily. Initially infused at a rate of 0.1 ml/minute for 30 minutes. Rate may be increased but should not exceed 100 ml/hour.

ADVERSE REACTIONS
Early reactions to fat overload:
CNS: headache, sleepiness, dizziness.
EENT: pressure over eyes.
GI: nausea, vomiting.
Hematologic: *hypercoagulability, thrombocytopenia in neonates* (rare).
Respiratory: dyspnea, cyanosis.
Skin: flushing, diaphoresis.
Other: hyperlipidemia, fever, chest and back pains, hypersensitivity reactions, irritation at infusion site.
Delayed reactions:
CNS: focal seizures.
CV: *shock.*
Hematologic: thrombocytopenia, leukopenia, leukocytosis.
Hepatic: transient increases in liver function test values, hepatomegaly.
Other: fever, splenomegaly, *fat accumulation in lungs.*

INTERACTIONS
None significant.

CONTRAINDICATIONS
Contraindicated in hyperlipidemia, lipid nephrosis, or acute pancreatitis accompanied by hyperlipidemia or in patients with severe egg allergies.

NURSING CONSIDERATIONS
• Use cautiously in patients with severe hepatic disease; pulmonary disease; anemia; or blood coagulation disorders, including thrombocytopenia; and in patients at risk for fat embolism.
• Also use cautiously in jaundiced or premature infants.
• **I.V. use:** Avoid rapid infusion, and use an infusion pump to regulate rate.
• Be aware that drug may be mixed with amino acid solution, dextrose, electrolytes, and vitamins in the same

I.V. container. Check with the pharmacist for acceptable proportions and compatibility information.
• Be aware that an in-line filter with pores of 1.2 micron or larger is sometimes used to remove particulate matter.
• Do not use fat emulsion if it separates or becomes oily.
• Lipids support bacterial growth, so change all I.V. tubing before each infusion. Check injection site daily. Report signs of inflammation or infection promptly.
• Monitor the patient for adverse reactions, especially during first half of infusion.
• Monitor serum lipid levels closely when the patient is receiving fat emulsion therapy. Lipemia must clear between dosing.
• Monitor hepatic function carefully in long-term use.
• Check platelet count frequently in neonates receiving fat emulsions I.V.
• Carefully monitor serum triglycerides and free fatty acids in infants, as ordered.
• Know that refrigeration is not necessary.
• Keep in mind that Intralipid and Liposyn differ mainly by their fatty acid components.

---

invert sugar
Travert

Pregnancy Risk Category: NR

HOW SUPPLIED
Injection: 5% and 10% with electrolytes

ACTION
Composed of equal amounts of dextrose and fructose; minimizes gluconeogenesis and promotes anabolism in patients who can't receive sufficient oral caloric intake.

---

*Liquid form contains alcohol.   *Common* reactions are in italics; *life-threatening,* in bold italics.
**May contain tartrazine.

ONSET, PEAK, DURATION
Onset and serum levels peak immediately after I.V. infusion. Duration unknown.

INDICATIONS & DOSAGE
Fluid replacement and caloric supplementation solution –
Adults and children: dosage depends on the patient's age, weight, and clinical need. I.V. infusion rate should not exceed 1 g/kg/hour. A single liter of 5% invert sugar yields 375 calories. Most patients receive 1 to 3 liters of 10% solution daily.

ADVERSE REACTIONS
CNS: confusion, unconsciousness in *hyperosmolar nonketotic syndrome.*
CV: increased pulse rate, precipitation or exacerbation of *CHF* in susceptible patients, hypertension, thrombophlebitis.
GU: glycosuria, osmotic diuresis.
Respiratory: *pulmonary edema.*
Other: hypervolemia, hyperglycemia, hyperosmolarity, sloughing with extravasation at infusion site.

INTERACTIONS
None significant.

CONTRAINDICATIONS
Contraindicated in patients in diabetic coma while blood glucose remains excessively high or in patients with intracranial or intraspinal hemorrhage, or in dehydrated patients with delirium tremens.

NURSING CONSIDERATIONS
• Use cautiously in patients with cardiac disease, hypertension, pulmonary disease, hypervolemia, renal insufficiency, or urinary tract obstruction.
• **I.V. use:** Take care to avoid extravasation, and change infusion sites regularly to avoid irritation with prolonged therapy.
• Check vital signs frequently and notify the doctor promptly if adverse reactions occur.
• Monitor the patient for signs of fluid overload, pulmonary edema, or CHF. Monitor blood pressure frequently.
• Monitor fluid intake and output and weight closely, especially in patients with renal function impairment.
• Monitor serum glucose levels closely. Prolonged therapy can cause decreased pancreatic insulin production and secretion. Rapid termination of long-term infusion may cause hypoglycemia from rebound hyperinsulinemia.

medium-chain triglycerides
M.C.T.◊

Pregnancy Risk Category: NR

HOW SUPPLIED
Oil: 960 ml (115 calories/15 ml)◊

ACTION
Source of rapidly hydrolyzable lipid.

ONSET, PEAK, DURATION
Unknown.

INDICATIONS & DOSAGE
Inadequate digestion or absorption of food fats –
Adults: 15 ml P.O. t.i.d. or q.i.d.

ADVERSE REACTIONS
CNS: reversible *coma* in susceptible patients (such as those with advanced hepatic cirrhosis).
GI: *nausea, vomiting, diarrhea, abdominal distention, cramps.*

INTERACTIONS
None significant.

CONTRAINDICATIONS
None reported.

NURSING CONSIDERATIONS
• Use cautiously in patients with hepatic cirrhosis and complications such as portacaval shunts or tendency to encephalopathy.
• To minimize GI adverse reactions, give smaller, more frequent doses with meals, mixed with salad dressing, or in chilled fruit juice.
• Do not use plastic containers or utensils to administer the drug.
• Keep in mind that drug is more easily absorbed than long-chain fats; not dependent on bile salts for emulsification.
• Know that drug's rapid metabolism provides quick energy.
• Keep in mind that drug provides 7.7 calories/ml. No essential fatty acids are provided.

allopurinol
colchicine
probenecid
sulfinpyrazone

COMBINATION PRODUCTS
COLBENEMID, PROBEN-C, PROBEN-ECID WITH COLCHICINE: probenecid 500 mg and colchicine 0.5 mg.

---

allopurinol
Alloremed‡, Capurate‡, Lopurin, Zyloprim

Pregnancy Risk Category: C

HOW SUPPLIED
Tablets (scored): 100 mg, 300 mg
Capsules: 100 mg‡, 300 mg‡

ACTION
Reduces uric acid production by inhibiting the biochemical reactions preceding its formation.

ONSET, PEAK, DURATION
Onset occurs within 2 or 3 days. Allopurinol levels peak in 0.5 to 2 hours; oxypurinol (active metabolite) levels in 4.5 to 5 hours. Effects persist for 1 to 2 weeks.

INDICATIONS & DOSAGE
Gout, primary or secondary to hyperuricemia; secondary to diseases such as acute or chronic leukemia, polycythemia vera, multiple myeloma, and psoriasis –
Dosage varies with severity of disease; can be given as single dose or divided, but doses larger than 300 mg should be divided.
Adults: mild gout, 200 to 300 mg P.O. daily; severe gout with large tophi, 400 to 600 mg P.O. daily. Same dosage for maintenance in secondary hyperuricemia.
Hyperuricemia secondary to malignancies –
Children under 6 years: 50 mg P.O. t.i.d.
Children 6 to 10 years: 300 mg P.O. daily or divided t.i.d.
Prevention of acute gouty attacks –
Adults: 100 mg P.O. daily; increase at weekly intervals by 100 mg without exceeding maximum dose (800 mg), until serum uric acid falls to 6 mg/100 ml or less.
Prevention of uric acid nephropathy during cancer chemotherapy –
Adults: 600 to 800 mg P.O. daily for 2 to 3 days, with high fluid intake.
Recurrent calcium oxalate calculi –
Adults: 200 to 300 mg P.O. daily in single or divided doses.
   In impaired renal function in adults: 200 mg P.O. daily if creatinine clearance is 10 to 20 ml/minute; 100 mg P.O. daily if less than 10 ml/minute; 100 mg P.O. more than 24 hours apart if less than 3 ml/minute.

ADVERSE REACTIONS
CNS: drowsiness, headache.
EENT: cataracts, retinopathy.
GI: nausea, vomiting, diarrhea, abdominal pain.
Hematologic: *agranulocytosis,* anemia, *aplastic anemia.*
Hepatic: altered liver function studies, *hepatitis.*
Skin: *rash, usually maculopapular; exfoliative,* urticarial, and purpuric lesions; *erythema multiforme;* severe furunculosis of nose; ichthyosis, *toxic epidermal necrolysis.*

INTERACTIONS

Amoxicillin, ampicillin, bacampicillin: increased possibility of skin rash. Avoid concomitant use.

Anticoagulants: potentiation of anticoagulant effect. Dosage adjustments may be necessary.

Antineoplastic agents: increased potential for bone marrow suppression. Monitor the patient carefully.

Chlorpropamide: possible increased hypoglycemic effect. Avoid concomitant use.

Diazoxide, diuretics, ethanol, mecamylamine, pyrazinamide: increased serum acid concentration. Adjust dosage of allopurinol.

Ethacrynic acid, thiazide diuretics: increased risk of allopurinol toxicity. Reduce dosage of allopurinol and closely monitor renal function.

Uricosuric agents: additive effect. May be used to therapeutic advantage.

Urine-acidifying agents (ammonium chloride, ascorbic acid, potassium or sodium phosphate): may increase the possibility of kidney stone formation. Monitor the patient carefully.

Xanthines: increased serum theophylline levels. Adjust dosage of theophyllines.

CONTRAINDICATIONS

Contraindicated in patients with hypersensitivity to the drug and in those with idiopathic hemochromatosis.

NURSING CONSIDERATIONS

● To minimize GI adverse reactions, administer with or immediately after meals.

● Monitor serum uric acid levels, as ordered, to evaluate drug's effectiveness.

● Monitor fluid intake and output; daily urine output of at least 2 liters and maintenance of neutral or slightly alkaline urine are desirable.

● Encourage the patient to drink plenty of fluids while taking this drug unless otherwise contraindicated.

● Periodically monitor CBC and hepatic and renal function, especially at start of therapy, as ordered.

● If renal insufficiency occurs at any time during treatment, be prepared to reduce dosage, as ordered.

● Be aware that allopurinol may predispose the patient to amoxicillin- or ampicillin-induced rash; drug may cause rash even weeks after discontinuation.

● Keep in mind that optimal benefits may require 2 to 6 weeks of therapy. Because acute gouty attacks may occur during this time, concurrent use of colchicine may be prescribed prophylactically.

● Because drug may cause drowsiness, advise the patient to refrain from driving car or performing hazardous tasks requiring mental alertness until CNS effects of the drug are known.

● If the patient is taking allopurinol for treatment of recurrent calcium oxalate stones, advise him to also reduce his dietary intake of animal protein, sodium, refined sugars, oxalate-rich foods, and calcium.

● Tell patient to discontinue at first sign of rash, which may precede severe hypersensitivity or other adverse reaction. Rash is more common in patients taking diuretics and in those with renal disorders. Tell the patient to report all adverse reactions immediately.

colchicine

Colchicine MR‡, Colgout‡,
Colsalide, Novocolchicine†

Pregnancy Risk Category: D

HOW SUPPLIED

Tablets: 0.5 mg (1/120 grain), 0.6 mg (1/100 grain) as sugar-coated granules

Injection: 1 mg (1/60 grain)/2 ml

---

*Liquid form contains alcohol.
**May contain tartrazine.
Common reactions are in italics; **life-threatening,** in bold italics.

ACTION
Unknown. As antigout agent, apparently decreases WBC motility, phagocytosis, and lactic acid production, decreasing urate crystal deposits and reducing inflammation. As antiosteolytic agent, apparently inhibits mitosis of osteoprogenitor cells and decreases osteoclast activity.

ONSET, PEAK, DURATION
Onset is 6 to 12 hours after I.V. administration; within 12 hours after oral administration. Levels peak in 0.5 to 2 hours. Duration unknown.

INDICATIONS & DOSAGE
Prevention of acute gout attacks as prophylactic or maintenance therapy –
Adults: 0.5 or 0.6 mg P.O. daily. Patients who normally have one attack per year or less should receive the drug only 1 to 4 days per week; patients who have more than one attack per year should receive the drug daily. In severe cases, 1 to 1.8 mg daily.
Prevention of gout attacks in patients undergoing surgery –
Adults: 0.5 to 0.6 mg P.O. t.i.d. 3 days before and 3 days after surgery.
Acute gout, acute gouty arthritis –
Adults: initially, 0.5 to 1.2 mg P.O., then 0.5 or 0.6 mg q 1 to 2 hours until pain is relieved; nausea, vomiting, or diarrhea ensues; or the maximum dosage of 10 mg is reached. Alternatively, 2 mg I.V. followed by 0.5 mg I.V. q 6 hours if necessary. (Note that some clinicians prefer to give a single I.V. injection of 3 mg.) Total I.V. dosage over 24 hours (one course of treatment) should not exceed 4 mg.

ADVERSE REACTIONS
CNS: peripheral neuritis.
GI: *nausea, vomiting, abdominal pain, diarrhea.*
Hematologic: *aplastic anemia and agranulocytosis with prolonged use;* nonthrombocytopenic purpura.
Skin: urticaria, dermatitis.
Other: alopecia, severe local irritation if extravasation occurs.

INTERACTIONS
Ethanol: may impair efficacy of colchicine prophylaxis. Don't use together.
Loop diuretics: may decrease efficacy of colchicine prophylaxis. Avoid concomitant use.
Phenylbutazone: may increase risk of leukopenia or thrombocytopenia. Avoid concomitant use.
Vitamin B$_{12}$: impaired absorption of vitamin B$_{12}$. Avoid concomitant use.

CONTRAINDICATIONS
Contraindicated in patients with serious cardiac disease, renal disease, or GI disorders, and in elderly or debilitated patients.

NURSING CONSIDERATIONS
• Use cautiously in elderly or debilitated patients or in patients with early manifestations of cardiac, renal, or GI disease.
• Obtain baseline laboratory studies, including CBC, prior to therapy, as ordered.
• **I.V. use:** Give by slow I.V. push over 2 to 5 minutes. Be sure to avoid extravasation because colchicine is very irritating to tissues. Don't dilute colchicine injection with dextrose 5% injection or any other fluid that might change pH of colchicine solution. If lower concentration of colchicine injection is needed, dilute with 0.9% sodium chloride solution or sterile water for injection and administer over 2 to 5 minutes by direct injection. Preferably, inject into the tubing of a free-flowing I.V. solution. However, don't inject if diluted solution becomes turbid.
• Do not administer I.M. or S.C.; severe local irritation occurs.
• Give with meals to reduce GI ef-

fects as maintenance therapy. May be used with uricosuric agents.
• Repeat baseline laboratory studies, including CBC, periodically, as ordered.
• Monitor fluid intake and output, and keep output at 2,000 ml daily.
• Know that after a full course of I.V. colchicine (4 mg), no more colchicine should be given by any route for at least 7 days. Colchicine is a toxic drug and fatalities have resulted from overdose.
• Keep in mind that the first sign of acute overdosage may be GI symptoms, followed by vascular damage, muscle weakness, and ascending paralysis. Delirium and seizures may occur without the patient losing consciousness.
• Discontinue drug as soon as gout pain is relieved or at the first sign of GI symptoms, as ordered.
• Be aware that colchicine has no effect on non-gouty arthritis.
• Store in tightly closed, light-resistant container.
• Instruct the patient how to take the drug.

---

probenecid
Benemid, Benn, Benuryl†, Probalan, Robenecid

Pregnancy Risk Category: NR

HOW SUPPLIED
Tablets: 500 mg

ACTION
Blocks renal tubular reabsorption of uric acid, increasing excretion, and inhibits active renal tubular secretion of many weak organic acids, such as penicillins and cephalosporins.

ONSET, PEAK, DURATION
Onset unknown. Serum levels peak in 2 to 4 hours; peak effects occur in 30 minutes for uricosuric effects and 2 hours for suppression of penicillin ex-

cretion. Duration unknown for uricosuric effects; effects persist for about 8 hours for suppression of penicillin excretion.

INDICATIONS & DOSAGE
Adjunct to penicillin therapy –
Adults and children over 50 kg: 500 mg P.O. q.i.d.
Children 2 to 14 years or 50 kg or under: initially, 25 mg/kg P.O., then 40 mg/kg in divided doses q.i.d.
Gonorrhea –
Adults: 3.5 g ampicillin P.O. with 1 g probenecid P.O. given together; or 1 g probenecid P.O. 30 minutes before dose of 4.8 million units of aqueous penicillin G procaine I.M., injected at two different sites.
Hyperuricemia of gout, gouty arthritis –
Adults: 250 mg P.O. b.i.d. for first week, then 500 mg b.i.d., to maximum of 2 g daily. Maintenance dosage should be reviewed every 6 months and reduced by increments of 500 mg if indicated.

ADVERSE REACTIONS
CNS: *headache,* dizziness.
CV: hypotension.
GI: anorexia, nausea, vomiting, sore gums, *gastric distress.*
GU: urinary frequency, renal colic.
Hematologic: **hemolytic anemia.**
Skin: dermatitis, pruritus.
Other: flushing, fever, alopecia.

INTERACTIONS
Ethanol: increased urate levels. Avoid use.
Indomethacin: decreased indomethacin excretion. Lower indomethacin dosages may be required.
Methotrexate: decreased methotrexate excretion. Lower methotrexate dosage may be required. Serum levels should be determined.
Oral antidiabetic agents: enhanced hypoglycemic effect. Monitor blood

---

glucose levels closely. Dosage adjustment may be required.
Salicylates: inhibited uricosuric effect of probenecid, causing urate retention. Do not use together.

CONTRAINDICATIONS
Contraindicated in patients with hypersensitivity to drug, uric acid kidney stones, or blood dyscrasias; in acute gout attack; and in children under 2 years.

NURSING CONSIDERATIONS
• Use cautiously in patients with peptic ulcer or renal impairment.
• To minimize GI distress, give with milk, food, or antacids. Continued disturbances might indicate need to lower dosage.
• Monitor periodic BUN and renal function tests in long-term therapy, as ordered.
• Force fluids to maintain minimum daily output of 2 to 3 liters. Alkalinize urine with sodium bicarbonate or potassium citrate, as ordered. These measures will prevent hematuria, renal colic, urate stone development, and costovertebral pain.
• Keep in mind that therapy is not initiated until acute attack subsides. Contains no analgesic or anti-inflammatory agent, and is of no value during acute gout attacks.
• Be aware that drug is typically preferred over sulfinpyrazone because probenecid produces fewer and less severe GI and hematologic adverse reactions.
• Be aware that drug is suitable for long-term use; no cumulative effects or tolerance reported.
• Know that drug is ineffective in patients with chronic renal insufficiency (glomerular filtration rate less than 30 ml/minute).
• Know that drug may increase frequency, severity, and length of acute gout attacks during first 6 to 12 months of therapy. Prophylactic colchicine or another anti-inflammatory agent is given during first 3 to 6 months.
• Be aware that drug may produce false-positive glucose tests with Benedict's solution or Clinitest, but not with glucose oxidase method (Clinistix, Diastix, Tes-Tape).
• Know that drug decreases urinary excretion of 17-ketosteroids, Bromsulphalein (BSP), aminohippuric acid, and iodine-related organic acids, interfering with laboratory procedures.
• Advise patients with gout to avoid all medications that contain aspirin, which may precipitate gout. Acetaminophen may be used for pain.
• Tell patient with gout to avoid alcohol; it increases urate level.
• Tell the patient with gout to limit intake of foods high in purine: anchovies, liver, sardines, kidneys, sweetbreads, peas, and lentils.
• Instruct the patient and his family that drug must be taken regularly as ordered or gout attacks may result. Tell him to visit the doctor regularly so uric acid can be monitored and dosage adjusted, if necessary. Lifelong therapy may be required in patients with hyperuricemia.

sulfinpyrazone
Anturan†, Anturane
Pregnancy Risk Category: NR

HOW SUPPLIED
Tablets: 100 mg
Capsules: 200 mg

ACTION
Blocks renal tubular reabsorption of uric acid, increasing excretion, and inhibits platelet aggregation.

ONSET, PEAK, DURATION
Onset unknown. Serum levels peak 1 to 2 hours after administration. Effects persist for 4 to 6 hours.

INDICATIONS & DOSAGE

Intermittent or chronic gouty arthritis—
Adults: 200 to 400 mg P.O. b.i.d. first week, then 400 mg P.O. b.i.d. Maximum dosage is 800 mg daily.

ADVERSE REACTIONS

CNS: dizziness, vertigo, tinnitus.
GI: *nausea, dyspepsia,* epigastric pain, blood loss, reactivation of peptic ulcerations.
Hematologic: *agranulocytosis, blood dyscrasia* (rare).
Skin: rash.

INTERACTIONS

Oral anticoagulants: increased anticoagulant effect and risk of bleeding. Use together cautiously.
Oral antidiabetic agents: increased effects. Monitor closely.
Probenecid: inhibited renal excretion of sulfinpyrazone. Use together cautiously.
Salicylates, aspirin: inhibited uricosuric effect of sulfinpyrazone. Do not use together.

CONTRAINDICATIONS

Contraindicated in patients with hypersensitivity to pyrazole derivatives (including oxyphenbutazone and phenylbutazone), active peptic ulcer, or symptoms of GI inflammation or ulceration.

NURSING CONSIDERATIONS

• Use cautiously in patients with healed peptic ulcer and in pregnant women.
• To minimize GI disturbances, give with milk, food, or antacids.
• Monitor periodic BUN, CBC, and renal function studies advised during long-term use, as ordered.
• Monitor fluid intake and output closely. Therapy, especially at start, may lead to renal colic and formation of uric acid stones until acid levels are normal (about 6 mg/dl).

• Force fluids to maintain minimum daily output of 2 to 3 liters. Alkalinize urine with sodium bicarbonate or other agent, as ordered.
• Know that drug is recommended for patients unresponsive to probenecid. Suitable for long-term use; neither cumulative effects nor tolerance develops.
• Be aware that drug contains no analgesic or anti-inflammatory agent and is of no value during acute gout attacks.
• Keep in mind that drug may increase frequency, severity, and length of acute gout attacks during first 6 to 12 months of therapy. Prophylactic colchicine or another anti-inflammatory agent is given during first 3 to 6 months.
• Know that lifelong therapy may be required in patients with hyperuricemia.
• Be aware that drug decreases urinary excretion of aminohippuric acid, interfering with laboratory test results.
• Keep in mind that alkalinizing agents are used therapeutically to increase sulfinpyrazone activity, preventing urolithiasis.
• Warn patients with gout not to take any aspirin-containing medications because these may precipitate gout. Acetaminophen may be used for pain.
• Instruct patients with gout to avoid foods high in purine: anchovies, liver, sardines, kidneys, sweetbreads, peas, and lentils.
• Instruct the patient and his family that drug must be taken regularly as ordered or gout attacks may result. Tell him to visit the doctor regularly so blood levels can be monitored and dosage adjusted if necessary.

---

chymopapain
collagenase
fibrinolysin and
    desoxyribonuclease
hyaluronidase
sutilains

COMBINATION PRODUCTS
None.

---

chymopapain
Chymodiactin

Pregnancy Risk Category: C

HOW SUPPLIED
Powder for injection: 4,000 units/vial, 10,000 units/vial; each unit of chymopapain also known as 1 picoKatal (pKat)

ACTION
Hydrolyzes noncollagenous proteins in the chondromucoprotein of the nucleus pulposus.

ONSET, PEAK, DURATION
Onset and peak unknown. Effects persist for at least 1 week.

INDICATIONS & DOSAGE
Herniated lumbar intervertebral disk—
Adults: 2,000 to 4,000 pKat units/disk injected intradiskally. Maximum dosage in patients with multiple disk herniation is 8,000 units.

ADVERSE REACTIONS
Systemic: *anaphylaxis, anaphylactoid reaction; paraplegia, cerebral hemorrhage, acute transverse myelitis,* nausea, headache, dizziness, leg weakness, paresthesia, numbness of legs and toes.

Other: *back pain, stiffness, back spasm.*

INTERACTIONS
Radiographic contrast media: potential adverse reactions when injected concomitantly with chymopapain. Avoid concurrent use.

CONTRAINDICATIONS
Contraindicated in patients with history of allergy to the drug, papaya, or papaya derivatives (such as meat tenderizers); in patients who have previously received an injection of chymopapain; and in those with severe spondylolisthesis in addition to spinal stenosis, severe progressing paralysis, or evidence of spinal cord tumor or a cauda equina lesion.

NURSING CONSIDERATIONS
• Know that a ChymoFAST test can detect hypersensitivity to this drug.
• Monitor patients very closely for anaphylactoid reaction (0.5% of patients). Can be immediate or delayed up to 1 hour after injection and can last for minutes to several hours or longer. Watch for hypotension and bronchospasm, possibly leading to laryngeal edema, arrhythmias, cardiac arrest, coma, and death. Other signs of allergic response include erythema, pilomotor erection, rash, pruritic urticaria, conjunctivitis, vasomotor rhinitis, angioedema, or various GI disturbances.
• Keep an I.V. line open to rapidly manage anaphylaxis. Keep epinephrine and steroids readily available.
• Keep in mind that drug should be used only by doctors qualified and experienced to perform laminectomy, diskectomy, or other spinal procedures, and who have received special-

---

ized training in chemonucleolysis. Drug shouldn't be injected in any region other than the lumbar spine. This drug is extremely toxic if injected into the subarachnoid space.

• Use within 60 minutes after reconstitution. Discard unused drug.

• Instruct the patient to anticipate delayed allergic reactions, such as rash, urticaria, or pruritus, which may occur as late as 15 days after injection. The patient should report these to the doctor immediately.

• Warn the patient that he may experience back pain or involuntary muscle spasm in the lower back for several days after injection. Reassure the patient that this is common and will not be chronic.

collagenase
Santyl

Pregnancy Risk Category: NR

HOW SUPPLIED
Ointment: 250 units/g

ACTION
An enzymatic debriding agent that hydrolyzes peptide bonds of undenatured and denatured collagen. The enzyme liquefies necrotic tissue without damaging granulation tissue.

ONSET, PEAK, DURATION
Unknown.

INDICATIONS & DOSAGE
To promote debridement of necrotic tissue in the treatment of severe burns and dermal ulcers (including decubitus ulcers) –

Adults and children: applied directly to wound once daily for hospitalized patients, once every other day for outpatients.

ADVERSE REACTIONS
Skin: pain and burning at application site, slight erythema in surrounding tissue.
Systemic: hypersensitivity reaction following prolonged use (more than 1 year) in conjunction with cortisone.

INTERACTIONS
Burrow's solution: may stop the enzymatic action of collagenase. Avoid concomitant use.

CONTRAINDICATIONS
Contraindicated in patients with hypersensitivity to any component of the drug and for application into major body cavities, such as the pleural or peritoneal cavity.

NURSING CONSIDERATIONS
• Use caution when applied near the eyes. Also use cautiously in debilitated patients because debridement may increase the risk of bacteremia.

• Maintain strict aseptic conditions when applying drug.

• If the lesion to be treated has been exposed to antiseptics, detergents, or heavy-metal ions incompatible with collagenase, the site should be carefully cleaned by repeated washings with 0.9% sodium chloride solution.

• Before each application, gently clean the wound with a gauze pad saturated with 0.9% sodium chloride buffer solution or hydrogen peroxide to remove necrotic material.

• Remove all excess ointment at the time of each dressing change. Also remove as much loosened detritus as can be done readily with forceps and scissors. Thick eschar may be crosshatched with a #10 scalpel blade.

• Apply directly to deep wounds with a sterile wooden tongue depressor or spatula. For shallow wounds, the ointment may be applied to a sterile gauze pad, which is then applied to the wound and properly secured. Restrict application to the wound site only,

---

avoiding application to healthy, surrounding skin. A sterile gauze pad should be placed over the wound.
• Know that when infection is present, a topical antibiotic can be used concomitantly. If the infection does not respond to this combined therapy, be aware that collagenase should be discontinued until the infection is resolved.
• Know that application of drug should be discontinued as soon as sufficient debridement of necrotic tissue has been achieved and granulation tissue has developed.
• Warn patient that mild pain and burning may be experienced at the site of drug application.

fibrinolysin and desoxyribonuclease
Elase

Pregnancy Risk Category: NR

HOW SUPPLIED
Powder for solution: 25 units fibrinolysin and 15,000 units desoxyribonuclease in 30-ml vial
Ointment: 30 units fibrinolysin and 20,000 units desoxyribonuclease in 30-g tube (with applicator)

ACTION
Fibrinolysin attacks fibrin of blood clots and fibrinous exudates; desoxyribonuclease attacks DNA. Combined enzymatic action debrides wound surfaces and promotes healing.

ONSET, PEAK, DURATION
Unknown.

INDICATIONS & DOSAGE
Debridement of inflammatory and infected lesions, including surgical wounds, ulcerative lesions, second- and third-degree burns, circumcision, episiotomy, abscesses, fistulas, and sinus tracts –
Adults and children: ointment ap-

plied to lesions daily to t.i.d. for as long as enzyme action is desired. Alternatively, solution prepared from powder applied topically as a liquid, spray, or wet dressing.
   For wet-to-dry dressing, mix 1 vial of Elase powder with 10 to 50 ml of 0.9% sodium chloride solution; saturate strips of fine gauze with solution. Pack ulcerated area with Elase gauze. Allow gauze to dry in contact with ulcerated lesion for about 6 to 8 hours. Dried gauze removed and repeated t.i.d. or q.i.d.
Mild-to-moderate cervicitis or vaginitis –
Adults: 5 ml ointment inserted intravaginally using applicator supplied, once daily h.s. for 5 days or until tube is empty.
Irrigation of infected wounds, empyema cavities, abscesses, otorhinolaryngologic wounds, subcutaneous hematomas –
Adults and children: dilute prepared solution and irrigate wound p.r.n., depending on extent and severity of wound.
   For solution as irrigating agent, drain cavity and replace Elase every 6 to 10 hours to reduce amount of by-product accumulation and to minimize loss of enzyme activity.

ADVERSE REACTIONS
Systemic: hyperemia with high doses, hypersensitivity reactions.

INTERACTIONS
None significant.

CONTRAINDICATIONS
Contraindicated in patients with hypersensitivity to the drug; not for parenteral use (fibrinolysin may be antigenic).

NURSING CONSIDERATIONS
• Anticipate removal of dense, dry eschar surgically before enzymatic debridement. Enzyme must be in con-

---

stant contact with substrate. Accumulated necrotic debris is removed periodically; the enzyme is replenished at least once daily.
• Prepare solution just before use and discard after 24 hours.
• Clean wound with water, 0.9% sodium chloride solution, or hydrogen peroxide and dry gently; cover with thin layer of Elase. Cover with nonadherent dressing.
• Ensure that wound-dressing techniques are performed carefully under aseptic conditions and that antibiotic therapy is instituted, as ordered.
• Change dressing at least once and preferably two to three times daily. Flush away necrotic debris and reapply ointment. Frequency of application may be more important than the amount of drug used.

---

hyaluronidase
Wydase

Pregnancy Risk Category: C

HOW SUPPLIED
Injection: 150 units/vial, 1,500 units/vial; 150 units/ml in 1-ml, 10-ml vials

ACTION
Hydrolyzes hyaluronic acid, promoting diffusion of fluids in tissues.

ONSET, PEAK, DURATION
Unknown.

INDICATIONS & DOSAGE
Adjunct to increase absorption and dispersion of other injected drugs –
Adults and children: 150 units added to solution containing other medication.
Hypodermoclysis –
Adults and children over 3 years: 150 units injected S.C. before clysis or injected into clysis tubing near needle for each 1,000 ml clysis solution.

Excretory urography when contrast medium is given S.C. –
Adults and children: with the patient in a prone position, 75 units S.C. over each scapula, followed by injection of contrast medium at same sites.

ADVERSE REACTIONS
Skin: rash, urticaria, irritation.

INTERACTIONS
Local anesthetics: increased potential for toxic local reaction. Use together cautiously.

CONTRAINDICATIONS
Contraindicated in patients with hypersensitivity to drug.

NURSING CONSIDERATIONS
• Perform a skin test for sensitivity, as ordered. Avoid injecting into diseased areas (may spread infection), and observe injection site for local reactions.
• Do not inject into acutely inflamed or cancerous areas.
• Be aware that drug is not recommended for I.V. use.
• For children, add 15 units to each 100 ml of solution. The drip rate should not exceed 2 ml/minute.
• Don't add to any solutions containing epinephrine and heparin. Hyaluronidase is incompatible with these drugs.
• In patients with hypodermoclysis, be prepared to adjust dosage, rate of injection, and type of solution according to the patient's response, as ordered.
• Avoid getting solution in eyes; if solution does get in eyes, flush with water at once.
• Protect from heat. Do not use cloudy or discolored solution.

---

sutilains
Travase

Pregnancy Risk Category: B

HOW SUPPLIED
Ointment: approximately 82,000 casein units/g

ACTION
Selectively digests necrotic soft tissue by proteolytic action, thus facilitating the removal of necrotic tissue and purulent exudate that impair the development of granulation tissue and delay wound healing.

ONSET, PEAK, DURATION
Onset occurs within 1 hour. Peak occurs during the first 6 hours. Effects persist for 8 to 12 hours.

INDICATIONS & DOSAGE
To promote debridement of necrotic tissue in the treatment of second- and third-degree burns and in conjunction with other measures to assist in the debridement of necrotic tissue in patients with decubitus ulcers, ulcers secondary to peripheral vascular disease, and incisional, traumatic, and pyogenic wounds—
Adults and children: applied directly to wound t.i.d. or q.i.d.

ADVERSE REACTIONS
Skin: pain, paresthesia, bleeding, and transient dermatitis at application site.

INTERACTIONS
Anti-infectives (such as benzalkonium chloride, hexachlorophene, nitrofurazone), detergents, preparations with high content of metallic ions (such as thimerosal, silver nitrate), iodine-containing preparations: decreased enzymatic activity of sutilains. Avoid concomitant use.

CONTRAINDICATIONS
Contraindicated in the treatment of wounds communicating with major body cavities, wounds containing exposed major nerves or nervous tissue, and fungating neoplastic ulcers.

NURSING CONSIDERATIONS
• Use caution when applied near the eyes. If ointment comes into contact with the eyes, the eyes must immediately be irrigated with copious amounts of sterile 0.9% sodium chloride solution or water.
• Because the use of sutilains ointment and resultant digestion of the eschar result in increased fluid and blood loss in the area treated, no more than 10% to 15% of the burned area should receive the ointment at one time.
• Maintain strict aseptic conditions when applying drug.
• Be aware that moisture is necessary for the drug's proteolytic activity, which appears to be greatest at a pH of between 6 and 6.8.
• Before each application, gently clean and moisten the wound with 0.9% sodium chloride solution.
• Apply the ointment in a thin layer (approximately ⅛″ [3 mm]) to cleaned, moistened necrotic tissue and the area extending ¼″ to ½″ inch beyond the tissue being debrided.
• Expect to apply a topical anti-infective agent following drug application.
• To ensure a moist environment, use wet, loose dressings to cover the area being treated.
• Expect sutilains to be discontinued if dissolution or sloughing does not occur after 24 to 48 hours of use as adjunctive topical therapy.
• Know that although pain caused by this drug can usually be managed with mild analgesics, occasionally pain may be severe enough to require discontinuation.
• Keep ointment refrigerated at 2° to 8° C (36° to 46° F).
• Warn the patient that pain may occur at the application site.

carboprost tromethamine
dinoprostone
methylergonovine maleate
oxytocin, synthetic injection
oxytocin, synthetic nasal
   solution

COMBINATION PRODUCTS
None.

---

carboprost tromethamine
Hemabate

Pregnancy Risk Category: C

HOW SUPPLIED
Injection: 250 mcg/ml

ACTION
A prostaglandin that produces strong, prompt contractions of uterine smooth muscle, possibly mediated by calcium and cAMP.

ONSET, PEAK, DURATION
Onset unknown. Serum levels peak in 15 to 60 minutes. Average time to abortion, 16 hours; elimination complete in 24 hours.

INDICATIONS & DOSAGE
To abort pregnancy between 13th and 20th weeks of gestation—
Adults: initially, 250 mcg deep I.M. Subsequent doses of 250 mcg administered at intervals of 1½ to 3½ hours, depending on uterine response. Dosage may be increased in increments to 500 mcg if contractility is inadequate after several 250-mcg doses. Total dosage should not exceed 12 mg.
Postpartum hemorrhage caused by uterine atony not managed by conventional methods—
Adults: 250 mcg by deep I.M. injection. Repeat doses administered at 15- to 90-minute intervals, as necessary. Maximum total dosage is 2 mg.

ADVERSE REACTIONS
GI: *vomiting, diarrhea,* nausea.
Other: *fever,* chills, flushing.

INTERACTIONS
None significant.

CONTRAINDICATIONS
Contraindicated in patients with hypersensitivity to drug, acute pelvic inflammatory disease, or active cardiac, pulmonary, renal, or hepatic disease.

NURSING CONSIDERATIONS
• Use cautiously in patients with history of asthma; hypotension; hypertension; cardiovascular, adrenal, renal, or hepatic disease; anemia; jaundice; diabetes; seizure disorders; or previous uterine surgery.
• Unlike other prostaglandin abortifacients, carboprost is administered by I.M. injection. Injectable form avoids risk of expelling vaginal suppositories, which may occur in the presence of profuse vaginal bleeding.
• Know that carboprost should be used only by trained personnel in a hospital setting.

---

dinoprostone
Prepidil, Prostin E$_2$

Pregnancy Risk Category: C

HOW SUPPLIED
Vaginal suppositories: 20 mg
Endocervical gel: 0.5 mg per application (2.5-ml syringe)

---

*Liquid form contains alcohol.   *Common* reactions are in italics; ***life-threatening,*** in bold italics.
**May contain tartrazine.

ACTION
A prostaglandin that produces strong, prompt contractions of uterine smooth muscle, possibly mediated by calcium and cAMP.

ONSET, PEAK, DURATION
Onset occurs within 10 minutes for suppositories, 15 to 30 minutes for gel. Peak unknown. Contractions persist for 2 to 6 hours following insertion of suppository. Average time to abortion is 17 hours for suppositories; unknown for gel.

INDICATIONS & DOSAGE
To abort second-trimester pregnancy; to evacuate uterus in missed abortion, intrauterine fetal deaths up to 28 weeks of gestation, or benign hydatidiform mole (suppository only) –
Adults: 20-mg suppository inserted high into posterior vaginal fornix. Repeated q 3 to 5 hours until abortion is complete.
Ripening of an unfavorable cervix in pregnant patients at or near term (gel only) –
Adults: contents of one syringe administered intravaginally; if cervix remains unfavorable after 6 hours, dosage repeated. No more than 1.5 mg (three applications) should be given per 24 hours.

ADVERSE REACTIONS
CNS: headache, *dizziness.*
CV: hypotension (in large doses).
GI: *nausea, vomiting, diarrhea.*
GU: vaginal pain, vaginitis.
Respiratory: *bronchospasm.*
Other: *nocturnal leg cramps, fever, shivering, chills, joint inflammation.*

INTERACTIONS
Ethanol: inhibited effectiveness of dinoprostone with high doses. Avoid concomitant use.

CONTRAINDICATIONS
• The gel form is contraindicated where prolonged contractions of the uterus are considered inappropriate and in patients with hypersensitivity to prostaglandins or constituents of the gel. Also contraindicated in patients with placenta previa or unexplained vaginal bleeding during this pregnancy and in whom vaginal delivery is not indicated (that is, because of vasa previa or active herpes genitalia).
• The suppository form is contraindicated in patients with hypersensitivity to the drug, acute pelvic inflammatory disease, and active cardiac, pulmonary, renal, or hepatic disease.

NURSING CONSIDERATIONS
• Use suppository form cautiously in patients with asthma; seizure disorders; anemia; diabetes; hypertension or hypotension; jaundice; CV, renal, or hepatic disease; scarred uterus; cervicitis; or acute vaginitis.
• Use gel form cautiously in patients with asthma or history of asthma, glaucoma or raised intraocular pressure, renal or hepatic dysfunction, and in patients with ruptured membranes.
• Administer only when critical care facilities are readily available.
• Just before use, warm dinoprostone suppositories in their wrapping to room temperature. After administration, patient should remain supine for 10 minutes.
• When used as an abortifacient, be prepared to pretreat the patient with an antiemetic and an antidiarrheal agent.
• When used for cervical ripening, have the patient lying on her back, with the cervix visualized using a speculum. Assist with insertion: using aseptic technique, catheter provided with the drug is used to administer the gel into the cervical canal just below the level of the internal os.
• Be aware that when gel form is

used, contents of the syringe are used for one patient only. Discard the syringe, catheter, and any unused drug after administration; do not attempt to administer the small amount of drug remaining in the catheter.

• Treat dinoprostone-induced fever (self-limiting and transient and occurs in approximately 50% of all patients) with water or alcohol sponging and increased fluid intake, not with aspirin.

• Check vaginal discharge regularly.

• Keep in mind that abortion should be complete within 30 hours when suppository form is used.

• Freeze suppositories at −20° C (−4° F).

---

methylergonovine maleate
Methergine

Pregnancy Risk Category: C

HOW SUPPLIED
Tablets: 0.2 mg
Injection: 0.2 mg/ml

ACTION
Increases motor activity of the uterus by direct stimulation.

ONSET, PEAK, DURATION
Onset occurs in 2 to 5 minutes after I.M. use, 5 to 10 minutes after oral use, immediate after I.V. use. Serum levels peak 30 minutes after oral use; unknown for other forms of administration. Effects persist for 3 hours or more after oral or I.M. use; 45 minutes after I.V. administration.

INDICATIONS & DOSAGE
Prevention and treatment of postpartum hemorrhage caused by uterine atony or subinvolution –
Adults: 0.2 mg I.M. q 2 to 4 hours; for excessive uterine bleeding or other emergencies, 0.2 mg I.V. over 1 minute while blood pressure and uterine contractions are monitored. After initial I.M. or I.V. dose, 0.2 mg P.O. q 6

to 8 hours for 2 to 7 days. Dosage decreased if severe cramping occurs.

ADVERSE REACTIONS
CNS: dizziness, headache, *seizures, CVA* with I.V. use.
CV: hypertension, *MI,* transient chest pain, palpitations, peripheral vasoconstriction, gangrene.
EENT: tinnitus.
GI: *nausea, vomiting.*
Respiratory: dyspnea.
Other: diaphoresis, hypersensitivity reactions, *uterine tetany.*

INTERACTIONS
Dopamine, I.V. oxytocin, regional anesthetics, vasoconstrictors: excessive vasoconstriction. Use together cautiously.

CONTRAINDICATIONS
Contraindicated in patients with hypertension, toxemia, or sensitivity to ergot preparations and in pregnant patients.

NURSING CONSIDERATIONS
• Use cautiously in patients with sepsis, obliterative vascular disease, or hepatic or renal disease and during last stage of labor.

• **I.V. use:** Keep in mind that drug should not be routinely administered I.V. because of the risk of severe hypertension and CVA. If it must be given by this route, administer slowly over 1 minute with careful blood pressure monitoring. I.V. dose may be diluted to 5 ml with 0.9% sodium chloride solution prior to administration. Contractions begin immediately after I.V. use and continue for up to 45 minutes.

• Monitor and record blood pressure, pulse rate, and uterine response; report any sudden change in vital signs, frequent periods of uterine relaxation, and character and amount of vaginal bleeding.

• Monitor contractions which may

---

*Liquid form contains alcohol.
**May contain tartrazine.

Common reactions are in italics; *life-threatening,* in bold italics.

continue 3 hours or more after P.O. or I.M. administration.
• Store in tightly closed, light-resistant containers. Discard if discolored.
• Store I.V. solutions below 8° C (46.4° F). Daily stock may be kept at room temperature for 60 to 90 days.

oxytocin, synthetic injection

Oxytocin, Pitocin, Syntocinon

Pregnancy Risk Category: NR

HOW SUPPLIED
Injection: 10 units/ml ampule or vial

ACTION
Causes potent and selective stimulation of uterine and mammary gland smooth muscle.

ONSET, PEAK, DURATION
Onset occurs 3 to 5 minutes after I.M. use, immediate after I.V. use. Peak unknown. Effects persist 1 hour after I.V. use, 2 to 3 hours after I.M. use.

INDICATIONS & DOSAGE
Induction or stimulation of labor –
Adults: initially, 1 ml (10 units) ampule in 1,000 ml of dextrose 5% injection or 0.9% sodium chloride solution I.V. infused at 1 to 2 milliunits/minute. Rate increased in increments of no more than 1 to 2 milliunits/minute at 15- to 30-minute intervals until normal contraction pattern is established. Rate decreased when labor is firmly established.
Reduction of postpartum bleeding after expulsion of placenta –
Adults: 10 to 40 units added to 1,000 ml of D_5W or 0.9% sodium chloride solution infused at rate necessary to control bleeding, usually 20 to 40 milliunits/minute. Also, 1 ml (10 units) can be given I.M. after delivery of the placenta.
Incomplete or inevitable abortion –
Adults: 10 units of oxytocin I.V. in 500 ml of 0.9% sodium chloride solution or dextrose 5% in 0.9% sodium chloride solution. Infuse at rate of 20 to 40 drops/minute.

ADVERSE REACTIONS
Maternal –
CNS: *subarachnoid hemorrhage* from hypertension; *seizures or coma* from water intoxication.
CV: *hypertension;* increased heart rate, systemic venous return, and cardiac output; *arrhythmias.*
GI: nausea, vomiting.
Hematologic: afibrinogenemia; may be related to postpartum bleeding.
Other: hypersensitivity reactions *(anaphylaxis),* tetanic uterine contractions, *abruptio placentae, impaired uterine blood flow,* pelvic hematoma, *increased uterine motility.*
Fetal –
CV: bradycardia, tachycardia, *PVCs.*
Hematologic: hyperbilirubinemia.
Respiratory: *anoxia, asphyxia.*

INTERACTIONS
Cyclopropane anesthetics: less pronounced bradycardia and hypotension. Use together cautiously.
Thiopental anesthetics: possible delayed induction. Use together cautiously.
Vasoconstrictors: severe hypertension if oxytocin is given within 3 to 4 hours of vasoconstrictor in patients receiving caudal block anesthetic. Avoid concomitant use.

CONTRAINDICATIONS
Contraindicated when cephalopelvic disproportion is present or when delivery requires conversion, as in transverse lie; in fetal distress when delivery isn't imminent, prematurity, and other obstetric emergencies; and in patients with severe toxemia, hypertonic uterine patterns, hypersensitivity to drug, total placenta previa, and vasoprevia.

NURSING CONSIDERATIONS

• Use with extreme caution during first and second stages of labor because cervical laceration, uterine rupture, and maternal and fetal death have been reported.

• Use with extreme caution, if at all, in patients with history of cervical or uterine surgery (including cesarean section), grand multiparity, uterine sepsis, traumatic delivery, or overdistended uterus and in invasive cervical carcinoma.

• **I.V. use:** Don't give by I.V. bolus injection. Administer by infusion only; give by piggyback infusion so the drug may be discontinued without interrupting the I.V. line. Use an infusion pump.

• Know that drug is not recommended for routine I.M. use. However, 10 units may be given I.M. after delivery of placenta to control postpartum uterine bleeding.

• Never give oxytocin simultaneously by more than one route.

• Be aware that drug is used to induce or reinforce labor only when pelvis is known to be adequate, when vaginal delivery is indicated, when fetal maturity is assured, and when fetal position is favorable. Should be used only in hospital where critical care facilities and doctor are immediately available.

• Monitor fluid intake and output. Antidiuretic effect may lead to fluid overload, seizures, and coma.

• Monitor and record uterine contractions, heart rate, blood pressure, intrauterine pressure, fetal heart rate, and character of blood loss every 15 minutes.

• Have magnesium sulfate (20% solution) available for relaxation of the myometrium.

• If contractions occur less than 2 minutes apart and if contractions above 50 mm Hg are recorded, or if contractions last 90 seconds or longer, stop infusion, turn the patient on her side, and notify the doctor.

• Oxytocin is not known to present a risk of fetal abnormalities when used as indicated.

oxytocin, synthetic nasal solution
Syntocinon

Pregnancy Risk Category: X

HOW SUPPLIED
Nasal solution: 40 units/ml

ACTION
Stimulates smooth muscle to facilitate ejection of milk from breasts.

ONSET, PEAK, DURATION
Onset occurs within a few minutes. Peak unknown. Effects persist for 20 minutes.

INDICATIONS & DOSAGE
Promotion of initial milk ejection—
Adults: 1 spray into one or both nostrils 2 or 3 minutes before breastfeeding or pumping breasts.

ADVERSE REACTIONS
None reported.

INTERACTIONS
None significant.

CONTRAINDICATIONS
Contraindicated in patients with hypersensitivity to the drug and during pregnancy.

NURSING CONSIDERATIONS
Instruct the patient to clear nasal passages first. With the patient's head in vertical position, hold squeeze bottle upright and eject solution into nostril.

---

*Liquid form contains alcohol.   *Common* reactions are in italics; ***life-threatening***, in bold italics.
**May contain tartrazine.

flavoxate hydrochloride
oxybutynin chloride
phenazopyridine hydrochloride

COMBINATION PRODUCTS
None.

---

flavoxate hydrochloride
Urispas

Pregnancy Risk Category: B

HOW SUPPLIED
Tablets: 100 mg

ACTION
Produces direct spasmolytic effect on smooth muscles of the urinary tract and provides some local anesthesia and analgesia.

ONSET, PEAK, DURATION
Onset and duration unknown. Levels peak within 2 hours.

INDICATIONS & DOSAGE
Symptomatic relief of dysuria, urinary frequency and urgency, nocturia, incontinence, and suprapubic pain associated with urologic disorders –
Adults and children over 12 years:
100 to 200 mg P.O. t.i.d. to q.i.d.

ADVERSE REACTIONS
CNS: *confusion* (especially in elderly patients), nervousness, dizziness, headache, drowsiness, difficulty concentrating.
CV: tachycardia, palpitations.
EENT: *dry throat, blurred vision,* disturbed eye accommodation.
GI: abdominal pain, constipation (with high doses), dry mouth, nausea, vomiting.
Skin: urticaria, dermatoses.
Other: fever.

INTERACTIONS
None significant.

CONTRAINDICATIONS
Contraindicated in patients with pyloric or duodenal obstruction, obstructive intestinal lesions or ileus, achalasia, GI hemorrhage, or obstructive uropathies of lower urinary tract.

NURSING CONSIDERATIONS
• Use cautiously in patients suspected of having glaucoma.
• Check history for other drug use before giving drugs with anticholinergic adverse reactions. Such reactions may be intensified by flavoxate.
• Warn patients to avoid hazardous activities, such as operating machinery or driving, until the CNS effects of the drug are known.
• Tell patients to contact the doctor if they experience adverse reactions to the drug or if symptoms do not improve.

---

oxybutynin chloride
Ditropan

Pregnancy Risk Category: B

HOW SUPPLIED
Tablets: 5 mg
Syrup: 5 mg/5 ml

ACTION
Produces a direct spasmolytic effect and an antimuscarinic (atropine-like) effect on urinary tract smooth muscles, increasing urinary bladder capacity and providing some local anesthesia and mild analgesia.

ONSET, PEAK, DURATION
Onset occurs in 30 to 60 minutes. Levels peak within 3 to 4 hours. Effects persist for 6 to 10 hours.

INDICATIONS & DOSAGE
Antispasmodic for uninhibited or reflex neurogenic bladder—
Adults: 5 mg P.O. b.i.d. to t.i.d., to maximum of 5 mg q.i.d.
Children over 5 years: 5 mg P.O. b.i.d., to maximum of 5 mg t.i.d.

ADVERSE REACTIONS
CNS: *drowsiness,* dizziness, insomnia. restlessness, impaired alertness.
CV: *palpitations, tachycardia.*
EENT: *transient blurred vision,* mydriasis, cycloplegia.
GI: nausea, vomiting, *constipation,* bloated feeling, *dry mouth.*
GU: impotence, *urinary hesitancy or urine retention.*
Skin: rash, urticaria, allergic reactions.
Other: decreased diaphoresis, fever, suppression of lactation, flushing.

INTERACTIONS
None significant.

CONTRAINDICATIONS
Contraindicated in patients with hypersensitivity to drug, myasthenia gravis, GI obstruction, glaucoma, adynamic ileus, megacolon, severe colitis, ulcerative colitis when megacolon is present, or obstructive uropathy; in elderly or debilitated patients with intestinal atony; and in hemorrhaging patients with unstable CV status.

NURSING CONSIDERATIONS
• Use cautiously in elderly patients and in patients with autonomic neuropathy, reflux esophagitis, and hepatic or renal disease.
• Before giving oxybutynin, anticipate confirmation of neurogenic bladder by cystometry and rule out partial intestinal obstruction in patients with diarrhea, especially those with colostomy or ileostomy.
• If urinary tract infection is present, administer antibiotics, as ordered.
• Be aware that drug may aggravate symptoms of hyperthyroidism, coronary artery disease, CHF, arrhythmias, tachycardia, hypertension, or prostatic hyperplasia.
• Periodically prepare patient for cystometry to evaluate response to therapy.
• To minimize tendency toward tolerance, be prepared to stop therapy periodically to determine whether patients can get along without it.
• Warn patients to avoid hazardous activities, such as operating machinery or driving, until CNS effects of the drug are known.
• Caution patients that using drug during very hot weather may precipitate fever or heatstroke because it suppresses diaphoresis.
• Advise patients to store the drug in tightly closed containers at 59° to 86° F (15° to 30° C).

---

phenazopyridine hydrochloride (phenylazo diamino pyridine hydrochloride)
Azo-Standard◇, Baridium◇, Di-Azo◇, Eridium◇, Geridium◇, Phenazo†, Phenazodine◇, Pyrazodine◇, Pyridiate◇, Pyridin◇, Pyridium, Pyronium†, Urodine◇, Urogesic◇, Viridium◇

Pregnancy Risk Category: B

HOW SUPPLIED
Tablets: 100 mg◇, 200 mg

ACTION
Unknown. Exerts local anesthetic action on urinary mucosa through unknown mechanism.

---

*Liquid form contains alcohol.   *Common* reactions are in italics; ***life-threatening,*** in bold italics.
**May contain tartrazine.

ONSET, PEAK, DURATION
Unknown.

INDICATIONS & DOSAGE
Pain with urinary tract irritation or infection–
Adults: 200 mg P.O. t.i.d.
Children: 12 mg/kg P.O. daily in 3 equally divided doses.

ADVERSE REACTIONS
CNS: headache, vertigo.
GI: nausea.
Skin: rash.

INTERACTIONS
None significant.

CONTRAINDICATIONS
Contraindicated in patients with glomerulonephritis, severe hepatitis, uremia, pyelonephritis during pregnancy, or renal insufficiency.

NURSING CONSIDERATIONS
• Advise patients that taking the drug with meals may minimize GI distress.
• Caution patients to stop taking drug and to notify the doctor immediately if skin or sclera becomes yellow-tinged. These signs may indicate accumulation caused by impaired renal excretion.
• Alert patient that drug colors urine red or orange. May stain fabrics.
• Tell diabetic patients that drug may alter Clinistix or Tes-Tape results. Use Clinitest for accurate urine glucose test results.

Gold salts

auranofin
aurothioglucose
gold sodium thiomalate

COMBINATION PRODUCTS
None.

auranofin
Ridaura

Pregnancy Risk Category: C

HOW SUPPLIED
Capsules: 3 mg

ACTION
Unknown. Anti-inflammatory effects in rheumatoid arthritis are probably caused by inhibition of sulfhydryl systems, which alters cellular metabolism. Auranofin may also alter enzyme function and immune response and suppress phagocytic activity.

ONSET, PEAK, DURATION
Onset occurs in 1 to 3 months, possibly 6 months. Serum levels peak within 2 hours. Effects may last for months after drug is discontinued.

INDICATIONS & DOSAGE
Rheumatoid arthritis –
Adults: 6 mg P.O. daily, either as 3 mg b.i.d. or 6 mg once daily. After 6 months, may be increased to 9 mg daily.

ADVERSE REACTIONS
GI: *diarrhea, abdominal pain, nausea, vomiting,* stomatitis, enterocolitis, anorexia, metallic taste, dyspepsia, flatulence.
GU: proteinuria, hematuria, nephrotic syndrome, glomerulonephritis.
Hematologic: *thrombocytopenia*
(with or without purpura), *aplastic anemia, agranulocytosis,* leukopenia, eosinophilia.
Hepatic: jaundice, elevated liver enzymes.
Respiratory: interstitial pneumonitis.
Skin: *rash, pruritus, dermatitis, exfoliative dermatitis.*

INTERACTIONS
Phenytoin: may increase phenytoin blood levels. Monitor for toxicity.

CONTRAINDICATIONS
Contraindicated in patients with history of severe gold toxicity, necrotizing enterocolitis, pulmonary fibrosis, exfoliative dermatitis, bone marrow aplasia, severe hematologic disorders or history of severe toxicity resulting from previous exposure to other heavy metals. Also contraindicated in patients with urticaria, eczema, colitis, severe debilitation, hemorrhagic conditions, or systemic lupus erythematosus and in patients who have recently received radiation therapy.

NURSING CONSIDERATIONS
• Use cautiously with other drugs that cause blood dyscrasias. Also use cautiously in patients who have preexisting renal, hepatic, or inflammatory bowel disease or skin rash or a history of bone marrow depression.
• Encourage patients to take drug as prescribed and not to alter dosage schedule.
• Tell patients to continue taking concomitant drug therapy, such as NSAIDs, if prescribed.
• Remind patients to see their doctor for monthly platelet counts. Know that auranofin should be discontinued if platelet count falls below 100,000/mm³, if hemoglobin drops

*Liquid form contains alcohol.   *Common* reactions are in italics; *life-threatening,* in bold italics.
**May contain tartrazine.

suddenly, if granulocytes are below 1,500/mm³, or if leukopenia (WBC count below 4,000/mm³) or eosinophilia (eosinophils > 75%) is present.

• Advise patients to have regular urinalysis. If proteinuria or hematuria is detected, discontinue drug because it can produce a nephrotic syndrome or glomerulonephritis, and notify doctor.

• Tell patients to continue taking drug if they experience mild diarrhea, and to contact the doctor immediately if blood is noted in stool. Diarrhea is the most common adverse reaction.

• Advise patients to report any rashes or other skin problems immediately. Pruritus in many instances precedes dermatitis; any pruritic skin eruption while patients are receiving auranofin should be considered a reaction to this drug until proven otherwise. Advise patient to stop therapy until reaction subsides and notify doctor.

• Advise patients that stomatitis is preceded in many instances by a metallic taste, which should be reported to the doctor immediately. Promote careful oral hygiene during therapy.

• Reassure patients that beneficial drug effect may be delayed as long as 3 months. However, if response is inadequate and maximum dose has been reached, expect the doctor to discontinue drug.

• Warn patients not to give the drug to others. Auranofin, like injectable gold preparations, should be prescribed only for selected rheumatoid arthritis patients.

---

aurothioglucose
Gold-50‡, Solganal

gold sodium thiomalate
Myochrysine

Pregnancy Risk Category: C

HOW SUPPLIED
aurothioglucose
Injection (suspension): 50 mg/ml in sesame oil with aluminum monostearate 2% and propylparaben 0.1% in a 10-ml container
gold sodium thiomalate
Injection: 25 mg/ml, 50 mg/ml with benzyl alcohol

ACTION
Unknown. Anti-inflammatory effects in rheumatoid arthritis are probably caused by inhibition of sulfhydryl systems, which alters cellular metabolism. Gold salts may also alter enzyme function and immune response and suppress phagocytic activity.

ONSET, PEAK, DURATION
Onset and duration unknown. Serum levels peak within 3 to 6 hours.

INDICATIONS & DOSAGE
Rheumatoid arthritis –
aurothioglucose
Adults: initially, 10 mg I.M., followed by 25 mg for second and third doses at weekly intervals. Then, 50 mg weekly until 1 g has been given. If improvement occurs without toxicity, 25 to 50 mg is continued at 3- to 4-week intervals indefinitely as maintenance therapy.
Children 6 to 12 years: ¼ usual adult dosage. Or 1 mg/kg I.M. once weekly for 20 weeks.
gold sodium thiomalate
Adults: initially, 10 mg I.M., followed by 25 mg in 1 week. Then, 25 to 50 mg weekly until 14 to 20 doses have been given. If improvement occurs without toxicity, 25 to 50 mg q 2 weeks for four doses; then, 25 to 50 mg q 3 weeks for four doses; then, 25 to 50 mg every month indefinitely as maintenance therapy. If relapse occurs during maintenance therapy, injections are resumed at weekly intervals.
Children: 1 mg/kg I.M. weekly for

---

20 weeks. If response is good, may be given q 3 to 4 weeks indefinitely.

ADVERSE REACTIONS
CNS: *dizziness,* syncope.
CV: bradycardia, hypotension.
EENT: corneal gold deposition, corneal ulcers.
GI: *metallic taste, stomatitis,* difficulty swallowing, nausea, vomiting.
GU: albuminuria, proteinuria, *nephrotic syndrome,* nephritis, acute tubular necrosis.
Hematologic: *thrombocytopenia* (with or without purpura), *aplastic anemia, agranulocytosis,* leukopenia, eosinophilia.
Hepatic: hepatitis, jaundice.
Skin: photosensitivity; *rash and dermatitis in 20% of patients* (may lead to fatal *exfoliative dermatitis* if drug is not stopped).
Other: *anaphylaxis, angioedema,* diaphoresis.

INTERACTIONS
None significant.

CONTRAINDICATIONS
Contraindicated in patients with hypersensitivity to the drug; in those with a history of severe toxicity from previous exposure to gold or other heavy metals, hepatitis, or exfoliative dermatitis; and in patients with severe uncontrollable diabetes, renal disease, hepatic dysfunction, uncontrolled heart failure, systemic lupus erythematosus, colitis, or Sjögren's syndrome. Also contraindicated in patients with urticaria, eczema, hemorrhagic conditions, or severe hematologic disorders and in those who have recently received radiation therapy.

NURSING CONSIDERATIONS
• Use with extreme caution, if at all, in patients with rash, marked hypertension, compromised cerebral or cardiovascular circulation, or history of renal or hepatic disease, drug allergies, or blood dyscrasias.
• Administer only under constant supervision of a doctor who is thoroughly familiar with drug's toxicities and benefits.
• Administer all gold salts I.M., as ordered, preferably intragluteally. Drug is pale yellow; don't use if it darkens.
• Immerse aurothioglucose (a suspension) vial in warm water and shake vigorously before injecting.
• When giving gold sodium thiomalate, have patients lie down and remain recumbent for 10 to 20 minutes after injection to minimize hypotension.
• Observe patients for 30 minutes after administration because of possible anaphylactoid reaction.
• Keep dimercaprol on hand to treat acute toxicity.
• Analyze urine for protein and sediment changes before each injection.
• Monitor CBC, including platelet count, before every second injection during therapy, as ordered.
• Monitor platelet counts if patients develop purpura or ecchymoses, as ordered.
• Know that gold therapy may alter liver function studies.
• Know that gold compounds are typically used only in active rheumatoid arthritis that has not responded adequately to salicylates, rest, and physical therapy. Some clinicians advocate earlier use before disease progression.
• Be aware that most adverse reactions are readily reversible if drug is stopped immediately.
• If adverse reactions are mild, keep in mind that some rheumatologists resume gold therapy after 2 to 3 weeks' rest.
• Inform patients that benefits of therapy may not appear for 3 to 4 months or longer.
• Advise patients that increased joint pain may occur for 1 to 2 days after

---

*Liquid form contains alcohol.
**May contain tartrazine.

Common reactions are in italics; ***life-threatening,*** in bold italics.

injection but usually subsides after a few injections.

• Advise patients to report any skin rashes or problems immediately. Pruritus precedes dermatitis in many instances; any pruritic skin eruption while patients are receiving gold therapy should be considered a reaction to therapy until proven otherwise. Advise patient to stop therapy until reaction subsides and notify doctor.

• Advise patients that stomatitis is preceded in many instances by a metallic taste, which should be reported to the doctor immediately. Promote careful oral hygiene during therapy.

• Tell patients to avoid sunlight and artificial ultraviolet light to minimize the risk of photosensitivity.

• Stress need for close medical follow-ups and frequent blood and urine tests during therapy.

coccidioidin
histoplasmin
mumps skin test antigen
tuberculin purified protein
   derivative
tuberculosis multiple-puncture
   tests

COMBINATION PRODUCTS
None.

---

coccidioidin
Spherulin

Pregnancy Risk Category: NR

HOW SUPPLIED
Injection: 1:100 dilution (1 ml), 1:10 dilution (0.5 ml)

ACTION
Causes a T-cell-mediated immune response.

ONSET, PEAK, DURATION
Onset may occur within 15 minutes. Reaction peaks within 24 to 48 hours. Duration not applicable.

INDICATIONS & DOSAGE
Suspected coccidioidomycosis –
Adults and children: 0.1 ml of 1:100 dilution intradermally into flexor surface of the forearm. In persons nonreactive to this form, test repeated using 1:10 dilution.

ADVERSE REACTIONS
Systemic: hypersensitivity reactions (vesiculation, ulceration, necrosis), *anaphylaxis,* Arthus reaction.

INTERACTIONS
None significant.

CONTRAINDICATIONS
Contraindicated in patients hypersensitive to thimerosal or in the presence of erythema nodosum.

NURSING CONSIDERATIONS
• Obtain history of allergies and reactions to skin tests prior to administering.
• Obtain history of any recent residence in or travel to endemic areas — southern California, Arizona, New Mexico, and western Texas.
• Keep epinephrine 1:1,000 available in case of hypersensitivity reaction.
• Give drug intradermally using tuberculin syringe with 26G or 27G ½″ needle; S.C. injection invalidates test. If erythema without induration appears when the test should be read, injection was probably S.C. Repeat test, as ordered.
• Read test at 24 and 48 hours. Induration of 5 mm or more indicates a positive reaction (cell-mediated immune response). Erythema does not indicate a delayed hypersensitivity reaction or a positive reaction.
• Be aware that if coccidioidomycosis is suspected because of clinical manifestations or X-ray findings and the 1:100 dilution is negative, the 1:10 dilution may be used.
• Test HIV-positive and high-risk patients for anergy, as ordered, to verify a negative reaction.
• Keep in mind that reactivity to this test may be depressed or suppressed for as long as 4 to 6 weeks in individuals who have received concurrent or recent immunization with certain vaccines (for example, measles or influenza), in those receiving corticosteroids or immunosuppressants, in severely malnourished patients, in patients with HIV, and in those who

---

*Liquid form contains alcohol.   *Common* reactions are in italics; *life-threatening,* in bold italics.
**May contain tartrazine.

have had viral infections (rubeola, influenza, mumps, and probably others).
• If severe reaction occurs, use cold packs or topical corticosteroids to relieve pain or itching.
• Tell patients not to wash off circle marked on skin for serial skin tests because it aids in reading test results.
• Advise patient that it is not necessary to cover the area with a bandage.

histoplasmin
Histolyn-CYL, Histoplasmin Diluted

Pregnancy Risk Category: NR

HOW SUPPLIED
Injection: vials containing 10 doses of 0.1 ml

ACTION
Causes a T-cell-mediated immune response.

ONSET, PEAK, DURATION
Onset may occur within minutes. Reaction peaks in 48 to 72 hours. Duration not applicable.

INDICATIONS & DOSAGE
To differentiate histoplasmosis from coccidioidomycosis, tuberculosis, sarcoidosis, or other mycotic or bacterial infections –
Adults and children: 0.1 ml intradermally into flexor surface of the forearm.

ADVERSE REACTIONS
Skin: urticaria, ulceration, or necrosis in highly sensitive patients.
Systemic: *anaphylaxis.*

INTERACTIONS
None significant.

CONTRAINDICATIONS
Contraindicated in patients known to be positive reactors.

NURSING CONSIDERATIONS
• Obtain history of allergies and reactions to skin tests prior to administering.
• Obtain history of any recent residence in or travel to endemic areas – Africa and central (Ohio Valley) and eastern United States.
• Give drug intradermally; use tuberculin syringe with 26G or 27G ½″ needle; S.C. injection invalidates test. If erythema without induration appears when test should be read, injection was probably S.C. Repeat test as ordered.
• Give tuberculin skin test concurrently with histoplasmin test.
• Read test within 24 to 48 hours. Induration of 5 mm or more indicates a positive reaction; erythema does not indicate a positive reaction. In some instances, maximum reactions may not be present until fourth day.
• Know that serologic titers are boosted in many instances by a previous skin test. Draw serologic sample before skin test or at least 96 hours after test administration, as ordered.
• Keep in mind that positive reaction may indicate past infection or mild subacute or chronic histoplasmosis or related fungal infection, such as coccidioidomycosis or blastomycosis.
• Test HIV-positive and high-risk patients for anergy to verify a negative reaction, as ordered.
• Keep in mind that reactivity to this test may be depressed or suppressed for as long as 4 to 6 weeks in individuals who have received concurrent or recent immunization with certain virus vaccines (for example, measles or influenza), in those who are receiving corticosteroids or immunosuppressants, in severely malnourished patients, in patients with HIV, and in those who have had viral infections (rubeola, influenza, mumps, and probably others).
• If severe reaction occurs, use cold

packs or topical corticosteroids to relieve pain and itching.

mumps skin test antigen
MSTA

Pregnancy Risk Category: NR

HOW SUPPLIED
Injection (suspension): 20 complement-fixing units/ml

ACTION
Causes a T-cell-mediated immune response.

ONSET, PEAK, DURATION
Onset may occur in minutes. Reaction peaks in 48 to 72 hours. Duration not applicable.

INDICATIONS & DOSAGE
To assess T-cell-mediated immunity –
Adults and children: 0.1 ml intradermally into flexor surface of the forearm.

ADVERSE REACTIONS
Systemic: hypersensitivity reactions (vesiculation, ulceration), *anaphylaxis,* Arthus reaction.

INTERACTIONS
None significant.

CONTRAINDICATIONS
Contraindicated in patients hypersensitive to eggs or egg products or to thimerosal.

NURSING CONSIDERATIONS
• Use cautiously in patients hypersensitive to feathers or chicken.
• Obtain history of allergies and reactions to skin tests prior to administering.
• Keep epinephrine 1:1,000 available in case of hypersensitivity reaction.
• Use tuberculin syringe with 26G or 27G ½″ needle.
• Read test at 48- and 72-hour intervals. Induration of 5 mm or more indicates a positive reaction (cell-mediated immune response). Erythema does not indicate a delayed hypersensitivity reaction.
• Keep in mind that reactivity to this test may be depressed or suppressed for as long as 4 to 6 weeks in individuals who have received concurrent or recent immunization with certain vaccines (for example, measles or influenza), in those receiving corticosteroids or immunosuppressants, in severely malnourished patients, in patients with HIV, and in those who have had viral infections (rubeola, influenza, mumps, and probably others).
• Know that mumps skin test antigen is used to assess T-cell function for immunocompetence, not exposure to mumps.
• If severe reaction occurs, use cold packs or topical corticosteroids to relieve pain or itching.
• Store vials in refrigerator.

tuberculin purified protein derivative (PPD)
Aplisol, PPD-stabilized Solution (Mantoux test), Tubersol

Pregnancy Risk Category: C

HOW SUPPLIED
Injection: 1 tuberculin unit (TU)/0.1 ml, 5 TU/0.1 ml, 250 TU/0.1 ml

ACTION
Causes a cell-mediated immune response.

ONSET, PEAK, DURATION
Onset unknown. Reaction peaks in 48 to 72 hours. Duration not applicable.

INDICATIONS & DOSAGE
Diagnosis of tuberculosis (past, latent, or current infection) –
Adults and children: initially, 1 TU for individuals suspected of being

---

*Liquid form contains alcohol.   *Common* reactions are in italics; *life-threatening,* in bold italics.
**May contain tartrazine.

highly sensitized or 5 TU for individuals not expected to be highly sensitized intradermally into flexor surface of the forearm. If negative, patient is retested with 250 TU. If still no response, the individual is nonreactive.

ADVERSE REACTIONS
Skin: pruritus, vesiculation.
Systemic: hypersensitivity reactions, *anaphylaxis,* Arthus reaction.
Other: pain, ulceration, necrosis.

INTERACTIONS
None significant.

CONTRAINDICATIONS
Contraindicated in known tuberculin-positive reactors; severe reactions may occur.

NURSING CONSIDERATIONS
• Obtain history of allergies and reactions to skin tests prior to administering.
• Keep epinephrine 1:1,000 available in case of hypersensitivity reaction.
• Give drug intradermally using tuberculin syringe with 26G or 26G ½" needle; S.C. injection invalidates test results. Bleb (6 to 10 mm in diameter) must form on skin upon intradermal injection.
• Read test within 48 to 72 hours. Induration of 15 mm or more indicates a significant reaction (formerly called positive reaction). Significance of reaction is determined by its size and by circumstances. For example, a reaction of 5 mm or more may be considered significant in patients who have had close contact with persons with known tuberculosis, in patients with HIV or at risk for HIV, or in patients with chest X-rays indicating old tuberculosis scars. A reaction of 10 mm or more may be considered significant in patients born in Asia, Africa, or Latin America; in HIV-negative I.V. drug users; in medically underserved low-income populations; in residents of long-term care facilities; or in high-risk patients, such as those with diabetes or renal failure, or in those receiving immunosuppressants. Induration of 5 mm or less in persons not belonging to these groups implies that infection is unlikely. Amount of induration—not erythema—at the site determines the significance of the reaction.
• If reaction is positive, anticipate further testing to confirm diagnosis. Report all known cases of tuberculosis to the appropriate public health agency.
• Never give initial test with second test strength (250 TU). Use only when patients have a negative response to a 5-TU PPD but have the clinical signs and symptoms of tuberculosis.
• When retesting, know that the first test will not exert a booster phenomenon. Test may be repeated immediately at a different site at least 5 cm from first site.
• Be aware that strongly positive tests can result in scarring at test site.
• If severe reaction occurs, use cold packs or topical corticosteroids to relieve pain and itching.
• Know that patients immunized with BCG vaccine should react positively.
• Test HIV-positive and high-risk patients for anergy to verify a negative reaction, as ordered.
• Keep in mind that reactivity to this test may be depressed or suppressed for as long as 4 to 6 weeks in individuals who have received concurrent or recent immunization with certain vaccines (for example, measles or influenza), in those receiving corticosteroids or immunosuppressants, in severely malnourished patients, in patients with HIV, and in those who have had viral infections (rubeola, influenza, mumps, and probably others).

tuberculosis multiple-puncture tests

Aplitest (dried purified protein derivative [PPD]), Mono-Vacc Test (liquid Old Tuberculin [OT]), Sclavo Test (dried PPD), Tine Test (dried OT, dried PPD)

Pregnancy Risk Category: C

HOW SUPPLIED
Test: 5 tuberculin units (TU)/device

ACTION
Causes a cell-mediated immune response.

ONSET, PEAK, DURATION
Onset unknown. Reaction peaks within 48 to 72 hours. Duration not applicable.

INDICATIONS & DOSAGE
Screening for tuberculosis –
Adults and children: clean skin thoroughly with alcohol; make skin taut on flexor surface of forearm and press points firmly into selected site. Hold device at injection site for about 3 seconds to ensure depositing of the dried tuberculin B in tissue lymph.

ADVERSE REACTIONS
Systemic: hypersensitivity reactions (vesiculation, ulceration, necrosis), *anaphylaxis.*

INTERACTIONS
Aminocaproic acid, corticosteroids: false-negative or insignificant reactions to tuberculosis multiple-puncture tests. Don't administer concomitantly.

CONTRAINDICATIONS
Contraindicated in known tuberculin-positive reactors.

NURSING CONSIDERATIONS
• Obtain history of allergies, especially to acacia (a stabilizer in the Tine Test), and reactions to skin tests prior to administering.
• Keep epinephrine 1:1,000 available in case of hypersensitivity reaction.
• Read test within 48 to 72 hours. Verify questionable or positive reactions by the Mantoux test. Induration of 1 to 2 mm indicates a significant reaction. Induration – not erythema – at the site determines the significance of the reaction.
• If vesiculation is present, interpret test as positive.
• Be alert that minimal bleeding can occur at the puncture site (rare). It does not interfere with interpretation of the test results.
• Know that false-positive reaction can occur in sensitive patients. False-negative reaction can occur from anergy or poor technique.
• Keep in mind that reactivity to this test may be depressed or suppressed for as long as 4 to 6 weeks in individuals who have received concurrent or recent immunization with certain vaccines (for example, measles or influenza), in those receiving corticosteroids or immunosuppressants, in severely malnourished patients, in patients with HIV, and in those who have had viral infections (rubeola, influenza, mumps, and probably others) or miliary tuberculosis.
• If severe reaction occurs, use cold packs or topical corticosteroids to relieve pain and itching.
• Report all cases of tuberculosis to the appropriate public health agency.

Liquid form contains alcohol.   *Common* reactions are in italics; ***life-threatening,*** in bold italics.
**May contain tartrazine.

Miscellaneous antagonists and antidotes

activated charcoal
aminocaproic acid
ammonia, aromatic spirits
deferoxamine mesylate
digoxin immune FAB (ovine)
dimercaprol
disulfiram
D-penicillamine
edetate calcium disodium
edetate disodium
flumazenil
ipecac syrup
nalmefene hydrochloride
naloxone hydrochloride
naltrexone hydrochloride
pralidoxime chloride
protamine sulfate
sodium cellulose phosphate
sodium polystyrene sulfonate
succimer
trientine hydrochloride

(See also Chapter 38, ANTICHOLINERGICS.)
(See also Chapter 40, ADRENERGIC
 BLOCKERS [SYMPATHOLYTICS].)

COMBINATION PRODUCTS
None.

---

activated charcoal
Actidose-Aqua◇, Charcoaide◇,
Charcocaps◇, Liqui-Char◇,
Supercha◇

Pregnancy Risk Category: NR

HOW SUPPLIED
Tablets: 200 mg‡◇, 300 mg‡◇, 325
mg◇, 650 mg◇
Capsules: 260 mg◇
Powder: 30 g◇, 50 g◇
Oral suspension: 0.625 g/5 ml◇, 0.83
g/5 ml◇, 1 g/5 ml◇, 1.25 g/5 ml◇

ACTION
An adsorbent that adheres to many
drugs and chemicals, inhibiting their
absorption from the GI tract.

ONSET, PEAK, DURATION
Onset immediate upon contact. Peak
and duration not applicable because
drug is not absorbed.

INDICATIONS & DOSAGE
Flatulence or dyspepsia –
Adults: 600 mg to 5 g P.O. t.i.d. after
meals.
Poisoning –
Adults: initially, 1 g/kg (30 to 100 g)
P.O. or 5 to 10 times the amount of
poison ingested as a suspension in 180
to 240 ml of water.
Children: 5 to 10 times estimated
weight of drug or chemical ingested.
Minimum dose is 30 g P.O. in 240 ml
of water to make a slurry. Given preferably within 30 minutes of poisoning. Larger dose is necessary if food
is in the stomach.
　　Commonly used for treating poisoning or overdosage with acetaminophen, aspirin, atropine, barbiturates,
dextropropoxyphene, digitalis glycosides, poisonous mushrooms, oxalic
acid, parathion, phenol, phenylpropanolamine, phenytoin, propantheline,
propoxyphene, strychnine, or tricyclic antidepressants.
　　Check with poison control center
for use in other types of poisonings or
overdoses.

ADVERSE REACTIONS
GI: black stools, nausea, constipation.

INTERACTIONS
Acetylcysteine, ipecac: render charcoal ineffective. Don't administer to-

---

gether, or lavage stomach until all charcoal is removed.

CONTRAINDICATIONS
None reported.

NURSING CONSIDERATIONS
• Give after emesis is complete because activated charcoal absorbs and inactivates syrup of ipecac.
• Mix powder form (most effective) with tap water to form consistency of thick syrup. Adding a small amount of fruit juice or flavoring will make mix more palatable.
• Give by nasogastric tube after lavage if necessary.
• Don't give in ice cream, milk, or sherbet, which reduce absorptive capacity.
• If patients vomit shortly after administration, be prepared to repeat dose.
• Space doses at least 1 hour apart from other drugs if treatment is for any indication other than poisoning.
• Follow treatment with stool softener or laxative, as ordered, to prevent constipation.
• Be aware that preparations made with sorbitol have a laxative effect that lessens the risk of severe constipation or fecal impaction.
• Warn patients that feces will be black.
• Be aware drug is not effective for all drugs and toxic substances.

---

aminocaproic acid
Amicar

Pregnancy Risk Category: C

HOW SUPPLIED
Tablets: 500 mg
Syrup: 250 mg/ml
Injection: 5 g/20 ml for dilution, 24 g/ 96 ml for infusion

ACTION
Inhibits plasminogen activator substances and, to a lesser degree, blocks antiplasmin activity by inhibiting fibrinolysis.

ONSET, PEAK, DURATION
Onset occurs within 1 hour. Levels peak within 2 hours after oral administration; unknown after I.V. administration. Effects persist for less than 3 hours after I.V. administration, unknown for oral administration.

INDICATIONS & DOSAGE
Excessive bleeding resulting from hyperfibrinolysis –
Adults: initially, 5 g P.O. or slow I.V. infusion, followed by 1 to 1.25 g hourly until bleeding is controlled. Maximum dosage is 30 g daily.

ADVERSE REACTIONS
CNS: dizziness, malaise, headache.
CV: hypotension, bradycardia, *arrhythmias* (with rapid I.V. infusion).
EENT: tinnitus, nasal stuffiness, conjunctival suffusion.
GI: nausea, cramps, diarrhea.
Hematologic: generalized thrombosis.
Skin: rash.
Other: malaise, myopathy.

INTERACTIONS
Estrogens, oral contraceptives: increased probability of hypercoagulability. Use together cautiously.

CONTRAINDICATIONS
Contraindicated in patients with active intravascular clotting or presence of disseminated intravascular coagulation unless heparin is used concomitantly. Injectable form is contraindicated in newborns.

NURSING CONSIDERATIONS
• Use cautiously in patients with cardiac, hepatic, or renal disease.
• **I.V. use:** Dilute solution with sterile

---

*Liquid form contains alcohol.   *Common* reactions are in italics; *life-threatening*, in bold italics.
**May contain tartrazine.

water for injection, 0.9% sodium chloride injection, D₅W, or Ringer's injection. Infuse slowly. Don't give by direct or intermittent injection.
• Monitor coagulation studies as ordered and heart rhythm and blood pressure. Notify the doctor of any change immediately.

ammonia, aromatic spirits◊
Pregnancy Risk Category: NR

HOW SUPPLIED
Solution: 30 ml◊, 60 ml◊, 120 ml◊; pints◊; gallons◊
Inhalant: 0.33 ml◊, 0.4 ml◊

ACTION
Irritates the sensory receptors in the nasal membranes, producing reflex stimulation of the respiratory centers.

ONSET, PEAK, DURATION
Onset immediate. Peak and duration unknown.

INDICATIONS & DOSAGE
Fainting –
Adults and children: inhaled as 2 to 4 ml P.O. diluted in at least 30 ml of water, p.r.n.

ADVERSE REACTIONS
EENT: irritation.

INTERACTIONS
None significant.

CONTRAINDICATIONS
None reported.

NURSING CONSIDERATIONS
• Avoid inhaling vapors when administering drug.
• Monitor patient closely for response.

deferoxamine mesylate
Desferal

Pregnancy Risk Category: C

HOW SUPPLIED
Powder for injection: 500 mg

ACTION
Chelates iron by binding ferric ions.

ONSET, PEAK, DURATION
Unknown.

INDICATIONS & DOSAGE
Adjunctive treatment of acute iron intoxication –
Adults and children: 1 g I.M. or I.V. followed by 500 mg I.M. or I.V. for two doses q 4 hours; then 500 mg I.M. or I.V. q 4 to 12 hours. Maximum dosage is 6 g in 24 hours.
Chronic iron overload from multiple transfusions –
Adults and children: 500 mg to 1 g I.M. daily and 2 g slow I.V. infusion in separate solution along with each unit of blood transfused. Maximum dosage is 6 g daily. Alternatively, 20 to 40 mg/kg via S.C. infusion pump daily.

ADVERSE REACTIONS
CV: tachycardia with long-term use.
EENT: blurred vision, cataracts, hearing loss.
GI: diarrhea and abdominal discomfort with long-term use.
GU: dysuria with long-term use.
Other: hypersensitivity reactions (cutaneous wheal formation, pruritus, rash, *anaphylaxis*); pain and induration at injection site; leg cramps, fever; after rapid I.V. administration – *erythema, urticaria, hypotension, shock.*

INTERACTIONS
Ascorbic acid: may enhance the effects of deferoxamine and increase tissue toxicity of iron. Use together

---

†Available in Canada only.   ‡Available in Australia only.   ◊Available OTC.

with extreme caution and close monitoring.

CONTRAINDICATIONS
Contraindicated in patients with severe renal disease or anuria.

NURSING CONSIDERATIONS
• Use cautiously in patients with impaired renal function.
• To reconstitute, add 2 ml of sterile water for injection to each ampule. Make sure drug is completely dissolved. Reconstituted solution is good for 1 week at room temperature. Protect from light.
• After reconstitution, add to 0.9% sodium chloride solution, D_5W, or lactated Ringer's solution and infuse at a rate not exceeding 15 mg/kg hourly.
• Have epinephrine 1:1,000 readily available to treat hypersensitivity reaction.
• Monitor fluid intake and output carefully.
• Warn patients that urine may be red.
• Advise patients to have regular eye examinations during long-term therapy.

---

digoxin immune FAB (ovine)
Digibind

Pregnancy Risk Category: C

HOW SUPPLIED
Injection: 40-mg vial

ACTION
Binds molecules of digoxin and digitoxin, making them unavailable for binding at site of action on cells.

ONSET, PEAK, DURATION
Onset variable but thought to occur within 30 minutes. Peak occurs at completion of I.V. infusion. Effects persist for 2 to 6 hours.

INDICATIONS & DOSAGE
Potentially life-threatening digoxin or digitoxin intoxication –
Adults and children: I.V. dosage varies according to the amount of digoxin or digitoxin to be neutralized. Each vial binds about 0.6 mg of digoxin or digitoxin. Average dosage is 6 vials (240 mg). However, if the toxicity resulted from acute digoxin ingestion and neither a serum digoxin level nor an estimated ingestion amount is known, 20 vials (800 mg) may be required. See package insert for complete, specific dosage instructions.

ADVERSE REACTIONS
CV: *CHF* and rapid ventricular rate (both caused by reversal of the digitalis glycoside's therapeutic effects).
Other: hypersensitivity reactions, hypokalemia.

INTERACTIONS
None reported.

CONTRAINDICATIONS
None.

NURSING CONSIDERATIONS
• Use cautiously in patients known to be allergic to ovine proteins. In these high-risk patients, skin testing is recommended because the drug is derived from digoxin-specific antibody fragments obtained from immunized sheep.
• **I.V. use:** Reconstitute 40-mg vial with 4 ml of sterile water for injection. Gently roll vial to dissolve the powder. Reconstituted solution contains 10 mg/ml. Drug may be given by direct injection if cardiac arrest seems imminent. Alternatively, dilute with 0.9% sodium chloride injection to an appropriate volume and give by intermittent infusion.
• Infuse the drug through a 0.22-micron membrane filter.
• Refrigerate powder for injection. Reconstitute drug immediately before

---

*Liquid form contains alcohol.
**May contain tartrazine.

Common reactions are in italics; **life-threatening,** in bold italics.

use. Reconstituted solutions may be refrigerated for 4 hours.
• Monitor potassium level closely, as ordered.
• Know that in most patients, signs of digitalis toxicity disappear within a few hours.
• Be aware that because drug will interfere with digitalis immunoassay measurements, standard serum digoxin levels will be misleading until drug is cleared from body (about 2 days).
• Know that drug is used only for life-threatening overdose in patients in shock or cardiac arrest; with ventricular arrhythmias, such as ventricular tachycardia or fibrillation; with progressive bradycardia, such as severe sinus bradycardia; or with second- or third-degree AV block not responsive to atropine.

---

dimercaprol
BAL in Oil

Pregnancy Risk Category: NR

HOW SUPPLIED
Injection: 100 mg/ml

ACTION
Forms complexes with heavy metals.

ONSET, PEAK, DURATION
Onset unknown. Levels peak within 30 to 60 minutes. Effects persist for 4 hours.

INDICATIONS & DOSAGE
Severe arsenic or gold poisoning –
Adults and children: 3 mg/kg deep I.M. q 4 hours for 2 days, then q.i.d. on third day, then b.i.d. for 10 days.
Mild arsenic or gold poisoning –
Adults and children: 2.5 mg/kg deep I.M. q.i.d. for 2 days, then b.i.d. on third day, then once daily for 10 days.
Mercury poisoning –
Adults and children: initially, 5 mg/

kg deep I.M., then 2.5 mg/kg daily or b.i.d. for 10 days.
Acute lead encephalopathy or lead level greater than 100 mcg/ml –
Adults and children: 4 mg/kg deep I.M., then q 4 hours with edetate calcium disodium (250 mg/m^2 I.M.). Use separate sites. Maximum dosage is 5 mg/kg per dose.

ADVERSE REACTIONS
CNS: pain or tightness in throat, chest, or hands; headache; paresthesia; muscle pain or weakness.
CV: *transient increase in blood pressure* (returns to normal in 2 hours), *tachycardia.*
EENT: blepharospasm, conjunctivitis, lacrimation, rhinorrhea, excessive salivation.
GI: *halitosis; nausea; vomiting; burning sensation in lips, mouth, and throat; abdominal pain.*
GU: *dysuria;* renal damage if alkaline urine not maintained.
Other: *fever (especially in children),* diaphoresis, pain in teeth, sterile abscess, pain at injection site, decreased iodine uptake.

INTERACTIONS
Iron: toxic metal complex formed; concurrent therapy contraindicated. Wait 24 hours after last dimercaprol dose.
^{131}I uptake thyroid tests: decreased. Don't schedule patient for this test during course of dimercaprol therapy.

CONTRAINDICATIONS
Contraindicated in patients with hepatic dysfunction (except postarsenical jaundice).

NURSING CONSIDERATIONS
• Use cautiously in patients with hypertension or oliguria.
• Know that safe use in pregnancy has not been established and drug should not be used unless judged by

doctor to be necessary to treat a life-threatening acute poisoning.
• Don't give I.V.; give by deep I.M. route only.
• Be careful not to let drug come in contact with skin because it may cause a skin reaction.
• Be aware that drug has an unpleasant, garlic-like odor.
• Know that solution with slight sediment is usable.
• Use ephedrine or antihistamine, as ordered, to prevent or relieve mild adverse reactions.
• Keep urine alkaline to prevent renal damage. Oral sodium bicarbonate may be ordered.
• Know that drug is ineffective in arsine gas poisoning.

disulfiram
Antabuse, Cronetal, Ro-Sulfiram-500

Pregnancy Risk Category: NR

HOW SUPPLIED
Tablets: 250 mg, 500 mg

ACTION
Blocks oxidation of ethanol at the acetaldehyde stage. Excess acetaldehyde produces a highly unpleasant reaction in the presence of even small amounts of ethanol.

ONSET, PEAK, DURATION
Onset occurs in 1 to 2 hours. Peak unknown. Effects persist for 14 days after drug discontinuation.

INDICATIONS & DOSAGE
Adjunct in management of chronic alcoholism –
Adults: 250 to 500 mg P.O. as a single dose in the morning for 1 to 2 weeks. Can be taken in evening if drowsiness occurs. Maintenance: 125 to 500 mg P.O. daily (average dosage 250 mg) until permanent self-control

is established. Treatment may continue for months or years.

ADVERSE REACTIONS
CNS: drowsiness, headache, fatigue, delirium, depression, neuritis, peripheral neuritis, polyneuritis.
EENT: optic neuritis.
GI: metallic or garlic aftertaste.
GU: impotence.
Skin: acneiform or allergic dermatitis.
Other: disulfiram reaction (precipitated by ethanol use), which may include flushing, throbbing headache, dyspnea, nausea, copious vomiting, diaphoresis, thirst, chest pain, palpitations, hyperventilation, hypotension, syncope, anxiety, weakness, blurred vision, confusion. *In severe reactions – respiratory depression, cardiovascular collapse, arrhythmias, MI, acute CHF, seizures, unconsciousness, or death.*

INTERACTIONS
Alfentanil: prolonged duration of effect. Closely monitor patient.
Anticoagulants: increased anticoagulant effect. Adjust dosage of anticoagulant.
Bacampicillin: lowered concentrations of ethanol and acetaldehyde.
CNS depressants: increased CNS depression. Use together cautiously.
Ethanol: precipitated disulfiram reaction. Do not use concomitantly.
Isoniazid: ataxia or marked change in behavior. Do not use concomitantly.
Metronidazole: psychotic reaction. Do not use concomitantly.
Midazolam: increased plasma levels of midazolam. Use together cautiously.
Paraldehyde: toxic levels of acetaldehyde. Do not use concomitantly.
Phenytoin: increased blood levels of phenytoin. Monitor phenytoin blood levels and expect the doctor to adjust phenytoin dosages.
Tricyclic antidepressants, especially

---

*Liquid form contains alcohol.   *Common* reactions are in italics; *life-threatening*, in bold italics.
**May contain tartrazine.

amitriptyline: transient delirium. Closely monitor the patient.

CONTRAINDICATIONS
Contraindicated during alcohol intoxication and within 12 hours of alcohol ingestion; in patients with hypersensitivity to disulfiram or to other thiuram derivatives used in pesticides and rubber vulcanization; and in patients with psychoses, myocardial disease, or coronary occlusion; and in patients receiving metronidazole, paraldehyde, alcohol, or alcohol-containing preparations.

NURSING CONSIDERATIONS
• Know that drug should not be administered during pregnancy.
• Use with extreme caution in patients with diabetes mellitus, hypothyroidism, seizure disorder, cerebral damage, nephritis or hepatic cirrhosis or insufficiency and with concurrent phenytoin therapy.
• Use only under close medical and nursing supervision. Never administer until the patient has abstained from alcohol for at least 12 hours. Patients should clearly understand consequences of disulfiram therapy and give permission for its use. Use drug only in patients who are cooperative, well motivated, and receiving supportive psychiatric therapy.
• Know that complete physical examination and laboratory studies, including CBC, SMA-12, and transaminase, should precede therapy and be repeated regularly, as ordered.
• Caution patient's family that disulfiram should never be given to the patient without his knowledge; severe reaction or death could result if the patient ingests alcohol.
• Warn patients to avoid all sources of alcohol (for example, sauces and cough syrups). Even external application of liniments, shaving lotion, and back-rub preparations may precipitate disulfiram reaction. Tell patients that

alcohol reaction may occur as long as 2 weeks after single dose of disulfiram; the longer patients remain on drug, the more sensitive they become to alcohol.
• Tell patients they should wear a bracelet or carry a card supplied by drug manufacturer identifying them as disulfiram user. *Note:* Mild reactions may occur in sensitive patients with blood alcohol levels of 5 to 10 mg/100 ml; symptoms are fully developed at 50 mg/100 ml; unconsciousness typically occurs at 125 to 150 mg/100 ml level. Reaction may last from 30 minutes to several hours or as long as alcohol remains in blood.
• Reassure patients that disulfiram-induced adverse reactions (unrelated to concomitant alcohol use), such as drowsiness, fatigue, impotence, headache, peripheral neuritis, and metallic or garlic taste, subside after about 2 weeks of therapy.

D-penicillamine
Cuprimine, Depen, D-Penamine‡

Pregnancy Risk Category: NR

HOW SUPPLIED
Tablets: 125 mg‡, 250 mg
Capsules: 125 mg, 250 mg

ACTION
Chelates heavy metals and may inhibit collagen formation. Unknown for rheumatoid arthritis.

ONSET, PEAK, DURATION
Onset and duration unknown. Peak levels occur in 1 hour.

INDICATIONS & DOSAGE
Wilson's disease –
Adults and children: 250 mg P.O. q.i.d. 30 to 60 minutes before meals. Dosage adjusted to achieve urinary copper excretion of 0.5 to 1 mg daily.
Cystinuria –
Adults: 250 mg to 1 g P.O. q.i.d. be-

fore meals. Dosage adjusted to achieve urinary cystine excretion of less than 100 mg daily when renal calculi are present, or 100 to 200 mg daily when no calculi are present. Maximum dosage is 4 g daily.

Children: 30 mg/kg P.O. daily divided q.i.d. before meals. Dosage adjusted to achieve urinary cystine excretion of less than 100 mg daily when renal calculi are present, or 100 to 200 mg daily when no calculi are present.

Rheumatoid arthritis –
Adults: initially, 125 to 250 mg P.O. daily, with increases of 125 to 250 mg q 1 to 3 months, if necessary. Maximum dosage is 1.5 g daily.

ADVERSE REACTIONS
EENT: tinnitus.
GU: *nephrotic syndrome, glomerulonephritis,* proteinuria.
Hepatic: hepatotoxicity.
Hematologic: *leukopenia, eosinophilia, thrombocytopenia, monocytosis, granulocytopenia,* elevated sedimentation rate, lupus-like syndrome.
Skin: friability, especially at pressure spots; wrinkling; erythema; urticaria; ecchymoses.
Other: reversible taste impairment, especially of salts and sweets; hair loss; myasthenia gravis syndrome with long-term use; *decreased pyridoxine (may cause optic neuritis),* decreased zinc and mercury. About one-third of patients develop allergic reactions *(rash, pruritus, fever), arthralgia, lymphadenopathy, or pneumonitis.*

INTERACTIONS
Antacids, oral iron: decreased effectiveness of D-penicillamine. Give at least 2 hours apart.

CONTRAINDICATIONS
Contraindicated in pregnant patients with cystinuria, in patients with previous penicillamine-related aplastic anemia or granulocytosis, and in rheumatoid arthritis patients with renal insufficiency.

NURSING CONSIDERATIONS
• Use with extreme caution, if at all, in patients with hypersensitivity to penicillin.
• Give dose on empty stomach to facilitate absorption, preferably 1 hour before or 3 hours after meals.
• Keep in mind patients should receive supplemental pyridoxine daily.
• If patients have a skin reaction, give antihistamines as prescribed. Handle patients carefully to avoid skin damage.
• Monitor CBC and renal and hepatic function every 2 weeks for the first 6 months, then monthly, as ordered.
• Monitor urinalysis regularly for protein loss.
• Report rash and fever (important signs of toxicity) to the doctor immediately.
• Withhold drug and notify the doctor if WBC count falls below 3,500/mm³ or platelet count falls below 100,000/mm³. A progressive decline in platelet or WBC count in three successive blood tests may necessitate temporary cessation of therapy, even if such counts are within normal limits.
• Tell patients that therapeutic effect may be delayed up to 3 months in treatment of rheumatoid arthritis.
• Tell patients to maintain adequate fluid intake, especially at night.
• Advise patients to report early signs of granulocytopenia: fever, sore throat, chills, bruising, and prolonged bleeding time.
• Reassure patients that taste impairment usually resolves in 6 weeks without changes in dosage.

---

edetate calcium disodium
Calcium Disodium Versenate,
Calcium EDTA

Pregnancy Risk Category: NR

MISCELLANEOUS ANTAGONISTS AND ANTIDOTES **1193**

HOW SUPPLIED
Injection: 200 mg/ml

ACTION
Forms stable, soluble complexes with metals, particularly lead.

ONSET, PEAK, DURATION
Onset occurs in 1 hour. Effects peak after 24 to 48 hours. Duration unknown.

INDICATIONS & DOSAGE
Acute lead encephalopathy or blood lead levels above 70 mcg/dl –
Adults and children: 1.5 g/m² I.V. or I.M. daily in divided doses at 12-hour intervals for 3 to 5 days, usually in conjunction with dimercaprol. A second course may be administered in 5 to 7 days.
Lead poisoning without encephalopathy or asymptomatic with blood levels greater than 70 mcg/dl –
Children: 1 g/m² I.V. or I.M. daily in divided doses.

ADVERSE REACTIONS
CNS: headache, paresthesia, numbness, fatigue (4 to 8 hours after infusion).
CV: *arrhythmias,* hypotension.
EENT: sneezing and nasal congestion (4 to 8 hours after infusion).
GI: anorexia, nausea, vomiting.
GU: proteinuria, hematuria; *nephrotoxicity with renal tubular necrosis leading to fatal nephrosis.*
Other: arthralgia, myalgia, hypercalcemia; sudden fever, chills, and excessive thirst (4 to 8 hours after infusion).

INTERACTIONS
None significant.

CONTRAINDICATIONS
Contraindicated in patients with anuria, hepatitis, and acute renal disease.

NURSING CONSIDERATIONS
• Use with extreme caution in patients with mild renal disease. Expect dosages to be reduced.
• **I.V. use:** Dilute with D₅W or 0.9% sodium chloride injection to a concentration of 2 to 4 mg/ml. Infuse one-half of the daily dose over 1 hour in asymptomatic patients or 2 hours in symptomatic patients. Give the rest of the infusion at least 6 hours later. Alternatively, give by slow infusion over at least 8 hours.
• Add procaine hydrochloride, as ordered, to I.M. solution to minimize pain. Watch for local reactions.
• Because I.V. use may increase intracranial pressure, do not administer by that route to treat lead encephalopathy. Give by I.M. route instead.
• Know that I.M. route preferred, especially for children and patients with lead encephalopathy.
• Force fluids to facilitate lead excretion, except in patients with lead encephalopathy.
• Monitor fluid intake and output, urinalysis, BUN, and ECGs daily, as ordered.
• To avoid toxicity, use with dimercaprol, as ordered.
• Do not confuse with edetate disodium, which is used to treat hypercalcemia.

---

edetate disodium
Disodium EDTA, Disotate, Endrate
Pregnancy Risk Category: NR

HOW SUPPLIED
Injection: 150 mg/ml

ACTION
Chelates with metals, such as calcium, to form a stable, soluble complex.

ONSET, PEAK, DURATION
Unknown.

INDICATIONS & DOSAGE

Hypercalcemic crisis –
Adults: 50 mg/kg by slow I.V. infusion added to 500 ml of D₅W or 0.9% sodium chloride solution administered over 3 or more hours. Maximum dosage is 3 g/day.
Children: 40 to 70 mg/kg by slow I.V. infusion, diluted to a maximum concentration of 30 mg/ml in D₅W or 0.9% sodium chloride solution administered over 3 or more hours. Maximum dosage is 70 mg/kg/day.
Digitalis-induced cardiac arrhythmias –
Adults and children: 15 mg/kg/hour I.V. with maximum daily dosage 60 mg/kg daily.

ADVERSE REACTIONS

CNS: circumoral paresthesia, numbness, headache, malaise, fatigue, muscle pain or weakness.
CV: hypertension, thrombophlebitis, orthostatic hypotension.
EENT: erythema.
GI: nausea, vomiting, diarrhea, anorexia, abdominal cramps.
GU: in excessive doses – nephrotoxicity with urinary urgency, nocturia, dysuria, polyuria, proteinuria, renal insufficiency, *renal failure, tubular necrosis.*
Skin: dermatitis.
Other: *severe hypocalcemia,* decreased magnesium, pain at site of infusion.

INTERACTIONS
None significant.

CONTRAINDICATIONS
Contraindicated in patients with hypersensitivity to drug, anuria, known or suspected hypocalcemia, significant renal disease, active or healed tubercular lesions, or history of seizures or intracranial lesions.

NURSING CONSIDERATIONS

• Use cautiously in patients with limited cardiac reserve, CHF, or hypokalemia.
• **I.V. use:** Dilute before use. Avoid rapid I.V. infusion; profound hypocalcemia may occur, leading to tetany, seizures, arrhythmias, and respiratory arrest. Not recommended for direct or intermittent injection. Avoid extravasation.
• Record I.V. site used, and avoid repeated use of the same site, which increases likelihood of thrombophlebitis.
• Keep I.V. calcium available to treat hypocalcemia.
• Keep patients in bed for 15 minutes after infusion to avoid orthostatic hypotension. Monitor blood pressure closely.
• Monitor ECG and renal function tests frequently, as ordered.
• Obtain serum calcium after each dose, as ordered.
• If generalized systemic reactions – fever, chills, back pain, emesis, muscle cramps, urinary urgency – occur 4 to 8 hours after infusion, report them to the doctor. Treatment is usually supportive. Symptoms generally subside within 12 hours.
• Don't use to treat lead toxicity; know that edetate calcium disodium should be used instead.
• Know that other drug treatments for hypercalcemia are safer and more effective than edetate disodium.

flumazenil
Romazicon

Pregnancy Risk Category: C

HOW SUPPLIED
Injection: 0.1 mg/ml in 5- and 10-ml multiple-dose vials

ACTION
Benzodiazepine antagonist that competitively inhibits the actions of ben-

---

*Liquid form contains alcohol.
**May contain tartrazine.   *Common* reactions are in italics; *life-threatening,* in bold italics.

zodiazepines on the gamma-aminobutyric acid-benzodiazepine receptor complex.

ONSET, PEAK, DURATION
Unknown.

INDICATIONS & DOSAGE
Complete or partial reversal of sedative effects of benzodiazepines after anesthesia or short diagnostic procedures (conscious sedation) –
Adults: initially, 0.2 mg I.V. over 15 seconds. If patient does not reach the desired level of consciousness after 45 seconds, dose is repeated. Repeated at 1-minute intervals until a cumulative dose of 1 mg has been given (initial dose plus four additional doses), if needed. Most patients respond after 0.6 to 1 mg of drug. In case of resedation, dosage may be repeated after 20 minutes; however, no more than 1 mg should be given at any one time and no more than 3 mg/hour.
Suspected benzodiazepine overdose –
Adults: initially, 0.2 mg I.V. over 15 seconds. If patient does not reach the desired level of consciousness after 30 seconds, 0.3 mg is administered over 30 seconds. If patient still does not respond adequately, 0.5 mg is administered over 30 seconds; 0.5-mg doses are repeated as needed at 1-minute intervals until a cumulative dose of 3 mg has been given. Most patients suffering from benzodiazepine overdose respond to cumulative doses between 1 and 3 mg; rarely, patients who respond partially after 3 mg may require additional doses. No more than 5 mg over 5 minutes should be given initially. Sedation that persists after this dosage is unlikely to be caused by benzodiazepines. In case of resedation, dosage may be repeated after 20 minutes; however, no more than 1 mg should be given at any one time and no more than 3 mg/hour.

ADVERSE REACTIONS
CNS: *dizziness, abnormal or blurred vision, headache, seizures,* fatigue, agitation, emotional lability.
CV: *arrhythmias,* cutaneous vasodilation.
GI: nausea, vomiting.
Other: *diaphoresis, pain at injection site.*

INTERACTIONS
Antidepressants; drugs that can cause seizures or arrhythmias: seizures or arrhythmias can develop after effect of benzodiazepine overdose is removed. Use flumazenil with caution in cases of mixed overdose.

CONTRAINDICATIONS
Contraindicated in patients hypersensitive to flumazenil or benzodiazepines; in patients who show evidence of serious cyclic antidepressant overdose; and in those who received benzodiazepine to treat a potentially life-threatening condition (such as status epilepticus).

NURSING CONSIDERATIONS
• Use cautiously in patients at high risk for developing seizures; patients who have recently received multiple doses of a parenteral benzodiazepine; patients displaying some signs of seizure activity; patients who may be at risk for unrecognized benzodiazepine dependence, such as intensive care unit patients; patients with head injury; psychiatric patients; and alcohol-dependent patients.
• **I.V. use:** Administer by direct injection or dilute with a compatible solution. Discard unused drug that has been drawn into a syringe or diluted within 24 hours.
• Administer drug into an I.V. line in a large vein with a free-flowing I.V. solution to minimize pain at the injection site. Compatible solutions include D_5W, lactated Ringer's injection, and 0.9% sodium chloride.

• Monitor patients closely for resedation that may occur after reversal of benzodiazepine effects because flumazenil's duration of action is shorter than that of all benzodiazepines. Duration of monitoring period depends on specific drug being reversed. Monitor closely after long-acting benzodiazepines, such as diazepam, or after high doses of short-acting benzodiazepines, such as 10 mg of midazolam. In most cases, severe resedation is unlikely in patients who fail to show signs of resedation 2 hours after a 1-mg dose of flumazenil.
• Know that dosage adjustments don't appear necessary in elderly patients.
• Be aware that safety and efficacy in children have not been established.
• Warn patients not to perform hazardous activities, such as operating heavy equipment or driving, within 24 hours of procedure because of resedation risk.
• Tell patients to avoid alcohol, CNS depressants, and OTC drugs for 24 hours.
• Give family members important instructions or provide patients with written instructions. Do not expect patients to recall information told to them in the postprocedure period because drug does not reverse the amnesic effects of benzodiazepines.

---

ipecac syrup
Pregnancy Risk Category: C

HOW SUPPLIED
Syrup*: 70 mg powdered ipecac/ml (contains glycerin 10% and alcohol 1% to 2.5%)◊

ACTION
Induces vomiting by acting locally on the gastric mucosa and centrally on the chemoreceptor trigger zone.

ONSET, PEAK, DURATION
Onset occurs in 20 to 30 minutes. Peak unknown. Effects persist for 20 to 25 minutes.

INDICATIONS & DOSAGE
To induce vomiting in poisoning –
Adults and children 12 years and older: 30 ml P.O., followed by 200 to 300 ml of water.
Children 6 months to 1 year: 5 ml P.O., followed by 100 to 200 ml of water or milk. If necessary, repeat dose once after 20 minutes.
Children 1 year to 12 years: 15 ml P.O., followed by about 200 ml of water or milk.

ADVERSE REACTIONS
CNS: depression.
CV: *arrhythmias,* bradycardia, hypotension, atrial fibrillation, or *fatal myocarditis* after ingestion of excessive dose.
GI: diarrhea.

INTERACTIONS
Activated charcoal: neutralized emetic effect. Don't give together; may give activated charcoal after vomiting.

CONTRAINDICATIONS
Contraindicated in semicomatose or unconscious patients, or those with severe inebriation, seizures, shock, or loss of gag reflex.

NURSING CONSIDERATIONS
• Unless advised otherwise by a poison control center, don't give after ingestion of petroleum distillates (for example, kerosene, gasoline) or volatile oils; retching and vomiting may cause aspiration and lead to bronchospasm, pulmonary edema, or aspiration pneumonitis. Vegetable oil will delay absorption of these substances. Don't give after ingestion of caustic substances, such as lye; additional in-

---

*Liquid form contains alcohol.   *Common* reactions are in italics; ***life-threatening,*** in bold italics.
**May contain tartrazine.

jury to the esophagus and mediastinum can occur.
• Keep in mind that stomach is usually emptied completely; vomitus also may contain some intestinal material.
• If two doses do not induce vomiting, be prepared for gastric lavage.
• Know that ipecac syrup usually induces vomiting within 20 to 30 minutes.
• In antiemetic toxicity, know that ipecac syrup is usually effective if less than 1 hour has passed since ingestion of antiemetic.
• Be aware that no systemic toxicity occurs with doses of 30 ml or less.
• Clearly indicate ipecac *syrup,* not single word "ipecac," to avoid confusion with fluidextract, which is 14 times more concentrated and, if inadvertently used instead of syrup, may cause death. Fluidextract is no longer commercially available in the United States.
• Be aware that ipecac syrup is now commonly abused by bulimics who binge and then purge.
• Recommend to parents that 1 oz (30 ml) of syrup be readily available in the home when child becomes 1 year old for immediate use in case of emergency.

---

nalmefene hydrochloride
Revex

Pregnancy Risk Category: B

HOW SUPPLIED
Injection: 100 mcg/ml, 1 mg/ml

ACTION
Blocks opioid receptors and thereby prevents or reverses the effects of opioids, including respiratory depression, sedation, and hypotension.

ONSET, PEAK, DURATION
Onset and peak occur almost immediately after I.V. administration. Duration varies, but usually is as long as most opioid analgesics. Low doses (1 mcg/kg) may last for 30 to 60 minutes; fully reversing doses (1 mg/70 kg) may last for many hours.

INDICATIONS & DOSAGE
Reversal of postoperative opioid effects –
Adults: use 100 mcg/ml dosage strength as follows: initially, 0.25 mcg/kg I.V., followed by 0.25-mcg/kg incremental doses at 2- to 5-minute intervals, p.r.n. A cumulative total dose above 1 mcg/kg does not provide additional therapeutic effect.
Management of opioid overdose –
Adults: use 1 mg/ml dosage strength as follows: initially, 0.5 mg/70 kg I.V., followed by 1 mg/70 kg in 2 to 5 minutes, p.r.n.

ADVERSE REACTIONS
CNS: *dizziness, headache,* somnolence, depression, agitation, nervousness, tremor, confusion, withdrawal syndrome, myoclonus.
CV: *tachycardia, hypertension or hypotension, vasodilation,* bradycardia, arrhythmias.
GI: *nausea, vomiting,* diarrhea, dry mouth.
GU: urine retention.
Skin: pruritus.
Other: *postoperative pain, fever, chills.*

INTERACTIONS
None known.

CONTRAINDICATIONS
Contraindicated in patients with hypersensitivity to the drug.

NURSING CONSIDERATIONS
• Use with extreme caution in patients with known physical dependence on opioids or following surgery involving high doses of opioids. Know that excessive doses of opioid antagonists in the postoperative setting has been associated with hypertension,

tachycardia, and excessive mortality in patients at high risk for cardiovascular complications.

• Use with caution in patients with CV disease and in those who are receiving potentially cardiotoxic drugs or who are breast-feeding.

• Be aware that nalmefene may not completely reverse buprenorphine-induced respiratory depression.

• **I.V. use:** Drug is supplied in two concentrations: an ampule with a blue label contains 1 ml at a concentration suitable for postoperative use (100 mcg/ml), and an ampule with a green label contains 2 ml at a concentration suitable for management of overdose (1 mg/ml). Check concentration carefully before administering drug.

• In postoperative cases where the patient is known to be at increased risk for CV complications, be aware that doctor may order drug to be diluted 1:1 with saline solution or sterile water and smaller initial and incremental doses of 0.1 mcg/kg.

• Be aware that patients with renal failure may require incremental doses to be given slowly (over 60 seconds) to minimize the hypertension and dizziness that has been reported following the abrupt administration of the drug to such patients.

• Know that a cumulative total dose above 1.5 mg/70 kg is unlikely to have an effect.

• Know that if drug cannot be administered I.V., a single 1-mg dose may produce therapeutic results within 5 to 15 minutes if administered I.M. or S.C.

• Monitor patient's respiratory depth and rate closely. Duration of action of the opioid may exceed that of nalmefene, causing the patient to relapse into respiratory depression. Keep patient under close observation until there is no reasonable risk of recurring respiratory depression.

• Know that nalmefene may produce acute withdrawal symptoms in pa-

tients with known physical dependence on opioids. If suspicion of opioid dependency is present, administer a test dose of 0.1 mg/70 kg I.V., as ordered. If no evidence of withdrawal occurs in 2 minutes, the recommended dose may be administered, as ordered.

naloxone hydrochloride
Narcan
Pregnancy Risk Category: B

HOW SUPPLIED
Injection: 0.4 mg/ml, 1 mg/ml

ACTION
Unknown. Thought to displace previously administered narcotic analgesics from their receptors (competitive antagonism). Has no pharmacologic activity of its own.

ONSET, PEAK, DURATION
Onset occurs in 1 to 2 minutes after I.V. use, 2 to 5 minutes after S.C. or I.M. use. Peak unknown. Duration depends on dose and route of administration. I.M. administration provides a more prolonged duration.

INDICATIONS & DOSAGE
Known or suspected narcotic-induced respiratory depression, including that caused by pentazocine and propoxyphene –
Adults: 0.4 to 2 mg I.V., S.C., or I.M. Repeated q 2 to 3 minutes, p.r.n. If no response is observed after 10 mg has been administered, the diagnosis of narcotic-induced toxicity should be questioned.
Postoperative narcotic depression –
Adults: 0.1 to 0.2 mg I.V. q 2 to 3 minutes, p.r.n.
Children: 0.005 to 0.01 mg/kg dose I.V. Repeated q 2 to 3 minutes, p.r.n.
Neonates (asphyxia neonatorum): 0.01 mg/kg I.V. into umbilical vein. May be repeated q 2 to 3 minutes.

---

*Liquid form contains alcohol.   *Common* reactions are in italics; *life-threatening*, in bold italics.
**May contain tartrazine.

ADVERSE REACTIONS
CV: tachycardia and hypertension with higher-than-recommended doses.
GI: nausea and vomiting with higher-than-recommended doses.
Other: tremors and withdrawal symptoms in narcotic-dependent patients with higher-than-recommended doses.

INTERACTIONS
None significant.

CONTRAINDICATIONS
Contraindicated in patients with hypersensitivity to the drug.

NURSING CONSIDERATIONS
• Use cautiously in patients with cardiac irritability and opiate addiction. Abrupt reversal of opiate-induced CNS depression may result in nausea, vomiting, diaphoresis, tachycardia, CNS excitement, and increased blood pressure.
• **I.V. use:** Be prepared to administer continuous I.V. infusion (necessary in many instances to control adverse effects of epidurally administered morphine). Adult concentration (0.4 mg) may be diluted by mixing 0.5 ml with 9.5 ml of sterile water or sodium chloride solution for injection to make neonatal concentration (0.02 mg/ml).
• Keep in mind that duration of action of the narcotic may exceed that of naloxone and patients may relapse into respiratory depression.
• Know that respiratory rate increases within 1 to 2 minutes.
• Be aware that drug is effective only in reversing respiratory depression caused by opiates, not against other drug-induced respiratory depression. Know that flumazenil should be used to treat respiratory depression caused by diazepam or other benzodiazepines.
• Be aware that patients who receive naloxone to reverse opioid-induced respiratory depression may exhibit tachypnea.
• Monitor respiratory depth and rate. Be prepared to provide oxygen, ventilation, and other resuscitation measures.

---

naltrexone hydrochloride
Re Via

Pregnancy Risk Category: C

HOW SUPPLIED
Tablets: 50 mg

ACTION
Unknown. Probably reversibly blocks the subjective effects of intravenously administered opioids by occupying opiate receptors in the brain.

ONSET, PEAK, DURATION
Onset occurs in 15 to 30 minutes. Effects peak after 12 hours. Effects persist about 24 hours.

INDICATIONS & DOSAGE
Adjunct for maintenance of opioid-free state in detoxified individuals –
Adults: initially, 25 mg P.O. If no withdrawal signs occur within 1 hour, an additional 25 mg is given. Once patient has been started on 50 mg q 24 hours, flexible maintenance schedule may be used. From 50 to 150 mg may be given daily, depending on the schedule prescribed.
Treatment of alcohol dependence –
Adults: 50 mg P.O. once daily.

ADVERSE REACTIONS
CNS: *insomnia, anxiety, nervousness, headache,* depression.
GI: *nausea, vomiting,* anorexia, *abdominal pain.*
Hepatic: hepatotoxicity.
Other: *muscle and joint pain.*

INTERACTIONS
None significant.

CONTRAINDICATIONS

Contraindicated in patients receiving opioid analgesics, in opioid-dependent patients, in patients in acute opioid withdrawal, and in those with positive urine screen for opioids or in acute hepatitis or liver failure. Also contraindicated in patients with hypersensitivity to drug.

NURSING CONSIDERATIONS

• Use cautiously in patients with mild hepatic disease or history of recent hepatic disease.

• Be aware that treatment for opioid dependency shouldn't begin until patients receive naloxone challenge, a provocative test of opioid dependency. If signs of opioid withdrawal persist after naloxone challenge, don't administer naltrexone.

• Keep in mind that patients must be completely free of opioids before taking naltrexone or severe withdrawal symptoms may occur. Patients who have been addicted to short-acting opioids, such as heroin and meperidine, must wait at least 7 days after the last opioid dose before starting naltrexone. Patients who have been addicted to longer-acting opioids, such as methadone, should wait at least 10 days.

• In an emergency, anticipate that patients receiving naltrexone may be given an opioid analgesic, but the dose must be higher than usual to surmount naltrexone's effect. Monitor for respiratory depression from the opioid; it may be longer and deeper.

• For patients being treated because of a history of opioid dependency and who are expected to be poor compliers, be prepared to try a flexible maintenance dosage regimen: 100 mg on Monday and Wednesday, 150 mg on Friday, as ordered.

• Know that naltrexone should be used only as part of a comprehensive rehabilitation program.

• Advise patients to carry a medical identification card. Warn them to tell medical personnel that they are taking naltrexone.

• Give patients names of nonopioid drugs that they can continue to take for pain, diarrhea, or cough.

pralidoxime chloride (pyridine-2-aldoxime methochloride; 2-PAM)
Protopam Chloride

Pregnancy Risk Category: C

HOW SUPPLIED

Injection: 1 g/20 ml in 20-ml vial without diluent or syringe; 1 g/20 ml in 20-ml vial with diluent, syringe, needle, and alcohol swab (emergency kit); 600 mg/2 ml auto-injector, parenteral

ACTION

Reactivates cholinesterase that has been inactivated by organophosphorus pesticides and related compounds, permitting degradation of accumulated acetylcholine and facilitating normal functioning of neuromuscular junctions.

ONSET, PEAK, DURATION

Onset and duration unknown. Levels peak within 5 to 15 minutes after I.V. administration; 10 to 20 minutes after I.M. administration; unknown after S.C. administration.

INDICATIONS & DOSAGE

Antidote for organophosphate poisoning—

Adults: 1 to 2 g in 100 ml of sodium chloride solution by I.V. infusion over 15 to 30 minutes. If pulmonary edema is present, give by slow I.V. push over 5 minutes. Repeated in 1 hour if muscle weakness persists. Additional doses may be given cautiously. I.M. or S.C. injection may be used if I.V. is not feasible.

---

*Liquid form contains alcohol.   *Common* reactions are in italics; *life-threatening,* in bold italics.
**May contain tartrazine.

Children: 20 to 40 mg/kg I.V. administered as for adults.
Cholinergic crisis in myasthenia gravis –
Adults: 1 to 2 g I.V., followed by 250 mg I.V. q 5 minutes as needed.

ADVERSE REACTIONS
CNS: dizziness, headache, drowsiness, excitement, manic behavior after recovery of consciousness.
CV: tachycardia.
EENT: blurred vision, diplopia, impaired accommodation, ***laryngospasm.***
GI: nausea.
Other: muscular weakness, muscle rigidity, hyperventilation.

INTERACTIONS
None significant.

CONTRAINDICATIONS
None.

NURSING CONSIDERATIONS
• Use with extreme caution in patients with myasthenia gravis (overdosage may precipitate myasthenic crisis).
• Initially, remove secretions, maintain patent airway, and institute artificial ventilation if needed. After dermal exposure to organophosphate, remove the patient's clothing and wash his skin and hair with sodium bicarbonate, soap, water, and alcohol as soon as possible. A second washing may be necessary. When washing the patient, wear protective gloves and clothes to avoid exposure.
• Draw blood for cholinesterase levels before giving pralidoxime.
• **I.V. use:** Give I.V. preparation slowly as diluted solution. Dilute with sterile water without preservatives.
• To ameliorate muscarinic effects and block accumulation of acetylcholine associated with organophosphate poisoning, give atropine 2 to 4 mg I.V. along with pralidoxine if cyanosis

is not present, as ordered. (If cyanosis is present, atropine should be given I.M.) Give atropine every 5 to 6 minutes, as ordered, until signs and symptoms of atropine toxicity (flushing, tachycardia, dry mouth, blurred vision, excitement, delirium, and hallucinations) appear; know that atropinization should be maintained for at least 48 hours.
• Observe patient for 48 to 72 hours if poison was ingested. Delayed absorption may occur from lower bowel. It is difficult to distinguish between toxic effects produced by atropine or by organophosphate compounds and those resulting from pralidoxime.
• Observe the patient with myasthenia gravis treated for overdose of cholinergic drugs closely for signs of rapid weakening. This patient can pass quickly from a cholinergic crisis to a myasthenic crisis, and requires more cholinergic drugs to treat the myasthenia. Keep edrophonium (Tensilon) available in such situations for establishing differential diagnosis.
• Know that drug should be used in hospitalized patients only; have respiratory and other supportive measures available. If possible, obtain accurate medical history and chronology of poisoning. Know that drug should be given as soon as possible after poisoning; treatment is most effective if initiated within 24 hours after exposure.
• Know that drug relieves paralysis of respiratory muscles but is less effective in relieving depression of respiratory center.
• Be aware that drug is not effective against poisoning due to phosphorus, inorganic phosphates, or organophosphates with no anticholinesterase activity.
• Caution the patient treated for organophosphate poisoning to avoid contact with insecticides for several weeks.

protamine sulfate
Pregnancy Risk Category: C

HOW SUPPLIED
Injection: 10 mg/ml

ACTION
A heparin antagonist that forms a physiologically inert complex with heparin sodium.

ONSET, PEAK, DURATION
Onset within 30 seconds to 1 minute. Peak unknown. Effects persist for 2 hours.

INDICATIONS & DOSAGE
Heparin overdose –
Adults: dosage based on venous blood coagulation studies, usually 1 mg for each 90 to 115 units of heparin. Give by slow I.V. injection over 10 minutes in doses not to exceed 50 mg.

ADVERSE REACTIONS
CV: fall in blood pressure, bradycardia.
Respiratory: dyspnea.
Other: transitory flushing, feeling of warmth, *anaphylaxis, anaphylactoid reactions.*

INTERACTIONS
None significant.

CONTRAINDICATIONS
Contraindicated in patients with hypersensitivity to drug.

NURSING CONSIDERATIONS
• Use cautiously after cardiac surgery.
• Calculate dosage carefully. One mg of protamine neutralizes 90 to 115 units of heparin depending on the salt (heparin calcium or heparin sodium) and the source of heparin (beef or pork).
• **I.V. use:** Administer slowly by direct I.V. injection. Have equipment available to treat shock.
• Monitor patients continually. Check vital signs frequently.
• Watch for spontaneous bleeding (heparin "rebound"), especially in patients undergoing dialysis and in those who have undergone cardiac surgery.
• Be aware that protamine sulfate may act as anticoagulant in very high doses.

sodium cellulose phosphate
Calcibind
Pregnancy Risk Category: C

HOW SUPPLIED
Powder: 2.5-g packets or 300-g bulk. Inorganic phosphate content approximately 34%; sodium content approximately 11%.

ACTION
Binds calcium in the GI tract and decreases the amount absorbed.

ONSET, PEAK, DURATION
Unknown.

INDICATIONS & DOSAGE
Absorptive hypercalciuria type I with recurrent calcium oxalate or calcium phosphate renal stones –
Adults: 15 g/day P.O. (5 g with each meal) in patients with urine calcium greater than 300 mg/day. When urine calcium declines to less than 150 mg/day, dosage reduced to 10 g/day (5 g with dinner, 2.5 g with two remaining meals).

ADVERSE REACTIONS
CNS: drowsiness, mood or mental changes, *seizures,* trembling.
GI: anorexia, nausea, vomiting, discomfort, diarrhea, dyspepsia.
GU: hyperoxaluria, hypomagnesuria.
Other: acute arthralgia.

---

*Liquid form contains alcohol.
**May contain tartrazine.
Common reactions are in italics; *life-threatening,* in bold italics.

INTERACTIONS
Calcium-containing products, dairy products: worsened hypercalcemia. Avoid use.
Magnesium-containing products: may bind drug. Separate doses by at least 1 hour.
Vitamin C: risk of nephrolithiasis. Avoid excessive intake.

CONTRAINDICATIONS
Contraindicated in patients with primary or secondary hyperparathyroidism, including renal hypercalciuria; hypomagnesemic states; bone disease; hypocalcemic states; normal or low intestinal absorption; renal excretion of calcium; or enteric hyperoxaluria.

NURSING CONSIDERATIONS
• Use cautiously in patients with CHF or ascites.
• Know that drug is recommended only for the type of absorptive hypercalciuria in which both intestinal calcium absorption and urine calcium remain abnormally high even with a calcium-restricted diet. When administered inappropriately it may cause hypocalciuria, which could stimulate parathyroid function and lead to parathyroid bone disease.
• Because of the difficulty involved in managing sodium cellulose phosphate therapy, keep in mind that many doctors prefer to treat hypercalciuria with a low-calcium diet, high fluid intake, and thiazides, when necessary.
• Advise patients to mix powder with 8 oz of fruit juice, water, or a soft drink and to take it with meals. Remind patients to refill glass, mix, and drink all of the fluid to get the full dose.
• Instruct patients to maintain a calcium-restricted diet and avoid all dairy products.
• Advise patients to restrict dietary intake of oxalates (found in spinach, rhubarb, chocolate, and tea). Patients

taking sodium cellulose phosphate may develop hyperoxaluria and hypomagnesuria, which predispose them to stone formation.
• Tell patients to avoid vitamin C because it can increase urine oxalate.
• Encourage fluid intake. Urine output should be at least 2 liters/day.
• Encourage a low-sodium diet because drug has 2 to 3 mEq of sodium/g. Tell patients to avoid salty foods and to avoid adding salt at the table.

---

sodium polystyrene sulfonate
Kayexalate, Resonium A, SPS
Pregnancy Risk Category: C

HOW SUPPLIED
Powder: 1-lb jar (3.5 g/teaspoon)
Suspension: 60 ml*, 120 ml*, 200 ml*, 480 ml*, 500 ml*

ACTION
Potassium-removing resin exchanges sodium ions for potassium ions in the intestine: 1 g of sodium polystyrene sulfonate is exchanged for 0.5 to 1 mEq of potassium. The resin is then eliminated. Much of the exchange capacity is used for cations other than potassium (calcium and magnesium) and possibly for fats and proteins.

ONSET, PEAK, DURATION
Unknown.

INDICATIONS & DOSAGE
Hyperkalemia –
Adults: 15 g P.O. daily to q.i.d. in water or sorbitol (3 to 4 ml/g of resin). Alternatively, mix powder with appropriate medium – aqueous suspension or diet appropriate for renal failure – and instill in nasogastric tube.
Or 30 to 50 g/100 ml of sorbitol q 6 hours as warm emulsion deep into sigmoid colon (20 cm). In persistent vomiting or paralytic ileus, high-re-

tention enema of sodium polystyrene sulfonate (30 g) suspended in 200 ml of 10% methylcellulose, 10% dextrose, or 25% sorbitol solution may be given.

Children: 1 g of resin P.O. or P.R. for each mEq of potassium to be removed.

Oral administration preferred because drug should remain in intestine for at least 6 hours.

ADVERSE REACTIONS

GI: *constipation,* fecal impaction (in elderly patients), anorexia, gastric irritation, nausea, vomiting, *diarrhea* (with sorbitol emulsions).
Other: *hypokalemia,* hypocalcemia, hypomagnesemia, sodium retention.

INTERACTIONS

Antacids and laxatives (nonabsorbable cation-donating types, including magnesium hydroxide): systemic alkalosis and reduced potassium exchange capability. Don't use together.

CONTRAINDICATIONS

Contraindicated in patients with hypokalemia or hypersensitivity to drug.

NURSING CONSIDERATIONS

• Use cautiously in patients with severe CHF, severe hypertension, or marked edema.
• Do not heat resin; this will impair the drug's effectiveness. Mix resin only with water or sorbitol for P.O. administration. Above all, *never* mix with orange juice (high potassium content) to disguise taste.
• Chill oral suspension for greater palatability.
• If sorbitol is given, mix with resin suspension.
• Consider solid form. Resin cookie and candy recipes are available; ask pharmacist or dietitian to supply.
• Know that premixed forms are available (SPS and others).
• If preparing manually, mix polystyrene resin only with water and sorbitol for rectal use. Do not use mineral oil for rectal administration to prevent impaction; ion exchange requires aqueous medium. Sorbitol content prevents impaction.
• Prepare rectal dose at room temperature. Stir emulsion gently during administration.
• Use #28 French rubber tube for rectal dose; insert 20 cm into sigmoid colon. Tape tube in place. Alternatively, consider a Foley catheter with a 30-ml balloon inflated distal to anal sphincter to aid in retention. This is especially helpful for patients with poor sphincter control (for example, after CVA). Use gravity flow. Drain returns constantly through Y-tube connection. Place patient in knee-chest position or with hips on pillow for a while if back-leakage occurs.
• After rectal administration, flush tubing with 50 to 100 ml of nonsodium fluid to ensure delivery of all medication. Flush rectum to remove the resin.
• Prevent fecal impaction in elderly patients by administering resin rectally, as ordered. Give cleansing enema before rectal administration. Explain to patients the need to retain enema—for 6 to 10 hours is ideal, but 30 to 60 minutes is acceptable.
• Watch for constipation in oral or nasogastric administration. Use sorbitol (10 to 20 ml of 70% syrup every 2 hours as needed) to produce one or two watery stools daily.
• Monitor serum potassium levels at least once daily, as ordered. Treatment may result in potassium deficiency. Treatment is usually stopped when potassium is reduced to 4 or 5 mEq/L.
• Watch for other signs of hypokalemia: irritability, confusion, arrhythmias, ECG changes, severe muscle weakness and sometimes paralysis, and digitalis toxicity in digitalized patients.

---

*Liquid form contains alcohol.   *Common* reactions are in italics; *life-threatening,* in bold italics.
**May contain tartrazine.

• If hyperkalemia is severe, know that doctor does not depend solely on polystyrene resin to lower serum potassium. Dextrose 50% with regular insulin I.V. push may be given.

• Monitor for symptoms of other electrolyte deficiencies (magnesium, calcium) because drug is nonselective. Monitor serum calcium in patients receiving sodium polystyrene therapy for more than 3 days. Supplementary calcium may be needed.

• Watch for sodium overload. Drug contains about 100 mg sodium/g. About ⅓ of resin's sodium is retained.

---

succimer
Chemet

Pregnancy Risk Category: C

HOW SUPPLIED
Capsules: 100 mg

ACTION
A chelating agent that forms water-soluble complexes with lead and increases its excretion in urine.

ONSET, PEAK, DURATION
Onset and duration unknown. Serum levels peak in 1 to 2 hours.

INDICATIONS & DOSAGE
Lead poisoning in children with blood lead levels above 45 mcg/dl–
Children: initially, 10 mg/kg or 350 mg/m^2 q 8 hours for 5 days. Dosage rounded as appropriate to nearest 100 mg (see chart). Then, frequency of administration decreased to q 12 hours for an additional 2 weeks of therapy.

Weight (kg)	Dose (mg)
8 to 15	100
16 to 23	200
24 to 34	300
35 to 44	400
>45	500

ADVERSE REACTIONS
CNS: *drowsiness, dizziness, sensory motor neuropathy, sleepiness, paresthesia, headache.*
CV: arrhythmias.
EENT: plugged ears, cloudy film in eyes, otitis media, watery eyes, sore throat, rhinorrhea, nasal congestion.
GI: *nausea, vomiting, diarrhea, loss of appetite,* abdominal cramps, hemorrhoidal symptoms, *metallic taste in mouth.*
GU: decreased urination, difficult urination, proteinuria.
Hematologic: increased platelet count, intermittent eosinophilia.
Respiratory: cough, head cold.
Skin: papular rash, herpetic rash, mucocutaneous eruptions, pruritus.
Other: *leg, kneecap, back, stomach, rib, or flank pain; flulike symptoms;* moniliasis; *elevated serum AST, ALT, alkaline phosphatase, or cholesterol levels.*

INTERACTIONS
None reported.

CONTRAINDICATIONS
Contraindicated in patients with hypersensitivity to the drug.

NURSING CONSIDERATIONS
• Use cautiously in patients with compromised renal function.
• Measure severity by initial blood lead level and by rate and degree of rebound of blood lead level. Severity of lead intoxication should be used as a guide for more frequent blood lead monitoring.
• Monitor serum transaminase before and at least weekly during therapy, as ordered. Transient mild elevations of serum transaminases have been observed. Patients with history of hepatic disease should be monitored more closely.
• Monitor patients at least once weekly for rebound blood lead levels, as ordered. Elevated blood lead levels

---

and associated symptoms may return rapidly after drug is discontinued because of redistribution of lead from bone to soft tissues and blood.
• Be aware that course of treatment lasts 19 days. Repeated courses may be necessary if indicated by weekly monitoring of blood lead levels.
• Know that a minimum of 2 weeks between courses is recommended unless high blood lead levels indicate need for immediate therapy.
• Know that false-positive results for ketones in urine using nitroprusside reagents (Ketostix) and falsely decreased levels of serum uric acid and CK have been reported.
• Know that concurrent administration of succimer with other chelating agents is not recommended. Patients who have received edetate calcium disodium with or without dimercaprol may use succimer as subsequent therapy after a 4-week interval.
• Tell parents of young children who cannot swallow capsules that capsule can be opened and its contents sprinkled on a small amount of soft food. Alternatively, medicated beads from capsule may be poured on a spoon; follow with flavored beverage, such as a fruit drink.
• Assisting parents with identifying and removing sources of lead in child's
environment is critical to successful therapy. Chelation therapy is not a substitute for preventing further exposure and should not be used to permit continued exposure.
• Tell patients to consult the doctor if rash occurs. Consider possibility of allergic or other mucocutaneous reactions each time drug is used.

trientine hydrochloride
Syprine

Pregnancy Risk Category: C

HOW SUPPLIED
Capsules: 250 mg

ACTION
Chelates copper and increases its urinary excretion.

ONSET, PEAK, DURATION
Unknown.

INDICATIONS & DOSAGE
Wilson's disease in patients who cannot tolerate penicillamine –
Adults: 750 to 1,250 mg P.O. daily in two, three, or four divided doses. Dosage may then be increased up to 2,000 mg daily, p.r.n.
Children age 12 and under: 500 to 750 mg P.O. daily in two, three, or four divided doses. Dosage may then be increased up to 1,500 mg daily, p.r.n.
The optimal long-term maintenance dosage should be determined q 6 to 12 months, according to serum copper analysis.

ADVERSE REACTIONS
Hematologic: iron-deficiency anemia.
Other: hypersensitivity reactions (rash), fever.

INTERACTIONS
Mineral supplements, including iron: may block trientine absorption. Administer at least 2 hours apart.

CONTRAINDICATIONS
Contraindicated in patients with hypersensitivity to the drug.

NURSING CONSIDERATIONS
• Patients (especially women) should be closely monitored for evidence of iron-deficiency anemia throughout therapy.
• Observe patients for signs of hypersensitivity reactions, such as skin rash.
• Tell patients to take trientine on an empty stomach at least 1 hour before

or 2 hours after meals, and at least 1 hour apart from any other drug, food, or milk.

• Tell patients to swallow capsules whole with water and not to open or chew them.

• If capsule is accidentally opened and contents spilled on skin, tell patients to wash site thoroughly. Exposure to capsule contents may cause contact dermatitis.

• Tell patients to take their temperature every night and report any fevers or skin eruptions, especially during the first month of therapy.

• Urge patients to faithfully follow trientine regimen and low-copper diet as prescribed.

abciximab
acetohydroxamic acid
alglucerase
aminoglutethimide
aprotinin
benzoyl peroxide cleansers
benzoyl peroxide creams
benzoyl peroxide gels
benzoyl peroxide lotions
calcipotriene
capsaicin
cisapride
clomiphene citrate
cysteamine bitartrate
diazoxide, oral
etretinate
finasteride
gallium nitrate
imiglucerase
isotretinoin
levocarnitine
levomethadyl acetate
   hydrochloride
masoprocol
mesalamine
mesna
methoxsalen
minoxidil (topical)
nimodipine
olsalazine sodium
pamidronate disodium
ritodrine hydrochloride
sodium benzoate and sodium
   phenylacetate
strontium 89 (⁸⁹SR) chloride
sulfasalazine
tiopronin
tretinoin
trilostane

COMBINATION PRODUCTS
None.

abciximab
ReoPro

Pregnancy Risk Category: C

HOW SUPPLIED
Injection: 2 mg/ml

ACTION
Binds to the glycoprotein 11b/111a
(GP11b/111a) receptor of human
platelets and inhibits platelet aggregation.

ONSET, PEAK, DURATION
Onset and peak occur almost immediately after I.V. infusion. Effects on
platelet aggregation persist for about
48 hours.

INDICATIONS & DOSAGE
*Adjunct to percutaneous transluminal
coronary angioplasty (PTCA) or atherectomy for the prevention of acute
cardiac ischemic complications in patients at high risk for abrupt closure of
the treated coronary vessel –*
Adults: 0.25 mg/kg as an I.V. bolus
administered 10 to 60 minutes before
start of PTCA or atherectomy, followed by a continuous I.V. infusion of
10 mcg/minute for 12 hours.

ADVERSE REACTIONS
CNS: hypoesthesia, confusion.
CV: *hypotension,* bradycardia, pe-
ripheral edema.
EENT: abnormal vision.
GI: *nausea, vomiting.*
Hematologic: bleeding, thrombocy-
topenia, anemia, leukocytosis.
Respiratory: pleural effusion, pleu-
risy, pneumonia.
Other: pain.

---

*Liquid form contains alcohol.   *Common* reactions are in italics; *life-threatening,* in bold italics.
**May contain tartrazine.

INTERACTIONS
Antiplatelet agents, heparin, NSAIDs, other anticoagulants, thrombolytics: increased risk of bleeding. Monitor patient closely.

CONTRAINDICATIONS
Contraindicated in patients with hypersensitivity to any component of the drug or to murine proteins; in those with active internal bleeding, recent (within 6 weeks) GI or GU bleeding of clinical significance, history of CVA within past 2 years or CVA with significant residual neurologic deficit, bleeding diathesis, thrombocytopenia (less than 100,000/mm³), recent (within 6 weeks) major surgery or trauma, intracranial neoplasm, intracranial arteriovenous malformation, intracranial aneurysm, severe uncontrolled hypertension, or history of vasculitis; when oral anticoagulants have been administered within past 7 days unless prothrombin time is equal to or less than 1.2 times control; or with use of I.V. dextran before PTCA or intent to use it during PTCA.

NURSING CONSIDERATIONS
• Use with caution in patients at increased risk for bleeding. Patients at risk include those who weigh less than 75 kg, are over age 65, have a history of GI disease, or are receiving thrombolytic agents. Conditions that also increase the patient's risk of bleeding include PTCA within 12 hours of onset of symptoms for acute MI, prolonged PTCA (lasting more than 70 minutes), or failed PTCA. Heparin used in conjunction with abciximab also may contribute to the risk of bleeding.
• Know that patients who are at risk for abrupt closure and thus would be candidates for abciximab therapy include those undergoing PTCA with at least one of the following conditions: unstable angina or a non-Q wave MI, an acute Q wave MI within 12 hours of onset of symptoms, the presence of two type B lesions in the artery to be dilated, the presence of one type B lesion in the artery to be dilated in a woman over age 65 or in a patient with diabetes, the presence of one type C lesion in the artery to be dilated, or angioplasty of an infarct-related lesion within 7 days of MI.
• Be aware that abciximab is intended for use with aspirin and heparin.
• Keep epinephrine, dopamine, theophylline, antihistamines, and corticosteroids readily available in case anaphylaxis occurs.
• **I.V. use:** Inspect solution for particulate matter before administration. If any visibly opaque particles are found, discard solution and obtain new vial. Withdraw the necessary amount of abciximab for I.V. bolus injection through a sterile, nonpyrogenic, low-protein-binding 0.2- or 0.22-micron filter into a syringe. The I.V. bolus should be administered 10 to 60 minutes before the procedure.
• Withdraw 4.5 ml of abciximab for continuous I.V. infusion through a sterile, nonpyrogenic, low-protein-binding 0.2-or 0.22-micron filter into a syringe. Inject into 250 ml of sterile 0.9% sodium chloride solution or 5% dextrose and infuse at a rate of 17 ml/hour for 12 hours via a continuous infusion pump equipped with an in-line filter. Discard the unused portion at the end of the 12-hour infusion.
• Administer abciximab in a separate I.V. line; no other medication should be added to the infusion solution.
• Monitor the patient closely for bleeding. Bleeding associated with therapy falls into two broad categories: that observed at the arterial access site used for cardiac catheterization and internal bleeding involving the GI or GU tract, or retroperitoneal sites.
• Institute bleeding precautions. Maintain patient on bed rest for 6 to 8 hours following sheath removal or

discontinuation of abciximab infusion, whichever is later. Minimize or avoid, if possible, arterial and venous punctures; I.M. injections; use of urinary catheters, nasogastric tubes, or automatic blood pressure cuffs; and nasotracheal intubation.

acetohydroxamic acid
Lithostat

Pregnancy Risk Category: X

HOW SUPPLIED
Tablets (scored): 250 mg

ACTION
Prevents formation of renal stones by inhibiting bacterial urease activity.

ONSET, PEAK, DURATION
Onset and duration unknown. Serum levels peak within 15 to 60 minutes.

INDICATIONS & DOSAGE
Urinary tract infection caused by kidney stones –
Adults: 250 mg P.O. t.i.d. or q.i.d. at 6- to 8-hour intervals when the stomach is empty. Maximum daily dosage is 1.5 g.
Children: 10 mg/kg/day P.O. in two or three divided doses.

ADVERSE REACTIONS
CNS: *mild headache, depression, anxiety, nervousness.*
CV: phlebitis, palpitations.
GI: *nausea, vomiting, diarrhea, constipation, anorexia.*
Hematologic: *hemolytic anemia.*
Skin: *nonpruritic, macular rash on arms and face.*
Other: alopecia, deep vein thrombosis, malaise.

INTERACTIONS
Methenamine: may produce synergistic effects.
Oral iron supplements: reduced absorption of acetohydroxamic acid.

Check with the doctor, who may request that iron be administered I.M.

CONTRAINDICATIONS
Contraindicated in patients whose physical state and disease are amenable to surgery and appropriate antibiotics, in patients whose urine is infected by nonurease-producing organisms, during pregnancy, and in patients with poor renal function.

NURSING CONSIDERATIONS
• Monitor CBC, including reticulocyte count, after 2 weeks of therapy, then at 3-month intervals for duration of treatment, as ordered. If laboratory findings indicate hemolytic anemia, discontinue drug and notify doctor.
• Anticipate using a reduced dosage in renal impairment.
• Be aware that a negative Coombs' test for hemolytic anemia has occurred in patients receiving acetohydroxamic acid.
• Keep in mind that patients may also be given methenamine to enhance response to acetohydroxamic acid.
• Monitor for skin rash, more common during prolonged use and with concomitant use of alcoholic beverages. The rash appears 30 to 45 minutes after ingestion of alcoholic beverages and disappears spontaneously in 30 to 60 minutes.
• Although skin rash doesn't usually require treatment, advise patients to avoid alcohol.

alglucerase
(glucocerebrosidase,
glucosylceramidase,
glucocerebrosidase-beta-
glucosidase)
Ceredase

Pregnancy Risk Category: C

HOW SUPPLIED
Injection: 10 IU/ml in 5 ml bottles, 80 IU/ml in 5-ml bottles

---

*Liquid form contains alcohol.   *Common* reactions are in italics; *life-threatening,* in bold italics.
**May contain tartrazine.

ACTION
Reduces glycolipid accumulation by acting as a catalyst for the hydrolysis of glucocerebroside to glucose and ceramide — part of the normal degradation pathway for lipids.

ONSET, PEAK, DURATION
Onset and duration unknown. Serum levels peak in 1 hour following I.V. administration.

INDICATIONS & DOSAGE
Long-term endogenous enzyme (glucosylceramidase) replacement therapy in confirmed Type I Gaucher's disease —
Adults and children: individualized dosage; initially, 2.5 units/kg I.V. three times weekly up to as much as 60 units/kg once a week or as infrequently as q 4 weeks. Infusion should run over 1 to 2 hours. Once response is established, dosage reduced for maintenance at 3- to 6-month intervals.

ADVERSE REACTIONS
GI: abdominal discomfort, nausea, vomiting.
Other: chills, slight fever, discomfort, burning, swelling at injection site.

INTERACTIONS
None significant.

CONTRAINDICATIONS
None.

NURSING CONSIDERATIONS
• Use cautiously in patients with symptoms of hypersensitivity to drug. Know that pre-treatment with antihistamines may be required. Also use cautiously in patients with androgen sensitive malignancies (e.g. prostate cancer) and patients with known prior allergies to hCG.
• **I.V. use:** To prepare solution, dilute appropriate amount of alglucerase with 0.9% sodium chloride solution to a final volume not to exceed 100 ml. Use an in-line particulate filter during administration. Because alglucerase is preservative-free, use immediately.
• Do not shake bottle. Shaking may denature the glycoprotein and render it biologically inactive.
• Monitor response parameters to use lowest effective dose.
• Be aware that alglucerase is purified from a large pool of human placental tissue collected from selected donors. Although the risk of viral contamination from slow-acting or latent viruses is believed to be remote, the risks and benefits of therapy must be carefully assessed before administration.
• Keep in mind that hemoglobin levels may normalize after 6 months of therapy. Improved mineralization may also occur after prolonged treatment.
• Store at 39° F (4° C). Do not use solution that is discolored or that contains particles.

aminoglutethimide
Cytadren

Pregnancy Risk Category: D

HOW SUPPLIED
Tablets: 250 mg

ACTION
Blocks conversion of cholesterol to delta-5-pregnenolone in the adrenal cortex, inhibiting the synthesis of adrenal steroids.

ONSET, PEAK, DURATION
Suprression of adrenal function occurs in 3 to 5 days. Time to peak concentration occurs in 1 ½ hours. Adrenal function usually returns to normal 1 ½ to 3 days after discontinuing drug, although recovery may take a year or longer after prolonged therapy.

INDICATIONS & DOSAGE

Suppression of adrenal function in Cushing's syndrome and adrenal cancer —

Adults: 250 mg q.i.d. at 6-hour intervals. Dosage may be increased in increments of 250 mg daily q 1 to 2 weeks to a maximum daily dosage of 2 g.

ADVERSE REACTIONS

CNS: *drowsiness,* headache, dizziness.
CV: hypotension, tachycardia.
GI: nausea, anorexia.
Hematologic: transient leukopenia, *agranulocytosis.*
Skin: *morbilliform rash,* pruritus, urticaria.
Other: fever, myalgia, adrenal insufficiency, masculinization, hirsutism, hypothyroidism.

INTERACTIONS

Dexamethasone, medroxyprogesterone: increased hepatic metabolism of these agents.
Ethanol: may potentiate the effects of aminoglutethimide.
Oral anticoagulants: decreased anticoagulant effect.

CONTRAINDICATIONS

Contraindicated in patients hypersensitive to the drug or glutethimide.

NURSING CONSIDERATIONS

• Perform baseline hematologic studies, as ordered.
• Monitor blood pressure frequently.
• Monitor CBC periodically, as ordered.
• Be aware that drug may cause adrenal hypofunction, especially under stressful conditions, such as surgery, trauma, or acute illness. Patients may need mineralocorticoid supplements to treat hyponatremia and orthostatic hypotension. Glucocorticoid replacement may also be necessary, especially in patients with breast cancer. Monitor such patients carefully.
• Know that drug may cause a decrease in thyroid hormone production. Monitor thyroid function studies.
• Warn patients to watch for signs of infection (fever, sore throat, fatigue) and bleeding (easy bruising, nosebleeds, bleeding gums, melena). Take temperature daily.
• Warn patients to avoid activities that require alertness and good motor coordination until CNS effects of the drug are known.
• Advise patients to stand up slowly to minimize orthostatic hypotension.
• Tell patients to report if rash persists for more than 8 days. Reassure patients that drowsiness, nausea, and loss of appetite usually diminish within 2 weeks after start of aminoglutethimide therapy, but advise them to notify the doctor if these symptoms persist.

aprotinin
Trasylol

Pregnancy Risk Category: B

HOW SUPPLIED

Injection: 10,000 KIU(kallikrein inactivator units)/ml (1.4 mg/ml) in 100-ml and 200-ml vials

ACTION

A naturally occurring protease inhibitor that acts as a systemic hemostatic agent, decreasing bleeding and turnover of coagulation factors. It inhibits fibrinolysis by affecting kallikrein and plasmin, prevents triggering of the contact phase of the coagulation pathway, and increases the resistance of platelets to damage from mechanical injury and high plasmin levels that occur during cardiopulmonary bypass.

ONSET, PEAK, DURATION

Unknown.

---

*Liquid form contains alcohol.   *Common* reactions are in italics; *life-threatening,* in bold italics.
**May contain tartrazine.

INDICATIONS & DOSAGE

To reduce blood loss or the need for transfusion in patients undergoing coronary artery bypass grafts –
Adults: started with 10,000 units test dose at least 10 minutes before the loading dose. If no allergic reaction is evident, anesthesia may be induced while the loading dose of 2 million units is given slowly over 20 to 30 minutes. When the loading dose is complete, sternotomy may be performed. Before bypass is initiated, the cardiopulmonary bypass circuit is primed with 2 million units of the drug by replacing an aliquot of the priming fluid with the drug. A continuous infusion at a rate of 500,000 units/hour is then given until the patient leaves the operating room.

ADVERSE REACTIONS

CV: *cardiac arrest, CHF, MI, heart failure, ventricular tachycardia,* atrial fibrillation, atrial flutter, hypotension, supraventricular tachycardia.
GU: nephrotoxicity
Respiratory: pneumonia, respiratory disorder, *bronchospasm.*
Other: hypersensitivity reactions, *anaphylaxis,* fever.

INTERACTIONS

None significant.

CONTRAINDICATIONS

Contraindicated in patients hypersensitive to beef because the drug is prepared from bovine lung.

NURSING CONSIDERATIONS

• Use drug cautiously and monitor patients closely for hypersensitivity reaction. Patients may experience anaphylaxis after the full therapeutic dose even if they remained asymptomatic after the test dose. If symptoms of hypersensitivity occur (skin eruptions, itching, dyspnea, nausea, tachycardia), discontinue the infusion immediately, make doctor aware, and provide supportive treatment.

• Obtain history of possible allergies. Patients with a history of allergies to drugs or other substances may be at higher risk of developing an allergic reaction to aprotinin.

• Be prepared to administer a test dose. Test dose is particularly important in patients who have previously received the drug because they have a higher risk of anaphylaxis. In such patients, pretreat with an antihistamine, as ordered.

• **I.V. use:** Keep in mind that aprotinin is incompatible with amino acids, corticosteroids, fat emulsions, heparin, and tetracyclines. Don't add any drugs to the I.V. container and use a separate I.V. line.

• Administer all doses through a central line.

• To avoid hypotension, make sure patients are supine when the loading dose is given.

• Monitor laboratory studies, as ordered. Aprotinin will prolong activated clotting time and PTT. It may increase CK and transaminase levels and may falsely prolong whole blood clotting times when determined by surface activation methods, such as the Hemachron method.

• Monitor patients for increased serum creatinine levels and other signs of nephrotoxicity. If nephrotoxicity occurs, it is usually mild and reversible.

• Store between 2° and 25° C (36° and 77° F). Protect from freezing.

---

benzoyl peroxide cleansers

Benzac W Wash 5, Benzac W Wash 10, Desquam-X 5 Wash, Desquam-X 10 Wash, Fostex 10% BPO Cleansing◇, Fostex 10% BPO Wash◇, Oxy-10 Wash◇, PanOxyl 5◇, PanOxyl 10◇

---

benzoyl peroxide creams
Acne-Aid◇, Clearasil Maximum Strength◇, Cuticura Acne◇ Fostex 10% BPO Tinted◇, Oxy 10 Cover◇

benzoyl peroxide gels
Ben-Aqua 5, Ben-Aqua 10, Benzac 5, Benzac W 2½, Benzac W 5, Benzac W 10, 5 Benzagel, 10 Benzagel, Buf-Oxal 10◇, Clear By Design◇, Del Aqua 5◇, Del Aqua 10◇, Desquam-E, Desquam-X 2.5, Desquam-X 5, Desquam-X 10, Fostex 5% BPO◇, Fostex 10% BPO◇, PanOxyl 5, PanOxyl 10, PanOxyl AQ 2½, PanOxyl AQ 5, PanOxyl AQ 10, Persa-Gel, Persa-Gel W 5%, Persa-Gel W 10%, Xerac BP5◇, Xerac BP10◇, Zeroxin-5, Zeroxin-10

benzoyl peroxide lotions
Acne-10◇, Ben-Aqua 5◇, Benoxyl 5◇, Benoxyl 10◇, Clearasil 10◇, Loroxide◇, Oxy 5◇, Oxy 10◇, Vanoxide◇

Pregnancy Risk Category: C

HOW SUPPLIED
Cream: 5%◇, 10%◇
Gel: 2.5%◇, 5%◇, 10%◇
Liquid cleanser: 5%, 10%◇
Lotion: 5%◇, 5.5%◇, 10%◇
Soap (bar): 5%◇, 10%◇

ACTION
Unknown. Has antimicrobial and comedolytic activity.

ONSET, PEAK, DURATION
Unknown.

INDICATIONS & DOSAGE
Acne –
Adults and children: apply once daily to t.i.d., depending on tolerance and effect.

ADVERSE REACTIONS
Skin: stinging on application, warmth, painful irritation, pruritus, vesicles, allergic contact dermatitis.

INTERACTIONS
Abrasives, medical soaps and cleansers, acne preparations and preparations containing peeling agents, topical alcohol preparations (including cosmetics, after-shave, cologne): cumulative irritation of skin or excessive drying of skin. Use together cautiously.

CONTRAINDICATIONS
Contraindicated in patients sensitive to the drug or any its components.

NURSING CONSIDERATIONS
• Be prepared to initiate therapy with 2.5% or 5% preparation; change to 10% strength after 3 to 4 weeks or as tolerance develops and directed by doctor.
• Know that patients with fair skin or patients living in very dry climates should begin with one application daily.
• Tell patients to wash face thoroughly 20 to 30 minutes before applying.
• Warn patients not to use near eyes, on mucous membranes, or on denuded or highly inflamed skin.
• Warn patients that drug may bleach hair or clothing.
• Tell patient to discontinue temporarily if dryness, redness, and peeling (occur 3 to 4 days after starting treatment) cause considerable discomfort and to check with doctor when drug should be resumed.
• Advise patients to discontinue use if painful irritation or vesicles develop and to notify doctor.

Liquid form contains alcohol.
**May contain tartrazine.
*Common reactions are in italics; **life-threatening,** in bold italics.*

calcipotriene
Dovonex

Pregnancy Risk Category: C

HOW SUPPLIED
Ointment: 0.005%

ACTION
A synthetic vitamin D₃ analogue that regulates the development and production of skin cells.

ONSET, PEAK, DURATION
Unknown.

INDICATIONS & DOSAGE
Moderate plaque psoriasis –
Adults: apply a thin layer to the affected area b.i.d. Rub in gently and completely.

ADVERSE REACTIONS
Skin: *burning, pruritus, irritation,* atrophy, dermatitis, dry skin, erythema, folliculitis, hyperpigmentation, peeling, rash, worsening of psoriasis.
Other: hypercalcemia.

INTERACTIONS
None significant.

CONTRAINDICATIONS
Contraindicated in patients hypersensitive to the drug or any components in the preparation. Also contraindicated in patients with hypercalcemia or evidence of vitamin D toxicity.

NURSING CONSIDERATIONS
• Use cautiously in breastfeeding patients.
• Use cautiously in elderly patients; they may experience more severe adverse skin reactions.
• Advise patients to apply only a thin layer of the ointment. Transient elevations of serum calcium have been reported, especially when excess dosage is applied.

• Advise patients not to use the drug on the face, in the eyes, orally, or vaginally. Tell them to wash their hands after applying the ointment.
• Tell patients to discontinue the drug and call the doctor if the drug irritates lesions or surrounding uninvolved skin.

capsaicin
Axsain◇, Zostrix◇, Zostrix-HP 0.075%

Pregnancy Risk Category: NR

HOW SUPPLIED
Cream: 0.025%◇ (Zostrix◇), 0.075%◇ (Axsain◇)

ACTION
Unknown. May deplete substance P, the principal neurotransmitter for pain, in peripheral type C sensory fibers.

ONSET, PEAK, DURATION
Unknown.

INDICATIONS & DOSAGE
Temporary relief of pain after herpes zoster infections, neuralgias, such as postsurgical pain and painful diabetic neuropathy; pain associated with osteoarthritis or rheumatoid arthritis –
Adults and children over 2 years: applied to affected areas not more than q.i.d.

ADVERSE REACTIONS
Skin: redness, *stinging or burning on application.*

INTERACTIONS
None significant.

CONTRAINDICATIONS
Contraindicated in patients hypersensitive to the drug.

NURSING CONSIDERATIONS
• Warn patient to avoid getting drug in eyes or on broken skin.
• Advise patient not to bandage area tightly after applying drug.
• Tell patients to wash hands after applying drug.
• Inform patient that transient burning or stinging with application is usually evident at initial therapy but will decrease with cautious use. However, this effect will persist in patients who use the drug less frequently than three times a day.
• Tell patients who are self-medicating with capsaicin to contact the doctor if symptoms persist beyond 2 to 4 weeks or resolve and shortly reappear.

cisapride
Propulsid

Pregnancy Risk Category: C

HOW SUPPLIED
Tablets: 10 mg

ACTION
Stimulates serotonin-4 (5-HT₄) receptors, enhancing the release of acetylcholine at the myenteric plexus and increasing GI motility.

ONSET, PEAK, DURATION
Onset occurs in 30 to 60 minutes. Plasma levels peak within 1 to 2 hours. Duration unknown.

INDICATIONS & DOSAGE
Symptoms of nocturnal heartburn caused by gastroesophageal reflux disease –
Adults: initially, 10 mg P.O. q.i.d. 15 minutes before meals and h.s. If response is inadequate, increased to 20 mg q.i.d.

ADVERSE REACTIONS
CNS: *headache.*
CV: tachycardia.

GI: *diarrhea, abdominal pain,* nausea, constipation, flatulence, dyspepsia.
GU: frequency, urgency, vaginitis.
Respiratory: rhinitis, sinusitis, cough.
Skin: rash, pruritus.
Other: flulike symptoms, pain, fever.

INTERACTIONS
Anticholinergics: decreased effectiveness of cisapride. Avoid concomitant use.
Anticoagulants: may increase clotting times. Monitor closely.
Benzodiazepines, ethanol: enhanced sedation. Avoid concomitant use.
Cimetidine, ranitidine: increased absorption of these agents; cimetidine increases cisapride levels. Use together cautiously.
Intraconazole, ketoconazole, I.V. miconazole, troleandomycin: increased cisapride levels which may cause ventricular arrhythmias. Avoid concomitant use.

CONTRAINDICATIONS
Contraindicated in patients hypersensitive to the drug. Also contraindicated in patients in whom increased GI motility may be harmful, such as those with mechanical obstruction, hemorrhage, or perforation of the GI tract.

NURSING CONSIDERATIONS
• Use cautiously in breastfeeding patients because small amounts of the drug are excreted in breast milk.
• Remind patients to avoid alcohol and sedatives while using this drug.
• Advise patients to immediately report any adverse effects to their doctor.

clomiphene citrate
Clomid, Serophene

Pregnancy Risk Category: NR

---

*Liquid form contains alcohol.   *Common* reactions are in italics; ***life-threatening,*** in bold italics.
**May contain tartrazine.

HOW SUPPLIED
Tablets: 50 mg

ACTION
Unknown. Appears to stimulate release of pituitary gonadotropins, follicle-stimulating hormone, and luteinizing hormone. This results in maturation of the ovarian follicle, ovulation, and development of the corpus luteum.

ONSET, PEAK, DURATION
Not clearly defined although ovulation usually occurs 4 to 10 days after last day of treatment; this period of time may vary by patient and for each cycle.

INDICATIONS & DOSAGE
To induce ovulation–
Adults: 50 to 100 mg P.O. daily for 5 days, starting any time; or 50 to 100 mg P.O. daily starting on day 5 of menstrual cycle (first day of menstrual flow is day 1). Repeated until conception occurs or until three courses of therapy are completed.

ADVERSE REACTIONS
CNS: headache, restlessness, insomnia, dizziness, light-headedness, depression, fatigue, tension.
CV: hypertension.
EENT: blurred vision, diplopia, scotoma, photophobia.
GI: nausea, vomiting, bloating, distention, increased appetite, weight gain.
GU: urinary frequency and polyuria; ovarian enlargement and cyst formation, which regress spontaneously when drug is stopped.
Skin: urticaria, rash, dermatitis.
Other: *hot flashes,* reversible alopecia, *breast discomfort, hyperglycemia.*

INTERACTIONS
None significant.

CONTRAINDICATIONS
Contraindicated during pregnancy and in patients with undiagnosed abnormal genital bleeding, ovarian cyst not due to polycystic ovarian syndrome, hepatic disease or dysfunction, uncontrolled thyroid or adrenal dysfunction, or presence of organic intracranial lesion (such as a pituitary tumor).

NURSING CONSIDERATIONS
• Tell patients there is a possibility of multiple births with this drug. Risk increases with higher doses.
• Teach patients to take and chart basal body temperature to ascertain whether ovulation has occurred.
• Reassure patients that ovulation generally occurs after the first course of therapy. If pregnancy does not occur, course of therapy may be repeated twice.
• Advise patients to stop drug and contact the doctor immediately if pregnancy is suspected because the drug may have teratogenic effect.
• Advise patients to stop drug and contact the doctor immediately if abdominal symptoms or pain occurs because these may indicate ovarian enlargement or ovarian cyst.
• Tell patients to report signs of impending visual toxicity – blurred vision, diplopia, scotoma, or photophobia – to the doctor immediately.
• Warn patients to avoid hazardous activities, such as driving or operating machinery, until CNS effects are known. Drug may cause dizziness or visual disturbances.

---

cysteamine bitartrate
Cystagon
Pregnancy Risk Category: C

HOW SUPPLIED
Capsules: 50 mg, 150 mg

ACTION
Reacts with cystine, thereby decreasing the cystine level in cells.

ONSET, PEAK, DURATION
Unknown.

INDICATIONS & DOSAGE
Management of nephropathic cystinosis —
Adults and children over age 12 and more than 110 lb: initially, one-fourth to one-sixth of the maintenance dosage, then increased gradually over 4 to 6 weeks to achieve maintenance dosage. Maintenance dosage is 2 g (free base) P.O. in four divided doses.
Children age 12 and under: initially, one-fourth to one-sixth of the maintenance dosage, then increased gradually over 4 to 6 weeks to achieve maintenance dosage. Maintenance dosage is 1.3 g/m² (free base) P.O. daily in four divided doses.

ADVERSE REACTIONS
CNS: *lethargy,* somnolence, encephalopathy, headache, seizures, ataxia, confusion, tremor, hyperkinesis, decreasing hearing, dizziness, jitteriness, nervousness, abnormal thinking, depression, emotional lability, hallucinations, nightmares.
CV: hypertension.
GI: *vomiting, anorexia, diarrhea,* nausea, abdominal pain, dyspepsia, constipation, gastroenteritis, duodenitis, duodenal ulcer.
Hepatic: abnormal liver function.
Hematologic: anemia, leukopenia.
Skin: *rash,* urticaria.
Other: *fever,* dehydration, bad breath.

INTERACTIONS
None known.

CONTRAINDICATIONS
Contraindicated in patients with hypersensitivity to the drug, cysteamine, or penicillamine.

NURSING CONSIDERATIONS
• Know that drug therapy should begin as soon as the diagnosis of nephropathic cystinosis has been confirmed by increased level of cystine in increased WBCs.
• Monitor patient for a rash. If one develops, notify the doctor because the drug will need to be withheld until the rash clears. The doctor may then restart the drug at a lower dosage and slowly titrate dosage to achieve therapeutic effect. However, if a severe rash (such as erythema multiforme bullosa or toxic epidermal necrolysis) develops, know that the drug should not be restarted.
• Monitor patient closely for adverse CNS or GI reactions. If any develop, notify the doctor because the dosage will need to be adjusted or the drug temporarily withheld.
• Monitor patient's CBC and liver function studies, as ordered, to detect adverse hematologic reactions. Notify the doctor if any laboratory abnormalities are present.
• Be aware that measurements of cystine level in leukocytes may be ordered because they are useful in determining adequate dosage and compliance. When the drug is well tolerated, the goal of therapy is to keep leukocyte cystine levels below 1 mmol/½ cystine/mg protein five to six hours after administration of the drug. Measurements should be done at least every 3 months.
• Know that patients with cystinosis taking cysteamine hydrochloride or phosphocysteamine solutions may be transferred to equimolar doses of the drug.
• Inform the patient and parents that dosage of cysteamine is based on the

---

*Liquid form contains alcohol.   *Common* reactions are in italics; ***life-threatening,*** in bold italics.
**May contain tartrazine.

patient's weight and that patient must follow doctor's directions exactly.
• Instruct the patient and parents that if a dose of the drug is missed, it should be taken as soon as possible. However, if it is within 2 hours of the next dose, patient should skip the missed dose and go back to the regular dosing schedule. Tell patient not to double the dose.
• Tell parents of a child under age 6 not to give the child the capsule to swallow because the child may choke or aspirate it. Instead, the capsule may be opened and the contents sprinkled on food or mixed in formula.
• Inform the patient or parent that supplements also will be given to replace electrolytes lost through the kidneys and that periodic blood tests will need to be performed to help determine the correct dosage of the drug. Compliance with these measures is extremely important for maximal effectiveness of the drug.
• Instruct the patient not to engage in hazardous activities (such as driving) until the drug's CNS effects are known.
• Advise patient and parents to store the drug in a dry place, away from light.

---

diazoxide, oral
Proglycem

Pregnancy Risk Category: C

HOW SUPPLIED
Capsules: 50 mg
Oral suspension: 50 mg/ml in 30-ml bottle

ACTION
Inhibits release of insulin from the pancreas and decreases peripheral utilization of glucose.

ONSET, PEAK, DURATION
Onset occurs in 1 hour. Peak unknown. Effects persist for 8 hours.

INDICATIONS & DOSAGE
Hypoglycemia from a variety of conditions resulting in hyperinsulinism—
Adults and children: 3 to 8 mg/kg P.O. daily, in three equally divided doses q 8 hours.
Infants and neonates: 8 to 15 mg/kg P.O. daily, in two or three equally divided doses q 8 to 12 hours.

ADVERSE REACTIONS
CV: arrhythmias.
EENT: diplopia.
GI: nausea, vomiting, anorexia, taste alteration.
Hematologic: leukopenia, thrombocytopenia.
Other: *severe hypertrichosis (hair growth) in 25% of adults and higher percentage of children; sodium and fluid retention, ketoacidosis and hyperosmolar nonketotic syndrome, hyperuricemia.*

INTERACTIONS
Alpha-adrenergic blockers: antagonism of diazoxide inhibition of insulin release. Avoid concomitant use.
Anticoagulants: increased anticoagulant effect. Adjust dosage of anticoagulant.
Antigout agents: increased serum uric acid. Adjust dosage of antigout agent.
Antihypertensive agents, peripheral vasodilators: additive hypotensive effects. Monitor blood pressure.
Beta-adrenergic blockers: increased hypotensive effect. Monitor blood pressure.
Hydantoin anticonvulsants: decreased anticonvulsant effects and decreased hyperglycemic effect of diazoxide. Don't use together.
Thiazide diuretics: may potentiate hyperglycemic, hyperuricemic, and hypotensive effects. Monitor appropriate laboratory values.

CONTRAINDICATIONS
Contraindicated in patients hypersensitive to the drug or other thiazides

---

and in patients with functional hypoglycemia.

NURSING CONSIDERATIONS
• Monitor urine regularly for glucose and ketones; report any abnormalities to the doctor.
• If not effective after 2 or 3 weeks, be prepared to stop drug.
• Know that drug's most important use is to manage hypoglycemia from hyperinsulinism in infants and children.
• Be aware that oral diazoxide does not significantly lower blood pressure in the dosages used to treat hypoglycemia.
• Explain importance of following dietary restrictions for successful therapy.
• Reassure patients that hair growth on arms and forehead is a common adverse reaction that subsides when drug treatment is completed.
• Advise patients to report to the doctor any adverse reactions, including excessive thirst, fruity breath odor, or urinary frequency.

---

etretinate
Tegison

Pregnancy Risk Category: X

HOW SUPPLIED
Capsules: 10 mg, 25 mg

ACTION
Unknown. Thought to inhibit ornithine decarboxylase, an enzyme that regulates cell growth and differentiation. May also block neutrophil migration into the epidermis.

ONSET, PEAK, DURATION
Onset and duration unknown. Peak concentration occurs in 2 to 6 hours.

INDICATIONS & DOSAGE
Severe recalcitrant psoriasis, including erythrodermia and generalized pustular types in patients unresponsive to standard therapy (topical tar plus UVB light, psoralens plus UVA light, systemic corticosteroids, and methotrexate)—
Adults: initially, 0.75 to 1 mg/kg P.O. daily in divided doses. Maximum initial dosage is 1.5 mg/kg daily. After initial response, maintenance dosage is 0.5 to 0.75 mg/kg daily.

ADVERSE REACTIONS
CNS: *benign intracranial hypertension (pseudotumor cerebri), fatigue, headache,* dizziness, lethargy.
CV: thrombosis, edema.
EENT: *eye pain, blurred vision, dry eyes,* photosensitivity, decreased night vision.
GI: *appetite change, nausea, sore tongue, chapped lips, dry mouth.*
Hematologic: **blood dyscrasia,** anemia, altered PT.
Hepatic: **hepatitis,** elevated liver enzymes.
GU: *WBCs in urine,* proteinuria, hematuria.
Respiratory: dyspnea.
Skin: *peeling, pruritus.*
Other: *bone pain, hypokalemia or hyperkalemia, hyperlipidemia.*

INTERACTIONS
Ethanol: increased risk of hypertriglyceridemia. Avoid concomitant use.
Hepatotoxic medications (including methotrexate): increased risk of hepatotoxicity. Monitor closely.
Tetracyclines: increased risk of pseudotumor cerebri. Avoid concomitant use.
Vitamin A: additive toxic effects. Avoid concomitant use.

CONTRAINDICATIONS
Contraindicated in patients who are pregnant, who intend to become pregnant, or who may not use reliable contraception during and after treatment (drug causes severe birth defects).

---

*Liquid form contains alcohol. *Common* reactions are in italics; **life-threatening,** in bold italics.
**May contain tartrazine.

NURSING CONSIDERATIONS

• Monitor liver function tests every 1 to 2 weeks for the first 1 to 2 months of therapy, and every 1 to 3 months thereafter, as ordered. Suspected hepatotoxicity requires discontinuation of drug.

• Monitor blood lipids every 1 to 2 weeks during treatment, as ordered.

• Know that significant residual blood levels of etretinate have been reported as long as 2.9 years after discontinuation of treatment. Consequently, the period of time after treatment during which pregnancy must be avoided to prevent teratogenicity is unknown.

• Be aware that women of childbearing age must not receive etretinate unless pregnancy is excluded by a pregnancy test within 2 weeks before initiating therapy. Therapy may begin on second or third day of next normal menstrual period.

• Monitor patient for pseudotumor cerebri. If symptoms occur, immediately check for papilledema. If present, discontinue drug immediately and notify doctor.

• Warn patients to use effective contraception for 1 month before therapy begins, during treatment, and for an indefinite time after treatment is discontinued.

• Advise patients to take drug with milk or fatty food to enhance absorption.

• Advise patients never to double the dose. Tell them to take a missed dose as soon as possible. If it's nearly time for the next dose, skip missed dose and resume schedule.

• Warn patients not to take vitamin A supplements, to avoid possible additive adverse reactions.

• Reassure patients that transient exacerbation of psoriasis is common during beginning of therapy.

• Advise patients to expect dry skin and possible difficulty tolerating contact lenses during treatment.

• Tell patients to avoid excess bright sun and to use a sunblock to prevent photosensitivity reactions.

• Advise patients to use ice or sugarless hard candy or gum for dry mouth and to check with the dentist if this continues beyond 2 weeks.

• Advise patients to report visual difficulties.

• Advise diabetic patients to monitor blood glucose closely. Adjustments of hypoglycemic medications may be necessary.

• Tell patients to report possible early signs of pseudotumor cerebri — headache, nausea and vomiting, and visual disturbances — to the doctor promptly.

---

finasteride
Proscar

Pregnancy Risk Category: X

HOW SUPPLIED
Tablets: 5 mg

ACTION
Competitively inhibits steroid 5α-reductase, an enzyme responsible for formation of the potent androgen 5α-dihydrotestosterone (DHT) from testosterone. Because DHT influences development of the prostate gland, decreasing levels of this hormone in adult males should relieve the symptoms associated with benign prostatic hyperplasia (BPH).

ONSET, PEAK, DURATION
Osnet unknown. Serum levels peak in 1 to 2 hours. Effects persist for 24 hours after single dose; about 2 weeks after withdrawal of therapy.

INDICATIONS & DOSAGE
Symptomatic BPH —
Adults: 5 mg P.O. daily.

ADVERSE REACTIONS
GU: impotence, decreased volume of ejaculate.

Other: decreased libido.

INTERACTIONS
Theophylline: may increase theophylline clearance and decrease theophylline half-life. Monitor theophylline levels.

CONTRAINDICATIONS
Contraindicated in patients hypersensitive to the drug. Know that although drug is not used in women, manufacturer indicates pregnancy as a contraindication.

NURSING CONSIDERATIONS
• Before therapy, know that patient should be evaluated for conditions that might mimic BPH, including hypotonic bladder; prostate cancer, infection, or stricture; or relevant neurologic conditions.
• Anticipate baseline and periodic digital rectal examinations. Drug will decrease serum prostate-specific antigen (PSA) levels, even in prostate cancer. However, in clinical trials, drug didn't appear to decrease the rate of prostate cancer detection.
• Carefully monitor patients who have a large residual urine volume or severely diminished urine flow. Know that these patients may not be candidates for finasteride therapy.
• Carefully evaluate sustained increases in serum PSA levels, which could indicate noncompliance with therapy.
• Be aware that although drug's elimination rate is decreased in elderly patients, dosage adjustments aren't necessary.
• Because it's impossible to identify which patients will respond to finasteride, know that a minimum of 6 months of therapy may be necessary.
• Keep in mind that the long-term effects on the complications of BPH, including acute urinary obstruction, and incidence of surgery are unknown.
• Warn women who are or may become pregnant not to handle crushed tablets because of risk of adverse effects on a male fetus.
• Caution patients whose sexual partner is or may become pregnant to discontinue drug or take precautions to avoid exposing her to his semen.
• Reassure patients that finasteride may decrease volume of ejaculate but doesn't appear to impair normal sexual function. However, impotence and decreased libido have occurred in less than 4% of patients.

---

gallium nitrate
Ganite

Pregnancy Risk Category: C

HOW SUPPLIED
Injection: 25 mg/ml

ACTION
Unknown. Appears to reduce hypercalcemia by inhibiting resorption of bone and reducing bone turnover in patients with increased bone turnover.

ONSET, PEAK, DURATION
Onset and peak unknown. Effects persist for 6 days.

INDICATIONS & DOSAGE
Symptomatic, unresponsive hypercalcemia caused by cancer—
Adults: 200 mg/m^2 as a continuous I.V. infusion daily for 5 consecutive days or until serum calcium is normal. Lower doses (100 mg/m^2) may be given to patients with mild hypercalcemia.

ADVERSE REACTIONS
CNS: lethargy, confusion.
CV: tachycardia, lower extremity edema, decreased mean systolic and diastolic blood pressures.
EENT: visual or hearing impairment, acute optic neuritis.
GI: nausea and vomiting, diarrhea, constipation.

---

*Liquid form contains alcohol. *Common* reactions are in italics; *life-threatening,* in bold italics.
**May contain tartrazine.

GU: *acute renal failure, increased BUN and creatinine levels.*
Hematologic: anemia, leukopenia.
Respiratory: dyspnea, crackles and rhonchi, pulmonary infiltrates, pleural effusion.
Other: *hypophosphatemia, hypocalcemia, decreased serum bicarbonate.*

INTERACTIONS

Nephrotoxic drugs, such as aminoglycosides or amphotericin B: increased risk of nephrotoxicity. Avoid concomitant use.

CONTRAINDICATIONS

Contraindicated in patients with severe renal impairment.

NURSING CONSIDERATIONS

• Make sure that patients are adequately hydrated, either with oral fluids or I.V. sodium chloride solution, as ordered, before using drug. Establish adequate urine flow (2 liters/day) before treatment. Diuretic therapy is not recommended before correction of hypovolemia. Avoid overhydration, especially in patients with decreased CV function.
• **I.V. use:** Dilute daily dose in 1 liter of 0.9% sodium chloride injection or D_5W. Discard unused portion (drug contains no preservatives).
• Know that rapid I.V. infusion or dosage over 200 mg/m² may increase risk of nephrotoxicity or cause nausea and vomiting.
• Monitor hydration status during infusion.
• Monitor BUN and serum creatinine levels, as ordered, during therapy. Discontinue drug if serum creatinine rises above 2.5 mg/dl and notify doctor.
• Carefully monitor fluid intake and output and renal function, as ordered. Short-term therapy with I.V. calcium may also be needed. Overdosage is usually treated with vigorous hydra-

tion, sometimes with diuretics, for 2 to 3 days.
• In patients who require treatment with a potentially nephrotoxic drug, such as an aminoglycoside, be prepared to discontinue gallium nitrate therapy and continue hydration for several days after administration of the nephrotoxic drug, as ordered. Monitor renal function closely.
• Monitor serum calcium levels, as ordered, and assess patients for signs of hypocalcemia, including a positive Chvostek's sign. If hypocalcemia occurs, discontinue drug and notify doctor. Treatment of hypocalcemia may be required.
• Be aware that transient hypophosphatemia is common. Patients may require oral phosphorus supplements.
• Advise patients to report hearing or vision problems. In early clinical trials, a few patients experienced hearing loss and optic neuritis after high-dose gallium nitrate therapy when combined with investigational antineoplastic agents.

imiglucerase

Cerezyme

Pregnancy Risk Category: C

HOW SUPPLIED

Injection: 200 units/vial

ACTION

Catalyzes the hydrolysis of glucocerebroside to glucose and ceramide (part of the normal degradation pathway for lipids) and thus prevents the sequelae of Gaucher's disease, which normally occur as a result of the accumulation of glucocerebroside.

ONSET, PEAK, DURATION

Onset and duration unknown. Levels peak in 1 hour.

INDICATIONS & DOSAGE
Long-term endogenous enzyme (gluco-sylceramidase) replacement therapy in confirmed Type I Gaucher's disease –
Adults and children: dosage individualized; initially, up to 60 U/kg I.V. administered over 1 to 2 hours. Frequency of dosing typically is once q 2 weeks, but may range from three times weekly to once monthly, depending on severity of the disease. Dosage may be reduced for maintenance therapy, at intervals of 3 to 6 months, while response parameters are carefully monitored.

ADVERSE REACTIONS
CNS: headache, dizziness.
CV: mild hypotension.
GI: nausea, abdominal discomfort.
GU: decreased urinary frequency.
Skin: pruritus, rash.
Other: hypersensitivity reaction.

INTERACTIONS
None known.

CONTRAINDICATIONS
None known.

NURSING CONSIDERATIONS
• Use with caution in patients who have exhibited symptoms of hypersensitivity to the product and in those who have previously been treated with alglucerase and who have developed antibody to alglucerase or exhibited symptoms of hypersensitivity to alglucerase.
• **I.V. use:** Reconstitute each vial with 5.1 ml of sterile water for injection USP. Inspect solution for particulate matter and discoloration before use; if either is present, do not use. Dilute solution further with 0.9% sodium chloride solution to a final volume of 100 to 200 ml. Because imiglucerase is preservative-free, use immediately. Administer by I.V. infusion over 1 to 2 hours.
• Know that when diluted to 50 ml,

imiglucerase has been shown to be stable for up to 24 hours when stored at 2° to 8° C (36° to 46° F).
• Monitor response parameters for doctor to determine lowest effective dosage.

---

isotretinoin
Accutane, Roaccutane‡

Pregnancy Risk Category: X

HOW SUPPLIED
Capsules: 10 mg, 20 mg, 40 mg

ACTION
Unknown. Thought to normalize keratinization, reversibly decrease size of sebaceous glands, and alter composition of sebum to a less viscous form that is less likely to cause follicular plugging.

ONSET, PEAK, DURATION
Onset and duration unknown. Plasma levels peak in about 3 hours.

INDICATIONS & DOSAGE
Severe recalcitrant nodular acne unresponsive to conventional therapy –
Adults and adolescents: 0.5 to 2 mg/kg P.O. daily in two divided doses for 15 to 20 weeks.

ADVERSE REACTIONS
CNS: headache, fatigue, *pseudotumor cerebri* (benign intracranial hypertension).
EENT: *conjunctivitis,* corneal deposits, dry eyes, visual disturbances.
GI: nonspecific GI symptoms, gum bleeding and inflammation, nausea, vomiting.
Hematologic: anemia, elevated platelet count.
Hepatic: elevated AST, ALT, and alkaline phosphatase levels.
Skin: *cheilosis, rash, dry skin,* peeling of palms and toes, skin infection, photosensitivity.
Other: *hypertriglyceridemia, muscu-*

---

loskeletal pain (skeletal hyperostosis), thinning of hair, hyperglycemia.

INTERACTIONS
Ethanol: increased risk of hypertriglyceridemia. Avoid concomitant use.
Tetracyclines: increased risk of pseudotumor cerebri. Avoid concomitant use.
Vitamin A, products containing vitamin A: increased toxic effects of isotretinoin. Don't use together without the doctor's permission.

CONTRAINDICATIONS
• Contraindicated in women of childbearing age unless patient has had a negative serum pregnancy test within 2 weeks before beginning therapy; will begin drug therapy on second or third day of next menstrual period; and will comply with stringent contraceptive measures for 1 month before therapy, during therapy, and for at least 1 month after therapy. *Severe fetal abnormalities may occur if used during pregnancy.*
• Also contraindicated in patients hypersensitive to parabens, which are used as preservatives.

NURSING CONSIDERATIONS
• Monitor baseline serum lipid studies and liver function tests prior to therapy, as ordered.
• Monitor serum lipid studies and liver function tests at regular intervals until response to drug is established, usually about 4 weeks.
• Monitor blood glucose regularly.
• Monitor CK levels in patients who participate in vigorous physical activity, as ordered.
• Know that most adverse reactions appear to be dose-related, occurring at dosages greater than 1 mg/kg daily. They are generally reversible when therapy is discontinued or dosage is reduced.
• Be aware that patients who experience headache, nausea and vomiting,

or visual disturbances should be screened for papilledema. Signs and symptoms of pseudotumor cerebri require immediate discontinuation of therapy and prompt neurologic intervention.
• Anticipate a second course of therapy, if needed, not to start for at least 8 weeks after completion of first course because improvement may continue after withdrawal of drug.
• Advise patients to take drug with or shortly after meals to ensure adequate absorption.
• Tell patients to immediately report any visual disturbances and bone, muscle, or joint pain.
• Warn patients that contact lenses may feel uncomfortable during isotretinoin therapy.
• Warn patients against using abrasives, medicated soaps and cleansers, acne preparations containing peeling agents, and topical alcohol preparations (including cosmetics, aftershave, cologne) because these agents cause cumulative irritation or excessive drying of skin.
• Tell patients to avoid prolonged exposure to the sun and to use sunblock. Drug may have additive effect if used with other agents that cause photosensitivity.

levocarnitine (L-carnitine)
Carnitor
Pregnancy Risk Category: B

HOW SUPPLIED
Tablets: 330 mg
Oral liquid: 100 mg/ml
Injection: 1 g/5 ml

ACTION
Facilitates transport of fatty acids into cellular mitochondria. The fatty acids are then used to produce energy.

ONSET, PEAK, DURATION
Unknown.

INDICATIONS & DOSAGE
Primary and secondary systemic carnitine deficiency–
Adults: 990 mg P.O. b.i.d. or t.i.d. Alternatively, 10 to 30 ml (1 to 3 g) of oral liquid daily.
Children: 50 to 100 mg/kg/day P.O. in divided doses.

All dosages depend on the clinical response. Higher dosages may be given. However, for children, maximum dosage is 3 g/day.
Acute and chronic treatment of secondary carnitine deficiency–
Adults: 50 mg/kg I.V. slowly over 2 to 3 minutes q 3 to 4 hours.

ADVERSE REACTIONS
GI: *nausea, vomiting, cramps, diarrhea.*
Other: body odor.

INTERACTIONS
D,L-carnitine (sold as vitamin B_T): inhibition of levocarnitine and possible deficiency. Avoid concomitant use.
Valproic acid: increased requirement for carnitine. Adjust dosage as ordered.

CONTRAINDICATIONS
None reported.

NURSING CONSIDERATIONS
• Give enteral liquid alone or dissolved in drinks or liquid food.
• Space doses evenly every 3 to 4 hours and give drug with or after meals, if possible.
• Use entire or partial contents of containers of liquid immediately after opening; discard any unused contents.
• Do not refrigerate solution.
• Monitor patient's tolerance during first week of therapy and after increasing dosage, as ordered.
• Monitor blood chemistries and plasma carnitine concentrations periodically, as ordered, as well as vital signs and patient's overall clinical condition.
• Tell patients to consume oral liquid slowly to minimize GI distress. If GI intolerance persists, dosage may have to be reduced.
• Warn patients to avoid "vitamin B_T" in health food stores. This will interact with the drug and render it ineffective.
• Caution patients not to share drug with others. Some people have used it to improve athletic performance.

---

levomethadyl acetate hydrochloride
ORLAAM
Controlled Substance Schedule II
Pregnancy Risk Category: C

HOW SUPPLIED
Oral solution: 10 mg/ml

ACTION
A synthetic opiate agonist structurally similar to methadone that suppresses symptoms of withdrawal in opiate-tolerant individuals by cross-substituting for opiate agonists. Long-term administration may produce sufficient tolerance to block the euphoric effects of opiate agonists.

ONSET, PEAK, DURATION
Onset and peak unknown. Effects persist for 48 to 72 hours.

INDICATIONS & DOSAGE
Opiate addiction–
Adults: dosage is highly individualized. Initially, 20 to 40 mg q 48 to 72 hours. Subsequent doses increased in increments of 5 to 10 mg at 48 to 72 hour intervals until steady state is reached, usually within 1 to 2 weeks. Most patients are stable on 60 to 90 mg three times a week.

---

*Liquid form contains alcohol.   *Common* reactions are in italics; *life-threatening*, in bold italics.
**May contain tartrazine.

ADVERSE REACTIONS

CNS: drowsiness, sedation.
CV: bradycardia, edema, prolonged QT interval.
EENT: blurred vision, rhinitis.
GI: *abdominal pain, diarrhea, constipation, dry mouth, nausea, vomiting.*
GU: *impotence, difficulty with ejaculation.*
Respiratory: *cough.*
Skin: *rash, diaphoresis.*
Other: yawning, arthralgia, asthenia, back pain, chills, flulike syndrome, malaise, abstinence syndrome with sudden withdrawal.

INTERACTIONS

Carbamazepine, phenobarbital, phenytoin, rifampin: increased hepatic enzyme activity; may increase levomethadyl's peak activity or shorten its duration of action. Monitor closely.
Cimetidine, erythromycin, ketoconazole: decreased hepatic enzyme activity; may decrease levomethadyl's peak activity or prolong its duration of action. Monitor closely.
Naloxone; pentazocine or other opioid agonist-antagonists: may precipitate abstinence syndrome. Don't use together.

CONTRAINDICATIONS

Contraindicated in patients hypersensitive to the drug.

NURSING CONSIDERATIONS

• Use cautiously in patients with cardiac conduction defects or with hepatic or renal failure.
• Be aware that levomethadyl is to be used only by certain licensed and approved clinics. There are no recognized clinical uses for the drug outside of addiction treatment programs. Levomethadyl may only be dispensed by treatment programs approved by the FDA, DEA, and designated state authority. By law, take-home doses are forbidden.
• If administering to women of child-

bearing age, anticipate monthly pregnancy tests. Patients should be switched to methadone if pregnancy occurs.
• Know that this drug should never be administered on a daily basis because of the risk of fatal overdose.
• Know that most patients can tolerate the 72-hour interval between weekly regimens. If withdrawal is a problem during the 72-hour interval, be prepared to increase the preceding dose or switch to an alternate-day schedule as ordered. Never give levomethadyl on 2 consecutive days; instead, give small supplemental doses of methadone. Consider the risk of drug diversion before giving patients take-home methadone.
• When used to replace methadone, keep in mind that the suggested initial dose is 1.2 to 1.3 times the daily methadone dose three times a week, not to exceed 120 mg. Adjust dosage according to clinical response as ordered. The crossover to methadone should be done in a single dose rather than decreasing doses of methadone and increasing doses of levomethadyl.

masoprocol
Actinex
Pregnancy Risk Category: B

HOW SUPPLIED
Cream: 10%

ACTION
Unknown. Has antiproliferative activity against keratinocytes in vitro.

ONSET, PEAK, DURATION
Unknown.

INDICATIONS & DOSAGE
Actinic (solar) keratoses –
Adults: a sufficient amount of cream to cover area b.i.d., in morning and evening, for 28 days.

ADVERSE REACTIONS
EENT: eye irritation.
Skin: *erythema, flaking, dryness, pruritus, burning, soreness,* bleeding, crusting, blistering, oozing, rash, irritation, stinging, tightness, tingling.

INTERACTIONS
None significant.

CONTRAINDICATIONS
Contraindicated in patients hypersensitive to the drug or any component of the formulation.

NURSING CONSIDERATIONS
• Drug contains sulfites, which may cause allergic reactions in sensitive individuals.
• Use cautiously near the eyes because drug may cause pain and burning if it comes into contact with them. If such contact occurs, rinse with plenty of water.
• Instruct patients to wash and dry the area, then gently massage in the cream (avoiding eyes and mucous membranes of nose and mouth) until evenly distributed; and to wash hands after applying drug with fingers. Tell them not to use occlusive dressings or to apply makeup or any other skin product without their doctor's approval.
• Explain to patients that local skin reactions will clear within 2 weeks of discontinuing drug. Local skin reactions are common but don't interfere with drug's effectiveness. However, if severe reactions occur, such as oozing or blistering, tell patients to discontinue drug and contact their doctor immediately.
• Warn patients to avoid unnecessary exposure to sun to prevent actinic (solar) keratoses. Advise patients to wear protective clothing and to use sunblock.
• Advise patient drug may stain clothing or fabrics.

mesalamine
Asacol, Pentasa, Rowasa
Pregnancy Risk Category: B

HOW SUPPLIED
Tablets (delayed release): 400 mg.
Capsules (controlled release): 250 mg
Rectal suspension: 4 g/60 ml
Suppositories: 500 mg

ACTION
Unknown. An active metabolite of sulfasalazine; probably acts topically by inhibiting prostaglandin production in the colon. Exact mechanism unknown.

ONSET, PEAK, DURATION
Onset and duration unknown. Peak levels occur within 3 to 6 hours.

INDICATIONS & DOSAGE
Active mild to moderate distal ulcerative colitis, proctitis, or proctosigmoiditis –
Adults: 800 mg P.O. (tablets) t.i.d. for total dose of 2.4 g/day for 6 weeks; 1 g P.O. (capsules) 4 times daily for a total dose of 4 g up to 8 weeks; 500 mg P.R. (suppository) b.i.d., or 4 g as a retention enema once daily (preferably h.s.). Rectal dosage form should be retained overnight (for about 8 hours). Usual course of therapy for rectal forms is 3 to 6 weeks.

ADVERSE REACTIONS
CNS: headache, dizziness, fatigue, malaise.
GI: abdominal pain, cramps, discomfort, flatulence, diarrhea, rectal pain, bloating, nausea, *pancolitis.*
Skin: itching, rash, urticaria, hair loss.
Other: wheezing, **anaphylaxis** (rare), fever.

INTERACTIONS
None significant.

*Liquid form contains alcohol.   *Common* reactions are in italics; *life-threatening*, in bold italics.
**May contain tartrazine.

CONTRAINDICATIONS
Contraindicated in patients hypersensitive to the drug, its components, or salicylates.

NURSING CONSIDERATIONS
• Use cautiously in patients with renal impairment. Problems have not been documented, but nephrotoxic potential from absorbed mesalamine exists.
• Monitor periodic renal function studies in patients on long-term therapy, as ordered.
• Because it contains potassium metabisulfite, keep in mind that mesalamine may cause hypersensitivity reactions in patients sensitive to sulfites.
• Instruct patients to carefully follow instructions supplied with medication.
• Instruct patients to discontinue drug if they experience a fever or rash. Patients intolerant of sulfasalazine may also be hypersensitive to mesalamine.

---

mesna
Mesnex

Pregnancy Risk Category: B

HOW SUPPLIED
Injection: 100 mg/ml

ACTION
Prevents ifosfamide-induced hemorrhagic cystitis by reacting with urotoxic ifosfamide metabolites.

ONSET, PEAK, DURATION
Unknown.

INDICATIONS & DOSAGE
Prophylaxis of hemorrhagic cystitis in patients receiving ifosfamide –
Adults: dosage varies with amount of ifosfamide administered. Usual dosage is 240 mg/m^2 as an I.V. bolus with administration of ifosfamide. Dosage repeated at 4 hours and 8 hours after administration of ifosfamide.

ADVERSE REACTIONS
GI: soft stools, nausea, vomiting, diarrhea, dysgeusia.
   Note: Because mesna is used concomitantly with ifosfamide and other chemotherapeutic agents, it is difficult to determine adverse reactions attributable solely to mesna.

INTERACTIONS
None significant.

CONTRAINDICATIONS
Contraindicated in patients hypersensitive to mesna or thiol-containing compounds.

NURSING CONSIDERATIONS
• **I.V. use:** Prepare I.V. solution by diluting commercially available ampules with D$_5$W solution, dextrose 5% and 0.9% sodium chloride injection, 0.9% sodium chloride injection, or lactated Ringer's solution to obtain a final solution of 20 mg mesna/ml.
• Do not mix mesna I.V. with cisplatin. Mesna I.V. is incompatible with cisplatin.
• Refrigerate diluted solutions after preparation and use within 6 hours. Diluted solutions are stable for 24 hours at room temperature. After opening ampule, discard any unused drug because it decomposes quickly into an inactive compound.
• Monitor urine samples daily in patients receiving mesna for hematuria.
• Know that mesna is not effective in preventing hematuria from other causes (such as thrombocytopenia).
• Although formulated to prevent hemorrhagic cystitis from ifosfamide, be aware that drug will not protect against other toxicities associated with ifosfamide therapy.
• Keep in mind that up to 6% of patients may not respond to drug's protective effects.
• Be aware that mesna may interfere with diagnostic tests for urine ketones.

---

methoxsalen (topical)
Oxsoralen-Ultra

Pregnancy Risk Category: C

HOW SUPPLIED
Lotion: 1%

ACTION
Unknown. May enhance melanogenesis, either directly or secondarily, to an inflammatory process.

ONSET, PEAK, DURATION
Unknown.

INDICATIONS & DOSAGE
To induce repigmentation in vitiligo; psoriasis –
Adults and children over 12 years: lotion applied to small, well-defined vitiliginous lesions. For optimum effect, the lotion should be applied about 1 to 2 hours before exposure to UV light. The treated area may be exposed to UV light for a limited time.

After exposure, wash lesions with soap and water and protect area with sunblock. Manufacturer recommends weekly treatment.

ADVERSE REACTIONS
Skin: edema, erythema, painful blistering, burning, peeling, pruritus.

INTERACTIONS
Photosensitizing agents: may increase methoxsalen toxicity. Don't use together.

CONTRAINDICATIONS
Contraindicated in patients sensitive to psoralen compounds and in patients with diseases associated with photosensitivity (such as porphyria, acute lupus erythematosus, xerodoma, or hydromorphic and polymorphic light eruptions). Also contraindicated in patients with melanoma, invasive squamous cell carcinoma, and aphakia.

NURSING CONSIDERATIONS
• Use cautiously in patients with familial history of sunlight allergy, GI diseases, or chronic infection.
• Be prepared to regulate therapy carefully. Overdosage or overexposure to light can cause serious burning or blistering.
• Protect patient's eyes and lips during light exposure treatments.
• Obtain monthly liver function tests for patients with vitiligo (especially at beginning of therapy), as ordered.
• Tell patients to avoid excessive sunlight during therapy.

minoxidil (topical)
Rogaine

Pregnancy Risk Category: C

HOW SUPPLIED
Topical solution: 2%

ACTION
Unknown. Stimulates hair growth, possibly by dilating arterial microcapillaries around hair follicles.

ONSET, PEAK, DURATION
Unknown.

INDICATIONS & DOSAGE
Male pattern baldness (alopecia androgenetica) of the vertex and scalp –
Adults: 1 ml of 2% solution applied to affected area b.i.d. Maximum daily dosage is 2 ml.

ADVERSE REACTIONS
CNS: headache, dizziness, faintness, light-headedness.
CV: edema, chest pain, hypertension, hypotension, palpitations, increased or decreased pulse rate.
EENT: sinusitis.
GU: urinary tract infection, renal calculi, urethritis.
Respiratory: bronchitis, upper respiratory infection.
Skin: irritant dermatitis, allergic con-

---

*Liquid form contains alcohol.   *Common* reactions are in italics; ***life-threatening***, in bold italics.
**May contain tartrazine.

tact dermatitis, eczema, hypertri-chosis, local erythema, pruritus, dry skin or scalp, flaking, alopecia, exacerbation of hair loss.
Other: back pain, tendinitis, edema, weight gain.

INTERACTIONS
Topical corticosteroids, petrolatum, topical retinoids, or other drugs that may enhance skin absorption: increased risk of systemic effects of minoxidil. Do not apply minoxidil with other drugs.

CONTRAINDICATIONS
Contraindicated in patients hypersensitive to the drug or any component of the solution.

NURSING CONSIDERATIONS
• Use cautiously in individuals over 50 years, and in those with cardiac, renal, or hepatic disease.
• Know that patients need to have normal, healthy scalps before beginning therapy, because absorption of drug through irritated skin may cause adverse systemic effects.
• Be aware that treatment is most likely to succeed in patients with balding area smaller than 4″ (10 cm) that developed within the past 10 years.
• Teach patients how to apply topical minoxidil. Hair and scalp should be thoroughly dry before application, and drug should not be applied to any other body areas. Tell patients not to use drug on irritated or sunburned scalp, or with any other medication on scalp. Tell patients to thoroughly wash hands after application.
• Warn patients to avoid inhaling any spray or mist from drug. They should avoid spraying around eyes, because solution contains alcohol and may be irritating.
• Teach patients to monitor pulse rate and body weight.
• Advise patients of need for medical

follow-ups 1 month after initiation of therapy and every 6 months thereafter.
• Advise patients that therapy will be prolonged and will continue for at least 4 months before clinical effects appear. About 40% of patients will see moderate to dense hair growth.
• Tell patients that discontinuing drug may result in loss of new hair growth. New hair growth is usually fine and may be colorless, but will resemble existing hair after continued treatment.

nimodipine
Nimotop

Pregnancy Risk Category: C

HOW SUPPLIED
Capsules: 30 mg

ACTION
Inhibits calcium ion influx across cardiac and smooth muscle cells, decreasing myocardial contractility and oxygen demand, and dilates coronary and cerebral arteries and arterioles.

ONSET, PEAK, DURATION
Onset and duration unknown. Peak effect occurs within 1 hour.

INDICATIONS & DOSAGE
Improvement of neurologic deficits in patients after subarachnoid hemorrhage from ruptured congenital aneurysms –
Adults: 60 mg P.O. q 4 hours for 21 days. Therapy begun within 96 hours after subarachnoid hemorrhage.
  In patients with hepatic failure, 30 mg P.O. q 4 hours for 21 days.

ADVERSE REACTIONS
CNS: headache.
CV: decreased blood pressure, flushing, edema.
Other: muscle cramps.

INTERACTIONS
Antihypertensives: possible enhanced hypotensive effect.
Calcium channel blockers: possible enhanced cardiovascular effects.

CONTRAINDICATIONS
None known.

NURSING CONSIDERATIONS
• Use cautiously in patients with hepatic failure.
• Know that nimodipine should be reserved for patients who are in good neurologic condition (for example, Hunt and Hess grades I to II).
• Monitor blood pressure and heart rate in all patients, especially at start of therapy.

olsalazine sodium
Dipentum

Pregnancy Risk Category: C

HOW SUPPLIED
Capsules: 250 mg

ACTION
Unknown. After oral administration, converts to 5-aminosalicylic acid (5-ASA or mesalamine) in the colon, where it has a local anti-inflammatory effect.

ONSET, PEAK, DURATION
Onset and duration unknown. Time to peak concentration is 1 hour.

INDICATIONS & DOSAGE
Maintenance of remission of ulcerative colitis in patients intolerant of sulfasalazine –
Adults: 500 mg P.O. b.i.d. with meals.

ADVERSE REACTIONS
CNS: headache, depression, vertigo, dizziness.
GI: *diarrhea,* nausea, abdominal pain, heartburn.

Skin: rash, itching.
Other: arthralgia.

INTERACTIONS
None significant.

CONTRAINDICATIONS
Contraindicated in patients hypersensitive to salicylates.

NURSING CONSIDERATIONS
• Use cautiously in patients with preexisting renal disease. Although problems have not been reported with this drug, the possibility of renal tubular damage from absorbed mesalamine or its metabolites must be considered.
• Regularly monitor BUN and creatinine levels and urinalysis in patients with preexisting renal disease, as ordered.
• Be aware that in clinical trials, 17% of all patients reported diarrhea during therapy. Although diarrhea appears dose-related, it is difficult to distinguish from worsening of disease symptoms. Exacerbation of disease has been noted with similar drugs.
• Teach patients to take drug in evenly divided doses and with food to minimize adverse GI reactions.

pamidronate disodium
Aredia

Pregnancy Risk Category: C

HOW SUPPLIED
Injection: 30 mg/vial

ACTION
An antihypercalcemic agent that inhibits resorption of bone. Adsorbs to hydroxyapatite crystals in bone and may directly block dissolution of calcium phosphate. Drug apparently doesn't inhibit bone formation or mineralization.

ONSET, PEAK, DURATION
Unknown.

---

*Liquid form contains alcohol.   *Common* reactions are in italics; *life-threatening,* in bold italics.
**May contain tartrazine.

INDICATIONS & DOSAGE

Moderate to severe hypercalcemia associated with cancer (with or without bone metastases) –
Adults: dosage depends on severity of hypercalcemia. Serum calcium levels should be corrected for serum albumin:

$$\text{Corrected serum} \atop \text{calcium (CCa)} \atop \text{(in mg/dl)} = \text{serum calcium} \atop \text{(in mg/dl)} + 0.8 (4 - \text{serum} \atop \text{albumin)} \atop \text{(in g/dl)}$$

Patients with moderate hypercalcemia (CCa levels of 12 to 13.5 mg/dl) may receive 60 to 90 mg by I.V. infusion over 4 hours. Patients with severe hypercalcemia (CCa levels over 13.5 mg/dl) may receive 90 mg by I.V. infusion over 4 hours. A miminum of 7 days should elapse before retreatment to allow for full response to the initial dose.
Moderate to severe Paget's disease –
Adults: 30 mg I.V. as a 4-hour infusion on 3 consecutive days for total dose of 90 mg. Cycle repeated, as needed.

ADVERSE REACTIONS
CNS: *seizures.*
CV: *fluid overload, hypertension.*
GI: *abdominal pain, anorexia, constipation, nausea, vomiting.*
GU: *urinary tract infection.*
Hematologic: *leukopenia, thrombocytopenia, anemia.*
Other: *hypophosphatemia, hypokalemia, hypomagnesemia, hypocalcemia, bone pain, fever, redness, swelling, pain.*

INTERACTIONS
None significant.

CONTRAINDICATIONS
Contraindicated in patients hypersensitive to the drug or to other biphosphonates, such as etidronate.

NURSING CONSIDERATIONS
• Use with extreme caution and consider the risks and benefits in patients with renal impairment.
• Assess hydration status prior to treatment. Know that drug should be used only after patients have been vigorously hydrated with sodium chloride solution. In patients with mild to moderate hypercalcemia, hydration alone may be sufficient.
• **I.V. use:** Reconstitute vial with 10 ml of sterile water for injection. After drug is completely dissolved, add to 1,000 ml of 0.45% or 0.9% sodium chloride injection or D_5W. Do not mix with infusion solutions that contain calcium, such as Ringer's injection or lactated Ringer's injection. Visually inspect for precipitate before administering.
• Give only by I.V. infusion. Animal studies have shown evidence of nephropathy when drug is given as a bolus.
• Because drug can cause electrolyte disturbances, carefully monitor serum electrolytes, especially calcium, phosphate, and magnesium, as ordered. Short-term administration of calcium may be necessary in patients with severe hypocalcemia. Also monitor creatinine level, CBC and differential, hematocrit, and hemoglobin, as ordered.
• Carefully monitor patients with pre-existing anemia, leukopenia, or thrombocytopenia during first 2 weeks of therapy.
• Monitor patient's temperature. In clinical trials, 27% of patients experienced an elevation of 1° C (1.8° F) for 24 to 48 hours after therapy.
• Solution is stable for 24 hours at room temperature.

ritodrine hydrochloride
Yutopar

Pregnancy Risk Category: B

---

†Available in Canada only.   ‡Available in Australia only.   ◇ Available OTC.

HOW SUPPLIED
Tablets: 10 mg
Injection: 10 mg/ml, 15 mg/ml

ACTION
A beta-receptor agonist that stimulates the beta$_2$-adrenergic receptors in uterine smooth muscle, inhibiting contractility.

ONSET, PEAK, DURATION
Onset occurs in 30 to 60 minutes after oral administration, 5 minutes after I.V. administration. Serum levels peak 30 to 60 minutes after oral administration in nonpregnant females; 60 minutes after I.V. administration in nonpregnant females. Duration unknown.

INDICATIONS & DOSAGE
Preterm labor —
Adults: dilute 150 mg (3 ampules) in 500 ml of fluid, yielding a final concentration of 0.3 mg/ml. Usual initial dose is 0.05 mg/minute I.V., gradually increased by 0.05 mg/minute q 10 minutes until desired result is obtained. Effective dosage usually ranges from 0.15 to 0.35 mg/minute.
  Note: I.V. infusion should be continued for 12 hours after contractions have stopped. Oral maintenance: 10 mg approximately 30 minutes before termination of I.V. therapy. Usual dosage for first 24 hours of maintenance is 10 mg P.O. q 2 hours. Thereafter, usual dosage is 10 to 20 mg P.O. q 4 to 6 hours. Total daily dosage should not exceed 120 mg.

ADVERSE REACTIONS
Intravenous:
CNS: nervousness, anxiety, headache.
CV: *dose-related alterations in blood pressure, palpitations,* **pulmonary edema,** *tachycardia,* ECG changes.
GI: nausea, vomiting.
Other: erythema, *hyperglycemia,* hypokalemia.

Oral:
CNS: tremors, nervousness.
CV: palpitations.
GI: nausea, vomiting.
Skin: rash.

INTERACTIONS
Beta-adrenergic blockers: may inhibit ritodrine's action. Avoid concurrent use.
Corticosteroids: may produce pulmonary edema in mother. Monitor patient closely.
Inhalation anesthetics: potentiated adverse cardiac effects, arrhythmias, and hypotension. Monitor patient closely.
Sympathomimetics: additive sympathomimetic effects. Use together cautiously.

CONTRAINDICATIONS
• Contraindicated in pregnant women before 20th week of pregnancy and in women with antepartum hemorrhage, eclampsia, intrauterine fetal death, chorioamnionitis, maternal cardiac disease, pulmonary hypertension, maternal hyperthyroidism, or uncontrolled maternal diabetes mellitus.
• Also contraindicated in patients hypersensitive to the drug or with preexisting maternal medical conditions that would seriously be affected by the known pharmacologic properties of this drug, such as hypovolemia, pheochromocytoma, or uncontrolled hypertension.

NURSING CONSIDERATIONS
• Use cautiously in patients with a sulfite sensitivity.
• **I.V. use:** Because cardiovascular responses are common and more pronounced during I.V. administration, closely monitor cardiovascular effects — including maternal pulse rate and blood pressure, and fetal heart rate. Maternal tachycardia of over 140 beats/minute or persistent respiratory rate of over 20 breaths/minute may be

---

*Liquid form contains alcohol.   *Common* reactions are in italics; **life-threatening,** in bold italics.
**May contain tartrazine.

a sign of impending pulmonary edema.
• Monitor blood glucose concentrations during infusion, especially in diabetic mother.
• Monitor amount of fluids administered I.V. to prevent circulatory overload.
• Discontinue drug if pulmonary edema develops and notify doctor.
• Don't use ritodrine I.V. if solution is discolored or contains a precipitate.

---

sodium benzoate and sodium phenylacetate
Ucephan

Pregnancy Risk Category: C

HOW SUPPLIED
Oral solution: 10 g sodium benzoate and 10 g sodium phenylacetate per 100 ml

ACTION
Activates metabolic pathways that are ineffective in patients with urea cycle enzymopathies, resulting in decreased ammonia formation.

ONSET, PEAK, DURATION
Onset and duration unknown. Serum levels peak within 1 hour.

INDICATIONS & DOSAGE
Prevention or treatment of hyperammonemia in patients with urea cycle enzymopathy –
Children: 2.5 ml/kg P.O. daily in three to six equally divided doses. Maximum daily dosage is 100 ml.

ADVERSE REACTIONS
GI: nausea, vomiting.

INTERACTIONS
Penicillin, probenecid: may impair renal excretion of conjugated metabolites. Monitor the patient for toxicity.

CONTRAINDICATIONS
Contraindicated in patients hypersensitive to sodium benzoate or sodium phenylacetate and in patients who have CHF or renal impairment.

NURSING CONSIDERATIONS
• Use cautiously in neonates with hyperbilirubinemia.
• Carefully measure required dosage because stock solution is very concentrated.
• Dilute each dose in 4 to 8 oz of infant formula or milk and administer with meals. Inspect mixture for compatibility if other liquids are used. Drug may precipitate in some solutions, especially acidic solutions such as fruit juice, depending on concentration and pH.
• Avoid getting solution on skin or clothing; lingering odor of drug may be offensive.
• Watch for salicylate-associated adverse reactions, including mild respiratory alkalosis and exacerbation of peptic ulcerations. Drug is structurally similar to salicylates.
• Know that drug may compete with bilirubin for binding sites on serum albumin.
• Be aware that drug is not intended as sole therapy for patients with urea cycle enzymopathies. It is most effective when combined with a low-protein diet and amino acid supplementation.

---

strontium 89 (^{89}Sr) chloride
Metastron

Pregnancy Risk Category: D

HOW SUPPLIED
Injection: 4 millicuries (mCi)/10 ml

ACTION
Acts as a calcium analogue that is actively taken up by bone, particularly in areas of active osteogenesis such as metastatic bone tumors. The drug lo-

cally irradiates tissue with beta radiation.

ONSET, PEAK, DURATION
Rapidly taken up by bone within hours of injection. Pain relief typically takes 7 to 20 days. Effects persist for 4 to 12 months.

INDICATIONS & DOSAGE
Relief of bone pain in patients with painful metastatic lesions –
Adults: 4 mCi by slow I.V. injection over 1 to 2 minutes.

ADVERSE REACTIONS
CV: cutaneous flushing with rapid injection.
Hematologic: *bone marrow suppression.*
Other: transient increase in pain ("flare" reaction).

INTERACTIONS
Calcium supplements: decreased effectiveness of strontium 89. Discontinue calcium supplements about 2 weeks before strontium 89 administration.
Cytotoxic agents: additive bone marrow suppression. Monitor closely.

CONTRAINDICATIONS
None.

NURSING CONSIDERATIONS
• Use cautiously in patients with platelet counts below 60,000/mm³ or WBC counts below 2,400/mm³.
• Follow institutional safety measures to minimize radiation exposure. Urinary excretion of radiation is greatest during the first 2 days after administration.
• Consider placing an indwelling urinary catheter in incontinent patients to minimize contamination of the environment with radiation.
• Frequently assess the degree of pain relief after administration of the drug. During the first week, a transient increase in pain may necessitate a dosage increase in concomitantly administered analgesics. Pain relief from strontium 89 usually occurs after 2 to 3 weeks. In clinical trials, over 75% of patients received substantial pain relief, allowing a reduction or elimination of opioid analgesics.
• Because the drug is a potential carcinogen, know that use should be restricted to patients with documented metastatic bone cancer.
• Because of the delayed onset of pain relief, be aware that this drug should not be used in patients with a short life expectancy.
• Teach patients proper radiation precautions; during the first few days of treatment, the patient should flush the toilet twice, wipe any spilled urine with a tissue that is subsequently flushed, and immediately launder any linens soiled with blood or urine. Make sure patients understand that the drug has a low level of radioactivity and that they will pose no risk to family members.
• Advise women of childbearing age to avoid becoming pregnant while taking this drug.

sulfasalazine (salazosulfapyridine, sulphasalazine)
Azulfidine, Azulfidine EN-Tabs, PMS Sulfasalazine E.C.†, Salazopyrin†‡, Salazopyrin EN-Tabs†‡, S.A.S., S.A.S.-Enteric

Pregnancy Risk Category: B

HOW SUPPLIED
Tablets: 500 mg with or without enteric coating
Oral suspension: 250 mg/5 ml

ACTION
Inhibits formation of dihydrofolic acid from PABA, decreasing bacterial folic acid synthesis.

---

*Liquid form contains alcohol.   *Common* reactions are in italics; ***life-threatening***, in bold italics.
**May contain tartrazine.

ONSET, PEAK, DURATION
Onset and duration unknown. Peak serum levels of parent drug occur within 1½ to 6 hours; peak levels of metabolites, within 12 to 24 hours.

INDICATIONS & DOSAGE
Mild to moderate ulcerative colitis, adjunctive therapy in severe ulcerative colitis, Crohn's disease –
Adults: initially, 3 to 4 g P.O. daily in evenly divided doses; usual maintenance dosage is 1.5 to 2 g P.O. daily in divided doses q 6 hours. Dosage may be started with 1 to 2 g, with a gradual increase in dosage to minimize adverse effects.
Children over age 2: initially, 40 to 60 mg/kg P.O. daily, divided into 3 to 6 doses; then 30 mg/kg daily in 4 doses. Dosage may be started at lower dose if GI intolerance occurs.

ADVERSE REACTIONS
CNS: headache, depression, *seizures,* hallucinations.
GI: *nausea, vomiting, diarrhea,* abdominal pain, anorexia, stomatitis.
GU: *toxic nephrosis with oliguria and anuria,* crystalluria, hematuria.
Hematologic: *agranulocytosis, aplastic anemia,* megaloblastic anemia, thrombocytopenia, leukopenia, *hemolytic anemia.*
Hepatic: jaundice, hepatotoxicity.
Skin: *erythema multiforme (Stevens-Johnson syndrome), generalized skin eruption, epidermal necrolysis, exfoliative dermatitis,* photosensitivity, urticaria, pruritus.
Other: *hypersensitivity reactions (serum sickness, drug fever, anaphylaxis*) oligospermia, infertility.

INTERACTIONS
Antibiotics: may alter action of sulfasalazine by altering internal flora. Monitor closely.
Digoxin: may reduce absorption of digoxin. Monitor closely.

Folic acid: absorption may be decreased. No intervention necessary.
Iron: lowered blood concentrations of sulfasalazine caused by iron chelation. Monitor closely.
Oral anticoagulants: increased anticoagulant effect. Monitor for bleeding.
Oral contraceptives: decreased contraceptive effectiveness and increased risk of breakthrough bleeding. Suggest a nonhormonal form of contraception.
Oral hypoglycemic agents: increased hypoglycemic effect. Monitor blood glucose levels.

CONTRAINDICATIONS
Contraindicated in patients with hypersensitivity to the drug or its metabolites, porphyria, or intestinal and urinary obstruction and in infants under 2 years of age.

NURSING CONSIDERATIONS
• Use cautiously and in reduced dosages in patients with impaired hepatic or renal function, severe allergy, bronchial asthma, and G6PD deficiency.
• Minimize adverse GI symptoms by spacing doses evenly and administering after food intake.
• Be aware that drug colors alkaline urine orange-yellow.
• Discontinue immediately if the patient shows signs and symptoms of hypersensitivity and notify doctor.
• Warn the patient to avoid direct sunlight and ultraviolet light to prevent photosensitivity reaction.

---

tiopronin
Thiola
Pregnancy Risk Category: C

HOW SUPPLIED
Tablets: 100 mg

ACTION

Forms a water-soluble chemical complex with cysteine in the urine, increasing cysteine solubility and preventing formation of urinary cysteine stones.

ONSET, PEAK, DURATION

Onset rapid. Peak unknown. Effects persist less than 10 hours.

INDICATIONS & DOSAGE

Prevention of urinary cysteine stone formation in patients with severe homozygous cysteinuria (urinary cysteine excretion exceeding 500 mg/day) unresponsive to other therapies –
Adults: 800 mg P.O. daily, divided t.i.d.
Children: 15 mg/kg P.O. daily, divided t.i.d.

ADVERSE REACTIONS

GI: hypogeusia.
Skin: rash, pruritus, wrinkling, friability.
Other: drug fever, lupus erythematosus-like reaction.

INTERACTIONS

None significant.

CONTRAINDICATIONS

Contraindicated in patients with a history of agranulocytosis, aplastic anemia, or thrombocytopenia.

NURSING CONSIDERATIONS

• Keep in mind that the following conservative measures to treat cysteinuria should be attempted before tiopronin is administered. Patients should drink at least 3 liters of fluid daily, including at least two 8-oz glasses of water at each meal and at bedtime. Urine output should be at least 3 liters daily, and urine pH should be 6.5 to 7. Excessive alkalization of urine may precipitate calcium stones. Urine pH should not exceed 7.

• Monitor CBC, platelet counts, hemoglobin, serum albumin, liver function tests, 24-hour urine protein, and routine urinalysis at 3- to 6-month intervals during treatment, as ordered.
• Frequently monitor urine cysteine during first 6 months of treatment to identify optimal dosage level and then at least every 6 months, as ordered.
• Inspect skin for rash. Generalized rash with mild pruritus that develops in first few months of therapy may be controlled with antihistamines and will disappear after discontinuing the drug. A rash accompanied by intense pruritus may appear on the trunk after 6 months of therapy. This rash disappears slowly after discontinuing drug.
• Drug fever may develop, especially during first month of therapy. Expect drug to be discontinued until fever subsides and to be reinstituted at lower dosages.
• Know that dosage is usually adjusted to keep urine cysteine levels below 250 mg/L.
• Be aware that studies indicate that about two-thirds of patients who cannot tolerate penicillamine will tolerate tiopronin.
• Whenever possible, have patients take tiopronin at least 1 hour before or 2 hours after meals.
• Advise patients to have annual abdominal X-ray to assess for presence of stones.
• Tell patients to report any signs or symptoms of hematologic abnormalities, including fever, sore throat, bleeding or bruising, and chills. Blood dyscrasias have been reported in patients receiving other drugs for cysteinuria.

tretinoin (vitamin A acid, retinoic acid)

Retin-A, StieVAA†

Pregnancy Risk Category: C

HOW SUPPLIED
Cream: 0.025%, 0.05%, 0.1%
Gel: 0.025%, 0.01%
Solution: 0.05%

ACTION
Inhibits comedones by increasing epidermal cell mitosis and turnover.

ONSET, PEAK, DURATION
Unknown.

INDICATIONS & DOSAGE
Acne vulgaris (especially grades I, II, and III) —
Adults and children: clean affected area and lightly apply solution once daily h.s.

ADVERSE REACTIONS
Skin: *feeling of warmth, slight stinging, local erythema, peeling,* chapping, swelling, blistering, crusting, temporary hyperpigmentation or hypopigmentation.

INTERACTIONS
Topical preparations containing sulfur, resorcinol, or salicylic acid: increased risk of skin irritation. Don't use together.

CONTRAINDICATIONS
Contraindicated in patients hypersensitive to any tretinoin component.

NURSING CONSIDERATIONS
• Use cautiously in patients with eczema.
• Know that relapses generally occur within 3 to 6 weeks after therapy is stopped.
• Instruct patients to clean area thoroughly before application and to avoid getting drug in eyes, mouth, or mucous membranes.
• Tell patients to wash face with mild soap no more than two or three times a day. Warn against using strong or medicated cosmetics, soaps, or other skin cleansers. Also advise patients to avoid topical products containing alcohol, astringents, spices, and lime because they may interfere with drug.
• Advise patients not to discontinue the drug if it causes transient exacerbation of inflammatory lesions. If severe local irritation develops, advise patient to discontinue temporarily and notify doctor. Dosage will be readjusted when application is resumed. Some redness and scaling are normal reactions.
• Warn patients that they may experience increased sensitivity to wind or cold temperatures.
• Instruct patients to minimize exposure to sunlight or ultraviolet rays during treatment. If patients become sunburned, delay therapy until sunburn subsides. Tell patients who can't avoid exposure to sunlight to use SPF 15 sunblock and to wear protective clothing.

---

trilostane
Modrastane

Pregnancy Risk Category: X

HOW SUPPLIED
Capsules: 30 mg, 60 mg

ACTION
Reversibly lowers elevated circulating levels of glucocorticoids by inhibiting the enzyme system essential for their production in the adrenal gland.

ONSET, PEAK, DURATION
Unknown.

INDICATIONS & DOSAGE
Adrenocortical hyperfunction in Cushing's syndrome —
Adults: 30 mg P.O. q.i.d. initially. May be increased at intervals of 3 to 4 days to maximum of 480 mg/day. Most patients respond to doses below 360 mg/day.

ADVERSE REACTIONS

CNS: headache, dizziness, light-headedness.

CV: *orthostatic hypotension.*

EENT: burning of oral and nasal membranes.

GI: *diarrhea, upset stomach,* nausea, flatulence, cramps, bloating.

Skin: flushing, rash.

Other: fever, fatigue, hot flashes, muscle aches, hyperkalemia.

INTERACTIONS

Aminoglutethimide, mitotane: may cause severe adrenocortical hypofunction.

Loop diuretics, thiazides: decreased potassium loss because trilostane inhibits aldosterone production.

CONTRAINDICATIONS

Contraindicated in patients with severe renal or hepatic disease.

NURSING CONSIDERATIONS

• Use cautiously in patients who are receiving other drugs that suppress adrenal function.

• Because the drug may cause orthostatic hypotension by suppressing aldosterone production, monitor blood pressure regularly in all patients.

• Be aware that trilostane may prevent normal response to physiologically stressful situation. Therefore, patients who develop a severe illness or need surgery may need to have this drug temporarily discontinued. Supplemental corticosteroids may be necessary.

• Trilostane is prescribed when surgery or pituitary radiation therapy is inappropriate or must be delayed. Explain to patients that the drug does not cure the underlying disease.

---

*Liquid form contains alcohol.   *Common* reactions are in italics; *life-threatening,* in bold italics.
**May contain tartrazine.

Appendices
and Index

Anesthetics: Local and topical ophthalmic

DRUG, INDICATIONS, DOSAGE	ADVERSE REACTIONS

Local

bupivacaine hydrochloride
(Marcain‡, Marcaine, Sensorcaine)
Dosages given are for the drug without epinephrine
and for adults. Volume listed below refers to the total
volume of anesthetic given, sometimes in incremental doses of 2 to 6 ml.
Epidural block —
0.25% solution: 10 to 20 ml (25 to 50 mg)
0.5% solution: 10 to 20 ml (50 to 100 mg)
0.75% solution: 10 to 20 ml (75 to 150 mg)
Caudal block —
0.25% solution: 15 to 30 ml (37.5 to 75 mg)
0.5% solution: 15 to 30 ml (75 to 150 mg)
Spinal block —
0.75% solution (in dextrose 8.25%): 1 to 1.6 ml (7.5
to 12 mg)
Peripheral nerve block —
0.25% solution: 5 ml (12.5 mg)
0.5% solution: 5 ml (25 mg)

Skin: dermatologic reactions.
Other: edema, *status asthmaticus, anaphylaxis, anaphylactoid reactions.*
Systemic effects from high
blood levels of the drug —
CNS: anxiety, nervousness,
seizures followed by drowsiness.
CV: bradycardia, hypotension,
myocardial depression, *arrhythmias, cardiac arrest.*
EENT: blurred vision, tinnitus.
GI: nausea, vomiting.
Respiratory: *respiratory
arrest.*

chloroprocaine hydrochloride
(Nesacaine, Nesacaine MPF)
Dosages given are for the drug without epinephrine
and for adults. Volume listed below refers to the total
volume of anesthetic given, sometimes in incremental doses·of 2 to 6 ml.
Infiltration and nerve block —
1% solution: 3 to 20 ml (30 to 200 mg)
2% solution: 2 to 40 ml (40 to 800 mg)
Caudal and epidural block —
2% to 3% solution: 15 to 25 ml (300 to 750 mg).
   May be repeated with smaller doses q 40 to 50 minutes. Dose and interval may be increased when combined with epinephrine. Maximum adult dosage is 800
mg or 11 mg/kg; when combined with epinephrine, maximum dosage is 1 g.

Skin: dermatologic reactions.
Other: edema, *status asthmaticus, anaphylaxis, anaphylactoid reactions.*
Systemic effects from high
blood levels of the drug —
CNS: anxiety, nervousness,
seizures followed by drowsiness.
CV: myocardial depression,
hypotension, *arrhythmias,
cardiac arrest.*
EENT: blurred vision, tinnitus.
GI: nausea, vomiting.
Respiratory: *respiratory
arrest.*

etidocaine hydrochloride
(Duranest)
Dosages given are for the drug without epinephrine
and for adults.
   Dose limit is 4 mg/kg or 300 mg per injection.
When combined with epinephrine, dose limit is 5.5
mg/kg or 400 mg per injection. May be repeated q 2
to 3 hours.
Peripheral nerve block —
1% solution: 5 to 40 ml (50 to 400 mg)

Skin: dermatologic reactions.
Other: edema, *status asthmaticus, anaphylaxis, anaphylactoid reactions.*
Systemic effects from high
blood levels of the drug —
CNS: anxiety, apprehension,
nervousness, *seizures* followed by drowsiness.

*Liquid form contains alcohol.   *Common* reactions are in italics; *life-threatening,* in bold italics.
**May contain tartrazine.

INTERACTIONS	NURSING CONSIDERATIONS
Beta-adrenergic blockers: enhanced sympathomimetic effects. Avoid concomitant use. *Chloroprocaine:* may lessen bupivacaine's action. Don't use together. *Cyclic antidepressants, MAO inhibitors:* severe, sustained hypertension when used with bupivacaine and epinephrine. Use with extreme caution. *Enflurane, halothane, isoflurane, related drugs:* arrhythmias when used with bupivacaine and epinephrine. Use with extreme caution.	● Contraindicated in children under 12 years and for spinal or topical anesthesia or paracervical block. Some solutions contain sulfites and should be avoided in patients with sulfite hypersensitivity. ● Should not be used for I.V. regional anesthesia (Bier block, Bier's anesthesia). ● The 0.75% solution should not be used for obstetrical surgery; lower concentrations are effective and less hazardous. ● Use cautiously in debilitated, elderly, or acutely ill patients and in patients with severe hepatic disease or drug allergies. ● Use solutions with epinephrine cautiously in patients with CV disorders and in body areas with limited blood supply (ears, nose, fingers, toes). ● Keep resuscitation equipment and drugs available. ● Don't use solution with preservatives for caudal or epidural block. ● Discard partially used vials without preservatives. ● Check solution for particles. ● Protect solutions containing epinephrine from light.
None significant.	● Contraindicated in patients with hypersensitivity to procaine, tetracaine, or other PABA derivatives and for spinal or topical anesthesia. Epidural and caudal blocks are contraindicated in patients with CNS disease. ● Use cautiously in debilitated, elderly, or acutely ill patients; in children; and in patients with drug allergies, paracervical block, or CV disease. ● Keep resuscitation equipment and drugs available. ● Don't use solution with preservatives for caudal or epidural block. ● Don't use discolored solution. ● Check solution for particles. ● Discard partially used vials without preservatives.
Cyclic antidepressants, MAO inhibitors, phenothiazines: severe, sustained hypertension or hypotension with etidocaine and epinephrine. Use with extreme caution. *Enflurane, halothane, isoflurane, related drugs:* arrhythmias when used with etidocaine and epinephrine. Use with extreme caution.	● Contraindicated in patients with inflammation or infection in puncture region, septicemia, severe hypertension, spinal deformities, or neurologic disorders; in children under 14 years; and for spinal anesthesia. Some solutions contain sulfites and should be avoided in patients with sulfite hypersensitivity. ● Use cautiously in debilitated, elderly, or acutely ill patients; in patients with severe shock, heart block, general drug allergies, or hepatic and renal disease; and as epidural block in obstetric patients.

Anesthetics: Local and topical ophthalmic *(continued)*

DRUG, INDICATIONS, DOSAGE	ADVERSE REACTIONS

Local *(continued)*

etidocaine hydrochloride *(continued)*
Central neural block (lower limbs, cesarean section, lumbar, epidural) —
1% solution: 10 to 30 ml (100 to 300 mg)
1.5% solution: 10 to 20 ml (150 to 300 mg)
Transvaginal block —
1% solution: 5 to 20 ml (50 to 200 mg)
Caudal block —
1% solution: 10 to 30 ml (100 to 300 mg)

CV: myocardial depression, hypotension, *arrhythmias, cardiac arrest.*
EENT: blurred vision, tinnitus.
GI: nausea, vomiting.
Respiratory: *respiratory arrest.*

---

lidocaine hydrochloride
[lignocaine hydrochloride]
(Dilocaine, Lidoject-1, Lidoject-2, Xylocaine)
Dosages given are for the drug without epinephrine and for adults. Volume listed below refers to the total volume of anesthetic given, sometimes in incremental doses of 2 to 6 ml.
For anesthesia other than spinal —
Maximum single dose is 4.5 mg/kg or 300 mg. With epinephrine, maximum dose is 7 mg/kg or 500 mg.
Caudal (obstetric) or epidural (thoracic) block —
1% solution: 20 to 30 ml (200 to 300 mg)
Epidural (lumbar anesthesia) block —
1.5% solution: 15 to 20 ml (225 to 300 mg)
2% solution: 10 to 15 ml (200 to 300 mg)
Spinal surgical anesthesia —
5% (with 7.5% dextrose): 1.5 to 2 ml (75 to 100 mg)
Caudal (surgery) block —
1.5% solution: 15 to 20 ml (225 to 300 mg)

Skin: dermatologic reactions.
Other: edema, *status asthmaticus, anaphylaxis, anaphylactoid reactions.*
Systemic effects from high blood levels of the drug —
CNS: anxiety, nervousness, *seizures* followed by drowsiness.
CV: myocardial depression, hypotension, *arrhythmias, cardiac arrest.*
EENT: blurred vision, tinnitus.
GI: nausea, vomiting.
Respiratory: *respiratory arrest.*

---

mepivacaine hydrochloride
(Carbocaine, Polocaine)
Dosages given are for the drug without levonordefrin. Dose and interval may be increased with levonordefrin. Volume listed below refers to the total volume of anesthetic given, sometimes in incremental doses of 2 to 6 ml.
Adults: maximum single dose is 7 mg/kg up to 550 mg. Not repeated more often than q 90 minutes. Maximum dosage is 1,000 mg daily.
Children: maximum dose is 6 mg/kg. In children under 3 years or weighing less than 14 kg, use 0.5% or 1.5% solution only.
Nerve block —
1% solution: 5 to 20 ml (50 to 200 mg)
2% solution: 5 to 20 ml (100 to 400 mg)
Transvaginal block or infiltration (maximum dose) —
1% solution: 20 ml (200 mg)
Paracervical block (obstetric) —
1% solution: 10 ml (100 mg). Give on each side (200 mg total) per 90-minute period.

Skin: dermatologic reactions.
Other: edema, *status asthmaticus, anaphylaxis, anaphylactoid reactions.*
Systemic effects from high blood levels of the drug —
CNS: anxiety, nervousness, *seizures* followed by drowsiness.
CV: myocardial depression, hypotension, *arrhythmias, cardiac arrest.*
EENT: blurred vision, tinnitus.
GI: nausea, vomiting.
Respiratory: *respiratory arrest.*

---

*Liquid form contains alcohol.   *Common* reactions are in italics; ***life-threatening,*** in bold italics.
**May contain tartrazine.

INTERACTIONS	NURSING CONSIDERATIONS
	• Use solutions with epinephrine cautiously in patients with CV disease and in body areas with limited blood supply (ears, nose, fingers, toes). • Don't use solution with preservatives for caudal or epidural block. • Keep resuscitation equipment and drugs available. • Check solution for particles.
Cyclic antidepressants, MAO inhibitors: severe, sustained hypertension when used with lidocaine and epinephrine. Use with extreme caution. *Enflurane, halothane, isoflurane, related drugs:* arrhythmias when used with lidocaine and epinephrine. Use with extreme caution.	• Contraindicated in patients with inflammation or infection in puncture region, septicemia, severe hypertension, spinal deformities, and neurologic disorders. • Use cautiously in debilitated, elderly, or acutely ill patients; in patients with severe shock, heart block, general drug allergies; in obstetric patients; and for paracervical block. • Dose and interval are increased with epinephrine. • Use solutions with epinephrine cautiously in patients with CV disorders and in body areas with limited blood supply (ears, nose, fingers, toes). • Don't use solution with preservatives for spinal, epidural, or caudal block. • Keep resuscitation equipment and drugs available. • Discard partially used vials without preservatives. • Check solution for particles.
Cyclic antidepressants, MAO inhibitors: severe, sustained hypertension when used with mepivacaine and levonordefrin. *Enflurane, halothane, isoflurane, related drugs:* arrhythmias when used with mepivacaine and levonordefrin. Use with extreme caution.	• Contraindicated in patients with sensitivity to methylparaben, in those with heart block, and for spinal anesthesia. • Use cautiously in debilitated, elderly, or acutely ill patients and for paracervical block. • Use solutions with levonordefrin cautiously in patients with CV disease and in body areas with limited blood supply (ears, nose, fingers, toes). • Monitor fetal heart rate when paracervical block is used in delivery. • Keep resuscitation equipment and drugs available.

Anesthetics: Local and topical ophthalmic (continued)

DRUG, INDICATIONS, DOSAGE	ADVERSE REACTIONS

Local (continued)

mepivacaine hydrochloride (continued)
Caudal and epidural block—
1% solution: 15 to 30 ml (150 to 300 mg)
1.5% solution: 10 to 25 ml (150 to 375 mg)
2% solution: 10 to 20 ml (200 to 400 mg)
Peripheral nerve block—
1% solution: 1 to 5 ml (10 to 50 mg)
2% solution: 1 to 5 ml (20 to 100 mg)

---

procaine hydrochloride
(Novocain)
Spinal anesthesia—
Adults: initial dose should not exceed 1 g.
  Before using, dilute 10% solution with 0.9% sodium chloride injection, sterile distilled water, or CSF. For hyperbaric technique, use dextrose solution.
Perineum: 0.5 ml 10% solution and 0.5 ml diluent injected at the L4 interspace.
Perineum and lower extremities: 1 ml 10% solution and 1 ml diluent injected at the L3 or L4 interspace.
Up to costal margin: 2 ml 10% solution and 1 ml diluent injected at the L2, L3, or L4 interspace.
Epidural block—
1.5% solution: 25 ml (375 mg)
Peripheral nerve block—
1% solution: 50 ml (500 mg)
2% solution: 25 ml (500 mg)
Infiltration—
350 to 600 mg in a 0.25% to 0.5% solution. Maximum initial dose is 1 g.

Skin: dermatologic reactions.
Other: edema, *status asthmaticus, anaphylaxis, anaphylactoid reactions.*
Systemic effects from high blood levels of the drug—
CNS: anxiety, nervousness, *seizures* followed by drowsiness.
CV: myocardial depression, hypotension, *arrhythmias,* *cardiac arrest.*
EENT: blurred vision, tinnitus.
GI: nausea, vomiting.
Respiratory: *respiratory arrest.*

---

tetracaine hydrochloride
(Pontocaine)
Dosage for adults varies according to the extent of the block as follows.
Low spinal (saddle) block in vaginal delivery—
2 to 5 mg as hyperbaric solution (in 10% dextrose).
Perineum and lower extremities: 5 to 10 mg.
Up to costal margin: 15 to 20 mg.

Skin: dermatologic reactions.
Other: edema, *status asthmaticus, anaphylaxis, anaphylactoid reactions.*
Systemic effects from high blood levels of the drug—
CNS: anxiety, nervousness, *seizures* followed by drowsiness.
CV: myocardial depression, hypotension, *arrhythmias,* *cardiac arrest.*
EENT: blurred vision, tinnitus.
GI: nausea, vomiting.
Respiratory: *respiratory arrest.*

---

*Liquid form contains alcohol.
**May contain tartrazine.

Common reactions are in italics; *life-threatening,* in bold italics.

Anesthetics, local and topical ophthalmic (continued)

INTERACTIONS	NURSING CONSIDERATIONS

| | • Don't use solution with preservatives for caudal or epidural block.
• Discard partially used vials without preservatives.
• Check solution for particles. |

| *Echothiophate iodide:* reduced hydrolysis of procaine. Use together cautiously.
Succinylcholine: prolonged neuromuscular blockade. Use together cautiously. | • Contraindicated in patients with traumatized urethras and in those with hypersensitivity to chloroprocaine, tetracaine, or other PABA derivatives.
• Contraindicated for obstetric use in patients with cephalopelvic disproportion, placenta previa, abruptio placentae, floating fetal head, and intrauterine manipulation.
• Use cautiously in hyperexcitable patients; in those with CNS disease, infection at puncture site, shock, profound anemia, cachexia, sepsis, hypertension, hypotension, GI hemorrhage, bowel perforation or strangulation, peritonitis, cardiac decompensation, massive pleural effusion, or increased intra-abdominal pressure; and in obstetric patients.
• Keep resuscitation equipment and drugs available.
• Use solution without preservatives for epidural block.
• Discard partially used vials without preservatives.
• Check solution for particles. |

| None significant. | • Contraindicated in patients with infection at injection site or CNS disease and in those with hypersensitivity to procaine or related agents.
• Saddle block is contraindicated in patients with cephalopelvic disproportion, placenta previa, abruptio placentae, intrauterine manipulation, and floating fetal head.
• Use cautiously in patients with shock, profound anemia, cachexia, hypertension, hypotension, peritonitis, cardiac decompensation, massive pleural effusion, increased intracranial pressure, and infection.
• Keep resuscitation equipment and drugs available.
• When CSF is added to powdered drug or drug solution during spinal anesthesia, solution may be cloudy. Don't use discolored or crystallized solutions.
• Protect from light; store in refrigerator. |

Anesthetics: Local and topical ophthalmic (continued)

DRUG, INDICATIONS, DOSAGE	ADVERSE REACTIONS

Topical ophthalmic

proparacaine hydrochloride
(AK-taine, Alcaine, Ophthaine, Ophthetic)
Anesthesia for tonometry, gonioscopy; removal of sutures or foreign bodies from cornea—
Adults and children: 1 to 2 drops of 0.5% solution instilled in eye just before procedure.
Anesthesia for cataract extraction, glaucoma surgery—
Adults and children: 1 drop of 0.5% solution instilled in eye q 5 to 10 minutes for five to seven doses.

EENT: conjunctival redness, transient eye pain.
Other: hypersensitivity reactions.

---

tetracaine
(Pontocaine Eye Ointment)
tetracaine hydrochloride
(Pontocaine)
Anesthesia for tonometry, gonioscopy; removal of corneal foreign bodies, suture removal from cornea; other diagnostic and minor surgical procedures—
Adults and children: 1 to 2 drops of 0.5% solution or a small strip (0.5 to 1 inch) of ointment in eye just before procedure.

EENT: transient stinging in eye 30 seconds after initial instillation, epithelial damage in excessive or long-term use.
Other: sensitization with repeated use (allergic skin rash, urticaria).

---

*Liquid form contains alcohol.
**May contain tartrazine.

Common reactions are in italics; ***life-threatening,*** in bold italics.

INTERACTIONS	NURSING CONSIDERATIONS
None significant.	• Use cautiously in patients with cardiac disease and hyperthyroidism. • Not for long-term use; may delay wound healing. • Warn patients not to rub or touch eye while cornea is anesthetized. This may cause corneal abrasion and greater discomfort when anesthesia wears off. • Warn patients with corneal abrasion that pain is relieved only temporarily. • Don't use discolored solution. • Store in tightly closed container. Refrigerate opened containers.
Cholinesterase inhibitors: prolonged ocular anesthesia and increased risk of toxicity. *Sulfonamides:* interference with sulfonamide antibacterial activity. Wait ½ hour after anesthesia before instilling sulfonamide.	• Contraindicated in patients with hypersensitivity to the drug. • Avoid long-term use. • Does not dilate the pupil, paralyze accommodation, or increase intraocular pressure. • Don't use discolored solution. Keep container tightly closed. • Warn patient not to touch or rub eye while cornea is anesthetized. This may cause corneal abrasion and greater discomfort when anesthesia wears off.

Cancer chemotherapy: Acronyms and protocols

Combination chemotherapy is well established for treatment of cancer. The chart below lists commonly used acronyms and protocols, including standard dosages for specific cancers.

ACRONYM & INDICATION	DRUG		DOSAGE
	Generic name	Trade name	
AA (Leukemia—AML, induction)	cytarabine (ara-C)	Cytosar-U	100 mg/m² daily by continuous I.V. infusion for 7 to 10 days
	doxorubicin	Adriamycin	30 mg/m² I.V., days 1 to 3
ABVD (Hodgkin's lymphoma)	doxorubicin	Adriamycin	25 mg/m² I.V., days 1 and 15
	bleomycin	Blenoxane	10 units/m² I.V., days 1 and 15
	vinblastine	Velban	6 mg/m² I.V., days 1 and 15
	dacarbazine	DTIC-Dome	375 mg/m² I.V., days 1 and 15 *Repeat cycle q 28 days.*
AC (Multiple myeloma)	doxorubicin	Adriamycin	30 mg/m² I.V., day 1
	carmustine	BiCNU	30 mg/m² I.V., day 1 *Repeat cycle q 21 to 28 days.*
AC (Bony sarcoma)	doxorubicin	Adriamycin	75 to 90 mg/m² by 96-hour continuous I.V. infusion
	cisplatin	Platinol	90 to 120 mg/m² I.V., day 6 *Repeat cycle q 28 days.*
AC (Breast cancer)	doxorubicin	Adriamycin	45 mg/m² I.V., day 1
	cyclophosphamide	Cytoxan	500 mg/m² I.V., day 1 *Repeat cycle q 28 days.*
AFM (Breast cancer)	doxorubicin	Adriamycin	25 mg/m² by continuous I.V. infusion, days 1 to 3
	fluorouracil (5-FU)	Adrucil	400 mg/m² I.V., days 1 to 5
	methotrexate	Folex	250 mg/m² I.V., day 18
	leucovorin calcium	Wellcovorin	15 mg/m² P.O. q 6 hours, days 19 to 20 *Repeat cycle q 21 days for four cycles.*
AP (Ovarian cancer, epithelial)	doxorubicin	Adriamycin	50 to 60 mg/m² I.V., day 1
	cisplatin	Platinol	50 to 60 mg/m² I.V., day 1 *Repeat cycle q 21 days.*
APE (EAP) (Gastric cancer)	doxorubicin	Adriamycin	20 mg/m² I.V. daily, days 1 and 7
	cisplatin	Platinol	40 mg/m² I.V. daily, days 2 and 8
	etoposide (VP-16)	VePesid	120 mg/m² I.V. daily, days 4, 5, and 6 *Repeat cycle q 8 weeks.*

Cancer chemotherapy: Acronyms and protocols *(continued)*

ACRONYM & INDICATION	DRUG		DOSAGE
	Generic name	Trade name	
ASHAP (Malignant lymphoma)	doxorubicin	Adriamycin	10 mg/m² daily by continuous I.V. infusion, days 1 to 4
	cisplatin	Platinol	25 mg/m² daily by continuous I.V. infusion days 1 to 4
	cytarabine (ara-C)	Cytosar-U	1,500 mg/m² I.V. immediately after completion of doxorubicin and cisplatin therapy
	methylprednisolone	Solu-Medrol	500 mg I.V. daily, days 1 to 5 *Repeat cycle q 21 to 25 days.*
BACON (Non-small-cell lung cancer)	bleomycin	Blenoxane	30 units I.V. q 6 weeks, day 2
	doxorubicin	Adriamycin	40 mg/m² I.V. q 4 weeks, day 1
	lomustine (CCNU)	CeeNU	65 mg/m² P.O. q 8 weeks, day 1
	vincristine	Oncovin	0.75 to 1 mg/m² I.V. q 6 weeks, day 2
	mechlorethamine (nitrogen mustard)	Mustargen	8 mg/m² I.V. q 4 weeks, day 1
BACOP (Malignant lymphoma)	bleomycin	Blenoxane	5 units/m² I.V. daily, days 15 and 22
	doxorubicin	Adriamycin	25 mg/m² I.V., days 1 and 8
	cyclophosphamide	Cytoxan	650 mg/m² I.V., days 1 and 8
	vincristine	Oncovin	1.4 mg/m² (2 mg maximum) I.V., days 1 and 8
	prednisone	Deltasone	60 mg/m² P.O., days 15 to 28 *Repeat cycle q 28 days.*
BCP (Multiple myeloma)	carmustine	BiCNU	75 mg/m² I.V., day 1
	cyclophosphamide	Cytoxan	400 mg/m² I.V., day 1
	prednisone	Deltasone	75 mg P.O., days 1 to 7 *Repeat cycle q 28 days.*
BEP (Genitourinary cancer)	bleomycin	Blenoxane	30 units I.V., days 2, 9, and 16
	etoposide (VP-16)	VePesid	100 mg/m², days 1 to 5
	cisplatin	Platinol	20 mg/m² I.V., days 1 to 5 *Repeat cycle q 21 days.*
BHD (Malignant melanoma)	carmustine	BiCNU	100 to 150 mg/m² I.V. q 6 weeks
	hydroxyurea	Hydrea	1,480 mg/m² P.O. q 3 weeks, days 1 to 5
	dacarbazine	DTIC-Dome	100 to 150 mg/m² I.V. q 3 weeks, days 1 to 5
CA (Breast cancer)	cyclophosphamide	Cytoxan	200 mg/m² P.O., days 3 to 6
	doxorubicin	Adriamycin	40 mg/m² I.V., day 1 *Repeat cycle q 21 to 28 days.*
CAE (ACE) (Small-cell lung cancer)	cyclophosphamide	Cytoxan	1 g/m² I.V., day 1
	doxorubicin	Adriamycin	45 mg/m² I.V., day 1
	etoposide (VP-16)	VePesid	50 mg/m² I.V., day 1 *Repeat cycle q 21 days.*

(continued)

Cancer chemotherapy: Acronyms and protocols *(continued)*

ACRONYM & INDICATION	DRUG		DOSAGE
	Generic name	Trade name	
CAF (FAC) (Breast cancer)	cyclophosphamide	Cytoxan	100 mg/m² P.O., days 1 to 14
	doxorubicin	Adriamycin	30 mg/m² I.V., days 1 and 8
	fluorouracil (5-FU)	Adrucil	400 to 500 mg/m² I.V., days 1 and 8 *Repeat cycle q 28 days.*
or	cyclophosphamide	Cytoxan	400 to 600 mg/m² I.V., day 1
	doxorubicin	Adriamycin	40 to 60 mg/m² I.V., day 1
	fluorouracil (5-FU)	Adrucil	400 to 600 mg/m² I.V., day 1 *Repeat cycle q 21 days.*
CAMP (Non-small-cell lung cancer)	cyclophosphamide	Cytoxan	300 mg/m² I.V., days 1 and 8
	doxorubicin	Adriamycin	20 mg/m² I.V., days 1 and 8
	methotrexate	Folex	15 mg/m² I.V., days 1 and 8
	procarbazine	Matulane	100 mg/m² P.O., days 1 to 10 *Repeat cycle q 28 days.*
CAP (Genitourinary cancer)	cisplatin	Platinol	60 mg/m² I.V., day 1
	doxorubicin	Adriamycin	40 mg/m² I.V., day 1
	cyclophosphamide	Cytoxan	400 mg/m² I.V., day 1 *Repeat cycle q 21 days.*
CAP (Non-small-cell lung cancer)	cyclophosphamide	Cytoxan	400 mg/m² I.V., day 1
	doxorubicin	Adriamycin	40 mg/m² I.V., day 1
	cisplatin	Platinol	60 mg/m² I.V., day 1 *Repeat cycle q 28 days.*
CAP (PAC) (Ovarian cancer, epithelial)	cisplatin	Platinol	50 mg/m² I.V., day 1
	doxorubicin	Adriamycin	50 mg/m² I.V., day 1
	cyclophosphamide	Cytoxan	500 mg/m² I.V., day 1 *Repeat cycle q 21 days for eight cycles.*
CAV (Small-cell lung cancer)	cyclophosphamide	Cytoxan	1,000 mg/m² I.V., day 1
	doxorubicin	Adriamycin	50 mg/m² I.V., day 1
	vincristine	Oncovin	1.4 mg/m² I.V., day 1 *Repeat cycle q 3 weeks.*
CAVE (Small-cell lung cancer)	cyclophosphamide	Cytoxan	750 mg/m² I.V., day 1
	doxorubicin	Adriamycin	50 mg/m² I.V., day 1
	vincristine	Oncovin	1.4 mg/m² I.V., day 1
	etoposide (VP-16)	VePesid	60 to 100 mg/m² I.V., days 1 to 3 *Repeat cycle q 21 days.*
CAVe (Hodgkin's lymphoma)	lomustine (CCNU)	CeeNU	100 mg/m² I.V., day 1
	doxorubicin	Adriamycin	60 mg/m² I.V., day 1
	vinblastine	Velban	5 mg/m² I.V., day 1 *Repeat cycle q 6 weeks for nine cycles.*

Cancer chemotherapy: Acronyms and protocols *(continued)*

ACRONYM & INDICATION	DRUG		DOSAGE
	Generic name	Trade name	
CC (Ovarian cancer, epithelial)	carboplatin	Paraplatin	300 mg/m² I.V., day 1
	cyclophosphamide	Cytoxan	600 mg/m² I.V., day 1 *Repeat cycle q 28 days.*
CD (DC) (Leukemia – ANLL, consolidation)	cytarabine (ara-C)	Cytosar-U	3,000 mg/m² I.V. q 12 hours for 6 days
	daunorubicin	Cerubidine	30 mg/m² I.V. daily for 3 days, after cytarabine therapy
CDC (Ovarian cancer, epithelial)	carboplatin	Paraplatin	300 mg/m² I.V., day 1
	doxorubicin	Adriamycin	40 mg/m² I.V., day 1
	cyclophosphamide	Cytoxan	500 mg/m² I.V., day 1 *Repeat cycle q 28 days.*
CF (Head and neck cancer)	cisplatin	Platinol	100 mg/m² I.V., day 1
	fluorouracil (5-FU)	Adrucil	1,000 mg/m² daily by continuous I.V. infusion, days 1 to 5 *Repeat cycle q 21 to 28 days.*
or	carboplatin	Paraplatin	400 mg/m² I.V., day 1
	fluorouracil (5-FU)	Adrucil	1,000 mg/m² daily by continuous I.V. infusion, days 1 to 5 *Repeat cycle q 21 to 28 days.*
CFL (Head and neck cancer)	cisplatin	Platinol	100 mg/m² I.V., day 1
	fluorouracil (5-FU)	Adrucil	600 to 800 mg/m² daily by continuous I.V. infusion, days 1 to 5
	leucovorin calcium	Wellcovorin	200 to 300 mg/m² I.V. daily, days 1 to 5 *Repeat cycle q 21 days.*
CFM (Breast cancer)	cyclophosphamide	Cytoxan	500 mg/m² I.V., day 1
	fluorouracil (5-FU)	Adrucil	500 mg/m² I.V., day 1
	mitoxantrone	Novantrone	10 mg/m² I.V., day 1 *Repeat cycle q 21 days.*
CFPT (Breast cancer)	cyclophosphamide	Cytoxan	150 mg/m² I.V., days 1 to 5
	fluorouracil (5-FU)	Adrucil	300 mg/m² I.V., days 1 to 5
	prednisone	Deltasone	10 mg P.O. t.i.d. for first 7 days of each course
	tamoxifen	Nolvadex	10 mg P.O. b.i.d. (daily through each course) *Repeat cycle q 6 weeks.*
CHAP (Ovarian cancer, epithelial)	cyclophosphamide	Cytoxan	300 to 500 mg/m² I.V., day 1
	altretamine	Hexalen	150 mg/m² P.O., days 1 to 7
	doxorubicin	Adriamycin	30 to 50 mg/m² I.V., day 1
	cisplatin	Platinol	50 mg/m² I.V., day 1 *Repeat cycle q 28 days.*

(continued)

Cancer chemotherapy: Acronyms and protocols (continued)

ACRONYM & INDICATION	DRUG		DOSAGE
	Generic name	Trade name	
ChIVPP (Hodgkin's lymphoma)	chlorambucil	Leukeran	6 mg/m² P.O., days 1 to 14 (10 mg/day maximum)
	vinblastine	Velban	6 mg/m² I.V., days 1 to 8 (10 mg/day maximum)
	procarbazine	Matulane	50 mg P.O., days 1 to 14 (150 mg/day maximum)
	prednisone	Deltasone	40 mg/m² P.O., days 1 to 14 (25 mg/m² for child)
CHOP (Malignant lymphoma)	cyclophosphamide	Cytoxan	750 mg/m² I.V., day 1
	doxorubicin	Adriamycin	50 mg/m² I.V., day 1
	vincristine	Oncovin	1.4 mg/m² (2 mg maximum) I.V., day 1
	prednisone	Deltasone	100 mg/m² P.O., days 1 to 5. *Repeat cycle q 21 days.*
CHOP-Bleo (Malignant lymphoma)	cyclophosphamide	Cytoxan	750 mg/m² I.V., day 1
	doxorubicin	Adriamycin	50 mg/m² I.V., day 1
	vincristine	Oncovin	2 mg I.V., days 1 and 5
	prednisone	Deltasone	100 mg P.O., days 1 to 5
	bleomycin	Blenoxane	15 units I.V., days 1 and 5. *Repeat cycle q 21 days.*
CISCA (Genitourinary cancer)	cyclophosphamide	Cytoxan	650 mg/m² I.V., day 1
	doxorubicin	Adriamycin	50 mg/m² I.V., day 1
	cisplatin	Platinol	70 to 100 mg/m² I.V., day 2. *Repeat cycle q 21 to 28 days.*
CMF (Breast cancer)	cyclophosphamide	Cytoxan	100 mg/m² P.O., days 1 to 14, or 400 to 600 mg/m² I.V., day 1
	methotrexate	Folex	40 to 60 mg/m² I.V., days 1 and 8
	fluorouracil (5-FU)	Adrucil	400 to 600 mg/m² I.V., days 1 and 8. *Repeat cycle q 28 days.*
CMFP (Breast cancer)	cyclophosphamide	Cytoxan	100 mg/m² P.O., days 1 to 14
	methotrexate	Folex	60 mg/m² I.V., days 1 and 8
	fluorouracil (5-FU)	Adrucil	700 mg/m² I.V., days 1 and 8
	prednisone	Deltasone	40 mg/m² P.O., days 1 to 14. *Repeat cycle q 28 days.*
CMFVP (Cooper's) (Breast cancer)	cyclophosphamide	Cytoxan	2 mg/kg P.O. daily
	methotrexate	Folex	0.75 mg/kg I.V. weekly
	fluorouracil (5-FU)	Adrucil	12 mg/kg I.V. weekly
	vincristine	Oncovin	0.025 mg/kg (2 mg/week maximum) I.V. weekly
	prednisone	Deltasone	0.75 mg/kg P.O. daily, days 1 to 21, then tapered

Cancer chemotherapy: Acronyms and protocols (continued)

ACRONYM & INDICATION	DRUG		DOSAGE
	Generic name	Trade name	
CMFVP (SWOG) (Breast cancer)	cyclophosphamide	Cytoxan	60 mg/m² P.O. daily for 1 year
	methotrexate	Folex	15 mg/m² I.V. weekly for 1 year
	fluorouracil (5-FU)	Adrucil	300 mg/m² I.V. weekly for 1 year
	vincristine	Oncovin	0.625 mg/m² I.V. weekly for 1 year
	prednisone	Deltasone	30 mg/m² P.O., days 1 to 14; 20 mg/m², days 15 to 28; 10 mg/m², days 29 to 42 *Repeat cycle q 42 days.*
CMV (Genitourinary [bladder] cancer)	vinblastine	Velban	4 mg/m² I.V., days 1 and 8
	methotrexate	Folex	30 mg/m² I.V., days 1 and 8
	cisplatin	Platinol	100 mg/m² I.V., 12 hours after methotrexate *Repeat cycle q 21 days.*
COAP (Leukemia – AML, induction)	cyclophosphamide	Cytoxan	100 mg/m² I.V. or P.O., days 1 to 5
	vincristine	Oncovin	2 mg/m² I.V., day 1
	cytarabine (ara-C)	Cytosar-U	100 mg/m² I.V., days 1 to 5
	prednisone	Deltasone	100 mg P.O., days 1 to 5
COB (Head and neck cancer)	cisplatin	Platinol	100 mg/m² I.V., day 1
	vincristine	Oncovin	1 mg I.V., days 2 and 5
	bleomycin	Blenoxane	30 units by continuous I.V. infusion, days 2 to 5 *Repeat cycle q 21 days.*
CODE (Small-cell lung cancer)	cisplatin	Platinol	25 mg/m² I.V. weekly for 9 weeks
	vincristine	Oncovin	1 mg/m² I.V., weeks 1, 2,4, 6, and 8
	doxorubicin	Adriamycin	25 mg/m² I.V, weeks 1, 3, 5, 7, and 9
	etoposide (VP-16)	VePesid	80 mg/m² I.V., weeks 1, 3, 5, 7, and 9
COMLA (Malignant lymphoma)	cyclophosphamide	Cytoxan	1,500 mg/m² I.V., day 1
	vincristine	Oncovin	1.4 mg/m² (2.5 mg maximum) I.V., days 1, 8, and 15
	methotrexate	Folex	120 mg/m² I.V., days 22, 29, 36, 43, 50, 57, 64, and 71
	leucovorin calcium	Wellcovorin	25 mg/m² P.O. q 6 hours for four doses, beginning 24 hours after each methotrexate dose
	cytarabine (ara-C)	Cytosar-U	300 mg/m² I.V., days 22, 29, 36, 43, 50, 57, 64, and 71 *Repeat cycle q 21 days.*
COP (Malignant lymphoma)	cyclophosphamide	Cytoxan	800 to 1,000 mg/m² I.V., day 1
	vincristine	Oncovin	1.4 mg/m² (2 mg maximum) I.V., day 1
	prednisone	Deltasone	60 mg/m² P.O., days 1 to 5 *Repeat cycle q 21 days.*

(continued)

Cancer chemotherapy: Acronyms and protocols (continued)

ACRONYM & INDICATION	DRUG		DOSAGE
	Generic name	Trade name	
COP-BLAM (Malignant lymphoma)	cyclophosphamide	Cytoxan	400 mg/m^2 I.V., day 1
	vincristine	Oncovin	1 mg/m^2 I.V., day 1
	prednisone	Deltasone	40 mg/m^2 P.O., days 1 to 10
	bleomycin	Blenoxane	15 mg I.V., day 14
	doxorubicin	Adriamycin	40 mg/m^2, day 1
	procarbazine	Matulane	100 mg/m^2, days 1 to 10
COPE (Small-cell lung cancer)	cyclophosphamide	Cytoxan	750 mg/m^2 I.V., day 1
	cisplatin	Platinol	20 mg/m^2 I.V., days 1 to 3
	etoposide (VP-16)	VePesid	100 mg/m^2 I.V., days 1 to 3
	vincristine	Oncovin	1.4 mg/m^2 I.V., day 3 *Repeat cycle q 21 days.*
COPP (Malignant lymphoma)	cyclophosphamide	Cytoxan	400 to 650 mg/m^2 I.V., days 1 and 8
	vincristine	Oncovin	1.4 to 1.5 mg/m^2 (2 mg maximum) I.V., days 1 and 8
	procarbazine	Matulane	100 mg/m^2 P.O., days 1 to 10 or 1 to 14
	prednisone	Deltasone	40 mg/m^2 P.O., days 1 to 14 *Repeat cycle q 28 days.*
CP (Ovarian cancer, epithelial)	cyclophosphamide	Cytoxan	1,000 mg/m^2 I.V., day 1
	cisplatin	Platinol	75 mg/m^2 I.V., day 1 *Repeat cycle q 21 days.*
CV (Small-cell lung cancer)	cisplatin	Platinol	50 mg/m^2 I.V., day 1
	etoposide (VP-16)	VePesid	60 mg/m^2 I.V., days 1 to 5 *Repeat cycle q 21 to 28 days.*
CV (Non-small-cell lung cancer)	cisplatin	Platinol	60 to 80 mg/m^2 I.V., day 1
	etoposide (VP-16)	VePesid	120 mg/m^2 I.V., days 4, 6, and 8 *Repeat cycle q 21 to 28 days.*
CVEB (Genitourinary cancer)	cisplatin	Platinol	40 mg/m^2 I.V., days 1 to 5
	vinblastine	Velban	7.5 mg/m^2 I.V., day 1
	etoposide (VP-16)	VePesid	100 mg/m^2 I.V., days 1 to 5
	bleomycin	Blenoxane	30 units I.V. weekly *Repeat cycle q 21 days.*
CVI (VIC) (Non-small-cell lung cancer)	carboplatin	Paraplatin	300 mg/m^2 I.V., day 1
	etoposide (VP-16)	VePesid	60 to 100 mg/m^2 I.V., day 1
	ifosfamide	Ifex	1.5 g/m^2 I.V., days 1, 3, and 5
	mesna	Mesnex	Dosage is 20% of ifosfamide dose, given immediately before and at 4 and 8 hours after ifosfamide infusion *Repeat cycle q 28 days.*

(continued)

Cancer chemotherapy: Acronyms and protocols *(continued)*

ACRONYM & INDICATION	DRUG		DOSAGE
	Generic name	Trade name	
CVP (Leukemia – CLL, blast crisis)	cyclophosphamide	Cytoxan	300 mg/m² P.O., days 1 to 5
	vincristine	Oncovin	1.4 mg/m² (2 mg maximum) I.V., day 1
	prednisone	Deltasone	100 mg/m² P.O., days 1 to 5 *Repeat cycle q 21 days.*
CVP (Malignant lymphoma)	cyclophosphamide	Cytoxan	400 mg/m² P.O., days 1 to 5
	vincristine	Oncovin	1.4 mg/m² (2 mg maximum) I.V., day 1
	prednisone	Deltasone	100 mg/m² P.O., days 1 to 5 *Repeat cycle q 21 days.*
CVPP (Hodgkin's lymphoma)	lomustine (CCNU)	CeeNU	75 mg/m² P.O., day 1
	vinblastine	Velban	4 mg/m² I.V., days 1 and 8
	procarbazine	Matulane	100 mg/m² P.O., days 1 to 14
	prednisone	Deltasone	30 mg/m² P.O., days 1 to 14 (cycles 1 and 4 only) *Repeat cycle q 28 days.*
CYADIC (Soft-tissue sarcoma)	cyclophosphamide	Cytoxan	600 mg/m² I.V., day 1
	doxorubicin	Adriamycin	15 mg/m² by continuous I.V. infusion, days 1 to 4
	dacarbazine	DTIC-Dome	250 mg/m² by continuous I.V. infusion, days 1 to 4 *Repeat cycle q 21 to 28 days.*
CYVADIC (Bony sarcoma)	cyclophosphamide	Cytoxan	600 mg/m² I.V., day 1
	vincristine	Oncovin	1.4 mg/m² (2 mg maximum) I.V., days 1 and 5
	doxorubicin	Adriamycin	50 mg/m² I.V., day 1
	dacarbazine	DTIC-Dome	250 mg/m² I.V., days 1 to 5 *Repeat cycle q 21 days.*
CYVADIC (Soft-tissue sarcoma)	cyclophosphamide	Cytoxan	500 mg/m² I.V., day 1
	vincristine	Oncovin	1.4 mg/m² (2 mg maximum) I.V., days 1 and 5
	doxorubicin	Adriamycin	50 mg/m² I.V., day 1
	dacarbazine	DTIC-Dome	250 mg/m² I.V., days 1 to 5 *Repeat cycle q 21 days.*
DC (Leukemia – pediatric AML, induction)	daunorubicin	Cerubidine	45 to 60 mg/m² I.V., days 1 to 3
	cytarabine (ara-C)	Cytosar-U	100 mg/m² I.V. or S.C. q 12 hours for 5 to 7 days
DCPM (Leukemia – pediatric AML, induction)	daunorubicin	Cerubidine	25 mg/m² I.V., day 1
	cytarabine (ara-C)	Cytosar-U	80 mg/m² I.V., days 1 to 3
	prednisone	Deltasone	40 mg/m² P.O. daily
	mercaptopurine (6-MP)	Purinethol	100 mg/m² P.O. daily

Cancer chemotherapy: Acronyms and protocols *(continued)*

ACRONYM & INDICATION	DRUG		DOSAGE
	Generic name	Trade name	
DCT (Leukemia – ANLL, induction)	daunorubicin	Cerubidine	60 mg/m² I.V., days 1 to 3
	cytarabine (ara-C)	Cytosar-U	200 mg/m² daily by continuous I.V. days 1 to 5
	thioguanine (6-TG)		100 mg/m² P.O. q 12 hours, days 1 to 5
DHAP (Hodgkin's lymphoma)	dexamethasone	Decadron	40 mg P.O. or I.V., days 1 to 4
	cisplatin	Platinol	100 mg/m² by continuous I.V. infusion, day 1
	cytarabine (ara-C)	Cytosar-U	2 g/m² I.V. q 12 hours for two doses, day 2 *Repeat cycle q 3 to 4 weeks.*
DTIC-ACTD (Malignant melanoma)	dacarbazine	DTIC-Dome	750 mg/m² I.V., day 1
	dactinomycin (actinomycin D)	Cosmegen	1 mg/m² I.V., day 1 *Repeat cycle q 28 days.*
DVP (Leukemia – ALL, induction)	daunorubicin	Cerubidine	45 mg/m² I.V., days 1 to 3 and 14
	vincristine	Oncovin	2 mg/m² (2 mg max.) I.V. weekly for 4 weeks
	prednisone	Deltasone	45 mg/m² P.O., for 28 to 35 days
EAP (Gastric cancer)	doxorubicin	Adriamycin	20 mg/m² I.V., days 1 and 7
	cisplatin	Platinol	40 mg/m² I.V., days 2 and 8
	etoposide (VP-16)	VePesid	120 mg/m² I.V., days 4, 5, and 6 *Repeat cycle q 21 days.*
EC (Small-cell lung cancer)	etoposide (VP-16)	VePesid	60 to 100 mg/m² I.V., days 1 to 3
	carboplatin	Paraplatin	400 mg/m² I.V., day 1 *Repeat cycle q 28 days.*
EDAP (Multiple myeloma)	etoposide (VP-16)	VePesid	100 to 200 mg/m² by continuous I.V. infusion, days 1 to 4
	dexamethasone	Decadron	40 mg/m² I.V. or P.O., days 1 to 5
	cytarabine (ara-C)	Cytosar-U	1,000 mg/m² I.V., day 5
	cisplatin	Platinol	20 mg by continuous I.V. infusion, days 1 to 4
ELF (Gastric cancer)	etoposide (VP-16)	VePesid	120 mg/m² I.V., days 1 to 3
	fluorouracil (5-FU)	Adrucil	500 mg/m² I.V., days 1 to 3
	leucovorin calcium	Wellcovorin	300 mg/m² I.V., days 1 to 3 *Repeat cycle q 21 to 28 days.*
EP (Small-cell or non-small-cell lung cancer)	cisplatin	Platinol	75 to 100 mg/m² I.V., day 1
	etoposide (VP-16)	VePesid	75 to 100 mg/m² I.V., days 1 to 3 *Repeat cycle q 21 to 28 days.*
ESHAP (Malignant lymphoma)	etoposide (VP-16)	VePesid	60 mg/m² I.V. over 30 to 60 minutes, days 1 to 4
	cisplatin	Platinol	25 mg/m² daily by continuous I.V., days 1 to 4
	cytarabine (ara-C)	Cytosar-U	2 g/m² I.V. immediately after completion of etoposide and cisplatin therapy
	methylprednisolone	Solu-Medrol	500 mg I.V. daily, days 1 to 4 *Repeat cycle q 21 to 28 days.*

Cancer chemotherapy: Acronyms and protocols (continued)

ACRONYM & INDICATION	DRUG		DOSAGE
	Generic name	Trade name	
EVA (Hodgkin's lymphoma)	etoposide (VP-16)	VePesid	100 mg/m² I.V., days 1 to 3
	vinblastine	Velban	6 mg/m² I.V., day 1
	doxorubicin	Adriamycin	50 mg/m² I.V., day 1 *Repeat cycle q 28 days.*
FAC (CAF) (Breast cancer)	fluorouracil (5-FU)	Adrucil	500 mg/m² I.V., days 1 and 8
	doxorubicin	Adriamycin	50 mg/m² I.V., day 1
	cyclophosphamide	Cytoxan	500 mg/m² I.V., day 1 *Repeat cycle q 21 days.*
FAM (Colon cancer; gastric cancer)	fluorouracil (5-FU)	Adrucil	600 mg/m² I.V., days 1, 8, 29, and 36
	doxorubicin	Adriamycin	30 mg/m² I.V., days 1 and 29
	mitomycin	Mutamycin	10 mg/m² I.V., day 1 *Repeat cycle q 8 weeks.*
FAM (Non-small-cell lung cancer)	fluorouracil (5-FU)	Adrucil	600 mg/m² I.V., days 1, 8, 28, and 36
	doxorubicin	Adriamycin	30 mg/m² I.V., days 1 and 28
	mitomycin	Mutamycin	10 mg/m² I.V., day 1 *Repeat cycle q 8 weeks.*
FAM (Pancreatic cancer)	fluorouracil (5-FU)	Adrucil	600 mg/m² I.V., days 1, 8, 29, 36, and 57
	doxorubicin	Adriamycin	30 mg/m² I.V., days 1, 29, and 57
	mitomycin	Mutamycin	10 mg/m² I.V., days 1 and 57
FAME (Gastric cancer)	fluorouracil (5-FU)	Adrucil	350 mg/m² I.V., days 1 to 5 and 36 to 40
	doxorubicin	Adriamycin	40 mg/m² I.V., days 1 and 36
	semustine (methyl CCNU)		150 mg/m² P.O., day 1 *Repeat cycle q 10 weeks.*
FAMTX (Gastric cancer)	fluorouracil (5-FU)	Adrucil	1,500 mg/m² I.V., day 1
	methotrexate	Folex	1,500 mg/m² I.V., day 1
	doxorubicin	Adriamycin	30 mg/m² I.V., day 15
	leucovorin calcium	Wellcovorin	20 to 25 mg P.O. q 6 hours for 8 doses, beginning 24 hours after each methotrexate dose
FCE (Gastric cancer)	fluorouracil (5-FU)	Adrucil	900 mg/m² by continuous I.V. infusion, days 1 to 5
	cisplatin	Platinol	20 mg/m² I.V., days 1 to 5
	etoposide (VP-16)	VePesid	90 mg/m² I.V., days 1, 3, and 5 *Repeat cycle q 21 days.*
F-CL (Breast cancer)	fluorouracil (5-FU)	Adrucil	500 mg/m² I.V. weekly, 1 hour after initiating leucovorin calcium infusion, for 6 weeks
	leucovorin calcium	Wellcovorin	500 mg/m² I.V., over 2 hours, weekly for 6 weeks *Two-week pause, then cycle repeated.*

(continued)

Cancer chemotherapy: Acronyms and protocols *(continued)*

ACRONYM & INDICATION	DRUG		DOSAGE
	Generic name	Trade name	
F-CL (Colon cancer)	fluorouracil (5-FU)	Adrucil	370 mg/m² I.V., days 1 to 5
	leucovorin calcium	Wellcovorin	200 mg/m² daily I.V., days 1 to 5, begun 15 minutes before fluorouracil infusion *Repeat cycle q 28 days.*
5 + 2 (Leukemia— ANLL, consolidation)	cytarabine (ara-C)	Cytosar-U	100 to 200 mg/m² by continuous I.V. infusion, days 1 to 5
	daunorubicin	Cerubidine	45 mg/m² I.V., days 1 and 2
FL (Genitourinary cancer) *or*	flutamide	Eulexin	250 mg P.O. t.i.d.
	leuprolide acetate	Lupron	1 mg S.C. daily
	flutamide	Eulexin	250 mg P.O. t.i.d.
	leuprolide acetate	Lupron Depot	7.5 mg I.M. q 28 days
FLe (Colon cancer)	levamisole	Ergamisol	50 mg P.O. t.i.d. for 3 days, repeated q 2 weeks for 1 year
	fluorouracil (5-FU)	Adrucil	450 mg/m² I.V. for 5 days, then, after a pause of 4 weeks, 450 mg/m² I.V. weekly for 48 weeks
FMS (Pancreatic cancer)	fluorouracil (5-FU)	Adrucil	600 mg/m² I.V., days 1, 8, 29, and 36
	mitomycin	Mutamycin	10 mg/m² I.V., day 1
	streptozocin	Zanosar	1 g/m² I.V., days 1, 8, 29, and 36 *Repeat cycle q 8 weeks.*
FMV (Colon cancer)	fluorouracil (5-FU)	Adrucil	10 mg/kg I.V., days 1 to 5
	semustine (methyl CCNU)		175 mg/m² P.O., day 1
	vincristine	Oncovin	1 mg/m² (2 mg maximum) I.V., day 1 *Repeat cycle q 35 days.*
FZ (Genitourinary cancer)	flutamide	Eulexin	250 P.O. t.i.d.
	goserelin acetate	Zoladex	3.6 mg implant S.C. q 28 days
HDMTX (high-dose methotrexate) (Bony sarcoma)	methotrexate sodium	Folex	12 g/m² I.V. (20 g maximum)
	leucovorin calcium	Wellcovorin	15 mg I.V. or P.O. q 6 hours for 10 doses, beginning 24 hours after methotrexate dose (serum methotrexate levels must be monitored) *Repeat cycle q 4 to 16 weeks.*
Hexa-CAF (Ovarian cancer, epithelial)	altretamine	Hexalen	150 mg/m² P.O., days 1 to 14
	cyclophosphamide	Cytoxan	150 mg/m² P.O., days 1 to 14
	methotrexate sodium	Folex	40 mg/m², days 1 and 8
	fluorouracil (5-FU)	Adrucil	600 mg/m² I.V., days 1 and 8 *Repeat cycle q 28 days.*

Cancer chemotherapy: Acronyms and protocols (continued)

ACRONYM & INDICATION	DRUG		DOSAGE
	Generic name	Trade name	
HiDAC (Leukemia – ANLL, consolidation)	cytarabine (ara-C)	Cytosar-U	3,000 mg/m² I.V. q 12 hours, days 1 to 6 or days 1, 3, and 5
IMF (Breast cancer)	ifosfamide	Ifex	1.5 g/m² I.V., days 1 and 8
	mesna	Mesnex	Dosage is 20% of ifosfamide dose, given immediately before and at 4 and 8 hours after ifosfamide infusion
	methotrexate	Folex	40 mg/m² I.V., days 1 and 8
	fluorouracil (5-FU)	Adrucil	600 mg/m² I.V., days 1 and 8 *Repeat cycle q 28 days.*
L-VAM (Genitourinary cancer)	leuprolide acetate	Lupron	1 mg S.C. daily
	vinblastine	Velban	1.5 mg/m² by continuous I.V. infusion, days 2 to 7
	doxorubicin	Adriamycin	50 mg/m² by 24-hour continuous I.V. infusion, day 1
	mitomycin	Mutamycin	10 mg/m² I.V., day 2 *Repeat VAM cycle q 28 days.*
MACC (Non-small-cell lung cancer)	methotrexate	Folex	40 mg/m² I.V., day 1
	doxorubicin	Adriamycin	40 mg/m² I.V., day 1
	cyclophosphamide	Cytoxan	400 mg/m² I.V., day 1
	lomustine (CCNU)	CeeNU	30 mg/m² P.O., day 1 *Repeat cycle q 21 days.*
MACOP-B (Malignant lymphoma)	methotrexate sodium	Folex	100 mg/m² I.V., weeks 2, 6, and 10; then 300 mg/m² I.V. for 4 hours, weeks 2, 6, and 10
	leucovorin calcium	Wellcovorin	15 mg P.O.q 6 hours for 6 doses, beginning 24 hours after methotrexate
	doxorubicin	Adriamycin	50 mg/m² I.V., weeks 1, 3, 5, 7, 9, and 11
	cyclophosphamide	Cytoxan	350 mg/m² I.V., weeks 1, 3, 5, 7, 9, and 11
	vincristine	Oncovin	1.4 mg/m² I.V. (2 mg maximum), weeks 2, 4, 8, 10, and 12
	bleomycin	Blenoxane	10 mg/m² I.V., weeks 4, 8, and 12
	prednisone	Deltasone	75 mg P.O. daily
MAID (Bony sarcoma)	mesna	Mesnex	Uroprotection 1.5 to 2.5 g/m² by continuous I.V. infusion, days 1 to 4
	doxorubicin	Adriamycin	15 mg/m² by continuous I.V. infusion, days 1 to 3
	ifosfamide	Ifex	1.5 to 2.5 g/m² by continuous I.V. infusion, days 1 to 3
	dacarbazine	DTIC-Dome	250 mg/m² by continuous I.V. infusion, days 1 to 3 *Repeat cycle q 21 to 28 days.*

(continued)

Cancer chemotherapy: Acronyms and protocols *(continued)*

ACRONYM & INDICATION	DRUG		DOSAGE
	Generic name	Trade name	
MAID (Soft-tissue sarcoma)	mesna	Mesnex	1.5 to 2.5 g/m² by continuous I.V. infusion, days 1 to 4
	doxorubicin	Adriamycin	15 mg/m² by continuous I.V. infusion, days 1 to 3
	ifosfamide	Ifex	1.5 to 2.5 g/m² by continuous I.V. infusion, days 1 to 3
	dacarbazine	DTIC-Dome	250 mg/m² by continuous I.V. infusion, days 1 to 3 *Repeat cycle q 21 to 28 days.*
MAP (Head and neck cancer)	mitomycin	Mutamycin	8 mg/m² I.V., day 1
	doxorubicin	Adriamycin	40 mg/m² I.V., day 1
	cisplatin	Platinol	60 mg/m² I.V., day 1 *Repeat cycle q 28 days.*
m-BACOD (Malignant lymphoma)	bleomycin	Blenoxane	4 units/m² I.V., day 1
	doxorubicin	Adriamycin	45 mg/m² I.V., day 1
	cyclophosphamide	Cytoxan	600 mg/m² I.V., day 1
	vincristine	Oncovin	1 mg/m² I.V., day 1
	dexamethasone	Decadron	6 mg/m² I.V., days 1 to 5
	methotrexate	Folex	200 mg/m² I.V., days 8 and 15
	leucovorin calcium	Wellcovorin	10 mg/m² P.O. q 6 hours for 8 doses, beginning 24 hours after each methotrexate dose *Repeat cycle q 21 days.*
m-BACOS (Malignant lymphoma)	doxorubicin	Adriamycin	50 mg/m² by 24-hour continuous I.V. infusion, day 1
	vincristine	Oncovin	1.4 mg/m² (2 mg maximum) I.V., day 1
	bleomycin	Blenoxane	10 units/m² I.V., day 1
	cyclophosphamide	Cytoxan	750 mg/m² I.V., day 1
	methotrexate	Folex	1 g/m² I.V., day 2
	leucovorin calcium	Wellcovorin	15 mg P.O. q 6 hours for 8 doses starting 24 hours after methotrexate dose
	methylprednisolone	Solu-Medrol	500 mg I.V., days 1 to 3 *Repeat cycle q 21 to 25 days.*
MBC (Head and neck cancer)	methotrexate	Folex	40 mg/m² I.M. or I.V., days 1 and 15
	bleomycin	Blenoxane	10 units I.M. or I.V. weekly
	cisplatin	Platinol	50 mg/m² I.V., day 1 *Repeat cycle q 21 days.*
MC (Leukemia – ANLL, consolidation)	mitoxantrone	Novantrone	12 mg/m² I.V. daily, days 1 and 2
	cytarabine (ara-C)	Cytosar-U	100 mg/m² daily by continuous I.V. infusion, days 1 to 5 *Repeat cycle q 28 days.*

Cancer chemotherapy: Acronyms and protocols (continued)

ACRONYM & INDICATION	DRUG		DOSAGE
	Generic name	Trade name	
MC (Leukemia – ANLL, induction)	mitoxantrone	Novantrone	12 mg/m² I.V., days 1 to 3 and 17 to 18
	cytarabine (ara-C)	Cytosar-U	100 mg/m² daily by continuous I.V. infusion, days 1 to 7 and 17 to 21
MF (Head and neck cancer)	methotrexate	Folex	125 to 250 mg/m² I.V., day 1
	fluorouracil (5-FU)	Adrucil	600 mg/m² I.V., beginning 1 hour after methotrexate dose
	leucovorin calcium	Wellcovorin	10 mg/m² I.V. or P.O. q 8 hours for 8 doses, beginning 24 hours after methotrexate dose *Repeat cycle weekly.*
MICE (ICE) (Small-cell and non-small-cell lung cancer)	mesna	Mesnex	Dosage is 20% of ifosfamide dose given I.V. immediately before and at 4 and 8 hours after ifosfamide infusion
	ifosfamide	Ifex	2,000 mg/m² I.V., days 1 to 3
	carboplatin	Paraplatin	300 to 350 mg/m² I.V., day 1
	etoposide (VP-16)	VePesid	60 to 100 mg/m² I.V., days 1 to 3
MINE (Malignant lymphoma)	mesna	Mesnex	1.3 to 1.5 g/m² I.V., days 1 to 3
	ifosfamide	Ifex	1.3 to 1.5 g/m² I.V., days 1 to 3
	mitoxantrone	Novantrone	8 to 10 mg/m² I.V., day 1
	etoposide (VP-16)	VePesid	65 to 80 mg/m² I.V., days 1 to 3
MM (Leukemia – ALL, maintenance)	mercaptopurine (6-MP)	Purinethol	50 mg/m² P.O. daily
	methotrexate sodium	Folex	20 mg/m² P.O. or I.V. weekly
MOF (Colon cancer)	fluorouracil (5-FU)	Adrucil	10 mg/kg/day I.V., days 1 to 5
	semustine (methyl CCNU)		175 mg/m² P.O., day 1
	vincristine	Oncovin	1 mg/m² (2 mg maximum) I.V., day 1 *Repeat cycle q 35 days.*
MOP (Pediatric brain tumors)	mechlorethamine (nitrogen mustard)	Mustargen	6 mg/m² I.V., days 1 and 8
	vincristine	Oncovin	1.4 mg/m² (2 mg maximum) I.V., days 1 and 8
	procarbazine	Matulane	100 mg/m² P.O., days 1 to 14 *Repeat cycle q 28 days.*
MOPP (Hodgkin's lymphoma)	mechlorethamine	Mustargen	6 mg/m² I.V., days 1 and 8
	vincristine	Oncovin	1.4 mg/m² (2 mg maximum) I.V., days 1 and 8
	procarbazine	Matulane	100 mg/m² P.O., days 1 to 14
	prednisone	Deltasone	40 mg/m² P.O., days 1 to 14 *Repeat cycle q 28 days.*

(continued)

Cancer chemotherapy: Acronyms and protocols *(continued)*

ACRONYM & INDICATION	DRUG		DOSAGE
	Generic name	Trade name	
MP (Multiple myeloma)	melphalan (L-phenylalanine mustard)	Alkeran	8 mg/m² P.O., days 1 to 4
	prednisone	Deltasone	40 mg/m² P.O., days 1 to 7 *Repeat cycle q 28 days.*
m-PFL (Genitourinary cancer)	methotrexate sodium	Folex	60 mg/m², day 1
	cisplatin	Platinol	25 mg/m² by continuous I.V. infusion, days 2 to 6
	fluorouracil (5-FU)	Adrucil	800 mg/m² by continuous I.V. infusion, days 2 to 6
	leucovorin calcium	Wellcovorin	500 mg/m² by continuous I.V. infusion, days 2 to 6 *Repeat cycle q 28 days for four cycles.*
M-2 (Multiple myeloma)	vincristine	Oncovin	0.03 mg/kg (2 mg maximum) I.V., day 1
	carmustine	BiCNU	0.5 mg/kg I.V., day 1
	cyclophosphamide	Cytoxan	10 mg/kg I.V, day 1
	melphalan (L-phenylalanine mustard)	Alkeran	0.25 mg/kg P.O., days 1 to 4
	prednisone	Deltasone	1 mg/kg, days 1 to 7, then tapered over next 14 days *Repeat cycle q 35 days.*
MV (Leukemia – AML, induction)	mitoxantrone	Novantrone	10 mg/m² I.V., days 1 to 5
	etoposide (VP-16)	VePesid	100 mg/m² I.V., days 1 to 5
MVAC (Genitourinary cancer)	methotrexate	Folex	30 mg/m² I.V., days 1, 15, and 22
	vinblastine	Velban	3 mg/m² I.V., days 2, 15, and 22
	doxorubicin	Adriamycin	30 mg/m² I.V., day 2
	cisplatin	Platinol	70 mg/m² I.V., day 2 *Repeat cycle q 28 days.*
MVP (Non-small-cell lung cancer)	mitomycin	Mutamycin	8 mg/m² I.V., days 1, 29, and 71
	vinblastine	Velban	4.5 mg/m² I.V., days 15, 22, and 29, then q 2 weeks
	cisplatin	Platinol	120 mg/m² I.V., days 1 and 29, then q 6 weeks
MVPP (Hodgkin's lymphoma)	mechlorethamine (nitrogen mustard)	Mustargen	6 mg/m² I.V., days 1 and 8
	vinblastine	Velban	6 mg/m² I.V., days 1 and 8
	procarbazine	Matulane	100 mg/m² P.O., days 1 to 14
	prednisone	Deltasone	40 mg/m² P.O., days 1 to 14 *Repeat cycle q 42 days for six cycles.*

Cancer chemotherapy: Acronyms and protocols (continued)

ACRONYM & INDICATION	DRUG		DOSAGE
	Generic name	Trade name	
NFL (Breast cancer)	mitoxantrone	Novantrone	12 mg/m² I.V., day 1
	leucovorin calcium	Wellcovorin	300 mg I.V., days 1 to 3
	fluorouracil (5-FU)	Adrucil	350 mg/m² I.V. given after leucovorin calcium, days 1 to 3
or	mitoxantrone	Novantrone	10 mg/m² I.V., day 1
	leucovorin calcium	Wellcovorin	100 mg/m² I.V., days 1 to 3
	fluorouracil (5-FU)	Adrucil	1,000 mg/m² by continuous I.V infusion given after leucovorin calcium, days 1 to 3 *Repeat cycle q 21 days.*
NOVP (Hodgkin's lymphoma)	mitoxantrone	Novantrone	10 mg/m² I.V., day 1
	vincristine	Oncovin	2 mg/m² I.V., day 8
	vinblastine	Velban	6 mg/m² I.V., day 1
	prednisone	Deltasone	100 mg P.O., days 1 to 5 *Repeat cycle q 21 days.*
OPEN (Malignant lymphoma)	vincristine	Oncovin	2 mg I.V., day 1
	prednisone	Deltasone	100 mg P.O. daily for 5 days
	etoposide (VP-16)	VePesid	100 mg/m² I.V. daily for 3 days
	mitoxantrone	Novantrone	10 mg/m² I.V., day 1
PCV (Pediatric brain tumors)	procarbazine	Matulane	60 mg/m² P.O., days 18 to 21
	lomustine (CCNU)	CeeNU	110 mg/m² P.O., day 1
	vincristine	Oncovin	1.4 mg/m² (2 mg maximum), days 8 and 29 *Repeat cycle q 6 to 8 weeks.*
PFL (Head and neck cancer; gastric cancer)	cisplatin	Platinol	25 mg/m² by continuous I.V. infusion, days 1 to 5
	fluorouracil (5-FU)	Adrucil	800 mg/m² by continuous I.V. infusion, days 2 to 5
	leucovorin calcium	Wellcovorin	500 mg/m² by continuous I.V. infusion, days 1 to 5 *Repeat cycle q 28 days.*
PFL (Non-small-cell lung cancer)	cisplatin	Platinol	25 mg/m² I.V., days 1 and 15
	fluorouracil (5-FU)	Adrucil	800 mg/m² by continuous I.V. infusion, days 1 to 5
	leucovorin calcium	Wellcovorin	500 mg/m² by continuous I.V. infusion, days 1 to 5 *Repeat cycle q 28 days.*
PFL + IFN (Head and neck cancer)	cisplatin	Platinol	100 mg/m² I.V., day 1
	fluorouracil (5-FU)	Adrucil	640 mg/m² by continuous I.V. infusion, days 1 to 5
	leucovorin calcium	Wellcovorin	100 mg P.O. q 4 hours, days 1 to 5
	interferon alfa-2b	Intron A	2×10^6 units/m² S.C., days 1 to 6

(continued)

Cancer chemotherapy: Acronyms and protocols *(continued)*

ACRONYM & INDICATION	DRUG		DOSAGE
	Generic name	Trade name	
ProMACE/ MOPP (Malignant lymphoma)	prednisone	Deltasone	60 mg/m² P.O., days 1 to 14
	methotrexate	Folex	1.5 g/m² I.V., day 14
	leucovorin calcium	Wellcovorin	50 mg/m² I.V. q 6 hours for 5 doses, beginning 24 hours after methotrexate dose
	doxorubicin	Adriamycin	25 mg/m² I.V., days 1 and 8
	cyclophosphamide	Cytoxan	650 mg/m² I.V., days 1 and 8
	etoposide (VP-16)	VePesid	120 mg/m² I.V., days 1 and 8 *Repeat cycle q 28 days; MOPP therapy to begin after the required number of ProMACE cycles are completed.*
ProMACE/ cytaBOM (Malignant lymphoma)	cyclophosphamide	Cytoxan	650 mg/m² I.V., day 1
	doxorubicin	Adriamycin	25 mg/m² I.V., day 1
	etoposide (VP-16)	VePesid	120 mg/m² I.V., day 1
	cytarabine (ara-C)	Cytosar-U	300 mg/m² I.V., day 8
	bleomycin	Blenoxane	5 mg/m² I.V., day 8
	vincristine	Oncovin	1.4 mg/m² I.V., day 8
	methotrexate	Folex	120 mg/m² I.V., day 8
	leucovorin calcium	Wellcovorin	25 mg/m² P.O. q 6 hours for 4 doses *Repeat cycle q 28 days.*
(pulse) VAC (Soft-tissue sarcoma)	vincristine	Oncovin	1.5 g/m² (2 mg maximum) I.V., day 1 or weekly, starting on day 1
	dactinomycin (actinomycin D)	Cosmegen	0.4 mg/m² I.V., day 1
	cyclophosphamide	Cytoxan	1,000 mg/m² I.V., day 1 *Repeat cycle q 3 to 4 weeks.*
PVB (Testicular cancer)	vinblastine	Velban	6 mg/m² I.V., days 1 and 2
	bleomycin	Blenoxane	30 units I.V. weekly
	cisplatin	Platinol	20 mg/m² I.V., days 1 to 5 *Repeat cycle q 21 to 28 days.*
7 + 3 (A + D) (Leukemia— AML, induction)	cytarabine (ara-C)	Cytosar-U	100 or 200 mg/m² by continuous I.V. infusion, days 1 to 7
	daunorubicin	Cerubidine	45 mg/m² I.V., days 1 to 3
TC (Leukemia— ANLL, maintenance)	thioguanine (6-TG)		40 mg/m² P.O. q 12 hours for 8 doses, days 1 to 4
	cytarabine (ara-C)	Cytosar-U	60 mg/m² S.C., day 5 *Repeat cycle weekly.*

Cancer chemotherapy: Acronyms and protocols (continued)

ACRONYM & INDICATION	DRUG		DOSAGE
	Generic name	Trade name	
T-10 (Pediatric bony sarcoma)	methotrexate	Folex	12 g/m² I.V. for 12 or 16 doses
	leucovorin calcium	Wellcovorin	15 mg I.V. or P.O. q 6 hours for 10 doses, each starting 20 hours after methotrexate dose
	doxorubicin	Adriamycin	30 mg/m² I.V. for 2 to 3 days
	cisplatin	Platinol	120 mg/m² I.V. for 1 day
	bleomycin	Blenoxane	15 units/m² I.V. for 2 days
	cyclophosphamide	Cytoxan	600 mg/m² I.V. for 2 days
	dactinomycin (actinomycin D)	Cosmegen	0.6 mg/m² I.V. for 2 days
VA (Wilms' tumor)	vincristine	Oncovin	1.5 mg/m² (2 mg maximum) weekly
	dactinomycin (actinomycin D)	Cosmegen	0.4 mg/m² q 2 weeks
VAB (Genitourinary cancer)	vinblastine	Velban	4 mg/m² I.V., day 1
	dactinomycin (actinomycin D)	Cosmegen	1 mg/m² I.V., day 1
	bleomycin	Blenoxane	30 units I.V. push, then 20 units/m² by continuous I.V. infusion, days 1 to 3
	cisplatin	Platinol	120 mg/m² I.V., day 4
	cyclophosphamide	Cytoxan	600 mg/m² I.V., day 1 *Repeat cycle q 21 days.*
VAC (Small-cell lung cancer)	vincristine	Oncovin	2 mg I.V., day 1
	doxorubicin	Adriamycin	50 mg/m² I.V., day 1
	cyclophosphamide	Cytoxan	750 mg/m² I.V., day 1 *Repeat cycle q 21 days for four cycles.*
VAC (Ovarian cancer, germ-cell)	vincristine	Oncovin	1.2 to 1.5 mg/m² (2 mg maximum) I.V. weekly for 10 to 12 weeks, or q 2 weeks for 12 doses
	dactinomycin (actinomycin D)	Cosmegen	0.3 to 0.4 mg/m² I.V., days 1 to 5
	cyclophosphamide	Cytoxan	150 mg/m² I.V., days 1 to 5 *Repeat cycle q 28 days.*
VAC (Wilms' tumor)	vincristine	Oncovin	1.5 mg/m² (2 mg maximum) weekly
	dactinomycin (actinomycin D)	Cosmegen	1.25 g/m² q 3 weeks
	cyclophosphamide	Cytoxan	1,000 mg/m² q 3 weeks
VAD (Multiple myeloma)	vincristine	Oncovin	0.4 mg by continuous I.V. infusion, days 1 to 4
	doxorubicin	Adriamycin	12 mg/m² by continuous I.V. infusion, days 1 to 4
	dexamethasone	Decadron	40 mg P.O. on days 1 to 4, 9 to 12, and 17 to 20 *Repeat cycle q 25 to 35 days.*

(continued)

Cancer chemotherapy: Acronyms and protocols *(continued)*

ACRONYM & INDICATION	DRUG		DOSAGE
	Generic name	Trade name	
VAP (VP + A) (Leukemia – pediatric ALL, induction)	vincristine	Oncovin	1.5 to 2 mg/m² (2 mg maximum) I.V. weekly for 4 weeks
	asparaginase	Elspar	10,000 units I.M., days 1 and 8 (other doses include 6,000 units/m² I.M. for 3 days/week or 25,000 units/m²)
	prednisone	Deltasone	40 mg/m² P.O., days 1 to 28, then tapered over 7 days
VATH (Breast cancer)	vinblastine	Velban	4.5 mg/m² I.V., day 1
	doxorubicin	Adriamycin	45 mg/m² I.V., day 1
	thiotepa	Thiotepa	12 mg/m² I.V., day 1
	fluoxymesterone	Halotestin	30 mg P.O. daily (through each course) *Repeat cycle q 21 days.*
VB (Genitourinary cancer)	vinblastine	Velban	3 to 4 mg/m² I.V., day 1
	methotrexate	Folex	30 to 40 mg/m² I.V., day 1 *Repeat cycle weekly.*
VBAP (Multiple myeloma)	vincristine	Oncovin	1 mg I.V., day 1
	carmustine	BiCNU	30 mg/m² I.V., day 1
	doxorubicin	Adriamycin	30 mg/m² I.V., day 1
	prednisone	Deltasone	100 mg P.O., days 1 to 4 *Repeat cycle q 21 days.*
VBC (Malignant melanoma)	vinblastine	Velban	6 mg/m² I.V., days 1 and 2
	bleomycin	Blenoxane	15 units/m² by continuous I.V. infusion, days 1 to 5
	cisplatin	Platinol	50 mg/m² I.V., day 5 *Repeat cycle q 28 days.*
VBP (Genitourinary cancer)	vinblastine	Velban	6 mg/m² I.V., days 1 and 2
	bleomycin	Blenoxane	30 units I.V. weekly
	cisplatin	Platinol	20 mg/m² I.V., days 1 to 5 *Repeat cycle q 21 to 28 days.*
VC (Small-cell lung cancer)	etoposide (VP-16)	VePesid	100 to 200 mg/m² I.V., days 1 to 3
	carboplatin	Paraplatin	50 to 125 mg/m² I.V., days 1 to 3 *Repeat cycle q 28 days.*

Cancer chemotherapy: Acronyms and protocols (continued)

ACRONYM & INDICATION	DRUG		DOSAGE
	Generic name	Trade name	
VCAP (Multiple myeloma)	vincristine	Oncovin	1 mg I.V., day 1
	cyclophosphamide	Cytoxan	100 mg/m² P.O., days 1 to 4
	doxorubicin	Adriamycin	25 mg/m² I.V., day 2
	prednisone	Deltasone	60 mg/m² P.O., days 1 to 4 *Repeat cycle q 28 days.*
VDP (Malignant melanoma)	vinblastine	Velban	5 mg/m² I.V., days 1 and 2
	dacarbazine	DTIC-Dome	150 mg/m² I.V., days 1 to 5
	cisplatin	Platinol	75 mg/m² I.V., day 5 *Repeat cycle q 21 to 28 days.*
VIP (Genitourinary cancer)	vinblastine	Velban	0.11 mg/kg I.V., days 1 and 2
	ifosfamide	Ifex	1.2 g/m² I.V., days 1 to 5
	cisplatin	Platinol	20 mg/m²I.V., days 1 to 5
	mesna	Mesnex	400 mg I.V. 15 minutes before ifosfamide, then 1.2 g by continuous I.V. infusion, days 1 to 5 *Repeat cycle q 3 weeks for four cycles.*
or	etoposide (VP-16)	VePesid	75 mg/m² I.V., days 1 to 5
	ifosfamide	Ifex	1.2 g/m² I.V., days 1 to 5
	cisplatin	Platinol	20 mg/m², days 1 to 5
	mesna	Mesnex	400 mg I.V. 15 minutes before ifosfamide, then 1.2 g by continuous I.V. infusion, days 1 to 5 *Repeat cycle q 3 weeks for four cycles.*
Wayne State (Head and neck cancer)	cisplatin	Platinol	100 mg/m² I.V. over 30 minutes, day 1
	fluorouracil (5-FU)	Adrucil	1,000 mg/m² by continuous I.V. infusion, days 1 to 4 or days 1 to 5 *Repeat cycle q 21 days.*

Avoiding medication errors

To ensure safe and effective drug therapy, you need a thorough understanding of a drug's pharmacokinetic and pharmacodynamic properties, as well as knowledge of correct administration techniques. Before administering any drug, you should be able to answer the following questions:

• What is the drug being used for?
• Is the dosage appropriate for this patient?
• Is the route of administration appropriate?
• What is the expected effect of the drug and how should this be monitored?
• How should any adverse reactions be managed?

For help, you can consult a variety of drug information sources, including the *American Hospital Formulary Service (AHFS)* and the *Physicians' Desk Reference (PDR)*. Please note, however, that the *PDR* merely compiles the FDA-approved package inserts for the various drug products selected by the manufacturer and may or may not include a given drug's most up-to-date clinical information. Your institution's pharmacist and pharmacy department's drug information center may be the best sources of updated information.

However, even when armed with all the necessary drug information, you are still vulnerable to medication errors. Such errors can result from problems or distraction at any point during drug prescription, dispensation, and administration. The following errors are most common: incorrectly transcribing a medication order onto a medication administration record (MAR), dispensing the wrong drug, administering the wrong dosage, using the wrong route of administration, and missing scheduled administration times.

These errors may interfere with therapeutic effectiveness, produce adverse reactions, and, at worst, threaten the patient's life.

The following guidelines also will help you avoid medication errors.

• Utilize the classic safeguards, known as the five "rights" of medication administration (checking to be sure it's the right drug, dose, patient, time, and route before administration).
• Regardless of its legal classification, no drug — including OTC products and placebos — should be administered to a patient unless ordered by a doctor.
• Remember that verbal orders for drug therapy can be accepted only by a registered nurse, *only in emergencies,* and only with extreme care to ensure accuracy.
• If possible, avoid using a patient's own medications, the composition and condition of which may be unknown. If, however, they must be used, be sure to obtain a doctor's written order authorizing it, and have the drugs identified by a pharmacist before administering them.
• Store drugs and preparations meant for external use separate from internal medications. Make sure that such products are clearly labeled "for external use only."
• Store all controlled substances under a double-lock system to limit access by unauthorized persons.
• When obtaining a drug from storage, check the drug name carefully. Pay particular attention to spelling — some dissimilar drugs

have similar spellings. Consult a reliable reference if you are unsure about a drug name, and don't hesitate to ask another nurse or the pharmacist for verification.

• Always read the label to identify a drug. Don't rely on the color, shape, or shelf location of a container for identification.

• Check the drug's label against the doctor's order and the patient's MAR three times before administration: when obtaining the drug, when preparing the dose, and when returning the drug to storage or discarding its container.

• Wash hands thoroughly before preparing or administering any medication.

• Prepare medications in a clean, distraction-free area.

• Never administer a medication prepared by another nurse.

• Clearly label liquid doses drawn up in a syringe with the drug name, concentration, date and time drawn up, and your initials.

• Ensure the accuracy of your dosage calculations by having another nurse or a pharmacist double-check them.

• Administer a drug as close as possible to the scheduled administration time specified by the doctor's order and institutional policy. Be especially punctual with drugs that must be maintained in adequate blood concentrations for optimal therapeutic effect, such as antibiotics, chemotherapeutic agents, and anticholinergics.

• Record the reason for any delayed or otherwise untimely administration in the nurses' notes and take other appropriate actions, as defined by your institution's procedures.

• Before administering any drug, double-check the patient's identity by reading his wristband and addressing him by name.

• If the patient expresses concern about a drug you are about to administer, double-check the drug and dosage information.

• If a patient refuses to take a medication, ask why. Often, your explanation of the drug's necessity and benefits will convince the patient to comply. If the patient still refuses, inform the patient care manager and doctor. Document the patient's noncompliance and your subsequent actions.

• Never administer a drug that looks discolored, in which a precipitate has formed, or that otherwise appears abnormal. Instead, notify the pharmacist of your concern and have him evaluate the drug.

• Always check the expiration date before administering any drug. Return all expired drugs to the pharmacy for disposal.

• Never leave medications at the patient's bedside unless this is permitted by hospital policy and specifically authorized by a doctor's written order. If the patient is allowed to self-medicate, make sure that he can do so correctly, and monitor usage carefully.

• When administering a drug p.r.n., make sure that sufficient time has passed since the last dose.

• Provide privacy when giving injections, suppositories, and enemas.

• Document all drug administration on the patient's chart.

• Always assess and record the patient's response after administering medications — especially after administering cardiac drugs and opioid analgesics.

• Discard used needles and syringes in proper disposal containers.

• Include any significant amounts of fluids used to deliver medications, such as I.V. piggyback fluid, in the patient's intake and output records, as applicable.

Index

t refers to a table; **boldface** refers to full-color photoguide

t refers to a table; **boldface** refers to full-color photoguide

t refers to a table; **boldface** refers to full-color photoguide

t refers to a table; **boldface** refers to full-color photoguide

t refers to a table; **boldface** refers to full-color photoguide

t refers to a table; **boldface** refers to full-color photoguide

t refers to a table; **boldface** refers to full-color photoguide

t refers to a table; **boldface** refers to full-color photoguide

t refers to a table; **boldface** refers to full-color photoguide

t refers to a table; **boldface** refers to full-color photoguide

Z

TABLE OF EQUIVALENTS

Metric system equivalents

Metric weight
1 kilogram = 1,000 grams (g or gm)
1 gram = 1,000 milligrams (mg)
1 milligram = 1,000 micrograms (μg or mcg)

0.6 g	= 600 mg
0.3 g	= 300 mg
0.1 g	= 100 mg
0.06 g	= 60 mg
0.03 g	= 30 mg
0.015 g	= 15 mg
.001 g	= 1 mg

Metric volume
1 liter (l or L) = 1,000 milliliters (ml)*
1 milliliter = 1,000 microliters (μl)

Household		Metric
1 teaspoon (tsp)	=	5 ml
1 tablespoon (T or tbs)	=	15 ml
2 tablespoons	=	30 ml
1 measuring cupful	=	240 ml
1 pint (pt)	=	473 ml
1 quart (qt)	=	946 ml
1 gallon (gal)	=	3,785 ml

Temperature conversions

FAHRENHEIT DEGREES	CENTIGRADE DEGREES	FAHRENHEIT DEGREES	CENTIGRADE DEGREES	FAHRENHEIT DEGREES	CENTIGRADE DEGREES
106.0	41.1	100.6	38.1	95.2	35.1
105.8	41.0	100.4	38.0	95.0	35.0
105.6	40.9	100.2	37.9	94.8	34.9
105.4	40.8	100.0	37.8	94.6	34.8
105.2	40.7	99.8	37.7	94.4	34.7
105.0	40.6	99.6	37.6	94.2	34.6
104.8	40.4	99.4	37.4	94.0	34.4
104.6	40.3	99.2	37.3	93.8	34.3
104.4	40.2	99.0	37.2	93.6	34.2
104.2	40.1	98.8	37.1	93.4	34.1
104.0	40.0	98.6	37.0	93.2	34.0
103.8	39.9	98.4	36.9	93.0	33.9
103.6	39.8	98.2	36.8	92.8	33.8
103.4	39.7	98.0	36.7	92.6	33.7
103.2	39.6	97.8	36.5	92.4	33.6
103.0	39.4	97.6	36.4	92.2	33.4
102.8	39.3	97.4	36.3	92.0	33.3
102.6	39.2	97.2	36.2	91.8	33.2
102.4	39.1	97.0	36.1	91.6	33.1
102.2	39.0	96.8	36.0	91.4	33.0
102.0	38.9	96.6	35.9	91.2	32.9
101.8	38.8	96.4	35.8	91.0	32.8
101.6	38.7	96.2	35.7	90.8	32.7
101.4	38.6	96.0	35.6	90.6	32.6
101.2	38.4	95.8	35.4	90.4	32.4
101.0	38.3	95.6	35.3	90.2	32.3
100.8	38.2	95.4	35.2	90.0	32.2

Weight conversions

1 oz = 30 g	1 lb = 453.6 g	2.2 lb = 1 kg

*1 ml = 1 cubic centimeter (cc); however, ml is the preferred measurement term today.

•